Principles and Practice
of Cancer Infectious Diseases

CURRENT CLINICAL ONCOLOGY

Maurie Markman, MD, Series Editor

For other titles published in this series, go to
www.springer.com/series/7631

Amar Safdar
Editor

Principles and Practice of Cancer Infectious Diseases

❄ Humana Press

Editor
Amar Safdar
Department of Infectious Diseases,
Infection Control, and Employee Health
The University of Texas
M.D. Anderson Cancer Center
Houston, TX
USA
amarsafdar@gmail.com

ISBN 978-1-60761-643-6   e-ISBN 978-1-60761-644-3
DOI 10.1007/978-1-60761-644-3
Springer New York Dordrecht Heidelberg London

Library of Congress Control Number: 2011928679

© Springer Science+Business Media, LLC 2011
All rights reserved. This work may not be translated or copied in whole or in part without the written permission of the publisher (Humana Press, c/o Springer Science+Business Media, LLC, 233 Spring Street, New York, NY 10013, USA), except for brief excerpts in connection with reviews or scholarly analysis. Use in connection with any form of information storage and retrieval, electronic adaptation, computer software, or by similar or dissimilar methodology now known or hereafter developed is forbidden.
The use in this publication of trade names, trademarks, service marks, and similar terms, even if they are not identified as such, is not to be taken as an expression of opinion as to whether or not they are subject to proprietary rights.
While the advice and information in this book are believed to be true and accurate at the date of going to press, neither the authors nor the editors nor the publisher can accept any legal responsibility for any errors or omissions that may be made. The publisher makes no warranty, express or implied, with respect to the material contained herein.

Printed on acid-free paper

Humana Press is part of Springer Science+Business Media (www.springer.com)

This book is dedicated for promoting excellence in care and well-being for the patients with cancer.

Preface

Patients with cancer are highly susceptible to infections. These infections are inclined to be difficult to prevent, diagnose, and treat. There are a variety of reasons for this which will be discussed in detail in the chapters of this book. The intent for this book is to provide a comprehensive review of the ever changing spectrum of the management of infectious diseases in this complex population of patients. The changes in patient demography, near-constant global migration of contagious infections, emerging resistance to standard antimicrobial therapy, and the impact of expanding repertoire of antineoplastic therapies including the anticancer biologics and stem cell transplantation have influenced these changes. This book will provide a detailed guide for assessment of risk factors for various infections, evaluating prognosis among susceptible oncology patients with complex issues related to management of opportunistic infections. Strategies to promote hosts' immune response underscore the future measures based on perspicacious insight in the disease pathogenesis; interaction between the pathogen and host's immune function and inflammatory response are given prominent discussion throughout the book. I hope the reader will become acquainted with common and less often encountered infections and importantly, develop a keen knowledge of conditions that might be mistaken as infectious diseases in patients undergoing treatment for neoplastic diseases.

Houston, TX, USA   Amar Safdar, MD

Contents

Part I Overview and Special Population

1. **Infections in Patients with Cancer: Overview** ... 3
   Amar Safdar, Gerald Bodey, and Donald Armstrong

2. **Infections in Hematopoietic Stem Cell Transplant Recipients** ... 17
   Georg Maschmeyer and Per Ljungman

3. **Infections in Patients with Hematologic Malignancies** ... 27
   Genovefa Papanicolaou and Jayesh Mehta

4. **Infections in Solid Tumor Patients** ... 39
   Alison G. Freifeld

5. **Infections in Patients with Hematologic Malignancies Treated with Monoclonal Antineoplastic Therapy** ... 47
   André Goy and Susan O'Brien

6. **Postsurgery Infections in Cancer Patients** ... 67
   Emilio Bouza, Almudena Burillo, Juan Carlos Lopez-Gutierrez, and José F. Tomás-Martinez

7. **Management of Infections in Critically Ill Cancer Patients** ... 87
   Henry Masur

Part II Clinical Syndromes

8. **Management of the Neutropenic Patient with Fever** ... 95
   Kenneth V.I. Rolston and Gerald P. Bodey

9. **Controversies in Empiric Therapy of Febrile Neutropenia** ... 105
   John R. Wingard

10. **Catheter-Related Infections in Cancer Patients** ... 113
    Iba Al Wohoush, Anne-Marie Chaftari, and Issam Raad

11. **Intravascular Device-Related Infections: Catheter Salvage Strategies and Prevention of Device-Related Infection** ... 123
    Nasia Safdar and Dennis G. Maki

12. **Pneumonia in the Cancer Patient** ... 143
    Scott E. Evans and Amar Safdar

| 13 | Noninfectious Lung Infiltrates That May Be Confused with Pneumonia in the Cancer Patient .... | 153 |

Rana Kaplan, Lara Bashoura, Vickie R. Shannon, Burton F. Dickey, and Diane E. Stover

| 14 | Mucosal Barrier Injury and Infections .... | 167 |

Nicole M.A. Blijlevens and J. Peter Donnelly

| 15 | Bacterial Colonization and Host Immunity .... | 175 |

Coralia N. Mihu, Karen J. Vigil, and Javier A. Adachi

| 16 | Neutropenic Enterocolitis and *Clostridium difficile* Infections .... | 181 |

Amar Safdar, Bruno P. Granwehr, Stephen A. Harold, and Herbert L. DuPont

| 17 | Management of Reactivation of Hepatitis B and Hepatitis C During Antineoplastic Therapy .... | 189 |

Marta Davila and Harrys A. Torres

| 18 | Management of Genitourinary Tract Infections .... | 195 |

Amar Safdar and Maurie Markman

| 19 | Central Nervous System Infections in Cancer Patients .... | 207 |

Victor Mulanovich and Amar Safdar

| 20 | Endocarditis in Oncology Patients .... | 219 |

Sara E. Cosgrove and Aruna Subramanian

| 21 | Skin Disorders Difficult to Distinguish from Infection .... | 233 |

Sharon Hymes, Susan Chon, and Ana Ciurea

Part III Major Etiologic Agents

| 22 | Overview of Invasive Fungal Disease in Oncology Patients .... | 257 |

Amar Safdar

| 23 | Diagnosis of Invasive Fungal Disease .... | 261 |

Dionissios Neofytos and Kieren Marr

| 24 | Invasive Candidiasis in Management of Infections in Cancer Patients .... | 273 |

Matteo Bassetti, Malgorzata Mikulska, Juan Gea-Banacloche, and Claudio Viscoli

| 25 | Management of Aspergillosis, Zygomycosis, and Other Clinically Relevant Mold Infections .... | 283 |

Konstantinos Leventakos and Dimitrios P. Kontoyiannis

| 26 | Cryptococcal Disease and Endemic Mycosis .... | 293 |

Johan A. Maertens and Hélène Schoemans

| 27 | Current Controversies in the Treatment of Fungal Infections .... | 301 |

Christopher D. Pfeiffer, John R. Perfect, and Barbara D. Alexander

28	**Fungal Drug Resistance and Pharmacologic Considerations of Dosing Newer Antifungal Therapies**........	317
	Russell E. Lewis and David S. Perlin	
29	**Immunotherapy for Difficult-to-Treat Invasive Fungal Diseases**........	331
	Brahm H. Segal, Amar Safdar, and David A. Stevens	
30	**Cytomegalovirus in Patients with Cancer**........	341
	Morgan Hakki, Per Ljungman, and Michael Boeckh	
31	**Epstein-Barr Virus, Varicella Zoster Virus, and Human Herpes Viruses-6 and -8**........	359
	Mini Kamboj and David M. Weinstock	
32	**Respiratory Viruses**........	371
	Roy F. Chemaly, Dhanesh B. Rathod, and Robert Couch	
33	**BK, JC, and Parvovirus Infections in Patients with Hematologic Malignancies**........	387
	Véronique Erard and Michael Boeckh	
34	**Antiviral Resistance and Implications for Prophylaxis**........	397
	Robin K. Avery	
35	**Management of Gram-Positive Bacterial Disease: *Staphylococcus aureus*, Streptococcal, Pneumococcal, and Enterococcal Infections**........	409
	Samuel Shelburne and Daniel M. Musher	
36	**Infections Caused by Aerobic and Anaerobic Gram-Negative Bacilli**........	423
	Kenneth V.I. Rolston, David E. Greenberg, and Amar Safdar	
37	**Listeriosis and Nocardiosis**........	435
	Heather E. Clauss and Bennett Lorber	
38	**Antibacterial Distribution and Drug–Drug Interactions in Cancer Patients**........	443
	Ursula Theuretzbacher and Markus Zeitlinger	
39	***Mycobacterium tuberculous* Infection**........	455
	Michael Glickman	
40	**Nontuberculous Mycobacterial Infections**........	463
	Amar Safdar	
41	**Parasitic Infections in Cancer Patients: Toxoplasmosis, Strongyloidiasis, and Other Parasites**........	469
	Brian G. Blackburn and José G. Montoya	
42	**Zoonoses in Cancer Patients**........	481
	Donald Armstrong	

Part IV Management of Antimicrobial Therapy

43 Antimicrobial Stewardship: Considerations for a Cancer Center 491
Coralia N. Mihu, Alla Paskovaty, and Susan K. Seo

44 Controversies in Antimicrobial Stewardship 499
Graeme N. Forrest

**45 Prevention of Antimicrobial Resistance: Current
and Future Strategies** 507
Cesar A. Arias and Adolf W. Karchmer

Part V Infection Prevention: Antimicorbial Prophylaxis and Immunization

**46 Antibacterial, Antifungal, and Antiviral Prophylaxis
in High-Risk Cancer and Stem Cell Transplant Population** 521
Marcio Nucci and John R. Wingard

47 Controversies in Antimicrobial Prophylaxis 533
Ben de Pauw and Marta Stanzani

**48 Infection Prevention – Protected Environment
and Infection Control** 541
J. Peter Donnelly

**49 Prevention of Tropical and Parasitic Infections:
The Immunocompromised Traveler** 551
Francesca F. Norman and Rogelio López-Vélez

**50 Prophylactic Vaccination of Cancer Patients
and Hematopoietic Stem Cell Transplant Recipients** 561
William Decker and Amar Safdar

Index 573

Contributors

Javier A. Adachi, M.D.
Department of Infectious Diseases, The University of Texas
M.D. Anderson Cancer Center, Houston, TX, USA

Barbara D. Alexander, M.D.
Department of Medicine, Division of Infectious Diseases and International Health,
Duke University Medical Center, Durham, NC, USA

Iba Al Wohoush, M.D.
Infectious Diseases, Infection Control, and Employee Health,
The University of Texas M.D. Anderson Cancer Center,
Houston, Texas, USA

Cesar A. Arias, M.D.
Department of Internal Medicine, Division of Infectious Diseases,
University of Texas Medical School at Houston, TX, USA

Donald Armstrong, M.D.
Department of Medicine, Infectious Disease Service, Memorial Sloan–Kettering
Cancer Center, New York, NY, USA

Robin K. Avery, M.D.
Department of Infectious Disease, Cleveland Clinic Foundation,
Lerner College of Medicine of Case Western Reserve University, Cleveland, OH, USA

Lara Bashoura, M.D.
Department of Pulmonary Medicine, The University of Texas
M.D. Anderson Cancer Center, Houston, TX, USA

Matteo Bassetti, M.D., Ph.D.
Division of Infectious Diseases, San Martino Hospital and University of Genoa,
Genoa, Italy

Brian G. Blackburn, M.D.
Department of Internal Medicine, Division of Infectious Diseases
and Geographic Medicine, Stanford University School of Medicine,
Stanford, CA, USA

Nicole M. A. Blijlevens, M.D.
Department of Haematology, Radboud University Nijmegen Medical Centre
& Nijmegen University Centre for Infectious Diseases, Nijmegen, The Netherlands

Gerald P. Bodey, M.D.
Department of Infectious Diseases, Infection Control, and Employee Health,
The University of Texas M.D. Anderson Cancer Center, Houston, TX, USA

Michael Boeckh, M.D.
Vaccine and Infectious Disease Division, University of Washington, Fred Hutchinson Cancer Research Center, Seattle, WA, USA

Emilio Bouza, M.D.
Clinical Microbiology and Infectious Diseases Department, Hospital General Universitario Gregorio Marañón, Universidad Complutense de Madrid; CIBER de Enfermedades Respiratorias (CIBERES), Madrid, Spain

Almudena Burrillo, M.D., Ph.D.
Clinical Microbiology Department, Hospital Universitario de Móstoles, Madrid, Spain

Anne-Marie Chaftari, M.D.
Department of Infectious Diseases, Infection Control, and Employee Health, The University of Texas M.D. Anderson Cancer Center, Houston, TX, USA

Roy F. Chemaly, M.D.
Department of Infectious Diseases, Infection Control, and Employee Health, The University of Texas M.D. Anderson Cancer Center, Houston, TX, USA

Susan Chon, M.D.
Department of Dermatology, The University of Texas M.D. Anderson Cancer Center, Houston, TX, USA

Ana Ciurea, M.D.
Department of Dermatology, The University of Texas M.D. Anderson Cancer Center, Houston, TX, USA

Heather E. Clauss, M.D.
Department of Infectious Diseases, Temple University Hospital, Philadelphia, PA, USA

Sara E. Cosgrove, M.D.
Division of Infectious Diseases, Johns Hopkins University School of Medicine, Baltimore, MD, USA

Robert Couch, M.D.
Department of Molecular Virology and Microbiology, Baylor College of Medicine, Center for Infection and Immunity Research, Houston, TX, USA

Marta Davila, M.D.
Department of Gastroenterology, Hepatology, and Nutrition, The University of Texas M.D. Anderson Cancer Center, Houston, TX, USA

William Decker, Ph.D.
Department of Blood and Marrow Transplantation, The University of Texas M.D. Anderson Cancer Center, Houston, TX, USA

Burton F. Dickey, M.D.
Department of Pulmonary Medicine, The University of Texas M.D. Anderson Cancer Center, Houston, TX, USA

J. Peter Donnelly, Ph.D.
Department of Haematology and Nijmegen Institute for Infection, Inflammation and Immunity, Radboud University Nijmegen Medical Centre, Nijmegen, The Netherlands

Herbert L. DuPont, M.D.
Department of Medicine, The University of Texas, School of Public Health,
Center for Infectious Diseases; Department of Internal Medicine, St. Luke's Episcopal
Hospital; Department of Microbiology and Immunology, Baylor College of Medicine,
Houston, TX, USA

Véronique Erard, M.D.
Médecin Adjointe, Infectiologie, HFR-Fribourg, Switzerland

Scott E. Evans, M.D.
Department of Pulmonary Medicine, The University of Texas
M.D. Anderson Cancer Center, Houston, TX, USA

Graeme N. Forrest, M.D.
Division of Infectious Disease, Portland VA Medical Center, Portland, OR, USA

Alison G. Freifeld, M.D.
Department of Medicine, University of Nebraska Medical Center,
Omaha, NE, USA

Juan Gea-Banacloche, M.D.
Experimental Transplantation and Immunology Branch,
National Cancer Institute, Bethesda, MD, USA

Michael Glickman, M.D.
Department of Medicine, Infectious Disease Service,
Memorial Sloan Kettering Cancer Center, New York, NY, USA

Andre Goy, M.D.
Hematology/Oncology, Internal Medicine, Hackensack University Medical Center,
Hackensack, NJ, USA

Bruno P. Granwehr, M.D.
Department of Infectious Diseases, The University of Texas
M.D. Anderson Cancer Center, Houston, TX, USA

David E. Greenberg, M.D.
Department of Infectious Diseases, National Institute of Allergy
and Infectious Diseases, Bethesda, MD, USA

Morgan Hakki, M.D.
Division of Infectious Diseases, Oregon Health & Science University,
Portland, OR, USA

Stephen A. Harold
Department of Medicine, The University of Texas, School of Public Health,
Center for Infectious Diseases, Houston, TX, USA

Sharone Hymes, M.D.
Department of Dermatology, The University of Texas
M.D. Anderson Cancer Center, Houston, TX, USA

Mini Kamboj, M.D.
Department of Medicine, Infectious Disease Service, Memorial Sloan-Kettering
Cancer Center, New York, NY, USA

Rana Kaplan, M.D.
Department of Medicine, Pulmonary Medicine Service,
Memorial Sloan–Kettering Cancer Center, New York, NY, USA

Adolf W. Karchmer, M.D.
Division of Infectious Diseases, Beth Israel Deaconess Medical Center, Boston, MA, USA

Dimitrios P. Kontoyiannis, M.D.
Department of Infectious Diseases, Infection Control, and Employee Health,
The University of Texas M.D. Anderson Cancer Center, Houston, TX, USA

Konstantinos Leventakos, M.D.
Department of Infectious Diseases, Infection Control, and Employee Health,
The University of Texas M.D. Anderson Cancer Center, Houston, TX, USA

Russell E. Lewis, Pharm. D.
Department of Infectious Diseases, Infection Control, and Employee Health,
The University of Texas M.D. Anderson Cancer Center, Houston, TX, USA

Per Ljungman, M.D.
Hematology Center, Karolinska University, Stockholm, Sweden

Juan Carlos Lopez-Gutierrez, M.D.
Department of Pediatric Surgery, Hospital Universitario Lu Paz,
Universidad Autonoma de Madrid, Spain

Rogelio López-Vélez, M.D.
Tropical Medicine and Clinical Parasitology Unit, Department of Infectious Diseases,
Ramón y Cajal Hospital, Instituto Ramón y Cajal de Investigación Sanitaria (IRYCIS),
Madrid, Spain

Bennett Lorber, M.D.
Department of Medicine, Section of Infectious Diseases,
Temple University School of Medicine, Philadelphia, PA, USA

Johan A. Maertens, M.D., Ph.D.
Department of Hematology, Acute Leukemia and Stem Cell Transplantation Unit,
University Hospitals Leuven, Leuven, Belgium

Dennis G. Maki, M.D.
Department of Medicine, University of Wisconsin Hospital and Clinics, Madison, WI, USA

Maurie Markman, M.D.
Department of Gynecologic Oncology, The University of Texas M.D. Anderson Cancer
Center, Houston, Texas, USA

Kieren Marr, M.D.
Division of Infectious Diseases, The Johns Hopkins Hospital, Baltimore, MD, USA

Georg Maschmeyer, M.D.
Department of Hematology, Oncology and Palliative Care, Klinikum Ernst von Bergmann,
Potsdam, Germany

Henry Masur, M.D.
Critical Care Medicine Department, Clinical Center, National Institutes of Health,
Bethesda, MD, USA

Jayesh Mehta, M.D.
Hematopoietic Stem Cell Transplant Program, Robert H. Lurie Comprehensive
Cancer Center, Northwestern University Medical Center, Chicago, IL, USA

Coralia N. Mihu, M.D.
Department of Infectious Diseases, Infection Control, and Employee Health,
The University of Texas M.D. Anderson Cancer Center, Houston, TX, USA

Malgorzata Mikulska, M.D.
Division of Infectious Diseases, San Martino Hospital and University of Genoa, Genoa, Italy

José G. Montoya, M.D.
Department of Internal Medicine, Division of Infectious Diseases and Geographic Medicine, Stanford University School of Medicine, Stanford, CA, USA;
Toxoplasma Serology Laboratory, Palo Alto Medical Foundation,
Palo Alto, CA, USA

Victor Mulanovich, M.D.
Infectious Diseases Department, The University of Texas
M.D. Anderson Cancer Center, Houston, TX, USA

Daniel M. Musher, M.D.
Departments of Medicine, Microbiology and Immunology, Baylor College of Medicine, Infectious Diseases Section, Veterans Affairs Medical Center, Houston, TX, USA

Dionissios Neofytos, M.D.
Division of Infectious Diseases, The Johns Hopkins Hospital, Baltimore, MD, USA

Francesca F. Norman, M.D.
Tropical Medicine and Clinical Parasitology Unit, Department of Infectious Diseases, Ramón y Cajal Hospital, Madrid, Spain

Marcio Nucci, M.D.
Department of Internal Medicine, Hematology Unit Head, Mycology Laboratory,
Hospital Universitário Clementino Fraga Filho – Federal University of Rio de Janeiro,
Rio de Janeiro, Brazil

Susan O'Brien, M.D.
Department of Leukemia, The University of Texas M.D. Anderson Cancer Center,
Houston, TX, USA

Genovefa Papanicolaou, M.D.
Infectious Diseases Service, Memorial Sloan-Kettering Cancer Center,
New York, NY, USA

Alla Paskovaty, Pharm.D.
Infectious Diseases Service, Memorial Sloan-Kettering Cancer Center, New York, NY, USA

Ben de Pauw, M.D.
Institute of Haematology and Clinical Oncology "Lorenzo e Ariosto Seràgnoli",
Sant'Orsola-Malpighi Hospital, University of Bologna, Bologna, Italy

John R. Perfect, M.D.
Department of Medicine, Division of Infectious Diseases and International Health,
Duke University Medical Center, Durham, NC, USA

David S. Perlin, Ph.D.
Department of Clinical Sciences and Administration, College of Pharmacy,
University of Houston, Texas Medical Center Campus, Houston, TX, USA;
Department of Infectious Disease, Infection Control, and Employee Health, The University
of Texas/M.D. Anderson Cancer Center, Houston, TX, USA

Christopher D. Pfeiffer, M.D.
Department of Medicine, Division of Infectious Diseases and International Health,
Duke University Medical Center, Durham, NC, USA

Issam Raad, M.D.
Department of Infectious Diseases, Infection Control, and Employee Health,
The University of Texas M.D. Anderson Cancer Center, Houston, TX, USA

Dhanesh B. Rathod, M.D.
Department of Infectious Diseases, Infection Control, and Employee Health,
The University of Texas M.D. Anderson Cancer Center, Houston, TX, USA

Kenneth V. I. Rolston, M.D.
Department of Infectious Diseases, Infection Control, and Employee Health,
The University of Texas M.D. Anderson Cancer Center, Houston, TX, USA

Amar Safdar, M.D.
Department of Infectious Diseases, Infection Control, and Employee Health,
The University of Texas M.D. Anderson Cancer Center, Houston, TX, USA

Nasia Safdar, M.D.
Section of Infectious Diseases, Department of Medicine, University of Wisconsin
Medical School, Madison, WI, USA

Hélène Schoemans, M.D.
Department of Hematology, Acute Leukemia and Stem Cell Transplantation Unit,
University Hospitals Leuven, Leuven, Belgium

Brahm H. Segal, M.D.
Department of Medicine and Immunology, Roswell Park Cancer Institute,
Department of Medicine, School of Medicine and Biomedical Sciences,
University of Buffalo, Elm & Carlton Streets, Buffalo, NY, USA

Susan K. Seo, M.D.
Infectious Diseases Service, Memorial Sloan-Kettering Cancer Center,
New York, NY, USA

Vickie R. Shannon, M.D.
Department of Pulmonary Medicine, The University of Texas
M.D. Anderson Cancer Center, Houston, TX, USA

Samuel Shelburne, M.D.
Department of Infectious Diseases, The University of Texas
M.D. Anderson Cancer Center, Houston, TX, USA

Marta Stanzani, M.D.
Institute of Haematology and Clinical Oncology "Lorenzo e Ariosto Seràgnoli",
Sant' Orsola-Malpighi Hospital, University of Bologna, Bologna, Italy

David A. Stevens, M.D.
Department of Medicine, Stanford University School of Medicine Division
of Infectious Diseases, Santa Clara Valley Medical Center, Saratoga, CA, USA

Diane E. Stover, M.D.
Department of Medicine, Pulmonary Medicine Service, Memorial Sloan-Kettering,
New York, NY, USA

Aruna Subramanian, M.D.
Division of Infectious Diseases, Johns Hopkins University School of Medicine,
Baltimore, MD, USA

Ursula Theuretzbacher, Ph.D.
Center for Anti-Infective Agents, Vienna, Austria

José Francisco Tomaś-Martinez, M.D.
Department of Hematology, The University of Texas M.D. Anderson International España,
Madrid, Spain

Harrys A. Torres, M.D.
Department of Infectious Diseases, Infection Control, and Employee Health,
The University of Texas M.D. Anderson Cancer Center, Houston, TX, USA

Karen J. Vigil, M.D.
University of Texas Health Science Center, Houston, TX, USA

Claudio Viscoli, M.D.
Division of Infectious Diseases, San Martino Hospital
and University of Genoa, Genoa, Italy

David M. Weinstock, M.D.
Department of Medical Oncology, Dana-Farber Cancer Institute, Boston, MA, USA

John R. Wingard, M.D.
Department of Medicine, University of Florida, Gainesville, FL, USA

Markus Zeitlinger, M.D.
Department of Clinical Pharmacology, Medical University of Vienna, Vienna, Austria

Part I
Overview and Special Population

Chapter 1
Infections in Patients with Cancer: Overview

Amar Safdar, Gerald Bodey, and Donald Armstrong

Abstract Patients with neoplastic disease are often highly susceptible to severe infections. The following factors influence the types, severity, and response to therapy of these infections: (1) Changing epidemiology of infections; (2) cancer- and/or treatment-associated neutropenia; (3) acquired immune deficiency states such as cellular immune defect; (4) recent development of new-generation diagnostic tools including widely available DNA amplification tests; (5) effective intervention for infection prevention; (6) empiric or presumptive therapy during high-risk periods; (7) availability of new classes of highly active antimicrobial drugs; (8) strategies to promote hosts' immune response; and (9) future measures. This introductory chapter intended for the reader to become familiar with the important historical milestones in the understanding and development in the field of infectious diseases in immunosuppressed patients with an underlying neoplasms and patients undergoing hematopoietic stem cell transplantation.

Keywords Cancer • Infection • Neutropenia • Immune defects • Diagnosis • Therapy

Patients with neoplastic disease are often highly susceptible to severe infections. These are inclined to be difficult to prevent, diagnose, and treat. There are a variety of reasons for this which will be discussed in detail in the chapters of this book. We will introduce this volume by reviewing the history and background of such infections, where we believe major advances have been made and what we believe will be necessary to effectively prevent and manage such infections in the future. The following factors influence the types, severity, and response to therapy of these infections: (1) Changing epidemiology of infections; (2) cancer- and/or treatment-associated neutropenia; (3) acquired immune deficiency states such as cellular immune defect; (4) recent development of new-generation diagnostic tools including widely available DNA amplification tests; (5) effective intervention for infection prevention; (6) empiric or presumptive therapy during high-risk periods; (7) availability of new classes of highly active antimicrobial drugs; (8) strategies to promote hosts' immune response; and (9) future measures.

Historical Perspective

The introduction of chemotherapeutic regimens has expanded the population at risk, since many of these agents affect host defenses, most often causing neutropenia. However, even in acute leukemia, the malignancy with the highest frequency of infection, very little was published about infectious complications until the second half of the twentieth century. The paucity of published data is illustrated by a book on acute leukemia, published in 1958, which made no mention of infectious complications [1]. Indeed, at that time, some physicians attributed fevers in leukemia patients to a general hypermetabolic condition caused by the neoplasm.

By the 1950s, several antineoplastic agents became available which caused at least transient improvement in some malignant diseases. Nitrogen mustard caused responses in Hodgkin disease, aminopterin caused responses in acute leukemia, and methotrexate cured choriocarcinoma in women. The subsequent use of multiple drug combinations in acute lymphocytic leukemia and Hodgkin disease represented major advances [2]. Another important advance was the use of platelet transfusions to control and prevent hemorrhage in acute leukemia patients with thrombocytopenia [3]. In an autopsy study, the frequency of hemorrhage as a cause of death in acute leukemia patients decreased from 67 to 37% due to the use of platelet transfusions [4]. Unfortunately, infection remained a major cause of death. There have been many reviews of the subjects over the years, some with international contributors and continuity which are references here [5–11].

A. Safdar (✉)
Department of Infectious Diseases, Infection Control, and Employee Health, The University of Texas M.D. Anderson Cancer Center, 1515 Holcombe Boulevard, Houston, TX 77030, USA
e-mail: amarsafdar@gmail.com

Epidemiological Factors

Exposures to organisms in the distant as well as recent past should be considered in patients with neoplastic disease. Latent infections may be activated in the presence of waning immunity whether it be due to the disease itself or to the treatment. The classic example of this is reactivation of latent tuberculous in patients with treatment-induced helper T-cell dysfunction. Additional latent infections which may be activated, for example, are histoplasmosis, coccidiomycosis, disease caused by the Herpes group of viruses, toxoplasmosis, strongyloidiasis, and others. These demand consideration and many such as TB, herpes simplex, and strongyloidiasis can be effectively treated prophylactically. Recent travel or residence and hospitalization may expose patients to organisms which may incubate such as malaria after travel to an endemic area or colonization due to drug-resistant bacteria such as *Klebsiella*, *Pseudomonas*, and *Stenotrophomonas* species acquired during a previous hospitalization. Questions to investigate epidemiologic factors should include exposures at home along with work, habits, and hobbies. Also, a detailed history of recent and remote travel and recreational activities may provide clues for an otherwise improbable diagnosis. All of these can be a source of infection, some of which can be avoided with appropriate patient education.

Hosts' Susceptibility

It is not surprising that the frequency of infection is related to the type of underlying malignancy and most infections occur in patients who are failing to respond to their cancer therapy. Surveys in the 1960s found that about 80% of patients with acute leukemia, 75% with lymphoma, but less than 40% of patients with metastatic carcinoma developed infection [12, 13]. There are a wide variety of factors that may impact on the susceptibility of cancer patients to infection [11]. Local factors such as tumor masses that may obstruct the bronchial tree or urinary tract and necrotic tumors in the gastrointestinal tract can result in infection. In an autopsy study of children with metastatic carcinoma, 80% of cases of pneumonia were associated with pulmonary metastases, aspiration, or tracheostomy [14]. Antibiotic therapy is often of limited efficacy in these types of tumors, unless the local predisposing factor can be removed.

Immunological Factors

Neutropenia is the most important predisposing factor and can be due to the disease or its therapy. While there were some reports of the role of neutropenia in infection, a detailed analysis of 52 patients with acute leukemia was published in 1966 [15]. This study demonstrated that the risk of infection was related to the degree and duration of neutropenia. The risk increased when the neutrophil count was less than 1,000/mm^3, but increased substantially when it was below 500/mm^3. Also, the risk of developing infection increased the longer the duration of neutropenia. One hundred percent of episodes of severe neutropenia (<100 PMN/mL) lasting 3 weeks or longer were accompanied by identifiable infection compared to 65% of episodes lasting one week. Neutropenia diminishes the likelihood of detecting characteristic manifestations of infection. One study compared physical findings of infection in a group of patients with severe neutropenia with a group with adequate neutrophil counts [16]. Only 8% of patients in the former group with pneumonia were able to produce purulent sputum compared to 84% in the latter group. Similarly, among patients with urinary tract infections, pyuria was found in 11 and 97%, respectively. In an autopsy study, it was demonstrated that many pulmonary infections were not detected on routine chest radiographs antemortem [17]. Likewise, among patients with gram-negative bacillary pneumonia, 85% of those with initially abnormal chest radiographs had >1,000 neutrophils/mL, whereas 81% with normal roentgenograms had <1,000 neutrophils/mL [18]. The lack of signs of infection in febrile neutropenic patients impairs the physician's ability to determine whether or not fever is due to infection. In one study of fever in neutropenic patients, physicians were required to conclude whether infection was present or not before instituting therapy [19]. The physician's initial diagnosis (infection or fever of unknown origin) was incorrect in 33% of the cases.

White blood cell (WBC) transfusions were initiated in an effort to improve the outcome of infections in severely neutropenic patients. Since it was difficult to collect sufficient neutrophils from normal donors, initially, patients with chronic myelogenous leukemia with high neutrophil counts were used as donors [20]. Later, the development of the continuous cell separating machine made it possible to collect adequate cells from normal donors [21]. Studies demonstrated that there was a direct relationship between the number of cells transfused and the increment in the recipient's neutrophil count. In one study of 128 neutropenic patients who had fever unresponsive to antibiotic therapy, 49% responded after WBC transfusions, including patients with pneumonia and gram-negative bacillary septicemia [22]. Unfortunately, potential adverse effects occurred in some recipients. In one study when WBC transfusions were administered with amphotericin B, 64% of patients developed acute dyspnea, respiratory deterioration, and new pulmonary infiltrates compared to only 6% of patients who did not receive amphotericin B [23]. Several other studies failed to observe this toxicity. Another potential adverse event primarily for bone marrow transplant recipients was acquisition of cytomegalovirus (CMV) infection [24]. Reports of graft-versus-host disease (GVHD) in a few recipients has led to routine irradiation transfused cells, but questions have been raised about adverse effects of radiation on the function of the transfused neutrophils. In a review of seven prospective randomized trials of WBC transfusions in neutropenic patients with infection, it was concluded that the transfusions were of some benefit in five studies but the number of patients in each study was small [25]. A problem with many was the ignoring of the number of neutrophils administered; hence, some patients received an inadequate dose. The use of WBC transfusions diminished by the 1980s because there was inadequate evidence of their efficacy from prospective comparative studies. However, there has been a resurgence of interest in increasing available neutrophils since recombinant myeloid growth factor granulocyte-colony-stimulating factor (G-CSF) has become available. Administration of G-CSF to donors improves the number of neutrophils collected as well as increases their activity against infection [26].

Protected Environment. Because of the risk of infection during periods of chemotherapy-induced neutropenia, efforts were made to provide a sterile environment for these patients. The first type of unit was a bed surrounded by a plastic canopy with filtered air (Fig. 1.1). Later, laminar air flow rooms were designed [27]. These units provided filtered air, sterile water supply, sterile room, specially prepared food, and toilet facilities. The patients were given specifically prepared "sterile" food and prophylactic oral and topical antibiotics. These rooms, air, food, and patients were carefully monitored for microbial contamination [28, 29]. The program reduced the frequency of infection and permitted the use of more intensive chemotherapy in the premyeloid growth factor era. Unfortunately, more intensive chemotherapy in this setting did not result in higher remission rates for several malignancies including acute leukemia [30], lymphoma [31], and sarcoma [32]. One review of protected environment entitled "Protected Environment are discomforting and expensive and do not offer meaningful protection" summarized the discussion as follows "The one constant in almost every controlled study is that life has not been prolonged, remission induction increased, nor remission prolonged" [8].

In the late 1940s and early 1950s, patients with neoplasms were originally found to be infected with organisms from the flora in their nasopharynx and the gastrointestinal tract due to neutropenia caused by their disease or subsequent therapy. Exceptions were those with cellular immune defects due to the neoplasm such as Hodgkin's disease, who might present with cryptococcosis or those with multiple myeloma who might present with pneumococcal septicemia because of their decreased production of normal immune globulins. In the neutropenic patient, the organisms invading from the nasopharynx were usually *Streptococcus pyogenes* or *Staphylococcus aureus* (penicillin susceptible). From the orointestinal tract, *Escherica coli* and *Klebsiella* or *Proteus* species were responsible; these bacteria were sensitive to most available antibiotics during early 1950s. Gradually, but steadily, resistance developed in most of the organisms except *S. pyogenes*. *S. aureus* resistant to penicillin and *Pseudomonas aeruginosa* resistant to all antimicrobials except polymyxin appeared in the late 1950s [4, 33, 34]. Antimicrobial resistance developed over the years among the orointestinal isolates and the Gram-positive cocci increased to become predominate by the 1980s with MRSA and penicillin-resistant

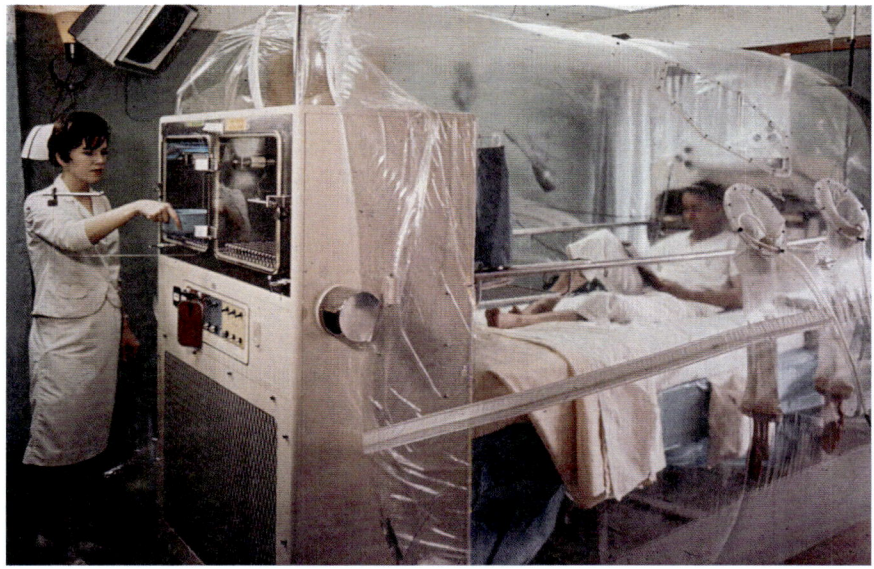

Fig. 1.1 First type of protective environment for severely neutropenic patients. Note, sleeves in the side of canopy to perform tasks on patient and chambers at the foot that irradiated items placed into unit

alpha streptococci appearing. Many of the effective anticancer treatment regimens result in neutropenia so that these types of infection remain a major problem in patients with neoplastic disease.

In contrast, patients with cellular immune defects due to their basic disease or its therapy are prey to a different array of organisms. Predisposing diseases include Hodgkin's disease, T lymphocyte lymphomas and leukemias, and hairy cell leukemia. Various transplantation procedures and GVHD along with treatments for them including cyclosporine, antithymocyte globulin, tacrolimus and adrenocorticosteroids induce defects which result in such opportunistic infections. The diseases are due to organisms from all categories including *Salmonella* spp., *Histoplasma capsulatum*, *Leishmania* spp., and CMV. In the early 1980s and with the advent of the AIDS epidemic, investigators with access to laboratories where T cells could be measured began systematic studies that revealed that patients with levels in the 200 range or lower would develop one or more of these opportunistic infections, especially PCP. It became apparent that as the T cells fell, it could be predicted which organisms would cause disease [8, 35]. Now with the measurements of endogenous cytokines, T-cell subset populations, and functional analysis, this is even more predictable and offers opportunities for treatment and prevention.

B-cell defects have been well described occurring in certain groups of patients with certain underlying neoplastic diseases such as multiple myeloma and chronic lymphocytic leukemia or those after bone marrow transplantation. In these instances, the organisms to be anticipated are *Streptococcus pneumoniae*, *Hemophilus influenzae*, *Neiseriae meningitimus,* or late after transplantation, Echoviruses. Vaccine studies in this group of patients and others are underway to try to achieve protection.

An altered integument allows access to a large variety of organisms to invade patients with neoplastic disease. Areas at risk include the entire orointestinal tract where chemotherapy-induced mucositis with ulcers allow organisms' entry into tissues and the bloodstream. Intravascular catheters allow direct entry into the bloodstream and other catheters such as bladder, intraperitoneal or intracranial devices are sources of infection especially in the neutropenic patient. In addition, life-threatening infections may result from infusion of blood products or transplanted organs. These may vary from HIV and HTLV-I [36] to *Salmonella* spp., *Candida* spp., and *Trypanasoma cruzi* among others.

Knowing the immunological defect in a patient with neoplastic disease suspected of having an infection is extremely important. From the clinical picture, the appropriate tests can be done to confirm the diagnosis, and if indicated, empiric therapy can be started. A fine example of this is the empiric therapy of the neutropenic patient with appropriate antibiotics for anticipated organisms in the clinical setting such as a particular hospital. In the early 1960s, a clinical study from the NCI documented the association of the fall of the neutrophil count with the rise of the severe infections [15]. An example of a population at risk for a specific infection due to an immune defect was the prevention of Pneumocystis pneumonia in children with acute lymphoblastic leukemia carried out at St. Judes Hospital in Memphis TN [37]. Almost 100% protection was achieved. Knowledge of the perturbations in immune function following bone marrow transplantation has enabled clinicians to use preemptive therapy for suspected infections such as those caused by CMV.

Finally, immune defects involving innate and adaptive immune responses may occur in patients who have received prolonged courses of chemotherapy, neoadjuvant antineoplastic monoclonal antibody therapy, or immunosuppressive agents for treatment of GVHD following allogeneic stem cell transplantation.

Diagnostic Evaluation of Infection

There have been remarkable advances in diagnostic tests for the evaluation of infection in the past five decades, especially in diagnostic microbiology allowing us to make earlier and more specific microbial diagnoses. Gram stains, invented in 1884 by Hans Christian Gram in Denmark, and variations on dye techniques are still routine and useful for early presumptive diagnoses, but immunological methods using direct fluorescent antibody stains have been developed and are regularly used especially for viruses. In unusual circumstances such as suspected polyoma virus infection, electron microscopy may be used. New culture methods include isolator lysis centrifugation tubes which are used for continuous around-the-clock monitoring employing a fluorescent carbon dioxide detection system. An automated broth system can be used for quantitation by colony counts of centrifuged sediments and these systems are more sensitive for the isolation of some fungi, mycobacteria and *Bartonella* species. In addition, the broth can be examined by nucleic acid probes and HPLC for rapid organism identification. Automated broth Minimum Inhibitory Concentration (MIC) antimicrobial susceptibility tests yield more rapid results which can be entered into online computer systems for clinicians and recorded for antimicrobial susceptibility patterns for hospital infection control. To help select antimicrobial regimens for empiric therapy, these data can also be available for local and national Health Departments as well as the hospital.

Polymerase chain reaction (PCR) techniques to recognize copies of nucleic acid fragments in various specimens have been developed and are being used. Many are undergoing FDA approval and some may be available only in special laboratories. These techniques may well replace earlier tests using antigen detection by poly or monoclonal antibodies and chemical tests for specific cellular elements such as arabinatol, beta D-glucan, or galactomanans of fungi.

Antibody tests are much easier to perform since the enzyme-linked antibody (ELISA) test has replaced the compliment fixation (CF) test, and for specificity, the Western blot has become the "gold standard". However, for cancer patients and those following allogeneic stem cell transplantation, serologic diagnosis may provide limited information regarding active versus remotely acquired disease. Furthermore, a negative serology cannot be interpreted with certainty due to potential defects in B-cell function.

Radiologic testing with CT scans and MRIs has better defined anatomic lesions for presumptive diagnoses, and recent advances in safe tissue sampling can be used by interventional radiology techniques for specific diagnoses. Bronchoalveolar lavages have virtually replaced open lung biopsies for investigating pulmonary lesions; however, similar to diagnostic reliability of serologic diagnosis, a negative BAL sample smear or culture dose not exclude the possibility of opportunistic lung infection. Radioactive labeling of the patient's own neutrophils and injecting them for localizing foci of infection can sometimes be helpful as can technetium scans. Efforts to localize infected sites using antibody for specific organisms are presently under study and this method could also offer treatment opportunities. Similarly, PET scan are now commonly used for tumor burden and disease recurrence monitoring; this new technology appears promising as an adjuvant diagnostic tool.

Pathogens of Interest

Most infections occurring in patients with nonhematological malignancies are caused by organisms commonly associated with the site of the tumor or nosocomial pathogens except when on chemotherapy. Infections in patients with hematological malignancies are usually caused by organisms that are prevalent in association with specific deficiencies in host defense mechanisms or are due to nosocomial pathogens. Only a few examples will be presented in this discussion, primarily focused on those infections prevalent in neutropenic patients.

Bacterial Infections

Early studies of infection in patients receiving chemotherapy for hematological malignancies found that *S. aureus* developed resistance to penicillin. It became the predominant cause of fatal infection in neutropenic patients [4]. Once effective antibiotics became available for treatment of penicillin-resistant *S. aureus*, gram-negative bacilli emerged as the most common cause of fatal infections. *Pseudonomas aeruginosa* became a major cause of infections, especially among neutropenic patients [29, 37, 38]. Although polymyxin B and colistin were very active in vitro against the pathogen, they were ineffective for therapy in neutropenic patients and were of limited benefit in other patients. Their efficacy in neutropenic patients depended upon the recovery from neutropenia. The availability of carbenicillin, the first β lactam with anti-pseudomonal activity, had a dramatic impact on the therapy of life-threatening *Pseudomonas* infections [39]. Other gram-negative bacilli emerged as significant pathogens, including *Klebiella* spp. and *Serratia marcescens*. Cephalothins were the first β lactam available for the treatment of some of these infections [40]. Over the years, multiplicity of antibiotics has been developed including potent broad-spectrum cephalosprosins, carbapenims, and fluoroquinolones [41]. Despite these important advances, bacterial infections remain a serious threat to cancer patients, due in large part to the ability of organisms to develop resistance to multiple antibiotics. Recent increase in nonpseudomonal nonfermentative Gram-negative bacteria such as *Stenotrophomonas maltophilia* has been associated with difficult-to-treat healthcare-associated infections; these bacteria may also cause less severe community-acquired infections [42]; high-dose trimethoprim-sulfamethoxazole remains the treatment of choice, although occasionally a multidrug-resistant organism poses a serious challenge [43]. Emergence and spread of extended-spectrum beta-lactamases (ESBL) *Enterobacteriaceae* and recently identified carbapenemases producing *Klebsiella* species (KPC) and spreading to other gram-negative disease-associated bacteria herald alarming limitation in choice for effective antimicrobial therapy against these new groups of MDR-gram-negative bacterial infections [44].

Listeria monocytogenes was one of the first bacterial infections reported as occurring more frequently in patients with cellular immune defects [8, 45] and it continues to be a problem [46]. It soon became apparent that *Salmonella* spp., *Nocardia asteroids*, and *Rhodococcus equi* were also opportunistic bacterial pathogens in this setting. *Mycobacterium hemphilum* [47] was thereafter established as a *Mycobacterium* to be anticipated in T-cell-deficient patients, in addition to the classic example of *M. tuberculous* [48] and subsequently *M. avium-intracellulare* complex.

Principles of Antibiotic Therapy in Neutropenic Patient

This discussion will be limited to general principles. Discussion of specific antibiotic therapies is presented in other chapters of this book. After multiple antibiotics became available and the potential for emergence of resistance became apparent, it became the standard practice to withhold antibiotic therapy in the febrile patient until the infecting pathogen was identified. However, early studies of antibiotic therapy for fever in neutropenic patients clearly indicated the importance of instituting antibiotic therapy promptly to neutropenic patients when they become febrile. It has been demonstrated that mortality rates increase substantially if therapy is not administered promptly. The choice of initial antibiotic therapy should provide broad-spectrum antibacterial coverage against gram-positive cocci and gram-negative bacilli. Most infections are caused by aerobic gram-negative bacilli and anaerobic infections tend to be uncommon. It is of critical importance for physicians caring for neutropenic patients to be aware of the common pathogens causing infections at their hospitals and their antimicrobial susceptibilities so that appropriate antibiotic regimens will be selected. Antibiotics that are bactericidal should be selected when possible. The greatest experience has been obtained with broad-spectrum β lactams and aminoglycosides. Aminoglycosides are less effective as single agents in neutropenic patients and should not be used alone [49].

Some studies have indicated that synergistic combinations that provide high serum cidal levels such as a β lactam plus an aminoglycoside are more effective than single agents [50]. However, aminoglycosides have potential nephrotoxicity, which are more prevalent in the elderly and patients with cancer such as multiple myeloma or cancer therapy induced reduced renal reserves.

Various regional, national, and international groups have met and are still meeting to study questions of treatment and how to conduct studies to evaluate treatment of bacterial infections. These have included The Infectious Diseases Society of America [51], The European Organization for Research and Treatment of Cancer [52], and The Immunocompromised Host Society [53]. For empirical antibacterial treatment, it is evident that regimens should be aimed at the most prevalent organisms with reliable knowledge of their susceptibility infecting the patient at a given hospital. It must be stressed that continued efforts at prevention, e.g., scrupulous hygiene, are most important.

Patients with fever of unknown origin that persists after several days of broad-spectrum of antibiotic therapy represent a difficult problem. Careful reevaluation and collection of additional appropriate diagnostic tests need to be performed and additional therapeutic measures should be considered. These may include other antibacterial, antifungal, or antiviral agents. Antifungal agents should be given serious consideration in these patients. Some investigators have advocated that antibiotic therapy be continued in patients with documented infections until the neutrophil count recovers. There is considerable evidence to indicate that this is unnecessary and can encourage superinfection. A more appropriate approach is to discontinue the therapeutic agents, watch carefully.

Mycobacterial Infections

Tuberculous is a well-recognized, albeit uncommon, complication even in patients with severe cellular immune defect [48]. Patients with solid organ cancer may be as susceptible to active *Mycobacterium tuberculous* infection as patients with hematologic malignancy and those undergoing hematopoietic stem cell transplantation [54]. It remains important to realize that tuberculous, being an indolent disease, may be mistaken for a slowly progressing neoplasm and may lead to unnecessary large excisions that can be avoided by initial fine needle aspiration and biopsy of the suspected mass [55].

Nontuberculous mycobacterial disease due to slow-growing mycobacteria is on the rise. Cancer patients with *Mycobacterium intracellulare* lung infections are often postmenopausal women [56], with a selective defect in interferon gamma production or presence of interferon gamma inhibitor [57, 58]. Rapidly growing mycobacterial (RGM) lung disease is uncommon and mostly seen in patients undergoing chemotherapy and in individuals with pervious pulmonary involvement with cancer [59]. *Mycobacterium chelonae* and *Mycobacterium fortuitum* were the prominent RGM associated with lung disease [59, 60]; recently, *Mycobacterium abscessus* has been a predominate RGM pulmonary pathogen [61]. *M. abscessus* infections are difficult-to-treat due to high level of drug-resistance [61] and issues related with drug intolerance. Patients with severe cellular immune defects have significantly poor outcome with disseminated RGM end-organ infection [62], with the exception of *Mycobacterium mucogenicum* catheter-associated infection that responds to prompt removal of the infected catheter and a short course of combination antimicrobial therapy [61].

Fungal Infections

Fungal infections emerged as a significant complication of patients with hematological malignancies after effective chemotherapy became available. The major predisposing factors to these infections were determined to be prolonged neutropenia and adrenocorticosteroid therapy, which interferes with macrophage function. These infections are also prevalent among HSCT recipients who develop graft vs. host disease and receive adrenocorticosteroid therapy.

As early as the mid-1950s, an increasing proportion of patients with acute leukemia developed fungal infections, predominantly candidiasis and aspergillosis [63]. In recent years, infections caused by Zygomycetes, *Fusrium* species, and *Scedasporium* species have become increasingly frequent [64, 65].

There are multiple species of *Candida*, with different antifungal susceptibilities and patterns of infection [56, 66–68]. Superficial candidiasis occurs in cancer patients receiving radiation therapy and those with impaired T-cell function. Infections involved the oropharynx, esophagus, larynx, urinary tract, and gastrointestinal tract and serve as the origin of disseminated infection, especially in those with neutropenia and long-term intravenous catheters. Disseminated infection is often difficult to diagnose because there may be few signs and symptoms except fever and progressive debilitation and the organism is often not cultured from blood specimens. About 10% percent of patients have multiple skin lesions [69]. There is a chronic form of disseminated candidiasis that occurs in neutropenic patients, which persists after neutrophil recovery and is characterized by persistent fever, debilitation, weight loss, and in some patients, hepatosplenomegaly and right upper quadrant pain [70–72].

Mortality rates have been as high as 70% among patients treated with amphotericin B. Fluconazole prophylaxis has been associated with a significant increase in drug-resistant *Candida krusei* and *Candida glabrata* breakthrough disseminated infections [73–75]. Other alternatives are lipid formulations of amphoterician B and echinocandins. Neutrophil recovery is a critical factor in recovery from candidiasis. Prolonged therapy with fluconazole has been effective for chronic candidiasis and recent experience suggests that anti-inflammatory agents may be useful.

Aspergillosis. The major sites of infection are the lungs and sinuses. Disseminated infection is uncommon. Infection is acquired by inhalation of spores and epidemics have occurred during construction in hospitals. The hyphae invade blood vessels causing thrombosis and infraction and can erode through facial planes, cartilage, and bone. Patients with pulmonary infection may present with symptoms suggesting acute pulmonary embolism. Characteristic nodular infiltrates can be detected on pulmonary CT scans "Halo sign" when radiographs are normal [76]. Culture specimens are often negative, but blood galactamannan tests are helpful in establishing the diagnosis and evaluating treatment response [77]. Sinus infections often present with black eschars on the nose or palate. Progressive infection causes proptosis, endophthalmitis, or cerebral infraction. Therapy consists of effective new *Aspergillus* active triazole-based drugs such as voriconazole and posaconazole, and echinocandins such as caspofungin and micafungin in combination or as a single agent [78]. Lipid formulations of amphoterician B are also used in combination with other mold-active drugs. Neutrophil recovery and discontinuation of systemic immunosuppressive therapy, especially adrenal costicosteroids, are important for recovery from the infection. Surgical resection of the infected tissue may benefit some patients and resection of residual cavitary lesions may be necessary to prevent pulmonary hemorrhage and late-recurring bacterial superinfections.

Patients at risk of developing cryptococcosis have impaired cellular immunity or are receiving adrenal corticosteroids; hence, patients with CLL or lymphoma or HSCT recipients are at greatest risk. Infection is acquired by inhalation of organisms; hence, the lung is the primary site of infection, although less than 40% of infected patients present with symptoms of pneumonia. The infection can progress rapidly leading to death. Over 50% of cancer patients develop meningitis and some have widely disseminated infection. The latex agglutination test detects cryptococcal antigen in cerebrospinal fluid or blood of infected patients [79]. Optimal treatment consists of initial systemic therapy with amphotericen B plus low-dose flucytosine [80]; for patients with mild-to-moderate infection, high-dose oral fluconazole may be given for maintenance therapy.

Zygomycosis, caused by molds of the order Mucorales, are increasing in frequency [81]. These infections share the same characteristics as aspergillosis, but mortality rates exceed 70% despite amphotericin B therapy. Newer azoles such as posaconazole may be effective therapy [82]. Over 80% of *Trichosporon* infections are disseminated and the organism can be cultured from blood specimens of most patients. Other infections include endophthalmitis, pneumonia, meningitis, and osteomyelitis [83]. Optimal therapy may be a combination of amphotericin B and fluconazole, but the mortality rate is high in neutropenic patients despite therapy; high-dose voriconazole may be effective in patients with disseminated or hepatosplenic *Trichosporon* species infection [84]. Breakthrough *Trichosporon* infection may occur in patients receiving mold-active drugs such as echinocandins or oral broad-spectrum triazoles [85, 86].

Fusarium spp. cause infections predominantly in the sinuses and lungs. Fusariosis like *Aspergillus* species infection are angioinvasive; pulmonary nodular or mass-like disease is indistinguishable from other mold infections [87]. About 75% of infections in neutropenic patients disseminate and the organism often can be cultured from blood specimens. Nearly half of patients are fungemic and up to 80% or more present may develop multiple (>10) nodular skin lesions that develop necrotic center; skin biopsy is diagnostic and should be performed promptly. Mortality remains high despite the availability of highly active triazole drugs against this organism [87].

Unresolved immune suppression continues to influence treatment response among cancer and hematopoietic stem cell transplant (HSCT) recipients with systemic fungal disease [88]. Various strategies including donor granulocyte transfusions in patients with severe neutropenia have not shown significant improvement in outcomes in recent clinical trials [89]. Combined therapy using effective antifungal agents plus recombinant cytokines to boost macrophage, helper, and cytotoxic lymphocyte functions have been explored; a nonrandomized study using granulocyte-macrophage colony-stimulating factor (GM-CSF) and interferon gamma (IFNγ) which were safe and appeared to have a favorable impact in patients receiving donor granulocyte transfusions [90]. Safety of IFNγ has been a concern due to potential cytokine-induced graft compromise and/or GVHD in recipients of allogeneic HSCT; these concerns were not observed in our patients with life-threatening fungal infections [91], although larger, randomized studies are needed to explore this important issue further. Similarly, drugs that may promote pathogen-directed immune capture by introducing configurational changes in these pathogens are being explored [92, 93].

Viral Infections

For many years, little attention was focused on viral infections in cancer patients due to the lack of rapid diagnostic tests and effective therapy. For example, only in recent years have community respiratory viral infections been recognized as potentially serious to immunocompromised patients. Table 1.1 lists most of these viral infections and available therapy. Many acute viral infections represent reactivation of long-standing latent infection.

Human herpes viruses are among the most common causes of viral infections in cancer patients and are associated with significant morbidity and mortality in severely immunocompromised hosts. Herpes simplex viruses cause oropharyngeal and esophageal disease and may disseminate to other organs. Reactivation of varicella-zoster virus occurs mainly in patients with leukemia and lymphoma and can result in localized infection (shingles), disseminated cutaneous infection, pneumonia, encephalitis, hepatitis, or small bowel disease [94]. CMV infection is most often due to reactivation of latent infection, but has also been attributed to transmission by white blood cell transfusions [24, 95]. It is a special risk to HSCT recipients who may receive infected tissue. CMV may cause hepatitis, meninoencephalitis, pneumonitis, or gastroenteritis [96, 97]. The disease has immunosuppressive effects that increase the risk of other infection. Prophylaxis or preemptive therapeutic strategies are necessary for patients undergoing stem cell transplantation [98]. Epstein–Barr virus can cause a fulminant fatal lymphoproliferative disorder in occasional patients following allogeneic stem cell transplantation. Immunocompromised cancer patients occasionally develop interstitial pneumonitis, encephalitis, or hepatitis due to human herpes virus 6 infections.

Progressive multifocal leukoencephalopathy is a demyelinating disease of the brain caused by the JC virus which occurs infrequently among patients with CLL and Hodgkin disease. The disease is due to reactivation of latent infection that is prevalent in normal adults. Symptoms include visual disturbances, speech defects, and mental deterioration leading to dementia and coma with 80% of patients dying within one year. Parvovirus B19 may cause anemia in cancer patients which may be followed by severe polyarthritis. Most patients have been infected with polyomavirus (BK) virus that persists in the genitourinary tract and is a major cause of hemorrhagic cystitis in HSCT recipients [99].

Community respiratory viral infections cause about 30% of respiratory infections in cancer patients during winter and spring and can be a serious threat to transplant recipients and patients with acute leukemia who may develop viral pneumonia or superinfection with bacteria or fungi [100, 101]. Epidemics have occurred in transplant and leukemia units. Some of these patients have very prolonged viral shedding after resolution of symptoms. Viruses causing infection include influenza A and B, respiratory syncytial virus (RSV), parainfluenza (PIV), and adenovirus. In stem cell transplant recipients following PIV and RSV infections, pulmonary obstructive defects were recently recognized; these may be severe and complete resolution may take longer than 12 months after the initial viral infection [102]. Novel respiratory viruses recently recognized to cause serious life-threatening disease include human metapneumovirus, human cornonavirus NL63 and HKU1, agent of severe acute respiratory syndrome (SARS), and human bocavirus [103, 104]. Adenovirus also causes gastrointestinal infection, hepatitis, hemorrhagic cystitis, pancreatitis, and encephalitis; fatal disseminated adenovirus infections are seen in adults and pediatric patients with profound cellular immune defects such as cordblood transplant recipients with GVHD [105].

Parasitic Infections

Neuro-hepatic toxoplasosis is more common in cancer and transplant recipients in the northeastern United States, whereas strongyloidiasis infestation rates are mostly seen in habitants of southeast and south-central US states. Similarly, amebiasis and giardiasis are infrequently seen in patients from rural residences who consume water from shallow contaminated wells. Latent *Toxoplasma gondii* infection is difficult to diagnose on the bases of travel, food consumption, or history of domestic feline exposure; serology may be diagnostic, although in patients with B-cell defects PCR analysis may be needed. Malaria is mostly seen in patients traveling to endemic regions without prophylaxis or receiving ineffective chemoprophylaxis due to drug-resistant strains of *Plasmodium* species. "Airport malaria" has also been seldom reported in patients who reside near airports with frequent international flights. Transfusion malaria has been observed in patients with neoplastic diseases and should be considered and explored in the presence of unexplained fever [106]. Chaga's disease has also been transmitted by transfusions

Table 1.1 Infections causing pneumonia in cancer patients based on the underlying immune defect

Immune defect	Bacteria	Fungi	Parasites	Viruses
Granulocytopenia	*Staphylococcus aureus*	*Aspergillus fumigatus;* and other *Aspergillus* spp.		Herpes simplex virus I and II
	Streptococcus pneumoniae	Non-*Aspergillus* hyalohyphomycosis		Varicella-zoster virus
	Streptococcus species	Such as *Pseudallescheria boydii, Fusarium solani.*		
	Pseudomonas aeruginosa	Mucorales (zygomycoses)		
	Enterobacteriaceae	Dematiaceous (black) fungi such as *Alternaria*		
	Escherichia coli	*Bipolaris, Curvularia, Scedosporium apiospermum*		
	Klebsiella species	*Scedosporium prolificans*		
	Stenotrophomonas maltophilia			
	Acinetobacter species			
Cellular immune Dysfunction	*Nocardia asteroides* complex	*Aspergillus* and non-*Aspergillus* filamentous molds	*Toxoplasma gondii*	Cytomegalovirus
	Salmonella typhimurium spp.	*Pneumocystis jiroveci (P. carini)*	*Microsporidium* spp.	Respiratory viruses
	Salmonella enteritidis	*Cryptococcus neoformans*	*Leishmania donovani*	Influenza A and Influenza B
	Rhodococcus equi	Endemic mycoses due to *Histoplasma capsulatum*	*Leishmania infantum*	Parainfluenza type-3
	Rhodococcus bronchialis	*Coccidioides immitis, Blastomyces dermatitidis*	*Strongyloides stercoralis*	Respiratory syncytial virus
	Listeria monocytogenes	*Penicillium marnefie*		Adenovirus
	Mycobacterium tuberculous			Varicella-zoster virus
	Nontuberculous mycobacteria			HHV 6
				JC and BK virus
				Parvovirus B19
				SARS-associated coronavirus?
				Paramyxovirus?
				Hantavirus?
Humoral immune Dysfunction Splenctomy	*Streptococcus pneumoniae*	*Pneumocystis jiroveci (P. carini)?*	*Giardia lamblia*	VZV
	Haemophilus influenzae		*Babesia microti*	Echovirus
	Neisseria meningitidis			Enterovirus
	Capnocytophaga canimorsus			
	Campylobacter			
Mixed defects	*Streptococcus pneumoniae*	*Pneumocystis jiroveci (P. carini)*	*Toxoplasma gondii*	Respiratory viruses
	Staphylococcus aureus	*Aspergillus* spp.	*Strongyloides stercoralis*	Influenza
	Haemophilus influenzae	*Candida* spp.		Parainfluenza
	Klebsiella pneumonia	*Cryptococcus neoformans*		Respiratory syncytial virus
	Pseudomonas aeruginosa	Mucorales (zygomycoses)		Adenovirus
	Acinetobacter spp.	Endemic mycoses (severe systemic dissemination)		VZV
	Enterobacter spp.			
	Stenotrophomonas maltophilia			
	Nocardia asteroides complex			
	Listeria monocytogenes			
	Legionella spp.			

Patients with mixed immune defects include recipients of allogeneic hematopoietic stem cell transplant; acute or chronic graft versus host disease; myelodysplastic syndrome; adult T-cell leukemia lymphoma; antineoplastic agents like cyclophosphamide, fludarabine, and HHV6: Human herpesvirus 6 *L. donovani* and *L. infantum* may lead to serious visceral leishmaniasis. *L. donovani* is seen in Africa and Asia, *L. infantum* is seen in Africa, Europe, Mediterranean, and Central and South America. VZV is rarely associated with systemic dissemination in patients with humoral immune defects, or even those with mixed immune dysfunctions. *Strongyloides stercoralis* may lead to serious, life-threatening hyperinfection syndrome in patients with marked cellular immune defects

causing fevers and pericardial effusions [107]. This disease may become more common as the number of potential donors coming from endemic areas increases and also the reduvid bug appears to be moving north into southwestern states. Screening donors may become necessary. A recent increase in fatal *Babesia* species infection reported since

November 2005 in the US has raised concerns of this rare intraerythrocytic parasite disease [108].

Hydated cyst due to *Echinococcus granulosus* and *E. multilocularis* and neurocycticercosis is difficult to distinguish from cystic brain tumor or bacterial or fungal brain abscess. Liver hydrated cyst may present as polymicrobial bacterial abscess in patients from the developing world.

End-Organ Infection

Septicemia including disseminated infection and pneumonia are the most common sites of infection; urinary tract, skin, and central nervous system infection occurs less commonly. The site of infection is often related to the site of the primary tumor, a metastasis, or a surgical procedure. Septicemia is most likely to occur in patients with impaired host defenses. The frequency of infection has been determined in several autopsy studies.

Pneumonia

The management of pneumonia in the cancer patient is often frustrating and difficult. The spectrum of potential pathogens is exceptionally broad including those that infect normal hosts and those that occur predominately in immunocompromised hosts; predisposing factors include deficiencies in host defense mechanisms such as neutropenia or hypo IgG, bronchial obstruction or ulceration due to tumor, mucosal damage due to chemotherapeutics agents, and the use of mechanical ventilation. Cancer patients may develop pulmonary infiltrates due to noninfectious causes such as hemorrhage, radiation pneumonitis, and leukoagglutinin reaction. Several neutropenia patients are unable to produce adequate inflammatory responses and thus may fail to produce persistent sputum, develop clinic signs and symptoms, or develop abnormalities on chest radiographs.

In a study of gram-negative bacillary pneumonia in cancer patients (most of whom had hematological malignances), only 64% had abnormal radiographs at the onset of their pneumonia and 20% never developed abnormalities [109]. Identification of the infecting pathogen is often difficult. Adequate sputum specimens are often not available. The diagnostic yield from invasive procedures such as bronchoalveolar lavage is suboptimal. Biopsies are often contraindicated because of the risk of hemorrhage due to thrombocytopenia or coagulopathies. The use of CT scans and blood tests such as galactomannon detection for Aspergillosis have improved diagnostic capabilities [76].

Abdominal Infections

A wide variety of infection agents may infect the gastrointestinal tract due to obstruction, ulceration, and other factors. This discussion will focus on two infections with potentially serious consequences in neutropenic patients: typhlitis and perianal infections. Typhlitis or neutropenic enterocolitis is characterized by well-demarcated ulcers, hemorrhage, and large masses of organisms with few inflammatory cells usually limited to the cecum, but can be more extensive. Computed tomography scans provide superior images of the intra-abdominal organs and may be able to diagnose subclinical small bowel perforations, infected collections, and pneumatosis intestinalis, a serious complication which requires intense bowel management and presents as surgical dilemma [110]. Bacteremia occurs in 70% of patients. Therapy consists of broad-spectrum antibiotics, and anti-*Candida* agents, bowel rest, and decompression are important [110].

Perianal infections are most common in patients with acute monocytic leukemias. The prominent symptoms are fever and pain on defecation. Lesions often arise adjacent to a hemorrhoids and are indurated and ulcerated, often with extensive necroses. It is important to evaluate for recrudescent Herpes virus infections and perirectal abscess. Evaluation of surgical intervention may be obtained if there is not a prompt response to antimicrobial therapy or if a drainable focus is identified.

Catheter-Related Infections

Most cancer patients receiving antineoplastic therapy have indwelling central venous access. Catheter infections are an important cause of delay in chemotherapy, hospitalization, cost of care, and deaths [111, 112]. Coagulase-negative *Staphylococcus* (CoNS) and other skin gram-positive bacteria are common pathogens. Catheter removal reduces risk of infection recurrences [113], and in patients with high-grade bacteremia or candidemia with or without hemodynamic compromise, the catheter should be removed immediately. A thorough evaluation for underlying endovascular infection such as septic thrombophlebitis may yield a source of persistent bacteremia, lack of complete response, and influence duration of systemic antimicrobial therapy. Factors that influence antimicrobial choice include (a) penetration of drug in the biofilm, (b) antimicrobial activity within the biofilm, and (c) activity against the nonplanktonic stationary phase of the microorganisms [114]. A detailed discussion of this important topic is presented in two chapters.

This introductory chapter intended for the reader to become familiar with the important historical milestones in the understanding and development in the field of infectious diseases in immunosuppressed patients with an underlying neoplasm and patients undergoing hematopoietic stem cell transplantation.

References

1. Dameshek W, Gunz F. Leukemia. 1st ed. New York: Grune & Stratten; 1958.
2. DeVita VT, Chu E. A history of cancer chemotherapy. Cancer Res. 2008;68:8643–53.
3. Gaydos LA, Freireich EJ, Mantel N. The quantitative relation between platelet count and hemorrhage in patients with acute leukemia. N Engl J Med. 1962;266:905–9.
4. Hersh EM, Bodey GP, Nies BA, et al. Causes of death in acute leukemia. A ten year study of 414 patients from 1954-1963. JAMA. 1965;193:105–9.
5. Armstrong D. Infections complicates of neoplastic diseases: diagnosis and management – part I. Clin Bull. 1976;6:135–41.
6. Armstrong D. Infections complicates of neoplastic diseases: diagnosis and management – part II. Clin Bull. 1977;7:13–20.
7. Armstrong D. Infections in patients with neoplastic disease. In: Verhoef J et al., editors. Infections in the immunocompromised host – Pathogenesis, prevention and therapy. New York: Elsevier/North Holland; 1980. p. 129–58.
8. Brown AE, Armstrong D, editors. Controversies in the management of infectious complications of neoplastic disease. New York: Yorke Medical Books; 1985. p. 1–424.
9. Armstrong D, Brown AE. Controversies in the management of infectious complications of neoplastic disease. Rev Infect Dis. 1993;17 Suppl 2:317–551.
10. Brown AE. White MH. Controversies in the management of immunocompromised patients. Clin Infect Dis. 1993;17 Suppl 2:317–551.
11. Safdar A, Armstrong D. Infectious morbidity in critically ill patients with cancer. Crit Care Clin. 2001;17:531–70.
12. Boggs DR, Frei III E. Clinical studies of fever and infection in cancer. Cancer. 1960;6:1240–53.
13. Raab SO, Hoeprich PD, Wintrob MM, et al. The clinical significance of fever in acute leukemia. Blood. 1960;16:1609–28.
14. Bodey GP, Hersh EM. The problem of infection in children with malignant disease. In: Neoplasia in childhood. Proceedings of the 12th Annual Clinical Conference at the University of Texas M. D. Anderson Hospital and Tumor Institute at Houston. Chicago, IL, Year Book Medical; 1969. p. 135–54.
15. Bodey GP, Buckley M, Sathe YS, et al. Quantitative relationship between circulating leukocytes and infection in patients with acute leukemia. Ann Intern Med. 1966;64:328–40.
16. Sickles EA, Greene WH, Wiernik PH. Clinical presentation of infection in granulocytopenic patients. Arch Intern Med. 1975;135:715–9.
17. Bodey GP, Powell Jr RD, Hersh EM, et al. Pulmonary complications of acute leukemia. Cancer. 1966;19:781–93.
18. Valdivieso M, Gil-Extremera B, Zornoza J, et al. Gram-negative bacillary pneumonia in the compromised host. Medicine. 1977;56:241–54.
19. Lawson RD, Gentry LO, Bodey GP, et al. Randomized study of tobramycin plus ticarcillin, tobramycin plus cephalothin and ticarcillin, or tobramycin plus mezlocillin in the treatment of infection in neutropenic patients with malignancies. Am J Med Sci. 1984;287:16–23.
20. Morse EE, Freireich EJ, Carbone PP, et al. The transfusion of leukocytes from donors with chronic myelogenous leukemia to patients with leukopenia. Transfusion. 1966;6:183–92.
21. Hester JP, Kellogg RM, Mulzet AP, et al. Principles of blood separation and component extraction in a disposable continuous-flow single-state channel. Blood. 1979;54:254–68.
22. Vallejos C, McCredie KB, Bodey GP, et al. White blood cell transfusions for control of infections in neutropenic patients. Transfusion. 1975;15:28–33.
23. Wright DG, Robichaud KJ, Pizzo PA, et al. Lethal pulmonary reactions associated with the combined use of amphotericin B and leukocyte transfusions. N Engl J Med. 1981;304:1185–9.
24. Winston DJ, Ho WG, Young LS, et al. Prophylactic granulocyte transfusions during human bone marrow transplantation. Am J Med. 1980;68:893–7.
25. Bishton M, Chopra R. The role of granulocyte transfusions in neurtropenic patients. Br J Haematol. 2004;127:501–8.
26. Anderlini P, Champlin RE. Biologic and molecular effects of granulocyte colony-stimulating factor in healthy individuals: recent findings and current challenges. Blood. 2008;111:1767–72.
27. Bodey GP, Hart JS, Freireich EJ, Frei III E. Studies of a patient isolator unit and prophylactic antibiotics in cancer chemotherapy. Cancer. 1968;22:1018–26.
28. Bodey GP, Rosenbaum B. Effect of prophylactic measures on the microbial flora of patients in protected environment units. Medicine. 1974;53:209–28.
29. Bodey GP, Rodriguez V. Infections in cancer patients on a protected environment - prophylactic antibiotic program. Am J Med. 1975;59:497–504.
30. Bodey GP, Gehan EA, Freireich EJ, Frei III E. Protected environment-prophylactic antibiotic program in the chemotherapy of acute leukemia. Am J Med Sci. 1971;252:138–51.
31. Bodey GP. Laminar air flow unit for patients undergoing cancer chemotherapy. In: Mirand EA, Back N, editors. Germ-Free Biology. New York, NY: Plenum Press; 1969. p. 19–26.
32. Bodey GP, Rodriguez V, Murphy WK, Burgess MA, Benjamin RS. Protected environment-prophylactic antibiotic program for malignant sarcomas: Randomized trial during remission induction chemotherapy. Cancer. 1981;47:2422–9.
33. Bodey GP. Epidemiological studies of Pseudomonas speices in patients with leukmeia. Am J Med Sci. 1970;260:82–6.
34. Schimpff SC, Young VM, Greene WH, et al. Origin of infection in acute nonlymphocytic leukemia. Significance of hospital acquisition of potential pathogens. Ann Intern Med. 1972;77:707–14.
35. Hughes WT, Kuhn S, Chaudhary S, et al. Successful chemoprophylaxis for *Pneumocystis carinii* pneumonitis. N Engl J Med. 1977;297:1419–26.
36. Minamoto GY, Gold JWM, Scheinberg DA, et al. Infection with human T-cell leukemia virus type 1 in patients with leukemia. N Engl J Med. 1988;318:219–22.
37. Whitecar Jr JP, Bodey GP, Luna M. Pseudomonas bacteremia in cancer patients. Am J Med Sci. 1970;260:216–23.
38. Schimpff SC, Greene WH, Young VM, et al. Significance of *Pseudomonas aeruginosa* in the patient with leukemia or lymphoma. J Infect Dis. 1974;130(Suppl):24–31.
39. Tapper ML, Armstrong D. Bactermeia due to *Pseudomonas aeruginosa* complicating neoplastic disease. A progress report. J Infect Dis. 1974;130 Suppl:14–23.
40. Bodey GP, Whitecar Jr JP, Middleman E, et al. Carbenicillin therapy of *Pseudomonas* infections. JAMA. 1971;218:62–6.
41. Middleman EA, Watanabe A, Kaizer H, Bodey GP. Antibiotic combinations for infections in neutropenic patients. Evaluation of carbenicillin plus either cephalothin or kanamycin. Cancer. 1972;30:573–9.
42. Aisenberg G, Rolston KV, Dickey BF, Kontoyiannis DP, Raad II, Safdar A. *Stenotrophomonas maltophilia* pneumonia in cancer patients without traditional risk factors for infection, 1997–2004. Eur J Clin Microbiol Infect Dis. 2007;26:13–20.

43. Safdar A, Rolston KV. *Stenotrophomonas maltophilia*: changing spectrum of a serious bacterial pathogen in patients with cancer. Clin Infect Dis. 2007;45:1602–9.
44. Sidjabat HE, Silveira FP, Potoski BA, et al. Interspecies spread of *Klebsiella pneumoniae* carbapenemase gene in a single patient. Clin Infect Dis. 2009;49:1736–8.
45. Louria DB, Hensle T, Armstrong D, et al. Listeriosis complicating malignant disease: a new association. Ann Intern Med. 1967;67:261–81.
46. Safdar A, Armstrong D. Listeriosis in patients at a comprehensive cancer center, 1955–1997. Clin Infect Dis. 2003;37:359–64.
47. Armstrong D, Kiehn T, Boone N, et al. *Mycobacterium haemophilum* infections – New York City metropolitan area, 1990–1991. MMWR Morb Mortal Wkly Rep. 1991;40:636–43.
48. Kaplan MH, Armstrong D, Rosen P. Tuberculosis complicating neoplastic disease. A review of 201 cases. Cancer. 1974;33:850–8.
49. Bodey GP, Middleman E, Umsawasdi T, et al. Infections in cancer patients – results with gentamicin sulfate therapy. Cancer. 1972;29:1697–701.
50. Klasterskly J, Vamecq G, Cappel R, et al. Effects of the combination of gentamicin and carbenicillin on the bactericidal activity of serum. J Infect Dis. 1972;125:183–6.
51. Hughes WT, Armstrong D, Bodey GP, et al. From the working committee, Infectious Diseases Society of America: guidelines for the use of antimicrobial agents in neutropenic patients with unexplained fever. J Infect Dis. 1990;161:381–96.
52. Viscoli C, for the European Organization for the Research and Treatment of Cancer. Management of infection in cancer patients: studies of the EORTC International Antimicrobial Therapy Group (IATG). Eur J Cancer. 2002;38:82–7.
53. Pizzo PA, Armstrong D, Bodey G, et al. From the Immunocompromised Host Society: the design, analysis, and reporting of the clinical trials on the empirical antibiotic management of the neutropenic patient. Report of a consensus panel. J Infect Dis. 1990;161:397–401.
54. De La Rosa GR, Jacobson KL, Rolston KV, Raad II, Kontoyiannis DP, Safdar A. *Mycobacterium tuberculosis* at a comprehensive cancer centre: active disease in patients with underlying malignancy during 1990-2000. Clin Microbiol Infect. 2004;10:749–52.
55. Aisenberg GM, Jacobson K, Chemaly RF, Rolston KV, Raad II, Safdar A. Extrapulmonary tuberculosis active infection misdiagnosed as cancer: *Mycobacterium tuberculosis* disease in patients at a Comprehensive Cancer Center (2001–2005). Cancer. 2005;104:2882–7.
56. Han XY, Tarrand JJ, Infante R, Jacobson KL, Truong M. Clinical significance and epidemiologic analyses of *Mycobacterium avium* and *Mycobacterium intracellulare* among patients without AIDS. J Clin Microbiol. 2005;43:4407–12.
57. Safdar A, White DA, Stover D, Armstrong D, Murray HW. Profound interferon gamma deficiency in patients with chronic pulmonary nontuberculous mycobacteriosis. Am J Med. 2002;113:756–9.
58. Safdar A, Armstrong D, Murray HW. A novel defect in interferon-gamma secretion in patients with refractory nontuberculous pulmonary mycobacteriosis. Ann Intern Med. 2003;138:521.
59. Rolston KV, Jones PG, Fainstein V, Bodey GP. Pulmonary disease caused by rapidly growing mycobacteria in patients with cancer. Chest. 1985;87:503–6.
60. Jacobson K, Garcia R, Libshitz H, Whimbey E, Rolston K, Abi-Said D, et al. Clinical and radiological features of pulmonary disease caused by rapidly growing mycobacteria in cancer patients. Eur J Clin Microbiol Infect Dis. 1998;17:615–21.
61. Han XY, Dé I, Jacobson KL. Rapidly growing mycobacteria: clinical and microbiologic studies of 115 cases. Am J Clin Pathol. 2007;128:612–21.
62. Ingram CW, Tanner DC, Durack DT, Kernodle Jr GW, Corey GR. Disseminated infection with rapidly growing mycobacteria. Clin Infect Dis. 1993;16:463–71.
63. Bodey GP. Fungal infections complicating acute leukemia. J Chronic Dis. 1966;19:667–87.
64. Roden MM, Zaoutis TE, Buchanan WL, et al. Epidemiology and outcome of zygomycosis: a review of 929 reported cases. Clin Infect Dis. 2005;41:634–53.
65. Kontoyiannis DP, Lionakis MS, Lewis RE, et al. Zygomycosis in a tertiary-care cancer center in the era of Aspergillus-active antifungal therapy: a case-control observational study of 27 recent cases. J Infect Dis. 2005;191:1350–60.
66. Singer C, Kaplan MH, Armstrong D. Bacteremia and fungemia complicating neoplastic disease. A study of 364 cases. Am J Med. 1977;62:731–42.
67. Whimbey E, Kiehn TE, Brannon P, Blevins A, Armstrong D. Bacteremia and fungemia in patients with neoplastic disease. Am J Med. 1987;82:723–30.
68. Safdar A, Perlin DS, Armstrong D. Hematogenous infections due to *Candida parapsilosis*: changing trends in fungemic patients at a comprehensive cancer center during the last four decades. Diagn Microbiol Infect Dis. 2002;44:11–6.
69. Bodey GP, Luna M. Skin lesions associated with disseminated candidiasis. JAMA. 1974;229:1466–8.
70. Bodey GP, DeJongh D, Isassi A, Freireich EJ. Hypersplenism due to disseminated candidiasis in a patient with acute leukemia. Cancer. 1969;26:417–20.
71. Ferreira RP, Yu B, Niki Y, Armstrong D. Detection of *Candida antigenuria* in disseminated candidiasis by immunoblotting. J Clin Microbiol. 1990;28:1075–8.
72. Horn R, Wong B, Kiehn TE, Armstrong D. Fungemia in a cancer hospital: changing frequency, earlier onset, and results of therapy. Rev Infect Dis. 1985;7:646–55.
73. Wingard JR. The use of fluconazole prophylaxis in patients with chemotherapy-induced neutropenia. Leuk Lymphoma. 1992;8:353–9.
74. Wingard JR, Merz WG, Rinaldi MG, Johnson TR, Karp JE, Saral R. Increase in *Candida krusei* infection among patients with bone marrow transplantation and neutropenia treated prophylactically with fluconazole. N Engl J Med. 1991;325:1274–7.
75. Safdar A, van Rhee F, Henslee-Downey JP, Singhal S, Mehta J. *Candida glabrata* and *Candida krusei* fungemia after high-risk allogeneic marrow transplantation: no adverse effect of low-dose fluconazole prophylaxis on incidence and outcome. Bone Marrow Transplant. 2001;28:873–8.
76. Greene RE, Schlamm HT, Oestmann JW, et al. Imaging findings in acute invasive pulmonary aspergillosis: clinical significance of the halo sign. Clin Infect Dis. 2007;44:373–9.
77. Maschmeyer G, Beinert T, Buchheidt D, et al. Diagnosis and antimicrobial therapy of lung infiltrates in febrile neutropenic patients: Guidelines of the infectious diseases working party of the German Society of Haematology and Oncology. Eur J Cancer. 2009;45:2462–72.
78. Marr KA, Boeckh M, Carter RA, Kim HW, Corey L. Combination antifungal therapy for invasive aspergillosis. Clin Infect Dis. 2004;39:797–802.
79. Fisher BD, Armstrong D. Cryptococcal interstitial pneumonia: value of antigen determination. N Engl J Med. 1977;97:1440–1.
80. White M, Cirrincione C, Blevins A, Armstrong D. Cryptococcal meningitis: outcome in patients with AIDS and patients with neoplastic disease. J Infect Dis. 1992;165:960–3.
81. Kontoyiannis DP, Wessel VC, Bodey GP, Rolston KVI. Zygomycosis in the 1990s in a tertiary-care cancer center. Clin Infect Dis. 2000;30:851–6.
82. Greenberg RN, Mullane K, van Burik JA, et al. Posaconazole as salvage therapy for zygomycosis. Antimicrob Agents Chemother. 2006;50:126–33.

83. Walsh TJ, Melcher GP, Rinaldi MG, Lecciones J, McGough DA, Kelly P, et al. *Trichosporon beigelii*, an emerging pathogen resistant to amphotericin B. J Clin Microbiol. 1990;28:1616–22.
84. Asada N, Uryu H, Koseki M, Takeuchi M, Komatsu M, Matsue K. Successful treatment of breakthrough *Trichosporon asahii* fungemia with voriconazole in a patient with acute myeloid leukemia. Clin Infect Dis. 2006;43:e39–41.
85. Bayramoglu G, Sonmez M, Tosun I, Aydin K, Aydin F. Breakthrough *Trichosporon asahii* fungemia in neutropenic patient with acute leukemia while receiving caspofungin. Infection. 2008;36:68–70.
86. Rieger C, Geiger S, Herold T, Nickenig C, Ostermann H. Breakthrough infection of *Trichosporon asahii* during posaconazole treatment in a patient with acute myeloid leukaemia. Eur J Clin Microbiol Infect Dis. 2007;26:843–5.
87. Torres HA, Raad II, Kontoyiannis DP. Infections caused by Fusarium species. J Chemother. 2003;15 Suppl 2:28–35.
88. Safdar A. Strategies to enhance immune function in hematopoietic transplantation recipients who have fungal infections. Bone Marrow Transplant. 2006;38:327–37.
89. Seidel MG, Peters C, Wacker A, Northoff H, Moog R, Boehme A, et al. Randomized phase III study of granulocyte transfusions in neutropenic patients. Bone Marrow Transplant. 2008;42:679–84.
90. Safdar A, Rodriguez GH, Lichtiger B, Dickey BF, Kontoyiannis DP, Freireich EJ, et al. Recombinant interferon gamma1b immune enhancement in 20 patients with hematologic malignancies and systemic opportunistic infections treated with donor granulocyte transfusions. Cancer. 2006;106:2664–71.
91. Safdar A, Rodriguez G, Ohmagari N, Kontoyiannis DP, Rolston KV, Raad II, et al. The safety of interferon-gamma-1b therapy for invasive fungal infections after hematopoietic stem cell transplantation. Cancer. 2005;103:731–9.
92. Safdar A, Rodriguez G, Rolston KV, O'Brien S, Khouri IF, Shpall EJ, et al. High-dose caspofungin combination antifungal therapy in patients with hematologic malignancies and hematopoietic stem cell transplantation. Bone Marrow Transplant. 2007;39:157–64.
93. Safdar A. Fungal cytoskeleton dysfunction or immune activation triggered by beta-glucan synthase inhibitors: potential mechanisms for the prolonged antifungal activity of echinocandins. Cancer. 2009;115:2812–5.
94. Armstrong D, Chmel H, Singer C, Tapper M, Rosen PP. Nonbacterial infections associated with neoplastic disease. Eur J Cancer. 1975;11 Suppl:79–94.
95. Nichols WG, Price TH, Gooley T, Corey L, Boeckh M. Transfusion-transmitted cytomegalovirus infection after receipt of leukoreduced blood products. Blood. 2003;101:4195–200.
96. Meyers JD, Flournoy N, Thomas ED. Cytomegalovirus infection and specific cell-mediated immunity after marrow transplant. J Infect Dis. 1980;142:816–24.
97. Boeckh M, Leisenring W, Riddell SR, et al. Late cytomegalovirus disease and mortality in recipients of allogeneic hematopoietic stem cell transplants: importance of viral load and T-cell immunity. Blood. 2003;101:407–14.
98. Goodrich JM, Mori M, Gleaves CA, et al. Early treatment with ganciclovir to prevent cytomegalovirus disease after allogeneic bone marrow transplantation. N Engl J Med. 1991;325:1601–7.
99. Arthur RR, Shah KV, Baust SJ, Santos GW, Saral R. Association of BK viruria with hemorrhagic cystitis in recipients of bone marrow transplants. N Engl J Med. 1986;315:230–4.
100. Kim YJ, Boeckh M, Englund JA. Community respiratory virus infections in immunocompromised patients: hematopoietic stem cell and solid organ transplant recipients, and individuals with human immunodeficiency virus infection. Semin Respir Crit Care Med. 2007;28:222–42.
101. Chemaly RF, Ghosh S, Bodey GP, Rohatgi N, Safdar A, Keating MJ, et al. Respiratory viral infections in adults with hematologic malignancies and human stem cell transplantation recipients: a retrospective study at a major cancer center. Medicine (Baltimore). 2006;85:278–87.
102. Erard V, Chien JW, Kim HW, Nichols WG, Flowers ME, Martin PJ, et al. Airflow decline after myeloablative allogeneic hematopoietic cell transplantation: the role of community respiratory viruses. J Infect Dis. 2006;193:1619–25.
103. Boeckh M. The challenge of respiratory virus infections in hematopoietic cell transplant recipients. Br J Haematol. 2008;143: 455–67.
104. Safdar A. Immune modulatory activity of ribavirin for serious human metapneumovirus disease: early i.v. therapy may improve outcomes in immunosuppressed SCT recipients. Bone Marrow Transplant. 2008;41:707–8.
105. La Rosa AM, Champlin RE, Mirza N, Gajewski J, Giralt S, Rolston KV, et al. Adenovirus infections in adult recipients of blood and marrow transplants. Clin Infect Dis. 2001;32:871–6.
106. Tapper ML, Armstrong D. Malaria complicating neoplastic disease. Arch Intern Med. 1976;136:807–10.
107. Grant IH, Gold JWM, Wittner M, et al. Transfusion-associated acute Chagas disease acquired in the United States. Ann Intern Med. 1989;111:849–51.
108. Gubernot DM, Lucey CT, Lee KC, Conley GB, Holness LG, Wise RP. Babesia infection through blood transfusions: reports received by the US Food and Drug Administration, 1997–2007. Clin Infect Dis. 2009;48:25–30.
109. Chang HY, Rodriguez V, Narboni G, Bodey GP, Luna MA, Freireich EJ. Causes of death in adults with acute leukemia. Medicine. 1976;55:259–68.
110. Williams N, Scott AD. Neutropenic colitis: a continuing surgical challenge. Br J Surg. 1997;84:1200–5.
111. Howell PB, Walters PE, Donowitz GR, Farr BM. Risk factors for infection of adult patients with cancer who have tunneled central venous catheters. Cancer. 1995;75:1367–75.
112. Rotstein C, Brock L, Roberts RS. The incidence of first Hickman catheter-related infection and predictors of catheter removal in cancer patients. Infect Control Hosp Epidemiol. 1995;16:451–8.
113. Raad I, Kassar R, Ghannam D, Chaftari AM, Hachem R, Jiang Y. Management of the catheter in documented catheter-related coagulase-negative staphylococcal bacteremia: remove or retain? Clin Infect Dis. 2009;49:1187–94.
114. Fux CA, Wilson S, Stoodley P. Detachment characteristics and oxacillin resistance of *Staphyloccocus aureus* biofilm emboli in an in vitro catheter infection model. J Bacteriol. 2004;186: 4486–91.

Chapter 2
Infections in Hematopoietic Stem Cell Transplant Recipients

Georg Maschmeyer and Per Ljungman

Abstract The risk of infection among allogeneic hematopoietic stem cell transplant (aHSCT) recipients is determined by patient age, underlying disease, the complications that occurred during preceding treatment regimens, the selected transplantation modality, and the severity of graft-versus-host disease. Immunological reconstitution after hematopoietic recovery has an impact on the type of posttransplant infectious complications, and infection-related mortality is significantly higher postengraftment than during the short posttransplant neutropenia. As different pathogenetic and epidemiological backgrounds of infections occur following aHSCT, three consecutive time periods posttransplant are separately described: the early posttransplant period (preengraftment, comprising 3 weeks), the intermediate posttransplant period (3 weeks to 3 months), and the late posttransplant period (later than day +90).

Keywords Allogeneic • Hematopoietic stem cell transplant • Early infection • CMV • Late infections • Graft-versus-host disease

during preceding treatment regimens, the selected transplantation modality, and the severity of graft-versus-host disease (GvHD) [1, 2]. In comparison with patients undergoing high-dose chemotherapy and autologous stem cell transplantation, recipients of aHSCT are at a much higher risk of infection also after hematopoietic reconstitution, due to delayed recovery of T-cell and B-cell functions. Immunological reconstitution after hematopoietic recovery has an impact on the type of posttransplant infectious complications [3, 4], and infection-related mortality is significantly higher postengraftment than during the short posttransplant neutropenia. After nonmyeloablative conditioning, there is a lower risk of severe and fatal infections in the early posttransplant period [5–9]. Because of different pathogenetic and epidemiological backgrounds of infections, three consecutive time periods posttransplant are separately described: the early posttransplant period (preengraftment, comprising 3 weeks), the intermediate posttransplant period (3 weeks to 3 months), and the late posttransplant period (later than day +90) (Fig. 2.1).

Introduction

Fever and Infection After Allogeneic Hematopoietic Stem Cell Transplant

The risk of infection among allogeneic hematopoietic stem cell transplant (aHSCT) recipients is determined by patient age, underlying disease, the complications that occurred

Early Posttransplant Period (Preengraftment; Earlier than Day +21)

Epidemiology of Infections During Neutropenia Posttransplant

Almost all patients receiving myeloablative conditioning regimens develop fever during neutropenia, and most of these febrile episodes are due to infections. The risk of severe bacterial or fungal infection in the early posttransplant period is markedly reduced when nonmyeloablative conditioning has been used. Clinical signs of infection apart from fever may be absent or discrete, and an infectious focus frequently will not be identified by clinical examination, microbiological, or imaging techniques. The differential diagnosis of noninfectious causes of fever, such as transfusion reactions,

G. Maschmeyer (✉)
Department of Hematology, Oncology and Palliative Care, Klinikum Ernst von Bergmann, Charlottenstrasse 72, 14467 Potsdam, Germany
e-mail: gmaschmeyer@klinikumevb.de

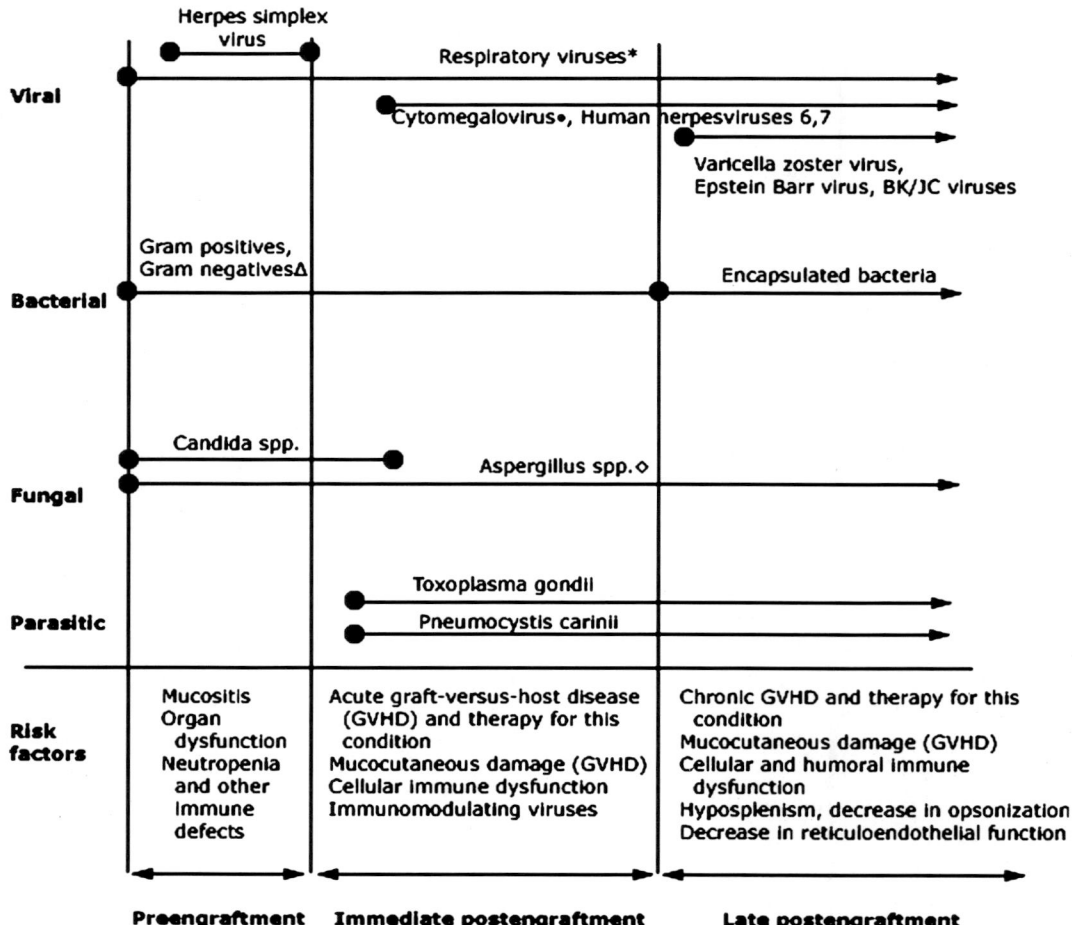

Fig. 2.1 Infections following allogeneic hematopoietic stem cell transplantation (from Up to Date v18.3, Anaissie E, Marr KA, Thorner AR, 2010)

drug-related adverse events, allergy, and acute GvHD, must be considered.

Infections in neutropenia after aHSCT may be life-threatening. Bacterial pathogens account for about 90% of infections during this phase. Epidemiological factors relevant for bacterial infections are shown in Table 2.1. Bacteremia, often related to central venous catheters (CVCs) and/or severe mucositis, occurs in up to 30% of patients after aHSCT, with the majority being caused by Gram-positive pathogens, predominantly coagulase-negative staphylococci, corynebacteria, and alpha-hemolytic streptococci [10–14]. Rarely, viridans streptococcal bacteremia may cause toxic shock and acute respiratory distress, potentially resulting in fatal outcome. Gram-negative infections are less frequent, but typically associated with higher morbidity and mortality. Gram-negative pathogens may enter the bloodstream via mucosal damage in the gastrointestinal tract of patients. Beyond that, fungal infection may occur in up to 15% of patients [15], and herpes simplex virus (HSV) infections emerge in this early posttransplant period unless acyclovir prophylaxis is given.

Table 2.1 Epidemiological aspects of bacterial infections after hematopoietic stem cell transplantation (HSCT)

- Similar spectrum as neutropenic patients after intensive chemotherapy
- Lower risk of severe and fatal infections early post-TxP after non-myeloablative conditioning
- Short neutropenia ± mucositis after autologous HSCT: infections comparable to other patients with short-term neutropenia, but Gram-positive pathogens more frequent
- Allogeneic HSCT: critical role of immune reconstitution
  - Slow after T-cell depletion
  - Slow after mismatched donor
  - Slow/absent with significant graft-versus-host disease
  - Chronic GvHD: functional asplenia

Diagnostic Procedures

- Afebrile patient.
  - Daily clinical exam + body temperature at least three times daily.
  Note: antipyretic medication (steroids; analgesics such as metamizole).

- Serum C-reactive protein (CRP) twice weekly.
- *Aspergillus* antigen (GM) ≥twice weekly.
• First fever.
  - Update physical exam, blood cultures, clinical chemistry, CRP, interleukin-6 (IL-6), and thoracic computed tomography (CT) scan; other measures according to clinical findings (see below).
• Persistent fever.
  - Update physical exam, blood cultures, clinical chemistry, CRP, IL-6, and thoracic CT scan; consider abdominal ultrasound or magnetic resonance imaging (MRI).
  - Check results of antigen testings.
• Fever + pulmonary infiltrates.
  - Bronchoscopy + bronchoalveolar lavage (BAL) => microscopy + culture for bacteria; test for *Mycobacterium tuberculous* (MTB), *Pneumocystis*, cytomegalovirus (CMV), respiratory viruses, adenovirus, *Aspergillus* + other fungi; check for *Aspergillus* GM; optional: *Aspergillus*-PCR and MTB-/*Pneumocystis*-PCR.
• Fever + signs of inflammation at CVC.
  - Blood cultures from peripheral vein and from CVC.
  - Follow-up cultures in case of cultures positive for *Staphylococcus aureus* and *Candida* spp.
• Fever accompanied by skin lesions.
  - Blood cultures.
  - Biopsy (=>histopathology and *nonfixated* =>microbiology).
• Neurological symptoms ± fever.
  - Cerebrospinal fluid (CSF) =>human herpes virus-6 (HHV-6); *Aspergillus* GM; CMV; HSV, VZV.
  - Fundoscopy.
  - Cranial MRI.
• Fever + abdominal symptoms.
  - *Clostridium difficile* toxins; noro-/rotaviruses; CMV; adenovirus; Epstein–Barr virus (EBV).
• Perianal infiltrate/abscess.
  - Beware of results from inappropriate microbiological diagnostics suggesting monomicrobial etiology.
• Fever + increasing "liver function tests" =>viral (hepatitis B virus (HBV), varicella zoster virus (VZV); CMV, etc.), *Candida*?
  - Liver ultrasound or CT or MRI (preferred) [16].
    NB: *Pneumocystis jiroveci* typically accompanied by lactate dehydrogenase rise

If causative microorganisms have been isolated from blood, urine, or CSF culture, follow-up cultures should be obtained to document microbiological eradication, whenever possible.

Since conventional chest radiography is insensitive and has a low negative predictive value for detecting pulmonary infiltrates in neutropenic patients, multislice or high-resolution CT of the lungs should be obtained early in neutropenic patients and particularly in those not responding to initial antimicrobial therapy [17]. Differential diagnoses to pulmonary infiltrates posttransplant are shown in Table 2.2.

Table 2.2 Pulmonary infections and noninfectious complications following allogeneic HSCT

	Early <90 days	Late (>90 days)
Infectious (pneumonia)	Bacterial, fungal, viral, protozoal pathogens	Bacterial, fungal, viral pathogens
Noninfectious	Pulmonary edema	Restrictive lung disease
	Idiopathic pneumonia syndrome	Constrictive bronchiolitis
	Diffuse alveolar hemorrhage	Lymphocytic interstitial pneumonitis
	Engraftment syndrome	
	Delayed pulmonary toxicity syndrome	
	Secondary pulmonary alveolar proteinosis, pulmonary veno-occlusive disease	

Antimicrobial Therapy in Patients with Neutropenic Fever After Allogeneic Stem Cell Transplantation

Fever of more than 38.2°C, or fever of 38.0°C lasting for an hour or longer, or that recurs within 24 h should give reason for immediate broad-spectrum antibacterial treatment. Microbiological identification of an underlying pathogen is achievable in about one third of all patients. Therefore, it has become an accepted clinical practice to initiate broad-spectrum antimicrobial treatment empirically, or preemptively in the presence of specific clinical or radiological signs or symptoms. For selection of empiric antibacterial therapy in patients with febrile neutropenia, local antimicrobial resistance pattern must be taken into account.

Initial empirical regimens should be active against enterobacteriaceae, *Pseudomonas aeruginosa*, *S. aureus*, and streptococci. Clinical trials that investigated single-agent regimens in patients with neutropenic fever included only few patients after allogeneic stem cell transplantation. Patients with severe mucositis should not be given single-agent ceftazidime because of the risk of bacteremia due to viridans streptococci, whereas piperacillin-tazobactam, imipenem, or meropenem appear appropriate.

In the case of skin infections or venous catheter infections, prompt addition of a glycopeptide antibiotic to the initial empiric regimen should be considered. Stopping the administration of glycopeptides should be considered, if no multiresistant Gram-positive bacteria have been identified.

In febrile neutropenic patients with pulmonary infiltrates, prompt preemptive addition of a systemic antifungal active against *Aspergillus* spp. is recommended [16].

Second-Line Empiric Antimicrobial Regimens in Patients with Neutropenic Fever After Allogeneic Stem Cell Transplantation

If a causative infectious agent has been identified, modification of the empirically started antibacterial therapy according to the in vitro susceptibility pattern should be considered. In case of clinical nonresponse after 72–96 h of full-dose antibacterial treatment, modification of the antimicrobial regimen must be discussed and diagnostic procedures be repeated. Particularly in patients given a prednisone equivalent at a dose of >2 mg/kg/day, broad-spectrum systemic antifungal treatment should be part of the second-line treatment.

Duration of Antimicrobial Treatment

Antimicrobial treatment may be discontinued if all of the following conditions are met: defervescence for at least 48 h, negative cultures, no clinical or radiological evidence of an infection, and neutrophil recovery to above 1,000/μL.

If infections have been microbiologically proven, it is advisable to repeat the initial diagnostic procedures, in order to document the microbiological response (e.g., blood cultures, CSF cultures, urine cultures, stool cultures, bronchial secretions in case of ventilated patients, smears). In some cases, narrowing the antimicrobial spectrum can be acceptable.

Early Fungal Infections After Allogeneic Stem Cell Transplantation

Epidemiological aspects of invasive fungal infections in transplant patients are listed in Table 2.3. In this patient population, the incidence rate of systemic mycoses can be as high as 15%, or higher under certain circumstances [15]. Increased risk is expected in patients with a previous history of invasive fungal infection, long-lasting severe neutropenia, previous episodes of prolonged neutropenia, severe skin and mucosal damages due to conditioning treatment, transplantation outside of a laminar air flow unit, age >45 years, intensive immunosuppression as part of the conditioning regimen or for prophylaxis, and/or treatment of GvHD [18]. Apart from specific local epidemiological conditions, *Candida* and *Aspergillus* species are predominant pathogens.

Fever unresponsive to broad-spectrum antibiotic treatment may be the only early symptom of a systemic fungal infection. In patients with pulmonary *Aspergillus* infection, pleuritic chest pain, cough, or hemoptysis may occur. Blood cultures may occasionally grow *Candida* species. *Aspergillus* spp. detected in clinical specimens (such as saliva or throat swabs) from neutropenic patients are likely to indicate incipient invasive infection. At the same time, even if moulds have been isolated from BAL specimens, it may be difficult to distinguish between contamination and true invasive pulmonary infection, whereas in cases of documented invasive pulmonary aspergillosis, cultures from BAL are often negative. Serial screening of blood samples for *Aspergillus* galactomannan or beta-D-glucan as well as for fungal DNA by polymerase chain reaction (PCR) may be helpful for early initiation of broad-spectrum systemic antifungal treatment.

Antifungal agents frequently used in this situation are liposomal amphotericin B and caspofungin, both being licensed for empirical treatment of refractory neutropenic fever. If, however, thoracic CT scan shows typical findings indicative of invasive aspergillosis, voriconazole might be the first choice, as in case of probable or proven aspergillosis. Antifungal treatment is continued at least until neutrophil recovery and resolution of clinical and radiological signs of infection.

Other mould infections such as zygomycosis and fusariosis are rare, but increasingly reported in patients post-aHSCT, and in case of suspected zygomycosis, liposomal amphotericin B would be the preferred choice.

Table 2.3 Risk factors of invasive fungal infection in patients after allogeneic SCT

Early fungal infection (<40 days after SCT)
- Previous history of invasive fungal infection
- Long-lasting neutropenia
- Advanced malignancy/previous neutropenia
- Severe skin and mucosal damages due to conditioning treatment
- Transplantation outside of LAF unit
- Age >45 years

Intensive immunosuppression as part of the conditioning regimen
- Immunosuppression as prophylaxis and/or treatment of GvHD

Late fungal infection (>40 days after SCT)
- Immunosuppression due to GvHD and its treatment (corticosteroid or other more intensive immunosuppressive treatments)
- Transplants from unrelated donors or family donors mismatched for HLA class I and/or class II antigens
- Cytomegalovirus infections and antiviral therapy
- Age >45 years

Early Viral Infections After Allogeneic Stem Cell Transplantation

Virus infections can occur during the period before hematopoietic engraftment. HSV reactivates frequently in this early period unless acyclovir prophylaxis is given, and the clinical symptoms are frequently uncharacteristic [19]. Acyclovir-resistant viruses have been reported in different patient series to occur in up to 10% and should be suspected if mucositis is prolonged in patients on acyclovir prophylaxis [20, 21]. Respiratory viral infections especially caused by RSV, parainfluenza, and influenza can occur early and are frequently due to nosocomial transmission within the transplant unit and therefore infection control procedures should be in place during times due to community outbreaks of these viruses [22–27]. Lower respiratory tract infection due to RSV and parainfluenza are associated with significant mortality. Patients, who are HBV DNA positive or HBsAg positive, before aHSCT are at risk for severe hepatitis and should be given prolonged antiviral prophylaxis [28–30].

Intermediate Posttransplant Period (3 Weeks to 3 Months)

Specific Epidemiology of Infections in the Intermediate Posttransplant Period

In the majority of allogeneic stem cell transplant recipients, infections emerge later than day +50 posttransplant. After hematopoietic reconstitution, a severe combined quantitative and functional deficiency in the T and B lymphocyte compartment persists. If T-cell depletion has been used, or if HLA-incompatibility between recipient and donor had to be accepted, immunodeficiency will be prolonged after transplantation. Immunodeficiency comprises impaired T helper cell function, immunoglobulin synthesis, and cytotoxic T cell response. Despite normalization of white blood cell counts, compromised granulocyte functions, primarily impairment of chemotaxis and phagocytosis, may persist.

Bacterial and Fungal Infections in the Intermediate Posttransplantation Period

In 14% of patients, bacteremia occurs after hematopoietic engraftment, with a mortality rate comparable to that before and after engraftment. Among blood culture isolates, Gram-positive pathogens (staphylococci in particular) are predominant, with the focus being identified in more than 50% of patients. Venous catheter infections are the cause for more than 30% of bacteremias, and fever and chills within the first hour after start of fluid infusion typically are indicating a catheter-related bacteremia. Other more frequent infections during the intermediate posttransplant period are pneumonias, preferably caused by *Streptococcus pneumoniae*, *Klebsiella* species, and *P. aeruginosa*, or by filamentous fungi such as *Aspergillus*. Among less frequent bacterial pathogens relevant during this period are *Listeria monocytogenes* and *Legionella pneumophila*. While listeriosis may origin from products made from unpasteurized milk, the latter typically is related to the use of showers or jacuzzis after the water has been resting in the pipes for a longer period of time. In patients who are treated with tumor necrosis factor antagonists such as infliximab, a dramatic increase in the risk of invasive fungal infections must be considered [31, 32]. Apart from aspergillosis, some rare forms of invasive mycosis caused by *Fusarium* spp., zygomycetes, resistant *Candida* spp., *Pseudallescheria boydii* (or its asexual form, *Scedosporium apiospermum*), and others may occur during this time period [33]. Typically, patients with fusariosis have skin lesions and positive blood cultures, while zygomycetes cause clinical syndromes resembling aspergillosis.

Viral Infections

Viruses are common causes of infections during the period from engraftment to day +90 after HSCT. The classic viral pathogen during this period is CMV called "the troll of transplantation." CMV reactivates in 60–70% of pretransplant seropositive patients and primary infections occur in up to one third of seronegative patients with seropositive donors [34]. Established end-organ CMV disease is still associated with significant morbidity and mortality. Therefore, preventive strategies either by antiviral prophylaxis or preemptive therapy should be used [35, 36]. Antiviral prophylaxis has been less used, but new antiviral agents might make this strategy more attractive. Monitoring with sensitive assays such as pp65 antigenemia or quantitative PCR in blood is indicated in all aHSCT recipients to allow early initiation of antiviral therapy with ganciclovir or valganciclovir [35].

Epstein-Barr Virus (EBV) also reactivates very frequently after aHSCT, but rarely causes end-organ disease [37]. However, EBV-driven posttransplant lymphoproliferative disease (PTLD) is a complication with high mortality unless treated [38–41]. This complication is more commonly seen in EBV seronegative patients receiving grafts from EBV seropositive donors and in patients having delayed immune reconstitution such as after a T-cell-depleted or HLA-mismatched stem cell transplantation. PTLD frequently causes unspecific symptoms frequently with fever and lymphadenopathy and is associated with high levels of EBV in blood [39, 40, 42–44]. Rituximab (anti CD20 antibody) given either as preemptive therapy or as therapy for established PTLD is most likely effective, although no controlled trial has been performed [45–49].

Adenovirus infections can cause multiorgan disease including pneumonia, encephalitis, hepatitis, gastroenteritis, and hemorrhagic cystitis. Severe adenovirus disease is more frequently seen in children especially after transplant procedures resulting in delayed reconstitution of the immune system such as haploidentical transplants or mismatched cord blood grafts and monitoring for adenovirus in blood might be indicated in such patients [50–57]. Cidofovir is a potentially effective antiviral agent, but is associated with nephrotoxicity [58–60].

Other viral pathogens potentially important during this period after HSCT are HHV-6 associated with encephalitis and bone marrow suppression [61–66], BK-virus infections associated with hemorrhagic cystitis [67, 68], and respiratory viruses.

Late Period After Allogeneic Stem Cell Transplantation (Later than Day +90)

Specific Epidemiology of Infections During the Late Posttransplant Period

In the late posttransplant period, immune reconstitution usually advances, particularly in patients who have received a transplant from an HLA-identical family donor. These patients often show full hematopoietic reconstitution and early immune reconstitution. If no relevant GVHD emerges, prophylactic immunosuppression will typically be discontinued. Patients with a CD4-count of >200/μL blood and normalized serum immunoglobulin levels can be considered as immunocompetent without an increased risk of opportunistic infections. However, in the case of chronic GvHD, which may occur in more than 30% of patients, a severe combined cellular and humoral immunodeficiency will persist for a prolonged period of time. Mucosal damage, functional deficiencies of granulocytes (especially impaired chemotaxis), functional asplenia, and qualitative as well as quantitative T- and B-cell deficiencies pave the way to a significantly increased susceptibility to infections in these patients. In particular, bacterial infections of the respiratory tract constitute a major cause of death [69]. Life-threatening infections are typically caused by encapsulated bacteria such as S. pneumoniae or Haemophilus influenzae. Sinusitis, otitis media, and pharyngitis may indicate such infections in the late posttransplant period. Patients among this risk group presenting with signs of infection should receive immediate antibacterial treatment.

An important pathogen of interstitial pneumonia in the late phase after allogeneic stem cell transplantation is P. jiroveci [70]. Without specific prophylaxis, about 30% of patients with chronic GvHD develop Pneumocystis pneumonia, which can take a fatal course in up to 15% of patients and prophylaxis given for at least 6 months (and longer in patients with chronic GvHD) is recommended to all patients. In regions with relatively high prevalence rates, mycobacterial infections should be taken into consideration as well [71, 72].

Late Viral Infections After Stem Cell Transplantation

Late-occurring CMV infection and disease have become more frequent during the last decade. These are associated with delayed and incomplete reconstitution of specific immunity, primarily of T-cells, and occur more commonly in patients experiencing severe GvHD [73, 74]. Prolonged monitoring and repeated antiviral therapy are needed in such patients, although toxicity from antiviral therapy and development of resistant CMV strains are important considerations [34, 36]. The possibility to reconstitute specific immunity by adoptive transfer of T-cells has been explored by several groups.

VZV is an important pathogen after HSCT. Primary varicella – chickenpox – occurring in seronegative patients is an important complication especially in children. Preventive measures should be taken after exposure and i.v. acyclovir therapy given if the infection develops. VZV can reactivate also early after aHSCT, but infections are more commonly seen during the late posttransplant period. The clinical manifestations vary from localized herpes zoster – shingles – to visceral disseminated disease associated with high mortality [75–77]. Visceral disease including CNS disease can occur without cutaneous manifestations and can therefore be difficult to diagnose. Early initiation of antiviral therapy with intravenous acyclovir is crucial when visceral or disseminated VZV disease is suspected. Localized shingles can often be treated with orally given valacyclovir or famciclovir [37]. In many centers, long-term prophylaxis given for at least one year after HSCT is used to prevent VZV reactivations [78, 79].

Respiratory viruses, especially influenza, can also be severe late after HSCT. Yearly vaccination against influenza is therefore recommended [80]. RSV and parainfluenza infections have been associated with late respiratory compromise presumably through immune-mediated mechanisms [81, 82].

HBV infection can reactivate in previously HBV-infected patients, especially during prolonged treatment for GvHD. Reactivation can result in a potentially severe acute hepatitis and patients should be carefully monitored, and if signs of HBV reactivation develop, be given antiviral therapy [28–30].

Late Fungal Infections After Stem Cell Transplant

Fungal infections during late transplant period are discussed in detail in Part III.

References

1. Walter E, Bowden RA. Infection in the bone marrow transplant recipient. Infect Dis Clin North Am. 1995;9:823–47.
2. Krüger WH, Bohlius J, Cornely OA, et al. Antimicrobial prophylaxis in allogeneic bone marrow transplantation. Guidelines of the infectious diseases working party (AGIHO) of the German Society of Haematology and Oncology. Ann Oncol. 2005;16:1381–90.
3. Tomblyn M, Chiller T, Einsele H, et al. Guidelines for preventing infectious complications among hematopoietic cell transplantation recipients: a global perspective. Biol Blood Marrow Transplant. 2009;15:1143–238.
4. Welniak LA, Blazar BR, Murphy WJ. Immunobiology of allogeneic hematopoietic stem cell transplantation. Annu Rev Immunol. 2007;25:139–70.
5. Aschan J. Risk assessment in haematopoietic stem cell transplantation: conditioning. Best Pract Res Clin Haematol. 2007;20:295–310.
6. Bachanova V, Brunstein CG, Burns LJ, et al. Fewer infections and lower infection-related mortality following non-myeloablative versus myeloablative conditioning for allotransplantation of patients with lymphoma. Bone Marrow Transplant. 2009;43:237–44.
7. Baron F, Storb R. Hematopoietic cell transplantation after reduced-intensity conditioning for older adults with acute myeloid leukemia in complete remission. Curr Opin Hematol. 2007;14:145–51.
8. Junghanss C, Marr KA, Carter RA, et al. Incidence and outcome of bacterial and fungal infections following nonmyeloablative compared with myeloablative allogeneic hematopoietic stem cell transplantation: a matched control study. Biol Blood Marrow Transplant. 2002;8:512–20.
9. Meijer E, Dekker AW, Lokhorst HM, Petersen EJ, Nieuwenhuis HK, Verdonck LF. Low incidence of infectious complications after nonmyeloablative compared with myeloablative allogeneic stem cell transplantation. Transpl Infect Dis. 2004;6:171–8.
10. Blijlevens NM, Donnelly JP, de Pauw BE. Prospective evaluation of gut mucosal barrier injury following various myeloablative regimens for haematopoietic stem cell transplant. Bone Marrow Transplant. 2005;35:707–11.
11. Collin BA, Leather HL, Wingard JR, Ramphal R. Evolution, incidence, and susceptibility of bacterial bloodstream isolates from 519 bone marrow transplant patients. Clin Infect Dis. 2001;33:947–53.
12. Kolbe K, Domkin D, Derigs HG, Bhakdi S, Huber C, Aulitzky WE. Infectious complications during neutropenia subsequent to peripheral blood stem cell transplantation. Bone Marrow Transplant. 1997;19:143–7.
13. Krüger W, Rüssmann B, Kröger N, et al. Early infections in patients undergoing bone marrow or blood stem cell transplantation – a 7 year single centre investigation of 409 cases. Bone Marrow Transplant. 1999;23:589–97.
14. Yuen KY, Woo PCY, Hui CH, et al. Unique risk factors for bacteraemia in allogeneic bone marrow transplant recipients before and after engraftment. Bone Marrow Transplant. 1998;21:1137–43.
15. Marr KA, Carter RA, Boeckh M, Martin P, Corey L. Invasive aspergillosis in allogeneic stem cell transplant recipients: changes in epidemiology and risk factors. Blood. 2002;100:4358–66.
16. Einsele H, Bertz H, Beyer J, et al. Infectious complications after allogeneic stem cell transplantation - Epidemiology and interventional therapy strategies. Ann Hematol. 2003;82 Suppl 2:S175–85.
17. Heussel CP, Kauczor HU, Heussel GE, et al. Pneumonia in febrile neutropenic patients and in bone marrow and blood stem-cell transplant recipients: use of high-resolution computed tomography. J Clin Oncol. 1999;17:796–805.
18. Barnes PD, Marr KA. Risks, diagnosis and outcomes of invasive fungal infections in haematopoietic stem cell transplant recipients. Br J Haematol. 2007;139:519–31.
19. Wade JC, Day LM, Crowley JJ, Meyers JD. Recurrent infection with herpes simplex virus after marrow transplantation: role of the specific immune response and acyclovir treatment. J Infect Dis. 1984;149:750–6.
20. Chakrabarti S, Pillay D, Ratcliffe D, Cane PA, Collingham KE, Milligan DW. Resistance to antiviral drugs in herpes simplex virus infections among allogeneic stem cell transplant recipients: risk factors and prognostic significance. J Infect Dis. 2000;181:2055–8.
21. Chen Y, Scieux C, Garrait V, et al. Resistant herpes simplex virus type 1 infection: an emerging concern after allogeneic stem cell transplantation. Clin Infect Dis. 2000;31:927–35.
22. Harrington RD, Hooton TM, Hackman RC, et al. An outbreak of respiratory syncytial virus in a bone marrow transplant center. J Infect Dis. 1992;165:987–93.
23. Ljungman P, Ward KN, Crooks BN, et al. Respiratory virus infections after stem cell transplantation: a prospective study from the infectious diseases working party of the European group for blood and marrow transplantation. Bone Marrow Transplant. 2001;28:479–84.
24. McCann S, Byrne JL, Rovira M, et al. Outbreaks of infectious diseases in stem cell transplant units: a silent cause of death for patients and transplant programmes. Bone Marrow Transplant. 2004;33:519–29.
25. Nichols WG, Corey L, Gooley T, Davis C, Boeckh M. Parainfluenza virus infections after hematopoietic stem cell transplantation: risk factors, response to antiviral therapy, and effect on transplant outcome. Blood. 2001;98:573–8.
26. Nichols WG, Guthrie KA, Corey L, Boeckh M. Influenza infections after hematopoietic stem cell transplantation: risk factors, mortality, and the effect of antiviral therapy. Clin Infect Dis. 2004;39:1300–6.
27. Machado CM. Influenza infections after hematopoietic stem cell transplantation. Clin Infect Dis. 2005;41:273–4.
28. Locasciulli A, Bruno B, Alessandrino EP, et al. Hepatitis reactivation and liver failure in haemopoietic stem cell transplants for hepatitis B virus (HBV)/hepatitis C virus (HCV) positive recipients: a retrospective study by the Italian group for blood and marrow transplantation. Bone Marrow Transplant. 2003;31:295–300.
29. Kitano K, Kobayashi H, Hanamura M, et al. Fulminant hepatitis after allogenic bone marrow transplantation caused by reactivation of hepatitis B virus with gene mutations in the core promotor region. Eur J Haematol. 2006;77:255–8.
30. Hsiao LT, Chiou TJ, Liu JH, et al. Extended lamivudine therapy against hepatitis B virus infection in hematopoietic stem cell transplant recipients. Biol Blood Marrow Transplant. 2006;12:84–94.
31. Hamadani M, Hofmeister CC, Jansak B, et al. Addition of infliximab to standard acute graft-versus-host disease prophylaxis following allogeneic peripheral blood cell transplantation. Biol Blood Marrow Transplant. 2008;14:783–9.
32. Marty FM, Lee SJ, Fahey MM, et al. Infliximab use in patients with severe graft-versus-host disease and other emerging risk factors of non-Candida invasive fungal infections in allogeneic hematopoietic stem cell transplant recipients: a cohort study. Blood. 2003;102:2768–76.
33. Marr KA, Carter RA, Crippa F, Wald A, Corey L. Epidemiology and outcome of mould infections in hematopoietic stem cell transplant recipients. Clin Infect Dis. 2002;34:909–17.
34. Boeckh M, Ljungman P. How we treat cytomegalovirus in hematopoietic cell transplant recipients. Blood. 2009;113:5711–9.
35. Ljungman P, de la Camara R, Cordonnier C, et al. Management of CMV, HHV-6, HHV-7 and Kaposi-sarcoma herpesvirus (HHV-8) infections in patients with hematological malignancies and after SCT. Bone Marrow Transplant. 2008;42:227–40.
36. Zaia J, Baden L, Boeckh MJ, et al. Viral disease prevention after hematopoietic cell transplantation. Bone Marrow Transplant. 2009;44:471–82.

37. Styczynski J, Reusser P, Einsele H, et al. Management of HSV, VZV and EBV infections in patients with hematological malignancies and after SCT: guidelines from the second European conference on infections in Leukemia. Bone Marrow Transplant. 2009;43:757–70.
38. Micallef IN, Chanabhai M, Gascoyne RD, et al. Lymphoproliferative disorders following allogeneic bone marrow transplantation: the Vancouver experience. Bone Marrow Transplant. 1998;22:981–7.
39. Juvonen E, Aalto SM, Tarkkanen J, et al. High incidence of PTLD after non-T-cell-depleted allogeneic haematopoietic stem cell transplantation as a consequence of intensive immunosuppressive treatment. Bone Marrow Transplant. 2003;32:97–102.
40. Sundin M, Le Blanc K, Ringden O, et al. The role of HLA mismatch, splenectomy and recipient Epstein–Barr virus seronegativity as risk factors in post-transplant lymphoproliferative disorder following allogeneic hematopoietic stem cell transplantation. Haematologica. 2006;91:1059–67.
41. Landgren O, Gilbert ES, Rizzo JD, et al. Risk factors for lymphoproliferative disorders after allogeneic hematopoietic cell transplantation. Blood. 2009;113:4992–5001.
42. Gartner BC, Schafer H, Marggraff K, et al. Evaluation of use of Epstein–Barr viral load in patients after allogeneic stem cell transplantation to diagnose and monitor posttransplant lymphoproliferative disease. J Clin Microbiol. 2002;40:351–8.
43. Greenfield HM, Gharib MI, Turner AJ, et al. The impact of monitoring Epstein–Barr virus PCR in paediatric bone marrow transplant patients: can it successfully predict outcome and guide intervention? Pediatr Blood Cancer. 2006;47:200–5.
44. Kinch A, Oberg G, Arvidson J, Falk KI, Linde A, Pauksens K. Post-transplant lymphoproliferative disease and other Epstein–Barr virus diseases in allogeneic haematopoietic stem cell transplantation after introduction of monitoring of viral load by polymerase chain reaction. Scand J Infect Dis. 2007;39:235–44.
45. Van Esser JW, Niesters HG, van der Holt B, et al. Prevention of Epstein–Barr virus-lymphoproliferative disease by molecular monitoring and preemptive rituximab in high-risk patients after allogeneic stem cell transplantation. Blood. 2002;99:4364–9.
46. Wagner HJ, Cheng YC, Huls MH, et al. Prompt versus preemptive intervention for EBV lymphoproliferative disease. Blood. 2004;103:3979–81.
47. Weinstock DM, Ambrossi GG, Brennan C, Kiehn TE, Jakubowski A. Preemptive diagnosis and treatment of Epstein–Barr virus-associated post transplant lymphoproliferative disorder after hematopoietic stem cell transplant: an approach in development. Bone Marrow Transplant. 2006;37:539–46.
48. Styczynski J, Einsele H, Gil L, Ljungman P. Outcome of treatment of Epstein–Barr virus-related post-transplant lymphoproliferative disorder in hematopoietic stem cell recipients: a comprehensive review of reported cases. Transpl Infect Dis. 2009;11:383–92.
49. Omar H, Hagglund H, Gustafsson-Jernberg A, et al. Targeted monitoring of patients at high risk of post-transplant lymphoproliferative disease by quantitative Epstein–Barr virus polymerase chain reaction. Transpl Infect Dis. 2009;11:393–9.
50. Shields AF, Hackman RC, Fife KH, Corey L, Meyers JD. Adenovirus infections in patients undergoing bone-marrow transplantation. N Engl J Med. 1985;312:529–33.
51. Flomenberg P, Babbitt J, Drobyski WR, et al. Increasing incidence of adenovirus disease in bone marrow transplant recipients. J Infect Dis. 1994;169:775–81.
52. Chakrabarti S, Mautner V, Osman H, et al. Adenovirus infections following allogeneic stem cell transplantation: incidence and outcome in relation to graft manipulation, immunosuppression, and immune recovery. Blood. 2002;100:1619–27.
53. Lion T, Baumgartinger R, Watzinger F, et al. Molecular monitoring of adenovirus in peripheral blood after allogeneic bone marrow transplantation permits early diagnosis of disseminated disease. Blood. 2003;102:1114–20.
54. Van Tol MJ, Kroes AC, Schinkel J, et al. Adenovirus infection in paediatric stem cell transplant recipients: increased risk in young children with a delayed immune recovery. Bone Marrow Transplant. 2005;36:39–50.
55. Feuchtinger T, Lang P, Handgretinger R. Adenovirus infection after allogeneic stem cell transplantation. Leuk Lymphoma. 2007;48:244–55.
56. Robin M, Marque-Juillet S, Scieux C, et al. Disseminated adenovirus infections after allogeneic hematopoietic stem cell transplantation: incidence, risk factors and outcome. Haematologica. 2007;92:1254–7.
57. Symeonidis N, Jakubowski A, Pierre-Louis S, Jaffe D, Pamer E, Sepkowitz K, et al. Invasive adenoviral infections in T-cell-depleted allogeneic hematopoietic stem cell transplantation: high mortality in the era of cidofovir. Transpl Infect Dis. 2007;9:108–13.
58. Ljungman P, Ribaud P, Eyrich M, et al. Cidofovir for adenovirus infections after allogeneic hematopoietic stem cell transplantation: a survey by the infectious diseases working party of the European group for blood and marrow transplantation. Bone Marrow Transplant. 2003;31:481–6.
59. Yusuf U, Hale GA, Carr J, et al. Cidofovir for the treatment of adenoviral infection in pediatric hematopoietic stem cell transplant patients. Transplantation. 2006;81:1398–404.
60. Neofytos D, Ojha A, Mookerjee B, et al. Treatment of adenovirus disease in stem cell transplant recipients with cidofovir. Biol Blood Marrow Transplant. 2007;13:74–81.
61. Drobyski WR, Dunne WM, Burd EM, et al. Human herpesvirus-6 (HHV-6) infection in allogeneic bone marrow transplant recipients: evidence of a marrow-suppressive role for HHV-6 in vivo. J Infect Dis. 1993;167:735–9.
62. Carrigan DR, Knox KK. Human herpesvirus 6 (HHV-6) isolation from bone marrow: HHV-6-associated bone marrow suppression in bone marrow transplant patients. Blood. 1994;84:3307–10.
63. Wang FZ, Linde A, Hagglund H, Testa M, Locasciulli A, Ljungman P. Human herpesvirus 6 DNA in cerebrospinal fluid specimens from allogeneic bone marrow transplant patients: does it have clinical significance? Clin Infect Dis. 1999;28:562–8.
64. Zerr DM, Gooley TA, Yeung L, et al. Human herpesvirus 6 reactivation and encephalitis in allogeneic bone marrow transplant recipients. Clin Infect Dis. 2001;33:763–71.
65. Zerr DM, Gupta D, Huang ML, Carter R, Corey L. Effect of antivirals on human herpesvirus 6 replication in hematopoietic stem cell transplant recipients. Clin Infect Dis. 2002;34:309–17.
66. Zerr DM, Corey L, Kim HW, Huang ML, Nguy L, Boeckh M. Clinical outcomes of human herpesvirus 6 reactivation after hematopoietic stem cell transplantation. Clin Infect Dis. 2005;40:932–40.
67. Leung AY, Suen CK, Lie AK, Liang RH, Yuen KY, Kwong YL. Quantification of polyoma BK viruria in hemorrhagic cystitis complicating bone marrow transplantation. Blood. 2001;98:1971–8.
68. Erard V, Kim HW, Corey L, et al. BK DNA viral load in plasma: evidence for an association with hemorrhagic cystitis in allogeneic hematopoietic cell transplant recipients. Blood. 2005;106:1130–2.
69. Chen CS, Boeckh M, Seidel K, et al. Incidence, risk factors, and mortality from pneumonia developing late after hematopoietic stem cell transplantation. Bone Marrow Transplant. 2003;32:515–22.
70. De Castro N, Neuville S, Sarfati C, et al. Occurrence of *Pneumocystis jiroveci* pneumonia after allogeneic stem cell transplantation: a 6-year retrospective study. Bone Marrow Transplant. 2005;36:879–83.
71. Cordonnier C, Martino R, Trabasso P, et al. Mycobacterial infection: a difficult and late diagnosis in stem cell transplant recipients. Clin Infect Dis. 2004;38:1229–36.
72. Erdstein AA, Daas P, Bradstock KF, Robinson T, Hertzberg MS. Tuberculous in allogeneic stem cell transplant recipients: still a problem in the 21st century. Transpl Infect Dis. 2004;6:142–6.

73. Boeckh M, Leisenring W, Riddell SR, et al. Late cytomegalovirus disease and mortality in recipients of allogeneic hematopoietic stem cell transplants: importance of viral load and T-cell immunity. Blood. 2003;101:407–14.
74. Hakki M, Riddell SR, Storek J, et al. Immune reconstitution to cytomegalovirus after allogeneic hematopoietic stem cell transplantation: impact of host factors, drug therapy, and subclinical reactivation. Blood. 2003;102:3060–7.
75. Locksley RM, Flournoy N, Sullivan KM, Meyers JD. Infection with varicella-zoster virus after marrow transplantation. J Infect Dis. 1985;152:1172–81.
76. Steer CB, Szer J, Sasadeusz J, Matthews JP, Beresford JA, Grigg A. Varicella-zoster infection after allogeneic bone marrow transplantation: incidence, risk factors and prevention with low-dose aciclovir and ganciclovir. Bone Marrow Transplant. 2000;25:657–64.
77. Martino R, Rovira M, Carreras E, et al. Severe infections after allogeneic peripheral blood stem cell transplantation: a matched-pair comparison of unmanipulated and CD34+ cell-selected transplantation. Haematologica. 2001;86:1075–86.
78. Boeckh M, Kim HW, Flowers ME, Meyers JD, Bowden RA. Long-term acyclovir for prevention of varicella zoster virus disease after allogeneic hematopoietic cell transplantation – a randomized double-blind placebo-controlled study. Blood. 2006;107:1800–5.
79. Erard V, Guthrie KA, Varley C, et al. One-year acyclovir prophylaxis for preventing varicella-zoster virus (VZV) disease following hematopoietic cell transplantation: no evidence of rebound VZV disease after drug discontinuation. Blood. 2007;110:3071–7.
80. Ljungman P, Cordonnier C, Einsele H, Englund J, Machado CM, Storek J, et al. Vaccination of hematopoietic cell transplant recipients. Bone Marrow Transplant. 2009;44:521–6.
81. Erard V, Chien JW, Kim HW, et al. Airflow decline after myeloablative allogeneic hematopoietic cell transplantation: the role of community respiratory viruses. J Infect Dis. 2006;193:1619–25.
82. Avetisyan G, Mattsson J, Sparrelid E, Ljungman P. Respiratory syncytial virus infection in recipients of allogeneic stem-cell transplantation: a retrospective study of the incidence, clinical features, and outcome. Transplantation. 2009;88:1222–6.

Chapter 3
Infections in Patients with Hematologic Malignancies

Genovefa Papanicolaou and Jayesh Mehta

Abstract Hematologic malignancies are a heterogeneous group of diseases with differing clinical manifestations, disease course, response to therapy, and long-term outcome. More intensive therapies are also being extended to older age groups and to patients with significant comorbidities, which were traditionally excluded from such treatment. These intensive treatment approaches are associated with multiple complications; infections from a wide variety of pathogenic and opportunistic organisms being amongst the commonest and the most serious. Infections affect quality of life, delay potentially saving chemotherapy and pose a substantial burden for the health care system and remain an important cause of death. In this chapter we outline the common immune defects and associated infections frequently seen in patients with hematologic malignancies.

Keywords Leukemia • Lymphoma • Multiple myeloma • Infections • Serious • Immune dysfunction • New chemotherapy • Old age

Introduction

Hematologic malignancies are a heterogeneous group of diseases with differing clinical manifestations, disease course, response to therapy, and long-term outcome. Response to therapy and long-term survival has improved significantly over the last few decades as a result of the development of more intensive and effective treatment approaches [1, 2]. These intensive treatment approaches are associated with multiple complications in patients with hematologic malignancies. Infections from a wide variety of pathogenic and opportunistic organisms are amongst the commonest and the most serious [2–5]. The availability of new, broad-spectrum antimicrobial agents has improved outcomes – but has also resulted in alterations in the types of infections seen. Hersh et al. noticed this trend almost half a century ago [6]. Over the study period, infections were amongst the major causes of death in 70% of the acute leukemia patients who died. Fatal staphylococcal infections declined by 85% over the period but fatal fungal infections tripled.

Microbiologically or clinically documented infection develops in 60–80% of patients undergoing induction chemotherapy for acute leukemia. Up to 50% of patients with chronic lymphocytic leukemia suffer from recurrent infections. Infections affect quality of life, delay potentially saving chemotherapy, pose a substantial burden for the health care system and remain an important cause of death for patients with hematologic malignancies [7–14].

Immune Host-Defects in Hematologic Malignancies

Under normal circumstances, the immune system consists of multiple layers that each contribute to protection against infection. Redundancy at the cellular and signaling level limits the potential for microbes to escape this defensive system, and modest compromise of one layer of immune defense may not be readily apparent. In patients with hematologic malignancies, the redundancy of the immune system has been severely compromised. Innate immune defenses like mucosal integrity, neutrophil and monocyte function, and numbers may be compromised as a result of cytotoxic therapy or steroids. In many cases, the underlying disease or therapy has compromised or even eliminated the adaptive immune system (i.e., antibody generation and T-cell responses). The underlying immune defect often plays a major role in defining the type and clinical presentation of many infections. For example, infection by *Streptococcus pneumoniae* often presents as fulminant sepsis in splenectomized patients [15, 16]. Community respiratory viruses causing self-limited upper respiratory infections in healthy individuals have been associated with high mortality in patients with leukemia [17]. Prevention of infection is

G. Papanicolaou (✉)
Infectious Diseases Service, Memorial Sloan-Kettering Cancer Center, New York, NY, USA
e-mail: papanicg@mskcc.org

Table 3.1 Infections control: close attention to all potential sources of infection [18]

Environment
- Ventilation and construction: *Aspergillus*
- Water: *Legionella pneumophila*
- Environmental surfaces: *Clostridium difficile,* VRE
- Invasive medical devices

Health care workers
- Hand washing
- Isolation technique
- Preemptive barrier precautions

Visitors

Contact with food, flowers, toys

Table 3.2 Role of host defenses on patient response: neutropenia significantly worsened response rates in patients with invasive aspergillosis [19]

Neutropenia status	Patient response to therapy		
	Aspergillus fumigatus	*Aspergillus terreus*	P value
No neutropenia	53% (8/15)	50% (4/8)	0.01
Neutropenia resolved	50% (4/8)	44% (4/9)	0.01
Persistent neutropenia	10% (1/10)	6% (1/15)	0.01

paramount for the most vulnerable patients. Close attention is paid to all potential sources of infection including the environment, health care workers, and visitors (Table 3.1) [18].

Immune recovery plays an important role on the outcome of infection (Table 3.2) [19–21].

A useful initial approach is the recognition of the major predisposing factors broadly classified as: (1) granulocytopenia and qualitative defects of phagocytes; (2) cellular immune dysfunction; (3) humoral immune dysfunction and (4) impaired mucosal integrity. More than one predisposing factors may be present at any given time. Classic associations between specific immune defects and types of infectious pathogens are helpful to guide the initial approach to the patient. Table 3.3 shows the predominant pathogens associated with major immune defects.

Neutropenia

Neutrophils are the first line of defense against pyogenic bacteria and fungi. The lack of inflammatory response due to the absence of neutrophils may result in rapid progression of infection in the absence of signs and symptoms. The relationship of granulocytopenia and risk of infection is well-established. It is widely appreciated that risk of infection increases very little until the granulocyte count drops below 500/mm^3 and rises rapidly as the count approaches 0 [22]. The severity and duration of neutropenia are important determinants of the type of infectious complications (Fig. 3.1).

Patients whose neutropenia persists for 10 days or longer are at high risk not only for acute bacterial infections, but also for secondary infections due to fungi and viruses. The risk of infection is more pronounced in patients who have a rapidly falling granulocyte count than in patients who have a prolonged stationary granulocyte count such a in myelodysplastic syndrome [23].

The bacterial pathogens isolated from neutropenic patients at the early stages of neutropenia tend to originate from the patients' endogenous flora. Gram-negative enteric organisms, α-hemolytic streptococci and enterococci are associated with oral and gastrointestinal mucositis. Skin related pathogens (staphylococci, coagulase negative staphylococci, and *Corynebacterium* spp.) are associated with line infections (Table 3.3).

The most common sites of infection are the bloodstream followed by lung and GI tract. Seeding of infection from the bloodstream may lead to localized abscesses that may become clinically apparent after neutrophil recovery (Fig. 3.2). Fever with mucositis and abdominal pain raises suspicion of neutropenic enterocolitis (typhlitis).

Since the mid-1980s, 60–70% of bacteremias associated with a single organism are caused by Gram-positive organisms [24–26] (Fig. 3.3). An increase in Gram-positive and polymicrobial infections is noted over the 15-year period of study.

The rise in the incidence of multiresistant organisms among patients with hematologic malignancies may reflect broader trends observed in nosocomial pathogens [27, 28].

The 30-day mortality rates for neutropenic patients with bacteremia approach 30% [13, 29, 30]. Polymicrobial bacteremia and fungemia have been associated with highest mortality rates [31]. Viridans streptococcal bacteremia has been associated with a toxic-shock-like syndrome with hypotension maculopapular rash palmar desquamation, and acute respiratory distress syndrome [32–34].

Persistent fever in a neutropenic patient despite broad spectrum antibiotics should raise suspicion for fungal infection. Prior to the implementation of preemptive antifungal therapy, up to 50% patients treated for leukemia were found to have a fungal infection at autopsy [35]. Empiric antifungal therapy has substantially reduced the incidence of fungal infections during neutropenia [36]. Only the minority of fungal infections is diagnosed antemortem (Fig. 3.4).

The likelihood of patients requiring systemic antifungals during neutropenia has changed over the years due to changes in our use of antifungal prophylaxis (Table 3.4).

The predominant fungal pathogens in neutropenic patients are shown on Table 3.3. *Candida* remains the most common yeast causing bloodstream infection (Fig. 3.5). In a recent study, the incidence of candidemia in patients with hematologic malignancies was approximately 20 episodes per 1,000

Table 3.3 Predominant pathogen association with selected host immune defects

Host defense	Bacteria	Fungi	Viruses	Other
Neutropenia	Gram-positive	*Candida* spp.		
	Staphylococci (CoNS, *S. aureus*)	*Aspergillus* spp.		
	Streptococci (α-hemolytic, Group D)	*Trichosporon* spp.		
	Anaerobes	*Fusarium* spp.		
	Anaerobic streptococci	*Mucor*		
	Clostridium spp.			
	Bacteroids spp.			
Cellular dysfunction	*Legionella*	*Cryptococcus*	Herpes viruses	*Toxoplasma*
	Salmonella	*Histoplasma*	VZV, CMV, HSV, HHV6, EBV	*Cryptosporidium*
	Nocardia	*Coccidioides*	Respiratory viruses	*Strongyloides*
	Mycobacteria (TB and atypical)	*Candida* spp.	Live virus vaccines	
	Live bacteria vaccine (BCG)	*Pneumocystis*		
Humoral dysfunction	Gram positive		Enteroviruses	
	S. pneumoniae		Live vaccine viruses	*Giardia*
	S. aureus			
	Gram-negative			
	H. influenzae			
	Neisseria spp.			
	Enteric organisms			
Anatomic disruption				
Upper GI	Mouth flora	*Candida*	Herpes simplex	
	α-Hemolytic streptococci			
	Anaerobic *Peptostreptococci*			
Lower GI	Gram-positive (Group D streptococci)	*Candida*		
	Enteric Gram-negative organisms			
	Anaerobes			
	Bacteroides, *Clostridium* spp., Group D streptococci			
Skin	Gram-positive	*Candida*		
	Staphylococci	*Aspergillus*		
	Corynebacterium spp.			
	Gram-negative			
	Pseudomonas spp.			
	Enteric Gram-negative			
	Mycobacteria			
	M. abscesses fortuitum, Mycobacterium chelonei			
Splenectomy	Gram-positive			*Babesia*
	S. pneumoniae			
	DF2 bacillus			
	Capnocytophaga canimorsus			
	Gram-negative			
	H. influenzae			
	Salmonella spp.			
	Neisseria meningitidis			

patient days despite antifungal prophylaxis. Non-albicans species predominated with *Candida tropicalis* and *Candida parapsilosis* accounting for 40% of all isolates. An increase in the frequency of fluconazole-resistant *Candida* species including *Candida glabrata* and *Candida krusei* has been noted in several studies possibly as a result of antifungal prophylaxis with fluconazole [37, 38]. A complication of candidemia is chronic disseminated candidiasis (hepatosplenic candidiasis). The only symptom may be persistent fever after resolution of neutropenia. Numerous target lesions in the liver and spleen may be apparent by CT imaging [39] (Fig. 3.6).

Infections by filamentous fungi, *Aspergillus* being the most common, are an important cause of mortality in patients

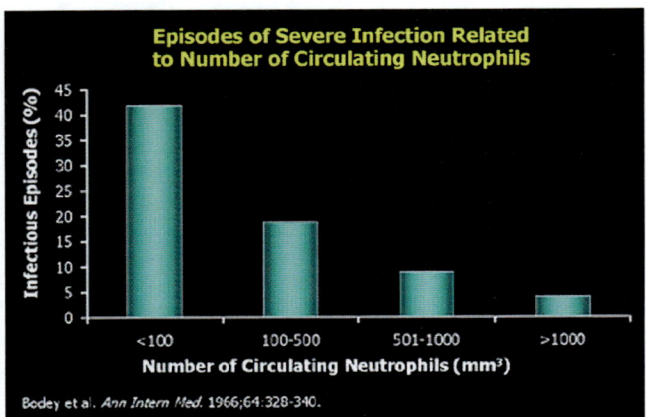

Fig. 3.1 Episodes of severe infection related to numbers of circulating neutrophils. Bodey et al. examined the occurrence of severe infection in 52 patients with acute leukemia treated at the National Institutes of Health from 1959 to 1963. The risk of developing severe infection at a given neutrophil count was calculated form the number of severe infections occurring per 1,000 days at each neutrophil count. When severe neutropenia was present 43 episodes of severe infection were observed per 1,000 days

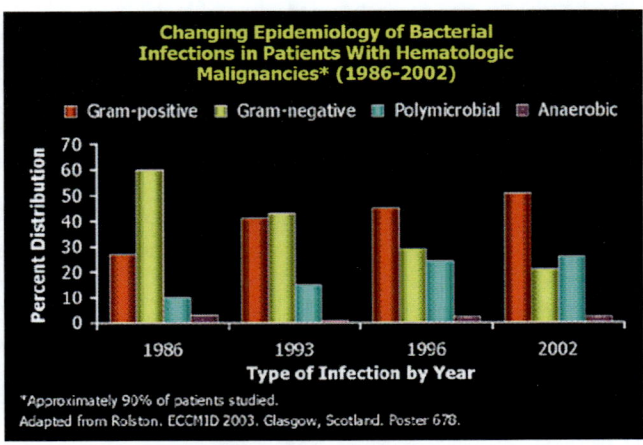

Fig. 3.3 Changing epidemiology of bacterial infections in patients with hematologic malignancies. An increase in Gram-positive and polymicrobial infections is noted over the 15-year period of study

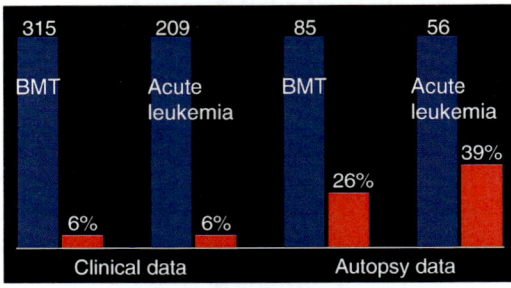

Fig. 3.4 The incidence of fungal infections is underestimated due to our inability to establish the diagnosis antemortem. *Left*: Number of patients dying after allogeneic bone marrow transplantation or induction/salvage therapy for acute leukemia (*blue bars*) over a 12-year period at the Royal Marsden Hospital, UK and percentage in whom fungal infections were clinically suspected (*red bars*). *Right*: Autopsy data: The subset of patients who had autopsy (*blue bars*) and percentage in whom fungus was detected (*red bars*)

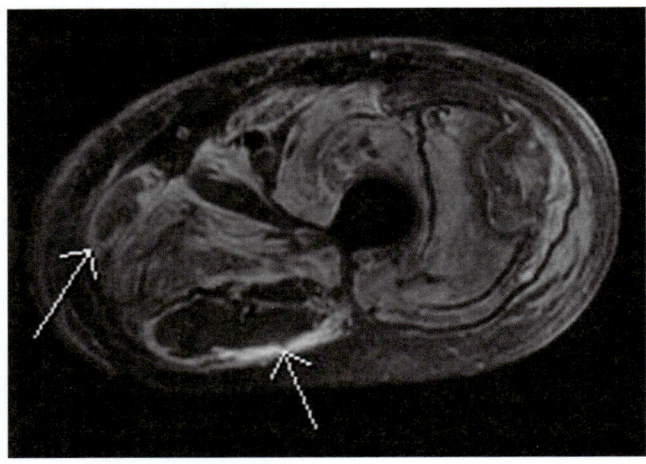

Fig. 3.2 MRI of thigh of a patient with lymphoma after neutrophil recovery form intensive chemotherapy. Multiple abscesses are shown in proximal/mid left. Diffuse edema and enhancement is noted in the muscles, along the fascia and subcutaneous issues. Aspirate of the abscess grew *Pseudomonas aeruginosa*

with hematologic malignancies [3, 40, 41]. The lungs are the most common site of infection followed by the sinuses. Aspergillosis of the central nervous system (CNS) may result from hematogenous dissemination with mortalities approaching 100% (Fig. 3.7) [42].

Zygomycosis is much less common than aspergillosis, but a rising trend has been noted increased use of prolonged antifungal prophylaxis with agents active against *Aspergillus*, such as voriconazole (Fig. 3.8) [43, 44].

Other molds previously thought to be contaminants or colonizers have been recognized to be causing invasive mycoses in severely immunosuppressed patients. Sinusitis with emerging fungal pathogens including Fusarium and dark-walled molds are being recognized with increasing frequency [45].

Qualitative Phagocyte Defects

Chemotaxis, cell activation, phagocytosis, and intra- or extracellular killing by oxygen-dependent and oxygen-independent pathways may be compromised in the presence of adequate cell numbers.

Intrinsic functional defects of granulocytes exist in patients with acute leukemia, myelodysplastic syndromes and preleukemic states [46]. From a clinical perspective such patients with borderline granulocyte count should be approached as if they had absolute neutropenia.

Table 3.4 Changes in the incidence of presumed/confirmed fungal infection with changes in antifungal prophylaxis

Stage of disease	Royal Marsden Hospital, UK, 1992–1995		Northwestern Memorial Hospital, Chicago, IL, 2002–2005	
	Antifungal prophylaxis	% of patients requiring systemic antifungal therapy	Antifungal prophylaxis	% of patient requiring systemic antifungal therapy
A. Acute Myelogenous Leukemia				
Within 6 weeks of induction	Nystatin	44%	Fluconazole	13%
Autograft in CR1	Nystatin	31%	Fluconazole	8%
Allograft in CR1	Nystatin	51%	Voriconoazole	15%
B. Multiple Myeloma				
Within 12 weeks of induction	None	4%	Fluconazole	0%
Early autograft	Nystatin	9%	Fluconazole	0%
Allograft for relapsed disease	Nystatin	67%	Voriconazole	0%

Percentage of patients requiring systemic antifungals during treatment for acute myelogenous leukemia (A) or multiple myeloma (B) over a 12-year period (Courtesy of Dr. Jayesh Mehta)

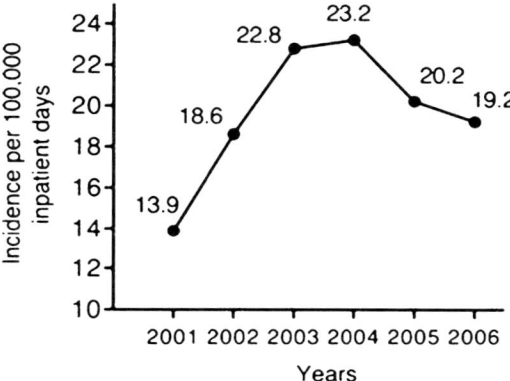

Fig. 3.5 Incidence of candidemia among patients with hematologic malignancies during 2001–2007 at the M.D Anderson Cancer Center. A slight decrease in the incidence of candidemia was observed during the last 2 years of the study. Seventy-six percent of infections were caused by non-albicans species. The attributable during the study period was 19%

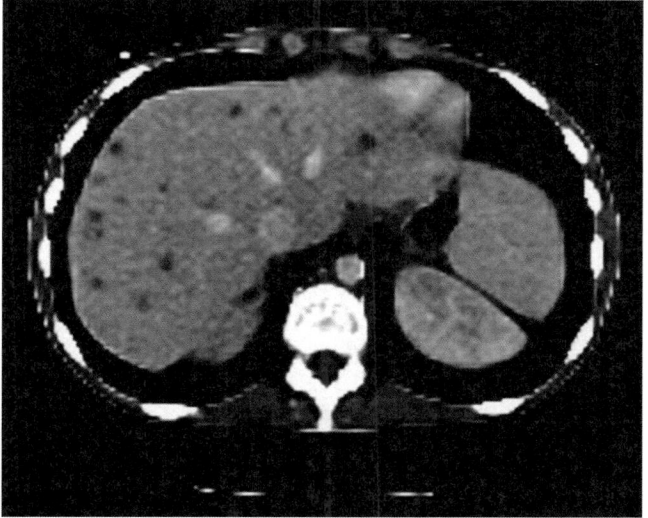

Fig. 3.6 Hepatosplenic candidiasis in a patient with acute myelogenous leukemia in remission. The patient developed persistent fever after four cycles of chemotherapy and associated prolonged neutropenia. CT of the abdomen: Multiple hypodense lesions in the liver. Liver biopsy showed granulomatous necrosis with yeast forms consistent with *Candida*

Leukemia and lymphoma are associated with intrinsic defects in monocyte function. Circulating monocytes are precursors for alveolar and lamina propria macrophages, the mucosal cells that play an important role in earliest defense against pulmonary and intestinal infection [47]. Although the exact relationship between circulating monocytes and infection has not been explored it is reasonable though to hypothesize that these cells would make an important contribution in the defense against bacterial or fungal infections.

Treatment modalities such chemotherapy, corticosteroids, radiation or growth factors may result in phagocyte dysfunction. The major effect of corticosteroids on granulocyte function appears to be impairment of chemotaxis which decreases localized inflammatory response. In vitro, steroids inhibit phagocytosis, microbicidal activity and antibody dependent cytotoxicity. In addition, a number of monocyte functions are impaired including chemotaxis, bactericidal activity, and production of interleukin-1 and TNF-α. Use of Corticosteroids predisposes to infections by pathogens that depend on phagocyte function such as *Staphylococcus aureus*, *Enterobacteriaceae*, and *fungi*. The risk of infection increases when the adult equivalent of prednisone 20–40 mg/day or higher is administered for longer than 4–6 weeks.

Steroids may also enhance susceptibility to infection though delay in wound healing, increased skin fragility, and impairment of lymphocyte function.

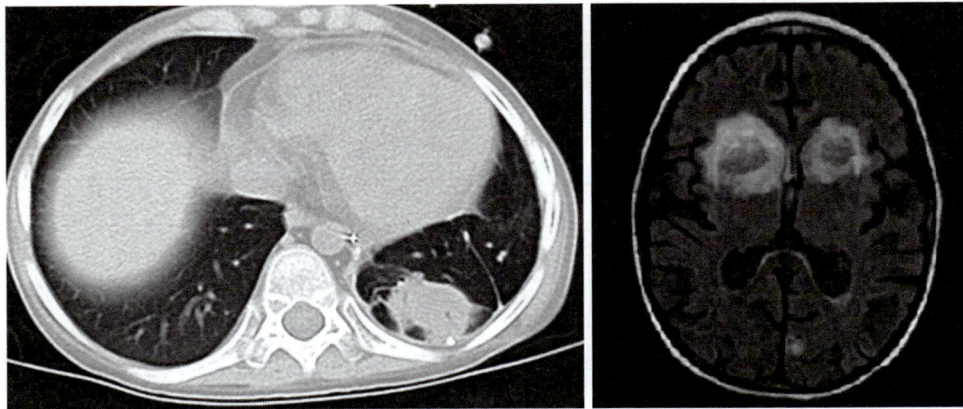

Fig. 3.7 Disseminated aspergillosis in a child with leukemia; *Left*: Chest CT demonstrating cavitary lesion. Biopsy showed septate hyphae. *Right*: MRI showing bilateral frontal lobe ring enhancing lesions

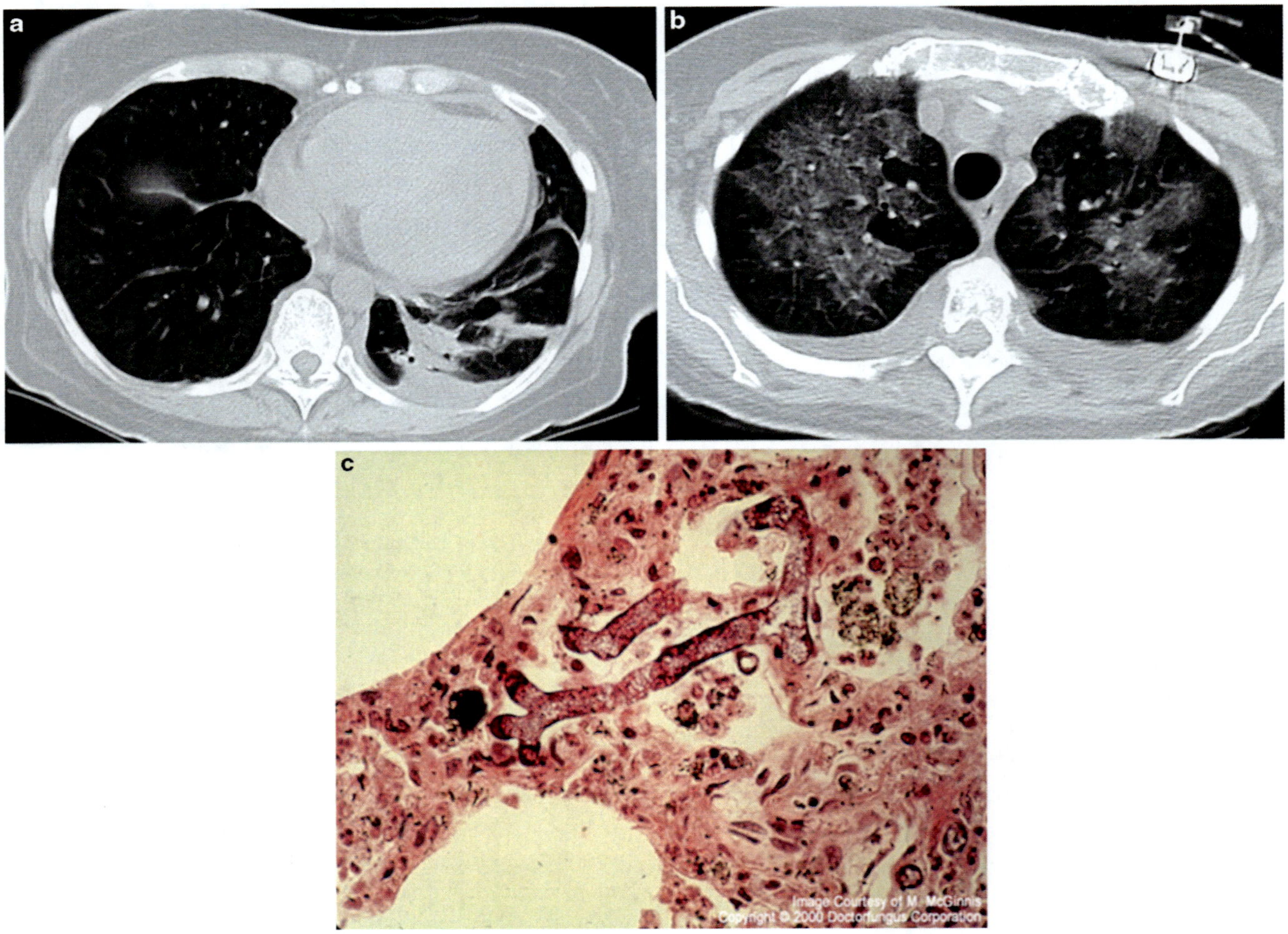

Fig. 3.8 Influenza and Mucor pneumonia in a heavily treated patient with lymphoma. Initially the patient presented with influenza infection and a left lung consolidation (**a**). Several weeks after empiric treatment with voriconazole the patient presented with respiratory distress and diffuse interstitial infiltrates (**b**). Sputum culture grew *Aspergillus* spp. and *Mucor* spp. Nasopharyngeal cultures were persistently positive for influenza A. Autopsy showed broad nonseptate hyphae consistent with zygomycosis (**c**)

Cellular Immune Dysfunction

Intrinsic defect in cellular immunity is the hallmark of immune dysfunction seen in lymphoma. T-cell function is required for macrophage activation and subsequent microbicidal activity. In the absence of functional T-cells, intracellular pathogens may survive and replicate inside macrophages. The pathogens causing infections in patients with impaired T-cell immunity include a broad array of intracellular bacteria, fungi, DNA viruses, and protozoa (Table 3.2).

Endemic fungi like *Histoplasma* or *Coccidioides*, or parasites like *Strongyloides stercoralis* may reactivate and cause severe disease during intense chemotherapy. A variety of opportunistic pathogens like atypical mycobacteria, Nocardia (Fig. 3.9), or toxoplasma may cause disseminated disease in patients with impaired T-cell immunity.

Lymphoreticular malignancy and corticosteroid therapy seem to be a major factor for infection by the opportunistic fungi *Cryptococcus* spp. and *Pneumocystis jiroveci* (Fig. 3.10).

The most common manifestation of cryptococcal infection is meningitis though primary pneumonia, fungemia, and cutaneous or visceral dissemination may occur.

Protective immunity against most viruses is highly dependent on virus-specific, MHC-restricted T-lymphocytes. Infections by the herpes viruses including herpes simplex (HSV), Varicella-zoster virus (VZV), and cytomegalovirus (CMV) are almost exclusively due to reactivation. HSV infections range from 15% among CLL patients treated with fludarabine to 90% of patients with acute leukemia. Mucocutaneous HSV disease will frequently present with an atypical appearance and can mimic other pathogens. The incidence of VZV infections ranges from 2% in patients with CML receiving imatinib to 10–15% in patients with CLL receiving fludarabine or alemtuzumab to 25% of patients with Hodgkin's lymphoma. More than 80% of VZV infections present with localized disease. Patients who are VZV naïve are at risk for primary infection with either wild type or vaccine strains and should be counseled about the risk of developing such an infection. T-cell depleting agents (e.g., alemtuzumab) and aggressive chemotherapy (e.g., hyper-CVAD and acute leukemia induction) appear to increase the incidence of CMV infection and disease [48].

Fulminant hepatitis B may occur during immunosuppression in patients with active hepatitis B [49, 50]. Disseminated disease caused by vaccination with live viruses such as varicella and polio and or bacteria such as BCG have been reported [51].

Humoral Immune Dysfunction

Multiple myeloma and chronic lymphocytic leukemia are associated with intrinsic defects in humoral immunity. Immunoglobulins and complement provide opsonic, lytic, and neutralizing activities essential for protection against bacterial pathogens. Impaired humoral immunity is a risk factor for recurrent infections from polysaccharide-encapsulated bacteria such as *S. pneumoniae*, *Haemophilus influenzae*, or *Neisseria* spp. Pyogenic infections by enteric Gram-negative organisms and staphylococci are also frequently encountered (Table 3.3).

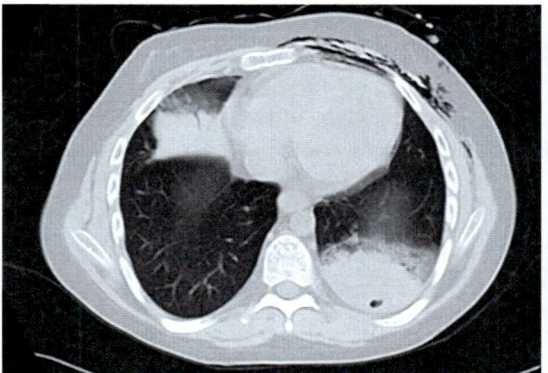
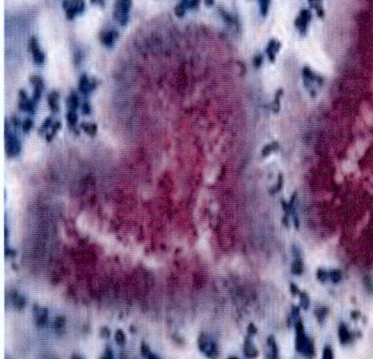
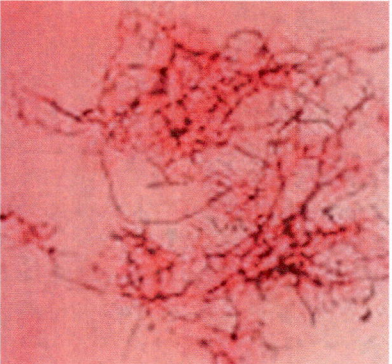

Fig. 3.9 Pulmonary nocardiosis in patients with lymphoma treated with high dose steroids, CT Chest (*right*) showed consolidation with cavitation in the right middle lobe and left lower lobe (*left*). At autopsy bilateral pneumonia and pulmonary abscesses were noted (*middle*) with colonies of filamentous micro-organisms morphologically consistent with *Nocardia* species (*right*)

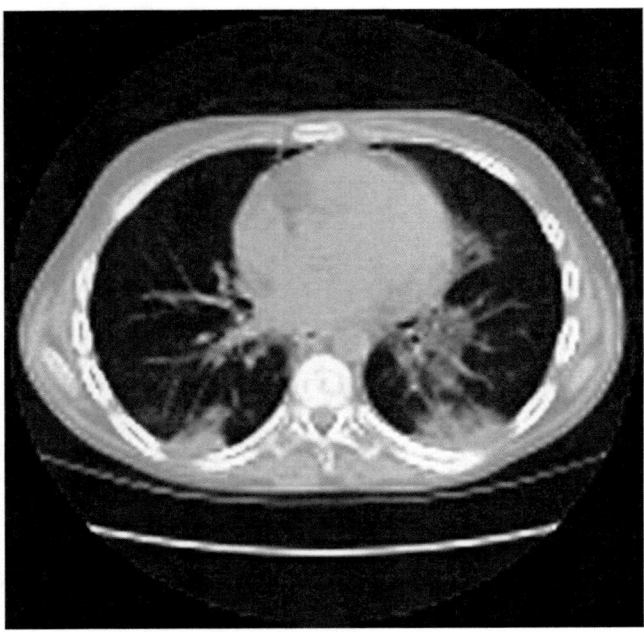

Fig. 3.10 Patient with lymphoma treated with Alemtuzumab and steroids presenting with shortness of breath. CT of chest showed nodular and interstitial infiltrates. Septate hyphae consistent with *Aspergillus* and *Pneumocystis* were noted at autopsy

The sites of infection are most frequently the upper respiratory tract, the urinary tract, or the skin. Septicemia occurs less frequently, but it does cause significant morbidity and mortality.

Normal humoral immune function is essential for the control of enteroviruses in the acute viremic phase. Chronic carriers of Hepatitis B are at risk for severe Hepatitis B reactivation after treatment with rituximab, a monoclonal antibody against B-cells [52]

Splenic Dysfunction

The spleen removes opsonized and non-opsonized microorganisms form the circulation and is the principal organ for the production of antibody to polysaccharide antigens. Splenectomized patients have decreased levels of IgM and properdin, and may be deficient in other phagocytosis promoting peptides. Splenectomized patients are highly vulnerable to bacterial infections by *S. pneumoniae* and *H. influenzae*, as well as *Neisseria* spp. and *Capnocytophaga canimorsus* (Table 3.2). Overwhelming infection after splenectomy occurs in 6.9% of post splenectomy patients with 50% of the infection-related deaths occurring within the first 3 months post splenectomy. Even overwhelming infection may present with subtle symptoms. Asplenic patients with underlying hematologic malignancy who present with fever should be managed initially as potentially septic.

Mucosal Impairment

Mucosal immunity of the gastrointestinal, sinopulmonary, and genitourinary tracts constitute the first line of host defense against invasion of these barriers by microorganisms. Oral and gastrointestinal mucositis is a frequent complication of treatment of patients with hematologic malignancies ranging from mild erythema and soreness to ulcerations with hemorrhage. The pathophysiology of mucositis is complex, involving initial damage by oxygen free radicals, followed by upregulation of proinflammatory cytokines and microvascular damage. This ultimately leads to ulceration, which is exacerbated by bacterial, viral, and fungal colonization [53–55]. In neutropenic patients, more than 80% of microbiologically documented infections are caused by organisms that are part of the endogenous flora and about one-half of the etiologic agents are acquired by the patients subsequent to hospital admission [56, 57].

Immune Defects in Specific Malignancies

The recognition of the principal immune defect enables us to assess the relative risk for specific pathogens. The predominant immune defects associated with most common hematologic malignancies and their treatments are listed on Table 3.5. Multiple immune deficits can coexist in the same patient.

Acute Leukemia

Severe and prolonged neutropenia and mucositis are the major immune defect in patients with acute leukemia undergoing intensive chemotherapy. Intensive induction chemotherapy or consolidation chemotherapy for acute leukemia are usually followed by 2–4 weeks or 8–12 days of neutropenia respectively. Fever develops in the vast majority of patients with neutropenia. An organism is identified in approximately 50% of the cases. The most common infections and causative agents during the neutropenic phase in acute leukemia are listed on Table 3.3.

Patients with acute lymphoblastic leukemia, hairy cell leukemia, and mycoses fungoides have an intrinsic impairment in cellular immunity. These patients are susceptible to opportunistic pathogens like *P. jiroveci* and reactivation of

Table 3.5 Predominant immune defects associated with common hematologic malignancies

Disease		Host defense impairment					
		Neutropenia	Phagocyte defects	Cellular immunity	Humoral immunity	Splenic dysfunction	Anatomic disruption
AML	Disease	+++	+	−	−	−	±
	Treatment	+++		+	+	−	+++
ALL	Disease	+++	+	+	−	−	±
	Treatment	+++		++	++	−	+++
Hairy cell leukemia	Disease	++*	+	±	±	−	±
	Treatment	++		+	++	If splenectomy	±
CLL	Disease	±	+	±	+++	±	±
	Treatment	++		++	++	++	+
CML	Disease	±	+	−	−		±
	Treatment	±		±	−		±
Myeloma	Disease	±	+	±	+++		±
	Treatment	± to ++		++	++		± to +
Lymphoma	Disease	−	+	+++	±	±	±
	Treatment	± to +++		++	++	If splenectomy	± to +++
MDS	Disease	++	+	−	±		±
	Treatment	++		+	−		

++ to +++: Significant; +: known; ±: not prominent;* also monocytopenia

latent viruses primarily varicella zoster and herpes simplex (Table 3.5) [58].

Chronic Lymphocytic Leukemia

In chronic lymphocytic leukemia, an intrinsic defect in the clonal B-cells leads to unbalanced immunoglobulin chain synthesis resulting in hypogammaglobulinemia. Impairments in cellular immunity, the complement system, and variable neutropenia depending on the extent of marrow involvement may also contribute to susceptibility to infections [59].

The incidence of infection correlates with the duration and the stage of disease as well as with the serum levels of immunoglobulins (particularly IgG). Up to 50% of patients with CLL experience recurrent infections [59]. The 25-year risk for severe infection was 26% in one cohort of 125 patients analyzed over 10 years [60]. In patients treated with conventional chemotherapy, infections are likely to be mainly bacterial; including *S. pneumoniae, S. aureus*, and enteric Gram-negative organisms. Opportunistic infections such as *Pneumocystis* and fungal infections are uncommon as cellular immunity is preserved in the early stages of disease [59].

Treatment with purine analogues (fludarabine and clofaradine) usually results in prolonged lymphopenia [59, 61]. Reactivation of HSV or VZV occurs approximately in 10–15% of patients treated with fludarabine [62–64]. The relative risk of infection related to cell-mediated immunity deficit is increased when fludarabine is combined with corticosteroids or alemtuzumab treatment [59, 61, 65]. The incidence of infection in patients treated with Alemtuzumab appears higher in pretreated patients compared to patients receiving alemtuzumab as first line single agent [66–74]. Although the majority or infections occur within the first 3 months of treatment some infections were reported up to 180 days post treatment [75, 76]. The addition of the anti B-cell antibody rituximab to nucleoside analogue based therapy does not appear to increase the risk of early or late infections [77, 78].

Myeloma

In multiple myeloma, the intrinsic immune deficits are a reduction in polyclonal immunoglobulin synthesis and a failure to make appropriate antibody responses post immunization. Cell-mediated immunity is intact unless patients are treated with corticosteroids of cytotoxic chemotherapy. The degree of humoral immunity impairment is related with the stage of disease [79]. Patients who have responded to chemotherapy and are in the "plateau phase" are at a low risk [80].

Infection is the most common cause of death among patients with multiple myeloma, accounting for 20–50% of all deaths. The sites of infections and causative pathogens are reviewed in Table 3.5. Most infections in newly diagnosed patients and during the first cycles of chemotherapy are caused by *S. pneumoniae, S. aureus* and *H. influenzae*, or *Neisseria* spp. In patients with renal failure, relapsed and/or refractory advanced disease, more than 90% of the infectious episodes are caused by Gram-negative bacilli or *S. aureus* [81]. Patients treated with bortezomib, particularly in combination with dexamethasone or cytotoxic agents, have a high incidence of varicella-zoster infections and prophylaxis with acyclovir is indicated [82]. An increased incidence of Aspergillosis has been reported after intensive chemotherapy and associated neutropenia [83].

Strategies for the prevention of infection in patients with myeloma include prophylactic antibiotics, passive immunization with polyclonal or specific immunoglobulins, and vaccinations.

Lymphoma

Impaired cellular immunity is the predominant intrinsic host immune defect in patients with Hodgkin's disease and non-Hodgkin's lymphomas. In addition, cytotoxic agents administered alone or in combination with steroids are major causes of impaired T-cell immunity. Fludarabine or Alemtuzumab (MabCampath®) result in profound and prolonged depletion of lymphocytes. Radiation can result in impaired T-cell immunity especially when given in combination with other immunosuppressive agents. Some degree of cellular dysfunction may persist even in patients who have been in remission for several years [84]. The most common sites and pathogens associated with impaired cellular immunity are reviewed in Table 3.3.

In patients with T-cell lymphoma, bacterial sepsis is the most common infectious complication and accounts for about 50% of all deaths [85, 86]. Cutaneous bacterial infections in particular due to *S. aureus* are the most common followed by cutaneous herpes simplex and VZV, bacteremia, bacterial pneumonia, and urinary tract infection [87]. In patients with T-cell lymphoma treated with alemtuzumab, CMV (CMV reactivation) is the most common viral infection followed by HSV and VZV [88, 89]. A high incidence of mold infections has also been reported [88]. Patients with HTLV-1 associated T-cell lymphoma are at increased risk of infection with *S. stercoralis* and possibly with *Mycobacterium tuberculous* and leprosy [90].

Summary

Over the last two decades, the increasing intensity of chemotherapeutic regimens and improved survival of patients with hematologic malignancies have lead to an increased population of highly immunocompromised individuals. Our evolving understanding of the immune system, sensitive diagnostic methods, and effective antiinfectives have led to an overall improvement in the incidence of infections and associated mortality. The relentless selective pressures on pathogens have led to shifts in the epidemiology of infections. A multidisciplinary team consisting of oncologists, infectious disease clinicians, and basic scientists is required to address the constantly evolving challenges of infections in patients with hematologic malignancies.

References

1. Burnett AK. Acute myeloid leukemia: treatment of adults under 60 years. Rev Clin Exp Hematol. 2002;6(1):26–45; discussion 86–7.
2. Koistinen P et al. Long-term outcome of intensive chemotherapy for adults with de novo acute myeloid leukaemia (AML): the nationwide AML-92 study by the Finnish Leukaemia Group. Eur J Haematol. 2007;78(6):477–86.
3. Chamilos G et al. Invasive fungal infections in patients with hematologic malignancies in a tertiary care cancer center: an autopsy study over a 15-year period (1989–2003). Haematologica. 2006;91(7):986–9.
4. Elonen E et al. Comparison between four and eight cycles of intensive chemotherapy in adult acute myeloid leukemia: a randomized trial of the Finnish Leukemia Group. Leukemia. 1998;12(7):1041–8.
5. Castaigne S et al. Randomized comparison of double induction and timed-sequential induction to a "3 + 7" induction in adults with AML: long-term analysis of the Acute Leukemia French Association (ALFA) 9000 study. Blood. 2004;104(8):2467–74.
6. Hersh EM et al. Causes of death in acute leukemia: a ten-year study of 414 patients from 1954–1963. JAMA. 1965;193:105–9.
7. Caggiano V et al. Incidence, cost, and mortality of neutropenia hospitalization associated with chemotherapy. Cancer. 2005;103(9):1916–24.
8. Dale DC. The benefits of haematopoietic growth factors in the management of gynaecological oncology. Eur J Gynaecol Oncol. 2004;25(2):133–44.
9. Darmon M et al. Impact of neutropenia duration on short-term mortality in neutropenic critically ill cancer patients. Intensive Care Med. 2002;28(12):1775–80.
10. Kuderer NM et al. Mortality, morbidity, and cost associated with febrile neutropenia in adult cancer patients. Cancer. 2006;106(10):2258–66.
11. Talcott JA et al. Risk assessment in cancer patients with fever and neutropenia: a prospective, two-center validation of a prediction rule. J Clin Oncol. 1992;10(2):316–22.
12. Rossini F. Prognosis of infections in elderly patients with haematological diseases. Support Care Cancer. 1996;4(1):46–50.
13. Elting LS et al. Outcomes of bacteremia in patients with cancer and neutropenia: observations from two decades of epidemiological and clinical trials. Clin Infect Dis. 1997;25(2):247–59.
14. Malik I, Hussain M, Yousuf H. Clinical characteristics and therapeutic outcome of patients with febrile neutropenia who present in shock: need for better strategies. J Infect. 2001;42(2):120–5.
15. Styrt B. Infection associated with asplenia: risks, mechanisms, and prevention. Am J Med. 1990;88(5N):33N–42.
16. Norris RP, Vergis EN, Yu VL. Overwhelming postsplenectomy infection: a critical review of etiologic pathogens and management. Infect Med. 1996;13:779–83.
17. Torres HA et al. Characteristics and outcome of respiratory syncytial virus infection in patients with leukemia. Haematologica. 2007;92(9):1216–23.
18. Zuccotti G, Sepkowitz KA. Management of infection in oncology patients: infection control. In: Wingard JR, Bowden RA, editors. Infections in oncology patients. Philadelphia, PA: Martin Dunitz; 2003.

19. Hachem RY et al. *Aspergillus terreus*: an emerging amphotericin B-resistant opportunistic mold in patients with hematologic malignancies. Cancer. 2004;101(7):1594–600.
20. Uzun O et al. Risk factors and predictors of outcome in patients with cancer and breakthrough candidemia. Clin Infect Dis. 2001;32(12):1713–7.
21. Anaissie EJ et al. Predictors of adverse outcome in cancer patients with candidemia. Am J Med. 1998;104(3):238–45.
22. Bodey GP et al. Quantitative relationships between circulating leukocytes and infection in patients with acute leukemia. Ann Intern Med. 1966;64(2):328–40.
23. Pizzo PA. Fever in immunocompromised patients. N Engl J Med. 1999;341(12):893–900.
24. Rolston KV et al. The spectrum of Gram-positive bloodstream infections in patients with hematologic malignancies, and the in vitro activity of various quinolones against Gram-positive bacteria isolated from cancer patients. Int J Infect Dis. 2006;10(3):223–30.
25. Safdar A et al. Changing trends in etiology of bacteremia in patients with cancer. Eur J Clin Microbiol Infect Dis. 2006;25(8):522–6.
26. Donowitz GR, et al. Infections in the neutropenic patient – new views of an old problem. Hematology Am Soc Hematol Educ Program. 2001;113–39.
27. Lautenbach E et al. Changes in the prevalence of vancomycin-resistant enterococci in response to antimicrobial formulary interventions: impact of progressive restrictions on use of vancomycin and third-generation cephalosporins. Clin Infect Dis. 2003;36(4):440–6.
28. Safdar N, Maki DG. The commonality of risk factors for nosocomial colonization and infection with antimicrobial-resistant *Staphylococcus aureus*, enterococcus, gram-negative bacilli, *Clostridium difficile*, and *Candida*. Ann Intern Med. 2002;136(11):834–44.
29. Gonzalez-Barca E et al. Prognostic factors influencing mortality in cancer patients with neutropenia and bacteremia. Eur J Clin Microbiol Infect Dis. 1999;18(8):539–44.
30. Pagano L et al. Bacteremia in patients with hematological malignancies. Analysis of risk factors, etiological agents and prognostic indicators. Haematologica. 1997;82(4):415–9.
31. Norgaard M et al. Risk of bacteraemia and mortality in patients with haematological malignancies. Clin Microbiol Infect. 2006;12(3):217–23.
32. Bochud PY et al. Bacteremia due to viridans streptococcus in neutropenic patients with cancer: clinical spectrum and risk factors. Clin Infect Dis. 1994;18(1):25–31.
33. Elting LS, Bodey GP, Keefe BH. Septicemia and shock syndrome due to viridans streptococci: a case-control study of predisposing factors. Clin Infect Dis. 1992;14(6):1201–17.
34. Tunkel AR, Sepkowitz KA. Infections caused by viridans streptococci in patients with neutropenia. Clin Infect Dis. 2002;34(11):1524–9.
35. Pizzo PA et al. Empiric antibiotic and antifungal therapy for cancer patients with prolonged fever and granulocytopenia. Am J Med. 1982;72(1):101–11.
36. Hughes WT et al. 1997 Guidelines for the use of antimicrobial agents in neutropenic patients with unexplained fever. Infectious Diseases Society of America. Clin Infect Dis. 1997;25(3):551–73.
37. Edmond MB et al. Nosocomial bloodstream infections in United States hospitals: a three-year analysis. Clin Infect Dis. 1999;29(2):239–44.
38. Pfaller MA et al. International surveillance of bloodstream infections due to *Candida* species: frequency of occurrence and in vitro susceptibilities to fluconazole, ravuconazole, and voriconazole of isolates collected from 1997 through 1999 in the SENTRY antimicrobial surveillance program. J Clin Microbiol. 2001;39(9):3254–9.
39. Anttila VJ et al. Hepatosplenic candidiasis in patients with acute leukemia: incidence and prognostic implications. Clin Infect Dis. 1997;24(3):375–80.
40. Kontoyiannis DP, Bodey GP. Invasive aspergillosis in 2002: an update. Eur J Clin Microbiol Infect Dis. 2002;21(3):161–72.
41. Pagano L et al. The epidemiology of fungal infections in patients with hematologic malignancies: the SEIFEM-2004 study. Haematologica. 2006;91(8):1068–75.
42. Walsh TJ, Hiemenz JW, Anaissie E. Recent progress and current problems in treatment of invasive fungal infections in neutropenic patients. Infect Dis Clin North Am. 1996;10(2):365–400.
43. Roden MM et al. Epidemiology and outcome of zygomycosis: a review of 929 reported cases. Clin Infect Dis. 2005;41(5):634–53.
44. Kontoyiannis DP et al. Zygomycosis in a tertiary-care cancer center in the era of *Aspergillus*-active antifungal therapy: a case-control observational study of 27 recent cases. J Infect Dis. 2005;191(8):1350–60.
45. Chandrasekar PH. Fungi other than *Candida* and *Aspergillus*. In: Bowden RA, editor. Infections in oncology patients. Philadelphia, PA: Martin Dunitz; 2003.
46. Bogomolski-Yahalom V, Matzner Y. Disorders of neutrophil function. Blood Rev. 1995;9(3):183–90.
47. Serbina NV et al. Monocyte-mediated defense against microbial pathogens. Annu Rev Immunol. 2008;26:421–52.
48. Wade JC. Viral infections in patients with hematological malignancies. Hematology Am Soc Hematol Educ Program. 2006;368–74.
49. Huang H et al. Lamivudine for the prevention of hepatitis B virus reactivation after high-dose chemotherapy and autologous hematopoietic stem cell transplantation for patients with advanced or relapsed non-Hodgkin's lymphoma single institution experience. Expert Opin Pharmacother. 2009;10(15):2399–406.
50. Uchiyama M, Tamai Y, Ikeda T. Low-dose acyclovir against reactivation of varicella zoster virus after unrelated cord blood transplantation. Int J Infect Dis. 2009;14(5):e451–2.
51. Waecker Jr NJ et al. Nosocomial transmission of Mycobacterium bovis bacille Calmette-Guerin to children receiving cancer therapy and to their health care providers. Clin Infect Dis. 2000;30(2):356–62.
52. Pei SN et al. Reactivation of hepatitis B virus following rituximab-based regimens: a serious complication in both HBsAg-positive and HBsAg-negative patients. Ann Hematol. 2009;89(3):255–62.
53. Gabriel DA et al. The effect of oral mucositis on morbidity and mortality in bone marrow transplant. Semin Oncol. 2003;30(6 Suppl 18):76–83.
54. Sonis ST. The biologic role for nuclear factor-kappaB in disease and its potential involvement in mucosal injury associated with antineoplastic therapy. Crit Rev Oral Biol Med. 2002;13(5):380–9.
55. Sonis ST et al. Perspectives on cancer therapy-induced mucosal injury: pathogenesis, measurement, epidemiology, and consequences for patients. Cancer. 2004;100(9 Suppl):1995–2025.
56. Schimpff SC et al. Origin of infection in acute nonlymphocytic leukemia. Significance of hospital acquisition of potential pathogens. Ann Intern Med. 1972;77(5):707–14.
57. Weinstock DM et al. Colonization, bloodstream infection, and mortality caused by vancomycin-resistant enterococcus early after allogeneic hematopoietic stem cell transplant. Biol Blood Marrow Transplant. 2007;13(5):615–21.
58. David DS et al. Visceral varicella-zoster after bone marrow transplantation: report of a case series and review of the literature. Am J Gastroenterol. 1998;93(5):810–3.
59. Ravandi F, Anaissie E, O'Brien S. Infections in chronic leukemias and other hematological malignancies. In: Wingard JR, Bowden RA, editors. Infections in oncology patients. Philadelphia, PA: Martin Dunitz; 2003.
60. Molica S, Levato D, Levato L. Infections in chronic lymphocytic leukemia. Analysis of incidence as a function of length of follow-up. Haematologica. 1993;78(6):374–7.
61. Tam CS et al. A new model for predicting infectious complications during fludarabine-based combination chemotherapy among patients with indolent lymphoid malignancies. Cancer. 2004;101(9):2042–9.

62. Anaissie EJ et al. Infection in patients with chronic lymphocytic leukemia treated with fludarabine. Ann Intern Med. 1998;129(7):559–66.
63. Lungman P. Viral infections: current diagnosis and treatment. Hematol J. 2004;5:S63–8.
64. Sandherr M et al. Antiviral prophylaxis in patients with haematological malignancies and solid tumours: Guidelines of the Infectious Diseases Working Party (AGIHO) of the German Society for Hematology and Oncology (DGHO). Ann Oncol. 2006;17(7):1051–9.
65. O'Brien SM et al. Results of the fludarabine and cyclophosphamide combination regimen in chronic lymphocytic leukemia. J Clin Oncol. 2001;19(5):1414–20.
66. Cavalli-Bjorkman N et al. Fatal adenovirus infection during alemtuzumab (anti-CD52 monoclonal antibody) treatment of a patient with fludarabine-refractory B-cell chronic lymphocytic leukemia. Med Oncol. 2002;19(4):277–80.
67. Kennedy B, Hillmen P. Immunological effects and safe administration of alemtuzumab (MabCampath) in advanced B-cLL. Med Oncol. 2002;19(Suppl):S49–55.
68. Rai KR et al. Alemtuzumab in previously treated chronic lymphocytic leukemia patients who also had received fludarabine. J Clin Oncol. 2002;20(18):3891–7.
69. Laurenti L et al. Cytomegalovirus reactivation during alemtuzumab therapy for chronic lymphocytic leukemia: incidence and treatment with oral ganciclovir. Haematologica. 2004;89(10):1248–52.
70. Rawstron AC et al. Early prediction of outcome and response to alemtuzumab therapy in chronic lymphocytic leukemia. Blood. 2004;103(6):2027–31.
71. Rieger K et al. Efficacy and tolerability of alemtuzumab (CAMPATH-1H) in the salvage treatment of B-cell chronic lymphocytic leukemia – change of regimen needed? Leuk Lymphoma. 2004;45(2):345–9.
72. Wendtner CM et al. Consolidation with alemtuzumab in patients with chronic lymphocytic leukemia (CLL) in first remission – experience on safety and efficacy within a randomized multicenter phase III trial of the German CLL Study Group (GCLLSG). Leukemia. 2004;18(6):1093–101.
73. Lin TS et al. Filgrastim and alemtuzumab (Campath-1H) for refractory chronic lymphocytic leukemia. Leukemia. 2005;19(7):1207–10.
74. Lundin J et al. Phase II trial of subcutaneous anti-CD52 monoclonal antibody alemtuzumab (Campath-1H) as first-line treatment for patients with B-cell chronic lymphocytic leukemia (B-CLL). Blood. 2002;100(3):768–73.
75. Keating MJ et al. Therapeutic role of alemtuzumab (Campath-1H) in patients who have failed fludarabine: results of a large international study. Blood. 2002;99(10):3554–61.
76. Keating MJ et al. Long-term follow-up of patients with chronic lymphocytic leukemia (CLL) receiving fludarabine regimens as initial therapy. Blood. 1998;92(4):1165–71.
77. Keating MJ et al. Early results of a chemoimmunotherapy regimen of fludarabine, cyclophosphamide, and rituximab as initial therapy for chronic lymphocytic leukemia. J Clin Oncol. 2005;23(18):4079–88.
78. Tam C et al. Early and late infectious consequences of adding rituximab to fludarabine and cyclophosphamide in patients with indolent lymphoid malignancies. Haematologica. 2005;90(5):700–2.
79. Blade, J, Rosinol L. Complications of multiple myeloma. Hematol Oncol Clin North Am. 2007;21(6):1231–46, xi.
80. Hargreaves RM et al. Immunological factors and risk of infection in plateau phase myeloma. J Clin Pathol. 1995;48(3):260–6.
81. Savage DG, Lindenbaum J, Garrett TJ. Biphasic pattern of bacterial infection in multiple myeloma. Ann Intern Med. 1982;96(1):47–50.
82. San Miguel JF et al. Bortezomib plus melphalan and prednisone for initial treatment of multiple myeloma. N Engl J Med. 2008;359(9):906–17.
83. Lortholary O et al. Invasive aspergillosis as an opportunistic infection in nonallografted patients with multiple myeloma: a European Organization for Research and Treatment of Cancer/Invasive Fungal Infections Cooperative Group and the Intergroupe Francais du Myelome. Clin Infect Dis. 2000;30(1):41–6.
84. Fisher RI et al. Persistent immunologic abnormalities in long-term survivors of advanced Hodgkin's disease. Ann Intern Med. 1980;92(5):595–9.
85. Dalton JA et al. Cutaneous T-cell lymphoma. Int J Dermatol. 1997;36(11):801–9.
86. Posner LE et al. Septicemic complications of the cutaneous T-cell lymphomas. Am J Med. 1981;71(2):210–6.
87. Axelrod PI, Lorber B, Vonderheid EC. Infections complicating mycosis fungoides and Sezary syndrome. JAMA. 1992;267(10):1354–8.
88. Thursky KA et al. Spectrum of infection, risk and recommendations for prophylaxis and screening among patients with lymphoproliferative disorders treated with alemtuzumab. Br J Haematol. 2006;132(1):3–12.
89. National Comprehensive Cancer Network. Clinical practice guidelines in oncology: prevention and treatment of cancer related infections (v.2.2009). Jenkintown, PA: NCCN; 2009.
90. Marshall BG et al. Increased inflammatory cytokines and new collagen formation in cutaneous tuberculous and sarcoidosis. Thorax. 1996;51(12):1253–61.

Chapter 4
Infections in Solid Tumor Patients

Alison G. Freifeld

Abstract Over 90% of the 1.4 million new cases of cancer diagnosed in the United States in 2008 were due to solid tumors, with predominant sites being lung, breast, prostate, colorectal, bladder, and uterine cancers. While it is clear to practicing oncologists that solid tumor patients are generally at lower risk for infection-related complications overall, infections are certainly not rare in this population. Common foci include intravascular catheter-related bacteremia, pneumonias, wound and skin/soft tissue infections, and fever associated with chemotherapy-induced neutropenia. Nonetheless, there is little published data examining the incidence or characteristics of infections in solid tumor patients. This is not only because infection is relatively uncommon in solid tumor patients but also because sites, pathogens, and severity will vary, to a large extent, with tumor location, natural history, and the type and intensity of anticancer therapy. This variability precludes a neat summary of all the bacterial, viral, and fungal infections that occur in the solid tumor group as a whole. Instead, observational series and anecdotal reports have lead to the recognition of patterns of infection that may be considered "typical" for specific solid tumor types, or that are associated with certain antitumor treatment regimens. The goal of this chapter is to familiarize the physician with these infection profiles, so they may identify and manage them promptly and effectively.

Keywords Infection • Neutropenia • Catheter-related infections • Postsurgical wound infections • Bacteremia • Colon cancer • Breast cancer • Lung cancer

Introduction

Over 90% of the 1.4 million new cases of cancer diagnosed in the United States in 2008 were due to solid tumors, with predominant sites being lung, breast, prostate, colorectal, bladder, and uterine cancers [1]. Hematologic malignancies accounted for less than 10% of new cancers in the same year (approximately 5% lymphomas, 3% leukemias, and 1.5% multiple myelomas), yet the levels of morbidity, mortality, and overall healthcare resource utilization among patients with hematologic cancers far exceed those for solid tumor patients [2, 3].

Duration of hospitalization and inpatient mortality tends to be significantly greater in leukemic patients with fever and neutropenia than for those with solid tumors [3]. In a recent multicenter European study, bloodstream infections were found to be nearly 3 times more common in lymphoma and leukemia patients with fever and neutropenia than in patients with solid tumors [4]. While it is clear to practicing oncologists that solid tumor patients are generally at lower risk for infection-related complications overall, infections are certainly not rare in this population. Common foci include intravascular catheter-related bacteremia, pneumonias, wound and skin/soft tissue infections, and fever associated with chemotherapy-induced neutropenia. Nonetheless, there is little published data examining the incidence or characteristics of infections in solid tumor patients. This is not only because infection is relatively uncommon in solid tumor patients but also because sites, pathogens, and severity will vary, to a large extent, with tumor location, natural history, and the type and intensity of anticancer therapy. This variability precludes a neat summary of all the bacterial, viral, and fungal infections that occur in the solid tumor group as a whole. Instead, observational series and anecdotal reports have led to the recognition of patterns of infection that may be considered "typical" for specific solid tumor types, or that are associated with certain antitumor treatment regimens. The goal of this chapter is to familiarize the physician with these infection profiles, so they may identify and manage them promptly and effectively.

Infection Risks and Pathogens

In the patient with hematologic malignancy, normal immune mediator cells are replaced by malignant clones that fail to perform protective immunologic tasks. Serial cycles of

A.G. Freifeld (✉)
Department of Medicine, University of Nebraska Medical Center, Omaha, NE 68198-5400, USA
e-mail: afreifeld@unmc.edu

intensive chemotherapy with corresponding prolonged periods of neutropenia further contribute to profound immunologic compromise that allow for opportunistic infections to advance. By contrast, defects in immune responses are far less frequent among solid tumor patients whose immune function is unaffected by the underlying disease, and less intensive cytoreductive therapies are more common.

Breeches in physical defense barriers are a common predisposing factor leading to infection in the solid tumor patient. Tumor infiltration across tissue planes with obstruction of a normally patent conduits of body secretions, such as colon, biliary tract, or bronchus, can lead to postobstructive infections. Tumor debulking or diagnostic surgeries with attendant anatomic disruptions and poor surgical wound healing will also contribute risks. Radiation therapy can also lead to tissue fragility and damage and impaired wound healing. Concurrent use of chemotherapy that enhances the radiosensitivity of tumors increases the chance of mucosal injury and neutropenia [5]. Disruptions of skin and mucous membrane integrity allow for skin and gastrointestinal commensals such as staphylococci, streptococci, enteric Gram-negative bacilli, and Candida species to gain access to surrounding tissue or to the bloodstream. These components of colonizing flora are common etiologies of infections in the solid tumor patient (Table 4.1).

Cytotoxic chemotherapy for solid tumors will often occur in repeated cycles, as with hematologic cancer treatments, but the attendant periods of chemotherapy-induced neutropenia are comparatively very mild (rarely yielding an absolute neutrophil count <100/mm^3) and brief, usually lasting a few days (and usually less than 1 week) with each cycle. Since the depth and duration of neutropenia are factors that dictate infection risk in cancer patients, it follows that solid tumor patients are less prone to documented invasive infections during neutropenia. This is particularly true in the case of invasive mold infections such as aspergillosis, which is vanishingly rare among solid tumor patients. Mold infections classically typically develop in the setting of profound (absolute neutrophils <100/mm^3) and prolonged neutropenia lasting more than 2 weeks and accordingly, they occur almost exclusively among patients with acute myeloid leukemia (AML) and very rarely in those with less intensively treated hematologic malignancies such as lymphoma and multiple myeloma, and almost never in solid tumor patients [6, 7]. Similarly, viral infections such as adenovirus, BK virus, or EBV-associated lymphoproliferative disorders, which take advantage of the immune dysregulation post allogeneic stem cell transplant, are distinctly rare in solid tumor patients. This is because the critical T-cell mechanisms controlling these infections are less profoundly impaired after chemotherapy for solid tumors compared with more intensive regimens given for acute leukemia or stem cell transplants [8]. In general, the spectrum of pathogens that commonly cause infections in solid tumor patients is narrower and more representative of "normal flora" than in patients undergoing treatment for hematologic malignancies. In the latter group, antibiotic resistant and hospital acquired pathogens such as Enterococcus, VRE, Pseudomonas, and beta-lactamase-producing Gram-negative bacilli are more likely to occur.

Infections Associated with Specific Cancers and Treatments (Table 4.2)

Lung Cancer

Cancer of the lung (small cell 10%, nonsmall cell 90%) was the leading cause of cancer mortality in the United States in 2009, resulting in 28% of all cancer deaths [1]. Surgical resection is a common initial approach to lung cancers, with adjuvant or neoadjuvant chemotherapy and/or radiation also being administered, depending on the location, extent, and tumor type. Despite aggressive multimodality approaches to management, infections are fairly uncommon after lung cancer surgery and/or chemotherapy. Among 1885 patients retrospectively reviewed from 1992 to 2003 in Japan, lung

Table 4.1 Comparison of common pathogens in solid tumor and hematologic malignancy patient groups

Pathogens	Solid tumor patients	Hematologic tumor patients (e.g., AML, stem cell transplant recipients)
Gram-positive bacteria	• Coagulase negative Staphylococci • Occasionally other Gram positives	• Coagulase negative Staphylococci • VRE and MRSA acquired in the hospital • Bacillus
Gram-negative bacteria	• Enteric Gram negatives	• Enteric Gram negatives • Pseudomonas and resistant Gram-negative bacilli acquired in the hospital
Fungi	• Occasional oral thrush	• Invasive candidiasis often prevented with prophylaxis but candidiasis associated with catheters occasionally occurs
	• Occasional candidemia associated with catheters	• Aspergillus and other molds occur almost exclusively in hematologic malignancy patients with GVHD and/or prolonged neutropenia

Table 4.2 Infectious complications associated with various solid tumor malignancies and treatment regimens

Solid tumor type	Potential infectious complications
Lung	Pneumonia
	Lung abscess
	COPD exacerbations
Breast	Skin/soft-tissue infections at surgical site
	Cellulitis in setting of lymphedema after axillary node dissection – now uncommon since sentinel node biopsy is standard of care
GI	Postoperative anastamotic leak or peritonitis
	Intra-abdominal abscess
	Hepatic abscess
Head and Neck	Wound infection due to surgical and/or radiation therapy tissue disruption
	Esophagitis initiated by radiation therapy, with fungal or viral superinfection
CNS	Temozolomide and steroids increase risk for *Pneumocystis jirovecii* pneumonia

cancer surgery was complicated by postoperative respiratory infections in fewer than 4%, with approximately 3% pneumonia cases and 1% having empyemas, usually with associated bronchopleural fistulas [9]. Multivariate analysis showed that age 75 years or older, decreased lung function as measured by FEV1%, advanced pathologic stage, and induction chemotherapy were independent risk factors for pneumonia. Pneumonia was also identified in only 5% of advanced lung cancer patients treated with cytotoxic chemotherapy alone, and again, older age and impaired pulmonary function were risk factors [10]. These risks are predictable since a significant proportion of patients with lung malignancy are of older age and have underlying chronic obstructive lung disease (COPD) as a consequence of prolonged cigarette smoking. Death due to pneumonia is distinctly uncommon, however, accounting for less than 1% of lung cancer mortality in a study of treatment-related toxicities during the 1990s [11].

Lung cancer is an important cause of nonresolving pneumonia in adults, often resulting from partial or complete obstruction of an airway by endobronchial tumor growth. Bacteria normally inhaled and then cleared by mucociliary action in the bronchial tree are, instead, trapped and overgrow distal to the blockage to cause a postobstructive pneumonia. Slow or delayed resolution of the infection despite seemingly adequate broad-spectrum antibiotic therapy is a hallmark of this process, in which mechanical clearance of pathogens is impaired [12]. In a study of 35 adults with nonresolving pneumonia, bronchoscopy revealed bronchoalveolar or adenocarcinoma as the cause in 4 (11%) [13]. Unlike simple pneumonias, segmental or lobar atelectasis is characteristic of postobstructive pneumonia as air is reabsorbed from portions of the lung distal to the obstructing lesion. Postobstructive pneumonias in the lung cancer patient are often polymicrobial. Oropharyngeal bacteria such as anaerobic and microaerophilic streptococci have traditionally been presumed to be the cause.

However, studies have suggested that *Staphylococcus aureus* and enteric Gram-negative bacilli are more prevalent contributors to respiratory infections in lung cancer patients, including postobstructive pneumonia and lung abscess [14, 15]. Alterations in oropharyngeal colonizing flora, with a transition from predominantly Gram-positive bacteria to Gram-negative enteric organisms, have been documented to occur commonly with the environmental pressures of illness, antibiotics, and/or chemotherapy in cancer patients; this change in oral flora is reflected in the bacterial profile of subsequent pneumonias in these patients [16]. Unless adequate treatment is provided, postobstructive pneumonias may progress to lung abscess or empyema. A broad spectrum antibiotic regimen, including Gram-negative, staphylococcal, and anaerobic coverage, should be instituted, with heed paid to the emergence of resistant bacteria in patients who have been in hospital settings. Clindamycin combined with a cephalosporin, piperacillin-tazobactam, or a carbapenem are acceptable antibiotic options. Effective therapy also requires relief of the obstruction by surgery, irradiation, and/or chemotherapy in order to allow drainage of the affected lung tissue.

Surgical resection is integral to the management of most nonsmall cell lung cancers, but postoperative infections, including empyema and pneumonia, appear to be rare [9]. Infection risk postoperatively is related to age older than 75 years, low FEV1%, advanced pathologic stage, and the use of induction chemotherapy. COPD is a common comorbid condition in lung cancer patients, and exacerbations may be frequent in the post-surgical stage or during chemo- or radiation therapy. Aspiration pneumonia, superinfection of necrotic tumor, and unusual opportunistic infections such as *Pneumocystis jerovicii* pneumonia or influenza pneumonia can also complicate lung cancer treatment [17]. Tuberculous infection with inflammation and scarring has been posited as a cofactor in the development of lung cancer, but proof of this concept has not been established [18]. In recent years, the coexistence of TB and lung cancer has been reported infrequently and exclusively from countries in southeast Asia, where TB is endemic [19, 20]. In these recent reports, it appears that coexisting respiratory TB does not appreciably alter the clinical course of lung cancer patients if antituberculous therapy is used properly.

Breast Cancer

Local skin and soft-tissue infections that involve the breast and/or arm are the most frequent infectious events seen in breast cancer patients, and these infections typically occur following surgery for tumor resection. For most women with stage I or II breast cancer, breast-conservation therapy (lumpectomy/partial mastectomy plus radiation therapy) is as effective as mastectomy and is now a common practice [21].

Breast cellulitis occurring months to years (226 days median time to onset) after breast-conservation therapy has been noted to occur in approximately 8% of women, as a novel complication of this approach. By contrast, the older surgical approach of modified radical mastectomy with axillary lymph node dissection was often complicated by chronic ipsilateral arm lymphedema and occasionally by recurrent bouts of streptococcal cellulitis in the affected arm [22]. The relatively long time period between breast conservation surgery and the onset of breast cellulitis has earned the moniker "delayed breast cellulitis" for this infection. Characterized by diffuse breast erythema, edema, tenderness, and warmth occurring more than 3 months after surgery, delayed breast cellulitis is generally responsive to prompt treatment with antistreptococcal antibiotics [23]. Antibiotic treatment should not be withheld in these patients' pending results of blood or tissue cultures, since a pathogen will rarely be isolated.

Colon Cancer

There is longstanding recognition that bloodstream infections due to certain gut organisms, particularly *Clostridium septicum* and *Streptococcus bovis*, may be harbingers of an occult colon cancer [24–26]. Tumor perforation through the colonic mucosa, typically in the ascending colon, is considered the point of entry for these pathogens. Rarely, myonecrosis with atraumatic gas gangrene may complicate *Clostridium septicum* sepsis, while endocarditis has been associated with *Streptococcus bovis* infections arising from occult colonic tumors [27, 28].

When sepsis or other serious infection due to these pathogens occurs without an obvious underlying etiology, there should be a high index of suspicion for associated colonic malignancy and colonoscopy is warranted.

Partial or complete bowel obstruction is a common presentation of primary colon cancer occurring in about 15–20% of patients at diagnosis [29, 30]. Fever and abdominal pain are typically associated with obstructing tumor masses. Bacterial translocation of enteric organisms from the gut lumen has been implicated as a possible source of fever and sepsis in patients with obstruction. In one clinicopathologic study, bacterial translocation to mesenteric nodes (identified by culture of biopsy specimens from surgery) occurred more frequently in colon cancer patients with large bowel obstruction than in those without obstruction (14 of 36 patients vs. 16 of 218 patients; $P<0.001$) [31]. Both aerobic and anaerobic bacteria were found to translocate in this study, and translocation of bacteria predisposed to postoperative septic complications including bacteremia and intra-abdominal abscess ($P<0.05$). Tumor perforation through the bowel wall with subsequent local intra-abdominal abscess formation is a very rare complication of intraluminal colon cancer [32]. Despite the frequency of obstructing colonic malignancies, only about 5% of patients have documented bacteremia or abscess in this setting [30, 32, 33].

Surgical resection is a mainstay of early colorectal cancer management. The incidence of postsurgical infections is approximately 10%, with most related to anastamotic leaks and intra-abdominal abscesses [33]. Nonetheless, in a comparison of 59 colon cancer patients with a leak or an abscess with 118 matched controls, the presence of leak or an abscess was not shown to impact the outcome at 5 years; however, these complications were associated with increased overall cancer-specific mortality and local recurrence in patients who underwent resection for rectal cancer [34]. Postoperative wound infection has also been found to be significantly more frequent in cases where the tumor site was the rectum rather than colon [35]. Wound infections after surgery for colorectal surgery are also decreased by the use of laparoscopic approach rather than open surgery, and by high-pressure washing of the wound before abdominal closure. Broad-spectrum antibiotic prophylaxis given before elective colorectal surgery is effective in reducing the incidence of postoperative surgical wound infections by at least 75% [36]. Single doses of regimens with broad spectrum activity against aerobic and anaerobic bacteria, such as ertapenem or a cephalosporin plus metronidazole, are as effective as multiple doses of antibiotics. It is essential to time antibiotic delivery to achieve maximal serum levels at the time of surgery, generally about 1–2 h prior to incision.

Other infrequent infection-related complications of surgical management include bacteremia, enterocutaneous or enterovaginal fistula, catheter infection, urinary tract infection, peritonitis, and pneumonia. An interesting observation made in the late 1980s was the finding that homologous blood transfusions given around the time of colorectal cancer surgery may be associated with a significant increase in the risk for developing wound infections or any of these other aforementioned infectious complications [33, 37]. However, larger retrospective follow-up studies failed to detect this link. Leukocytes depletion of blood products by filtration (now routine) appears to significantly lower the risk of infection and other complications in patients undergoing gastrointestinal surgery [37, 38].

Bevacizumab, an antibody that targets vascular endothelial growth factor (VGEF), inhibits tumor growth by inhibiting angiogenesis. In combination with chemotherapy, bevacizumab appears to extend progression-free survival and overall survival in patients with advanced colorectal malignancies. Rare, but important adverse effects of the antiangiogenesis antibody include gastrointestinal perforation and poor wound healing [39]. Clearly, serious infectious complications, such as sepsis or wound infection, may ensue from these unusual adverse effects of bevacizumab therapy (Table 4.3).

Table 4.3 Monoclonal antibodies used to treat solid tumors and their potential infectious complications

Bevacizumab	Poor wound healing, colon perforation, with intra-abdominal sepsis
Trastuzumab	infection

GU Cancers

Urogenital cancers including renal cell, prostate, and urothelial bladder cancer are typically treated with cytoreductive chemotherapy and/or special surgical interventions, although infectious complications occur infrequently. Fewer than 5% of urogenital cancer patients were noted to develop a documented infection during chemotherapy-related neutropenia in one large study [40]. Typically, those infections were associated with mechanical abnormalities such as urinary diversion or hydronephrosis or during severe neutropenia, when the absolute white blood cell count fell below 500/mm^3. Antimicrobial prophylaxis for standard chemotherapy regimens in this setting is therefore not recommended. The use of antimicrobial prophylaxis prior to "clean-contaminated" urologic surgery for diagnosis (i.e., prostate biopsy) or tumor resection is somewhat controversial because of the paucity of good clinical trial data. However, it is generally recommended that patients undergoing prostate biopsy, transurethral resection of bladder tumor, or manipulation of bowel segments for urinary diversion in patients with bladder cancer receive a brief course of antibiotic prophylaxis to decrease infectious complications [41–43].

An ileal conduit or a neobladder (ureterosigmoidostomy) is typically created to provide urinary diversion following cystectomy for bladder cancer. Bacteriuria is an expected finding in patients with an ileal neobladder, with at least 80% developing bacterial growth in urine cultures at some point. This must be distinguished from a true urinary tract infection because simple bacteriuria does not require antibiotic treatment. True urinary tract infection, with attendant fever and malaise and urinary bacterial concentrations of >10^5/ml, affects a significant proportion of patients following urinary diversion. Symptoms from the lower urinary tract may not be prominent in this group, so clinical suspicion is key to the diagnosis [44].

Antibiotics appropriate for urinary bacterial isolates should be administered for a 14-day course. Notably, the level of white blood cells in the urine may not correlate with the presence or absence of bacterial growth in urine cultures in samples from ileal conduits, suggesting that neutrophil inflammatory responses of ileal mucosa to the presence of bacteria differ from those of the bladder [45].

Percutaneous renal radiofrequency (RF) ablation is a well-established minimally invasive therapeutic option for the treatment of selected patients with renal cell carcinoma. Major complications are rare and include hematuria, internal hemorrhage, and unintended thermal injury to the ureter or other organs during ablation. Several patients with ileal conduits who underwent percutaneous renal RF ablation and developed infectious complications have been described: a renal abscess and a calyceal-cutaneous fistula [46]. Postablation syndrome characterized by low-grade fever (without infectious etiology), pain, and malaise following the procedure is reported in about one third of patients [47].

Bacillus Calmette-Guerin (BCG) is a live attenuated strain of *Mycobacterium bovis* that has been used to treat bladder carcinoma since 1976, and has been associated with disease eradication in more than two thirds of patients with early stage disease [48]. The precise mechanisms of action are unknown, but intravesical instillation of BCG triggers a variety of local immune responses, which appear to induce antitumor activity. Due to its success, BCG bladder instillation is widely employed. Although the mycobacterial strain is attenuated, side effects include fever (2.9%), granulomatous pneumonitis and/or hepatitis (0.7%), sepsis (0.4%), and a variety of local and disseminated BCG infections [49, 50]. A number of cases of mycotic vascular infections of large arteries secondary to *M. bovis* infection after intravesical BCG therapy have been reported, especially involving the abdominal aorta [51, 52]. Psoas and pancreatic abscesses, vertebral osteomyelitis, and aortoduodenal fistula have also been reported [53–55]. BCG sepsis or vascular infection is characterized by high fevers, chills, hypotension, and confusion occurring beyond the first day or two after installation. Disseminated intravascular coagulopathy, respiratory failure, and hepatic dysfunction may occur as well. Documentation of positive blood cultures is rare and treatment should be started based upon clinical suspicion. Treatment of serious *M. bovis* infections is with isoniazid (INH) and rifampin (RIF) for at least 6 months. The addition of prednisone 40 mg daily until fever resolves has been advocated to reduce the inflammatory component and may improve survival [49, 50].

CNS Cancer

The prolonged use of high-dose corticosteroids and radiotherapy in patients with primary brain tumors yields severe lymphocyte depletion that increases the risk of life-threatening opportunistic infections, particularly due to *Pneumocystis jerovici* pneumonia (known generally as "PCP") [56, 57].

Tapering of corticosteroid doses appears to be a predisposing factor for the development of (or "unmasking" of) Pneumocystis pneumonia symptoms in these patients [58]. Patients frequently present with nonspecific symptoms, such as a dry cough, slowly progressive dyspnea, and high fevers without clear etiology. Unlike patients with HIV/AIDS, cancer patients with PCP are more likely to present with the abrupt onset of dyspnea and hypoxia. Chest X-ray may be normal during the early stages of PCP, but typical diffuse bilateral interstitial infiltrates subsequently develop in most cases. Definitive diagnosis requires demonstration of *P. jiroveci* cysts in the sputum or bronchoalveolar lavage by silver stain or other method. Trimethoprim-sulfamethoxazole at high doses is the mainstay of treatment for PCP.

Temozolomide, an oral alkylating agent, has emerged as an important therapeutic advance in the management of malignant gliomas in the past decade. However, opportunistic infections have been observed due to profound lymphopenia that accompanies temozolomide long-term use, probably exacerbated by concurrent corticosteroid administration. *Pneumocystis jeroveci* pneumonia is a well-described adverse effect of temozolomide treatment for brain tumors, and prophylaxis with inhaled pentamidine or twice weekly oral trimethoprim-sulfamethoxazole is recommended during concomitant temozolomide and radiotherapy, or when CD4 lymphocyte counts decrease below 200/mm^3 [59]. Rare cases of cryptococcal meningitis, listeria brain abscess, and disseminated strongyloidiasis have also been reported in association with temozolomide therapy [57, 60, 61].

Summary

Infectious complications are considerably less frequent among solid tumor patients than those with hematologic malignancies. Nonetheless, they are not rare and the clinician must be aware of the syndromes and pathogens that are particularly associated with specific cancers and treatment regimens. It is emphasized that antimicrobial prophylaxis is rarely indicated in patients being treated with routine chemotherapy regimens. Instead, a heightened sense of suspicion and appropriate microbiologic and/or radiographic testing are the key to evaluating fever and diagnosing infections in the solid tumor population.

References

1. Jemal A, Siegel R, Ward E, Hao Y, Xu J, Thun MJ. Cancer statistics, 2009. CA Cancer J Clin. 2009;59:225–49.
2. Kuderer NM, Dale DC, Crawford J, Cosler LE, Lyman GH. Mortality, morbidity, and cost associated with febrile neutropenia in adult cancer patients. Cancer. 2006;106:2258–66.
3. Caggiano V, Weiss RV, Rickert TS, Linde-Zwirble WT. Incidence, cost, and mortality of neutropenia hospitalization associated with chemotherapy. Cancer. 2005;103:1916–24.
4. Klastersky J, Ameye L, Maertens J, Georgala A, Muanza F, Aoun M, et al. Bacteraemia in febrile neutropenic cancer patients. Int J Antimicrob Agents. 2007;30 Suppl 1:S51–9.
5. Spira A, Ettinger DS. Multidisciplinary management of lung cancer. N Engl J Med. 2004;350:379–92.
6. Cornillet A, Camus C, Nimubona S, Gandemer V, Tattevin P, Belleguic C, et al. Comparison of epidemiological, clinical, and biological features of invasive aspergillosis in neutropenic and nonneutropenic patients: a 6-year survey. Clin Infect Dis. 2006;43:577–84.
7. Pagano L, Caira M, Candoni A, Offidani M, Fianchi L, Martino B, et al. The epidemiology of fungal infections in patients with hematologic malignancies: the SEIFEM-2004 study. Haematologica. 2006;91:1068–75.
8. Mackall CL. T-cell immunodeficiency following cytotoxic antineoplastic therapy: a review. Stem Cells. 2000;18:10–8.
9. Shiono S, Yoshida J, Nishimura M, Hagiwara M, Hishida T, Nitadori J, et al. Risk factors of postoperative respiratory infections in lung cancer surgery. J Thorac Oncol. 2007;2:34–8.
10. Lee JO, Kim DY, Lim JH, Seo MD, Yi HG, Kim YJ, et al. Risk factors for bacterial pneumonia after cytotoxic chemotherapy in advanced lung cancer patients. Lung Cancer. 2008;62:381–4.
11. Ohe Y, Yamamoto S, Suzuki K, Hojo F, Kakinuma R, Matsumoto T, et al. Risk factors of treatment-related death in chemotherapy and thoracic radiotherapy for lung cancer. Eur J Cancer. 2001;37:54–63.
12. Kyprianou A, Hall CS, Shah R, Fein AM. The challenge of nonresolving pneumonia. Knowing the norms of radiographic resolution is key. Postgrad Med. 2003;113:79,82, 85–8, 91–2.
13. Feinsilver SH, Fein AM, Niederman MS, Schultz DE, Faegenburg DH. Utility of fiberoptic bronchoscopy in nonresolving pneumonia. Chest. 1990;98:1322–6.
14. Perlman LV, Lerner E, D'Esopo N. Clinical classification and analysis of 97 cases of lung abscess. Am Rev Respir Dis. 1969;99:390–8.
15. Yamada Y, Sekine Y, Suzuki H, Iwata T, Chiyo M, Nakajima T, et al. Trends of bacterial colonisation and the risk of postoperative pneumonia in lung cancer patients with chronic obstructive pulmonary disease. Eur J Cardiothorac Surg. 2010;37:752–7.
16. Los R, Rybojad P, Gozdziuk K, Malm A. Dynamics of nasopharyngeal colonization by gram-negative rods in patients with resectable lung cancer during short-term hospitalization. New Microbiol. 2008;31:507–12.
17. Seo SK. Infectious complications of lung cancer. Oncology (Williston Park). 2005;19:185–94; discussion 195–6, 199–203, 207–8.
18. Limas C, Japaze H, Garcia-Bunuel R. "Scar" carcinoma of the lung. Chest. 1971;59:219–22.
19. Dacosta NA, Kinare SG. Association of lung carcinoma and tuberculosis. J Postgrad Med. 1991;37:185–9.
20. Cha SI, Shin KM, Lee JW, Lee SY, Kim CH, Park JY, et al. The clinical course of respiratory tuberculosis in lung cancer patients. Int J Tuberc Lung Dis. 2009;13:1002–7.
21. Fisher B, Anderson S, Redmond CK, Wolmark N, Wickerham DL, Cronin WM. Reanalysis and results after 12 years of follow-up in a randomized clinical trial comparing total mastectomy with lumpectomy with or without irradiation in the treatment of breast cancer. N Engl J Med. 1995;333:1456–61.
22. Simon MS, Cody RL. Cellulitis after axillary lymph node dissection for carcinoma of the breast. Am J Med. 1992;93:543–8.
23. Indelicato DJ, Grobmyer SR, Newlin H, Morris CG, Haigh LS, Copeland III EM, et al. Delayed breast cellulitis: an evolving complication of breast conservation. 2006;66:1339–46.
24. Wentling GK, Metzger PP, Dozois EJ, Chua HK, Krishna M. Unusual bacterial infections and colorectal carcinoma–Streptococcus bovis and Clostridium septicum: report of three cases. Dis Colon Rectum. 2006;49:1223–7.
25. Mirza NN, McCloud JM, Cheetham MJ. Clostridium septicum sepsis and colorectal cancer – a reminder. World J Surg Oncol. 2009;7:73.
26. Chew SS, Lubowski DZ. Clostridium septicum and malignancy. ANZ J Surg. 2001;71:647–9.
27. El-Masry S. Spontaneous gas gangrene associated with occult carcinoma of the colon: a case report and review of literature. Int Surg. 2005;90:245–7.
28. Vaska VL, Faoagali JL. Streptococcus bovis bacteraemia: identification within organism complex and association with endocarditis and colonic malignancy. Pathology. 2009;41:183–6.

29. Phillips RK, Hittinger R, Fry JS, Fielding LP. Malignant large bowel obstruction. Br J Surg. 1985;72:296–302.
30. Lee YM, Law WL, Chu KW, Poon RT. Emergency surgery for obstructing colorectal cancers: a comparison between right-sided and left-sided lesions. J Am Coll Surg. 2001;192:719–25.
31. Sagar PM, MacFie J, Sedman P, May J, Mancey-Jones B, Johnstone D. Intestinal obstruction promotes gut translocation of bacteria. Dis Colon Rectum. 1995;38:640–4.
32. Tsai HL, Hsieh JS, Yu FJ, Wu DC, Chen FM, Huang CJ, et al. Perforated colonic cancer presenting as intra-abdominal abscess. Int J Colorectal Dis. 2007;22:15–9.
33. Heiss MM, Mempel W, Jauch KW, Delanoff C, Mayer G, Mempel M, et al. Beneficial effect of autologous blood transfusion on infectious complications after colorectal cancer surgery. Lancet. 1993;342:1328–33.
34. Eberhardt JM, Kiran RP, Lavery IC. The impact of anastomotic leak and intra-abdominal abscess on cancer-related outcomes after resection for colorectal cancer: a case control study. Dis Colon Rectum. 2009;52:380–6.
35. Nakamura T, Onozato W, Mitomi H, Sato T, Hatate K, Naioto M, et al. Analysis of the risk factors for wound infection after surgical treatment of colorectal cancer: a matched case control study. Hepatogastroenterology. 2009;56:1316–20.
36. Nelson RL, Glenny AM, Song F. Antimicrobial prophylaxis for colorectal surgery. Cochrane Database Syst Rev. 2009;(1): CD001181.
37. Tartter PI, Mohandas K, Azar P, Endres J, Kaplan J, Spivack M. Randomized trial comparing packed red cell blood transfusion with and without leukocyte depletion for gastrointestinal surgery. Am J Surg. 1998;176:462–6.
38. Skanberg J, Lundholm K, Haglind E. Effects of blood transfusion with leucocyte depletion on length of hospital stay, respiratory assistance and survival after curative surgery for colorectal cancer. Acta Oncol. 2007;46:1123–30.
39. Welch S, Spithoff K, Rumble RB, Maroun J, the Gastrointestinal Cancer Disease Site Group. Bevacizumab combined with chemotherapy for patients with advanced colorectal cancer: a systematic review. Ann Oncol. 2010;21:1152–62.
40. Matsumoto T, Takahashi K, Tanaka M, Kumazawa J. Infectious complications of combination anticancer chemotherapy for urogenital cancers. Int Urol Nephrol. 1999;31:7–14.
41. Wolf Jr JS, Bennett CJ, Dmochowski RR, Hollenbeck BK, Pearle MS, Schaeffer AJ, et al. Best practice policy statement on urologic surgery antimicrobial prophylaxis. J Urol. 2008;179:1379–90.
42. Bootsma AM, Laguna Pes MP, Geerlings SE, Goossens A. Antibiotic prophylaxis in urologic procedures: a systematic review. Eur Urol. 2008;54:1270–86.
43. Yamamoto S, Shima H. Controversies in antimicrobial prophylaxis for urologic surgery: more up-to-date evidence is needed. Nat Clin Pract Urol. 2008;5:588–9.
44. Falagas ME, Vergidis PI. Urinary tract infections in patients with urinary diversion. Am J Kidney Dis. 2005;46:1030–7.
45. Suriano F, Gallucci M, Flammia GP, Musco S, Alcini A, Imbalzano G, et al. Bacteriuria in patients with an orthotopic ileal neobladder: urinary tract infection or asymptomatic bacteriuria? BJU Int. 2008;101:1576–9.
46. Wah TM, Irving HC. Infectious complications after percutaneous radiofrequency ablation of renal cell carcinoma in patients with ileal conduit. J Vasc Interv Radiol. 2008;19:1382–5.
47. Carrafiello G, Lagana D, Ianniello A, Dionigi G, Novario R, Recaldini C, et al. Post-radiofrequency ablation syndrome after percutaneous radiofrequency of abdominal tumours: one centre experience and review of published works. Australas Radiol. 2007;51:550–4.
48. Nieder AM, Brausi M, Lamm D, O'Donnell M, Tomita K, Woo H, et al. Management of stage T1 tumors of the bladder: International Consensus Panel. Urology. 2005;66:108–25.
49. Lamm DL, van der Meijden PM, Morales A, Brosman SA, Catalona WJ, Herr HW, et al. Incidence and treatment of complications of bacillus Calmette-Guerin intravesical therapy in superficial bladder cancer. J Urol. 1992;147:596–600.
50. Koya MP, Simon MA, Soloway MS. Complications of intravesical therapy for urothelial cancer of the bladder. J Urol. 2006;175:2004–10.
51. Seelig MH, Oldenburg WA, Klingler PJ, Blute ML, Pairolero PC. Mycotic vascular infections of large arteries with Mycobacterium bovis after intravesical bacillus Calmette-Guerin therapy: case report. J Vasc Surg. 1999;29:377–81.
52. Harding GE, Lawlor DK. Ruptured mycotic abdominal aortic aneurysm secondary to Mycobacterium bovis after intravesical treatment with bacillus Calmette-Guerin. J Vasc Surg. 2007;46:131–4.
53. Mavrogenis AF, Sakellariou VI, Tsiodras S, Papagelopoulos PJ. Late Mycobacterium bovis spondylitis after intravesical BCG therapy. Joint Bone Spine. 2009;76:296–300.
54. Soylu A, Ince AT, Polat H, Yasar N, Ciltas A, Ozkara S, et al. Peritoneal tuberculosis and granulomatous hepatitis secondary to treatment of bladder cancer with Bacillus Calmette-Guerin. Ann Clin Microbiol Antimicrob. 2009;8:12.
55. Alvarez-Mugica M, Gomez JM, Vazquez VB, Monzon AJ, Rodriguez JM, Robles LR. Pancreatic and psoas abscesses as a late complication of intravesical administration of bacillus Calmette-Guerin for bladder cancer: a case report and review of the literature. J Med Case Reports. 2009;3:7323.
56. Sepkowitz KA. Opportunistic infections in patients with and patients without Acquired Immunodeficiency Syndrome. Clin Infect Dis. 2002;34:1098–107.
57. Ganiere V, Christen G, Bally F, Guillou L, Pica A, de Ribaupierre S, Stupp R. Listeria brain abscess, Pneumocystis pneumonia and Kaposi's sarcoma after temozolomide. Nat Clin Pract Oncol. 2006;3:339–43; quiz following 343.
58. Slivka A, Wen PY, Shea WM, Loeffler JS. Pneumocystis carinii pneumonia during steroid taper in patients with primary brain tumors. Am J Med. 1993;94:216–9.
59. Su YB, Sohn S, Krown SE, Livingston PO, Wolchok JD, Quinn C, et al. Selective CD4+ lymphopenia in melanoma patients treated with temozolomide: a toxicity with therapeutic implications. J Clin Oncol. 2004;22:610–6.
60. Choi JD, Powers CJ, Vredenburgh JJ, Friedman AH, Sampson JH. Cryptococcal meningitis in patients with glioma: a report of two cases. J Neurooncol. 2008;89:51–3.
61. Aregawi D, Lopez D, Wick M, Scheld WM, Schiff D. Disseminated strongyloidiasis complicating glioblastoma therapy: a case report. J Neurooncol. 2009;94:439–43.

Chapter 5
Infections in Patients with Hematologic Malignancies Treated with Monoclonal Antineoplastic Therapy

André Goy and Susan O'Brien

Abstract The advent of monoclonal antibody therapy heralded a new era in oncology. In 1997, rituximab became the first monoclonal antibody for the treatment of cancer following its approval for patients with B-cell non-Hodgkin's lymphoma. The potential risks of any pharmacotherapy should be considered alongside the obvious benefits. Recently, concerns have emerged over the possible increase in infectious complications associated with monoclonal antibodies compared with traditional chemotherapy. Due to the nature of the malignancies that they target, most of the monoclonal antibodies currently in use for the treatment of hematologic cancers are directed at specific surface markers on B or T cells. Consequently, the risk of infectious complications with these monoclonal antibodies is of particular concern and a comprehensive review of these complications is presented in this chapter.

Keywords Infections • Rituximab • Alemtuzuma • Daclizuma • CMV • Viral hepatitis

Introduction

The advent of monoclonal antibody therapy heralded a new era in oncology. In 1997, rituximab became the first monoclonal antibody for the treatment of cancer following its approval for patients with B-cell non-Hodgkin's lymphoma (NHL). The majority of monoclonal antibodies used in oncology bind to cell surface receptors present on malignant cells. It was hoped that the development of monoclonal antibodies would result in a more favorable tolerability profile than that offered by systemic cytotoxic chemotherapies by providing a more targeted therapy. Since rituximab, several monoclonal antibodies have demonstrated efficacy as well as relatively good tolerability profiles in a range of solid and hematologic tumor types. Hence, eight other monoclonal antibody therapies have subsequently received approval for the treatment of various cancers (four in hematologic malignancies) and over 100 are currently in clinical development [1].

The potential risks of any pharmacotherapy should be considered alongside the obvious benefits. Recently, concerns have emerged over the possible increase in infectious complications associated with monoclonal antibodies compared with traditional chemotherapy [2–4]. Due to the nature of the malignancies that they target, most of the monoclonal antibodies currently in use for the treatment of hematologic cancers are directed at specific surface markers on B or T cells [5]. Consequently, the risk of infectious complications with these monoclonal antibodies is of particular concern.

Interaction of Monoclonal Antibodies with the Immune System

Common targets for monoclonal antibodies in hematologic malignancies include CD20, CD33, CD52, and the α-chain of the interleukin-2 receptor (IL-2Rα), also known as the CD25 antigen. CD52 is a panlymphocytic cell surface antigen expressed on normal and malignant B- and T-lymphocytes, natural killer cells, but also macrophages and monocytes with relatively high density [5]. CD20 and IL-2R expressions are more limited, with CD20 expressed mainly on pre-B and mature B lymphocytes with weak expression on a subset of T cells and IL-2R expressed only on activated lymphocytes (Fig. 5.1) [5–8]. The CD33 antigen is expressed on most hematopoietic stem cells, on mature and immature myeloid cells, and on erythroid, megakaryocytic, and multipotent progenitors, but not on lymphoid cells [9, 10]. Monoclonal antibodies targeting these receptors can lead to the depletion of normal as well as malignant cells [11, 12]. As outlined in Fig. 5.1, B and T cells are an integral part of the immune system and are essential for the activation of humoral and cell-mediated immunity.

A. Goy (✉)
Hematology/Oncology, Internal Medicine, Hackensack University Medical Center, 20 Prospect Avenue, Suite 400, Hackensack, NJ 07601, USA
e-mail: agoy@humed.com

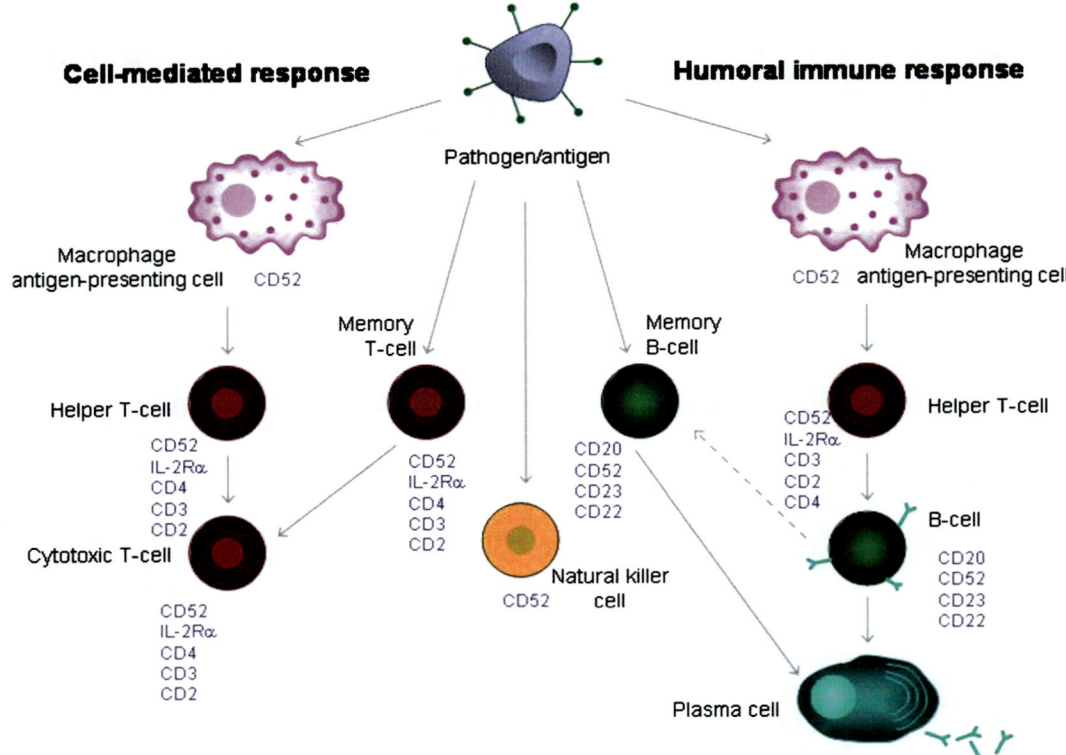

Fig. 5.1 Schematic overview of immune response and cell surface receptor targets for monoclonal antibody therapy

One monoclonal antibody, infliximab, does not bind to a cell surface receptor; rather it binds with high affinity to the soluble and transmembrane forms of tumor necrosis factor (TNF)-α. TNF-α plays an important role in immunity by activating a number of immune cells and inducing the local inflammatory response. Infliximab inhibits TNF-α binding to the cellular receptors [13], and a single dose results in a sharp and substantial decline in the levels of C-reactive protein and IL-6 [14].

Treatment of patients with a monoclonal antibody directed against CD20, CD33, CD52, IL-2Rα, or TNF-α, therefore, may compromise the immune system and increase the risk of opportunistic and nonopportunistic infections, such as pneumonia and reactivation of hepatitis B virus (HBV) [11, 15–17]. Immunosuppression resulting from the depletion of the body's reserve of B and T cells through monoclonal antibody therapy can be profound and prolonged [18]. Moreover, patients with hematologic malignancies are already at risk of infection as a result of immune dysfunction inherent in the underlying disease process and other risk factors such as prior cytotoxic chemotherapy. In addition, it is important to note that polymorphisms of leukocyte IgG receptors (FcγR) may also predispose patients to a higher risk of infection, although precise relationships are unclear [19]. For example, the FcγRIIa-R/R131 genotype has been linked to greater susceptibility to *Streptococcus pneumoniae* [20, 21], while other studies have reported no such association [22], and the FcγRIIa-R/R131–FcγRIIIb-NA2/NA2 genotype combination has been shown to be associated with high frequencies of meningococcal disease [23].

The aim of this chapter is to evaluate the incidence of infectious complications associated with the monoclonal antibodies most commonly used for the treatment of hematologic malignancies. A summary of the current evidence for the risk of infectious complications associated with monoclonal antibodies in hematologic malignancies is given in Table 5.1.

Anti-CD20 Antibodies

Rituximab

Rituximab was the first treatment of its kind to be approved for a hematologic malignancy and is perhaps the most comprehensively studied monoclonal antibody. The combination of rituximab with chemotherapy regimens has revolutionized the treatment of patients with indolent and aggressive B-cell NHL, providing the first improvement in overall survival vs. chemotherapy alone in 30 years [3, 24–30]. As a result, rituximab in combination with chemotherapy has become the

Table 5.1 Infections and associated complications reported during monoclonal antibody therapy for hematological malignancies

Treatment	Target	Infection complications	Overall infection rate
Rituximab	CD20	Bacterial infections, e.g., sepsis	≈30%
		Fungal infections, e.g., *Pneumocystis*	
		Viral infections, e.g., CMV/HBV/HCV/TB reactivation, VZV and PML	
Tositumumab	CD20	Bacterial infections, e.g., sepsis, pneumonia	13–45%
		Viral infections, e.g., herpes zoster, herpes simplex II	
Ibritumomab tiuxetan	CD20	Bacterial infections, e.g., sepsis, pneumonia	≈29%
		Viral infections	
Alemtuzumab	CD52	Bacterial infections	>50%
		Fungal infections	
		Viral infections, e.g., CMV infection/reactivation	
Gemtuzumab ozogamicin	CD33	Bacterial infections	28–36% (grade 3/4)
		Fungal infections, e.g., pulmonary aspergillosis	
Lumiliximab	CD23	Bacterial infections, e.g., pneumonia	15%
		Viral infections, e.g., parainfluenza virus	
Inotuzumab ozogamicin	CD22	Unknown	More data needed
Zanolimumab	CD4	Bacterial infections	49%; more data needed
		Fungal infections	
		Viral infections	
Muromonab-CD3	CD3	Bacterial infections	21–50%
Siplizumab	CD2	Viral infections, e.g., EBV	More data needed
Denileukin diftitox	IL-2R	Bacterial infections; more data needed	≈30%
Daclizumab	IL-2Rα	Bacterial infections	95%
		Fungal infections	
		Viral infections, e.g., CMV reactivation, respiratory viral infections, EBV	
Basiliximab	IL-2Rα	Bacterial infections	>75%
		Invasive fungal infections	
		Viral infections, e.g., CMV reactivation	
Tocilizumab	IL-6	Bacterial infections, e.g., pneumonia	More data needed
		Viral infections, e.g., herpes zoster	
Infliximab	TNFα	Bacterial infections, e.g., TB, *Listeria*	≈80%
		Invasive fungal infections, e.g., endemic mycoses, *Candida*	

CMV cytomegalovirus; *EBV* Epstein–Barr virus; *HBV* hepatitis B virus; *HCV* hepatitis C virus; *VZV* varicella zoster virus; *PML* progressive multifocal leukoencephalopathy; *TB* tuberculous

new standard of care in aggressive CD20-positive B-cell NHL [31]. Rituximab has recently been shown to improve progression-free survival in patients with previously untreated or relapsed chronic lymphocytic leukemia (CLL) [32, 33] and has demonstrated efficacy in patients with HIV1-associated B-cell NHL [34] and posttransplant lymphoproliferative disorder [35].

Rituximab binds to the CD20 antigen on B lymphocytes leading to cell lysis, which may be mediated by complement-dependent cytolysis (CDC), antibody-dependent cell-mediated cytotoxicity (ADCC), and/or direct induction of apoptosis [36, 37]. It has also been suggested that killing of malignant B cells by rituximab may result in a "vaccinal" effect, i.e., priming of lymphoma antigen-specific T-cell responses, leading to antilymphoma immunity that remains long after the initial antibody-induced cytotoxicity [38, 39]. The relative importance of each of these mechanisms to the therapeutic effects of rituximab needs further clarification; however, there is convincing evidence that direct induction of apoptosis by rituximab may occur before other proposed mechanisms (e.g., ADCC) are triggered [40]. ADCC is considered to be of particular interest as response to rituximab appears to depend on patients' FcγR genotype [41–43]. The observation that rituximab-induced B-cell depletion still occurs in mice that lack certain complement factors indicates that the exact role of CDC remains to be determined [44].

Rituximab-induced B-cell depletion is rapid and sustained, with peripheral B-cell depletion occurring 24–48 h after the first administration of rituximab in patients with relapsed low-grade B-cell NHL and persisting for 6–9 months after the completion of therapy [18]. Normalization of B cell counts appears to result from repopulation with naïve B cells, which exhibit a deficiency in expression of CD27, a memory B cell surface marker [45]. In addition to inducing B-cell depletion, rituximab treatment is associated with significantly reduced circulating immunoglobulin levels (IgM and IgG), persisting for 5–11 months after rituximab administration and falling below the normal range in 14% of patients [18]. More research examining the effects of rituximab on the immune system is needed, although early evidence has indicated that T cells are minimally affected and protective titers against immunized pathogens generally appear to be preserved [46].

The most common side effects of rituximab treatment typically occur during the first infusion and can include fever, chills, nausea, itching, cough, throat swelling, hypotension, and transient bronchospasm [15]. Occurrence of these reactions depends on the rate of rituximab infusion, but they usually develop within 30–120 min from the start of infusion [36, 47]. Tumor lysis syndrome (TLS) is a rare but potentially fatal adverse event observed within 12–24 h of the first infusion of rituximab in patients with a high number of circulating tumor cells (>25,000/mm^3) or high tumor load; TLS prophylaxis is recommended in high-risk patients [15, 36].

Prolonged or delayed secondary hypogammaglobulinemia can arise as a result of rituximab retreatment, prolonged scheduling (especially in the maintenance setting in indolent B-cell NHL), or after high-dose therapy following stem cell transplantation [48–51]. Rituximab has also been associated with an impaired secondary humoral response to recall antigens [52] and an altered B-cell repertoire during immunologic reconstitution [53]. In a study of patients with B-cell NHL who received rituximab as an adjuvant to autologous SCT, recovery of memory B cells was delayed and exhibited abnormal cell marker expression and function, indicating that naive B cells may fail to differentiate into plasma cells [53]. Expansion of functionally immature B cells and decreased memory B cells may contribute to an immunodeficient state in patients recovering from rituximab-mediated B-cell depletion, particularly following repeated treatment [54]. Evidence suggests that this immunodeficiency may lead to infectious complications associated with rituximab.

Rituximab is increasingly being used for long-term maintenance therapy with delayed relapse and increased progression-free survival. A rational maintenance schedule has been proposed as single infusions of rituximab 375 mg/m^2 given every 3–4 months to maintain serum levels above the threshold for response of 25 μg/mL [55], the 3-month schedule is being used in ongoing clinical studies such as the Eastern Cooperative Oncology Group (ECOG) 4402 (RESORT) study [39]. Other rituximab schedules for maintenance therapy have been shown to provide significant benefit in patients with lymphoma, including 4 weekly infusions every 6 months and single infusions every 2–3 months [56]. Such long-term maintenance treatment raises added concerns of prolonged exposure and B-cell depletion in increasing the risk of infectious adverse events.

Rituximab-Associated Infection

Randomized controlled trials performed to date have provided conflicting evidence on the incidence of infection in patients treated with rituximab plus chemotherapy vs. chemotherapy alone. A pooled analysis of data from 356 rituximab-treated patients indicated an overall incidence of infection of approximately 30%, with bacterial infection accounting for 19% of cases and viral infection accounting for 10% [15]. In an interim analysis of an open-label, Phase II trial investigating 6 cycles of dose-dense rituximab 12×375 mg/m^2 plus CHOP-14 (R-CHOP-14) in elderly patients with diffuse large B-cell lymphoma (DLBCL), 7 of the first 20 patients (35%) developed grade 3/4 infections and there were seven cases of interstitial pneumonia, some of which were related to CMV reactivation [57]. Compare this with another randomized trial of 6 vs. 8 cycles of "standard" R-CHOP-14 in elderly patients where the rate of grade 3/4 infection was 28 and 35%, respectively, and it appears that the rate of infection may be increased by using dose-dense rituximab. By contrast, lower rates of grade 3/4 neutropenia (17.5%) and grade 3/4 infections (16%) were observed in a phase II, open-label study of R-CHOP administered every 14 days for the treatment of patients with DLBCL who were younger than 70 years [58]. Therefore, the risk of infection appears to be greater in elderly patients than their younger counterparts.

Randomized controlled Phase III trials performed in patients with a variety of indolent and aggressive lymphomas have failed to demonstrate a significant increase in the infection rate in patients treated with rituximab-based regimens (Table 5.2). Similar conclusions were drawn from a meta-analysis of four randomized controlled trials [30] and a retrospective analysis of infection rates in 160 patients with CLL following fludarabine–cyclophosphamide treatment with or without rituximab [59]. Interestingly, adding rituximab to CHOP therapy has generated confounding evidence for myelosuppression, with some Phase III trials reporting no differences between the groups [3, 29, 60, 61] and others reporting a significantly increased risk of granulocytopenia in the rituximab arms [26, 62].

Studies investigating the impact of long-term maintenance therapy with rituximab on risk of infection have also yielded inconsistent findings. In a recent meta-analysis of five randomized controlled maintenance trials, the risk of both infection and neutropenia was significantly increased during rituximab maintenance therapy in patients with lymphoma [63]. Updated data from a European Organization for the Research and Treatment of Cancer (EORTC) Intergroup trial of rituximab in remission induction and maintenance, with a median follow-up of 6 years, also described how rituximab maintenance was associated with a significant increase in grade 3/4 infections: 9.7 vs. 2.4% ($p=0.01$). Seven of 167

Table 5.2 Infection rates in published phase III randomized controlled trials comparing treatment with vs. without rituximab

Treatment	Type of malignancy	Infection-related death rate (%)	Overall grade 3/4 infection rate (%)	Reference
Rituximab+CHOP ($n=202$)	DLBCL	NR	12	Coiffier et al. [31];
CHOP ($n=197$)		NR	20	Feugier et al. [3]
Rituximab+CHOP-like chemotherapy ($n=404$)	DLBCL	0.74	7	Pfreundschuh
CHOP-like chemotherapy ($n=403$)		0.25	8	et al. [29]
Rituximab+CHOP ($n=267$)	DLBCL	3.0	17	Habermann
CHOP ($n=279$)		2.5	16	et al. [61]
Rituximab+CHOP-14 ($n=578$)	Aggressive B-cell NHL	NR	31	Pfreundschuh
CHOP-14 ($n=570$)		NR	30	et al. [28]
Rituximab+CHOP ($n=99$)	HIV1-associated NHL	15	NR	Kaplan et al. [2].
CHOP ($n=50$)		2	NR	
Rituximab+CVP ($n=162$)	FL	NR	NR	Marcus et al. [197]
CVP ($n=159$)		NR	NR	
Rituximab+CHOP ($n=223$)	FL	1.8	5	Hiddemann
CHOP ($n=205$)		2.0	7	et al. [26]
Rituximab+MCP ($n=105$)	FL	NR	7	Herold et al. [25]
MCP ($n=96$)		NR	8	
Rituximab+CHVP-IFN ($n=175$)	FL	NR	3.4	Salles et al. [198]
CHVP-IFN ($n=183$)		NR	1.1	
Rituximab+CHOP ($n=234$)	FL	0.4	NR	van Oers et al. [60]
CHOP ($n=231$)		0.4	NR	
Rituximab+FCM ($n=66$)	FL and MCL	NR	1.4	Forstpointner
FCM ($n=62$)		NR	1.8	et al. [24]
Rituximab+CHOP ($n=62$)	MCL	6	5	Lenz et al. [62]
CHOP ($n=60$)		3	6	

CHVP-IFN cyclophosphamide, doxorubicin, etoposide, prednisolone, interferon-α2a; *CHOP* cyclophosphamide, doxorubicin, vincristine, prednisone, given in a 21-day cycle; *CHOP-14* CHOP given in a 14-day cycle; *CVP* cyclophosphamide, vincristine, prednisone; *DLBCL* diffuse large B-cell lymphoma; *FCM* fluradabine, cyclophosphamide, mitoxantrone; *FL* follicular lymphoma; *MCL* mantle cell lymphoma; *MCP* mitoxantrone, chlorambucil, prednisolone; *NHL* non-Hodgkin's lymphoma; *NR* not reported

patients discontinued rituximab maintenance because of toxicity, which was mostly recurrent infection [64]. However, other results from long-term rituximab therapy have contradicted these findings. No increased risk of major infection was observed over 5 years in patients with relapsed follicular lymphoma in a prospective single-arm study of autologous stem cell transplant combined with in vivo rituximab graft purging and posttransplant rituximab maintenance [49] and only mild infectious toxicity was seen in patients with relapsed B-CLL treated for 1–3.5 years [65].

In patients with HIV1-associated conditions, the addition of rituximab to standard treatment regimens has been associated with increased neutropenia and a higher rate of infectious complications compared with standard therapy alone, particularly in patients with low CD4 cell counts (<50 cells/μL). In a Phase III study comparing cyclophosphamide, doxorubicin, vincristine, and prednisone (CHOP) with or without rituximab, Kaplan and colleagues [2] observed a trend towards greater risk of neutropenia (62 vs. 48%), febrile neutropenia (31 vs. 24%), and treatment-related infectious diseases (13 vs. 2%) in patients with HIV1-associated lymphoma receiving R-CHOP vs. those receiving CHOP. Treatment-related infection led to the death of 8 of the 22 patients (36%) in the R-CHOP group who had a CD4 count of <50 cells/μL compared with 5 of the 77 patients (6%) with CD4 counts of ≥50 cells/μL. HIV1-related opportunistic infections in the R-CHOP group included *Candida albicans* ($n=1$), *Pneumocystis carinii* pneumonia (PCP; $n=3$), cytomegalovirus (CMV; $n=2$), esophageal candidiasis ($n=1$), and *Mycobacterium avium* ($n=1$); there were no opportunistic infections in the CHOP group. Spina and colleagues conducted a pooled analysis of three studies in 74 patients with HIV1-associated B-cell NHL, three-quarters of whom were receiving concurrent highly active antiretroviral therapy [66]. Adding rituximab to cytotoxic therapy resulted in grade 3/4 neutropenia in 78% of patients and a high rate of infectious complications (31%) including CMV retinitis ($n=3$), cryptosporidiosis ($n=3$), pulmonary tuberculous ($n=2$), PCP ($n=1$), and salmonellosis ($n=1$).

Certain infectious complications should be particularly borne in mind when initiating rituximab therapy. These include reactivation of HBV and hepatitis C virus (HCV), CMV infection, and progressive multifocal leukoencephalopathy (PML). Routine serologic screening, particularly for HBV and CMV, should be conducted prior to initiation of rituximab therapy and patients be carefully monitored for development of viral infections throughout treatment [67]. Prophylaxis with lamuvidine to prevent HBV reactivation is recommended throughout treatment and for at least 6 months after completion of therapy as late reactivations have occurred [68]. Prophylaxis for other viral infections is generally not recommended due to the toxicity associated with antiviral agents. Standard of care for the treatment of viral infections includes lamuvidine for HBV reactivation and ganciclovir for CMV.

Hepatitis B and C

Reactivation of HBV is a well-recognized complication of chemotherapy in inactive carriers, i.e., those testing positive for the HBV surface antigen (HBsAg), as well as in patients with chronic HBV infection. Reactivation occurs spontaneously in 14–50% of these individuals, and the rate could be even higher in patients with hematologic malignancies. HBV reactivation is therefore a concern in patients treated with immunosuppressant therapy such as rituximab, particularly in regions where HBV is endemic. In a review of 64 cases of viral infection after rituximab treatment for patients with lymphoma, HBV infection was the most commonly observed infection, occurring in 25 patients (39%), 13 of whom died as a result of hepatic failure [17] (Fig. 5.2). Among these 25 infected individuals, 13 had HBV reactivation (HBsAg positive) and eight had developed primary HBV infection (HBsAg-negative); the HBsAg status prior to rituximab therapy was unknown in the remaining four patients. More recently, Yeo and colleagues analyzed the rate of HBV reactivation among 104 patients with CD20-positive DLBCL who underwent chemotherapy with or without rituximab [69]. Among 46 patients who were HBsAg-negative and HBV-positive, 25 were treated with CHOP and the remainder with R-CHOP. HBV reactivation occurred in five R-CHOP-treated patients, but in none of those treated with CHOP alone. Notably, reactivation occurred up to 170 days following the last dose of R-CHOP, in line with previous reports of late HBV reactivation [68], suggesting that administration of antiviral therapy should continue for at least 6 months after completion of chemotherapy. Prophylactic lamivudine has been shown to reduce the risk of HBV reactivation in HBV carriers receiving rituximab-containing regimens for lymphoma [70–72]. Once HBV is reactivated, lamivudine treatment is much less effective – over 50% of

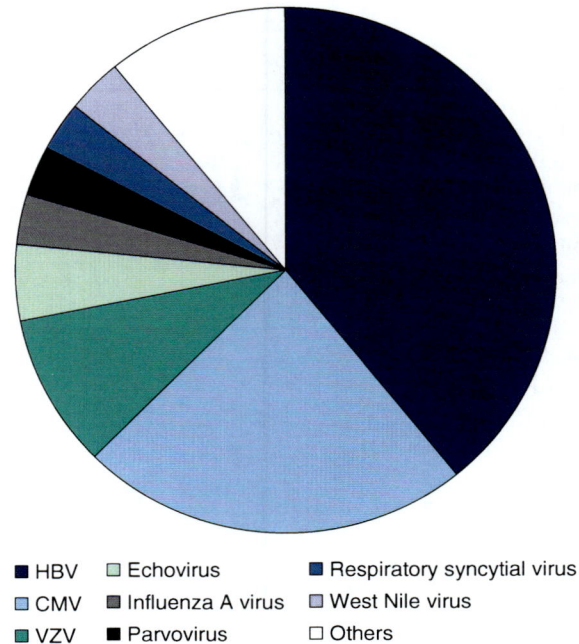

Fig. 5.2 Rituximab-related viral infections in patients with lymphoma ($n=64$) [17]. *HBV* hepatitis B virus; *CMV* cytomegalovirus; *VZV* varicella zoster virus

such patients died in one report – illustrating the importance of preemptive treatment [17].

The incidence of HCV reactivation is less well defined. Most HCV-infected individuals experience chronic infection that may potentially lead to cirrhosis and hepatocellular carcinoma. HCV infection is now known to be associated with B-cell lymphoproliferative disorders, including mixed cryoglobulinemia, B-cell NHL, marginal zone lymphoma (splenic, nodal and extranodal), small lymphocytic lymphoma/CLL, lymphoplasmacytic lymphoma, and DLBCL [73, 74]. The direct role of HCV infection in the genesis of these B-cell lymphoproliferative disorders remains unclear, but epidemiologic and molecular observations have recently suggested that HCV may be the causative agent in some cases of B-cell NHL [75]. Reactivation or worsening of HCV in patients receiving chemotherapy or immunochemotherapy has also been reported [76], although this appears to be much less common than HBV reactivation. Nonetheless, careful monitoring of these patients, which can reveal increased HCV RNA load during or after chemotherapy, is recommended [77].

Cytomegalovirus

CMV is a major cause of morbidity and mortality in immunocompromised individuals [78, 79]. CMV infection has been less widely reported than HBV infection in rituximab-treated patients; however, Aksoy and colleagues [17] did identify 15 cases of this challenging infection in their literature review, including one patient who had received rituximab alone to treat lymphoma 10 years after a kidney transplant and would therefore be immunosuppressed [80]. In a study of 46 patients with relapsed indolent or high-risk aggressive B-cell NHL, of whom 17 received rituximab before autologous hematopoietic stem cell transplantation (HSCT), Lee and colleagues [81] reported CMV infection in three rituximab-treated patients, two of whom developed CMV disease. The risk of developing CMV infection after autologous HSCT was higher in rituximab-treated patients (17.6 vs. 0%; $p = 0.045$, two-sided Fisher's exact test). Nevertheless, all patients with CMV disease recovered after ganciclovir and CMV-specific immunoglobulin therapy.

Progressive Multifocal Leukoencephalopathy

PML — a rare and devastating neurologic disease involving areas of demyelination in the central nervous system — is classically associated with profound immunosuppression. PML is caused by reactivation of the latent JC virus (JCV) that is present in up to 80% of adults, leading to the death of myelin-producing oligodendrocytes. A state of immunodeficiency is the main risk factor for JCV reactivation and development of PML, with the most common causes comprising HIV infection, hematologic malignancy, and post-transplant immunosuppressive therapy [82]. There is no specific antiviral treatment currently available for PML; successful treatment of PML with cidofovir appears to be limited to isolated cases [83–86]. If the accompanying underlying immune deficit can be reversed, PML mortality is in excess of 95% [87].

Isolated cases of PML have been reported among patients undergoing rituximab treatment after autologous peripheral blood stem cell transplantation. PML has recently been reported in patients treated with rituximab-based chemoimmunotherapy for lymphomas as well as for rheumatologic diseases [88]. The first two cases of PML were reported by Goldberg and colleagues [78] in patients with lymphoma who had undergone high-dose therapy followed by stem cell transplantation. More cases have since been reported, including a series of 52 cases of PML in patients with lymphoma, most of whom had been treated with cytotoxic chemotherapy plus rituximab [89].

Hence, while the risk of PML associated with rituximab remains uncertain because of confounding factors, particularly the complicated immunosuppressive regimens used in hematological cancers and prior stem cell transplantation, careful prescribing and continued vigilance are warranted with this agent [88].

Other Infections

Other infections anecdotally associated with rituximab administration include varicella zoster virus [90, 91], PCP [92–94], adenovirus [95], parvovirus B19, [96, 97] and bronchiolitis obliterans with organizing pneumonia (BOOP) [98, 99]. These occur at greatly reduced frequency compared with the infections discussed above. Among 64 cases of severe viral infection, Aksoy and colleagues reported six cases of varicella zoster virus infection compared with 25 cases of HBV. Isolated cases of enteroviral [100, 101] and echoviral infections [102, 103] have also been observed in patients undergoing treatment with rituximab.

Late Neutropenia

Late-onset neutropenia (LON) has been reported with rituximab-containing chemotherapy in patients with hematological cancers such as follicular lymphoma and NHL, particularly in those receiving autologous HSCT and high-dose regimens [104–106]. LON is generally an infrequent adverse effect of standard-dose chemotherapy, although it may be more common following high-dose chemotherapy and stem cell transplantation [105]. Rituximab-induced LON appears to be associated with a lack of granulopoiesis in the bone marrow that occurs when B-cell depletion in peripheral blood is maximal [107]. Although the exact mechanism of rituximab-induced LON is unclear, it has been proposed that it may be related to excessive B-cell recovery stimulated by increased serum levels of the cytokine BAFF [107], and that disruptions in stromal-derived factor-1 levels during rapid B-cell expansion reduce neutrophil migration from the bone marrow [108]. LON has also been attributed to rituximab-induced reactivation of parvovirus B19 infection [109]. This adverse effect has been reported to occur at least 4 weeks after the last dose of treatment, but can be resolved with granulocyte colony-stimulating factor [106] or intravenous immunoglobulin.

Other Approved Indications

Rituximab is also approved for the treatment of moderate-to-severe rheumatoid arthritis (RA) as B cells are believed to act at multiple sites during the pathogenesis of this disease. Similar to what is seen in B-cell NHL patients, significant and sustained peripheral B-cell depletion occurs in patients with RA, generally lasting for at least 6 months with subsequent gradual recovery. In a meta-analysis of data from three randomized clinical trials, a greater incidence of serious infections was observed with rituximab compared with placebo (2.3 vs. 1.5%), although the difference was not statistically significant [110]. The serious infections reported with rituximab comprised bronchopneumonia (one fatality), septic arthritis, pyelonephritis, gastroenteritis, epiglottitis, cellulitis, and acute hepatitis B.

Anti-CD20 Radioimmunoconjugates

Radioimmunoconjugates combine the targeted action of an antibody with the cytotoxic activity of a radioisotope, the latter conferring particular clinical benefit in radiosensitive hematologic cancers such as B-cell NHL [37]. Two radioimmunoconjugates are currently approved for the treatment of patients with CD20 antigen-expressing relapsed or refractory, low-grade or follicular NHL, including patients with rituximab-refractory disease: ^{131}I-tositumomab [111] and ibritumomab tiuxetan [112]. These agents are associated with reversible, radiation-related myelosuppression that has a late-onset and sometimes results in severe cytopenia, particularly neutropenia. With both radioimmunoconjugates, B-cell counts fall soon after treatment (median time to nadir of 4–7 weeks), with recovery to normal range occurring after approximately 6 months [113, 114]. There are no apparent clinical consequences of the transient B-cell depletion and no significant reductions in T cells or serum immunoglobulin levels [113, 114].

Tositumomab

Tositumomab is a murine antibody that results in very low rates of complete response when administered as monotherapy. In order to improve its efficacy, tositumomab has been conjugated with iodine-131 (^{131}I) to give ^{131}I-tositumomab.

Although grade 3/4 neutropenia has been reported to occur in almost two thirds of patients with B-cell NHL treated with ^{131}I-tositumomab, resultant infections are generally mild [111]. Infection rates of 13–45% have been observed in studies of patients with relapsed or refractory B-cell NHL [115–117]. Serious infections are uncommon, with an overall rate of 4.3% recorded in the ^{131}I-tositumomab safety database [118]. Indeed, grade 3/4 infections were observed in only 2% of 89 patients with follicular B-cell NHL treated with ^{131}I-tositumomab after initial therapy with CHOP [119]. In previously untreated patients with advanced follicular lymphoma, grade 3/4 hematologic toxicities were reported in 45% of these patients, with grade 4 neutropenia in 5% of patients and no infection-related hospitalizations [113].

Ibritumomab Tiuxetan

Ibritumomab tiuxetan is also a murine antibody, which, in its therapeutic form, is conjugated with yttrium-90 (^{90}Y). Treatment with ibritumomab tiuxetan requires two IV infusions of low-dose rituximab (250 mg/m^2) to be given before administration of ^{90}Y-ibritumomab tiuxetan on Day 1 and Day 7, 8, or 9 of the treatment schedule in order to deplete circulating B cells and improve biodistribution of the radioisotope and preferential delivery to tumor sites.

Available evidence suggests that ^{90}Y-ibritumomab tiuxetan may be associated with a similar rate of infection to rituximab. In an analysis of five clinical studies in which 349 patients with relapsed low-grade B-cell NHL were treated with ^{90}Y-ibritumomab tiuxetan, infection was reported in 29% of patients, including grade 3/4 infections in 5% [120]. Hospitalization as a result of infection was necessary in 7% of patients due to febrile neutropenia (2%), urinary tract infections (1%), sepsis (1%), pneumonia (1%), cellulitis or abscess (1%), and gastroenteritis or diarrhea (<1%). In a randomized study in 414 patients that compared consolidation with ^{90}Y-ibritumomab tiuxetan vs. no further treatment after first-line therapy, grade 3/4 infections were observed in 7.9% of patients in the consolidation arm, 7.4% of whom required hospitalization [121].

Second-Generation Anti-CD20 Antibodies

A number of second-generation anti-CD20 monoclonal antibodies are currently in development for the treatment of hematologic malignancies subdivided into those with engineered Fc portions and those with engineered Fab regions (Table 5.3). Research focuses on either making antibodies with a greater degree of humanization, more efficient binding, or antibodies that can target other CD20 epitopes. This may translate into improving infusion-related adverse effects, improving efficacy, overcoming rituximab resistance, and exploring the effects of combining anti-CD20 antibodies. Ofatumumab (HuMaxCD20) is in the most advanced stage of clinical development with phase III trials ongoing in several hematologic malignancies.

Anti-CD52 Antibodies

Alemtuzumab

Alemtuzumab is a humanized monoclonal antibody currently approved for the treatment of B-cell CLL [122]. Cellular immune reconstitution is significantly affected by

Table 5.3 Anti-CD20 monoclonal antibodies in development [37, 39]

Therapy	Stage of development	Details
Fc-engineered anti-CD20 monoclonal antibodies		
AME-133v	Phase I/II: follicular relapsed/refractory B-cell NHL	• Novel engineered anti-CD20 antibody with increased affinity to the FcγRIIIa (CD16) vs. rituximab • Tenfold increase in cytotoxicity vs. rituximab in preclinical studies
PRO131921 (rhuMAb v114)	Phase I/II: indolent B-cell NHL relapsed/refractory to rituximab; relapsed/refractory CLL Phase II: FL relapsed/refractory to rituximab	• Fc-engineered humanized anti-CD20 monoclonal antibody • 30-fold greater binding to low-affinity variant of FcγRIIIa vs. rituximab • ↑ADCC (two to tenfold in vitro) and ↑CDC
GA-101	Phase I/II: CD20+ malignancies (including DLBCL, CLL, B-cell NHL)	• Third generation, glycol-engineered type II humanized IgG1 anti-CD20 monoclonal antibody and a modified elbow hinge • 50-fold higher binding affinity to FcγRIIIa vs. rituximab • Engineered to ↑ADCC (10–100-fold in vitro), ↓CDC, and strongly induce apoptosis vs. rituximab
Fab-engineered anti-CD20 monoclonal antibodies		
Ofatumumab (HuMaxCD20)	Phase III: relapsed and untreated CLL; FL; rituximab-refractory FL Phase II: relapsed/progressive DLBCL	• Fully human IgG1$_K$ monoclonal antibody targeting a novel epitope of CD20 • Activity in cells with low CD20 expression (CLL) • Slower rate of disassociation from antigen and therefore higher potency for CDC vs. rituximab
Veltuzumab (IMMU-106/hA20)	Phase I/II: untreated or relapsed B-cell NHL and CLL	• Humanized anti-CD20 monoclonal antibody with CDRs of murine origin and 90% of human framework regions identical to epratuzumab (anti-CD22 IgG1 antibody) • Induces apoptosis of B cells and mediates ADCC and CDC
Ocrelizumab (PRO70769)	Phase II: B-cell NHL	• Fully humanized IgG1 anti-CD20 monoclonal antibody • ↑ADCC vs. rituximab

CDR complementarity-determining regions; *CLL* chronic lymphocytic lymphoma; *DLBCL* diffuse large B-cell lymphoma; *FL* follicular lymphoma; *NHL* non-Hodgkin's lymphoma

alemtuzumab treatment, with prolonged depletion of major blood lymphocyte subsets (including NK, T-, and B-cells), which may be sustained for over 9 months after the last treatment dose [123]. While it is effective for the treatment of CLL [4], alemtuzumab has been shown to be associated with diverse infectious complications [11]. Infections are also reported when alemtuzumab is used off-label for the treatment of acute rejection in organ transplant patients [124].

Alemtuzumab-Associated Infection

To date, two randomized controlled trials have investigated the efficacy and safety of alemtuzumab in patients with CLL [125, 126]. As with rituximab, alemtuzumab treatment appears to be associated with CMV reactivation. Both randomized trials reported a higher rate of CMV reactivation in patients treated with alemtuzumab compared with patients in the other arm of the trial (Table 5.4). In the trial comparing alemtuzumab and chlorambucil as first-line treatment for CLL [125], asymptomatic CMV (confirmed by polymerase chain reaction [PCR] testing) was confirmed in 52% of alemtuzumab-treated patients and 7.5% of those treated with chlorambucil, with symptomatic CMV reactivation occurring in 16 and 0% of patients, respectively. Symptomatic infections and asymptomatic CMV PCR positivity were managed successfully with standard therapies. In a consolidation study by the German CLL Study Group in which patients who had responded to treatment with fludarabine alone or in combination with cyclophosphamide subsequently received a standard dose of alemtuzumab or observation, alemtuzumab was associated with a higher rate of infectious complications [126]. Indeed, the trial was closed early after 7 of 11 patients in the active-treatment group discontinued treatment as a result of serious infections. These included one life-threatening pulmonary aspergillosis infection, three cases of CMV reactivation, two cases of CMV pneumonia, one herpes zoster infection, and one reactivation of pulmonary tuberculous. Only two episodes of infection were observed in the control group.

CMV reactivation rates in Phase II studies of single-agent alemtuzumab in patients with pretreated CLL have varied from 1 to 22% [122, 127–132]. In these studies, grade 3/4 infections included disseminated viral infection, systemic *Candida* spp. infection, mycobacterial reactivation, invasive fungal infection, *Listeria* meningitis, and PCP, the latter occurring primarily in patients not receiving antiviral prophylaxis. Alemtuzumab has also been used in combination

Table 5.4 Alemtuzumab infections in phase III clinical trials in patients with CLL

Setting	Hillmen et al. [125]		Wendtner et al. [126]	
	First-line CLL		CLL in first remission	
Treatment	Alemtuzumab	Chlorambucil	Alemtuzumab (30 mg IV TIW for 12 weeks)	Observation
No. of patients	149	148	11	10
Grade 3/4 neutropenia, %	41	25	64	0
Viral infection	CMV (symptomatic 16%; asymptomatic 52%)	CMV (asymptomatic 7.5%)	Bronchitis (9%), CMV reactivation (27%), CMV infection (18%), herpes zoster (9%), gastroenteritis (9%), HHV/HSV-6 (9%), sinusitis (9%)	Herpes zoster (10%), sinusitis (10%)
Bacterial infection	Bacteremia (3%), sepsis (1%), bronchopneumonia (0.7%), tuberculous (0.7%)	*Listeria monocytogenes* (0.7%), pneumonia (0.7%)	Tuberculous (9%)	–
Other infections	*Candida albicans* (0.7%)	NR	Aspergillosis (9%)	–

CLL B-cell chronic lymphocytic leukemia; *CMV* cytomegalovirus; *HHS* human herpes virus; *HSV* herpes simplex virus; *NR* not reported

with rituximab in patients with CLL. In a pilot study, Nabhan and colleagues [133] reported no treatment-related mortality and no CMV reactivation in 12 patients treated with escalating doses of alemtuzumab. Others, however, have reported serious toxicity with this combination [103, 134]. Faderl and colleagues [103] reported that 52% of patients ($n=25$) experienced one or more infection, including pneumonia ($n=5$) and sinusitis ($n=3$), while seven patients in the Minnie Pearl study experienced opportunistic infection, including five patients with CMV, one of whom died [134].

Alemtuzumab has been shown to have limited efficacy and considerable toxicity in NHL, as demonstrated by the results of a multicenter Phase II trial in 50 patients with advanced low-grade NHL who had previously been treated with chemotherapy [135]. Opportunistic infections occurred in seven patients, nine patients had bacterial septicemia, and three patients died as a result of infectious complications. CMV reactivation was also reported in one of ten patients with pretreated peripheral T-cell lymphoma following treatment with low-dose alemtuzumab [136]. The response rate reported in this study was similar to that previously reported with higher, more toxic doses [137, 138].

Gallamini and colleagues [139] observed a CMV reactivation rate of 9% in 24 patients with peripheral T-cell lymphoma who were treated with first-line alemtuzumab combined with CHOP; invasive aspergillosis was diagnosed in further two patients and bacterial infectious complications in three patients. Similar results were observed in the study by Lundin and colleagues [140], in which 4 of 41 patients with CLL experienced CMV reactivation. One patient who was allergic to cotrimoxazole and therefore did not receive prophylaxis developed PCP. However, a much higher CMV reactivation rate (31%) was observed in a phase II study of 16 patients with relapsed peripheral T-cell lymphoma treated with alemtuzumab plus dexamethasone, cisplatin, and cytarabine (A-DHAP) [141].

Although mycobacteria are rarely reported to cause infection after alemtuzumab treatment, infection with *Mycobacterium haemophilum*, a fastidious tuberculous mycobacterium, has been reported in two patients who experienced cutaneous lesions during alemtuzumab treatment [142]. Both infections were successfully treated using standard regimens. Viral infections have been anecdotally associated with alemtuzumab, including polyoma viruria in 21 of 58 T cell-depleted HSCT patients [143] and polyoma viremia in 6 of 54 highly HLA-sensitized renal transplant recipients [144]. HBV reactivation has been observed in two subjects with CLL and occult HBV infection who developed a virologic and biochemical flare of HBV following immunotherapy with alemtuzumab [145]. Pure red cell aplasia secondary to parvovirus B19 infection has also occurred in a number of patients undergoing alemtuzumab treatment [146, 147].

Alemtuzumab-Associated Infection: Prophylaxis

With a significant incidence of bacterial, fungal, and viral infectious complications expected as a result of the significant lymphopenia seen with alemtuzumab treatment, prophylactic PCP antibiotics (e.g., cotrimoxazole) and anti-herpes viral therapies (e.g., valacyclovir) are mandated. In addition, antifungal prophylaxis is often administered. As CMV reactivation is commonly reported during treatment with alemtuzumab, a recent randomized study investigated the efficacy of valganciclovir compared with valacyclovir prophylaxis in patients receiving any alemtuzumab-based regimen for the treatment of hematological malignancies [148]. None of the 20 patients receiving valganciclovir developed CMV reactivation compared with 7 of 20 patients receiving valacyclovir ($p=0.004$). Hence, using valganciclovir prophylaxis appears to prevent CMV reactivation during treatment with alemtuzumab.

Anti-CD33 Antibodies

Gemtuzumab Ozogamicin

Gemtuzumab ozogamicin is an antibody-drug conjugate (ADC) consisting of a semisynthetic derivative of calicheamicin, a potent cytotoxic antibiotic, linked to a humanized anti-CD33 monoclonal antibody. Gemtuzumab ozogamicin is internalized by target cells that express the CD33 surface antigen, and hydrolysis results in intracellular release of the cytotoxin [10]. This agent was first approved by the US Food and Drug Administration in 2000 for recurrence of acute myeloid leukemia (AML) in patients aged ≥60 years. Toxicities associated with gemtuzumab ozogamicin are primarily related to its myelosuppressive effects; in particular, neutropenia occurs in almost all patients undergoing this treatment [149] and hepatic veno-occlusive disease (VOD) (also known as sinusoidal obstructive syndrome [SOS]) has been reported at a rate up to 14% in patients undergoing allogeneic bone marrow transplant [150].

In a pooled analysis of three studies, the rate of neutropenia was high following gemtuzumab ozogamicin monotherapy for patients with AML who had failed prior treatment [16]. The vast majority of patients in this study had grade 3/4 neutropenia (97%) and thrombocytopenia (99%), although neutropenia would also be a characteristic of AML. Grade 3/4 infection occurred in 40 of the 142 patients (28%) and included sepsis in 16% and pneumonia in a further 7% of patients. A higher rate of sepsis was observed in a pilot study of combined gemtuzumab ozogamicin, idarubicin, and cytarabine in patients with refractory AML [151]. In this study, grade 3/4 sepsis occurred in 10 of 14 patients (71%), similar to the 63% grade 3/4 sepsis reported in the study of cytarabine, gemtuzumab ozogamicin, cyclosporine, and liposome-encapsulated daunorubicin in patients with refractory AML [152].

In a study in which 53 treatment-naïve or primary refractory/relapsed, poor-prognosis elderly patients with AML were treated with gemtuzumab ozogamicin, cytarabine, and granulocyte colony-stimulating factor, all 53 patients experienced grade 3/4 neutropenia [153]. In total, 19 patients (36%) had grade 3/4 infections, including bacterial sepsis ($n=13$) and pulmonary aspergillosis ($n=6$); the treatment-related mortality rate was 13%, with four patients dying as a result of infection. Similarly, in a study of 277 patients with CD33-positive AML who were treated with first-line gemtuzumab ozogamicin, sepsis and pneumonia occurred in 17 and 8% of patients, respectively [154]. In this study, 44 patients (16%) died within 28 days of the last dose of gemtuzumab ozogamicin, with infection being cited as the cause of death in 13 of these patients.

Anti-CD23 Antibodies

Lumiliximab

Lumiliximab is a chimeric macaque-human anti-CD23 monoclonal antibody that appears to induce apoptosis of CLL cells and CD23-expressing B cells [155]. In a phase I study of patients with CLL, lumiliximab was associated with a grade 3/4 infection rate of 15%, but the incidence and severity of infections were not related to the lumiliximab dose and there was no evidence of significant myelosuppression or cellular immune suppression [156].

Anti-CD22 Antibodies

Inotuzumab Ozogamicin

Inotuzumab ozogamicin (CMC-544) is an ADC combining a humanized anti-CD22 monoclonal antibody (IgG4 type) with the potent cytotoxic antibiotic, calicheamicin [157]. CD22 was chosen as a rational target for ADC therapy as the receptor is internalized following antibody binding facilitating the intracellular delivery of the cytotoxic. There have been no reports of infectious complications with inotuzumab ozogamicin treatment when administered as a single agent or in combination with rituximab in early phase I and II clinical trials [158–161]. However, grade 3–4 neutropenia has been reported in 12–31% of these patients, so further clinical development will elucidate whether the myelosuppressive effects associated with this agent will translate into an increased risk of infection.

Anti-CD4 Antibodies

Zanolimumab

Zanolimumab, a fully human monoclonal cytotoxic IgG1$_\kappa$ antibody targeting the CD4 molecule on T cells, is currently being investigated for the treatment of CD4+ malignancies such as cutaneous T-cell lymphomas (CTCL) and noncutaneous peripheral T-cell lymphomas (PTCL) [5, 162, 163]. In two phase II studies, 49% of patients with CTCL treated with zanolimumab developed infections (mainly skin or upper respiratory tract infections), although the majority were considered to be mild and unrelated to treatment [164]. A phase III efficacy trial of IV zanolimumab administered once weekly for 12 weeks is ongoing in patients with mycosis fungoides (MF)-type CTCL or Sezary Syndrome who are intolerant to or do not respond to treatment with bexarotene and one other standard therapy [162]. Data from this trial may provide more information on the toxicity, and specifically the risk of infection, associated with this agent.

Anti-CD3 Antibodies

Muromonab

Muromonab-CD3 (OKT3) is a murine IgG2a immunoglobulin used in transplant rejection that has also been used to treat steroid-resistant GVHD [165]. Muromonab-CD3 binds the CD3 molecule adjacent to the T-cell receptor, leading to nonspecific T-cell activation with cytokine release followed by transient but marked lymphocyte depletion and reemergence of CD3-negative T cells [166]. This lymphocyte depletion and T-cell receptor modulation result in immunosuppression and an increased risk of infection. High rates of opportunistic bacterial infection (21–50%) have been reported with muromonab in clinical trials of patients with transplant rejection [167–169].

Anti-CD2 Antibodies

Siplizumab

Siplizumab is a humanized anti-CD2 monoclonal antibody currently in phase I clinical development for the treatment of patients with relapsed/refractory CD2-positive T-cell lymphoma/leukemia, including T cell large granular lymphocyte (LGL) leukemia [170]. However, a phase I dose-escalation study had to be prematurely terminated after 14% of patients developed EBV-induced B-cell lymphoproliferative disease (LPD) [171]. Although T-cell counts were depleted in all patients, those who developed EBV-LPD had a significantly greater reduction in NK cells and CD2 expression on T cells.

Anti-Interleukin-2 Receptor Antibodies

Denileukin Diftitox

Denileukin diftitox (DAB389IL-2), a recombinant fusion protein consisting of IL-2 combined with the enzymatically active domain of diptheria toxin, is approved for the treatment of CTCL in patients with the CD25 component of the IL-2 receptor [172]. Denileukin difitox has also demonstrated efficacy in PTCL, B-cell NHL, CLL, and GVHD. After binding to the IL-2 receptor, denileukin diftitox is internalized via endocytosis and acts by inhibiting protein synthesis resulting in cell death. Results from three large phase III, randomized, double-blind, placebo-controlled trials conducted in patients with CTCL indicated that treatment with denileukin diftitox did not increase infection complications compared with placebo [173, 174]. In addition, when patients with relapsed/refractory B-cell NHL were treated with a combination of denileukin diftitox and rituximab in a phase II trial, myelotoxicity was reported to be uncommon [175]. However, in phase II studies of denileukin diftitox in patients with CLL, grade 3/4 neutropenia and infections (mainly bacterial, e.g., pneumonia) were reported in approximately 30% of patients [176, 177].

Daclizumab

Daclizumab and basiliximab are chimeric anti-IL-2Rα monoclonal antibodies approved for the prevention of renal allograft rejection, which act by blunting the antigenic challenge response. Both have also been used for the treatment of steroid-refractory graft versus host disease (GVHD).

Although the use of daclizumab in the treatment of leukemia and lymphoma has been limited to date, it has been used for the treatment of GVHD. Treatment of GVHD with daclizumab has been associated with high rates of infectious mortality, although this may, in part, be attributed to the underlying disease and prior therapies received by the patients. This theory is supported by the results of a randomized comparison of standard corticosteroids vs. corticosteroids plus daclizumab for the upfront treatment of acute GVHD, in which similar rates of grade 4/5 infections were seen in both arms (16% with corticosteroids alone vs. 25% with combination therapy; $p=0.34$) [6]. The study was, however, halted after a planned interim analysis showed significantly worse 100-day survival in the group receiving corticosteroids plus daclizumab compared with those receiving standard corticosteroids alone (77 vs. 94%; $p=0.02$). The higher mortality rate in the combination arm was attributed by the authors to both GVHD- and relapse-related deaths.

Perales and colleagues [178] reported a high rate of opportunistic infections in a retrospective review of 57 patients who underwent allogeneic HSCT and treatment with daclizumab for steroid-refractory acute GVHD. Opportunistic infections occurred in 95% of patients; 75% of patients died following treatment with daclizumab. Causes of death

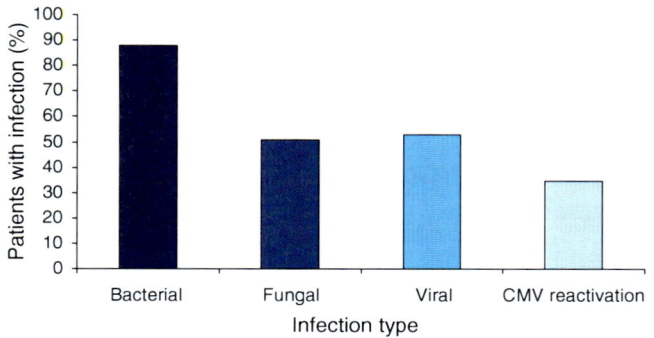

Fig. 5.3 Infection rates in a retrospective review of 57 patients who underwent an allogeneic hematopoetic stem cell transplant and treatment with daclizumab for steroid-refractory acute graft versus host disease (GVHD) [178]. *CMV* cytomegalovirus

included active GVHD and infection (79%), active GVHD (5%), chronic GVHD (2%), and relapse (14%). Bacterial, fungal, and viral infections occurred in 50 (88%), 29 (51%), and 30 (53%) patients, respectively, with CMV reactivation occurring in 35% of patients (Fig. 5.3). In another study of 12 patients undergoing nonmyeloablative allogeneic hematopoietic cell transplantation, daclizumab was associated with a rate of CMV reactivation of 87% and respiratory viral infections occurred in 42% of patients, including one fatal case of parainfluenza-3 infection and 1 case of Epstein–Barr virus-associated posttransplant lymphoproliferative disorder [179]. Willenbacher and colleagues [180] also reported a high infection rate in patients with corticosteroid-refractory GVHD undergoing daclizumab therapy. Fourteen out of 16 patients acquired infections during daclizumab treatment and three infection-related deaths were recorded.

Daclizumab has also been used to treat GVHD in children, but no treatment-related infections were reported [181, 182].

Basiliximab

Evidence for infection among patients with GVHD who were treated with basiliximab is limited, but appears to show a comparable rate and range of infectious complications to that seen with daclizumab. In a retrospective evaluation of 34 patients with refractory grade III/IV GVHD who received basiliximab, 19 infectious deaths were reported, 8 of which resulted from bacterial sepsis, 4 from CMV, and 6 from invasive fungal infection [183]. A high rate of infection was also seen in a prospective Phase II study of basiliximab in patients with steroid-refractory acute GVHD [184]. Ten of 23 patients developed bacterial infections, 4 of which led to deaths from sepsis. In addition, CMV reactivation was reported in five patients, two patients had invasive fungal infections, and 1 developed cerebral toxoplasmosis.

Anti-Interleukin-6-Receptor Antibodies

Tocilizumab

Tocilizumab is a humanized antihuman IL-6 receptor antibody that specifically blocks IL-6 cell-to-cell signaling. Tozilizumab was developed and is pending FDA approval for the treatment of patients with moderate-to severe RA. In addition to being a key proinflammatory cytokine in the pathogenesis of RA, IL-6 is involved in cell proliferation and survival [185, 186]. Hence, tocilizumab may be useful in the treatment of IL-6-related malignancies. Initial research has shown that IL-6 is involved in angiogenesis in several cancers, including multiple myeloma [187], and IL-6 expression is often elevated in patients with glioma [188]. Indeed, a recent study has shown tocilizumab to have an antitumor effect in glioma cells in vitro [186]. Clinical phase II/III and long-term trials in patients with RA have shown that neutropenia and infections (bacterial and viral) are commonly reported to occur with tocilizumab, with serious infections including pneumonia, gastroenteritis, upper respiratory tract infection, herpes zoster, and sepsis [189–191].

Anti-TNFα Monoclonal Antibodies

Infliximab

Infliximab was approved in November 1999 for the treatment of RA, but has also shown a therapeutic benefit in steroid-refractory GVHD. However, in this setting infliximab appears to increase the risk of infection compared with standard therapy. In a prospective trial of infliximab for the prophylaxis of acute GVHD in 19 patients undergoing myeloablative allogeneic stem cell transplantation for hematologic malignancies, significantly more bacterial and invasive fungal infections were observed compared with a matched control group of 30 patients contemporaneously undergoing treatment ($p=0.01$ and $p=0.02$, respectively) [192]. In a retrospective analysis of patients with severe steroid-refractory acute GVHD undergoing treatment with infliximab, 23 of the 32 patients (72%) developed one or more infectious episodes [193]. In total, seven patients developed septicemia (5 Gram-positive and 2 Gram-negative infections), two patients had septic shock, and seven patients had pneumonia. In addition, there were 13 cases of CMV reactivation, 4 cases of infectious enteritis, 2 invasive mycoses (candidemia and pulmonary aspergillosis), and one patient developed encephalitis. Marty and colleagues [194] undertook

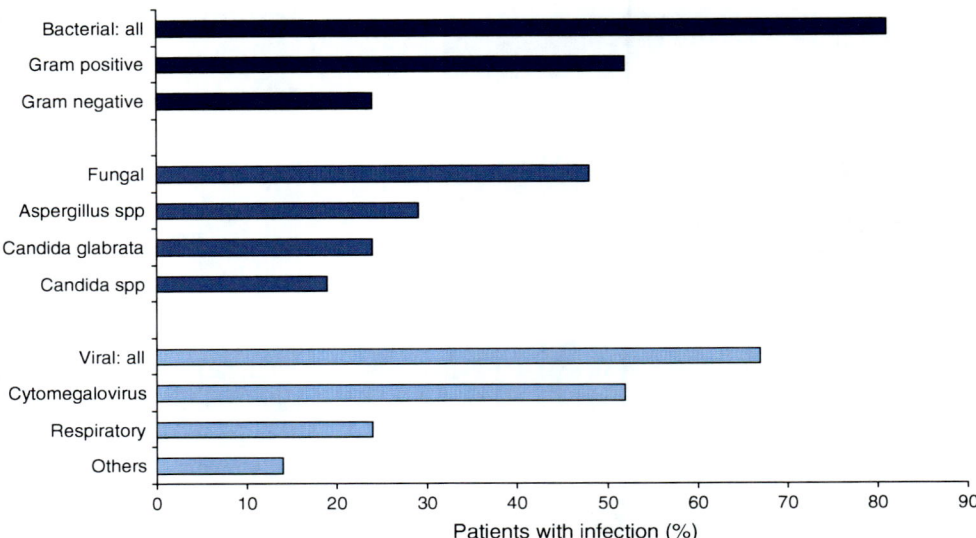

Fig. 5.4 Infections in patients treated with infliximab: retrospective analysis of 134 patients with acute GVHD [195]

a retrospective analysis of 264 patients with severe GVHD, in order to determine if this population was at an increased risk of non-*Candida* spp. invasive fungal infections. Of 11 infliximab recipients, 5 (45%) developed an invasive fungal infection compared with 5 such fungal infections among 42 patients (12%) who did not receive infliximab (adjusted hazard ratio 13.6; $p=0.004$). These data led the authors to conclude that infliximab administration was associated with a significantly increased risk of non-*Candida* spp. invasive fungal infections in patients with severe GVHD disease.

Couriel and colleagues [195] performed a retrospective evaluation of 134 patients with steroid-refractory GVHD, 21 of whom received infliximab therapy. Ten patients (48%) had 18 fungal infections, including *Aspergillus* spp. in 7 and *Candida* spp. in 10; 17 patients (81%) had bacterial infections, including 32 Gram-positive and 8 Gram-negative infections; and 14 patients (67%) had viral infections, primarily CMV reactivation (Fig. 5.4).

HLA-DR Antibody

Apolizumab (Hu1D10)

Apolizumab, a humanized monoclonal antibody against a polymorphic epitope on HLA-DRβ, has demonstrated evidence for therapeutic activity in 1D10-positive NHL when administered in combination with granulocyte colony-stimulating factor (G-CSF) [196]. The combination was well tolerated in this small pilot study, but further research is needed to clarify its effects.

Summary

Monoclonal antibodies have had an enormous impact on the treatment of patients with hematologic malignancies, improving response rates and survival for many. As with any oncology treatment, however, the benefits of therapy must be balanced against the risks. The ability of monoclonal antibodies to bind to specific antigens on malignant hematologic cells may provide a targeted therapy, but also leads to depletion of non-malignant immune cells, which in turn may increase the risk of infectious complications. The different targets of each of the monoclonal antibodies described in this chapter result in differences in the risks of infection, but the reactivation of latent infections such as HBV and CMV is a particular problem for many. The infectious complications associated with the most commonly used antibodies are now better understood, allowing physicians to anticipate these events, to monitor patients for early signs of infection, and to give prophylaxis where possible or treat when necessary, further improving outcomes for this patient population.

References

1. Oldham RK, Dillman RO. Monoclonal antibodies in cancer therapy: 25 years of progress. J Clin Oncol. 2008;26:1774–7.
2. Kaplan LD, Lee JY, Ambinder RF, Sparano JA, Cesarman E, Chadburn A, et al. Rituximab does not improve clinical outcome in a randomized phase 3 trial of CHOP with or without rituximab in patients with HIV-associated non-Hodgkin lymphoma: AIDS-Malignancies Consortium Trial 010. Blood. 2005;106:1538–43.
3. Feugier P, Van Hoof A, Sebban C, Solal-Celigny P, Bouabdallah R, Ferme C, et al. Long-term results of the R-CHOP study in the treatment of elderly patients with diffuse large B-cell lymphoma:

a study by the Groupe d'Etude des Lymphomes de l'Adulte. J Clin Oncol. 2005;23:4117–26.
4. Robak T. Alemtuzumab for B-cell chronic lymphocytic leukemia. Expert Rev Anticancer Ther. 2008;8:1033–51.
5. Castillo J, Winer E, Quesenberry P. Newer monoclonal antibodies for hematological malignancies. Exp Hematol. 2008;36:755–68.
6. Lee SJ, Zahrieh D, Agura E, MacMillan ML, Maziarz RT, McCarthy Jr PL, et al. Effect of up-front daclizumab when combined with steroids for the treatment of acute graft-versus-host disease: results of a randomized trial. Blood. 2004;104:1559–64.
7. Tkaczuk J, Yu CL, Baksh S, Milford EL, Carpenter CB, Burakoff SJ, et al. Effect of anti-IL-2Ralpha antibody on IL-2-induced Jak/STAT signaling. Am J Transplant. 2002;2:31–40.
8. Hultin LE, Hausner MA, Hultin PM, Giorgi JV. CD20 (pan-B cell) antigen is expressed at a low level on a subpopulation of human T lymphocytes. Cytometry. 1993;14:196–204.
9. Sperr WR, Florian S, Hauswirth AW, Valent P. CD 33 as a target of therapy in acute myeloid leukemia: current status and future perspectives. Leuk Lymphoma. 2005;46:1115–20.
10. Giles F, Estey E, O'Brien S. Gemtuzumab ozogamicin in the treatment of acute myeloid leukemia. Cancer. 2003;98:2095–104.
11. Martin SI, Marty FM, Fiumara K, Treon SP, Gribben JG, Baden LR. Infectious complications associated with alemtuzumab use for lymphoproliferative disorders. Clin Infect Dis. 2006;43:16–24.
12. Rituxan US Prescribing Information. http://www.fda.gov/cder/foi/label/2008/103705s5256lbl.pdf. Accessed on May, 2009.
13. Knight DM, Trinh H, Le J, Siegel S, Shealy D, McDonough M, et al. Construction and initial characterization of a mouse-human chimeric anti-TNF antibody. Mol Immunol. 1993;30:1443–53.
14. Charles P, Elliott MJ, Davis D, Potter A, Kalden JR, Antoni C, et al. Regulation of cytokines, cytokine inhibitors, and acute-phase proteins following anti-TNF-alpha therapy in rheumatoid arthritis. J Immunol. 1999;163:1521–8.
15. Kimby E. Tolerability and safety of rituximab (MabThera). Cancer Treat Rev. 2005;31:456–73.
16. Sievers EL, Larson RA, Stadtmauer EA, Estey E, Lowenberg B, Dombret H, et al. Efficacy and safety of gemtuzumab ozogamicin in patients with CD33-positive acute myeloid leukemia in first relapse. J Clin Oncol. 2001;19:3244–54.
17. Aksoy S, Harputluoglu H, Kilickap S, Dede DS, Dizdar O, Altundag K, et al. Rituximab-related viral infections in lymphoma patients. Leuk Lymphoma. 2007;48:1307–12.
18. McLaughlin P, Grillo-Lopez AJ, Link BK, Levy R, Czuczman MS, Williams ME, et al. Rituximab chimeric anti-CD20 monoclonal antibody therapy for relapsed indolent lymphoma: half of patients respond to a four-dose treatment program. J Clin Oncol. 1998;16:2825–33.
19. van Sorge NM, van der Pol WL, van de Winkel JG. FcgammaR polymorphisms: implications for function, disease susceptibility and immunotherapy. Tissue Antigens. 2003;61:189–202.
20. Sanders LA, van de Winkel JG, Rijkers GT, Voorhorst-Ogink MM, de Haas M, Capel PJ, et al. Fc gamma receptor IIa (CD32) heterogeneity in patients with recurrent bacterial respiratory tract infections. J Infect Dis. 1994;170:854–61.
21. Yee AM, Phan HM, Zuniga R, Salmon JE, Musher DM. Association between FcgammaRIIa-R131 allotype and bacteremic pneumococcal pneumonia. Clin Infect Dis. 2000;30:25–8.
22. Moens L, Van Hoeyveld E, Verhaegen J, De Boeck K, Peetermans WE, Bossuyt X. Fcgamma-receptor IIA genotype and invasive pneumococcal infection. Clin Immunol. 2006;118:20–3.
23. Fijen CA, Bredius RG, Kuijper EJ. Polymorphism of IgG Fc receptors in meningococcal disease. Ann Intern Med. 1993;119:636.
24. Forstpointner R, Dreyling M, Repp R, Hermann S, Hanel A, Metzner B, et al. The addition of rituximab to a combination of fludarabine, cyclophosphamide, mitoxantrone (FCM) significantly increases the response rate and prolongs survival as compared with FCM alone in patients with relapsed and refractory follicular and mantle cell lymphomas: results of a prospective randomized study of the German Low-Grade Lymphoma Study Group. Blood. 2004;104:3064–71.
25. Herold M, Haas A, Srock S, Neser S, Al Ali KH, Neubauer A, et al. Rituximab added to first-line mitoxantrone, chlorambucil, and prednisolone chemotherapy followed by interferon maintenance prolongs survival in patients with advanced follicular lymphoma: an East German Study Group Hematology and Oncology Study. J Clin Oncol. 2007;25:1986–92.
26. Hiddemann W, Kneba M, Dreyling M, Schmitz N, Lengfelder E, Schmits R, et al. Frontline therapy with rituximab added to the combination of cyclophosphamide, doxorubicin, vincristine, and prednisone (CHOP) significantly improves the outcome for patients with advanced-stage follicular lymphoma compared with therapy with CHOP alone: results of a prospective randomized study of the German Low-Grade Lymphoma Study Group. Blood. 2005;106:3725–32.
27. Marcus R, Imrie K, Solal-Celigny P, Catalano JV, Dmoszynska A, Raposo JC, et al. Phase III study of R-CVP compared with cyclophosphamide, vincristine, and prednisone alone in patients with previously untreated advanced follicular lymphoma. J Clin Oncol. 2008;26:4579–86.
28. Pfreundschuh M, Schubert J, Ziepert M, Schmits R, Mohren M, Lengfelder E, et al. Six versus eight cycles of bi-weekly CHOP-14 with or without rituximab in elderly patients with aggressive CD20+ B-cell lymphomas: a randomised controlled trial (RICOVER-60). Lancet Oncol. 2008;9:105–16.
29. Pfreundschuh M, Trumper L, Osterborg A, Pettengell R, Trneny M, Imrie K, et al. CHOP-like chemotherapy plus rituximab versus CHOP-like chemotherapy alone in young patients with good-prognosis diffuse large-B-cell lymphoma: a randomised controlled trial by the MabThera International Trial (MInT) Group. Lancet Oncol. 2006;7:379–91.
30. Schulz H, Bohlius JF, Trelle S, Skoetz N, Reiser M, Kober T, et al. Immunochemotherapy with rituximab and overall survival in patients with indolent or mantle cell lymphoma: a systematic review and meta-analysis. J Natl Cancer Inst. 2007;99:706–14.
31. Coiffier B, Lepage E, Briere J, Herbrecht R, Tilly H, Bouabdallah R, et al. CHOP chemotherapy plus rituximab compared with CHOP alone in elderly patients with diffuse large-B-cell lymphoma. N Engl J Med. 2002;346:235–42.
32. Hallek M, Fingerle-Rowson G, Fink A, Busch R, Mayer J, Hensel M. Immunochemotherapy with fludarabine (F), cyclophosphamide (C), and rituximab (R) (FCR) versus fludarabine and cyclophosphamide (FC) improves response rates and progression-free survival (PFS) of previously untreated patients (pts) with advanced chronic lymphocytic leukemia (CLL). Blood. 2008;112(Suppl. 11):Abstract 325.
33. Robak T, Moiseev SI, Dmoszynska A, Solal-Celigny P, Warzocha K, Loscertales J. Rituximab, fludarabine, and cyclophosphamide (R-FC) prolongs progression-free survival in relapsed or refractory chronic lymphocytic leukemia (CLL) compared with FC alone: final results from the international randomized phase III REACH trial. Blood. 2008;112(Suppl. 11):Abstract LBA1.
34. Ezzat H, Filipenko D, Vickars L, Galbraith P, Li C, Murphy K, et al. Improved survival in HIV-associated diffuse large B-cell lymphoma with the addition of rituximab to chemotherapy in patients receiving highly active antiretroviral therapy. HIV Clin Trials. 2007;8:132–44.
35. Oertel SH, Verschuuren E, Reinke P, Zeidler K, Papp-Vary M, Babel N, et al. Effect of anti-CD 20 antibody rituximab in patients with post-transplant lymphoproliferative disorder (PTLD). Am J Transplant. 2005;5:2901–6.
36. Rituxan US Prescribing Information. http://www.fda.gov/cder/foi/label/2008/103705s5256lbl.pdf. Accessed on May, 2009.

37. Cheson BD, Leonard JP. Monoclonal antibody therapy for B-cell non-Hodgkin's lymphoma. N Engl J Med. 2008;359:613–26.
38. Hilchey SP, Hyrien O, Mosmann TR, Livingstone AM, Friedberg JW, Young F, et al. Rituximab immunotherapy results in the induction of a lymphoma idiotype-specific T-cell response in patients with follicular lymphoma: support for a "vaccinal effect" of rituximab. Blood. 2009;113:3809–12.
39. Bello C, Sotomayor EM. Monoclonal antibodies for B-cell lymphomas: rituximab and beyond. Hematology Am Soc Hematol Educ Program. 2007;2007:233–42.
40. Byrd JC, Kitada S, Flinn IW, Aron JL, Pearson M, Lucas D, et al. The mechanism of tumor cell clearance by rituximab in vivo in patients with B-cell chronic lymphocytic leukemia: evidence of caspase activation and apoptosis induction. Blood. 2002;99:1038–43.
41. Cartron G, Dacheux L, Salles G, Solal-Celigny P, Bardos P, Colombat P, et al. Therapeutic activity of humanized anti-CD20 monoclonal antibody and polymorphism in IgG Fc receptor FcgammaRIIIa gene. Blood. 2002;99:754–8.
42. Weng WK, Levy R. Two immunoglobulin G fragment C receptor polymorphisms independently predict response to rituximab in patients with follicular lymphoma. J Clin Oncol. 2003;21:3940–7.
43. Ghielmini M, Rufibach K, Salles G, Leoncini-Franscini L, Leger-Falandry C, Cogliatti S, et al. Single agent rituximab in patients with follicular or mantle cell lymphoma: clinical and biological factors that are predictive of response and event-free survival as well as the effect of rituximab on the immune system: a study of the Swiss Group for Clinical Cancer Research (SAKK). Ann Oncol. 2005;16:1675–82.
44. Uchida J, Hamaguchi Y, Oliver JA, Ravetch JV, Poe JC, Haas KM, et al. The innate mononuclear phagocyte network depletes B lymphocytes through Fc receptor-dependent mechanisms during anti-CD20 antibody immunotherapy. J Exp Med. 2004;199:1659–69.
45. Sidner RA, Book BK, Agarwal A, Bearden CM, Vieira CA, Pescovitz MD. In vivo human B-cell subset recovery after in vivo depletion with rituximab, anti-human CD20 monoclonal antibody. Hum Antibodies. 2004;13:55–62.
46. Pescovitz MD. Rituximab, an anti-cd20 monoclonal antibody: history and mechanism of action. Am J Transplant. 2006;6:859–66.
47. Dillman RO, Hendrix CS. Unique aspects of supportive care using monoclonal antibodies in cancer treatment. Support Cancer Ther. 2003;1:38–48.
48. Cabanillas F, Liboy I, Pavia O, Rivera E. High incidence of non-neutropenic infections induced by rituximab plus fludarabine and associated with hypogammaglobulinemia: a frequently unrecognized and easily treatable complication. Ann Oncol. 2006;17:1424–7.
49. Hicks LK, Woods A, Buckstein R, Mangel J, Pennell N, Zhang L, et al. Rituximab purging and maintenance combined with auto-SCT: long-term molecular remissions and prolonged hypogammaglobulinemia in relapsed follicular lymphoma. Bone Marrow Transplant. 2008;43:701–8.
50. Miles SA, McGratten M. Persistent panhypogammaglobulinemia after CHOP-rituximab for HIV-related lymphoma. J Clin Oncol. 2005;23:247–8.
51. Walker AR, Kleiner A, Rich L, Conners C, Fisher RI, Anolik J, et al. Profound hypogammaglobulinemia 7 years after treatment for indolent lymphoma. Cancer Invest. 2008;26:431–3.
52. van der Kolk LE, Baars JW, Prins MH, van Oers MH. Rituximab treatment results in impaired secondary humoral immune responsiveness. Blood. 2002;100:2257–9.
53. Nishio M, Fujimoto K, Yamamoto S, Endo T, Sakai T, Obara M, et al. Delayed redistribution of CD27, CD40 and CD80 positive B cells and the impaired in vitro immunoglobulin production in patients with non-Hodgkin lymphoma after rituximab treatment as an adjuvant to autologous stem cell transplantation. Br J Haematol. 2007;137:349–54.
54. Anolik JH, Friedberg JW, Zheng B, Barnard J, Owen T, Cushing E, et al. B cell reconstitution after rituximab treatment of lymphoma recapitulates B cell ontogeny. Clin Immunol. 2007;122:139–45.
55. Gordan LN, Grow WB, Pusateri A, Douglas V, Mendenhall NP, Lynch JW. Phase II trial of individualized rituximab dosing for patients with CD20-positive lymphoproliferative disorders. J Clin Oncol. 2005;23:1096–102.
56. Vidal L, Gafter-Gvili A, Leibovici L, Dreyling M, Ghielmini M, Hsu Schmitz SF, et al. Rituximab maintenance for the treatment of patients with follicular lymphoma: systematic review and meta-analysis of randomized trials. J Natl Cancer Inst. 2009;101:248–55.
57. Pfreundschuh M, Zeynalova S, Poeschel V, Haenel M, Schmitz N, Hensel M, et al. Dose-dense rituximab improves outcome of elderly patients with poor-prognosis diffuse large b-cell lymphoma (DLBCL): results of the DENSE-R-CHOP-14 trial of the German High-Grade Non-Hodgkin Lymphoma Study Group (DSHNHL). Blood. 2007;110:Abstract 789.
58. Rueda A, Sabin P, Rifa J, Llanos M, Gomez-Codina J, Lobo F, et al. R-CHOP-14 in patients with diffuse large B-cell lymphoma younger than 70 years: a multicentre, prospective study. Hematol Oncol. 2008;26:27–32.
59. Tam C, Seymour JF, Brown M, Campbell P, Scarlett J, Underhill C, et al. Early and late infectious consequences of adding rituximab to fludarabine and cyclophosphamide in patients with indolent lymphoid malignancies. Haematologica. 2005;90:700–2.
60. van Oers MH, Klasa R, Marcus RE, Wolf M, Kimby E, Gascoyne RD, et al. Rituximab maintenance improves clinical outcome of relapsed/resistant follicular non-Hodgkin lymphoma in patients both with and without rituximab during induction: results of a prospective randomized phase 3 intergroup trial. Blood. 2006;108:3295–301.
61. Habermann TM, Weller EA, Morrison VA, Gascoyne RD, Cassileth PA, Cohn JB, et al. Rituximab-CHOP versus CHOP alone or with maintenance rituximab in older patients with diffuse large B-cell lymphoma. J Clin Oncol. 2006;24:3121–7.
62. Lenz G, Dreyling M, Hoster E, Wormann B, Duhrsen U, Metzner B, et al. Immunochemotherapy with rituximab and cyclophosphamide, doxorubicin, vincristine, and prednisone significantly improves response and time to treatment failure, but not long-term outcome in patients with previously untreated mantle cell lymphoma: results of a prospective randomized trial of the German Low Grade Lymphoma Study Group (GLSG). J Clin Oncol. 2005;23:1984–92.
63. Aksoy S, Dizdar O, Hayran M, Harputluoglu H. Infectious complications of rituximab in patients with lymphoma during maintenance therapy: a systematic review and meta-analysis. Leuk Lymphoma. 2009;50:357–65.
64. van Oers MH, Glabbeke MV, Baila L, Giurgia L, Klasa R, Marcus RE. Rituximab maintenance treatment of relapsed/resistant follicular non-Hodgkin's lymphoma: long-term outcome of the EORTC 20981 phase III randomized Intergroup study. Blood. 2008;112:Abstract 836.
65. Srock S, Schriever F, Neubauer A, Herold M, Huhn D. Long-term treatment with rituximab is feasible in selected patients with B-CLL: response-adjusted low-dose maintenance treatment with rituximab in patients with relapsed B-CLL, who achieved a partial or minimal response to prior rituximab therapy. Leuk Lymphoma. 2007;48:905–11.
66. Spina M, Jaeger U, Sparano JA, Talamini R, Simonelli C, Michieli M, et al. Rituximab plus infusional cyclophosphamide, doxorubicin, and etoposide in HIV-associated non-Hodgkin lymphoma: pooled results from 3 Phase 2 trials. Blood. 2005;105:1891–7.
67. Sandherr M, Einsele H, Hebart H, Kahl C, Kern W, Kiehl M, et al. Antiviral prophylaxis in patients with haematological malignancies and solid tumours: Guidelines of the Infectious Diseases Working Party (AGIHO) of the German Society for Hematology and Oncology (DGHO). Ann Oncol. 2006;17:1051–9.

68. Perceau G, Diris N, Estines O, Derancourt C, Levy S, Bernard P. Late lethal hepatitis B virus reactivation after rituximab treatment of low-grade cutaneous B-cell lymphoma. Br J Dermatol. 2006;155:1053–6.
69. Yeo W, Chan TC, Leung NW, Lam WY, Mo FK, Chu MT, et al. Hepatitis B virus reactivation in lymphoma patients with prior resolved hepatitis B undergoing anticancer therapy with or without rituximab. J Clin Oncol. 2009;27:605–11.
70. He YF, Li YH, Wang FH, Jiang WQ, Xu RH, Sun XF, et al. The effectiveness of lamivudine in preventing hepatitis B viral reactivation in rituximab-containing regimen for lymphoma. Ann Hematol. 2008;87:481–5.
71. Tsutsumi Y, Tanaka J, Kawamura T, Miura T, Kanamori H, Obara S et al. Possible efficacy of lamivudine treatment to prevent hepatitis B virus reactivation due to rituximab therapy in a patient with non-Hodgkin's lymphoma. Ann Hematol. 2004;83:58–60.
72. Yeo W, Chan PK, Ho WM, Zee B, Lam KC, Lei KI, et al. Lamivudine for the prevention of hepatitis B virus reactivation in hepatitis B s-antigen seropositive cancer patients undergoing cytotoxic chemotherapy. J Clin Oncol. 2004;22:927–34.
73. Besson C, Canioni D, Lepage E, Pol S, Morel P, Lederlin P, et al. Characteristics and outcome of diffuse large B-cell lymphoma in hepatitis C virus-positive patients in LNH 93 and LNH 98 Groupe d'Etude des Lymphomes de l'Adulte programs. J Clin Oncol. 2006;24:953–60.
74. Viswanatha DS, Dogan A. Hepatitis C virus and lymphoma. J Clin Pathol. 2007;60:1378–83.
75. Fiorilli M, Mecucci C, Farci P, Casato M. HCV-associated lymphomas. Rev Clin Exp Hematol. 2003;7:406–23.
76. Hsieh CY, Huang HH, Lin CY, Chung LW, Liao YM, Bai LY, et al. Rituximab-induced hepatitis C virus reactivation after spontaneous remission in diffuse large B-cell lymphoma. J Clin Oncol. 2008;26:2584–6.
77. Ennishi D, Terui Y, Yokoyama M, Mishima Y, Takahashi S, Takeuchi K, et al. Monitoring serum hepatitis C virus (HCV) RNA in patients with HCV-infected CD20-positive B-cell lymphoma undergoing rituximab combination chemotherapy. Am J Hematol. 2008;83:59–62.
78. Goldberg SL, Pecora AL, Alter RS, Kroll MS, Rowley SD, Waintraub SE, et al. Unusual viral infections (progressive multifocal leukoencephalopathy and cytomegalovirus disease) after high-dose chemotherapy with autologous blood stem cell rescue and peritransplantation rituximab. Blood. 2002;99:1486–8.
79. Vancikova Z, Dvorak P. Cytomegalovirus infection in immunocompetent and immunocompromised individuals - a review. Curr Drug Targets Immune Endocr Metabol Disord. 2001;1:179–87.
80. Suzan F, Ammor M, Ribrag V. Fatal reactivation of cytomegalovirus infection after use of rituximab for a post-transplantation lymphoproliferative disorder. N Engl J Med. 2001;345:1000.
81. Lee MY, Chiou TJ, Hsiao LT, Yang MH, Lin PC, Poh SB, et al. Rituximab therapy increased post-transplant cytomegalovirus complications in non-Hodgkin's lymphoma patients receiving autologous hematopoietic stem cell transplantation. Ann Hematol. 2008;87:285–9.
82. Calabrese LH, Molloy ES, Huang D, Ransohoff RM. Progressive multifocal leukoencephalopathy in rheumatic diseases: evolving clinical and pathologic patterns of disease. Arthritis Rheum. 2007;56:2116–28.
83. Viallard JF, Lazaro E, Lafon ME, Pellegrin JL. Successful cidofovir therapy of progressive multifocal leukoencephalopathy preceding angioimmunoblastic T-cell lymphoma. Leuk Lymphoma. 2005;46:1659–62.
84. De Luca A, Ammassari A, Pezzotti P, Cinque P, Gasnault J, Berenguer J, et al. Cidofovir in addition to antiretroviral treatment is not effective for AIDS-associated progressive multifocal leukoencephalopathy: a multicohort analysis. AIDS. 2008;22:1759–67.
85. Kraemer C, Evers S, Nolting T, Arendt G, Husstedt IW. Cidofovir in combination with HAART and survival in AIDS-associated progressive multifocal leukoencephalopathy. J Neurol. 2008;255:526–31.
86. Waggoner J, Martinu T, Palmer SM. Progressive multifocal leukoencephalopathy following heightened immunosuppression after lung transplant. J Heart Lung Transplant. 2009;28:395–8.
87. Berger JR. Progressive multifocal leukoencephalopathy. Curr Neurol Neurosci Rep. 2007;7:461–9.
88. Boren EJ, Cheema GS, Naguwa SM, Ansari AA, Gershwin ME. The emergence of progressive multifocal leukoencephalopathy (PML) in rheumatic diseases. J Autoimmun. 2008;30:90–8.
89. Carson KR, Evens AM, Richey EA, Habermann TM, Focosi D, Seymour JF, et al. Progressive multifocal leukoencephalopathy following rituximab therapy in HIV negative patients: a report of 57 cases from the Research on Adverse Drug Event and Reports (RADAR) project. Blood. 2009;113(20):4834–40.
90. Bermudez A, Marco F, Conde E, Mazo E, Recio M, Zubizarreta A. Fatal visceral varicella-zoster infection following rituximab and chemotherapy treatment in a patient with follicular lymphoma. Haematologica. 2000;85:894–5.
91. McIlwaine LM, Fitzsimons EJ, Soutar RL. Inappropriate antidiuretic hormone secretion, abdominal pain and disseminated varicella-zoster virus infection: an unusual and fatal triad in a patient 13 months post rituximab and autologous stem cell transplantation. Clin Lab Haematol. 2001;23:253–4.
92. Chang H, Yeh HC, Su YC, Lee MH. Pneumocystis jiroveci pneumonia in patients with non-Hodgkin's lymphoma receiving chemotherapy containing rituximab. J Chin Med Assoc. 2008;71:579–82.
93. Kolstad A, Holte H, Fossa A, Lauritzsen GF, Gaustad P, Torfoss D. Pneumocystis jirovecii pneumonia in B-cell lymphoma patients treated with the rituximab-CHOEP-14 regimen. Haematologica. 2007;92:139–40.
94. Venhuizen AC, Hustinx WN, van Houte AJ, Veth G. van der GR. Three cases of Pneumocystis jirovecii pneumonia (PCP) during first-line treatment with rituximab in combination with CHOP-14 for aggressive B-cell non-Hodgkin's lymphoma. Eur J Haematol. 2008;80:275–6.
95. Iyer A, Mathur R, Deepak BV, Sinard J. Fatal adenoviral hepatitis after rituximab therapy. Arch Pathol Lab Med. 2006;130:1557–60.
96. Sharma VR, Fleming DR, Slone SP. Pure red cell aplasia due to parvovirus B19 in a patient treated with rituximab. Blood. 2000;96:1184–6.
97. Isobe Y, Sugimoto K, Shiraki Y, Nishitani M, Koike K, Oshimi K. Successful high-titer immunoglobulin therapy for persistent parvovirus B19 infection in a lymphoma patient treated with rituximab-combined chemotherapy. Am J Hematol. 2004;77:370–3.
98. Biehn SE, Kirk D, Rivera MP, Martinez AE, Khandani AH, Orlowski RZ. Bronchiolitis obliterans with organizing pneumonia after rituximab therapy for non-Hodgkin's lymphoma. Hematol Oncol. 2006;24:234–7.
99. Soubrier M, Jeannin G, Kemeny JL, Tournadre A, Caillot N, Caillaud D, et al. Organizing pneumonia after rituximab therapy: two cases. Joint Bone Spine. 2008;75:362–5.
100. Padate BP, Keidan J. Enteroviral meningoencephalitis in a patient with non-Hodgkin's lymphoma treated previously with rituximab. Clin Lab Haematol. 2006;28:69–71.
101. Quartier P, Tournilhac O, Archimbaud C, Lazaro L, Chaleteix C, Millet P, et al. Enteroviral meningoencephalitis after anti-CD20 (rituximab) treatment. Clin Infect Dis. 2003;36:e47–9.
102. Archimbaud C, Bailly JL, Chambon M, Tournilhac O, Travade P, Peigue-Lafeuille H. Molecular evidence of persistent echovirus 13 meningoencephalitis in a patient with relapsed lymphoma after an outbreak of meningitis in 2000. J Clin Microbiol. 2003;41:4605–10.

103. Faderl S, Thomas DA, O'Brien S, Garcia-Manero G, Kantarjian HM, Giles FJ, et al. Experience with alemtuzumab plus rituximab in patients with relapsed and refractory lymphoid malignancies. Blood. 2003;101:3413–5.
104. Hirayama Y, Kohda K, Konuma Y, Hirata Y, Kuroda H, Fujimi Y, et al. Late onset neutropenia and immunoglobulin suppression of the patients with malignant lymphoma following autologous stem cell transplantation with rituximab. Intern Med. 2009;48:57–60.
105. Nitta E, Izutsu K, Sato T, Ota Y, Takeuchi K, Kamijo A, et al. A high incidence of late-onset neutropenia following rituximab-containing chemotherapy as a primary treatment of CD20-positive B-cell lymphoma: a single-institution study. Ann Oncol. 2007;18:364–9.
106. Fukuno K, Tsurumi H, Ando N, Kanemura N, Goto H, Tanabashi S, et al. Late-onset neutropenia in patients treated with rituximab for non-Hodgkin's lymphoma. Int J Hematol. 2006;84:242–7.
107. Terrier B, Ittah M, Tourneur L, Louache F, Soumelis V, Lavie F, et al. Late-onset neutropenia following rituximab results from a hematopoietic lineage competition due to an excessive BAFF-induced B-cell recovery. Haematologica. 2007;92:e20–3.
108. Dunleavy K, Hakim F, Kim HK, Janik JE, Grant N, Nakayama T, et al. B-cell recovery following rituximab-based therapy is associated with perturbations in stromal derived factor-1 and granulocyte homeostasis. Blood. 2005;106:795–802.
109. Klepfish A, Rachmilevitch E, Schattner A. Parvovirus B19 reactivation presenting as neutropenia after rituximab treatment. Eur J Intern Med. 2006;17:505–7.
110. Salliot C, Dougados M, Gossec L. Risk of serious infections during rituximab, abatacept and anakinra treatments for rheumatoid arthritis: meta-analyses of randomised placebo-controlled trials. Ann Rheum Dis. 2009;68:25–32.
111. Bexxar (^{90}Y-labeled ibritumomb tiuxetan) US Prescribing Information. http://www.us.gsk.com/products/assets/us_bexxar.pdf. Accessed on May, 2009.
112. Zevalin (^{131}I-labeled tositumomab) US Prescribing Information. http://www.zevalin.com/pdf/Zevalin_PI_website.pdf. Accessed on May, 2009.
113. Kaminski MS, Tuck M, Estes J, Kolstad A, Ross CW, Zasadny K, et al. ^{131}I-tositumomab therapy as initial treatment for follicular lymphoma. N Engl J Med. 2005;352:441–9.
114. Witzig TE, Flinn IW, Gordon LI, Emmanouilides C, Czuczman MS, Saleh MN, et al. Treatment with ibritumomab tiuxetan radioimmunotherapy in patients with rituximab-refractory follicular non-Hodgkin's lymphoma. J Clin Oncol. 2002;20:3262–9.
115. Kaminski MS, Estes J, Zasadny KR, Francis IR, Ross CW, Tuck M, et al. Radioimmunotherapy with iodine (131)I tositumomab for relapsed or refractory B-cell non-Hodgkin lymphoma: updated results and long-term follow-up of the University of Michigan experience. Blood. 2000;96:1259–66.
116. Vose JM, Wahl RL, Saleh M, Rohatiner AZ, Knox SJ, Radford JA, et al. Multicenter phase II study of iodine-131 tositumomab for chemotherapy-relapsed/refractory low-grade and transformed low-grade B-cell non-Hodgkin's lymphomas. J Clin Oncol. 2000;18:1316–23.
117. Davis TA, Kaminski MS, Leonard JP, Hsu FJ, Wilkinson M, Zelenetz A, et al. The radioisotope contributes significantly to the activity of radioimmunotherapy. Clin Cancer Res. 2004;10:7792–8.
118. Horning SJ, Younes A, Jain V, Kroll S, Lucas J, Podoloff D, et al. Efficacy and safety of tositumomab and iodine-131 tositumomab (Bexxar) in B-cell lymphoma, progressive after rituximab. J Clin Oncol. 2005;23:712–9.
119. Press OW, Unger JM, Braziel RM, Maloney DG, Miller TP, Leblanc M, et al. Phase II trial of CHOP chemotherapy followed by tositumomab/iodine I-131 tositumomab for previously untreated follicular non-Hodgkin's lymphoma: five-year follow-up of Southwest Oncology Group Protocol S9911. J Clin Oncol. 2006;24:4143–9.
120. Witzig TE, White CA, Gordon LI, Wiseman GA, Emmanouilides C, Murray JL, et al. Safety of yttrium-90 ibritumomab tiuxetan radioimmunotherapy for relapsed low-grade, follicular, or transformed non-Hodgkin's lymphoma. J Clin Oncol. 2003;21:1263–70.
121. Morschhauser F, Radford J, Van Hoof A, Vitolo U, Soubeyran P, Tilly H, et al. Phase III trial of consolidation therapy with yttrium-90-ibritumomab tiuxetan compared with no additional therapy after first remission in advanced follicular lymphoma. J Clin Oncol. 2008;26:5156–64.
122. Keating MJ, Flinn I, Jain V, Binet JL, Hillmen P, Byrd J, et al. Therapeutic role of alemtuzumab (Campath-1H) in patients who have failed fludarabine: results of a large international study. Blood. 2002;99:3554–61.
123. Lundin J, Porwit-MacDonald A, Rossmann ED, Karlsson C, Edman P, Rezvany MR, et al. Cellular immune reconstitution after subcutaneous alemtuzumab (anti-CD52 monoclonal antibody, CAMPATH-1H) treatment as first-line therapy for B-cell chronic lymphocytic leukaemia. Leukemia. 2004;18:484–90.
124. Peleg AY, Husain S, Kwak EJ, Silveira FP, Ndirangu M, Tran J, et al. Opportunistic infections in 547 organ transplant recipients receiving alemtuzumab, a humanized monoclonal CD-52 antibody. Clin Infect Dis. 2007;44:204–12.
125. Hillmen P, Skotnicki AB, Robak T, Jaksic B, Dmoszynska A, Wu J, et al. Alemtuzumab compared with chlorambucil as first-line therapy for chronic lymphocytic leukemia. J Clin Oncol. 2007;25:5616–23.
126. Wendtner CM, Ritgen M, Schweighofer CD, Fingerle-Rowson G, Campe H, Jager G, et al. Consolidation with alemtuzumab in patients with chronic lymphocytic leukemia (CLL) in first remission - experience on safety and efficacy within a randomized multicenter Phase III trial of the German CLL Study Group (GCLLSG). Leukemia. 2004;18:1093–101.
127. O'Brien SM, Kantarjian HM, Thomas DA, Cortes J, Giles FJ, Wierda WG, et al. Alemtuzumab as treatment for residual disease after chemotherapy in patients with chronic lymphocytic leukemia. Cancer. 2003;98:2657–63.
128. Ferrajoli A, O'Brien SM, Cortes JE, Giles FJ, Thomas DA, Faderl S, et al. Phase II study of alemtuzumab in chronic lymphoproliferative disorders. Cancer. 2003;98:773–8.
129. Fiegl M, Hopfinger G, Jaeger G. Alemtuzumab is effective in the treatment of patients with advanced, heavily pretreated B-cell chronic lymphocytic leukemia. Blood. 2003;102(Suppl. 2):Abstract 5157.
130. Moreton P, Kennedy B, Lucas G, Leach M, Rassam SM, Haynes A, et al. Eradication of minimal residual disease in B-cell chronic lymphocytic leukemia after alemtuzumab therapy is associated with prolonged survival. J Clin Oncol. 2005;23:2971–9.
131. Osuji NC, Del GI, Matutes E, Wotherspoon AC, Dearden C, Catovsky D. The efficacy of alemtuzumab for refractory chronic lymphocytic leukemia in relation to cytogenetic abnormalities of p53. Haematologica. 2005;90:1435–6.
132. Rai KR, Freter CE, Mercier RJ, Cooper MR, Mitchell BS, Stadtmauer EA, et al. Alemtuzumab in previously treated chronic lymphocytic leukemia patients who also had received fludarabine. J Clin Oncol. 2002;20:3891–7.
133. Nabhan C, Patton D, Gordon LI, Riley MB, Kuzel T, Tallman MS, et al. A pilot trial of rituximab and alemtuzumab combination therapy in patients with relapsed and/or refractory chronic lymphocytic leukemia (CLL). Leuk Lymphoma. 2004;45:2269–73.
134. Hainsworth JD, Vazquez ER, Spigel DR, Raefsky E, Bearden JD, Saez RA, et al. Combination therapy with fludarabine and rituximab followed by alemtuzumab in the first-line treatment of patients with chronic lymphocytic leukemia or small lymphocytic lymphoma: a phase 2 trial of the Minnie Pearl Cancer Research Network. Cancer. 2008;112:1288–95.
135. Lundin J, Osterborg A, Brittinger G, Crowther D, Dombret H, Engert A, et al. CAMPATH-1H monoclonal antibody in therapy for previously treated low-grade non-Hodgkin's lymphomas: a phase II multicenter study. European Study Group of CAMPATH-1H Treatment in Low-Grade Non-Hodgkin's Lymphoma. J Clin Oncol. 1998;16:3257–63.

136. Zinzani PL, Alinari L, Tani M, Fina M, Pileri S, Baccarani M. Preliminary observations of a Phase II study of reduced-dose alemtuzumab treatment in patients with pretreated T-cell lymphoma. Haematologica. 2005;90:702–3.
137. Enblad G, Hagberg H, Erlanson M, Lundin J, MacDonald AP, Repp R, et al. A pilot study of alemtuzumab (anti-CD52 monoclonal antibody) therapy for patients with relapsed or chemotherapy-refractory peripheral T-cell lymphomas. Blood. 2004;103:2920–4.
138. Lundin J, Hagberg H, Repp R, Cavallin-Stahl E, Freden S, Juliusson G, et al. Phase 2 study of alemtuzumab (anti-CD52 monoclonal antibody) in patients with advanced mycosis fungoides/Sezary syndrome. Blood. 2003;101:4267–72.
139. Gallamini A, Zaja F, Patti C, Billio A, Specchia MR, Tucci A, et al. Alemtuzumab (Campath-1H) and CHOP chemotherapy as first-line treatment of peripheral T-cell lymphoma: results of a GITIL (Gruppo Italiano Terapie Innovative nei Linfomi) prospective multicenter trial. Blood. 2007;110:2316–23.
140. Lundin J, Kimby E, Bjorkholm M, Broliden PA, Celsing F, Hjalmar V, et al. Phase II trial of subcutaneous anti-CD52 monoclonal antibody alemtuzumab (Campath-1H) as first-line treatment for patients with B-cell chronic lymphocytic leukemia (B-CLL). Blood. 2002;100:768–73.
141. Kim SJ, Kim K, Kim BS, Suh C, Huh J, Ko YH, et al. Alemtuzumab and DHAP (A-DHAP) is effective for relapsed peripheral T-cell lymphoma, unspecified: interim results of a phase II prospective study. Ann Oncol. 2009;20:390–2.
142. Kamboj M, Louie E, Kiehn T, Papanicolaou G, Glickman M, Sepkowitz K. Mycobacterium haemophilum infection after alemtuzumab treatment. Emerg Infect Dis. 2008;14:1821–3.
143. Chakrabarti S, Osman H, Collingham K, Milligan DW. Polyoma viruria following T-cell-depleted allogeneic transplants using Campath-1H: incidence and outcome in relation to graft manipulation, donor type and conditioning. Bone Marrow Transplant. 2003;31:379–86.
144. Vo AA, Wechsler EA, Wang J, Peng A, Toyoda M, Lukovsky M, et al. Analysis of subcutaneous (SQ) alemtuzumab induction therapy in highly sensitized patients desensitized with IVIG and rituximab. Am J Transplant. 2008;8:144–9.
145. Iannitto E, Minardi V, Calvaruso G, Mule A, Ammatuna E, Di Trapani R, et al. Hepatitis B virus reactivation and alemtuzumab therapy. Eur J Haematol. 2005;74:254–8.
146. Crowley B, Woodcock B. Red cell aplasia due to parvovirus b19 in a patient treated with alemtuzumab. Br J Haematol. 2002;119:279–80.
147. Herbert KE, Prince HM, Westerman DA. Pure red-cell aplasia due to parvovirus B19 infection in a patient treated with alemtuzumab. Blood. 2003;101:1654.
148. O'Brien S, Ravandi F, Riehl T, Wierda W, Huang X, Tarrand J, et al. Valganciclovir prevents cytomegalovirus reactivation in patients receiving alemtuzumab-based therapy. Blood. 2008;111:1816–9.
149. Leopold LH, Berger MS, Feingold J. Acute and long-term toxicities associated with gemtuzumab ozogamicin (Mylotarg) therapy of acute myeloid leukemia. Lymphoma. 2002;2 (Suppl 1): S29–34.
150. McKoy JM, Angelotta C, Bennett CL, Tallman MS, Wadleigh M, Evens AM, et al. Gemtuzumab ozogamicin-associated sinusoidal obstructive syndrome (SOS): an overview from the research on adverse drug events and reports (RADAR) project. Leuk Res. 2007;31:599–604.
151. Alvarado Y, Tsimberidou A, Kantarjian H, Cortes J, Garcia-Manero G, Faderl S, et al. Pilot study of Mylotarg, idarubicin and cytarabine combination regimen in patients with primary resistant or relapsed acute myeloid leukemia. Cancer Chemother Pharmacol. 2003;51:87–90.
152. Apostolidou E, Cortes J, Tsimberidou A, Estey E, Kantarjian H, Giles FJ. Pilot study of gemtuzumab ozogamicin, liposomal daunorubicin, cytarabine and cyclosporine regimen in patients with refractory acute myelogenous leukemia. Leuk Res. 2003;27:887–91.
153. Fianchi L, Pagano L, Leoni F, Storti S, Voso MT, Valentini CG, et al. Gemtuzumab ozogamicin, cytosine arabinoside, G-CSF combination (G-AraMy) in the treatment of elderly patients with poor-prognosis acute myeloid leukemia. Ann Oncol. 2008;19:128–34.
154. Larson RA, Sievers EL, Stadtmauer EA, Lowenberg B, Estey EH, Dombret H, et al. Final report of the efficacy and safety of gemtuzumab ozogamicin (Mylotarg) in patients with CD33-positive acute myeloid leukemia in first recurrence. Cancer. 2005;104:1442–52.
155. Pathan NI, Chu P, Hariharan K, Cheney C, Molina A, Byrd J. Mediation of apoptosis by and antitumor activity of lumiliximab in chronic lymphocytic leukemia cells and CD23+ lymphoma cell lines. Blood. 2008;111:1594–602.
156. Byrd JC, O'Brien S, Flinn IW, Kipps TJ, Weiss M, Rai K, et al. Phase 1 study of lumiliximab with detailed pharmacokinetic and pharmacodynamic measurements in patients with relapsed or refractory chronic lymphocytic leukemia. Clin Cancer Res. 2007;13:4448–55.
157. DiJoseph JF, Goad ME, Dougher MM, Boghaert ER, Kunz A, Hamann PR, et al. Potent and specific antitumor efficacy of CMC-544, a CD22-targeted immunoconjugate of calicheamicin, against systemically disseminated B-cell lymphoma. Clin Cancer Res. 2004;10:8620–9.
158. Advani A, Gine E, Gisselbrech C, Rohatiner A, Rosen S, Smith M, et al. Preliminary report of a phase I study of CMC-544, an antibody-targeted chemotherapy agent, in patients with B-cell non-Hodgkin's lymphoma (NHL). Blood. 2005;106:Abstract 230.
159. Fayad L, Patel H, Verhoef G, Czuczman M, Foran J, Gine E, et al. Clinical activity of the immunoconjugate CMC-544 in B-cell malignancies: preliminary report of the expanded maximum tolerated dose (MTD) cohort of a phase I study. Blood. 2006;108:Abstract 2711.
160. Fayad L, Patel H, Verhoef G, Smith MR, Johnson PW, Czuczman M, et al. Safety and clinical activity of the anti-CD22 immunoconjugate inotuzumab ozogamicin (CMC-544) in combination with rituximab in follicular lymphoma or diffuse large B-cell lymphoma: preliminary report of a phase 1/2 study. Blood. 2008;112:Abstract 266.
161. Tobinai K, Ogura M, Hatake K, Kobayashi Y, Watanabe T, Uchida T, et al. Phase I and pharmacokinetic study of inotuzumab ozogamicin (CMC-544) as a single agent in Japanese patients with follicular lymphoma pretreated with rituximab. Blood. 2008;112:Abstract 1565.
162. Duvic M, Kim Y, Korman NJ, Boh E, Lerner A, Heffernan MP, et al. Zanolimumab, a fully human monoclonal antibody: early results of an ongoing trial in patients with CD4+ mycosis fungoides (MF) type CTCL (stage Ib-IVB) who are refractory or intolerant to targretin and one other standard therapy. Blood. 2006;110:Abstract 2731.
163. d'Amore F, Radford J, Jerkeman M, Relander T, Tilly H, Osterborg A, et al. Zanolimumab (HuMax-CD4TM), a fully human monoclonal antibody: efficacy and safety in patients with relapsed or treatment-refractory non-cutaneous CD4+ T-cell lymphoma. Blood. 2007;110:Abstract 3409.
164. Kim YH, Duvic M, Obitz E, Gniadecki R, Iversen L, Osterborg A, et al. Clinical efficacy of zanolimumab (HuMax-CD4): two phase 2 studies in refractory cutaneous T-cell lymphoma. Blood. 2007;109:4655–62.
165. Knop S, Hebart H, Gscheidle H, Holler E, Kolb HJ, Niederwieser D, et al. OKT3 muromonab as second-line and subsequent treatment in recipients of stem cell allografts with steroid-resistant acute graft-versus-host disease. Bone Marrow Transplant. 2005;36:831–7.
166. Gea-Banacloche JC, Weinberg GA. Monoclonal antibody therapeutics and risk for infection. Pediatr Infect Dis J. 2007;26:1049–52.
167. Brock MV, Borja MC, Ferber L, Orens JB, Anzcek RA, Krishnan J, et al. Induction therapy in lung transplantation: a prospective, controlled clinical trial comparing OKT3, anti-thymocyte globulin, and daclizumab. J Heart Lung Transplant. 2001;20:1282–90.

168. Sevmis S, Emiroglu R, Karakayali F, Yagmurdur MC, Dalgic A, Moray G, et al. OKT3 treatment for steroid-resistant acute rejection in kidney transplantation. Transplant Proc. 2005;37:3016–8.
169. Chow FY, Polkinghorne K, Saunder A, Kerr PG, Atkins RC, Chadban SJ. Historical controlled trial of OKT3 versus basiliximab induction therapy in simultaneous pancreas-renal transplantation. Nephrology (Carlton). 2003;8:212–6.
170. Alekshun TJ, Sokol L. Diseases of large granular lymphocytes. Cancer Control. 2007;14:141–50.
171. O'Mahony D, Morris JC, Stetler-Stevenson M, Matthews H, Brown MR, Fleisher T, et al. EBV-related lymphoproliferative disease complicating therapy with the anti-CD2 monoclonal antibody, siplizumab, in patients with T-cell malignancies. Clin Cancer Res. 2009;15:2514–22.
172. Duvic M, Talpur R. Optimizing denileukin diftitox (Ontak®) therapy. Future Oncol. 2008;4:457–69.
173. Negro-Vilar A, Dziewanowska Z, Groves ES, Stevens V, Zhang JK, Prince M, et al. Efficacy and safety of denileeukin diftitox (Dd) in a phase II, double-blind, placebo-controlled study of CD25+ patients with cutaneous T-cell lymphoma (CTCL). J Clin Oncol. 2007;25:4475.
174. Negro-Vilar A, Prince HM, Duvic M, Richardson S, Sun Y, Acosta M. Efficacy and safety of denileukin diftitox (Dd) in cutaneous T-cell lymphoma (CTCL) patients: integrated analyisis of three large phase III trials. J Clin Oncol. 2008;26:4665.
175. Dang NH, Fayad L, McLaughlin P, Romaguara JE, Hagemeister F, Goy A, et al. Phase II trial of the combination of denileeukin diftitox and rituximab for relapsed/refractory B-cell non-Hodgkin lymphoma. Br J Haematol. 2007;138:502–5.
176. Lilly M, Kuriakose P, Turturro F, Berdeja J, Kerr R, Surendranathan A, et al. A phase II study of denileeukin diftitox (Ontak) in patients with fludarabine-refractory B-cell chronic lymphocytic leukemia. J Clin Oncol. 2005;23:5975.
177. Frankel AE, Surendranathan A, Black JH, White A, Ganjoo K, Cripe LD. Phase II clinical studies of denileukin diftitox diphtheria toxin fusion protein in patients with previously treated chronic lymphocytic leukemia. Cancer. 2006;106:2158–64.
178. Perales MA, Ishill N, Lomazow WA, Weinstock DM, Papadopoulos EB, Dastigir H, et al. Long-term follow-up of patients treated with daclizumab for steroid-refractory acute graft-vs-host disease. Bone Marrow Transplant. 2007;40:481–6.
179. Srinivasan R, Chakrabarti S, Walsh T, Igarashi T, Takahashi Y, Kleiner D, et al. Improved survival in steroid-refractory acute graft versus host disease after non-myeloablative allogeneic transplantation using a daclizumab-based strategy with comprehensive infection prophylaxis. Br J Haematol. 2004;124:777–86.
180. Willenbacher W, Basara N, Blau IW, Fauser AA, Kiehl MG. Treatment of steroid refractory acute and chronic graft-versus-host disease with daclizumab. Br J Haematol. 2001;112:820–3.
181. Teachey DT, Bickert B, Bunin N. Daclizumab for children with corticosteroid refractory graft-versus-host disease. Bone Marrow Transplant. 2006;37:95–9.
182. Rodriguez V, Anderson PM, Trotz BA, Arndt CA, Allen JA, Khan SP. Use of infliximab-daclizumab combination for the treatment of acute and chronic graft-versus-host disease of the liver and gut. Pediatr Blood Cancer. 2007;49:212–5.
183. Funke VA, de Medeiros CR, Setubal DC, Ruiz J, Bitencourt MA, Bonfim CM, et al. Therapy for severe refractory acute graft-versus-host disease with basiliximab, a selective interleukin-2 receptor antagonist. Bone Marrow Transplant. 2006;37:961–5.
184. Schmidt-Hieber M, Fietz T, Knauf W, Uharek L, Hopfenmuller W, Thiel E, et al. Efficacy of the interleukin-2 receptor antagonist basiliximab in steroid-refractory acute graft-versus-host disease. Br J Haematol. 2005;130:568–74.
185. Park JY, Pillinger MH. Interleukin-6 in the pathogenesis of rheumatoid arthritis. Bull NYU Hosp Jt Dis. 2007;65 Suppl 1:S4–10.
186. Kudo M, Jono H, Shinriki S, Yano S, Nakamura H, Makino K, et al. Antitumor effect of humanized anti-interleukin-6 receptor antibody (tocilizumab) on glioma cell proliferation. J Neurosurg. 2009;111:219–25.
187. Dankbar B, Padro T, Leo R, Feldmann B, Kropff M, Mesters RM, et al. Vascular endothelial growth factor and interleukin-6 in paracrine tumor-stromal cell interactions in multiple myeloma. Blood. 2000;95:2630–6.
188. Samaras V, Piperi C, Korkolopoulou P, Zisakis A, Levidou G, Themistocleous MS, et al. Application of the ELISPOT method for comparative analysis of interleukin (IL)-6 and IL-10 secretion in peripheral blood of patients with astroglial tumors. Mol Cell Biochem. 2007;304:343–51.
189. Nishimoto N, Hashimoto J, Miyasaka N, Yamamoto K, Kawai S, Takeuchi T, et al. Study of active controlled monotherapy used for rheumatoid arthritis, an IL-6 inhibitor (SAMURAI): evidence of clinical and radiographic benefit from an x ray reader-blinded randomised controlled trial of tocilizumab. Ann Rheum Dis. 2007;66:1162–7.
190. Nishimoto N, Miyasaka N, Yamamoto K, Kawai S, Takeuchi T, Azuma J, et al. Study of active controlled tocilizumab monotherapy for rheumatoid arthritis patients with an inadequate response to methotrexate (SATORI): significant reduction in disease activity and serum vascular endothelial growth factor by IL-6 receptor inhibition therapy. Mod Rheumatol. 2009;19:12–9.
191. Nishimoto N, Miyasaka N, Yamamoto K, Kawai S, Takeuchi T, Azuma J. Long-term safety and efficacy of tocilizumab, an anti-interleukin-6 receptor monoclonal antibody, in monotherapy, in patients with rheumatoid arthritis (the STREAM study): evidence of safety and efficacy in a 5-year extension study. Ann Rheum Dis. 2008;68:1580–4.
192. Hamadani M, Hofmeister CC, Jansak B, Phillips G, Elder P, Blum W, et al. Addition of infliximab to standard acute graft-versus-host disease prophylaxis following allogeneic peripheral blood cell transplantation. Biol Blood Marrow Transplant. 2008;14:783–9.
193. Patriarca F, Sperotto A, Damiani D, Morreale G, Bonifazi F, Olivieri A, et al. Infliximab treatment for steroid-refractory acute graft-versus-host disease. Haematologica. 2004;89:1352–9.
194. Marty FM, Lee SJ, Fahey MM, Alyea EP, Soiffer RJ, Antin JH, et al. Infliximab use in patients with severe graft-versus-host disease and other emerging risk factors of non-Candida invasive fungal infections in allogeneic hematopoietic stem cell transplant recipients: a cohort study. Blood. 2003;102:2768–76.
195. Couriel D, Saliba R, Hicks K, Ippoliti C, de Lima M, Hosing C, et al. Tumor necrosis factor-α blockade for the treatment of acute GVHD. Blood. 2004;104:649–54.
196. Rech J, Repp R, Rech D, Stockmeyer B, Dechant M, Niedobitek G, et al. A humanized HLA-DR antibody (hu1D10, apolizumab) in combination with granulocyte colony-stimulating factor (filgrastim) for the treatment of non-Hodgkin's lymphoma: a pilot study. Leuk Lymphoma. 2006;47:2147–54.
197. Marcus R, Imrie K, Belch A, Cunningham D, Flores E, Catalano J, et al. CVP chemotherapy plus rituximab compared with CVP as first-line treatment for advanced follicular lymphoma. Blood. 2005;105:1417–23.
198. Salles G, Mounier N, de Guibert S, Morschhauser F, Doyen C, Rossi JF, et al. Rituximab combined with chemotherapy and interferon in follicular lymphoma patients: results of the GELA-GOELAMS FL2000 study. Blood. 2008;112:4824–31.

Chapter 6
Postsurgery Infections in Cancer Patients

Emilio Bouza, Almudena Burillo, Juan Carlos Lopez-Gutierrez, and José F. Tomás-Martinez

Abstract Many different infections may occur after surgical events in patients with solid tumors, though infections of the operative site are the most common nosocomial infections in any surgical patient. Also frequent are infections of the lower respiratory tract, related or not to endotracheal intubation; of the urinary tract, usually related to the need for bladder or other urinary catheters; and bloodstream infections, mainly related to the use of intravascular catheters. This chapter reviews and discusses surgical site infections (SSI) produced after surgery for the most common tumors paying special attention to incidence, common clinical presentations and risk factors, diagnostic alertness, therapeutic principles, and particular aspects of prophylaxis if pertinent. Due to the existing variety of tumors and surgical procedures, we first address – from head to limbs – the most common tumors requiring surgery in adults and end the chapter with a section in which SSI are described in child cancer and compared to the situation in adults.

Keywords Neoplasms • Postoperative complications • Infection

Introduction

Many different infections may occur after surgical events in patients with solid tumors, though infections of the operative site are the most common nosocomial infections in any surgical patient [1]. Also frequent are infections of the lower respiratory tract, related or not to endotracheal intubation; of the urinary tract, usually related to the need for bladder or other urinary catheters; and bloodstream infections, mainly related to the use of intravascular catheters. These and other infections distant to the surgical site will be discussed in several other chapters of this book.

The general pathogenic mechanisms, therapeutic principles, and preventive measures for surgical site infections (SSIs) accepted for noncancer patients also generally apply to patients with solid tumors. This chapter reviews and discusses SSI produced after surgery for the most common tumors paying special attention to incidence, common clinical presentations and risk factors, diagnostic alertness, therapeutic principles, and particular aspects of prophylaxis if pertinent. Due to the existing variety of tumors and surgical procedures, we first address – from head to limbs – the most common tumors requiring surgery in adults and end the chapter with a section in which SSIs are described in child cancer and compared to the situation in adults.

Brain Cancer

Complications of cerebral spinal fluid (CSF) leakage and infections usually account for over half of all neurosurgery complications. Infections following brain cancer resection include superficial wound infection, subgaleal fluid collection infection, meningitis, and brain abscess. Other infections, such as postoperative pulmonary infections, may present in up to 25% of patients [2].

As with any other type of brain surgery, postoperative fever in patients with brain cancer may be caused by local inflammation induced by the surgical insult, tumor-associated fever, brain hemorrhage, central fever, or postoperative meningeal syndrome and is not always attributable to infection. In cases of SSI, fever onset usually occurs later than 72 h postsurgery.

Incidence

After a craniotomy, without the implant of a biomaterial, the incidence of infection is estimated at 0.3–5% depending on

E. Bouza (✉)
Clinical Microbiology and Infectious Diseases Department,
Hospital General Universitario Gregorio Marañón, Universidad Complutense de Madrid, Dr. Esquerdo 46, 28007 Madrid, Spain
and
CIBER de Enfermedades Respiratorias (CIBERES), 28007 Madrid, Spain
e-mail: ebouza@microb.net

the type of surgery, the presence of risk factors, the surgeon's skills, or the use of antibiotic prophylaxis, etc. [3–6]. In a recent study addressing this issue, McClelland and Hall examined the incidence of postoperative central nervous system infection after 2,111 neurosurgical procedures at their institution during a 15-year period [7], but the proportion of infections occurring in patients with cancer was not specified.

The incidence of infection among patients with a ventricular shunt [8] has steadily fallen with estimates in recent series running at 1.6–2.6% [7, 9].

Risk Factors

In the previously mentioned study by McClelland and Hall [7], the neurosurgical procedures associated with the highest rates of postoperative infection were CSF shunting (1.6%), followed by Ommaya reservoir placement (1.4%) and craniotomy for a mass, tumor, and/or lesion (1.1%). The risk factors for SSI following neurosurgery in cancer patients are prior neurosurgery, chemotherapy, radiotherapy, prolonged use of corticosteroids, a history of prior wound infection, prolonged intraoperative time, and the placement of a gliadel (BCNU) chemotherapy wafer into the brain tumor cavity [10, 11].

Risk factors for meningitis include CSF leak, concomitant incision infection, male sex, and duration of surgery [4].

The age groups most susceptible to ventricular shunt infection are infants under 1 year of age and elderly patients. Infections of a ventriculoatrial shunt are also more frequent than those of a ventriculoperitoneal shunt. The reimplantation of a shunt in the presence of an active infection at another anatomical site has also been linked to a greater infection risk.

Risk factors for postoperative pulmonary infection include type of surgery performed, prolonged mechanical ventilation over 48 h, time spent in the intensive care unit over 3 days, reduced level of consciousness, duration of surgery over 6 h, and previous chronic lung disease [2].

Etiology

The most common causative agents of superficial and deep-seated postneurosurgery infections are *Staphylococcus aureus* and Gram-negative bacilli, especially *Pseudomonas aeruginosa* and *Enterobacter* species [3, 4, 7]. *Propionibacterium acnes* is a rare but life-threatening cause of brain abscess or meningitis following neurosurgery [12]. If a foreign body is in place, such as a bone plate or a ventriculoperitoneal shunt, then coagulase-negative staphylococci are the most common cause of neurosurgical infection. Rarely, anaerobes such as anaerobic streptococci can provoke a deep-seated infection if the sinuses are entered during surgery.

Diagnosis

Craniotomy infection is frequently accompanied by osteomyelitis of the skull plate and manifests as a painful tumefaction with a purulent wound secretion, generally appearing within the first week of surgery.

Meningitis usually appears 7–10 days after surgery. It is more common after surgery performed at the suboccipital level and may occur in the absence of fever [4, 13]. Headache is the most constant clinical factor. CSF examination is of limited diagnostic value because cyto-biochemical variables may be normal or difficult to interpret. A positive Gram stain is obtained in a low proportion of cases (30–50%), and thus culture results need to be awaited. Prolonged incubation is recommended so that slow-growing microorganisms are not missed. Blood cultures may prove positive in a high proportion of patients, especially if the causal agent is *S. aureus* (64–100%).

Treatment

The drugs of choice for empirical therapy of deep-seated brain infection include intravenous vancomycin or linezolid for Gram-positive bacteria and meropenem or cefepime for Gram negatives. Osteomyelitis of the skull plate may require removal of the bone plate followed by placement of a titanium prosthesis. Radionecrosis of surrounding bone may lead to recurrent infection and chronic osteomyelitis despite the best of resection procedures.

Prevention

Antibiotic prophylaxis in craniotomy has proven effective in preventing SSI even in low-risk patients [3]. However prophylaxis does not clearly prevent meningitis and tends to select out antibiotic-resistant microorganisms [4]. The pathogenesis of postoperative meningitis is different from that of SSI in that the causative microorganisms are not acquired during the intraoperative period, but rather, later on as a consequence of a CSF leak.

Postoperative Infections Following Non-Neurosurgical Head and Neck Cancer Interventions

Patients undergoing head and neck oncologic surgery carry a high risk of complications [14]. These patients often have significant comorbidities and show a high anesthesia and surgery risk. An SSI in these patients can have devastating effects [15] leading to wound breakdown, mucocutaneous fistulae, esthetic and functional sequelae, and often severe sepsis and death. It can also prolong hospital stay and increase costs [16] and may delay the administration of radiotherapy or chemotherapy following surgery, which will increase the risk of tumor recurrence [17].

Incidence

Rates of SSI reported after clean-contaminated head and neck surgery range from 11 to 87% [16–22], and there is little doubt that bacterial contamination following the opening of the mucosal barriers increases the risk of SSI due mainly to the high bacterial load in saliva and mucosal surfaces [23].

Risk Factors

The main preoperative risk factors for SSI after head and neck surgery are age, previous radiotherapy, underlying diseases such as diabetes mellitus, an advanced tumor clinical stage, previous surgery, cigarette smoking, and alcohol consumption [22, 24–28]. Poor oral hygiene increases the risk of bacterial contamination of the surgical field [29].

Patients with laryngeal and hypopharyngeal tumors show a higher incidence of SSI [19].

Operative factors include technical skills of the surgeons, the extent of resection, methods of reconstruction, duration of surgery, and volume of blood transfused.

The following situations place patients with head or neck tumors at a higher risk of postoperative infection: total laryngectomy [24], stage III and IV tumors, composite resections, and flap reconstruction [22].

Performing a neck dissection appears to contribute to a higher incidence of infection [24], and skull base tumors present numerous surgery-related problems because of the involvement of functional structures, difficult access, and the creation of large defects after removal [20, 30, 31].

Postoperative factors include chemotherapy and exposure of tissues and prosthetic material to saliva and tracheal secretions. The impact of tracheotomy either before or after surgery on the incidence of SSI is still under debate [19, 24, 32, 33], but extending prophylaxis to exceed 48 h is also associated with an increased risk of infection [18, 19, 22, 32, 34].

In a retrospective review of 1,693 patients with cancer of the oral cavity, SSI occurred in 19.8% [35]. Wound infection also affected 69 out of 111 patients (62.1%) after oral and oropharynx cancer surgery with an immediate reconstruction [36].

Etiology

SSI in patients with head and neck tumors is commonly polymicrobial, and the role of individual microorganisms in its pathogenesis is difficult to assess. Etiologic agents frequently involved include microorganisms commonly found in oral flora such as staphylococci, streptococci, and anaerobic bacteria. However, when infections occur in patients already receiving antibiotics, resistant pathogens tend to predominate. These organisms include methicillin-resistant *S. aureus* (MRSA), Gram-negative rods, mainly *Enterobacteriaceae* and *P. aeruginosa*, and *Candida* species [23, 37].

Radionecrosis of the mandible may result in osteomyelitis, usually of polymicrobial cause.

Diagnosis

Diagnosis of infection is usually made on a clinical basis and a practical approach is to consider as infected any wound graded 4+ or above in the following scale: 0: no erythema, 1+: less than 1 cm of erythema, 2+: less than 5 cm of erythema and induration, 3+: greater than 5 cm of erythema and induration, 4+: purulent drainage, and 5+: wound breakdown with mucocutaneous fistula [29].

For a microbiological diagnosis, only specimens obtained during surgical examination of the wound or via radiology-guided puncture are considered valid since samples of wound secretions or from drainage tubes are often contaminated and results are not predictive of the bacteriologic findings in surgical samples [38].

Treatment

As in any SSI, surgical debridement is key in the treatment of these patients.

Empirical antibiotic treatment should be started in patients with cellulitis or systemic inflammatory response syndrome. There is no scientific evidence supporting one over another regimen recommended for empirical treatment. The antimicrobial selected should be active against commensal aerobes and anaerobes of the upper airways and against *P. aeruginosa* (meropenem or imipenem, piperacillin-tazobactam). In the context of a high incidence of MRSA, a glucopeptide or linezolid should be added.

Prevention

There is general agreement that perioperative antimicrobial prophylaxis should be given to patients undergoing clean-contaminated surgery for head and neck cancer. Rates of infection before prophylaxis could be as high as 87%, and after antimicrobial prophylaxis it may be reduced to below 10% [17, 29, 33, 39, 40]. There is still controversy regarding the drug of choice and the length of prophylaxis, but common recommendations include cephazolin or the combination of clindamycin with gentamicin [41]. Alternatives include amoxicillin-clavulanate [40], ampicillin/sulbactam [37, 42], and piperacillin-tazobactam [43].

In a prospective and comparative study involving 53 consecutive patients scheduled to receive either 1 or 3 day of antibiotic prophylaxis for major head or neck surgery, incidence of infection was not related to the duration of antibiotic prophylaxis [44].

Topical antibiotics have been advocated either alone or in combination with systemic therapy, but there is no clear evidence of their clinical benefits and the ecological implications of their use are a cause of serious concern [45–49].

A microorganism of particular importance is MRSA, which may colonize patients before surgery or be acquired in the postoperative period. A systematic search for MRSA colonization is mandatory in countries in which MRSA is a significant pathogen and for all major head and neck surgery procedures. Screening must be performed 7–10 days before surgery because if present, the time needed for MRSA decolonization before surgery is around 5 days [50]. In such a situation, the patient should be decolonized with topical mupirocin or other agents and with daily use of antiseptic soap while isolated in an individual room. In this case, surgical prophylaxis must include an antimicrobial agent active against MRSA such as vancomycin or teicoplanin [51].

In patients who acquire MRSA infection after surgery, contact isolation is also mandatory and antimicrobial therapy must include an agent active against MRSA such as the glycolipopeptides (vancomycin, teicoplanin, and daptomycin), linezolid, or other agents.

MRSA-infected patients require prolonged ICU stay and overall intrahospital stay, extra intensive care and medical care as well as additional costly antibiotics [51].

In a recent report from a maxillofacial unit in the United Kingdom, 14% of patients admitted for definitive treatment for previously untreated oral and oropharyngeal squamous cell carcinoma showed MRSA colonization and the two main risk factors were stage of cancer and free flap [52]. Compared to patients infected with methicillin-sensitive *S. aureus*, the MRSA group was associated with significantly longer hospitalization periods and intervals between admission and MRSA detection, as well as a significantly greater likelihood of a need for intravenous hyperalimentation, prior antibiotic use, and co-isolation of other pathogens [53].

Surgical Site Infections Following Breast Cancer Interventions

Infections following surgery for breast cancer include SSI from lumpectomy, mastectomy, and axillary lymph and node dissection. Breast expanders or implants can likewise become infected with pathogens commonly associated with a foreign device. Myocutaneous flaps can develop necrosis, fail to engraft or become infected. Rarely, chest wall infection (ribs and cartilage) can develop, especially if a mesh is present. Infection may lead to significant morbidity for the patient, delay in adjuvant treatments such as radiotherapy, and increased costs of care if the patient requires supplementary treatment due to infection [54–56].

In patients with postsurgical lymphedema, lymphangitis and erysipelas may develop, although these are not very frequent.

Incidence

The incidence of SSI after breast cancer surgery ranges from 0.8 to 30% [57–61] depending on the duration of surgery, underlying patient comorbidities, definitions used for infection, and other perioperative therapy. SSI has been reported in approximately 2.8% of mastectomy patients according to the most recent report by the National Healthcare Safety Network (NHSN) issued in 2008.

Risk Factors

The risk factors for SSI following breast cancer surgery are the same as for other body sites, including hematoma or seroma formation, prolonged surgical drains, lymphedema, prior chemotherapy or radiation therapy, reoperation for recurrence or to achieve better tumor-free margins, reconstructive surgery with implants, suboptimal prophylactic antibiotic dosing, smoking, a history of a previous SSI or postmastectomy wound infection, and skin flap necrosis

[56–59, 62–66]. The subset of patients undergoing immediate breast reconstruction is at a higher risk of infection [67, 68]. Knowledge of specific risk factors for SSI is essential to create a SSI risk stratification index specifically for breast operations.

Etiology

S. aureus is the most common pathogen followed by betahemolytic streptococci, enteric Gram-negative bacilli and, occasionally, rapidly growing mycobacteria [69]. *Pseudomonas* spp. may be found when infection of the cartilage of the costochondral junction is involved.

Diagnosis

According to the Centers for Disease Control (CDC), an SSI is diagnosed in the following situations: purulent drainage from the incision with or without laboratory confirmation; at least one of the following signs or symptoms of infection: pain or tenderness, localized swelling, redness, or heat, and incision deliberately opened by a surgeon; or an abscess or other evidence of infection involving the deep incision found on direct examination, during reoperation or by histopathologic or radiologic examination. A microbiological examination is only one of the criteria used for a diagnosis of SSI and is neither indispensable nor sufficient for a valid diagnosis.

Sometimes, patients who have undergone partial mastectomy, breast biopsy, or axillary lymph node excision shortly thereafter present with clinical signs (most notably erythema and edema) suggestive of infectious mastitis or inflammatory breast cancer. Representative histologic sections of involved skin usually reveal dilated dermal vessels with no specific evidence of infection or cancer. The hypothesis is that this might be due to interruption of lymph vessels. Although antibiotic therapy is generally ineffective, clinical findings resolve with time (from 2 months to 1 year). This condition should be considered in the differential diagnosis when this circumscribed patient population has such intervention-related symptoms [70].

Treatment

Mild incisional cellulitis can be treated with oral antibiotics, but nonresponding or extensive soft-tissue infection requires intravenous therapy. A minority of breast wound infections progress to a fully developed abscess. The pointing, fluctuant, and exquisitely tender mass of a breast abscess usually becomes apparent 1–2 weeks postoperatively and occurs at a lumpectomy, mastectomy, or axillary incision site. When there is uncertainty regarding the diagnosis (as may be the case with deep-seated abscesses after lumpectomy), ultrasound imaging may be helpful, but the complex mass that is visualized can appear identical to a consolidated seroma or hematoma. Aspiration may also confirm the diagnosis, but sampling error can mislead the clinician. Definitive management of an abscess requires incision and drainage; curative aspiration of purulent material is rarely successful, and the abscess generally reemerges. Usually incision and drainage can be accomplished by reopening the original surgical wound; the resulting cavity must be left open to heal by secondary intention. When recurrent cancer is a concern, it is prudent to perform a biopsy of the abscess cavity wall.

Prevention

In a review of antibiotic prophylaxis to prevent SSI after breast cancer surgery, it was shown that the infection risk is effectively reduced [68]. In this review, seven randomized controlled trials of pre- and perioperative antibiotics for patients undergoing surgery for breast cancer were included, with a total of 1,924 patients. Although there is no consensus as to the antibiotic of choice, additional postoperative doses are not recommended [61].

Suboptimal prophylactic antibiotic dosing is a potentially modifiable risk factor for SSI after breast operation [65]. Local infiltration of an anesthetic agent has been found to be associated with substantially reduced odds of SSI (odds ratio, OR 0.4; 95% confidence interval [CI] 0.1–0.9) [65].

Prevention of arm lymphedema and avoidance of any trauma to the arm are important prophylactic measures. Sentinel lymph node biopsy reduces the rate of axillary lymph node dissection and should thus reduce the incidence of lymphedema and erysipelas.

Infections Following Lung Cancer Interventions

The great majority of patients presenting with lung cancer are inoperable, and this disease is therefore very largely incurable [71].

Surgery-related infections following lung cancer resection include pneumonia, empyema, SSI, and bronchopleural fistula (BPF) formation. Extensive chest wall resections (defined as resection of at least one rib, and/or part of the sternum) can provoke a wide variety of complications, particularly, complicated wound healing [72].

Incidence

Pneumonia and acute respiratory distress syndrome (ARDS) are responsible for most postoperative deaths, accounting for 22–67% of all deaths following surgery [73, 74].

The incidence of postoperative pneumonia remains at 2–30% [72, 73, 75–78] and empyema complicates 6–10% of interventions [79].

BPF remains one of the most feared complications following surgery and affects between 2–12% of cases [77, 79, 80], usually as a late complication (10–45 days after surgery). Its associated mortality is around 60%.

SSI occurs less frequently (1–5%) [72, 75–78, 81].

Risk Factors

Risk factors for postoperative pneumonia include moderate to severe chronic obstructive pulmonary disease (COPD), perioperative/intraoperative airway colonization with a potential pathogen, age over 70 years, a high body mass index, the type and extent of resection, a high postoperative pain score, and type of prophylaxis [71, 73, 77, 78, 82].

BPF is most common following a right-sided pneumonectomy [71]. It is likelier if the residual bronchial stump is of larger diameter and if its blood supply has been reduced by surgical dissection. It is also more common with pleural space infection and empyema, which need prompt drainage to prevent the development of a stump infection [71, 73].

Etiology

Microorganisms causing postoperative pneumonia are Gram-negative bacteria and *Candida albicans* in 75% of patients [83], being acquired postoperatively from the patient's oral cavity and upper respiratory tract [83]. Most common causative pathogens include *Haemophilus influenzae*, *S. aureus*, Enterobacteriaceae, *Streptococcus pneumoniae*, *Aspergillus fumigatus*, MRSA, and *P. aeruginosa* [73].

Empyema due to chest tube placement is usually due to *S. aureus* (including MRSA) originating from skin colonization. Occasionally, enteric Gram-negative bacilli, alpha-hemolytic streptococci and *Candida* species cause empyema, especially if a BPF or esophageal anastomosis leak is present.

Diagnosis

The usefulness of procalcitonin (PCT) in the early detection of infection after thoracic surgery was evaluated by Falcoz et al. [84]. These authors found that the best cutoff value for detection of infection was 1 ng/mL, with an area under the ROC curve of 92% (95% CI 0.87–0.96). Thus, in patients with no postoperative infection, a steadily decreasing PCT level or a level <1 ng/mL is reassuring and may be helpful in deciding upon a safe early discharge.

In patients with suspected posterior mediastinitis, transesophageal endosonography with fine-needle aspiration of posterior mediastinal lesions is an effective and relatively noninvasive way to detect mediastinitis and provides material for culture to identify the etiologic agent [85].

Treatment

The mainstay of treatment is surgical drainage of pockets of fluid collection and appropriate antimicrobial therapy for 3–6 weeks. BPF may close spontaneously in time, but subsequent reoperation is frequently required. Chronic drainage of pleural fluid collections is necessary to prevent recurrent empyema and pneumonia.

Prevention

Antibiotic prophylaxis during surgery is effective at reducing the incidence of SSI and of postoperative pneumonia in these patients [82]. The antibiotics recommended for cardiothoracic procedures are cefazolin or cefuroxime, and alternatives are vancomycin or clindamycin [86].

Infections Following Surgery for Esophageal Cancer

Incidence

Major infections, including pneumonia, intra-abdominal or intrathoracic abscesses, sepsis or SSI requiring intervention, have been estimated to affect around 15–20% of patients undergoing esophageal surgery for cancer [87, 88]. Mediastinitis caused by anastomotic leaks is the most severe complication after esophagectomy and the major source of morbidity and mortality. It is characterized by local intrathoracic reactions (mediastinitis) and sepsis, and its incidence has been estimated at around 10% [81, 88].

Risk Factors

To determine risk factors for complications after esophageal resection for cancer, a prospective, nationwide, population-based study was conducted in Sweden in 2001–2003. Among 275 patients undergoing surgical resection for esophageal or cardiac cancer, 122 (44%) had at least one predefined complication. Thus, operations by low-volume surgeons (<5 operations annually) were followed by more anastomotic leakages than those conducted by higher-volume surgeons (OR 7.86; 95% CI 2.13–29.00). Hand-sewn and stapled anastomoses were associated with a similar risk of anastomotic leakage. Among the patients with cardiac cancer, a transthoracic approach resulted in more respiratory complications compared to a transhiatal (abdominal only) approach (OR 4.78; 95% CI 1.66–13.76). Older age, adjuvant oncologic therapy, and higher preoperative bleeding volume were related to a non-significantly greater risk of complications, while no influence of sex or tumor stage was found [88]. Other risk factors for complications include liver cirrhosis and cervical anastomosis [87].

Diagnosis

For successful management, early diagnostic workup is mandatory in every disturbance of the normal postoperative course. This includes direct endoscopic inspection of the anastomosis to evaluate the viability of the anastomosed organs and the size of leaks.

Treatment

According to the site and clinical classifications of the leak, the spectrum of therapeutic options ranges from simple drainage procedures, endoscopic interventions, and stent implantation to reoperation or discontinuity resection. In any case, the treatment goal must be immediate and should achieve sufficient drainage of the leakage and hindrance of further contamination across the leakage caused by gut contents. Also mandatory, is the early initiation of supportive systemic strategies according to pathophysiologic principles of sepsis [89]. The use of broad-spectrum antibiotics, such as piperacillin-tazobactam or a carbapenem, is recommended in these patients.

Turkyilmaz et al. recently presented a treatment algorithm for esophagogastric anastomotic leaks in their excellent review of this topic [90].

Prevention

The CDC's Guideline for Prevention of Surgical Site Infection, 1999 recommends several measures to reduce the SSI risk [91]. In patients with esophageal cancer and esophageal stenosis, the esophageal floral often switches to the fecal type. Thus, antimicrobial prophylaxis with the drugs used in colorectal surgery is recommended [92] such as a single dose of a third generation cephalosporin (ceftriaxone 2 g) and a nitroimidazole (metronidazole 1 g).

Intra-Abdominal Infections and Surgical Site Infections in Patients Undergoing GI Tract Interventions for Malignant Diseases

The main infections following gastrointestinal cancer surgery besides SSI are peritonitis, intra-abdominal abscess, and sepsis. Abdominal wall mesh infection may occur in patients requiring hernia repair following abdominal surgery for colorectal cancer. Enterocutaneous fistulas require prolonged bowel rest, and frequently, future bowel repair. Perineum infections can occur after abdominal perineal resection, as well as a presacral abscess, and much less frequently sacral osteomyelitis [93–95].

Postoperative infection in intra-abdominal cancer patients is clearly linked to a poorer prognosis and a higher mortality [96–100].

Incidence

The overall incidence of superficial or deep SSI after surgery for gastrointestinal cancers is 4.1% in patients receiving antimicrobial prophylaxis [101]. Figures in gastric cancer (2.8–18.7%), colon cancer (5.2–14.5%), and hepatic/biliary/pancreatic cancers (4.9%) are variable.

The incidence of space/organ SSI after surgery is higher in hepatic/biliary/pancreatic cancer (14.7%) than esophageal cancer (8.4%; $p=0.02$), gastric cancer (1.5–7.9%), or colon cancer (1.4–11.1%) [101–110].

Risk Factors

Risk factors for infection after surgery for intestinal cancer include advanced age, overweight, patient comorbidities, preoperative radiotherapy, emergency surgery, extended operation time, and combined organ resection [93, 95, 102–104, 109, 111–116]. Laparoscopic surgery for colorectal cancer is associated with a lower incidence of SSI than open colectomy [106, 117–119].

Table 6.1 Microorganisms isolated after laparotomy

Organism	Solomkin [127][a]	Mosdell [128][b]	Organism	Solomkin [127][a]	Mosdell [128][b]
Aerobic and facultative Gram positives			Aerobic and facultative Gram positives		
Escherichia coli	56.8	68.4	Streptococci	35.8	25.9
Enterobacter spp.	13.5	6.1	Enterococci	23.5	10.5
Klebsiella spp.	15.4	17	*Staphylococcus aureus* or *S. epidermidis*	10.5	10.5
Pseudomonas aeruginosa	14.8	19.1	Anaerobes		
Proteus spp.	6.2	2.7	*Bacteroides fragilis*	22.8	44.5
Serratia marcescens	1.2	4.1	*Bacteroides* spp.	21	–
Morganella spp.	1.2	–	*Clostridium* spp.	17.9	5.8
Citrobacter spp.	3.1	3.4	Peptococci/streptococci	7.4	16
Other	3.7	7.5	*Fusobacterium* spp.	6.2	5.1

Adapted from refs. [127, 128]
[a]Percentage of patients
[b]Percentage of abscesses

Risk factors for infection after resection of hepatic/biliary/pancreatic tumors include age older than 65 years, preoperative chemotherapy, type of surgery, the use of drainage tubes, the use of nonabsorbable silk sutures and bile leak, intraoperative bowel injury, blood loss >2,000 mL, and poor postoperative blood glucose control [120–126].

Etiology

Predominant pathogens include enteric Gram-negative bacilli, enteric anaerobes, enterococci, *S. aureus* (including MRSA), and *Candida* species, usually as part of a polymicrobial infection. The microorganisms isolated in patients with postsurgical peritonitis are shown in Table 6.1.

Diagnosis

Early focus identification by clinical, laboratory, and radiologic examination is of major importance. Sonography plays a minor role in the detection of intra-abdominal abscesses in patients undergoing colorectal surgery; computerized tomography (CT) and gallium scans are more helpful [129].

Treatment

Broad-spectrum antibiotics and sometimes also antifungals, occasionally for prolonged periods of time, along with surgical debridement and drainage, are needed for successful management. Postoperative infections are caused by more-resistant flora, which may include *P. aeruginosa*, *Enterobacter* spp., *Proteus* spp., MRSA, enterococci, and *Candida* spp. For these infections, complex multidrug regimens are recommended [130] since adequate empirical therapy is important to reduce mortality. Local nosocomial resistance patterns should guide empirical treatment, and treatment should be thereafter altered on the basis of the results of a thorough microbiologic workup of infected fluid.

These regimens include piperacillin/tazobactam; broad-spectrum carbapenems, including imipenem/cilastatin, meropenem, and doripenem; third- or fourth-generation cephalosporins plus metronidazole; and ciprofloxacin plus metronidazole. The regimen may be further broadened in selected patients to provide coverage of *Enterococcus*, yeast, and resistant gram-positive cocci.

In the case of progressive cancer, when the patient is no longer a surgery candidate, lifelong antimicrobial therapy may be needed to prevent further spread of infection. Aggressive radiation therapy may induce radiation colitis with perforation and fistula formation, which may require resection and a colostomy.

For severe intra-abdominal infection complicating colorectal disease, laparostomy may be useful in extreme circumstances [131].

Prevention

Antibiotic prophylaxis is effective to prevent postoperative SSI in patients with a gastrointestinal tumor [101, 132]. Prolonged antibiotic prophylaxis longer than 24 h does not reduce the SSI risk after elective gastric and colorectal surgery [133].

In a recently published meta-analysis, the oral and intravenous use of antibiotics covering aerobic and anaerobic bacteria is recommended prior to colorectal surgery, as antibiotics delivered within this framework reduced the risk of SSI by at least 75% [134]. In this meta-analysis, no statistically significant differences were detected when comparing short-and long-term duration of prophylaxis, or single dose vs. multiple dose antibiotics.

Supplemental perioperative oxygenation is beneficial in preventing SSI in patients undergoing colorectal surgery [135].

The administration of an immunonutrition diet preoperatively supplemented with two or more nutrients including glutamine, arginine, omega-3 polyunsaturated fatty acids, and ribonucleic acids has been identified as protective against the development of SSI (OR=0.41, $p<0.001$) [136, 137].

Infections Following Surgery for Genital and Urinary Tract Neoplasms

Genital and urinary tract neoplasms include a variety of tumors that are treated using different techniques and approaches.

In the case of gynecologic procedures, the risk of infection is directly related to the contaminating load of genital flora during surgery. Surgical procedures in the gynecologic oncology patient frequently leave behind large raw surfaces, such as in pelvic node dissection, extrafascial radical hysterectomy, pelvic exenteration, and debulking operations. The resulting rough areas, despite meticulous hemostasis, may lead to fluid collections and hematomas deep in the pelvis. Further, when bowel resection with or without primary anastomosis is part of the procedure, despite bowel preparation and a careful aseptic technique, fecal contamination frequently occurs. It is not surprising that the incidence of infected pelvic collections is higher in patients with gynecologic malignancies than in any other group of cancer patients, with the exception of patients with colorectal cancer.

The most serious type of infection after a hysterectomy is vaginal cuff infection. The cuff, created from the vaginal vault when the uterus is removed, is virtually always contaminated with vaginal flora and highly susceptible to postoperative infections. Vaginal cuff infections are more frequent after vaginal hysterectomy, but can also occur after abdominal hysterectomy. Cuff infections may be complicated by pelvic cellulitis and abscess formation [138]. In patients with pelvic exenteration, intestinal fistula formation is an uncommon but very serious complication [139].

Prostate cancer is the most common noncutaneous malignancy diagnosed in men older than 60 years. Advances in techniques, instrumentation, and surgical and perioperative management have made resection of the prostate a relatively safe procedure. Endoscopic extraperitoneal radical prostatectomy (EERPE) is a further advance in minimal invasive surgery as it overcomes the limitations of laparoscopic (transperitoneal) radical prostatectomy by the strictly extraperitoneal route of access, combining the advantages of minimal invasive surgery with those of an extraperitoneal procedure. The incidence of most complications directly correlates with the surgeon's experience.

Incidence

Brooker et al. [140] reported on 496 gynecologic oncology patients detecting an overall infection rate of 11%, excluding uncomplicated urinary tract infections (UTIs). The surgical infectious morbidity rate was 15%. By cancer site, rates of postoperative infection were 22% for cervical cancer, 12% for vulvar cancer, 12% for uterine cancer, and 11% for ovarian cancer. More recently, Iatrakis et al. [141] reported similar surgical infectious morbidities in a series of 1,180 gynecologic oncology patients.

After radical hysterectomy in patients with cervical or endometrial cancer, the incidence of SSI ranges from 3 to 20% [142, 143] and of vaginal cuff infection from 0.5 to 10% [142, 144]. SSI is more common in laparotomy patients while vaginal cuff infection occurs more frequently in patients undergoing a laparoscopic procedure. However, some studies have shown no differences in outcomes and costs of endometrial cancer treatment via traditional laparotomy, standard laparoscopy, and robotic techniques [145].

In urologic surgery (including radical or partial nephrectomy, nephroureterectomy, radical prostatectomy, and radical cystectomy), the incidence of postoperative infectious complications (SSI and UTI) ranges from <1–7% [146–149]. The incidence of postoperative UTI after transurethral resection of the prostate is around 5% [150].

Risk Factors

The patient's ultimate susceptibility to infection is influenced by factors inherent to the host, factors related to treatment, and factors associated with the malignant process [151]. Host factors include altered vaginal flora and microbial virulence, poor nutritional status, advanced age, comorbidities, and immunosuppression. Treatment-related factors include previous invasive diagnostic tests, adjuvant therapy with chemotherapy, radiotherapy or steroids, and complex surgical procedures (type of surgery, duration of the intervention) [143]. Tumor related-factors include malignancy-associated immunosuppression, microvascular alterations, necrotic tumor, and obstructive lesions.

The gamut of invasive diagnostic and therapeutic procedures that patients undergo increases the likelihood of infectious complications [151]. These procedures include cystoscopy, sigmoidoscopy, needle or incisional biopsy or both, conization, laparoscopy, dilatation and curettage, and invasive radiography. Any tumor that obstructs natural elimination pathways, such as the pulmonary, gastrointestinal, or urologic tracts, can also induce infection. Following urologic surgery, the most important risk factor for SSI is preoperative colonization of the urinary tract with bacteria (i.e., significant bacteriuria) [152]. Other risk factors are age [153] and patient comorbidities [148].

Etiology

The indigenous flora of the genital tract has long been considered a determining factor for postoperative infection [154]. However, though most infections in patients with gynecologic malignancies arise from the endogenous flora of the lower genital tract, especially anaerobic bacteria such as *Prevotella* spp., *Bacteroides* spp., and peptostreptococci, a significant percentage of infectious organisms are acquired during hospitalization. The most common isolates in such cases include *P. aeruginosa*, *Escherichia coli*, *Klebsiella pneumoniae*, *C. albicans*, and several *Enterobacteriaceae* [140].

Antibiotic prophylaxis in urologic patients with preoperative urinary tract bacterial colonization selects for more resistant pathogens that postoperatively cause UTI [152].

Diagnosis

Most wound infections become apparent 4–6 days postoperatively.

Posthysterectomy pelvic cellulitis presents with fever and lower pelvis pain, with an indurated and often exquisitely painful vaginal cuff 2–5 days after surgery. Postoperative pelvic abscesses of the vaginal cuff, pelvic floor, and sidewalls, or at the site of intra-abdominal blood or fluid collections, tend to present more than 5 days after the surgical procedure and may not manifest until after the patient has been discharged from the hospital. The clinical presentation of the patient with a pelvic abscess includes low-grade fever with mild-to-moderate abdominal pain and a pelvic mass.

Treatment

The preferred treatment for wound infections, whether superficial or deep, is still adequate drainage. No systemic antibiotics are usually administered, except to immunosuppressed patients, patients with an implanted prosthetic device (e.g., a mesh, infusion pumps), or patients with extensive cellulitis. Once the wound is clean, usually within 4–5 days, the wound edges can be reapproximated using skin tape (modified delayed secondary closure). Continued wet-to-dry dressing changes may result in adequate healing by secondary intention [155].

Management of postoperative pelvic abscess includes optimizing the patient's general status, antibiotic administration, and abscess drainage. Empiric antibiotic therapy should be directed against the microorganisms most likely to be recovered from the abscess. Surgical drainage is indicated for the treatment of postsurgical pelvic abscesses that fail to respond to maximal antibiotic therapy [151]. Percutaneous drainage of pelvic collections under ultrasound or CT guidance has proven to be a safe and effective alternative to open surgical drainage. A simple, well-defined abscess can be treated successfully by percutaneous drainage in more than 90% of cases. Even in patients in whom abscess elimination is not accomplished by percutaneous drainage, this maneuver facilitates subsequent surgery by diminishing the local inflammatory response.

Prevention

Today, the incidence of postoperative pelvic abscess with the use of prophylactic antibiotics is 1–4% for vaginal hysterectomy and 0.1% for abdominal hysterectomy. The American College of Obstetricians and Gynecologists has just issued its updated antibiotic prophylaxis guidelines for gynecologic procedures [156].

In these guidelines, level A recommendations (based on consistent scientific evidence) are single-dose antimicrobial prophylaxis given preoperatively to patients undergoing hysterectomy or elective suction curettage abortion, and *no* such prophylaxis in patients undergoing diagnostic laparoscopy. Level B recommendations (based on limited or inconsistent scientific evidence) include no antibiotic prophylaxis for hysteroscopic surgery.

The American Urological Association (AUA) recently published their guidelines for antimicrobial prophylaxis in urologic surgery [157]. These guidelines provide information on antimicrobial agents used for specific procedures, the duration of antimicrobial therapy, and doses. Antimicrobial prophylaxis is recommended for most urologic operations, including transurethral endoscopic, open or laparoscopic procedures, as well as extracorporeal shock wave lithotripsy. For some procedures, such as those not accessing the urinary tract, these guidelines endorse antimicrobial prophylaxis only in patients with a high risk of infection. Several issues remain to be addressed, especially operations in which bowel segments are grafted. These are classified as clean-contaminated operations in the CDC guidelines for the prevention of SSI [91] but as contaminated in the Japanese Urological Association (JUA) guidelines. In addition, the choice of antibiotics and optimal duration of antimicrobial prophylaxis for bowel segment procedures have yet to be determined. Another unresolved issue is whether laparoscopic operations require the same antimicrobial prophylaxis regimens as open surgery procedures [158].

Infections Following Limb Interventions in Cancer Patients

Bone and soft-tissue sarcomas account for only about 2% of all malignancies. Their treatment aims to both cure the patient and preserve the functionality of the affected body part. Several techniques of reconstruction have been advocated and have gained popularity following malignant tumor resection due to the introduction of allografts, tumor prostheses, composite allograft prostheses, or the technique of arthrodesis.

Endoprostheses are of established use to reconstruct defects following bone tumor resection. The long-term durability of reconstruction is excellent, with long-term limbsalvage achieved in 91% of patients at 20 years postsurgery. The main reasons for secondary amputation are locally recurrent disease and deep periprosthetic infection. Infection remains one of the greatest threats for early failure of a reconstruction using an endoprosthesis [159]. Most series of patients undergoing reconstructions show a periprosthetic infection rate of approximately 10% [160, 161]. Infection most frequently occurs within 12 months of the last surgical procedure. However, the risk of infection is life-long [162]. Risk factors for infection are preoperative radiotherapy and a tumor size over 5 cm [163]. The most common pathogenic organism is coagulase-negative *Staphylococcus*. The most effective treatment for deep infection is two-stage revision, with local treatments being of little use to cure a deep infection. Research is on-going into surface treatments with silver and other materials to help reduce infection rates. Jeys and Grimer have recently published an excellent review on the outcome of the use of endoprostheses in limb salvage surgery for the treatment of bone tumors [161].

Antibiotic prophylaxis is warranted in all patients undergoing surgery for limb cancer. When the patient requires major limb amputation, antibiotic prophylaxis has been shown to significantly reduce the rate of stump infection [164].

Emerging Prevention and Management Trends for Cancer Surgery Infections

In the near future, it is anticipated that we will continue to see developments in minimally invasive procedures. Laparoscopic surgery and video-assisted thoracoscopy have rapidly expanded in a number of applications. The net effect of the minimally invasive surgical strategy is that the surgical wound, as the origin of so many infectious complications in the past, will be far smaller and that the frequency and severity of SSI will most likely be reduced. Minimally invasive techniques should reduce the risks of bacterial contamination of the abdominal cavity, the pleural space, and the joint spaces manipulated in the operative procedure. Following surgery, workup of infection is most commonly prompted by fever. However, the presence of fever as a predictive factor for postoperative infections has been examined many times in the literature, and almost all studies have demonstrated its lack of sensitivity (14–60%) and specificity (69–80%), both in adult and pediatric patients [165–168]. Unnecessary workups initiated because of fever increase hospital costs, unnecessarily worry patients, and prolong hospital stay. Notwithstanding, the timing of postoperative fever is significant. Hence, fever that begins beyond the fifth postoperative day is much more likely to indicate a clinically significant infection [169].

In a growing number of reports, a relationship between intraoperative body temperature and the risk of postoperative SSI is starting to emerge. Thus, close attention paid to normothermia in the operating room, routine body temperature measurements during surgery, and correction of low body temperatures could reduce the number of SSI.

Evolving issues in the prevention of SSI also include tight adherence to prophylactic antibiotic guidelines, and good glycemic control and supplemental oxygenation during surgery [135, 170–173].

General risk factors for surgery and preventive measures apply to all types of procedure [91].

Postoperative Infections in Children with Cancer

Survival rates in children with cancer have improved dramatically over the past 30 years. Identifying biological and genetic characteristics as risk factors for the various tumors has led to changes in treatment using risk-based management as the template for care. Refinements in surgery, chemotherapy, and radiation therapy have been particularly helpful [174]. Surgery plays a pivotal role in treating most childhood cancers. Whether surgically removing a tumor, supporting nonsurgical treatment such as chemotherapy, or performing reconstructive surgery, the pediatric surgeon contributes to the comprehensive care of each child.

Despite significant advances in supportive care during the last years, infection remains a major cause of therapy-associated morbidity and death. Pediatric cancer patients have an increased risk of potentially life-threatening infectious complications due to their underlying illnesses and aggressive anticancer treatment. Rates of septicemia and its mortality are significantly higher in malignant hematologic disease than in solid tumors [175]. Major factors associated with the occurrence of postoperative infections in children with cancer include length of the surgical procedure and surgical procedure category (class I-clean, class II clean-contaminated, class III-contaminated, and class IV dirty-infected). Minor factors include age, myelosuppressive therapy with preoperative anemia, neutropenia or lymphopenia, bone marrow transplant, remote infection, obesity, malnutrition, central venous access devices, chemotherapy and radiotherapy [176], type of tumor [168], disease state (primary active, recurrent active, primary remission, or secondary remission) [10, 177, 178], operation room (intensive care unit vs. operating room), emergency operation, extensive surgery [178], length of intervention [168], surgical bleeding, external drains [121], and reoperation.

Risk Factors

Age

Infections in a pediatric oncologic surgery unit show a very different pattern to infections in adults. In children, it is widely accepted that surgery-related risk factors are more important than those related to the physiologic status of the patient. In general, children show a better overall success rate of surgery and lower mortality than adults. Death from infection is only 1% in children. Both neonates and children with cancer show a lower incidence of postsurgical infection (2–4%) and a lower surgery-related mortality [179–182].

Malignant neonatal tumors are rare and comprise 2% of childhood malignancies. This is an interesting group of tumors because their natural history and response to treatment differ from those seen in older children. Histologic type distributions (neuroblastoma 60%, mesenchymal tumors 15%, and brain tumors 10%) also differ considerably to those seen in older children such that oncologists are often faced with diagnostic, therapeutic and ethical challenges. A given neoplasm can be extremely malignant in an older child, while the same tumor type in a newborn may be generally well circumscribed and show benign biological behavior. Most patients undergo surgical resection and approximately 50% of neonates receive chemotherapy administered at a 30–50% reduced dose. Hematologic toxicities and infections are the main therapeutic complications. Nosocomial infection in newborns with solid tumors is significantly related to gender, birth weight, and the use of a central venous catheter (CVC) [183, 184]. Other devices including artificial ventilation, an umbilical artery catheter, umbilical venous catheter, and urinary catheter are not significant risk factors [185, 186].

Type of Tumor

Brain tumors are sometimes associated with abscess formation. Intrasellar or parasellar tumors are among the brain tumors that most frequently develop bacterial abscesses as the result of direct migration of flora from the paranasal sinuses. Intraparenchymal posterior fossa neoplasms harboring intratumoral abscesses are rare and, in such cases, a bloodstream route of spread has to be considered. All meningiomas with this complication reported have been parasagittally located.

SSI is not uncommon following abdominal cancer surgery and can be associated with serious morbidity, mortality, and increased resource utilization [187]. Our experience suggests that laparotomy infections in children are related more to factors inherent to the surgical procedure than to the overall physiologic status of the patient.

Surgery for colorectal tumors has returned some of the highest rates of infectious complications, but fortunately these tumors rarely appear in children.

The prognosis for children with bone sarcoma treated with limb-sparing surgery has improved considerably over the past 20 years, but this has also meant an increase in the number of complications requiring treatment. Limb-sparing wide excision is now as effective as amputation for treating limb sarcoma. Limb reconstruction traditionally involved allografting, but current reconstructive procedures include the use of a microvascular-free fibula flap, associated with a lower infection rate (around 15%) than traditional allograft reconstruction (even considering that vancomycin-supplemented allografts restore bone stock and provide sound fixation with a low incidence of further infection) [188]. If an endoprosthesis is used, it should be a "growing endoprosthesis" that requires revision to an adult prosthesis around the time of skeletal maturity. Gaur et al. report a SSI incidence of 16.5% and orthopedic device infection incidence of 21.3% in children and young adults with bone malignancies undergoing limb-sparing surgery [189]. Nonunion of the allograft-host junction after bone transplantation is not uncommon, and its treatment is frequently problematic. The greater the number of surgical procedures, the worse is the outcome. The rate of nonunions significantly increases in patients who receive chemotherapy as compared to patients not given chemotherapy. In order, the allograft types associated with the highest rates of infection and nonunion to the lowest rates are alloarthrodesis, intercalary, osteoarticular, and alloprostheses. The fracture rate is also higher in children with infection and nonunions than in those without infection or nonunions [189, 190].

Other Risk Factors

Minimally invasive surgery (MIS). Thoracoscopic and laparoscopic techniques play a major role in pediatric surgery. MIS is already established in pediatric oncology surgical treatment. So far in our experience, MIS is performed in every fourth patient and has proved to be an excellent approach in diagnostic interventions and tumor biopsies, whereas its efficacy is more limited in tumor resections [191]. Further factors (tumor recurrence, trocar site recurrence, tumor growth, and dissemination after CO_2 insufflation) still need to be assessed. Despite several reports on MIS procedures at several institutions, no significant differences have been found in the incidence of superficial or deep SSI, and at present surgeons are attempting to perform more oncological procedures as minimally invasive procedures.

Robot-assisted surgery represents an improvement over MIS that will most likely be increasingly utilized. Children as young as 5 months and as small as 20 lb have successfully undergone robotic surgery. Initial experience indicates that the robotic system is associated with an acceptable risk for SSI. Technologic advances in surgery will continue to be evaluated from an infection control viewpoint as the operating room remains a dynamic environment undergoing rapid change and innovation.

Neutropenia. Severe neutropenia is defined as an absolute neutrophil count (ANC) $<0.5 \times 10^9$/L or a decreasing leukocyte count $<1.0 \times 10^9$/L with no differential count available. In pediatric patients with SSI, the proportion of patients with neutropenia at the onset of infection is around 25%.

Therapy-induced neutropenia is the most important risk factor for infection in pediatric patients with hematologic cancer, but other factors, such as alterations in skin/mucosal barriers, and defects in cell-mediated or humoral immunity, also contribute to the risk of infection [192, 193]. The management of pediatric oncology patients with fever and neutropenia assumes that all patients are at risk of bacteremia, and therefore generally involves hospitalization and broad-spectrum parenteral antibiotics.

The incidence of postoperative SSI has been estimated at 3% in nonimmunocompromised children with a preoperative ANC under 1,000/mL, similar to the overall SSI rate in children with normal ANC. Thus, the cancelation of an elective surgery procedure in children with an ANC under 1,000/mL is not warranted on the grounds of concern about postoperative infection.

CVCs. Neutropenia is recognized as a risk factor for infection and compromised wound healing. The placement of a CVC in neutropenic children is associated with substantial infectious morbidity [179, 194]. In our recent experience (5 years), among children diagnosed with acute lymphocytic leukemia or aplastic anemia and a low ANC who receive a CVC, the removal of a port is more likely than the removal of a Hickman catheter for any reason including infection [195, 196]. When possible, CVC, particularly ports, should be avoided in the presence of neutropenia. Other authors have reported no differences in the risk of infection between tunneled catheters and implanted ports [194] or attributed a significantly higher rate of bloodstream infection to the use of Hickman catheters compared to implantable ports (4.6 vs. 1.45 episodes per 1,000 catheter-days) [197].

Despite the management benefits offered by permanent CVC, it is clear that children with a CVC show an increased rate of infection and their use should be carefully contemplated. The most important consideration is that fever >39.5°C in a child with a CVC is likely to be associated with a documented infection irrespective of the neutrophil count [194].

Nutrition. The frequencies of superficial, deep, and organ/space SSI in children with cancer who fail to thrive have been well documented. Preoperative enteral immunonutrition appears to be effective for preventing SSI in children with cancer and malnutrition [198]. Nutrition via a nasogastric tube or by means of a gastrostomy in children with cancer has several advantages. Gastrostomy is rarely associated with more than minor complications (the most frequent complication is inflammation during periods of neutropenia), it is cosmetically more acceptable than the nasogastric tube and it improves nutrition at a far lower cost than parenteral nutrition. In selected cases in which bone marrow transplantation or intensive treatment protocols are planned, gastrostomy should be considered before malnutrition develops to avoid surgical infection complications.

Blood transfusion. Perioperative blood transfusion carries numerous potential risks for the transmission of infective diseases, and immunosuppression will promote the occurrence of postoperative infectious complications. The link between perioperative blood transfusion and postoperative septic complications worldwide has not been well documented.

In conclusion, the accurate identification of risk factors is essential to design strategies aimed at preventing potentially devastating postsurgery infections in children [199]. In every pediatric oncology center, a team comprising surgeons, anesthesiologists, operating room nurses, oncologists, microbiologists, pharmacists, postoperative inpatient and clinical nurses, infection control professionals, and healthcare epidemiologists, among others is directly responsible for the prevention of nosocomial infections. Hospital guidelines for postoperative infection control in pediatric cancer patients have to be defined, personnel roles and processes should be standardized, and we should also try to encourage communication/education among health care professionals.

References

1. Tetteroo GW, Wagenvoort JH, Bruining HA. Role of selective decontamination in surgery. Br J Surg. 1992;79(4):300–4.
2. Sogame LC, Vidotto MC, Jardim JR, Faresin SM. Incidence and risk factors for postoperative pulmonary complications in elective intracranial surgery. J Neurosurg. 2008;109(2):222–7.
3. Korinek AM, Golmard JL, Elcheick A, Bismuth R, van Effenterre R, Coriat P, et al. Risk factors for neurosurgical site infections after craniotomy: a critical reappraisal of antibiotic prophylaxis on 4,578 patients. Br J Neurosurg. 2005;19(2):155–62.
4. Korinek AM, Baugnon T, Golmard JL, van Effenterre R, Coriat P, Puybasset L. Risk factors for adult nosocomial meningitis after craniotomy: role of antibiotic prophylaxis. Neurosurgery. 2008;62 Suppl 2:532–9.
5. Bohman LE, Gallardo J, Hankinson TC, Waziri AE, Mandigo CE, McKhann II GM, et al. The survival impact of postoperative infection in patients with glioblastoma multiforme. Neurosurgery. 2009;64(5):828–34. discussion 834–5.
6. Huo L, Bi C, Fang J, Wang Y, Zhang M, Chen F. Microsurgical treatment and prevention of postoperative complications for the fourth ventricle tumors in adults. Zhong Nan Da Xue Xue Bao Yi Xue Ban. 2009;34(7):642–5.
7. McClelland III S, Hall WA. Postoperative central nervous system infection: incidence and associated factors in 2111 neurosurgical procedures. Clin Infect Dis. 2007;45(1):55–9.
8. Gardner P, Leipzig T, Phillips P. Infections of central nervous system shunts. Med Clin North Am. 1985;69(2):297–314.
9. Federico G, Tumbarello M, Spanu T, Rosell R, Iacoangeli M, Scerrati M, et al. Risk factors and prognostic indicators of bacterial meningitis in a cohort of 3580 postneurosurgical patients. Scand J Infect Dis. 2001;33(7):533–7.
10. Angerpointner TA, Schmidt P, Donhauser U, Haas R, Bender-Gotze C. Postoperative course in children with malignant tumors following preoperative chemotherapy. Klin Padiatr. 1989;201(3):209–12.
11. Greene JN, Nicoonahad N. Complications of surgery in cancer patients. In: Greene JN, editor. Infections in cancer patients. New York: Marcel Dekker; 2004. p. 373–8.
12. Nisbet M, Briggs S, Ellis-Pegler R, Thomas M, Holland D. *Propionibacterium acnes*: an under-appreciated cause of postneurosurgical infection. J Antimicrob Chemother. 2007;60(5):1097–103.
13. Zarrouk V, Vassor I, Bert F, Bouccara D, Kalamarides M, Bendersky N, et al. Evaluation of the management of postoperative aseptic meningitis. Clin Infect Dis. 2007;44(12):1555–9.
14. Simo R, French G. The use of prophylactic antibiotics in head and neck oncological surgery. Curr Opin Otolaryngol Head Neck Surg. 2006;14(2):55–61.
15. Grandis JR, Snyderman CH, Johnson JT, Yu VL, D'Amico F. Postoperative wound infection. A poor prognostic sign for patients with head and neck cancer. Cancer. 1992;70(8):2166–70.
16. Penel N, Lefebvre JL, Cazin JL, Clisant S, Neu JC, Dervaux B, et al. Additional direct medical costs associated with nosocomial infections after head and neck cancer surgery: a hospital-perspective analysis. Int J Oral Maxillofac Surg. 2008;37(2):135–9. Epub 2007 Nov 19.
17. Weber RS, Callender DL. Antibiotic prophylaxis in clean-contaminated head and neck oncologic surgery. Ann Otol Rhinol Laryngol Suppl. 1992;155:16–20.
18. Barry B, Lucet JC, Kosmann MJ, Gehanno P. Risk factors for surgical wound infections in patients undergoing head and neck oncologic surgery. Acta Otorhinolaryngol Belg. 1999;53(3):241–4.
19. Penel N, Lefebvre D, Fournier C, Sarini J, Kara A, Lefebvre JL. Risk factors for wound infection in head and neck cancer surgery: a prospective study. Head Neck. 2001;23(6):447–55.
20. Ganly I, Patel SG, Singh B, Kraus DH, Bridger PG, Cantu G, et al. Complications of craniofacial resection for malignant tumors of the skull base: report of an International Collaborative Study. Head Neck. 2005;27(6):445–51.
21. Ganly I, Patel SG, Singh B, Kraus DH, Bridger PG, Cantu G, et al. Craniofacial resection for malignant paranasal sinus tumors: report of an International Collaborative Study. Head Neck. 2005;27(7):575–84.
22. Lotfi CJ, Cavalcanti Rde C, Costa e Silva AM, Latorre Mdo R, Ribeiro Kde C, Carvalho AL, et al. Risk factors for surgical-site infections in head and neck cancer surgery. Otolaryngol Head Neck Surg. 2008;138(1):74–80.
23. Barry B. Pharyngeal flora in patients undergoing head and neck oncologic surgery. Acta Otorhinolaryngol Belg. 1999;53(3):237–40.
24. Coskun H, Erisen L, Basut O. Factors affecting wound infection rates in head and neck surgery. Otolaryngol Head Neck Surg. 2000;123(3):328–33.
25. Penel N, Fournier C, Lefebvre D, Roussel-Delvallez M, Sarini J, Kara A, et al. Previous chemotherapy as a predictor of wound infections in nonmajor head and neck surgery: results of a prospective study. Head Neck. 2004;26(6):513–7.
26. Schwartz SR, Yueh B, Maynard C, Daley J, Henderson W, Khuri SF. Predictors of wound complications after laryngectomy: a study of over 2000 patients. Otolaryngol Head Neck Surg. 2004;131(1):61–8.
27. Fusconi M, Gallo A, Vitiello C, Pagliuca G, Pulice G, de Vincentiis M. Clean-contaminated neck surgery: risk of infection by intrinsic and extrinsic factors. Arch Otolaryngol Head Neck Surg. 2006;132(9):953–7.
28. Valentini V, Cassoni A, Marianetti TM, Mitro V, Gennaro P, Ialongo C, et al. Diabetes as main risk factor in head and neck reconstructive surgery with free flaps. J Craniofac Surg. 2008;19(4):1080–4.
29. Tabet JC, Johnson JT. Wound infection in head and neck surgery: prophylaxis, etiology and management. J Otolaryngol. 1990;19(3):197–200.
30. Kryzanski JT, Annino Jr DJ, Heilman CB. Complication avoidance in the treatment of malignant tumors of the skull base. Neurosurg Focus. 2002;12(5):e11.
31. Brown SM, Anand VK, Tabaee A, Schwartz TH. Role of perioperative antibiotics in endoscopic skull base surgery. Laryngoscope. 2007;117(9):1528–32.
32. Penel N, Fournier C, Lefebvre D, Lefebvre JL. Multivariate analysis of risk factors for wound infection in head and neck squamous cell carcinoma surgery with opening of mucosa. Study of 260 surgical procedures. Oral Oncol. 2005;41(3):294–303.
33. Johnson JT, Myers EN, Thearle PB, Sigler BA, Schramm Jr VL. Antimicrobial prophylaxis for contaminated head and neck surgery. Laryngoscope. 1984;94(1):46–51.
34. Arriaga MA, Kanel KT, Johnson JT, Myers EN. Medical complications in total laryngectomy: incidence and risk factors. Ann Otol Rhinol Laryngol. 1990;99(8):611–5.
35. Liu SA, Wong YK, Poon CK, Wang CC, Wang CP, Tung KC. Risk factors for wound infection after surgery in primary oral cavity cancer patients. Laryngoscope. 2007;117(1):166–71.

36. Belusic-Gobic M, Car M, Juretic M, Cerovic R, Gobic D, Golubovic V. Risk factors for wound infection after oral cancer surgery. Oral Oncol. 2007;43(1):77–81. Epub 2006 Jun 27.
37. Callender DL. Antibiotic prophylaxis in head and neck oncologic surgery: the role of gram-negative coverage. Int J Antimicrob Agents. 1999;12 Suppl 1:S21–5. discussion S26-7.
38. Becker GD. Ineffectiveness of closed suction drainage cultures in the prediction of bacteriologic findings in wound infections in patients undergoing contaminated head and neck cancer surgery. Otolaryngol Head Neck Surg. 1985;93(6):743–7.
39. Becker GD, Parell GJ. Cefazolin prophylaxis in head and neck cancer surgery. Ann Otol Rhinol Laryngol. 1979;88(2 Pt 1):183–6.
40. Skitarelic N, Morovic M, Manestar D. Antibiotic prophylaxis in clean-contaminated head and neck oncological surgery. J Craniomaxillofac Surg. 2007;35(1):15–20. Epub 2007 Feb 12.
41. Antimicrobial prophylaxis for surgery. Treat Guidel Med Lett. 2009;7(82):47–52.
42. Johnson JT, Kachman K, Wagner RL, Myers EN. Comparison of ampicillin/sulbactam versus clindamycin in the prevention of infection in patients undergoing head and neck surgery. Head Neck. 1997;19(5):367–71.
43. Simons JP, Johnson JT, Yu VL, Vickers RM, Gooding WE, Myers EN, et al. The role of topical antibiotic prophylaxis in patients undergoing contaminated head and neck surgery with flap reconstruction. Laryngoscope. 2001;111(2):329–35.
44. Liu SA, Tung KC, Shiao JY, Chiu YT. Preliminary report of associated factors in wound infection after major head and neck neoplasm operations – does the duration of prophylactic antibiotic matter? J Laryngol Otol. 2008;122(4):403–8. Epub 2007 Apr 20.
45. Ramos Macias A, de Miguel Martinez I, del Canizo Fernandez-Roldan A, Ibanez Perez R, Benito Garcia L. Changes in the flora of the oral cavity after oral topical antibiotics. Importance in antimicrobial prophylaxis in surgery of the neck and head. Acta Otorrinolaringol Esp. 1990;41(5):347–50.
46. Kirchner JC, Edberg SC, Sasaki CT. The use of topical oral antibiotics in head and neck prophylaxis: is it justified? Laryngoscope. 1988;98(1):26–9.
47. Grandis JR, Vickers RM, Rihs JD, Yu VL, Johnson JT. Efficacy of topical amoxicillin plus clavulanate/ticarcillin plus clavulanate and clindamycin in contaminated head and neck surgery: effect of antibiotic spectra and duration of therapy. J Infect Dis. 1994;170(3):729–32.
48. Grandis JR, Vickers RM, Rihs JD, Yu VL, Wagner RL, Kachman KK, et al. The efficacy of topical antibiotic prophylaxis for contaminated head and neck surgery. Laryngoscope. 1994;104(6 Pt 1):719–24.
49. Elledge ES, Whiddon Jr RG, Fraker JT, Stambaugh KI. The effects of topical oral clindamycin antibiotic rinses on the bacterial content of saliva on healthy human subjects. Otolaryngol Head Neck Surg. 1991;105(6):836–9.
50. Miyake M, Ohbayashi Y, Iwasaki A, Ogawa T, Nagahata S. Risk factors for methicillin-resistant Staphylococcus aureus (MRSA) and use of a nasal mupirocin ointment in oral cancer inpatients. J Oral Maxillofac Surg. 2007;65(11):2159–63.
51. Watters K, O'Dwyer TP, Rowley H. Cost and morbidity of MRSA in head and neck cancer patients: what are the consequences? J Laryngol Otol. 2004;118(9):694–9.
52. Rogers SN, Proczek K, Sen RA, Hughes J, Banks P, Lowe D. Which patients are most at risk of methicillin resistant Staphylococcus aureus: a review of admissions to a regional maxillofacial ward between 2001 and 2005. Br J Oral Maxillofac Surg. 2008;46(6):439–44. Epub 2008 Jun 13.
53. Shiomori T, Miyamoto H, Udaka T, Okochi J, Hiraki N, Hohchi N, et al. Clinical features of head and neck cancer patients with methicillin-resistant Staphylococcus aureus. Acta Otolaryngol. 2007;127(2):180–5.
54. Coello R, Glenister H, Fereres J, Bartlett C, Leigh D, Sedgwick J, et al. The cost of infection in surgical patients: a case-control study. J Hosp Infect. 1993;25(4):239–50.
55. Landes G, Harris PG, Lemaine V, Perreault I, Sampalis JS, Brutus JP, et al. Prevention of surgical site infection and appropriateness of antibiotic prescribing habits in plastic surgery. J Plast Reconstr Aesthet Surg. 2008;61(11):1347–56. Epub 2008 Jun 16.
56. Olsen MA, Chu-Ongsakul S, Brandt KE, Dietz JR, Mayfield J, Fraser VJ. Hospital-associated costs due to surgical site infection after breast surgery. Arch Surg. 2008;143(1):53–60. discussion 61.
57. Leinung S, Schonfelder M, Winzer KJ, Schuster E, Gastinger I, Lippert H, et al. Wound infection and infection-promoting factors in breast cancer surgery – a prospective multicenter study on quality control. Zentralbl Chir. 2005;130(1):16–20.
58. Ruvalcaba-Limon E, Robles-Vidal C, Poitevin-Chacon A, Chavez-Macgregor M, Gamboa-Vignolle C, Vilar-Compte D. Complications after breast cancer surgery in patients treated with concomitant preoperative chemoradiation: a case-control analysis. Breast Cancer Res Treat. 2006;95(2):147–52. Epub 2005 Dec 1.
59. Vitug AF, Newman LA. Complications in breast surgery. Surg Clin North Am. 2007;87(2):431–51. x.
60. Penel N, Yazdanpanah Y, Chauvet MP, Clisant S, Giard S, Neu JC, et al. Prevention of surgical site infection after breast cancer surgery by targeted prophylaxis antibiotic in patients at high risk of surgical site infection. J Surg Oncol. 2007;96(2):124–9.
61. Throckmorton AD, Boughey JC, Boostrom SY, Holifield AC, Stobbs MM, Hoskin T, et al. Postoperative prophylactic antibiotics and surgical site infection rates in breast surgery patients. Ann Surg Oncol. 2009;16(9):2464–9.
62. Morris DM, Robbins K. The effect of method of biopsy and timing of mastectomy on the development of postmastectomy nosocomial wound infection. J La State Med Soc. 1988;140(8):37–41.
63. Tran CL, Langer S, Broderick-Villa G, DiFronzo LA. Does reoperation predispose to postoperative wound infection in women undergoing operation for breast cancer? Am Surg. 2003;69(10):852–6.
64. Felippe WA, Werneck GL, Santoro-Lopes G. Surgical site infection among women discharged with a drain in situ after breast cancer surgery. World J Surg. 2007;31(12):2293–9. discussion 2300–1.
65. Olsen MA, Lefta M, Dietz JR, Brandt KE, Aft R, Matthews R, et al. Risk factors for surgical site infection after major breast operation. J Am Coll Surg. 2008;207(3):326–35.
66. Sorensen LT, Horby J, Friis E, Pilsgaard B, Jorgensen T. Smoking as a risk factor for wound healing and infection in breast cancer surgery. Eur J Surg Oncol. 2002;28(8):815–20.
67. Mortenson MM, Schneider PD, Khatri VP, Stevenson TR, Whetzel TP, Sommerhaug EJ, et al. Immediate breast reconstruction after mastectomy increases wound complications: however, initiation of adjuvant chemotherapy is not delayed. Arch Surg. 2004;139(9):988–91.
68. Cunningham M, Bunn F, Handscomb K. Prophylactic antibiotics to prevent surgical site infection after breast cancer surgery. Cochrane Database Syst Rev. 2006;2:CD005360.
69. Blancas D, Santin M, Olmo M, Alcaide F, Carratala J, Gudiol F. Group B streptococcal disease in nonpregnant adults: incidence, clinical characteristics, and outcome. Eur J Clin Microbiol Infect Dis. 2004;23(3):168–73.
70. Loprinzi CL, Okuno S, Pisansky TM, Steriof S, Gaffey TA, Morton RF. Postsurgical changes of the breast that mimic inflammatory breast carcinoma. Mayo Clin Proc. 1996;71(6):552–5.
71. Spiro SG, Douse J, Read C, Janes S. Complications of lung cancer treatment. Semin Respir Crit Care Med. 2008;29(3):302–17.

72. Busch E, Verazin G, Antkowiak JG, Driscoll D, Takita H. Pulmonary complications in patients undergoing thoracotomy for lung carcinoma. Chest. 1994;105(3):760–6.
73. Belda J, Cavalcanti M, Ferrer M, Serra M, Puig de la Bellacasa J, Canalis E, et al. Bronchial colonization and postoperative respiratory infections in patients undergoing lung cancer surgery. Chest. 2005;128(3):1571–9.
74. Seo SK. Infectious complications of lung cancer. Oncology (Williston Park). 2005;19(2):185–94. discussion 195–6, 199–203, 207–8.
75. Patel RL, Townsend ER, Fountain SW. Elective pneumonectomy: factors associated with morbidity and operative mortality. Ann Thorac Surg. 1992;54(1):84–8.
76. Deslauriers J, Ginsberg RJ, Piantadosi S, Fournier B. Prospective assessment of 30-day operative morbidity for surgical resections in lung cancer. Chest. 1994;106(6 Suppl):329S–30.
77. Yano T, Yokoyama H, Fukuyama Y, Takai E, Mizutani K, Ichinose Y. The current status of postoperative complications and risk factors after a pulmonary resection for primary lung cancer. A multivariate analysis. Eur J Cardiothorac Surg. 1997;11(3):445–9.
78. Stephan F, Boucheseiche S, Hollande J, Flahault A, Cheffi A, Bazelly B, et al. Pulmonary complications following lung resection: a comprehensive analysis of incidence and possible risk factors. Chest. 2000;118(5):1263–70.
79. Deschamps C, Bernard A, Nichols III FC, Allen MS, Miller DL, Trastek VF, et al. Empyema and bronchopleural fistula after pneumonectomy: factors affecting incidence. Ann Thorac Surg. 2001;72(1):243–7. discussion 248.
80. Sonobe M, Nakagawa M, Ichinose M, Ikegami N, Nagasawa M, Shindo T. Analysis of risk factors in bronchopleural fistula after pulmonary resection for primary lung cancer. Eur J Cardiothorac Surg. 2000;18(5):519–23.
81. Pezzella AT, Adebonojo SA, Hooker SG, Mabogunje OA, Conlan AA. Complications of general thoracic surgery. Curr Probl Surg. 2000;37(11):733–858.
82. Schussler O, Dermine H, Alifano M, Casetta A, Coignard S, Roche N, et al. Should we change antibiotic prophylaxis for lung surgery? Postoperative pneumonia is the critical issue. Ann Thorac Surg. 2008;86(6):1727–33.
83. Sok M, Dragas AZ, Erzen J, Jerman J. Sources of pathogens causing pleuropulmonary infections after lung cancer resection. Eur J Cardiothorac Surg. 2002;22(1):23–7. discussion 27–9.
84. Falcoz PE, Laluc F, Toubin MM, Puyraveau M, Clement F, Mercier M, et al. Usefulness of procalcitonin in the early detection of infection after thoracic surgery. Eur J Cardiothorac Surg. 2005;27(6):1074–8.
85. Fritscher-Ravens A, Schirrow L, Pothmann W, Knofel WT, Swain P, Soehendra N. Critical care transesophageal endosonography and guided fine-needle aspiration for diagnosis and management of posterior mediastinitis. Crit Care Med. 2003;31(1):126–32.
86. ASHP Therapeutic Guidelines on Antimicrobial Prophylaxis in Surgery. American society of health-system pharmacists. Am J Health Syst Pharm. 1999;56(18):1839–88.
87. Gonzalez-Gonzalez JJ, Sanz-Alvarez L, Marques-Alvarez L, Navarrete-Guijosa F, Martinez-Rodriguez E. Complications of surgical resection of esophageal cancer. Cir Esp. 2006;80(6):349–60.
88. Viklund P, Lindblad M, Lu M, Ye W, Johansson J, Lagergren J. Risk factors for complications after esophageal cancer resection: a prospective population-based study in Sweden. Ann Surg. 2006;243(2):204–11.
89. Bartels H, Siewert JR. Therapy of mediastinitis in patients with esophageal cancer. Chirurg. 2008;79(1):30–7.
90. Turkyilmaz A, Eroglu A, Aydin Y, Tekinbas C, Muharrem Erol M, Karaoglanoglu N. The management of esophagogastric anastomotic leak after esophagectomy for esophageal carcinoma. Dis Esophagus. 2009;22(2):119–26.
91. Mangram AJ, Horan TC, Pearson ML, Silver LC, Jarvis WR. Guideline for prevention of surgical site infection, 1999. Hospital Infection Control Practices Advisory Committee. Infect Control Hosp Epidemiol. 1999;20(4):250–78. quiz 279–80.
92. Bricard H, Deshayes JP, Sillard B, Lefrancois C, Delassus P, Lochu T, et al. Antibiotic prophylaxis in surgery of the esophagus. Ann Fr Anesth Reanim. 1994;13(5 Suppl):S161–8.
93. Luna-Perez P, Rodriguez-Ramirez S, Vega J, Sandoval E, Labastida S. Morbidity and mortality following abdominoperineal resection for low rectal adenocarcinoma. Rev Invest Clin. 2001;53(5):388–95.
94. Kressner U, Graf W, Mahteme H, Pahlman L, Glimelius B. Septic complications and prognosis after surgery for rectal cancer. Dis Colon Rectum. 2002;45(3):316–21.
95. Bullard KM, Trudel JL, Baxter NN, Rothenberger DA. Primary perineal wound closure after preoperative radiotherapy and abdominoperineal resection has a high incidence of wound failure. Dis Colon Rectum. 2005;48(3):438–43.
96. Schwarz RE, Karpeh MS, Brennan MF. Factors predicting hospitalization after operative treatment for gastric carcinoma in patients older than 70 years. J Am Coll Surg. 1997;184(1):9–15.
97. Parc Y, Frileux P, Schmitt G, Dehni N, Ollivier JM, Parc R. Management of postoperative peritonitis after anterior resection: experience from a referral intensive care unit. Dis Colon Rectum. 2000;43(5):579–87. discussion 587–9.
98. Nespoli A, Gianotti L, Bovo G, Brivio F, Nespoli L, Totis M. Impact of postoperative infections on survival in colon cancer patients. Surg Infect (Larchmt). 2006;7 Suppl 2:S41–3.
99. Eberhardt JM, Kiran RP, Lavery IC. The impact of anastomotic leak and intra-abdominal abscess on cancer-related outcomes after resection for colorectal cancer: a case control study. Dis Colon Rectum. 2009;52(3):380–6.
100. Tsujimoto H, Ichikura T, Ono S, Sugasawa H, Hiraki S, Sakamoto N, et al. Impact of postoperative infection on long-term survival after potentially curative resection for gastric cancer. Ann Surg Oncol. 2009;16(2):311–8.
101. Uchiyama K, Takifuji K, Tani M, Ueno M, Kawai M, Ozawa S, et al. Prevention of postoperative infections by administration of antimicrobial agents immediately before surgery for patients with gastrointestinal cancers. Hepatogastroenterology. 2007;54(77):1487–93.
102. Jesus Hernandez-Navarrete M, Arribas-Llorente JL, Solano-Bernad VM, Misiego-Peral A, Rodriguez-Garcia J, Fernandez-Garcia JL, et al. Quality improvement program of nosocomial infection in colorectal cancer surgery. Med Clin (Barc). 2005;125(14):521–4.
103. Ichikawa D, Kurioka H, Yamaguchi T, Koike H, Okamoto K, Otsuji E, et al. Postoperative complications following gastrectomy for gastric cancer during the last decade. Hepatogastroenterology. 2004;51(56):613–7.
104. Kim J, Mittal R, Konyalian V, King J, Stamos MJ, Kumar RR. Outcome analysis of patients undergoing colorectal resection for emergent and elective indications. Am Surg. 2007;73(10):991–3.
105. Kobayashi M, Mohri Y, Tonouchi H, Miki C, Nakai K, Kusunoki M. Randomized clinical trial comparing intravenous antimicrobial prophylaxis alone with oral and intravenous antimicrobial prophylaxis for the prevention of a surgical site infection in colorectal cancer surgery. Surg Today. 2007;37(5):383–8. Epub 2007 Apr 30.
106. Nakamura T, Mitomi H, Ihara A, Onozato W, Sato T, Ozawa H, et al. Risk factors for wound infection after surgery for colorectal cancer. World J Surg. 2008;32(6):1138–41.
107. Sah BK, Zhu ZG, Chen MM, Yan M, Yin HR, Zhen LY. Gastric cancer surgery and its hazards: post operative infection is the most important complication. Hepatogastroenterology. 2008;55(88):2259–63.
108. Iversen LH, Bulow S, Christensen IJ, Laurberg S, Harling H. Postoperative medical complications are the main cause of early death after emergency surgery for colonic cancer. Br J Surg. 2008;95(8):1012–9.

109. Lo CH, Chen JH, Wu CW, Lo SS, Hsieh MC, Lui WY. Risk factors and management of intra-abdominal infection after extended radical gastrectomy. Am J Surg. 2008;196(5):741–5.
110. Lohsiriwat V, Lohsiriwat D. Antibiotic prophylaxis and incisional surgical site infection following colorectal cancer surgery: an analysis of 330 cases. J Med Assoc Thai. 2009;92(1):12–6.
111. Park JM, Jin SH, Lee SR, Kim H, Jung IH, Cho YK, et al. Complications with laparoscopically assisted gastrectomy: multivariate analysis of 300 consecutive cases. Surg Endosc. 2008;22(10):2133–9.
112. Tsujinaka S, Konishi F, Kawamura YJ, Saito M, Tajima N, Tanaka O, et al. Visceral obesity predicts surgical outcomes after laparoscopic colectomy for sigmoid colon cancer. Dis Colon Rectum. 2008;51(12):1757–65. discussion 1765–7 Epub 2008 Jul 4.
113. Ojima T, Iwahashi M, Nakamori M, Nakamura M, Naka T, Ishida K, et al. Influence of overweight on patients with gastric cancer after undergoing curative gastrectomy: an analysis of 689 consecutive cases managed by a single center. Arch Surg. 2009;144(4):351–8. discussion 358.
114. Nickelsen TN, Jorgensen T, Kronborg O. Lifestyle and 30-day complications to surgery for colorectal cancer. Acta Oncol. 2005;44(3):218–23.
115. Moyes LH, Leitch EF, McKee RF, Anderson JH, Horgan PG, McMillan DC. Preoperative systemic inflammation predicts postoperative infectious complications in patients undergoing curative resection for colorectal cancer. Br J Cancer. 2009;100(8):1236–9.
116. Riedl S, Wiebelt H, Bergmann U, Hermanek Jr P. Postoperative complications and fatalities in surgical therapy of colon carcinoma. Results of the German multicenter study by the Colorectal Carcinoma Study Group. Chirurg. 1995;66(6):597–606.
117. Bilimoria KY, Bentrem DJ, Merkow RP, Nelson H, Wang E, Ko CY, et al. Laparoscopic-assisted vs. open colectomy for cancer: comparison of short-term outcomes from 121 hospitals. J Gastrointest Surg. 2008;12(11):2001–9.
118. Aziz O, Constantinides V, Tekkis PP, Athanasiou T, Purkayastha S, Paraskeva P, et al. Laparoscopic versus open surgery for rectal cancer: a meta-analysis. Ann Surg Oncol. 2006;13(3):413–24.
119. Tan LG, See JY, Wong KS. Necrotizing fasciitis after laparoscopic colonic surgery: case report and review of the literature. Surg Laparosc Endosc Percutan Tech. 2007;17(6):551–3.
120. Benzoni E, Lorenzin D, Baccarani U, Adani GL, Favero A, Cojutti A, et al. Resective surgery for liver tumor: a multivariate analysis of causes and risk factors linked to postoperative complications. Hepatobiliary Pancreat Dis Int. 2006;5(4):526–33.
121. Spunt SL, Lobe TE, Pappo AS, Parham DM, Wharam Jr MD, Arndt C, et al. Aggressive surgery is unwarranted for biliary tract rhabdomyosarcoma. J Pediatr Surg. 2000;35(2):309–16.
122. Kemeny MM. How many patients and how many complications does it take to decide if a drug is safe to use before surgery? J Clin Oncol. 2009;27(11):1917–8. author reply 1918.
123. Togo S, Matsuo K, Tanaka K, Matsumoto C, Shimizu T, Ueda M, et al. Perioperative infection control and its effectiveness in hepatectomy patients. J Gastroenterol Hepatol. 2007;22(11):1942–8.
124. Togo S, Kubota T, Takahashi T, Yoshida K, Matsuo K, Morioka D, et al. Usefulness of absorbable sutures in preventing surgical site infection in hepatectomy. J Gastrointest Surg. 2008;12(6):1041–6.
125. Kobayashi S, Gotohda N, Nakagohri T, Takahashi S, Konishi M, Kinoshita T. Risk factors of surgical site infection after hepatectomy for liver cancers. World J Surg. 2009;33(2):312–7.
126. Ambiru S, Kato A, Kimura F, Shimizu H, Yoshidome H, Otsuka M, et al. Poor postoperative blood glucose control increases surgical site infections after surgery for hepato-biliary-pancreatic cancer: a prospective study in a high-volume institute in Japan. J Hosp Infect. 2008;68(3):230–3.
127. Solomkin JS, Dellinger EP, Christou NV, Busuttil RW. Results of a multicenter trial comparing imipenem/cilastatin to tobramycin/clindamycin for intra-abdominal infections. Ann Surg. 1990;212(5):581–91.
128. Mosdell DM, Morris DM, Voltura A, Pitcher DE, Twiest MW, Milne RL, et al. Antibiotic treatment for surgical peritonitis. Ann Surg. 1991;214(5):543–9.
129. Lin CM, Hung GU, Chao TH, Lin WY, Wang SJ. The limited use of ultrasound in the detection of abdominal abscesses in patients after colorectal surgery: compared with gallium scan and computed tomography. Hepatogastroenterology. 2005;52(61):79–81.
130. Solomkin JS, Mazuski JE, Baron EJ, Sawyer RG, Nathens AB, DiPiro JT, et al. Guidelines for the selection of anti-infective agents for complicated intra-abdominal infections. Clin Infect Dis. 2003;37(8):997–1005.
131. Bailey CM, Thompson-Fawcett MW, Kettlewell MG, Garrard C, Mortensen NJ. Laparostomy for severe intra-abdominal infection complicating colorectal disease. Dis Colon Rectum. 2000;43(1):25–30.
132. Glenny AM, Song F. Antimicrobial prophylaxis in colorectal surgery. Qual Health Care. 1999;8(2):132–6.
133. Suehiro T, Hirashita T, Araki S, Matsumata T, Tsutsumi S, Mochiki E, et al. Prolonged antibiotic prophylaxis longer than 24 hours does not decrease surgical site infection after elective gastric and colorectal surgery. Hepatogastroenterology. 2008;55(86–87):1636–9.
134. Nelson RL, Glenny AM, Song F. Antimicrobial prophylaxis for colorectal surgery. Cochrane Database Syst Rev. 2009;1:CD1181.
135. Al-Niaimi A, Safdar N. Supplemental perioperative oxygen for reducing surgical site infection: a meta-analysis. J Eval Clin Pract. 2009;15(2):360–5.
136. Horie H, Okada M, Kojima M, Nagai H. Favorable effects of preoperative enteral immunonutrition on a surgical site infection in patients with colorectal cancer without malnutrition. Surg Today. 2006;36(12):1063–8. Epub 2006 Dec 25.
137. Zheng Y, Li F, Qi B, Luo B, Sun H, Liu S, et al. Application of perioperative immunonutrition for gastrointestinal surgery: a meta-analysis of randomized controlled trials. Asia Pac J Clin Nutr. 2007;16 Suppl 1:253–7.
138. Huang JY, Ziegler C, Tulandi T. Cervical stump necrosis and septic shock after laparoscopic supracervical hysterectomy. J Minim Invasive Gynecol. 2005;12(2):162–4.
139. Miller B, Morris M, Gershenson DM, Levenback CL, Burke TW. Intestinal fistulae formation following pelvic exenteration: a review of the University of Texas M. D. Anderson Cancer Center experience, 1957–1990. Gynecol Oncol. 1995;56(2):207–10.
140. Brooker DC, Savage JE, Twiggs LB, Adcock LL, Prem KA, Sanders CC. Infectious morbidity in gynecologic cancer. Am J Obstet Gynecol. 1987;156(2):513–20.
141. Iatrakis G, Sakellaropoulos G, Georgoulias N, Chadjithomas A, Kourounis G, Tsionis C, et al. Gynecologic cancer and surgical infectious morbidity. Clin Exp Obstet Gynecol. 1998;25(1–2):36–7.
142. Kuoppala T, Tomas E, Heinonen PK. Clinical outcome and complications of laparoscopic surgery compared with traditional surgery in women with endometrial cancer. Arch Gynecol Obstet. 2004;270(1):25–30.
143. Wu K, Zhang WH, Zhang R, Li H, Bai P, Li XG. Analysis of postoperative complications of radical hysterectomy for 219 cervical cancer patients. Zhonghua Zhong Liu Za Zhi. 2006;28(4):316–9.
144. Kietpeerakool C, Lattiwongsakorn W, Srisomboon J. Incidence and predictors of febrile morbidity after radical hysterectomy and pelvic lymphadenectomy for early stage cervical cancer patients. Asian Pac J Cancer Prev. 2008;9(2):213–6.
145. Bell MC, Torgerson J, Seshadri-Kreaden U, Suttle AW, Hunt S. Comparison of outcomes and cost for endometrial cancer staging via traditional laparotomy, standard laparoscopy and robotic techniques. Gynecol Oncol. 2008;111(3):407–11.
146. Rassweiler J, Seemann O, Schulze M, Teber D, Hatzinger M, Frede T. Laparoscopic versus open radical prostatectomy: a

146. comparative study at a single institution. J Urol. 2003;169(5): 1689–93.
147. Colombo Jr JR, Haber GP, Jelovsek JE, Nguyen M, Fergany A, Desai MM, et al. Complications of laparoscopic surgery for urological cancer: a single institution analysis. J Urol. 2007;178(3 Pt 1):786–91.
148. Fairey A, Chetner M, Metcalfe J, Moore R, Todd G, Rourke K, et al. Associations among age, comorbidity and clinical outcomes after radical cystectomy: results from the Alberta Urology Institute radical cystectomy database. J Urol. 2008;180(1):128–34. discussion 134.
149. Constantinides CA, Tyritzis SI, Skolarikos A, Liatsikos E, Zervas A, Deliveliotis C. Short- and long-term complications of open radical prostatectomy according to the Clavien classification system. BJU Int. 2009;103(3):336–40.
150. Wendt-Nordahl G, Bucher B, Hacker A, Knoll T, Alken P, Michel MS. Improvement in mortality and morbidity in transurethral resection of the prostate over 17 years in a single center. J Endourol. 2007;21(9):1081–7.
151. Adam RA, Adam YG. Infectious diseases in gynecologic oncology: an overview. Obstet Gynecol Clin North Am. 2001;28(4): 847–68.
152. Hamasuna R, Betsunoh H, Sueyoshi T, Yakushiji K, Tsukino H, Nagano M, et al. Bacteria of preoperative urinary tract infections contaminate the surgical fields and develop surgical site infections in urological operations. Int J Urol. 2004;11(11):941–7.
153. Krogh J, Jensen JS, Iversen HG, Andersen JT. Age as a prognostic variable in patients undergoing transurethral prostatectomy. Scand J Urol Nephrol. 1993;27(2):225–9.
154. Larsen B, Galask RP. Vaginal microbial flora: practical and theoretic relevance. Obstet Gynecol. 1980;55(5 Suppl):100S–13.
155. Hudspeth AS. Elimination of surgical wound infections by delayed primary closure. South Med J. 1973;66(8):934–6.
156. ACOG Committee on Practice Bulletins. ACOG practice bulletin No. 104: antibiotic prophylaxis for gynecologic procedures. Obstet Gynecol. 2009;113(5):1180–9.
157. Wolf Jr JS, Bennett CJ, Dmochowski RR, Hollenbeck BK, Pearle MS, Schaeffer AJ. Best practice policy statement on urologic surgery antimicrobial prophylaxis. J Urol. 2008;179(4): 1379–90.
158. Yamamoto S, Shima H. Controversies in antimicrobial prophylaxis for urologic surgery: more up-to-date evidence is needed. Nat Clin Pract Urol. 2008;5(11):588–9.
159. Hardes J, Gebert C, Schwappach A, Ahrens H, Streitburger A, Winkelmann W, et al. Characteristics and outcome of infections associated with tumor endoprostheses. Arch Orthop Trauma Surg. 2006;126(5):289–96.
160. Szendroi M, Vizkelety T. Results with endoprostheses and bone transplantation in surgery for bone tumors. Orv Hetil. 1992; 133(34):2141–6.
161. Jeys L, Grimer R. The long-term risks of infection and amputation with limb salvage surgery using endoprostheses. Recent Results Cancer Res. 2009;179:75–84.
162. Jeys LM, Grimer RJ, Carter SR, Tillman RM, Abudu A. Post operative infection and increased survival in osteosarcoma patients: are they associated? Ann Surg Oncol. 2007;14(10):2887–95.
163. Cannon CP, Ballo MT, Zagars GK, Mirza AN, Lin PP, Lewis VO, et al. Complications of combined modality treatment of primary lower extremity soft-tissue sarcomas. Cancer. 2006;107(10): 2455–61.
164. McIntosh J, Earnshaw JJ. Antibiotic prophylaxis for the prevention of infection after major limb amputation. Eur J Vasc Endovasc Surg. 2009;37(6):696–703.
165. Payman BC, Dampier SE, Hawthorn PJ. Postoperative temperature and infection in patients undergoing general surgery. J Adv Nurs. 1989;14(3):198–202.
166. Vermeulen H, Storm-Versloot MN, Goossens A, Speelman P, Legemate DA. Diagnostic accuracy of routine postoperative body temperature measurements. Clin Infect Dis. 2005;40(10):1404–10.
167. Kendrick JE, Numnum TM, Estes JM, Kimball KJ, Leath CA, Straughn Jr JM. Conservative management of postoperative fever in gynecologic patients undergoing major abdominal or vaginal operations. J Am Coll Surg. 2008;207(3):393–7.
168. Hendershot E, Chang A, Colapinto K, Gerstle JT, Malkin D, Sung L. Postoperative fevers in pediatric solid tumor patients: how should they be managed? J Pediatr Hematol Oncol. 2009;31(7): 485–8.
169. Dellinger EP. Should we measure body temperature for patients who have recently undergone surgery? Clin Infect Dis. 2005;40(10):1411–2.
170. Tan JA, Naik VN, Lingard L. Exploring obstacles to proper timing of prophylactic antibiotics for surgical site infections. Qual Saf Health Care. 2006;15(1):32–8.
171. Kao LS, Meeks D, Moyer VA, Lally KP. Peri-operative glycaemic control regimens for preventing surgical site infections in adults. Cochrane Database Syst Rev. 2009;3:CD006806.
172. Quinn A, Hill AD, Humphreys H. Evolving issues in the prevention of surgical site infections. Surgeon. 2009;7(3):170–2.
173. Qadan M, Akca O, Mahid SS, Hornung CA, Polk Jr HC. Perioperative supplemental oxygen therapy and surgical site infection: a meta-analysis of randomized controlled trials. Arch Surg. 2009;144(4):359–66. discussion 366–7.
174. Miller SD, Andrassy RJ. Complications in pediatric surgical oncology. J Am Coll Surg. 2003;197(5):832–7.
175. Aledo A, Heller G, Ren L, Gardner S, Dunkel I, McKay SW, et al. Septicemia and septic shock in pediatric patients: 140 consecutive cases on a pediatric hematology-oncology service. J Pediatr Hematol Oncol. 1998;20(3):215–21.
176. Springfield DS. Surgical wound healing. Cancer Treat Res. 1993;67:81–98.
177. Hillmann A, Ozaki T, Rube C, Hoffmann C, Schuck A, Blasius S, et al. Surgical complications after preoperative irradiation of Ewing's sarcoma. J Cancer Res Clin Oncol. 1997;123(1):57–62.
178. Seseke F, Rebmann S, Zoller G, Lakomek M, Ringert RH. Risk factors for perioperative complications in renal surgery for Wilms' tumor. Aktuelle Urol. 2007;38(1):46–51.
179. Haupt R, Romanengo M, Fears T, Viscoli C, Castagnola E. Incidence of septicaemias and invasive mycoses in children undergoing treatment for solid tumours: a 12-year experience at a single Italian institution. Eur J Cancer. 2001;37(18):2413–9.
180. Ritchey ML, Shamberger RC, Haase G, Horwitz J, Bergemann T, Breslow NE. Surgical complications after primary nephrectomy for Wilms' tumor: report from the National Wilms' Tumor Study Group. J Am Coll Surg. 2001;192(1):63–8. quiz 146.
181. Urrea M, Rives S, Cruz O, Navarro A, Garcia JJ, Estella J. Nosocomial infections among pediatric hematology/oncology patients: results of a prospective incidence study. Am J Infect Control. 2004;32(4):205–8.
182. Chittmittrapap S, Imvised T, Vejchapipat P. Resection for primary liver tumors in children: an experience of 52 cases at one institution. J Med Assoc Thai. 2008;91(8):1206–11.
183. Raymond J, Aujard Y. Nosocomial infections in pediatric patients: a European, multicenter prospective study. European Study Group. Infect Control Hosp Epidemiol. 2000;21(4):260–3.
184. Wisplinghoff H, Seifert H, Tallent SM, Bischoff T, Wenzel RP, Edmond MB. Nosocomial bloodstream infections in pediatric patients in United States hospitals: epidemiology, clinical features and susceptibilities. Pediatr Infect Dis J. 2003;22(8):686–91.
185. Paulus SC, van Saene HK, Hemsworth S, Hughes J, Ng A, Pizer BL. A prospective study of septicaemia on a paediatric oncology unit: a three-year experience at The Royal Liverpool Children's Hospital, Alder Hey, UK. Eur J Cancer. 2005;41(14):2132–40.

186. Haut C. Oncological emergencies in the pediatric intensive care unit. AACN Clin Issues. 2005;16(2):232–45.
187. Castagnola E, Conte M, Parodi S, Papio F, Caviglia I, Haupt R. Incidence of bacteremias and invasive mycoses in children with high risk neuroblastoma. Pediatr Blood Cancer. 2007;49(5):672–7.
188. Bertermann O, Marcove RC, Rosen G. Effect of intensive adjuvant chemotherapy on wound healing in 69 patients with osteogenic sarcomas of the lower extremities. Recent Results Cancer Res. 1985;98:135–41.
189. Gaur AH, Liu T, Knapp KM, Daw NC, Rao BN, Neel MD, et al. Infections in children and young adults with bone malignancies undergoing limb-sparing surgery. Cancer. 2005;104(3):602–10.
190. Trampuz A, Zimmerli W. Antimicrobial agents in orthopaedic surgery: prophylaxis and treatment. Drugs. 2006;66(8):1089–105.
191. Spurbeck WW, Davidoff AM, Lobe TE, Rao BN, Schropp KP, Shochat SJ. Minimally invasive surgery in pediatric cancer patients. Ann Surg Oncol. 2004;11(3):340–3.
192. Laws HJ, Kobbe G, Dilloo D, Dettenkofer M, Meisel R, Geisel R, et al. Surveillance of nosocomial infections in paediatric recipients of bone marrow or peripheral blood stem cell transplantation during neutropenia, compared with adult recipients. J Hosp Infect. 2006;62(1):80–8. Epub 2005 Oct 19.
193. Gaur AH, Flynn PM, Shenep JL. Optimum management of pediatric patients with fever and neutropenia. Indian J Pediatr. 2004;71(9):825–35.
194. Simon A, Fleischhack G, Hasan C, Bode U, Engelhart S, Kramer MH. Surveillance for nosocomial and central line-related infections among pediatric hematology-oncology patients. Infect Control Hosp Epidemiol. 2000;21(9):592–6.
195. Basford TJ, Poenaru D, Silva M. Comparison of delayed complications of central venous catheters placed surgically or radiologically in pediatric oncology patients. J Pediatr Surg. 2003;38(5):788–92.
196. Simon A, Bode U, Beutel K. Diagnosis and treatment of catheter-related infections in paediatric oncology: an update. Clin Microbiol Infect. 2006;12(7):606–20.
197. Adler A, Yaniv I, Steinberg R, Solter E, Samra Z, Stein J, et al. Infectious complications of implantable ports and Hickman catheters in paediatric haematology-oncology patients. J Hosp Infect. 2006;62(3):358–65. Epub 2006 Jan 10.
198. Neville HL, Lally KP. Pediatric surgical wound infection. Semi Pediatr Infect Dis. 2001;12(2):124–9.
199. Lejus C. Anaesthetic particularities for children with tumours. Ann Fr Anesth Reanim. 2006;25(4):424–31. Epub 2005 Nov 28.

Chapter 7
Management of Infections in Critically Ill Cancer Patients

Henry Masur

Abstract Advances in critical care medicine have enabled cancer patients to survive aggressive medical and surgical therapies that they could not have tolerated a decade ago. For patients whose goals can be met by ICU support, the diagnostic and empiric therapeutic approach will be far different than when patients are more stable in other hospital areas: evaluations must be completed rapidly while patients are able to tolerate such testing, and empiric therapy must be broad and promptly administered. Oncologists and infectious disease specialists need to be actively involved in evaluating cancer patients in the ICU and in developing their management plans due to the enhanced knowledge they are likely to have of the patient's history prior to the ICU, their knowledge of the underlying disease and life-threatening process, and their expertise in drug selection and monitoring.

Keywords Critical Care • ICU • Infection

Introduction

The past decade has witnessed dramatic improvement in prognosis for patients with many types of cancer. This improvement is due to aggressive management of medical and surgical approaches that can induce remissions and cures if patients can be kept alive despite the complications of their neoplastic process and if they can be kept alive despite the organ dysfunction brought about by their therapies. Critical care services clearly provide benefit to cancer patients with life-threatening complications [1–10].

A substantial fraction of cancer patients spend time in intensive care units due to complications arising from their disease or the antineoplastic therapy. Infections are responsible for a high percentage of such admissions and are a common complication of patients admitted to the ICU for noninfectious processes.

Cancer patients are admitted to the ICU for neutropenic fever with hypotension, catheter-related infections, pneumonia, gastrointestinal infections, urinary tract infections, and central nervous system infections, all of which are discussed in detail in Chaps. 1–6. The treatment of specific pathogens follows the recommendations detailed in Sects. 3 and 4. Patients in the ICU, however, require some special considerations.

Role of Oncologist and Infectious Disease Specialist in ICU

ICUs can be intimidating environments due to the complexity of equipment and the frenetic pace of staff activity. Some ICU staff take special pride in their ability to manage patients using the resources available to them in the ICU. Oncologists and infectious disease specialists must recognize, however, that they are likely to know the underlying disease, the patient's prior history, and the subtleties of infection management better than the ICU staff in some situations.

In some hospitals, oncologists and infectious disease specialists cease to follow patients regularly in the ICU. While there is no study proving the utility of having oncologists and infectious disease providers carefully evaluating patients in the ICU and taking an active role in management, it is likely that the specialized knowledge and continuity of care will result in improved outcome.

Oncologists and infectious disease experts must learn how to read the flow sheets and charts in the ICU and should communicate in person at least daily to the ICU physicians and nurses. An area of special attention should be drug selection, drug doses, drug interactions, and drug toxicities. Given the complex management required in the ICU, the oncology and infectious disease providers need to review drugs daily, assuring that the right drug, the right dose, the right time, and

H. Masur (✉)
Critical Care Medicine Department, Clinical Center, National Institutes of Health, Bethesda, MD 20892, USA
e-mail: hmasur@cc.nih.gov

the right monitoring are documented in the record, i.e., have in fact been selected and administered, rather than relying on verbal reports on rounds that may or may not be accurate. They also need to assist the ICU staff in assuring that the correct tests are ordered, are received by the laboratory, and are acted upon as soon as results are available. The infectious disease specialist interacting with the microbiology laboratory can often provide accurate information well before the intensivist might have received the helpful test results.

For prevention of complications, oncology and infectious disease teams can also assist ICU providers to be certain that the invasive equipments, such as intravenous catheters, are inspected daily and removed promptly when no longer needed, and that drugs are discontinued when the situation no longer warrants the use of these agents.

Critical Care Utilization: Does ICU Care Meet the Patient's Goals?

Before any patient is brought to the ICU, especially a patient with cancer, realistic planning should have taken place about the role of the ICU in achieving the patient's goals. Some patients have such a dismal prognosis from their underlying disease that intensive interventions in the ICU have virtually no likelihood in achieving the patient's goals. Some patients are willing to tolerate certain intervention, but are unwilling to undergo intubation and mechanical ventilation.

Too often, patients are brought to the ICU without a clear understanding of what can realistically be achieved, and what should be done that will meet the patient's wishes. Such planning is important before the need for critical care interventions occurs [11–13].

Critical Care Utilization: Does Critical Care Benefit Cancer Patients with Life-Threatening Complications?

As the therapeutic options for patients with cancer have expanded, and as critical care services have improved, it is clear that many patients with cancer survive their ICU admission to be discharged from the hospital for meaningful periods of time [1–8]. This is more likely to occur in ICUs that have extensive experience dealing with cancer patients. While there are some specific syndromes that continue to have very poor prognoses, such as diffuse alveolar hemorrhage, studies have shown that it is difficult in this rapidly evolving area to make meaningful generalizations that do not take into account many individual specifics [14–20].

Thus, the literature to date supports using ICUs to support patients through life-threatening complications despite their underlying disease and making individual decisions to limit care based on specific scenarios related to the underlying disease, the life-threatening complication, relevant comorbidities, and patient goals. Specifically, an underlying cancer should be considered no differently in deciding whether to use critical care services than other underlying diseases: each patient must be evaluated using the same general types of parameters.

A variety of scoring systems, including Simplified Acute Physiology Score (SAPS) II and APACHE II, have been assessed for patients with various types of cancer [21–24]. These scoring systems have yielded conflicting results about their ability to predict outcome in patients with various forms of cancer. There have also been conflicting results related to the impact of parameters of immunity/inflammation, such as neutropenia, and the impact of bacterial or fungal processes, which is not unexpected given the complex nature of variables related to the specific pathogen, the specific host defense defect, and the era when the study was performed.

There is extensive literature documenting improved prognosis for cancer patients in ICUs over the past decade [5, 15, 25]. This is undoubtedly due to a wide variety of issues related to improved patient selection, improved anticancer therapy, and improved critical care capabilities.

Providers need to keep in mind that these systems are intended to assess patient groups, and not individual patients. Moreover, with the development of new antimicrobial agents, new immunosuppressive drugs, and new critical care support modalities, many studies using various scoring systems are not contemporaneous enough to be relevant.

Diagnostic Approach

Cancer patients, especially those with substantial immunosuppression, require aggressive attempts to establish the precise cause of any infectious process that is severe enough to bring them to the ICU. While patients who are immunosuppressed are well recognized to require prompt and aggressive diagnostic approaches, those in the ICU deserve special attention.

By definition, such patients are unlikely to have a favorable prognosis if the correct diagnosis is not established promptly. It is well known that failure to institute appropriate therapy promptly reduces the likelihood for a successful outcome with bacterial, fungal, and viral processes.

It is also important to recognize that the window of opportunity to perform certain diagnostic testing may be very limited. Patients may quickly become too hypotensive to be safely moved for imaging studies. Patients with respiratory compromise may become so hypoxic that it is unsafe to perform bronchoscopic or surgical procedures to obtain pulmonary secretions or lung tissue. Thus, aggressive attempts to obtain appropriate studies and appropriate specimens take on an added sense of urgency.

Also important is for clinicians to take a broad approach to the differential diagnosis. When patients appear with febrile syndromes, healthcare providers dealing with cancer patients often leap to the assumption that infection is the only likely cause of the life-threatening disorder. Neutropenic patients or patients receiving high-dose corticosteroids who develop fever and diffuse pulmonary infiltrates may have pulmonary edema due to myocardial dysfunction (related to atherosclerotic disease or chemotherapeutic toxicities), drug toxicity, cryptogenic organizing pneumonia, radiation pneumonitis, or transfusion-associated lung injury. Patients with fever and hypotension may have bacterial or fungal sepsis, but they may also have febrile neutropenia of unknown cause in addition to adrenal insufficiency, myocardial ischemia, hyperthyroidism, or pericardial tamponade.

Thus, when cancer patients are admitted to the ICU, there is an urgency to consider a broad range of potential causes for their syndrome and to rapidly obtain the tests that are most likely to be diagnostic.

Given the narrow window of opportunity, diagnostic samples must be processed for the full range of potential pathogens. While with more stable patients there may be some valid reasons to be more cost conscious in ordering diagnostic tests, in most situations in the ICU, diagnostic and therapeutic approaches need to be comprehensive since the margin for error is so small.

Therapy

For patients in ICUs who appear to have microbial cause for their ICU admission or for a complication of their ICU stay that was initiated due to a noninfectious process, empiric therapy must be broad and must be delivered promptly.

Many consultants fail to grasp the difference between treating immunologically normal patients who are stable, as opposed to unstable patients, especially those with significant immunosuppression. First, the empiric regimen must be broad and must be active against all causes that are logically plausible. Many providers are reluctant to start "too many" antimicrobials for fear of creating resistance or drug-related toxicities. However, the primary goal in the ICU is to save the patient's life from the imminent threat rather than potential or hypothetical threats. Thus, several antibacterial and antifungal agents may be appropriate to start. As soon as the diagnosis is established, some of the multiple drugs can be discontinued or modified. Thus, "polypharmacy" may be dismissed by some providers as dangerous, when in fact the danger is failing to institute effective therapy promptly.

In choosing therapeutic regimens, clinicians often focus primarily on bacteria; however, especially for immunosuppressed patients, fungi and viruses need to be important considerations. Clinicians should keep in mind that for ICU-related blood stream infections, Candida is the fourth most common pathogen. Thus, for sepsis, antifungal therapy should be a prime consideration for initial therapy and should likely be a consideration for certain intraabdominal and genitourinary infections. Therapy for molds may also be appropriate initially in certain patient populations presenting with certain syndromes. Also, as CMV, VZV, HSV, Influenza, RSV, Adenovirus, and other viruses are more commonly documented as causing life-threatening disease, initial empiric therapy with antiviral agents needs to be a consideration.

Once a regimen is chosen, all providers must participate in assuring that the right drug at the right dose is administered promptly. Every member of the ICU staff should be well acquainted with the correlation between time to administration of antibiotic or antifungal and survival [26–32].

ICUs are complex organizations: many have difficulty assuring that the important antimicrobials are administered within the first hour after a regimen is ordered. Some physicians appear to believe that once they enter an order into the computer, their responsibility ends. The entire ICU team and consultants must make certain that the correct orders are entered and that the chain of responsibility from the pharmacy to the bedside nurse to the patient functions such that the patient receives the drug promptly.

Pharmacokinetics in the ICU must also be attended to. Critically ill patients are different from many other kinds of patients. Their volumes of distribution may be acutely altered due to aggressive fluid resuscitation, heart failure, or renal failure. Their renal or hepatic function may be compromised. They may have complex drug interactions. These issues must be carefully followed by subject-matter experts. Measurement of serum drug levels is especially important in the ICU where pharmacokinetics may not be as predictable as in more stable patients.

For cancer patients who are receiving chemotherapy or immunosuppressive therapies, critical illness may be a reason to reduce the doses of drugs or to temporarily or permanently discontinue the cancer therapies. Critically ill patients may not absorb oral agents if drugs are not available by parenteral route. Critically ill patients may not be able to survive the toxicities of these drugs. Such decisions must be carefully made. Orders for such agents are probably best entered not by the intensivists, who are usually unfamiliar with the doses and agents, but by the primary team managing the cancer.

Prevention of Infectious Complications

When patients enter ICUs for any reasons, there is an appropriate concern that infectious complications will occur involving invasive devices, surgical wounds, loss of ability to protect the airway, superinfection with virulent organisms, and multiple other factors. While patients often will survive only if they are monitored invasively, intubated and placed on mechanical ventilation, or administered very broad-spectrum antimicrobial therapy, there are many interventions that can reduce the likelihood of infectious complications.

Section 5 reviews some interventions that are likely to be useful. However, as stated above, removing invasive devices and antimicrobial therapies promptly when they are not needed will go a long way towards improving patient outcome.

Critical care units generally maintain a high degree of focus and adherence to infection control practices related to proper isolation, hand hygiene, staff immunization, and careful epidemiological monitoring to look for outbreaks and trends. When the patients involved are immunocompromised, such focus is especially important. Adherence to infection control practices is important by not only for the ICU staff, but for consultants and families as well.

Summary

Cancer patients can clearly benefit from critical care services, although decisions to admit them to ICUs or to continue to offer supportive care need to be individualized based on patient wishes, the prognosis for the underlying disease, and the prognosis for the life-threatening complication that makes them ICU candidates. Infections are well known to be frequent causes for ICU admission and to be frequent complications in patients admitted to ICUs for noninfectious complications. Oncologists and infectious disease specialists must be active members of the ICU team if patient outcome is to be optimized.

Acknowledgments Disclaimer: The opinions and assertions contained herein are those of the authors and are not to be construed as official or as reflecting the views of the Department of Defense, the Department of the Navy, or the naval services at large.
Disclaimer: The opinions or assertions contained herein are the private views of the authors and are not to be construed as official or as reflecting the views of the U.S. Department of the Army or the U.S. Department of Defense.

References

1. Darmon M, Azoulay E. Critical care management of cancer patients: cause for optimism and need for objectivity. Curr Opin Oncol. 2009;21:318–26.
2. Azoulay E, Afessa B. The intensive care support of patients with malignancy: do everything that can be done. Intensive Care Med. 2006;32:3–5.
3. Soares M, Azoulay E. Critical care management of lung cancer patients to prolong life without prolonging dying. Intensive Care Med 2009.
4. Soares M. Salluh JI, Azoulay E. Noninvasive ventilation in patients with malignancies and hypoxemic acute respiratory failure: A still pending question. J Crit Care; 2009.
5. Pene F, Percheron S, Lemiale V, et al. Temporal changes in management and outcome of septic shock in patients with malignancies in the intensive care unit. Crit Care Med. 2008;36:690–6.
6. Larche J, Azoulay E, Fieux F, et al. Improved survival of critically ill cancer patients with septic shock. Intensive Care Med. 2003;29:1688–95.
7. Benoit DD, Vandewoude KH, Decruyenaere JM, Hoste EA, Colardyn FA. Outcome and early prognostic indicators in patients with a hematologic malignancy admitted to the intensive care unit for a life-threatening complication. Crit Care Med. 2003;31:104–12.
8. Lamia B, Hellot MF, Girault C, et al. Changes in severity and organ failure scores as prognostic factors in onco-hematological malignancy patients admitted to the ICU. Intensive Care Med. 2006;32:1560–8.
9. Park HY, Suh GY, Jeon K, et al. Outcome and prognostic factors of patients with acute leukemia admitted to the intensive care unit for septic shock. Leuk Lymphoma. 2008;49:1929–34.
10. Thakkar SG, Fu AZ, Sweetenham JW, et al. Survival and predictors of outcome in patients with acute leukemia admitted to the intensive care unit. Cancer. 2008;112:2233–40.
11. Investigators TSP. A controlled trial to improve care for seriously ill hospitalized patients. The study to understand prognoses and preferences for outcomes and risks of treatments (SUPPORT). The SUPPORT Principal Investigators. Jama 1995;**274**:1591-8.
12. Angus DC, Barnato AE, Linde-Zwirble WT, et al. Use of intensive care at the end of life in the United States: an epidemiologic study. Crit Care Med. 2004;32:638–43.
13. Curtis JR, Rubenfeld GD. Introducing the concept of managing death in the ICU. In: Curtis JR, Rubenfeld GD, eds. Managing death in the intensive care unit. New York: Oxford University Press; 2001:3.
14. Thiery G, Azoulay E, Darmon M, et al. Outcome of cancer patients considered for intensive care unit admission: a hospital-wide prospective study. J Clin Oncol. 2005;23:4406–13.
15. Brenner H. Long-term survival rates of cancer patients achieved by the end of the 20th century: a period analysis. Lancet. 2002;360:1131–5.
16. Ferra C, Marcos P, Misis M, et al. Outcome and prognostic factors in patients with hematologic malignancies admitted to the intensive care unit: a single-center experience. Int J Hematol. 2007;85:195–202.
17. Massion PB, Dive AM, Doyen C, et al. Prognosis of hematologic malignancies does not predict intensive care unit mortality. Crit Care Med. 2002;30:2260–70.
18. Lecuyer L, Chevret S, Thiery G, Darmon M, Schlemmer B, Azoulay E. The ICU trial: a new admission policy for cancer patients requiring mechanical ventilation. Crit Care Med. 2007;35:808–14.
19. Soubani AO, Kseibi E, Bander JJ, et al. Outcome and prognostic factors of hematopoietic stem cell transplantation recipients admitted to a medical ICU. Chest. 2004;126:1604–11.
20. Rabbat A, Chaoui D, Montani D, et al. Prognosis of patients with acute myeloid leukaemia admitted to intensive care. Br J Haematol. 2005;129:350–7.
21. Merz TM, Schar P, Buhlmann M, Takala J, Rothen HU. Resource use and outcome in critically ill patients with hematological malignancy: a retrospective cohort study. Crit Care. 2008;12:R75.
22. Benoit DD, Hoste EA, Depuydt PO, et al. Outcome in critically ill medical patients treated with renal replacement therapy for acute renal failure: comparison between patients with and those without haematological malignancies. Nephrol Dial Transplant. 2005;20:552–8.
23. den Boer S, de Keizer NF, de Jonge E. Performance of prognostic models in critically ill cancer patients - a review. Crit Care. 2005;9:R458–63.
24. Beck DH, Smith GB, Pappachan JV, Millar B. External validation of the SAPS II, APACHE II and APACHE III prognostic models in South England: a multicentre study. Intensive Care Med. 2003;29:249–56.

25. Gondos A, Bray F, Hakulinen T, Brenner H. Trends in cancer survival in 11 European populations from 1990 to 2009: a model-based analysis. Ann Oncol. 2009;20:564–73.
26. Kumar A, Roberts D, Wood KE, et al. Duration of hypotension before initiation of effective antimicrobial therapy is the critical determinant of survival in human septic shock. Crit Care Med. 2006;34:1589–96.
27. Miner JR, Heegaard W, Mapes A, Biros M. Presentation, time to antibiotics, and mortality of patients with bacterial meningitis at an urban county medical center. J Emerg Med. 2001;21:387–92.
28. Proulx N, Frechette D, Toye B, Chan J, Kravcik S. Delays in the administration of antibiotics are associated with mortality from adult acute bacterial meningitis. Qjm. 2005;98:291–8.
29. Funk D, Sebat F, Kumar A. A systems approach to the early recognition and rapid administration of best practice therapy in sepsis and septic shock. Curr Opin Crit Care. 2009;15:301–7.
30. Marchaim D, Kaye KS, Fowler VG, et al. Case-control study to identify factors associated with mortality among patients with methicillin-resistant Staphylococcus aureus bacteraemia. Clin Microbiol Infect 2009.
31. Garey KW, Rege M, Pai MP, et al. Time to initiation of fluconazole therapy impacts mortality in patients with candidemia: a multi-institutional study. Clin Infect Dis. 2006;43:25–31.
32. Morrell M, Fraser VJ, Kollef MH. Delaying the empiric treatment of candida bloodstream infection until positive blood culture results are obtained: a potential risk factor for hospital mortality. Antimicrob Agents Chemother. 2005;49:3640–5.

Part II
Clinical Syndromes

Chapter 8
Management of the Neutropenic Patient with Fever

Kenneth V.I. Rolston and Gerald P. Bodey

Abstract Neutrophils provide protection against a wide variety of common and opportunistic bacterial and fungal pathogens. Consequently, the frequency and severity of infections caused by these organisms is increased in patients with neutropenia. At most cancer treatment centers, Gram-positive organisms are isolated more frequently from neutropenic patients with documented bacterial infections than Gram-negative bacilli, although institutional and regional differences occur as do periodic shifts in the spectrum of bacterial infections. *Candida* spp. and *Aspergillus* spp. remain the most common fungal pathogens in this setting, although a number of opportunistic fungal pathogens have emerged. The prompt administration of empiric, broad-spectrum, parenteral antibiotics in the hospital when a neutropenic patient becomes febrile is the standard of care. Over the past decade, it has become possible to reliably identify "low-risk" neutropenic patients both in adult and pediatric patient populations. Infection prevention (prophylaxis), infection control, and antimicrobial stewardship are important aspects in the overall management of the febrile neutropenic patient.

Keywords Neutropenia • Antimicrobial therapy • Low-risk • Febrile neutropenia • Fungal infection • Bacterial infection

Introduction

Neutrophils provide protection against a wide variety of common and opportunistic bacterial and fungal pathogens (Fig. 8.1). Consequently, the frequency and severity of infections caused by these organisms is increased in patients with neutropenia. The currently accepted definition of neutropenia is an absolute neutrophil count (ANC) of $\leq 500/mm^3$ [1]. At most cancer treatment centers, Gram-positive organisms (coagulase-negative staphylococci, *Staphylococcus aureus*, *Enterococcus* spp., *viridans* group streptococci) are isolated more frequently from neutropenic patients with documented bacterial infections than Gram-negative bacilli (*Escherichia coli*, *Klebsiella* spp., *Pseudomonas aeruginosa*), although institutional and regional differences occur as do periodic shifts in the spectrum of bacterial infections [2–4] (Fig. 8.2). *Candida* spp. and *Aspergillus* spp. remain the most common fungal pathogens in this setting, although a number of opportunistic fungal pathogens have emerged [5]. The prompt administration of empiric, broad-spectrum, parenteral antibiotics in the hospital when a neutropenic patient becomes febrile is the standard of care [1]. Over the past decade, it has become possible to reliably identify "low-risk" neutropenic patients both in adult and pediatric patient populations [6–8]. Carefully selected low-risk patients can be safely treated with oral or parenteral antibiotics without hospitalization or after a short period (~48 h) of hospitalization [9–12]. Patients failing to respond to appropriate antibacterial therapy frequently harbor fungal infections and should receive empiric or preemptive antifungal therapy while a diagnosis of a fungal infection is being pursued [13]. The overall duration of therapy will depend on several factors including the nature, anatomical site, and severity of infection, and recovery of the neutrophil count to normal levels [1]. Infection prevention (prophylaxis), infection control, and antimicrobial stewardship are important aspects in the overall management of the febrile neutropenic patient.

Epidemiology of Infections in Neutropenic Patients

Bacterial infections generally occur during the initial phases of neutropenic fever, whereas fungal infections are more common in patients with prolonged neutropenia. Table 8.1 provides a list of bacterial and fungal pathogens that cause infections in neutropenic patients. Recent epidemiologic surveys have

---

K.V.I. Rolston (✉)
Department of Infectious Diseases, Infection Control, and Employee Health, The University of Texas M.D. Anderson Cancer Center, 1515 Holcombe Boulevard, Houston, TX 77030, USA
e-mail: krolston@mdanderson.org

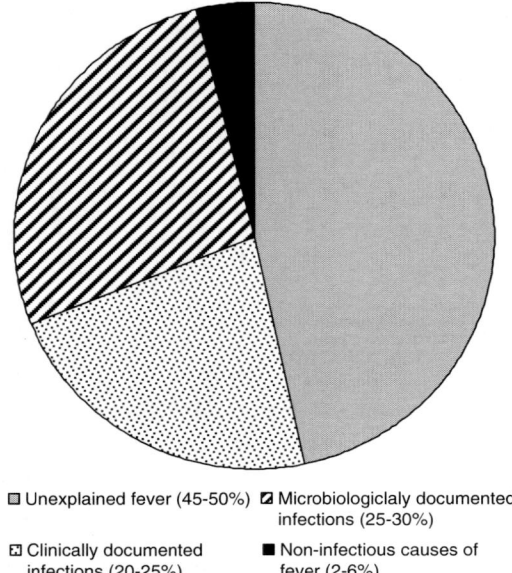

Fig. 8.1 Nature of febrile episodes in neutropenic patients. Data from recent surveys at The University of Texas M. D. Anderson Cancer Center, 2007–2008

Table 8.1 Common bacterial pathogens in neutropenic patients

Organism	Comment
Gram-positive	
Coagulase-negative staphylococci	>90% Methicillin resistant
Staphylococcus aureus	>50% Methicillin resistant
viridans group streptococci	~60% Penicillin non-susceptible
Enterococcus species	15–25% Vancomycin resistant
Bacillus species	10% Vancomycin resistant
Streptococcus Groups A, B, C, G, F	Penicillin/vancomycin tolerance
Streptococcus pneumoniae	~60% Penicillin non-susceptible
Corynebacterium species	Beta-lactam resistant
Stomatococcus mucilaginosus	Frequently causes meningitis
Gram-negative	
Escherichia coli	ESBL, increasing quinolone resistance
Klebsiella species	ESBL, carbapenamase (KPC)
Other *Enterobacteriace*	ESBL, multiple resistance mechanisms
Pseudomonas aeruginosa	Multidrug-resistant strains
Stenotrophomonas aeruginosa	Multidrug-resistant strains
Pseudomonas non-*aeruginosa* species	
Acinetobacter species	Multidrug-resistant strains
Anaerobes	
Bacteroides species	
Clostridium species	

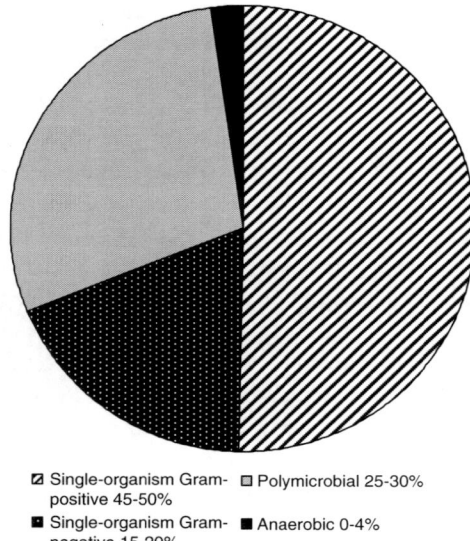

Fig. 8.2 Distribution of bacterial infections in neutropenic cancer patients. Data from recent surveys at The University of Texas M. D. Anderson Cancer Center, 2007–2008

demonstrated predominance of Gram-positive organisms over Gram-negative bacteria [2, 3]. The proportion of infections cause by Gram-positive organisms has been reported to be as high as 75–80% at some cancer treatment centers. However, both the Surveillance and Control of Pathogens of Epidemiologic Importance (SCOPE) and the European Organization for Research and Treatment of Cancer (EORTC) studies focus only on single-organism (monomicrobial) bacteremias. These data paint an incomplete picture because bacteremias cause only 20–30% of infection in cancer patients and other sites of infection, such as the lung, urinary tract, gastrointestinal tract, and skin/skin structure sites are not uncommon [4]. Although Gram-positive bacteria are the predominant organisms isolated from blood, Gram-negative organisms predominate at most other sites (e.g., pneumonia, neutropenic enterocolitis, perirectal infections, UTI's). Another critical piece of information missing from the SCOPE and EORTC studies is the proportion of infections that are polymicrobial. Data from our institution document that polymicrobial infections have more than doubled in frequency since the early 1980s and currently account for 25–30% of all bacterial infections [4, 14–16]. Additionally, approximately 80% of polymicrobial infections have a Gram-negative component and approximately 33% are caused exclusively by multiple species of Gram-negative bacilli [15]. When all sites of infection are taken into account and monomicrobial as well as polymicrobial infections are included in the overall spectrum, a substantially different epidemiologic picture emerges in which the proportion of monomicrobial Gram-positive infections falls sharply from approximately 80 to <50%. This can have a significant impact on the choice of agents used for antimicrobial prophylaxis and for empiric therapy in such patients.

Gram-positive organisms colonizing the skin are isolated frequently. These include coagulase-negative staphylococci, *Staphylococcus aureus*, *Bacillus* spp., and *Corynebacterium* spp. Gram-positive organisms arising from the oro-pharynx and upper airways include *viridans* group streptococci (VGE), *Streptococcus pneumoniae*, and *Stomatococcus mucilaginosus*, whereas *Enterococcus* spp. arise primarily from the intestinal tract. Gram-negative organisms are represented frequently by the Enterobacteriaceae (*Escherichia coli*, *Klebsiella* spp., *Enterobacter* spp.) and *Pseudomonas aeruginosa*, with *Acinetobacter* spp. and *Stenotrophomonas maltophilia* being reported with increasing frequency at some institutions [17, 18]. Strict anaerobes are seldom isolated from neutropenic patients. Rapidly growing mycobacteria are also uncommon but occasionally cause catheter-related infections in neutropenic patients [19].

Candida spp. are still the most common fungi isolated from neutropenic patients and cause infections ranging from superficial lesions (e.g., thrush and esophagitis) to deep, systemic candidiasis [20]. Most cancer treatment centers have reported a decline in the proportion of infections caused by *Candida albicans* and an increase in the proportion caused by other *Candida* species (*C. tropicalis*, *C. glabrata*, *C. parapsilosis*, etc.) [21, 22]. *Aspergillus* spp. are second in frequency among fungal pathogens in neutropenic patients [5]. They also cause a range of infections, including localized infections such as sinusitis, cutaneous aspergillosis, and aspergilloma (fungus ball), and invasive pulmonary or disseminated diseases frequently involving the central nervous system [23].

Many centers have reported an increase in the frequency of fungal infections caused by Zygomycetes, in part related to the use of agents such as voriconazole [24, 25]. These infections are often indistinguishable from aspergillosis, with the rhino-central form being particularly devastating. A large number of other opportunistic fungal pathogens have emerged in this patient population. They include *Fusarium* spp., *Trichosporon beigelii*, *Blastoschizomyces capitatus*, and *Scedosporium* spp. [5].

Viral infections are not common as a result of neutropenia, but are seen more often in patients with impaired cellular immunity. It is important to remember that such patients do develop neutropenia, and viral infections may then need to be considered [1, 13].

Initial Assessment of the Neutropenic Patient

A complete history and physical examination are essential. Historical information of interest should include details about antineoplastic therapy, the use of antimicrobial prophylaxis, travel history and potential exposure to sick contacts, and previous episodes of infection and their treatment. Underlying comorbid conditions such as diabetes, chronic lung disease, cardiac and hepatic problems, and recent surgeries should also be noted as they might have an impact on the nature and severity of infection and the risk of complications developing during a febrile episode.

The inflammatory response is often blunted in neutropenic patients resulting in a paucity of signs and symptoms usually associated with infections. Consequently, the physical examination should focus on the detection of subtle signs, particularly at frequently infected sites including the skin, oro-pharynx, gastro-intestinal tract, perineum, and larynx. Although fever is the most common manifestation of infection in neutropenic patients, some patients may harbor a serious infection without mounting a febrile response, especially if they are receiving corticosteroids or other immunosuppressive agents.

Standard laboratory investigations include blood and urine cultures and cultures of other sites (e.g., respiratory specimens, CSF, wounds, etc.) when indicated. Obtaining blood for culture simultaneously from a peripheral vein and from each lumen of a catheter, if a multilumen catheter is in place, is recommended. In patients with diarrhea, two stool specimens for the detection of *C. difficile* toxins should be obtained. Stool cultures for bacterial pathogens are of limited value. Patients with a pulmonary infiltrate might require a bronchoscopy to obtain adequate specimens for microbiologic evaluation as very few will have a productive cough. Nasal specimens are adequate for detecting the presence of community respiratory viruses, especially in the winter season.

Routine chest radiography is not recommended and should be done only in patients with respiratory signs and symptoms. CT scans of the chest and other areas (sinuses, abdomen, pelvis) should be performed as clinically indicated, and are generally more informative than routine radiographic imaging. Other laboratory tests include complete blood cell and differential counts, a serum electrolyte panel, levels of blood urea nitrogen, and serum creatinine and hepatic panel – serum bilirubin and liver enzymes. These investigations should be repeated as indicated clinically.

Risk Assessment and Risk-Based Therapy

It has long been recognized that not all neutropenic patients have the same risk of developing serious infections and/or complications. However, our ability to identify low-risk patients reliably was quite limited until recently, leading to the practice of administering hospital-based empiric antibiotic therapy to all febrile neutropenic patients [26]. With a greater

Table 8.2 The MASCC risk-index for low-risk neutropenic patients[*]

Clinical characteristic	Score
Burden of illness – no symptoms or mild symptoms	5
Burden of illness – moderate symptoms	3
Absence of hypotension	5
Absence of chronic lung disease	4
Solid tumor/no previous fungal infection	4
Absence of dehydration	3
Outpatient status at onset of fever	3
Age < 60 years	2

MASCC Multinational Association for Supportive Care in Cancer
[*]Highest possible score = 26. A score of 21 or more indicates low-risk status [6]

Table 8.3 Treatment options for low-risk febrile neutropenic patients

- Hospital-based parenteral or oral antibiotics
- Initial stabilization in hospital (24–48 h) followed by early discharge on outpatient parenteral or oral antibiotic regimen
- Outpatient antibiotics (parenteral → oral, or oral, if tolerated) for the entire febrile episode

Table 8.4 Frequently used antibiotic regimens in low-risk febrile neutropenic patients

Parenteral regimens
  Aztreonam + clindamycin
  Ciprofloxacin + clindamycin
  Ceftriaxone ± amikacin
  Ertapenem ± amikacin
  Ceftazidime or cefepime

Oral regimens
  Ciprofloxacin + amoxicillin/clavulanate, or azithromycin, or clindamycin, or linezolid
  Moxifloxacin ± agents listed above

understanding of the syndrome of "febrile neutropenia," several investigators have developed reliable risk-prediction rules in recent years. The most widely accepted of these is the risk-index developed by the Multinational Association for Supportive Care in Cancer (MASCC) [6]. This risk-index was developed by assigning integer weights to seven characteristics to develop an index score (Table 8.2). A score of 21 or greater identified low-risk patients with a positive predictive value of 91%. This index now forms the basis for most clinical trials in low-risk neutropenic adult patients. Separate, but similar risk-prediction rules have been developed for pediatric oncology patients [27]. Many institutions have developed simple clinical criteria to identify low-risk patients without having to calculate a risk-index score. This might be a more practical method in busy clinical settings. There is uniform agreement that patients who are not classified to be low-risk should be hospitalized for the administration of prompt, empiric, parenteral, broad-spectrum antibiotic therapy [1].

Several different approaches have recently been evaluated in low-risk, febrile neutropenic patients, including early discharge after a short period of hospitalization, and treatment of the entire febrile episode without hospitalization. All these options are discussed in detail below.

Empiric Antibiotic Therapy in Low-Risk Patients

The various treatment options for low-risk febrile neutropenic patients are listed in Tables 8.3 and 8.4. Despite the development of accurate risk-prediction rules, the availability of suitable oral antimicrobial agents and the emergence of home health care agencies capable of delivering outpatient antibiotic therapy, many clinicians are still not comfortable with this approach (KR – personal observations).

Many clinicians prefer to admit low-risk febrile neutropenic patients to the hospital for an initial 24–48 h "stabilization period" followed by early discharge on oral or parenteral regimens. This approach has been demonstrated to be successful in various clinical trials both in adult and pediatric patients [9, 10, 28]. Table 8.5 summarizes the results achieved in some of these trials. The results of the pilot study conducted by Talcott et al. were disappointing since 9 of 30 patients (30%) required readmission to the hospital and 4 (13.3%) developed serious medical complications [29]. These results brought into question the criteria used to identify low-risk patients, particularly the inclusion of patients with leukemia with the potential to develop prolonged neutropenia [30, 31]. Better results were achieved by investigators from the United Kingdom who only enrolled patients with solid tumors and lymphoma with an anticipated duration of neutropenia of 7 days or less [10]. Early discharge on oral ciprofloxacin and amoxicillin/clavulanate was associated with a much lower readmission rate (7.6%), the regimen was well tolerated, and there were no deaths among patients enrolled on this trial. Investigators from the Institute Jules Bordet in Belgium also used this approach (i.e., early discharge on oral ciprofloxacin plus amoxicillin/clavulanate) in 79 patients, mainly with solid tumors [9]. No complications occurred, and the overall success rate was 96%, with only three patients needing to be readmitted. In a similar study, children presenting with fever and neutropenia were assigned to receive oral cefuroxime 24–36 h after hospitalization if categorized to be low-risk [28]. Seventy-four (95%) of 78 patients treated in this manner had a positive response.

Table 8.5 Outpatient management of low-risk febrile neutropenic patients after a short hospital stay

References	Type of study and patient population	Antibiotic regimens	% Response to initial regimen ± No readmission
Talcott et al. [28]	Open-label, pilot study of 30 low-risk patients	IV mezlocillin + gentamicin or IV ceftazidime	70
Innes et al. [10]	Randomized study comparing oral outpatient therapy ($n=66$) to parenteral inpatient therapy ($n=60$) after 24 h of hospitalization	IV gentamicin + piperacillin/tazobactam vs. PO ciprofloxacin + amoxicillin/clavulanate	90 84.8
Klastersky et al. [9]	Open-label study of oral, outpatient antibiotics in 79 low-risk patients	Ciprofloxacin + amoxicillin/clavulanate	96
Santolaya et al. [27]	Prospective, randomized comparisons of hospital-based ($n=71$) and ambulatory ($n=78$) antibiotic therapy in low-risk pediatric patients following 24–36 h of hospitalization	IV ceftriaxone + teicoplanin (hospital-based treatment) PO cefuroxime (ambulatory treatment)	94 95

Ambulatory Management of the Entire Febrile Episode

A significant proportion of patients cared for at cancer treatment centers, such as The University of Texas M. D. Anderson Cancer Center (MDACC), come from other countries, are uninsured, or pay out-of-pocket. Even a short hospital stay can have a significant financial impact for such patients. In the early 1980s, approximately 90 patients with solid tumors who developed fever while being neutropenic refused hospital admission. They were treated with oral antibiotics (TMP/SMX plus rifampin or clindamycin) as outpatients. Most responded to these regimens with no serious complications or deaths (K. Rolston – unpublished data). This experience served as background data for formal trials of outpatient antibiotic treatment of febrile neutropenic patients at this institution. To date, three randomized trials at MDACC have evaluated this approach (i.e., outpatient treatment of the entire febrile episode) along with a few trials conducted at other institutions [32–35]. Institutional pathways in place at MDACC and small pilot studies have added to this experience which is summarized in Table 8.6 [36–38]. These studies demonstrated that both parenteral and oral regimens are safe and effective with response rates ranging from 80 to 95%. Many patients not responding to the initial regimens responded to alternative outpatient regimens [Table 8.3]. Among the few patients requiring hospitalization, none had serious complications, none required care in the intensive care unit, and there were no infection-related deaths. A recently published meta-analysis concluded that "oral antibiotics may be safely offered to neutropenic patients with fever who are at low-risk for mortality" [39].

Empiric Antibiotic Therapy in Patients Not Classified as Low-Risk

Standard therapy for neutropenic patients not considered to be low-risk includes the prompt administration of parenteral, broad-spectrum antibiotic therapy with close monitoring in the hospital [1]. The various treatment options are listed in Table 8.6. Until the availability of broad spectrum beta-lactams (extended spectrum cephalosporins, carbapenems), the combination of an antipseudomonal beta-lactam and an aminoglycoside was the most frequently used regimen, resulting in response rates of ~70% [1]. The potential advantages of such combination regimens include broad coverage against most pathogens seen in this setting (including anaerobes), possible synergy resulting in rapid bactericidal activity, and the potential for reducing the emergence of resistant organisms. The major disadvantages are increased oto- and nephrotoxicity, and suboptimal activity against many Gram-positive organisms. With the emergence of resistant Gram-positive organisms (coagulase-negative staphylococci, MRSA, viridans group streptococci, *Corynebacterium jeikeium*) as frequent pathogens in neutropenic patients, the inclusion of vancomycin and later linezolid into the initial regimen became common place [1, 13, 40]. Several studies, however, have demonstrated that the initial use of an agent like vancomycin is not associated with superior outcomes when compared to the use of this agent after isolation of a resistant Gram-positive pathogen [41–43]. These data and the association of increased vancomycin usage with the selection of VRE and staphylococci with reduced susceptibility to vancomycin have led to the recommendation by many experts and societies that vancomycin

Table 8.6 Outpatient antibiotic therapy of low-risk, febrile neutropenic patients: The M. D. Anderson experience

References	Type of study and patient population	Antibiotic regimens	% Response to initial regimen
Rubenstein et al. [33]	Randomized trial of IV vs. PO outpatient regimen. 83 episodes, all adult	IV – aztreonam + clindamycin PO – ciprofloxacin + clindamycin	95 88
Rolston et al. [34]	Randomized trial of IV vs. PO outpatient regimens 179 episodes, all adults	IV aztreonam + clindamycin PO ciprofloxacin + amoxicillin/clavulanate	87 90
Mullen et al. [35]	Randomized trial of IV vs. PO regimens in pediatric patients, 75 episodes	IV ceftazidime PO ciprofloxacin	94 80
Rolston et al. [36]	Open label, pilot study of oral quinolone monotherapy in adult, 40 episodes	PO gatifloxacin	95
Rolston et al. [37]	Open label, pilot study of oral quinolone monotherapy in adults, 21 episodes	PO moxifloxacin	95
Escalante et al. [38]	257 episodes, adult patients enrolled on institutional outpatient pathways	IV ceftazidime + clindamycin PO ciprofloxacin + amoxicillin/clavulanate	80[a]
Elting et al. [11]	529 episodes, adult patients enrolled on institutional outpatient pathways	PO ciprofloxacin + amoxicillin/clavulanate	80

IV intravenous, *PO* oral
[a]Combined response rate for parenteral and oral regimens, as individual response rates were not mentioned

should only be included in the initial regimen at institutions that have a high rate of isolation of resistant Gram-positive pathogens [1, 44].

With the availability of truly broad-spectrum agents since the 1980s, empiric monotherapy became an option in this patient population. Many prospective randomized studies have demonstrated that monotherapy with agents such as ceftazidime, cefepime, imipenem, meropenem, and piperacillin/tazobactam are associated with response rates similar to those associated with various comparator combination regimens [1, 5, 45]. A recently published meta-analysis showed that monotherapy regimens are as effective as combination regimens with similar mortality rates, similar rates of bacterial and fungal superinfections, and are associated with lower rates of treatment failures and fewer adverse events [46].

The same group has published an analysis linking cefepime monotherapy with a higher all cause mortality than other agents [47]. Ceftazidime is associated with substantial resistance against most Gram-positive and many Gram-negative pathogens at many institutions and may not be suitable for empiric monotherapy. At least one meta-analysis has reported lower response rates with ceftazidime, and this agent has largely been replaced by cefepime in general practice. The weight of current data/opinion supports the use of empiric monotherapy for most neutropenic patients with fever, selecting suitable agents based on local epidemiology and susceptibility/resistance patterns. In today's economic environment, monotherapy may represent the most cost-effective option. Figure 8.3 provides an algorithm for the management of various subsets (risk-groups) of febrile neutropenic patients.

Evaluation of Response and Duration of Therapy

The median time to defervescence in low-risk patients is approximately 2 days, and it is approximately 5 days in patients not classified as low-risk [48–50]. Persistence of fever for 3–5 days in otherwise stable patients does not necessarily indicate failure of the initial regimen. However, persistence of fever beyond 3–5 days should lead to a full reevaluation of the patient including a search for drainable and/or removable focus of infection or the development of a superinfection. A change of the initial regimen is recommended at this stage, and this may consist of additional antibacterial agents depending on the gaps in the original regimens, or the administration of antifungal or antiviral agents, if indicated [51].

The duration of therapy continues to engender considerable debate with opinion almost evenly split between two different approaches. Some authors advocate continuation of antibiotic therapy in all patients until the resolution of neutropenia (ANC > 500/mm^3) regardless of whether or not an infection was documented during the febrile episode [1, 13, 51]. Others recommend administration of therapy for 4 days after resolution of signs and symptoms (including microbiologic or radiographic evidence if present initially), with a

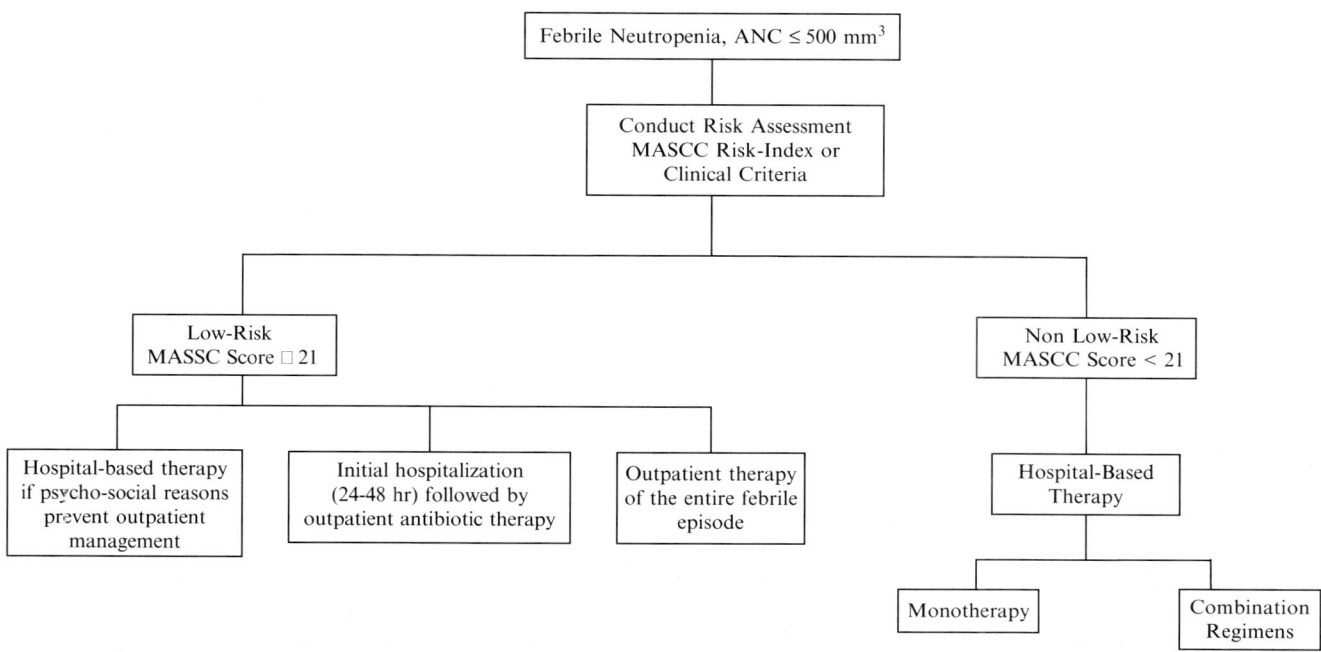

Fig. 8.3 Algorithm for the management of febrile neutropenic patients. Adapted from reference numbers [1, 6, 8–11, 13, 25, 26, 28, 29, 35]

minimum of 7 days treatment, regardless of whether or not the patient has persistent neutropenia. The former approach may result in needless administration of antibiotics to many patients potentially increasing costs, toxicity, and the development of bacterial or fungal superinfections. The latter approach requires careful observation of the patient after discontinuation of therapy. The ultimate decision of when to stop therapy often needs to be individualized and depends on several factors such as (1) the patient's risk group, (2) the presence of a documented infection, (3) the nature of the underlying malignancy (solid tumor or hematologic malignancy), (4) the need for additional chemotherapy or invasive procedures, and (5) the persistence of neutropenia. These and other controversial issues in the management of febrile neutropenic patients are discussed in detail in Chap. 9.

Antimicrobial Stewardship

Antimicrobial agents are used with greater frequency and for a larger number of indications (prophylaxis, empiric therapy, targeted therapy, maintenance therapy) in cancer patients than in most other patient populations [52]. This has led to an increase in the emergence of resistant pathogens [53]. Additionally, the development of novel agents is at an all time low, mandating the judicious use of currently available agents – termed antimicrobial stewardship. The various components of an effective antimicrobial stewardship program are listed in Table 8.7 and include a multidisciplinary antibiotic stewardship team (MAST), institutional guidelines/pathways, formulary restrictions, clearance for the use of selected agents, and de-escalation or streamlining of therapy when appropriate [54]. Antibiotic stewardship programs have already been successful at several cancer treatment centers, and in the opinion of this investigator, will soon become mandatory at most institutions [55–57].

Summary

Neutropenic patients continue to develop infections despite improvements in supportive care of the cancer patient, and the implementation of preventive and infection control strategies. The spectrum of infection undergoes periodic changes with the emergence of newer opportunistic pathogens and/or the development of resistance among recognized pathogens. Empiric antibiotic therapy remains the standard of care. However, not all febrile neutropenic patients have the same risk of developing severe infections or serious medical complications. Low-risk patients can now be reliably identified early on in the febrile episode and can be treated with a short period of hospitalization, or entirely as outpatients. Very little change has occurred in the management of moderate to high-risk febrile neutropenic

Table 8.7 Antibiotic regimens commonly used in febrile neutropenic patients not classified as low-risk

Combination regimens with vancomycin[a]
  Vancomycin + cefepime or ceftazidime[b]
  Piperacillin/tazobactam
  Imipenem or meropenem
  Aztreonam[c]
  Ciprofloxacin (or other quinolone)[d]

Combination regimens without vancomycin
  Aminoglycoside + cefepime or ceftazidime[b]
  Piperacillin/tazobactam
  Imipenem or meropenem
  Quinolone[d]

Monotherapy
  Cefepime or ceftazidime[b]
  Piperacillin/tazobactam
  Imipenem or meropenem

[a]Vancomycin is occasionally replaced by linezolid
[b]Ceftazidime not useful at many institutions due to the emergence of resistant pathogens
[c]Aztreonam used primarily in patients with severe beta-lactam allergy
[d]Quinolones should not be used if patients have received prophylaxis with these agents

patients over the past decade. Antimicrobial stewardship has become an important strategy in the overall management of these patients since new drug development has declined appreciably. It is hoped that antimicrobial stewardship and strict adherence to infection control measures will reduce the selection and spread of multi-drug-resistant organisms, which are posing serious therapeutic challenges to clinicians caring for these high-risk patients.

References

1. Hughes WT, Armstrong D, Bodey GP, et al. Guidelines for the use of antimicrobial agents in neutropenic patients with cancer. Clin Infect Dis. 2002;34:730–51.
2. Wisplinghoff H, Seifert H, Wenzel RP, Edmond MB. Current trends in the epidemiology of nosocomial bloodstream infections in patients with hematological malignancies and solid neoplasms in hospitals in the United States. Clin Infect Dis. 2003;36:1103–10.
3. Klastersky J, Ameye L, Maertens J, et al. Bacteremia in febrile neutropenic cancer patients. Internat J Antimicrob Agents. 2007;30S:551–9.
4. Yadegarynia D, Tarrand J, Raad I, Rolston K. Current spectrum of bacterial infections in cancer patients. Clin Infect Dis. 2003;37:1144–5.
5. Chamilos G, Luna M, Lewis RE, et al. Invasive fungal infections in patients with hematologic malignancies in a tertiary care cancer center: an autopsy study over a 15-year period (1989–2003). Haematologica. 2006;91:986–9.
6. Klastersky J, Paesmans M, Rubenstein E, et al. The MASCC Risk Index: a multinational scoring system to predict low-risk febrile neutropenic cancer patients. J Clin Oncol. 2000;18:3038–51.
7. Talcott JA, Finberg R, Mayer RJ, et al. The medical course of cancer patients with fever and neutropenia. Clinical identification of a low-risk subgroup at presentation. Arch Intern Med. 1988;148:2561–8.
8. Rolston K. New trends in patient management: risk-based therapy for febrile patients with neutropenia. Clin Infect Dis. 1999;29:515–21.
9. Klastersky J, Paesmans M, Georgala A, et al. Outpatient oral antibiotics for febrile neutropenic cancer patients using a score predictive for complications. J Clin Oncol. 2006;24:4129–34.
10. Innes HE, Smith DB, O'Reilly SM, et al. Oral antibiotics with early hospital discharge compared with in-patient intravenous antibiotics for low-risk febrile neutropenia in patients with cancer: a prospective randomized controlled single centre study. Br J Cancer. 2003;89:43–9.
11. Elting LS, Lu C, Escalante CP, et al. Outcomes and cost of outpatient or inpatient management of 712 patients with febrile neutropenia. J Clin Oncol. 2008;26:606–11.
12. Cherif H, Johansson E, Björklholm M, Kalin M. The feasibility of early hospital discharge with oral antimicrobial therapy in low risk patients with febrile neutropenia following chemotherapy for hematologic malignancies. Haematolgia. 2006;91:215–22.
13. Rolston KVI, Bodey GP. Infections in patients with cancer. In: Kufe DW, Bast Jr RC, Hait WN, Hong WK, Pollock RE, Weichselbaum RR, Holland JF, Frei III E, editors. Cancer Medicine, e7. Hamilton, ON: BC Decker; 2006. p. 2222–45.
14. Rolston KVI, Bodey GP, Safdar A. Polymicrobial infection in patients with cancer: an underappreciated and underreported entity. Clin Infect Dis. 2007;45:228–33.
15. Elting LS, Bodey GP, Fainstein V. Polymicrobial septicemia in the cancer patient. Medicine. 1986;65:218–25.
16. Adachi JA, Yadegarynia D, Rolston K. Spectrum of polymicrobial bacterial infection in patients with cancer, 1975–2002. (Abstract 4). American Society for Microbiology. Polymicrobial Diseases. Lake Tahoe, NV, Oct. 19–23, 2003.
17. Rolston KVI, Tarrand JJ. *Pseudomonas aeruginosa* – still a frequent pathogen in patients with cancer: 11-year experience from a comprehensive cancer center. Clin Infect Dis. 1999;29:463–4.
18. Safdar A, Rolston KV. *Stenotrophomonas maltophilia*: changing spectrum of a serious bacterial pathogen in patients with cancer. Clin Infect Dis. 2007;45:1602–9.
19. Han XY, Dé I, Jacobson KL. Rapidly growing mycobacteria. Clinical and Microbiologic studies of 115 cases. Am J Clin Pathol. 2007;128:612–21.
20. Abi-Said D, Anaissie E, Uzun O, Raad I, Pinzcowski H, Vartivarian S. The epidemiology of hematogenous candidiasis caused by different *Candida* species. Clin Infect Dis. 1997;24:1122–8.
21. Hachem R, Hanna H, Kontoyiannis D, Jiang Y, Raad I. The changing epidemiology of invasive candidiasis. *Candida glabrata* and *Candida krusei* as the leading causes of Candidemia in hematologic malignancy. Cancer. 2008;112:2493–9.
22. Mullen CA, Abd El-Baki H, Samir H, Tarrand JJ, Rolston KV. Non-albicans *Candida* is the most common cause of candidemia in pediatric cancer patients. Support Care Cancer. 2003;11:321–5.
23. Patterson TF, Kirkpatrick WR, White M, et al. Invasive aspergillosis: disease spectrum, treatment practices, and outcomes. Medicine. 2000;79:250–60.
24. Trifilio SM, Bennett CL, Yarnold PR, et al. Breakthrough zygomycosis after voriconazole administration among patients with hematolgic malignancies who receive hematopoietic stem-cell transplants or intensive chemotherapy. Bone Marrow Transplant. 2007;39:425–9.
25. Marty FM, Cosimi LA, Baden LR. Breakthrough zygomycosis after voriconazole treatment in recipients of hematopoietic stem-cell transplants. N Engl J Med. 2004;350:950–2.
26. Klastersky J. Management of fever in neutropenic patients with different risks of complications. Clin Infect Dis. 2004;39:S32–7.
27. Santolaya ME, Alvarez AM, Avilés CL, et al. Prospective evaluation of a model of prediction of invasive bacterial infection risk among children with cancer, fever and neutropenia. Clin Infect Dis. 2002;35:678–83.

28. Santolaya ME, Alvarez AM, Avilés CL, et al. Early hospital discharge followed by outpatient management versus continued hospitalization of children with cancer, fever, and neutropenia at low risk for invasive bacterial infection. J Clin Oncol. 2004;22:3784–9.
29. Talcott JA, Whalen A, Clark J, Rieker PP, Finberg R. Home antibiotic therapy for low-risk cancer patients with fever and neutropenia: a pilot study of 30 patients based on a validated prediction rule. J Clin Oncol. 1994;12:107–14.
30. Kern KV. Risk assessment and treatment of low-risk patients with febrile neutropenia. Clin Infect Dis. 2006;15:533–40.
31. Rolston KVI. Prediction of neutropenia. Int J Antimicrob Agents. 2000;16:113–5.
32. Hidalgo M, Hornedo J, Lumbreras JM, et al. Outpatient therapy with oral ofloxacin for patients with low risk neutropenia and fever. Cancer. 1999;85:213–9.
33. Rubenstein EB, Rolston K, Benjamin RS, et al. Outpatient treatment of febrile episodes in low risk neutropenic cancer patients. Cancer. 1993;71:3640–6.
34. Rolston K, Rubenstein E, Elting L, Escalante E, Manzullo E, Bodey GP. Ambulatory management of febrile episodes in low-risk neutropenic patients [abstract LM81]. In: Program and Abstract of the 35th Interscience Conference on Antimicrobial Agents and Chemotherapy, American Society for Microbiology (Washington, DC). 1995.
35. Mullen CA, Petropoulos D, Roberts WM, et al. Outpatient treatment of febrile neutropenia in low risk pediatric cancer patients. Cancer. 1999;86:126–34.
36. Rolston KVI, Manzullo EF, Elting LS, et al. Once daily, oral, outpatient quinolone monotherapy for low-risk cancer patients with fever and neutropenia. Cancer. 2006;106:2489–94.
37. Rolston KVI, Frisbee-Hume SE, Patel S, Manzullo EF, Benjamin RS. Oral moxifloxacin for outpatient treatment of low-risk, febrile neutropenic patients. Support Care Cancer. 2009;18(1):89–94.
38. Escalante CP, Weiser MA, Manzullo E, et al. Outcomes of treatment pathways in outpatient treatment of low risk febrile neutropenic cancer patients. Support Care Cancer. 2004;12:657–62.
39. Vidal L, Paul M, Ben Dor I, Soares-Weiser K, Leibovici L. Oral versus intravenous antibiotic treatment for febrile neutropenia in cancer patients: a systematic review and meta-analysis of randomized trials. J Antimicrob Chemother. 2004;54:29–37.
40. Jaksic B, Martinelli G, Perez-Oteyza J, Hartman CS, Leonard LB, Tack KJ. Efficacy and safety of linezolid compared with vancomycin in a randomized, double-blind study of febrile neutropenic patients with cancer. Clin Infect Dis. 2006;42:597–607.
41. Cinetta A, Kern WV, De Bock R, et al. Vancomycin versus placebo for treating persistent fever in patients with neutropenic cancer receiving piperacillin-tazobactam monotherapy. Clin Infect Dis. 2003;37:382–9.
42. Rubin M, Hathorn JW, Marshall D, Gress J, Steinberg SM, Pizzo PA. Gram-positive infections and the use of vancomycin in 550 episodes of fever and neutropenia. Ann Intern Med. 1988;108:30–5.
43. Ramphal R, Bolger M, Oblon DJ, et al. Vancomycin is not an essential component of the initial empiric treatment regimen for febrile neutropenic patients receiving ceftazidime: a randomized prospective study. Antimicrob Agents Chemother. 2003;36:1062–7.
44. Segal BH, Freifeld AG, Baden LR, et al. Prevention and treatment of cancer-related infections. J Natl Compr Canc Netw. 2008;6:122–74.
45. Viscoli C, Cometta A, Kern WV, et al. Piperacillin-tazobactam monotherapy in high-risk febrile and neutropenic cancer patients. Clin Microbiol Infect. 2006;12:212–6.
46. Paul M, Soares-Weiser K, Leibovici L. Beta lactam monotherapy versus beta lactam-aminoglycoside combination therapy for fever with neutropenia: systematic review and meta-analysis. Br Med J. 2003;326:1111–9.
47. Yahav D, Paul M, Fraser A, Sarid N, Leibovici L. Efficacy and safety of cefepime: a systematic review and meta-analysis. Lancet Infect Dis. 2007;7:338–48.
48. Elting LS, Rubenstein EB, Rolston K, et al. Time to clinical response: an outcome of antibiotic therapy of febrile neutropenia with implications for quality and cost of care. J Clin Oncol. 2000;18:3699–706.
49. Pizzo PA, Robichard KJ, Gill FA. Duration of empiric antibiotic therapy in granulopenic patients with cancer. Am J Med. 1979;67:194–9.
50. Corey L, Boeckh M. Persistent fever in patients with neutropenia. N Engl J Med. 2002;346:222–4.
51. Sipsas NV, Bodey GP, Kontoyiannis DP. Perspectives for the management of febrile neutropenic patients with cancer in the 21st Century. Cancer. 2005;103:1103–13.
52. Rolston KVI. Challenges in the treatment of infections caused by gram-positive and gram-negative bacteria in patients with cancer and neutropenia. Clin Infect Dis. 2005;40:S246–52.
53. Bad Bugs, No Drugs. Infectious Diseases Society of America. http://www.idsociety.org/pa/IDSA_Paper4_final_web.pdf. Accessed July 2004.
54. Dellit TH, Owens RC, McGowan JE, et al. Infectious Diseases Society of America and the Society for Healthcare Epidemiology of America Guidelines for developing an institutional program to enhance antimicrobial stewardship. Clin Infect Dis. 2007;44:159–77.
55. Metjian TA, Prasad PA, Kogon A, Coffin SE, Zaoutis TE. Evaluation of an antimicrobial stewardship program at a pediatric teaching hospital. Pediatr Infect Dis J. 2008;27:106–11.
56. Paskovaty A, Pflomm JM, Myke N, Seo SK. A multidisciplinary approach to antimicrobial stewardship: evolution into the 21st century. Int J Anticrob Agents. 2005;25:1–10.
57. Adachi J, Perego C, Vigil K, Mulanovich V, Chemaly R, Rolston K. Antibiotic stewardship initiative in the intensive care unit (ICU): evidence from a quality improvement project supporting the development of a multidisciplinary antimicrobial stewardship team (MAST). [Abst. #08-059]. In: Programs and abstracts of the Multinational Association for Supportive Care in Cancer (MASCC/ISOO) 2008 International Symposium, Houston, Texas, June 26–28, 2008.

Chapter 9
Controversies in Empiric Therapy of Febrile Neutropenia

John R. Wingard

Abstract Antineoplastic chemotherapy regimens induced myelosuppression was quickly recognized as a major limitation to the full utility of cytotoxic drug regimens targeting cancer. Measures taken to mitigate harm from myelosuppression have led to a number of controversies over the years. The first controversy faced by clinicians was whether or not empiric antibiotic therapy for febrile neutropenia is appropriate. The concerns was that fever may be due to noninfectious causes, inappropriate antibiotic use might lead to emergence of resistance or superinfections by resistant organisms, the patient might experience toxicities (the antibiotics of those days had considerable toxicity), and the drugs were costly. This controversy was eventually resolved in favor of empiric antibiotics through a series of studies. Today, there are yet other controversies about empiric therapy of febrile neutropenia. These include questions as to whether there is an optimal antibiotic regimen, persistent concerns about resistance, questions as to what are the causes for fevers that have no apparent explanation, quandaries about the role for empiric antifungal therapy, and the unresolved issues as to why some patients become quite ill while others are less affected. Other controversies as to optimal management of venous catheters, etiology of neutropenic enterocolitis (typhlitis), the role for antimicrobial prophylaxis, and antibiotic resistance are addressed in other chapters and will not be covered here.

Keywords Febrile neutropenia • Empiric therapy • Optimal antibiotic regimen • Drug resistance • Empiric antifungal therapy

Introduction

In the 1950s, antineoplastic chemotherapy regimens were first introduced into clinical practice and myelosuppression was quickly recognized as a major limitation to the full utility of cytotoxic drug regimens targeting cancer. Measures taken to mitigate harm from myelosuppression have led to a number of controversies over the years.

The first controversy faced by clinicians was whether or not empiric antibiotic therapy for febrile neutropenia is appropriate. Basic infectious disease principles for management of fever of unknown origin at the time dictated that antibiotics should be administered only after evaluation documented an infection and the therapy should narrowly target a specific pathogen. The reasoning was that fever may be due to noninfectious causes, inappropriate antibiotic use might lead to emergence of resistance or superinfections by resistant organisms, the patient might experience toxicities (the antibiotics of those days had considerable toxicity), and the drugs used were costly. This controversy was eventually resolved in favor of empiric antibiotics through a series of studies. Careful study of the epidemiology (most fevers are due to bacterial infections which can be documented if sufficient time lapses), elucidation of the natural history of febrile neutropenia (bacterial infections, especially by Gram negative organisms, progress rapidly and are associated with high mortality and morbidity if treatment is delayed), and evaluation of the efficacy of interventions (empiric antibiotics result in reductions in infectious morbidity and mortality) provided the basis for current concepts of empiric therapy febrile neutropenia. That controversy was resolved.

Today, there are yet other controversies about empiric therapy of febrile neutropenia. These include questions as to whether there is an optimal antibiotic regimen, persistent concerns about resistance, questions as to what are the causes for fevers that have no apparent explanation, quandaries about the role for empiric antifungal therapy, and the unresolved issues as to why some patients become quite ill while others are less affected. Other controversies as to optimal management of venous catheters, etiology of

J.R. Wingard (✉)
Department of Medicine, University of Florida, Box 103633, 1376 Mowry Road Ste. 145, Gainesville, FL 32610-3633, USA
e-mail: john.wingard@medicine.ufl.edu

neutropenic enterocolitis (typhlitis), the role for antimicrobial prophylaxis, and antibiotic resistance are addressed in other chapters and will not be covered here.

Is There One "Best" Antibiotic Regimen?

Randomized trials have demonstrated multiple effective antibiotic regimens. Guidelines have been formulated to codify best practices [1–5]. Several crucial principles have emerged over the years. Patients can be stratified into groups at "low" and "high" risk for serious complications and different evaluation and management approaches should be pursued. Even though Gram positive bacteria are the most common bloodstream isolates, the empiric regimen must principally target Gram negative bacteria since they remain the most virulent pathogens except in isolated settings with high rates of *Staphylococcus aureus* infections. Monotherapy options are as effective as combination regimens and may be associated with less serious toxicity. The empiric antibiotic choices should take into consideration the impact of whether or not antibiotic prophylaxis had been used. With all that is known about empiric therapy, there remain several unanswered questions.

Recently, concerns have been raised about dangers with cefepime. Two meta-analyses from one group have noted increased mortality with cefepime when compared to other β lactams [6, 7]. The meta-analyses showed cefepime to offer comparable response rates, infection-related mortality, and similar rates for other infection-related endpoints to other antibiotic regimens. Thus, the explanation for the apparent higher mortality rate is not clear. Several important points should be pointed out. The individual trials (in contrast to the meta-analyses) were not set up as primary tests of mortality differences. All-cause mortality was not uniformly reported in the various trials. Stratification of patients for neoplastic and comorbidity factors known to influence mortality was not done in the individual trials; thus, it is possible that inadvertent imbalance of risk factors (for mortality) may have been present and may explain this observation rather than some adverse event due to cefepime. This matter is being reviewed by the FDA. For now, many experts believe this to be a reliable and safe option for febrile neutropenia, pending more information.

Adjuvant use of growth factors to bolster neutrophil recovery, while appealing conceptually, has not been consistently shown to be helpful as an adjunct to antibiotic therapy for febrile neutropenia. In a meta-analysis, mortality was not affected [8], although there was a marginal benefit in infection-related mortality and shorter times to neutrophil recovery and hospital discharge. So, today, the adjuvant role of G-CSF remains uncertain and is generally not recommended.

So, is there truly one "best" antibiotic regimen? The answer is yes and no. Clearly, the choice should be governed by both patient factors and local antibiotic susceptibilities. The key is to choose a regimen that is active against the organisms that are the cause of infection, since 30-day mortality is much higher in patients with Gram negative bacteremia if the first choice is not active against the infecting organism. Thus, although there may be a "best" regimen for a given patient in a given setting, the best regimen may differ for a different patient (with different risk factors) in the same setting, or a patient with similar risk factors in a different setting.

If the Cultures Are Negative, What is the Cause of Febrile Neutropenia?

In many febrile neutropenic patients, infection is not clearly documented. The etiology of unexplained fever is poorly understood. Sometimes, it is merely a slow clinical response to an infection, and given sufficient time, defervescence will occur without change in the empiric antibiotic regimen. Pro-inflammatory cytokines released because of tissue damage from the cytotoxic antineoplastic therapy is the most likely noninfectious cause [9]. Other possible noninfectious causes include fever from certain drugs, transfusion of blood products, and the malignancy itself.

In some cases the fever is due to an infection, but the burden of organisms is below the threshold of detectability in current cultural systems. The routine use of empiric antibiotics has exacerbated the challenge of detection of pathogens, since intervention occurs much earlier in the course of infection preventing the number of organisms from reaching a peak that otherwise would occur if no intervention took place. Thus, many cases of culture negative fevers represent infections, yet they are in an early phase that cannot be documented by currently available diagnostic testing (and clinical evaluation).

It is known that if the volume of blood drawn for blood cultures is small, the likelihood of isolating an organism is less than with larger volumes [10, 11]. Studies have been performed to determine the optimal volume, balancing detection, and waste considerations. Retrospective studies found that two blood culture sets of 20 mL each inoculated into automated culture systems detect 80–90% of bloodstream pathogens; three or four sets during the first 24 h are necessary to detect more than 96% [10, 11]. Unfortunately, such studies have not examined separately the group of neutropenic patients to determine if bacterial load and optimal volumes are similar to the entire group of hospitalized patients. One important characteristic about neutropenic patients that may make them different is that institution of empiric antibiotics at first fever renders the usual recommendation for several samplings during the first 24 h moot since the antibiotics alter the organism load. This matter is in need of more study in febrile neutropenia.

It is known that antibiotics interfere with the organism being isolated from blood cultures, suppressing viable organisms to below the threshold of positivity. Resins added to the culture media can inactivate antibiotics and may improve the sensitivity of cultures in patients receiving antibiotics [12, 13]. However, the added advantage of resin blood culture media systems over conventional blood culture systems has been questioned [14]. Cell wall deficient bacteria can be induced by antibiotics that act on the cell wall and because of fragility they may not be easily identified by commercial blood culture systems. They are also occasional causes of unexplained fevers and in one series of neutropenic BMT patients, accounted for 25% of culture negative fevers [15].

Bacteria have been detected in blood samples from febrile neutropenic patients with negative blood cultures in studies using a eubacterial approach with PCR technology to detect 16S rRNA gene amplification. Up to 10–25% of culture negative febrile neutropenia may be due to bacteria detected by such assays [16, 17]. Although PCR diagnostic assays are increasingly assuming important roles in clinical microbiology for detection of many infectious pathogens, unfortunately, issues about suboptimal sensitivity, automation of the technology, and interpretation make this technology not suitable for this clinical application at present [18–20].

Similar molecular detection assays for fungi indicate fungi to be uncommon causes of FUO early in febrile neutropenia [17], but fungal DNA [21–26] as well as fungal proteins such as β-glucan and galactomannan [27–31] have been found to be present in a higher proportion of persistently febrile patients later in neutropenia.

These various observations indicate that even in the face of negative cultures many episodes of febrile neutropenia are truly infectious. Future studies are needed to improve our ability to detect organisms in culture negative patients so that targeting of antibiotics can be achieved.

Can Acute Phase Protein Responses Distinguish Infected Patients from Noninfected Patients?

A variety of inflammatory proteins and cytokines increase during febrile episodes. Various studies have examined the utility of these to attempt to distinguish fever due to infection from noninfectious causes.

C reactive protein (CRP) has been examined in chemotherapy and BMT patients. In BMT patients, the heights of CRP and temperature elevation were higher in fevers due to infection compared to fever due to GVHD [32, 33]. However, low sensitivities have been noted and other studies have not found CRP levels to reliably predict infection [34, 35]. Levels of interleukins-6 (IL6) and IL8 have been found to be elevated and in some studies these are useful to distinguish infection from noninfection [34, 35]. Procalcitonin (PCT) also has been evaluated and found to distinguish infection from noninfection [35]. In a meta-analysis PCT levels were more sensitive (88% [95% confidence interval [CI], 80–93%] vs. 75% [95% CI, 62–84%]) for CRP levels in differentiating bacterial infections from other causes of fever [36]. PCT levels were also more specific (81% [95% CI, 67–90%] vs. 67% [95% CI, 56–77%]) than CRP levels. A more recent review of procalcitonin studies in neutropenic infections also found promise in procalcitonin levels to distinguish infection from noninfection [37], but not superior to IL6 or CRP [37]. Several studies also suggest promise of such markers to predict outcome of the infection [38, 39]. At present, a lack of standard definitions, heterogeneity of study populations studied, and small numbers of patients make the true utility of such markers of infection not well established.

Is There Still a Role for Empiric Antifungal Therapy?

"Maintaining guidelines that dictate treatment of a population in which >90% of patients do not have invasive fungal disease is not justifiable...." [40].

Although invasive fungal disease is not a problem in short-term neutropenia (<7 days), prolonged neutropenia is associated with a risk for both invasive *Candida* and *Aspergillus* infections. It is undeniable that empiric antifungal therapy has dramatically reduced morbidity and mortality from invasive *Candida* and *Aspergillus* infections in patients with prolonged neutropenia. Since persistent fever is often the only manifestation of Candidemia, coupled with improved outcomes when therapy is begun early in the course of infection [41, 42], early therapy is crucial in patients with invasive fungal disease to minimize fungal deaths. The routine initiation of empiric antifungal therapy after 3–7 days of persistent fever has become widely practiced and endorsed by multiple expert consensus panels [1–5].

Amphotericin B was initially used but subsequently lipid formulations of amphotericin B, itraconazole, and caspofungin have also been shown to be effective. Although voriconazole has been studied, the pivotal randomized trial failed to demonstrate noninferiority and it has not received FDA approval for this indication. Notwithstanding, many experts feel that it is an acceptable option for empiric antifungal therapy based on its safety and efficacy demonstrated in documented *Candida* and *Aspergillus* infections in randomized trials of first-line therapy.

Generally, clinicians choose the "best" antifungal based on patient characteristics, weighing issues of activity of the agent against the suspected pathogen, safety, and cost.

Yet, the randomized trials that established the benefits for empiric antifungal therapy had few patients, data for several of the important endpoints were not significantly different due to limited statistical power, there was considerable heterogeneity of patients and treatments, and the use of antifungal prophylactic agents in some of the patients meant its impact could not be adequately assessed (discussed in [43, 44]). Moreover the use of myeloid growth factors and in the HSCT setting, optimization of stem cell content in the hematopoietic graft have led to shorter neutropenic episodes, raising the concern that empiric antifungal therapy may not be needed in many settings in which it was evaluated before these advances. Moreover, the use of azole prophylaxis has been widely adopted in high-risk patients, and the need for empiric antifungal therapy in patients receiving antifungal prophylaxis has not been evaluated.

The problem with giving antifungal therapy empirically to all patients with persistent fever is that most patients with persistent fever do not have invasive fungal disease. Thus, de Pauw's complaint above [40] rings true. Persistent fever is not a reliable guide for whom antifungal therapy is needed. Too many patients needlessly are exposed to drugs that are toxic, may interact with other drugs in potentially deleterious ways, and are costly. Moreover, overuse of any antimicrobial agent increases the risk for resistance, and that development ultimately may thwart the effectiveness of the drug. Its use encourages the risk that an inadequate course of therapy may be given to those who are truly infected since a diagnosis is not made and therapy is typically stopped at neutrophil recovery, whereas a longer course of therapy is needed for real infections.

Several strategies have been explored to better target antifungal therapy to those with a higher likelihood of invasive fungal disease. The first is the appearance of clinical signs and symptoms other than the mere presence of fever. For *Candida*, occasionally polyarthralgias or polymyalgias, new onset of azotemia, or maculopapular erythematous skin lesions may herald fungemia; the onset of such clinical manifestations are strong clues to Candidemia. For *Aspergillus*, the onset of respiratory, sinus, or orbital symptoms or signs are manifestations of *Aspergillus* pneumonia or sinusitis, the most common presentations of Aspergillosis. Radiologically, the appearance of dense nodules, a halo sign, cavitary infiltrate, boney erosion of sinus walls all strongly suggest invasive mold infection [42]. Although such clinical and radiologic manifestations are quite useful when present, they are not universally present and often are not manifested early during the course of infection.

The use of fungal biomarkers has been evaluated. Two diagnostic assays detecting fungal cell wall proteins have been FDA licensed. The β-glucan assay detects several fungal genera that include the most likely fungal pathogens, *Candida* and *Aspergillus*, along with several others (*Trichosporon* and *Fusarium*), but does not detect *Zygomycetes* and *Cryptococcus*. Sensitivity and specificity were 70 and 87%, respectively [28, 29]. A second assay is the serum galactomannan assay, which detects *Aspergillus* (but not *Candida*, *Zygomycetes* and most other fungal pathogens) [30, 31, 45, 46]. Data submitted to the FDA indicated sensitivity and specificity to exceed 80 and 80%, respectively. In practice, the sensitivity has been variable in different patient populations and generally somewhat less, with a sensitivity of only 71% with specificity of 89% in a meta-analysis [47]. Moreover, clinicians often forget that patients must be serially tested (typically 2–3 times weekly) over the period of risk rather than at a single point in time to achieve such sensitivity. A variety of conditions have been identified that affect the performance of these two tests, including the use of antimold prophylaxis (false negative) and the use of certain antibiotics such as piperacillin-tazobactam (false positive).

The ideal biomarker would detect infection at its earliest manifestation, at time of incipient invasion or tissue damage, even before the occurrence of clinical signs and symptoms. The serologic and PCR fungal assays are generally positive early in the course of infection and test positivity often antedates positive blood cultures and clinical signs and symptoms.

Evaluation of using a combination of fever, screening for presence of more specific clinical symptoms and signs, and serial monitoring of the galactomannan biomarker was performed in a pilot study in patients with hematologic malignancies and patients undergoing hematopoietic stem cell transplant [48]. Patients all received fluconazole prophylaxis to eliminate *Candida* from consideration so that the focus could be on Aspergillosis. No empiric antifungal therapy could be instituted unless some proof of definitive invasive fungal disease was documented. A total of 136 neutropenic episodes were assessed. Patients who met any of several clinical or biomarker criteria were evaluated with a CT scans and bronchoscopy. This strategy was able to detect a number of cases quite early, even while the patient was afebrile, in some cases and this provided an opportunity for accurate diagnosis, early intervention, and spared many patients from receiving unneeded therapy that would have been treated using persistent fever as the trigger for empiric antifungal therapy.

PCR fungal assays are also under development. Several have been evaluated in clinical settings and they too hold promise for even more sensitive detection. In one pilot study [25], a nested PCR that detects *Candida*, *Aspergillus*, *Trichosporon*, and *Cryptococcus* species and culture was evaluated in 42 neutropenic patients with cancer. Sequential blood samples were tested and infection was confirmed by culture. Infection was noted in 26 of the 31 PCR-positive samples and in none of the 52 PCR-negative ones. Among the PCR-positive samples, the second sample was PCR-positive 1–8 days before the culture results were available. In one trial, empirical antifungal therapy (with liposomal amphotericin B after 120 h of febrile neutropenia) was compared with either PCR-triggered or empirical antifungal therapy (after 120 h of febrile neutropenia) after allogeneic HSCT [49]. A total of 409 patients were studied in a randomized trial. A higher percentage of patients in the PCR screening arm received antifungal therapy (57 vs. 37%, $p<0.0001$). Slightly fewer patients in the PCR arm developed proven invasive fungal disease (12 vs. 16 cases). Mortality at 30 days was superior in the PCR arm at the end of the screening period of 30 days (1.5 vs. 6.3%, $p=0.015$), but the survival at 100 days was similar. Other studies have evaluated PCR assays for *Aspergillus* (reviewed in [50]).

Although molecular testing holds enormous promise, as yet there are formidable obstacles to its use in clinical practice that include variable sensitivity and specificity, limited per test positivity, lack of standardized reagents and targets, issues regarding false positives and negatives, and lack of validation in multiple centers. Moreover, there is no licensed PCR as yet.

Certainly the use of fungal diagnostics holds enormous appeal and may allow targeting of treatment to those truly in need while sparing others from therapy that may cause toxicity and is costly. Further, antibiotic stewardship would be expected to reduce the risk of emergence of drug resistance. The replacement of empiric therapy with targeted therapy is a high priority for clinical research.

Why Do some People Get Sicker than Others?

The age-old question as to why one patient gets infected while another with the same degree of immune compromise and same exposure to potential pathogens does not still puzzle us today. Unraveling some of the intricacies of the innate and acquired immunities in recent years has provided some clues. We now know that polymorphisms of immune response genes explain important differences in both likelihood of invasive infection and how serious an infection is once it occurs. Two examples have received considerable attention. Mannose binding lectin (MBL) is a molecule that is part of the innate immune response system that is responsible for recognizing a broad range of viral, bacterial, and fungal pathogens and is key in activating complement and facilitating phagocytosis. Mutations in the MBL gene occur in 10–30% of the general population and can lead to lower serum levels of MBL. Coupled with neutropenia, MBL deficiency has been associated with more severe and more prolonged febrile neutropenic episodes in several studies [51–56] and after HSCT [57–60]. Recently, low levels of MBL were associated with a risk for neutropenic *Aspergillus* infections in patients with multiple myeloma undergoing autologous HSCT [61]. Toll-like receptors are also important pattern recognition receptors for microbial pathogens. Polymorphisms in TLR molecules have also been implicated in the risk for infection in immunocompromised patients [62–64]. Lipopolysaccharide binding protein promoter variants have also been associated with the risk for Gram negative bacteremia after HSCT [65]. Cytokine polymorphisms also influence the risk of infection [66]. These various observations suggest that polymorphisms of various pro-inflammatory and anti-inflammatory molecules and cytokines may explain much of the variability in susceptibility to infection and severity of infection.

Identification of certain immune polymorphisms holds the promise that molecular profiles of patients could allow customization of an anti-infective strategy for each individual patient. Prophylaxis would be appropriate for some patients who could be identified in advance as at high risk for infection or serious sequelae of infection, while monitoring for infection and treating only should an infection occur would be best for others at lower risk.

What Does the Future Hold?

Historically, neutropenia and mucosal injury are the major factors that have influenced the risk for neutropenic infections and the epidemiology of febrile neutropenia. The increasing use of purine analogs and monoclonal antibodies in the therapy of lymphohematopoietic diseases impairs other arms of the host immunity and exposes the neutropenic patient to a wider array of potential opportunists not seen historically. In particular, various series are today reporting much higher risks for serious infections by the herpesviruses (especially cytomegalovirus and varicella zoster virus) and molds in less intensively treated patients than historically seen. As new antineoplastic therapies emerge with novel mechanisms of action, one can expect an evolving epidemiology of infectious complications.

Historically, we have used group characteristics to ascertain the likelihood of infection by various pathogens. We have tailored our antimicrobial strategies for groups of patients sharing common treatment and disease characteristics. We have made enormous strides in minimizing the threat of infectious complications using such group identifiers. The use of genetic testing to identify individual variability in immune response genes of individual patients in advance will allow us to develop customized approaches that may be even more effective.

References

1. Freifeld AG, Bow EJ, Sepkowitz KA, et al. Clinical practice guidelines for the use of antimicrobial agents in neutropenic patients with cancer: 2010 update by the infections diseases society of America. Clin Infect Dis. 2011;52(4):e56–93.
2. Segal BH, Freifeld AG, Baden LR, et al. Prevention and treatment of cancer-related infections. J Natl Compr Canc Netw. 2008;6(2):122–74.
3. Link H, Böhme A, Cornely OA, et al. Antimicrobial therapy of unexplained fever in neutropenic patients – guidelines of the Infectious Diseases Working Party (AGIHO) of the German Society of Hematology and Oncology (DGHO), Study Group Interventional Therapy of Unexplained Fever. Ann Hematol. 2003;82 Suppl 2:S105–17.
4. Infectious Diseases Society of Taiwan; Hematology Society of Taiwan; Medical Foundation in Memory Dr. Deh-Lin Cheng; Foundation of Professor Wei-Chuan Hsieh for Infectious Diseases Research and Education; CY Lee's Research Foundation for Pediatric Infectious Diseases and Vaccine. Guidelines for the use of antimicrobial agents in patients with febrile neutropenia in Taiwan. J Microbiol Immunol Infect. 2005;38(6):455–7.
5. Masaoka T. Evidence-based recommendations for antimicrobial use in febrile neutropenia in Japan: executive summary. Clin Infect Dis. 2004;39 Suppl 1:S49–52.
6. Yahav D, Paul M, Fraser A, et al. Efficacy and safety of cefepime: a systematic review and meta-analysis. Lancet Infect Dis. 2007;7(5):338–48.
7. Paul M, Yahav D, Fraser A, Leibovici L. Empirical antibiotic monotherapy for febrile neutropenia: systematic review and meta-analysis of randomized controlled trials. J Antimicrob Chemother. 2006;57(2):176–89.
8. Clark OA, Lyman GH, Castro AA, et al. Colony-stimulating factors for chemotherapy-induced febrile neutropenia: a meta-analysis of randomized controlled trials. J Clin Oncol. 2005;23(18):4198–214.
9. Oude Nijhuis CS, Daenen SM, Vellenga E, et al. Fever and neutropenia in cancer patients: the diagnostic role of cytokines in risk assessment strategies. Crit Rev Oncol Hematol. 2002;44(2):163–74.
10. Cockerill 3rd FR, Wilson JW, Vetter EA, et al. Optimal testing parameters for blood cultures. Clin Infect Dis. 2004;38(12):1724–30.
11. Lee A, Mirrett S, Reller LB, Weinstein MP. Detection of bloodstream infections in adults: how many blood cultures are needed? J Clin Microbiol. 2007;45(11):3546–8.
12. Spaargaren J, van Boven CP, Voorn GP. Effectiveness of resins in neutralizing antibiotic activities in bactec plus Aerobic/F culture medium. J Clin Microbiol. 1998;36(12):3731–3.
13. Flayhart D, Borek AP, Wakefield T, et al. Comparison of BACTEC PLUS blood culture media to BacT/Alert FA blood culture media for detection of bacterial pathogens in samples containing therapeutic levels of antibiotics. J Clin Microbiol. 2007;45(3):816–21.
14. Levin PD, Yinnon AM, Hersch M, Rudensky B. Impact of the resin blood culture medium on the treatment of critically ill patients. Crit Care Med. 1996;24(5):797–801.
15. Woo PC, Wong SS, Lum PN, et al. Cell-wall-deficient bacteria and culture-negative febrile episodes in bone-marrow-transplant recipients. Lancet. 2001;357(9257):675–9.
16. Ley BE, Linton CJ, Bennett DM, et al. Detection of bacteraemia in patients with fever and neutropenia using 16S rRNA gene amplification by polymerase chain reaction. Eur J Clin Microbiol Infect Dis. 1998;17(4):247–53.
17. Xu J, Moore JE, Millar BC, et al. Improved laboratory diagnosis of bacterial and fungal infections in patients with hematological malignancies using PCR and ribosomal RNA sequence analysis. Leuk Lymphoma. 2004;45(8):1637–41.
18. Ammann RA, Zucol F, Aebi C, et al. Real-time broad-range PCR versus blood culture. A prospective pilot study in pediatric cancer patients with fever and neutropenia. Support Care Cancer. 2007;15(6):637–41.
19. Woo PC, Lau SK, Teng JL, et al. Then and now: use of 16S rDNA gene sequencing for bacterial identification and discovery of novel bacteria in clinical microbiology laboratories. Clin Microbiol Infect. 2008;14(10):908–34.
20. Dreier J, Störmer M, Kleesiek K. Real-time polymerase chain reaction in transfusion medicine: applications for detection of bacterial contamination in blood products. Transfus Med Rev. 2007;21(3):237–54.
21. Yamikami Y, Hashimoto A, Yamagata E, et al. Evaluation of PCR for detection of DNA specific for *Aspergillus* species in sera of patients with various forms of pulmonary aspergillosis. J Clin Microbiol. 1998;36(12):3619–23.
22. Hebart H, Löffler J, Reitze H, et al. Prospective screening by a panfungal polymerase chain reaction assay in patients at risk for fungal infections: implications for the management of febrile neutropenia. Br J Haematol. 2000;111(2):635–40.
23. Skladny H, Buchheidt D, Baust C, et al. Specific detection of *Aspergillus* species in blood and bronchoalveolar lavage samples of immunocompromised patients by two-step PCR. J Clin Microbiol. 1999;37(12):3865–71.
24. Morace G, Pagano L, Sanguinetti M, et al. PCR-restriction enzyme analysis for detection of Candida DNA in blood from febrile patients with hematological malignancies. J Clin Microbiol. 1999;37(6):1871–5.
25. Lin MT, Lu HC, Chen WL. Improving efficacy of antifungal therapy by polymerase chain reaction – based strategy among febrile patients with neutropenia and cancer. Clin Infect Dis. 2001;33:1621–7.
26. Lass-Flörl C, Aigner J, Gunsilius E, et al. Screening for *Aspergillus* spp. using polymerase chain reaction of whole blood samples from patients with haematological malignancies. Br J Haematol. 2001;113(1):180–4.
27. Jordanides NE, Allan EK, McLintock LA, et al. A prospective study of real-time panfungal PCR for the early diagnosis of invasive fungal infection in haemato-oncology patients. Bone Marrow Transplant. 2005;35(4):389–95.
28. Odabasi Z, Mattiuzzi G, Estey E, et al. Beta-D-glucan as a diagnostic adjunct for invasive fungal infections: validation, cutoff development, and performance in patients with acute myelogenous leukemia and myelodysplastic syndrome. Clin Infect Dis. 2004;39:199–205.
29. Ostrosky-Zeichner L, Alexander BD, Kett DH, et al. Multicenter clinical evaluation of the (1->3) beta-D-glucan assay as an aid to diagnosis of fungal infections in humans. Clin Infect Dis. 2005;41:654–9.
30. Maertens J, Verhaegen J, Lagrou K, et al. Screening for circulating galactomannan as a noninvasive diagnostic tool for invasive Aspergillosis in prolonged neutropenic patients and stem cell transplantation recipients: a prospective validation. Blood. 2001;97:1604–10.
31. Marr KA, Balajee SA, McLaughlin L, et al. Detection of galactomannan antigenemia by enzyme immunoassay for the diagnosis of invasive aspergillosis: variables that affect performance. J Infect Dis. 2004;190:641–9.
32. Arber C, Passweg JR, Fluckiger U, Pless M, Gregor M, Tichelli A, et al. C-reactive protein and fever in neutropenic patients. Scand J Infect Dis. 2000;32(5):515–20.
33. de Bel C, Gerritsen E, de Maaker G, Moolenaar A, Vossen J. C-reactive protein in the management of children with fever after allogeneic bone marrow transplantation. Infection. 1991;19(2):92–6.
34. Engel A, Mack E, Kern P, Kern WV. An analysis of interleukin-8, interleukin-6 and C-reactive protein serum concentrations to predict fever, gram-negative bacteremia and complicated infection in neutropenic cancer patients. Infection. 1998;26(4):213–21.

35. von Lilienfeld-Toal M, Dietrich MP, Glasmacher A, Lehmann L, Breig P, Hahn C, Schmidt-Wolf IG, Marklein G, Schroeder S, Stuber F. Markers of bacteremia in febrile neutropenic patients with hematological malignancies: procalcitonin and IL-6 are more reliable than C-reactive protein. Eur J Clin Microbiol Infect Dis. 2004;23(7):539–44. Epub 2004 Jun 22.
36. Simon L, Gauvin F, Amre DK, Saint-Louis P, Lacroix J. Serum procalcitonin and C-reactive protein levels as markers of bacterial infection: a systematic review and meta-analysis. Clin Infect Dis. 2004;39(2):206–17.
37. Sakr Y, Sponholz C, Tuche F, Brunkhorst F, Reinhart K. The role of procalcitonin in febrile neutropenic patients: review of the literature. Infection. 2008;36(5):396–407.
38. Persson L, Soderquist B, Engervall P, Vikerfors T, Hansson LO, Tidefelt U. Assessment of systemic inflammation markers to differentiate a stable from a deteriorating clinical course in patients with febrile neutropenia. Eur J Haematol. 2005;74(4):297–303.
39. von Lilienfeld-Toal M, Schneider A, Orlopp K, Hahn-Ast C, Glasmacher A, Stuber F. Change of procalcitonin predicts clinical outcome of febrile episodes in patients with hematological malignancies. Support Care Cancer. 2006;14(12):1241–5.
40. de Pauw BE. Between over- and undertreatment of invasive fungal disease. Clin Infect Dis. 2005;41(9):1251–3.
41. Morrell M, Fraser VJ, Kollef MH. Delaying the empiric treatment of Candida bloodstream infection until positive blood culture results are obtained: a potential risk factor for hospital mortality. Antimicrob Agents Chemother. 2005;49:3640–5.
42. Greene RE, Schlamm HT, Oestmann JW, et al. Imaging findings in acute invasive pulmonary aspergillosis: clinical significance of the halo sign. Clin Infect Dis. 2007;44(3):373–9.
43. Wingard JR. Empirical antifungal therapy in febrile neutropenic patients. Clin Infect Dis. 2004;39 Suppl 1:S38–43.
44. Wingard JR. New approaches to invasive fungal infections in acute leukemia and hematopoietic stem cell transplant patients. Best Pract Res Clin Haematol. 2007;20(1):99–107.
45. Hope WW, Walsh TJ, Denning DW. Laboratory diagnosis of invasive aspergillosis. Lancet Infect Dis. 2005;5:609–22.
46. Alexander BD, Pfeiffer RM. Contemporary tools for diagnosis and managment of invasive mycoses. Clin Infect Dis. 2006;43:S15–27.
47. Pfeiffer CD, Fine JP, Safdar N. Diagnosis of invasive aspergillosis using a galactomannan assay: a meta-analysis. Clin Infect Dis. 2006;42(10):1417–27.
48. Maertens J, Theunissen K, Verhoef G, et al. Galactomannan and computed tomography-based preemptive antifungal therapy in neutropenic patients at high risk for invasive fungal infection: a prospective feasibility study. Clin Infect Dis. 2005;41:1242–50.
49. Hebart H, Klingspor L, Klingebiel T, et al. A prospective randomized controlled trial comparing PCR-based and empirical treatment with liposomal amphotericin B in patients after Allo-SCT. Bone Marrow Transplant. 2009;43(7):553–61.
50. Donnelly JP. Polymerase chain reaction for diagnosing invasive aspergillosis: getting closer but still a ways to go. Clin Infect Dis. 2006;42(4):487–9.
51. Peterslund NA, Koch C, Jensenius JC, Thiel S. Association between deficiency of mannose-binding lectin and severe infections after chemotherapy. Lancet. 2001;358(9282):637–8.
52. Neth O, Hann I, Turner MW, Klein NJ. Deficiency of mannose-binding lectin and burden of infection in children with malignancy: a prospective study. Lancet. 2001;358(9282):614–8.
53. Vekemans M, Robinson J, Georgala A, et al. Low mannose-binding lectin concentration is associated with severe infection in patients with hematological cancer who are undergoing chemotherapy. Clin Infect Dis. 2007;44(12):1593–601.
54. Mølle I, Steffensen R, Thiel S, Peterslund NA. Chemotherapy-related infections in patients with multiple myeloma: associations with mannan-binding lectin genotypes. Eur J Haematol. 2006;77(1):19–26.
55. Schlapbach LJ, Aebi C, Otth M, et al. Serum levels of mannose-binding lectin and the risk of fever in neutropenia pediatric cancer patients. Pediatr Blood Cancer. 2007;49(1):11–6.
56. Schlapbach LJ, Aebi C, Otth M, et al. Deficiency of mannose-binding lectin-associated serine protease-2 associated with increased risk of fever and neutropenia in pediatric cancer patients. Pediatr Infect Dis J. 2007;26(11):989–94.
57. Mullighan CG, Heatley S, Doherty K, et al. Mannose-binding lectin gene polymorphisms are associated with major infection following allogeneic hemopoietic stem cell transplantation. Blood. 2002;99(10):3524–9.
58. Mølle I, Peterslund NA, Thiel S, Steffensen R. MBL2 polymorphism and risk of severe infections in multiple myeloma patients receiving high-dose melphalan and autologous stem cell transplantation. Bone Marrow Transplant. 2006;38(8):555–60.
59. Mullighan CG, Heatley SL, Danner S, et al. Mannose-binding lectin status is associated with risk of major infection following myeloablative sibling allogeneic hematopoietic stem cell transplantation. Blood. 2008;112(5):2120–8.
60. Mølle I, Ostergaard M, Melsvik D, Nyvold CG. Infectious complications after chemotherapy and stem cell transplantation in multiple myeloma: implications of Fc gamma receptor and myeloperoxidase promoter polymorphisms. Leuk Lymphoma. 2008;49(6):1116–22.
61. Anaissie EJ, Zhao W, Wen Y et al. Deficiency of mannose-binding lectin is a risk factor for invasive pulmonary aspergillosis in patients with multiple myeloma: an analysis of 482 patients. Blood. 2008;112(11):249; Abstract 667.
62. Bochud PY, Chien JW, Marr KA, et al. Toll-like receptor 4 polymorphisms and aspergillosis in stem-cell transplantation. N Engl J Med. 2008;359(17):1766–77.
63. Woehrle T, Du W, Goetz A, et al. Pathogen specific cytokine release reveals an effect of TLR2 Arg753Gln during Candida sepsis in humans. Cytokine. 2008;41(3):322–9.
64. Wurfel MM, Gordon AC, Holden TD, et al. Toll-like receptor 1 polymorphisms affect innate immune responses and outcomes in sepsis. Am J Respir Crit Care Med. 2008;178(7):710–20.
65. Chien JW, Boeckh MJ, Hansen JA, Clark JG. Lipopolysaccharide binding protein promoter variants influence the risk for Gram-negative bacteremia and mortality after allogeneic hematopoietic cell transplantation. Blood. 2008;111(4):2462–9.
66. Seo KW, Kim DH, Sohn SK, et al. Protective role of interleukin-10 promoter gene polymorphism in the pathogenesis of invasive pulmonary aspergillosis after allogeneic stem cell transplantation. Bone Marrow Transplant. 2005;36(12):1089–95.

Chapter 10
Catheter-Related Infections in Cancer Patients

Iba Al Wohoush, Anne-Marie Chaftari, and Issam Raad

Abstract Central venous catheters (CVCs) play a major role in the management of high-risk patients, particularly cancer patients, and are mainly used for the administration of anti-cancer agents, antibiotics, and blood products. Catheter-related blood stream infection (CRBSI) rates are influenced by patient-related factors, such as type and severity of the illness, by catheter-related factors, and institutional factors (e.g., bed size and academic affiliation). Catheter-related infections could be local, such as exit site, tunnel, and pocket infections; or systemic such as catheter-related bloodstream infection. Many diagnostic methods have been developed, some of which require catheter removal, whereas others do not. Strategies for prevention and management of CRBSI are presented in this chapter.

Keywords Indwelling catheter-related blood stream infection • Infection prevention • Pathogenesis • Bacterial infection • Fungal infections • Biofilm

Introduction

Central venous catheters (CVCs) play a major role in the management of high-risk patients, particularly cancer patients, and are mainly used for the administration of anti-cancer agents, antibiotics, and blood products.

Before the introduction of CVCs into medical practice, patients with cancer received chemotherapeutic agents through a small, peripheral venous catheter. This practice resulted in several complications such as extravasation and thrombosis of the peripheral vein, which interfered with the administration of the anti-cancer agents. CVCs are considered to be a revolutionary step in the care of cancer and critically ill patients, since their use is not accompanied with such complications. However the infectious complications associated with the use of CVC are a major concern. In critically ill patients, CVCs are the leading source of bloodstream infections and are associated with substantial morbidity, mortality, and economical burden.

More than 150 million catheters are purchased annually by hospitals and clinics in the United States [1]. The majority of these devices are peripheral venous catheters, but more than five million CVCs are inserted annually [1]. Each year in the United States, CVCs may cause an estimated 80,000 catheter-related bloodstream infections and, as a result, up to 28,000 deaths among patients in intensive care units [2]. The median rate of catheter-related bloodstream infection in intensive care units of all types ranges from 1.8 to 5.2 per 1,000 catheter-days [3]. Given that the average cost of care for a patient is $45,000, such infections could cost up to $2.3 billion annually [2]. Catheter-related blood stream infection (CRBSI) rates are influenced by patient-related factors, such as type and severity of the illness, by catheter-related factors, and institutional factors (e.g., bed size and academic affiliation).

Pathogenesis

In order to diagnose, prevent, and manage CRBSI appropriately, the physician must have a complete understanding of the pathogenesis of CRBSI. The most common causative pathogens for CRBSI are coagulase-negative staphylococci, *Staphylococcus aureus*, *Enterococci*, and *Candida* species; less commonly are gram negative bacilli and micrococcus. The microorganisms that colonize the catheter surfaces may follow any of the following routes. Firstly, the skin organisms may migrate from the insertion site to the surface of the catheter, particularly the external one [4–6]; short-term nontunneled noncuffed catheters are usually colonized through this route. The second route is direct contamination of the catheter hub by contact with hands or contaminated devices; this route is particularly important in the long-term catheters such as tunneled catheters and ports [7, 8]. The third path, which is a rare form of catheter colonization, is hematogenous spread of the microorganisms from another site of infection. Lastly and rarely is infusate contamination [9, 10].

I. Al Wohoush (✉)
Infectious Diseases, Infection Control, and Employee Health,
The University of Texas M.D. Anderson Cancer Center,
Houston, Texas, USA
e-mail: IAAL@mdanderson.org

Clinical Manifestations and Definitions

Catheter-related infections could be local, such as exit site, tunnel, and pocket infections; or systemic such as catheter-related bloodstream infection [11].

Local Catheter-Related Infections

The presence of local inflammatory signs, such as erythema, warmth, tenderness, and purulent exudates, suggests a local catheter infection. However, neutropenic patients may not develop these symptoms when they have a catheter-related infection. Furthermore, the insertion of some catheters (e.g., PICC) may be associated with similar symptoms due to secondary mechanical irritation. As a conclusion, local inflammatory signs are unreliable for establishing the diagnosis of catheter-related infection because of their low specificity and sensitivity, and must be paired with microbiological confirmation to reach a final diagnosis. Finally, it is worth mentioning that all of the local catheter-related infections (i.e., exit site, tunnel, and pocket infections) could be associated with a CRBSI. In other words, their presence does not necessarily predict a CRBSI; and more tests are needed to establish a diagnosis of CRBSI. The following are the most commonly used definitions of local catheter-related infections.

Exit-Site Infection

Characterized by inflammatory changes within 2 cm of the catheter exit site.

Tunnel Infection

The afore-mentioned inflammatory signs, erythema >2 cm from the exit site and along the subcutaneous tract of a tunneled catheter.

Pocket Infection

The pocket of a totally implantable catheter is infected and filled with purulent exudates; possibly complicated by necrosis of the overlying skin or pocket rupture.

Systemic Catheter Infections (CRBSI)

Any patient with a CVC who has signs and symptoms of infection such as fever, chills, or hypotension and does not have any obvious source of infection (except for the catheter) should undergo microbiological testing to determine if CRBSI is the underlying cause of his symptoms. Probable CRBSI can be diagnosed by one or more positive blood cultures, along with the above signs and symptoms, and with no apparent source for the bacteremia (except for the catheter). The infectious diseases society of America IDSA has suggested one of the following methods to confirm the Diagnosis of CRBSI [11]: Positive quantitative or semiquantitative culture of the catheter; a ratio of 3:1 between quantitative blood cultures drawn simultaneously from a CVC and a peripheral vein; or differential time to positivity. All of the mentioned methods will be explained in detail later in this chapter.

Diagnosis of CRBSI

The clinical signs and symptoms of sepsis are unreliable in reaching a correct diagnosis of CRBSI. Safdar and Maki evaluated the role of inflammation as a diagnostic indicator of CRBSI with short-term catheters. Their study showed that inflammation at the insertion site was rarely present and had a very poor sensitivity ($\leq 3\%$) for predicting CRBSI [12]. Therefore microbiological confirmation is always required for the diagnosis of CRBSI.

Many diagnostic methods have been developed, some of which require catheter removal, whereas others do not. The latter types of these diagnostic tests are preferable since the catheter can remain in place.

Diagnostic Tests Without Catheter Removal

Comparative Quantitative Blood Culture

This method involves obtaining paired blood cultures drawn concomitantly from the CVC and the peripheral vein. A large ratio of CFU from the catheter blood culture to CFU from the peripheral culture is indicative of a CRBSI. Since the studies have reported different cut-off points for a positive diagnosis ranging from two to tenfold [13–15], the IDSA accepted a CFU that is threefold or higher from the CVC drawn blood culture vs. peripheral vein culture is indicative of CRBSI. In a recent study where fivefold was the cut-off point, sensitivity, specificity, and positive predictive value were found to be 62, 93, and 92% respectively [16]. In a meta-analysis of studies of diagnostic tests, this method was found to be the most accurate for the diagnosis of CRBSI; sensitivity and specificity for short-term catheter were 75 and 97% respectively and for long-term catheters, 93 and 100% respectively [17]. However, the use of this method is limited because it is labor intensive and expensive. Single quantitative or qualitative blood cultures, where the blood is drawn through the catheter alone, are unreliable for the diagnosis of CRBSI due to low positive predictive values [17].

Differential Time to Positivity

The differential time to positivity is defined as the difference between the times a blood culture drawn from the catheter and a simultaneous blood drawn from a peripheral vein become positive [18]. Through this simple technique, blood cultures are drawn simultaneously or within 15–20 min, from the CVC and the peripheral vein. They are then placed in an automatic positive detector that records culture positivity every 15 min according to changes in fluorescence related to microbial growth. Several studies indicated that definite diagnosis of CRBSI is established when the blood culture drawn from the CVC becomes positive at least 2 h earlier than blood culture drawn from the peripheral vein [18–20]. In a study of 235 neutropenic patients with febrile neutropenia, DTP had 82% sensitivity and 88% specificity in the diagnosis of CRBSI.

Raad et al. [21] evaluated the DTP in 191 cases of CRBSI. The sensitivity and specificity for this method in short-term catheters were 81 and 92% respectively. On the other hand, the sensitivity and specificity for DTP in long-term catheters were 93 and 75% respectively. In a recent study comparing quantitative blood cultures and differential time to positivity in pediatric patients, DTP was significantly more sensitive and mildly less specific, with a higher diagnostic accuracy compared to quantitative blood cultures [22]. The limitation of this study is that the cultures drawn from catheters may be falsely negative if antibiotics are given intraluminally and also does not evaluate patients with positive CVC cultures and negative peripheral blood cultures.

Diagnostic Tests with Catheter Removal

Many methods that require catheter removal have been improved to diagnose CRBSI (Table 10.1).

Semiquantitative Roll-Plate Catheter Culture

The semiquantitative catheter culture, which is also known as the roll-plate method, is one of the most studied diagnostic techniques. In this method, the distal segment of the catheter is cut and rolled against a blood agar plate at least four times before the plate is incubated overnight [23, 24]. Catheters are considered to be colonized if at least 15 CFU/catheter tip segments are grown [25], but the diagnosis of CRBSI is only established if a peripheral blood culture yields the same organism as in the catheter tip culture [26–33]. In a recent study, a sensitivity of 78% and a specificity of 88% have been reported using the roll-plate catheter culture as a diagnostic tool for CRBSI in short-term catheters [34]. Even more, the pooled sensitivity and specificity for roll-plate catheter cultures in 14 trials involving short-term catheters were found to be 84 and 85% respectively [23]. Bouza et al. reported a specificity and sensitivity of more than 90% for both short-term, and long-term catheters; the limitation for their study is that they defined the long-term catheters as those with only 7 days of dwell time or more [35]. However, the sensitivity from different studies using the roll plate as a diagnostic technique in long-term catheters (more than 30 days of dwell time) was found to be ranging from 45 to 75% [6, 26]. The difference between the sensitivity and specificity for roll plate between the short-term and long-term catheters is justified by the fact that the short-term catheters are mainly colonized on the external surface of the catheter, while the long-term catheters are predominantly colonized in the lumen of the catheter. Given the fact that this method retrieves free-floating (nonbiofilm) microorganisms only from the external surface of the catheter, therefore false negative results can be expected in long-term catheters where organisms mainly colonize the intraluminal surface of the catheters. Hence the roll-plate method is mainly useful in short term catheters.

Table 10.1 Comparison of diagnostic methods of catheter related blood stream infection

Diagnostic method	Diagnosis criteria	Disadvantages
Without catheter removal		
Simultaneous quantitative blood cultures	CFU blood culture drawn through CVC >3 times CFU drawn simultaneously from peripheral vein	Labor intensive and expensive
Differential time to positivity	Blood culture drawn through CVC turns positive at least 2 h before blood culture drawn simultaneously from peripheral vein	Cultures drawn from catheters may be falsely negative if the antibiotics are given intraluminally and also does not evaluate patients with positive CVC cultures and negative peripheral blood cultures
With catheter removal		
Semiquantitative CVC tip cultures	>15 CFU/mL from CVC tip	Cultures only the organisms on the external surface and does not culture organisms embedded in the biofilm
Quantitative CVC tip cultures	>100 CFU/mL from CVC tip	May over release the biofilm microorganisms that might not be clinically relevant; whereas, relevant planktonic organisms might be killed

Quantitative Catheter Segment Culture

To overcome the roll-plate limitation of missing the organisms colonizing the catheters' lumen, several methods such as centrifugation, vortexing, and sonication have been used [36–38]. The catheter segments are immersed in broth and flushed, followed by serial dilutions and surface plating on blood agar. A count of greater than or equal 100 CFU is considered to be associated with infection. The diagnosis of CRBSI is established if a peripheral blood culture yielded the same organism grown from the catheter tip culture [39]. Brun-Buisson et al. suggested a modified version of this method where the segments are vortexed rather than flushed. He reported a sensitivity of 97.5% and specificity of 88% [40]. Raad et al. compared the roll-plate culture with the catheter sonication method, and yielded sensitivities of 78 and 93% respectively and specificities of 88 and 94% respectively [34]. Widmer and Frei compared the sonication with the roll-plate method in short-term catheters and found similar sensitivities and specificities [41]. However, for long-term catheters, the sonication method was found to have higher sensitivity than the roll-plate method [6]. The pooled sensitivity and specificity of quantitative catheter segment culture for short-term catheters were 82 and 89% respectively, and 83 and 97% for long-term catheters [23]. The disadvantage of this method is that it releases the biofilm microorganisms that might not be clinically relevant; whereas, relevant planktonic organisms might be killed.

Prevention of Catheter-Related Infections

An ounce of prevention is worth a pound of cure, and this is completely true in medical practice. Not only CRBSIs may require the removal of the catheter consequently interfering with the treatment plan but also they are associated with high morbidity and mortality rates, as well increase cost of care. Therefore, the prevention of CRBSI is of paramount importance (Table 10.2). Successful preventive strategies should focus on controlling all factors that could lead to the colonization of CVC by microorganisms. Traditional measures for the prevention of catheter-related infections, recommended by the healthcare infection control practices advisory committee (HICPAC) guidelines, include education of health care workers on proper catheter insertion and maintenance, routine monitoring of institutional rates of CRBSI, hand hygiene, use of a dedicated infusion therapy team, use of sterile dressings, avoidance of femoral insertion, and removal of the vascular catheter as soon as possible [2]. In the next section, we will review major strategies for the prevention of catheter-related infections.

Maximal Sterile Barrier

The following five evidence-based procedures are recommended by the CDC and identified as having the greatest effect on the rate of CRBSI: hand washing, using full-barrier precautions during the insertion of CVC, cleaning the skin with chlorhexidine, avoiding the femoral site if possible, and removing unnecessary catheters. These five elements are particularly important in nontunneled catheters and PICCs, which are usually inserted out of the operating room; and hence, their insertion may not be subject to the strict sterile atmosphere of an operating room. Pronovost et al. [42] reported a decrease of median rate of catheter-related infections from 2.7/1,000 catheter-days at baseline to 0 within the first 3 months of applying the mentioned five elements, and a reduction in the rate of CRBSI of 66% at 16–18 months after implementation.

Other studies reported a decrease in the rate of CRBSI from 0.5/1,000 to 0.02/1,000 catheter-days after applying the maximal sterile barrier precautions consisting of wearing sterile gown, gloves and cap, and using a large drape during the insertion of catheters.

Tunneling

Tunneling the catheters creates a fibrous tissue around the dacron cuff (which is used to anchor the catheter in place), and this tissue will act as a barrier against the migration of microorganisms. A recent study comparing the tunneled and nontunneled catheters showed that the infection rate was 1.9 per catheter-days in the nontunneled group vs. 0.7 per catheter-days in the tunneled catheter group. Another study comparing these two groups failed to demonstrate a difference between them, and showed a rate of 0.22/1,000 catheter-days was reported in the nontunneled catheter group vs. 0.20/1,000 catheter-days in the tunneled group. More studies are needed to prove the efficacy of tunneled catheters in preventing catheter-related infections; especially since tunneling a catheter is a surgical procedure that may cost an additional $2,500.

Antimicrobial Coating of Catheters

Coating the catheters with antibiotics leads to a slow release of the antibiotics that prevent the adherence of the microorganisms to the catheter surfaces and preclude the initial formation of the biofilm [43]. Many generations and types of antibiotic-coated catheters were studied with different rates of success in preventing catheter-related infections.

Table 10.2 Prevention of catheter related blood stream infection

	Method	Advantages	Disadvantages
Maximal sterile barrier	Hand washing, using full-barrier precautions during the insertion of central venous catheter, cleaning the skin with chlorhexidine, avoiding the femoral site if possible, and removing unnecessary catheters	It lowers the rates of CRBSI	It requires continuous staff education and reinforcement. Role of all components have not been determined
Catheter tunneling	It creates a fibrous tissue around the dacron cuff, which acts as a barrier against the migration of microorganisms	The tunneled catheters are long-term ones	Costly, requires surgical procedure or interventional radiology for insertion and efficacy still not proven completely
Antiseptic catheters. First and second generation	They are coated only on the external surface of the catheter using CHX-SSD in first generation. External and luminal surfaces are impregnated in the second generation	Can lower the incidence of CRBSI in short-term catheters	Failed to show a decrease in CRBSI in long-term catheters. Inferior efficacy to CVC impregnated with minocycline-rifampin
Antibiotics-impregnated catheters	It is a polyurethane and silicone catheter impregnated with minocycline and rifampin on both the external and luminal surfaces of the catheter	It decreases the incidence of CRBSI significantly. It is not associated with increased resistance for minocycline or rifampin	It has no effect on catheter-related candidemia
Antimicrobial lock solution	The catheter lumen is filled with 2–3 mL of a combination of anticoagulant and an antimicrobial agent	Using EDTA with minocycline may have a synergistic activity against methicillin resistant staphylococci, gram negative bacilli, and *Candida albicans*	Use of vancomycin is associated with increased risk for resistance. Vancomycin has no coverage against gram negative bacteria. And limited activity against organisms embedded in the biofilm

Antiseptic Catheters

These catheters are impregnated with chlorhexidine and silver sulfadiazine. Two generations were developed in order to lower the rates of CRBSIs. The first generation of the chlorhexidine-silver sulfadiazine was coated only on the external surface of the catheter. Different prospective randomized clinical trials [2, 6, 27–38, 44–48] have evaluated this generation of chlorhexidine-sulfadiazine catheters, and most of them showed a reduction in the CRBSI but only two trials reported a significant reduction in CRBSI [49, 50]. It is estimated that the use of these catheters in patients at high risk for catheter-related infection can save $68–391 per insertion [51]. Several studies failed to show a decrease in catheter-related infections in long-term catheters. This lack of long-term efficacy is based on the limited antimicrobial durability of these catheters (around 7 days in serum) and the fact that only the outer surface of the catheter was impregnated, consequently providing no protection against luminal colonization [44]. As a conclusion, the first generation of the chlorhexidine-sulfadiazine impregnated catheters can reduce the risk of catheter-related infection in short-term catheters, but cannot reduce the risk of CRBSI in long-term catheters.

The second generation of these catheters was impregnated on the external and the luminal surfaces of the catheter. In one study, the use of these catheters decreased the catheter colonization from 11/1,000 to 3.6/1,000 catheter-days; but failed to decrease the rate of CRBSI's [52]. Three subsequent studies also failed to prove a decrease in the rate of CRBSIs [53–55]. The use of these catheters might be cost effective in high-risk patients such as ICU patients, burn patients, and other patient populations in which the rate of infection exceeds 3.3/1,000 catheter-days [4].

Antibiotic-Coated Catheter

The only FDA approved antibiotic-coated catheter is a polyurethane catheter impregnated with minocycline and rifampin on both the external and luminal surfaces of the catheter. Two trials demonstrated that the use of minocycline-rifampin coated catheters is associated with lower rates of CRBSIs compared to the use of uncoated catheters [56, 57]. A prospective, randomized, double blinded study comparing the first generation of chlorhexidine-sulfadiazine coated catheters and minocycline-rifampin coated catheters showed that Minocycline-rifampin coated catheters were 12-fold less likely to be associated with CRBSI and threefold less likely to be colonized [56, 58]. In a recent study, Wright et al. showed a reduction in ICU stay and ICU mortality after the introduction of antibiotic-coated catheters, but reported an increase in rifampin resistance among Staphylococcus epidermis isolates [59]. However, data from MD Anderson cancer center concluded that after 4 years, and more than 24,000 catheter-days, of using antibiotic-coated catheters in stem cell transplant patients, staphylococcus isolates remained highly susceptible to minocycline and rifampin [60]. Raad et al. reported in a 7-year study that the resistance to tetracycline and rifampin decreased 44 and 56% respectively among coagulase negative staphylococci; similarly, the resistance patterns to tetracycline and rifampin among MRSA clinical isolates had a significant decrease of 42 and 67% respectively. Several other studies have shown that the risk of minocycline and rifampin is very low [61, 62]. The risk to develop minocycline and rifampin resistance is low because both require different mutation mechanisms at a cumulative frequency of approximately $1:10^{12}$ bacteria. Such bacterial concentrations are only found in the gastrointestinal tract and are unlikely to be observed in the surrounding subcutaneous environment of the catheters. Moreover, antibiotics delivered by antibiotic-coated catheters are not detectable in the blood [63].

The authors recently suggested that it is mandatory to combine the maximal sterile barrier precautions and antimicrobial-impregnated catheters to achieve the desired goal of "zero tolerance" [64]. The use of the aseptic techniques bundle, including maximal sterile barrier precautions, prevents contamination of the CVC. However, the use of antimicrobial-coated CVC will prevent biofilm colonization of the external and the internal surfaces of the CVCs during the insertion and subsequently during the time it remains in place.

Antimicrobial Lock Solutions

Heparin has been used as an antithrombotic agent in catheters after several studies showed that heparin can reduce the catheter-related infections [65]. However, subsequent studies showed that heparin is as effective as saline in preventing phlebitis and enhances the staphylococcal biofilm formation [66]. Therefore, a novel technology was developed, in which the catheter lumen is flushed and filled with 2–3 mL of a solution that is usually a combination of an anticoagulant and an antimicrobial agent such as vancomycin. Few studies showed a decrease in the rate of CRBSI after using heparin-vancomycin as a lock solution [67, 68], other studies failed to show a significant benefit [69, 70]. However, using Vancomycin prophylactically should be avoided to minimize the risk of emergence of vancomycin-resistant organisms, besides it does not cover for gram negative bacteria and *Candida* species. Chelators as EDTA have an anticoagulant activity similar to heparin and have been found to enhance the activity of antimicrobial drugs against organisms in the biofilm [71–74]. Raad et al. used EDTA with minocycline as prophylaxis in three patients [75], and showed a synergistic activity against methicillin-resistant staphylococci, gram negative bacilli, and *Candida albicans* and a cidal effect against bacteria in the biofilm.

Management of Catheter-Related Blood Stream Infections

Antibiotic therapy for CRBSIs should be initiated empirically. The decision to remove the catheter has to be made cautiously since it is often assumed to be the source of infection, and there is tendency to remove the catheter even before determining whether it is the source of infection or not. The above decisions depend mainly on the type of the organism causing the CRBSI (Table 10.3). Usually vancomycin is the recommended drug for the empirical treatment for CRBSI, with the exceptions of hospital with predominance of MRSA, or when vancomycin MIC >2, in which case other agents such as Daptomycin should be used [5, 6].

Coagulative Negative Staphylococci

Coagulative negative Staphylococci (CoNS) are the most common cause of CRBSI, but at the same time they are a common colonizer of the human skin. Most patients have a benign clinical course; however occasionally, patients may develop frank sepsis with poor outcome [76–78]. A definite diagnosis of CoNS bacteremia requires at least two positive blood cultures, one of them obtained from a peripheral vein. CoNS bacteremia is treated with antibiotics for 5–7 days if the catheter is removed, and for 10–14 days in combination with antibiotic lock therapy if the catheter is still in place.

Table 10.3 Management of catheter related blood stream infection according to the causative agent

	CoNS	*S. aureus*	Enterococci	Gram negative	Candida Spp.
Catheter removal	Occasionally	Yes	Yes	Yes	Yes
Alternative for catheter removal	Antibacterial lock solution				ETOH lock solution
	Exchange over a guide wire for a new antimicrobial-impregnated catheter				
Duration of treatment	5–7 days if catheter is removed	14 days	7–14 days	7–14 days	14 days
	10–14 days + antimicrobial lock if catheter is retained				

Staphylococcus aureus

S. aureus is associated with a high rate of complications [79], most commonly septic thrombosis of large veins [80] which mainly occurs among patients with solid tumors [81]. The most serious complication associated with *S. aureus* CRBSI is endocarditis, thus it is always necessary for every patient with *S. aureus* bacteremia and a persistent fever or bacteremia to undergo a transesophageal echocardiography to exclude endocarditis [11, 82].

Many prospective studies have shown that removal of the CVC in patients with *S. aureus* CRBSI is associated with a more rapid response to therapy and a lower relapse rate [79, 83, 84]. Therefore, it is essential to remove the catheter in every patient with *S. aureus* CRBSI unless there is a major contraindication (i.e., no another venous access) [85, 86]. The type of antibiotics used should be based on the susceptibility of *S. aureus*. Semisynthetic antistaphylococcal penicillin or first generation cephalosporins are the first choice for patients with methicillin sensitive *S. aureus*, while vancomycin and daptomycin are the drugs of choice in patients with methicillin resistant *S. aureus* CRBSI [83, 84].

The usual duration of treatment of *S. aureus* CRBSI is 4–6 weeks, but it can be shortened (>14 days) if the patient is not diabetic, not immunocompromised, has no prosthetic intravascular device, has no complications associated with *S. aureus* CRBSI, and the catheter is removed [85].

Gram Negative Bacilli

Gram negative bacilli are not the usual suspects in CRBSI. However, gram negative bacillary CRBSI caused by organisms such as *Klebsiella pneumoniae*, Enterobacter spp., Pseudomonas spp., Acinetobacter spp., and Stenotrophomonas species have been reported [87, 88]. The empiric gram negative coverage should only be considered in specific groups of patients such as, neutropenic patients, severely ill patients with sepsis, or patients known to be colonized with these pathogens [81, 89, 90]. Hanna et al. showed that CRBSI caused by gram negative bacilli was associated with high rate of relapse if the catheter was not removed, whereas CVC removal was associated with only 1% risk of relapse [88]. Management of gram negative CRBSI consists of removing the CVC and treating with active antibiotics against gram negative bacilli such as gentamicin, amikacin, or ceftazidime [89, 91].

Candida Species

Catheter-related candidemia may be associated with serious complications such as septic thrombosis and endocarditis [92, 93]; therefore, rapid diagnosis and treatment are essential in the management of catheter-related candidemia.

Candida empiric coverage should be used in septic patients with any of the following risk factors: total parenteral nutrition, prolonged broad spectrum antibiotics, hematological malignancy, bone marrow transplant, femoral catheterization, and Candida colonization at multiple sites.

Several studies evaluated the impact of catheter removal on the outcome of the candidemia, and showed that catheter removal is associated with a better outcome [94–97]. Another study showed that catheter retention was found to be an independent variable risk of death in multivariate analysis independent of persistent neutropenia [95].

Raad et al. showed that CVC retention more than 72 h after the onset of candidemia is associated with poor outcome in patients with catheter-related candidemia [98]. Therefore, the catheter should be removed within the first 72 h in case of CRBSI due to Candida, and antifungal agents should be administered for at least 14 days according to the IDSA guidelines [91]. A recent study showed that fluconazole was shown to be equal in efficacy to amphotericin B in the treatment of candidemia with a better safety profile [99]. More recent studies showed that Echinocandin such as caspofungin and anidulafungin are equivalent or superior to fluconazole for the treatment of CRBSI due to Candida [99]. Fluconazole or any Echinocandins are considered as a first line in the treatment of CRBSI due to Candida.

Micrococcus

Micrococcus species have the ability to adhere to medical devices and cause associated infections, particularly CRBSIS [100]. These infections are more likely to persist in patients with prior hemodialysis, the absence of prior GCSF therapy, longer catheter retention intervals, and longer catheter dwell time [101]. A recent study showed that 100% of Micrococcus isolates were susceptible to vancomycin, 95% to trimethoprim-sulfamethoxazole, 84% to rifampin, and 41% to oxacillin [102].

Exchange over a Guide Wire

Catheter removal is required in almost all cases of CRBSI. However, in some instances (e.g., no another vascular access) removing the catheter may jeopardize the patient safety. Thus exchanging the infected catheter over a guide wire was suggested as an alternative method in treatment.

A recent study showed that exchanging the infected catheter with an uncoated one may result in a cross infection in the new catheter. Hence, exchanging the infected catheter with a minocycline-rifampin (M/R) impregnated catheter seemed to prevent the "cross infection." Authors have showed that exchanging the infected catheters with those M/R impregnated was associated with lower morbidity and mortality rates when compared to those of uncoated catheters. An improved overall response rate, risk of mechanical failure and infection recurrence were also noted [103].

References

1. Maki DG, Mermel LA. Infections due to infusion therapy. In: Bennet JV, Brachaman PS, editors. Hospital infections. Philadelphia: Lippincott-Raven; 1998. p. 689–724.
2. O'Grady NP, Alexander M, Dellinger EP, et al. Guidelines for the prevention of intravascular catheter related infections. MMWR Recomm Rep. 2002;51:1–29.
3. National Nosocomial Infections Surveillance System. National nosocomial infections (NNIS) system report, data summary from January 1992 through June 2004, issued October 2004. Am J Infect Control. 2004;32:470–85.
4. Maki DG, Stolz SM, Wheeler S, Mermel LA. Prevention of central venous catheter-related bloodstream infection by use of an antiseptic impregnated catheter: a randomized controlled trial. Ann Intern Med. 1997;127:257–66.
5. Mermel LA, McCormick RD, Springman SR, Maki DG. The pathogenesis and epidemiology of catheter-related infection with pulmonary artery Swan-Ganz catheters: a prospective study utilizing molecular subtyping. Am J Med. 1991;91(Suppl 3B):197S–205.
6. Raad I, Costerton W, Sabharwal U, Sacilowski M, Anaissie E, Bodey GP. Ultrastructural analysis of indwelling vascular catheters: a quantitative relationship between luminal colonization and duration of placement. J Infect Dis. 1993;168:400–7.
7. Stiges-Serra A, Puig P, Linares J, et al. Hub colonization as the initial step in an outbreak of catheter-related sepsis due to coagulase negative staphylococci during parenteral nutrition. J Parenter Enteral Nutr. 1984;8:668–72.
8. Salzman MB, Isenberg HD, Shapiro JF, et al. A prospective study of the catheter hub as the portal of entry for microorganisms causing catheter-related sepsis in neonates. J Infect Dis. 1993;167:487–90.
9. Centers for Disease Control. Nosocomial bacteremia associated with intravenous fluid therapy. MMWR. 1971;20 (Suppl 9):S1–2.
10. Maki DG, Rhame FS, Mackel DC, et al. Nation-wide epidemic of septicemia caused by contaminated intravenous products. Am J Med. 1976;60:471–85.
11. Mermel LA, Farr BM, Sherertz RJ, et al. Guidelines for the management of intravascular catheter related infections. Clin Infect Dis. 2001;32:1249–72.
12. Safdar N, Maki DG. Inflammation at the insertion site is not predictive of catheter-related bloodstream infection with short-term, non-cuffed central venous catheters. Crit Care Med. 2002;30:2632–5.
13. Chatzinikolau I, Hanna H, Hachem R, Alakech B, Tarrabd J, Raad I. Differential quantitative blood culture for the diagnosis of catheter related blood stream infections associated with short and long term catheters: a prospective study. Diagn Microbial Infect Dis. 2004;50:167–72.
14. Douard MC, Clementi E, Arlet G, et al. Negative catheter-tip culture and diagnosis of catheter-related bacteraemia. Nutrition. 1994;10:397–404.
15. Capdevila JA, Planes AM, Palomar M, et al. Value of differential quantitative blood cultures in the diagnosis of catheter-related sepsis. Eur J Clin Microbiol Infect Dis. 1992;11:403–7.
16. Douard MC, Arlet G, Longuet P, et al. Diagnosis of venous access port-related infections. Clin Infect Dis. 1999;29:1197–202.
17. Flynn PM, Shenep JL, Barrett FF. Differential quantitation with a commercial blood culture tube for diagnosis of catheter-related infection. J Clin Microbiol. 1988;26:1045–6.
18. Blot F, Schmidt E, Nitenberg G, et al. Earlier positivity of central venous versus peripheral-blood cultures is highly predictive of catheter-related sepsis. J Clin Microbiol. 1998;36:105–9.
19. Blot F, Nitenberg G, Chachaty E, et al. Diagnosis of catheter related bacteraemia: a prospective comparison of the time to positivity of hub-blood versus peripheral-blood cultures. Lancet. 1999;354:1071–7.
20. Raad I, Hanna HA, Alakech B, Chatzinikolaou I, Johnson MM, Tarrand J. Differential time to positivity: a useful method for diagnosing catheter-related bloodstream infections. Ann Intern Med. 2004;140:18–25.
21. Raad I, Hanna HA, Alakech B, et al. Differential time to positivity: a useful method for diagnosing catheter-related bloodstream infections. Ann Intern Med. 2004;140:18–25.
22. Acuna M, O'Ryan M, Cofre J, Alvarez I, Benadof D, Rodriguez P, et al. Differential time to positivity and quantitative cultures for noninvasive diagnosis of catheter related blood stream infection in children. Pediatr Infect Dis J. 2008;27:681–5.
23. Safdar N, Fine JP, Maki DG. Meta-analysis: methods for diagnosing intravascular device-related bloodstream infection. Ann Intern Med. 2005;142:451–66.
24. Hanna R, Raad II. Diagnosis of catheter-related bloodstream infection. Curr Infect Dis Rep. 2005;7:413–9.
25. Maki DG, Weise CE, Sarafin HW. A semiquantitative culture method for identifying intravenous-catheter-related infection. N Engl J Med. 1977;296:1305–9.
26. Rello J, Gatell JM, Almirall J, Campistol JM, Gonzalez J, Puig de la Bellacasa J. Evaluation of culture techniques for identification of catheter-related infection in hemodialysis patient. Eur J Clin Microbiol Infect Dis. 1989;8:620–2.
27. Gutierrez J, Leon C, Matamoros R, Nogales C, Martin E. Catheter related bacteraemia and fungaemia. Reliability of two methods for catheter culture. Diagn Microbiol Infect Dis. 1992;15:575–8.
28. Cercenado E, Ena J, Rodriguez-Creixems M, Romero I, Bouza E. A conservative procedure for the diagnosis of catheter-related infections. Arch Intern Med. 1990;150:1417–20.
29. Rello J, Coll P, Prats G. Laboratory diagnosis of catheter-related bacteraemia. Scand J Infect Dis. 1991;23:583–8.
30. Aufwerber E, Ringertz S, Ransjo U. Routine semiquantitative cultures and central venous catheter-related bacteraemia. APMIS. 1991;99:627–30.
31. Raad II, Sabbagh MF, Rand KH, Sherertz RJ. Quantitative tip culture methods and the diagnosis of central venous catheter-related infections. Diagn Microbiol Infect Dis. 1992;15:13–20.
32. Collignon PJ, Soni N, Pearson IY, Woods WP, Munro R, Sorrell TC. Is semiquantitative culture of central vein catheter tips useful in the diagnosis of catheter-associated bacteraemia? J Clin Microbiol. 1986;24:532–5.
33. Widmer AF, Nettleman M, Flint K, Wenzel RP. The clinical impact of culturing central venous catheters. A prospective study. Arch Intern Med. 1992;152:1299–302.
34. Raad II, Sabbagh MF, Rand KH, Sheretz RJ. Quantitative tip culture methods and the diagnosis of central venous catheter related infections. Diagn Microbiol Infect Dis. 1992;15:13–20.
35. Bouza E, Alvarado N, Alcala L, et al. A prospective, randomized, and comparative study of 3 different methods for the diagnosis of intravascular catheter colonization. Clin Infect Dis. 2005;40:1096–100.
36. Bjornson HS, Colley R, Bower RH, Duty VP, Schwartz-Fulton JT, Fischer JE. Association between microorganism growth at the catheter insertion site and colonization of the catheter in patients receiving total parenteral nutrition. Surgery. 1982;92:720–7.

37. Brun-Buisson C, Abrouk F, Legrand P, Huet Y, Larabi S, Rapin M. Diagnosis of central venous catheter-related sepsis. Critical level of quantitative tip culture. Arch Intern Med. 1987;147:873–7.
38. Sherertz R, Raad I, Belani A, et al. Three-year experience with sonicated vascular catheter cultures in a clinical microbiology laboratory. J Clin Microbiol. 1990;28:76–82.
39. Cleri DJ, Corrado ML, Seligman SJ. Quantitative culture of intravenous catheters and other intravascular inserts. J Infect Dis. 1980;141:781–6.
40. Brun-Buisson C, Abrouk F, Legrand P, et al. Diagnosis of central venous catheter related sepsis. A prospective study. Arch Intern Med. 1987;147:873–7.
41. Widmer AF, Frei R. Diagnosis of central venous catheter related infection: comparison of the roll plate and sonication technique in 1000 catheters [abstract K-2036]. In: Paper presented at the 43rd annual interscience conference on antimicrobial agents and chemotherapy, Chicago, 14–17 Sept 2003.
42. Pronovost P, Needham D, Berenholtz S, et al. An intervention to decrease catheter-related bloodstream infections in the ICU. N Eng J Med. 2006;355:2725–32.
43. Veenstra DL, Saint S, Saha S, Lumley T, Sullivan SD. Efficacy of antiseptic-impregnated central venous catheters in preventing catheter related bloodstream infection: a meta-analysis. JAMA. 1999;281:261–7.
44. Mermel LA. Prevention of intravascular catheter related infections. Ann Intern Med. 2000;132:391–402. Erratum, Ann Inter Med 2000;133:5.
45. Widmer AF, Frei R. Diagnosis of central-venous catheter-related infection: comparison of the roll-plate and sonication technique in 1000 catheters [abstract K-2036]. In: 43rd annual interscience conference on antimicrobial agents chemotherapy, Chicago, 14–17 Sept 2003.
46. Spencer RC, Kristinsson KG. Failure to diagnose intravascular associated infection by direct Gram staining of catheter segments. J Hosp Infect. 1986;7:305–6.
47. Crnich CJ, Maki DG. The promise of novel technology for the prevention of intravascular device-related bloodstream infection. I. Pathogenesis and short-term devices. Clin Infect Dis. 2002;34:1232–42.
48. Maki DG, Ringer M, Alvarado CJ. Prospective randomized trial of povidone-iodine, alcohol, and chlorhexidine for prevention of infection associated with central venous and arterial catheters. Lancet. 1991;338:339–43.
49. Pemberton LB, Ross V, Cuddy P, Kremer H, Fessler T, McGurk E. No difference in catheter sepsis between standard and antiseptic central venous catheters: a prospective randomized trial. Ann Intern Med. 1997;127:257–66.
50. Collin GR. Decreasing catheter colonization through the use of an antiseptic-impregnated catheter: a continuous quality improvement project. Chest. 1999;54:868–72.
51. Veenstra DL, Saint S, Sullivan SD. Cost-effectiveness of antiseptic-impregnated central venous catheters for the prevention of catheter-related bloodstream infection. JAMA. 1999;282(6):554–60.
52. Brun-Buisson C, Doyon F, Sollet JP, Cochard JF, et al. Prevention of intravascular catheter-related infection with newer chlorhexidine-silver sulfadiazine-coated catheters: a randomized controlled trial. Intensive Care Med. 2004;30(5):837–43.
53. Brun-Buisson C, Doyon F, Sollet JP, Cochard JF, Cohen Y, Nitenberg G. Prevention of intravascular catheter-related infection with newer chlorhexidine-silver sulfadiazine-coated catheters: a randomized controlled trial. Intensive Care Med. 2004;30:837–43.
54. Rupp ME, Lisco SJ, Lipsett PA, et al. Effect of a second-generation venous catheter impregnated with chlorhexidine and silver sulfadiazine on central catheter-related infection. A randomized, controlled trial. Ann Intern Med. 2005;143:570–80.
55. Ostendorf T, Meinhold A, Harter C, et al. Chlorhexidine and silver-sulfadiazine coated central venous catheters in haematological patients – a double-blind, randomized, prospective, controlled trial. Support Care Cancer. 2005;13:993–1000.
56. Raad I, Darouiche R, Dupuis J, et al. Central venous catheters coated with minocycline and rifampin for the prevention of catheter-related colonization and bloodstream infections. A randomized, double-blind trial. The Texas Medical Center Catheter Study Group. Ann Intern Med. 1997;127(4):267–74.
57. Hanna H, Benjamin R, Chatzinikolaou I, et al. Long-term silicone central venous catheters impregnated with minocycline and rifampin decrease rates of catheter-related bloodstream infection in cancer patients: a prospective randomized clinical trial. J Clin Oncol. 2004;22(15):3163–71.
58. Darouiche RO, Raad II, Heard SO, Thornby JI, Wenker OC, Gabrielli A, et al. Comparison of two anti-microbial impregnated central venous catheters. N Engl J Med. 1999;340:1–8.
59. Wright F, Heyland D, Drover J, McDonald S, Zoutman D. Antibiotic-coated central lines: Do they work in the critical care settings? Clin Intensive Care. 2001;12(1):21–8.
60. Chatzinikolau I, Hanna H, Graviss L, Chaiban G, Perego C, Arbuckle R, et al. Clinical experience with minocycline and rifampin-impregnated central venous catheters in bone marrow transplantation recipients: efficacy and low risk of developing staphylococcal resistance. Infect Control Hosp Epidemiol. 2003;24(12):961–3.
61. Sampath LA, Tambe SM, Modak SM. In vitro and in vivo efficacy of catheters impregnated with antiseptics or antibiotics: evaluation of the risk of bacterial resistance to the antimicrobials in the catheters. Infect Control Hosp Epidemiol. 2001;22(10):640–6.
62. Munson El, Heard SO, Doern GV. In vitro exposure of bacteria to antimicrobial impregnated-central venous catheters doesn't not directly lead to the emergence of antimicrobial resistance. Chest. 2004;126:1628–35.
63. Raad I, Darouiche R, Dupis J, Abi-Said D, Gabrielli A, Hachem R, et al. Central venous catheters coated with minocycline and rifampin for the prevention of catheter related colonization and bloodstream infections. A randomized, Double Blind Trial. Ann Intern Med. 1997;127:267–74.
64. Raad I. Zero tolerance for catheter-related bloodstream infections: the unnegotiable objective. Infect Control Hosp Epidemiol. 2008;29:952–3.
65. Randolph AG, Cook DJ, Gonzales CA, Andrew M. Benefit of heparin in central venous and pulmonary artery catheters: meta-analysis of randomized controlled trials. Chest. 1998;113:165–71.
66. Shanks RM, Donegan NP, Graber ML, et al. Heparin stimulates *Staphylococcus aureus* biofilm formation. Infect Immun. 2005;73:4596–606.
67. Henrickson KJ, Axtell RA, Hoover SM, et al. Prevention of central venous catheter-related infections and thrombotic events in immunocompromised children by the use of vancomycin/ ciprofloxacin/ heparin flush solution: a randomized, multicenter, double-blind trial. J Clin Oncol. 2000;18:1269–78.
68. Garland JS, Henrickson KJ, Maki DG. A prospective randomized trial of vancomycin-heparin lock for prevention of catheter-related bloodstream infection in an NNICU [abstract 1734]. In: 2002 annual meeting of the Pediatric Academic Societies, Baltimore, 4–7 May 2002.
69. Rackoff WR, Weiman M, Jacobowski D, et al. A randomized, controlled trial of the efficacy of a heparin and vancomycin solution in preventing central venous catheter infections in children. J Pediatr. 1995;127:147–51.
70. Daghistani D, Horn M, Rodriguez Z, Schoenike S, Toledano S. Prevention of indwelling central venous catheter sepsis. Med Pediatr Oncol. 1996;26:405–8.

71. Dogra GK, Herson H, Hutchison B, et al. Prevention of tunneled hemodialysis catheter-related infections using catheter-restricted filling with gentamicin and citrate: a randomized controlled study. J Am Soc Nephrol. 2002;13:2133–9.
72. Bleyer AJ, Mason L, Russell G, Raad II, Sherertz RJ. A randomized, controlled trial of a new vascular catheter flush solution (minocycline-EDTA) in temporary hemodialysis access. Infect Control Hosp Epidemiol. 2005;26:520–4.
73. Raad I, Hanna H, Jiang Y, et al. Comparative activities of daptomycin, linezolid, and tigecycline against catheter-related methicillin-resistant *Staphylococcus* bacteremic isolates embedded in biofilm. Antimicrob Agents Chemother. 2007;51:1656–60.
74. Raad I, Chatzinikolaou I, Chaiban G, et al. In vitro and ex vivo activity of minocycline and EDTA against microorganisms embedded in biofilm on catheter surfaces. Antimicrob Agents Chemother. 2003;47:3580–5.
75. Raad I, Buzaid A, Rhyne J, Hachem R, Darouiche R, Safar H, et al. Minocycline and ethlenediaminetetraacetate for the prevention of recurrent vascular catheter infections. Clin Infect Dis. 1997;25:149–51.
76. Christensen GD, Bison AL, Parisi JT, et al. Nosocomial septicemia due to multiply antibiotic-resistant staphylococcus epidermis. Ann Intern Med. 1982;96:1–10.
77. Sattler FR, Foderaro JB, Aber RC. Staphylococcus epidermis bacteremia associated with vascular catheter: an important cause of febrile morbidity in hospitalized patients. Infect Control. 1984;5: 279–83.
78. Engelhard D, Elishoov H, Strauss N, et al. Nosocomial coagulase negative staphylococcal infections in bone marrow transplantation recipients with central vein catheter. Transplantation. 1996;61:430–4.
79. Fowler VG, Sanders LL, Sexton DJ, et al. Outcome of *Staphylococcus aureus* bacteraemia according to compliance with recommendations of infectious disease specialists: experience with 244 patients. Clin Infect Dis. 1998;27:478–86.
80. Ghanem GA, Boktour M, Warneke C, et al. Catheter-related *Staphylococcus aureus* bacteremia in cancer patients: high rate of complications with therapeutic implications. Medicine. 2007;86:54–60.
81. Abdelkefi A, Ben Romdhane N, Kriaa A, et al. Prevalence of inherited prothrombotic abnormalities and central venous catheter-related thrombosis in haematopoietic stem cell transplants recipients. Bone Marrow Transplant. 2006;36:885–9.
82. Fowler Jr VG, Olsen MK, Corey R, et al. Clinical identifiers of complicated *Staphylococcus aureus* bacteraemia. Arch Intern Med. 2003;163:2066–71.
83. Raad I, Darouiche R, Vazquez J, et al. Efficacy and safety of weekly dalbavancin in the treatment of catheter-related bloodstream infections due to Gram-positive pathogens. Clin Infect Dis. 2005;40:374–8.
84. Carpenter CF, Chambers HF. Daptomycin: another novel agent for treating infection due to drug-resistant Gram-positive pathogens. Clin Infect Dis. 2004;38:994–1000.
85. Malanoski GJ, Samore MH, Pefanis A, Karchmer AW. *Staphylococcus aureus* catheter-associated bacteremia. Minimal effective therapy and unusual infectious complications associated with arterial sheath catheters. Arch Intern Med. 1995;155:1161–6.
86. Fowler Jr VG, Justice A, Moore C, et al. Risk factors for hematogenous complications of intravascular catheter-associated *Staphylococcus aureus* bacteremia. Clin Infect Dis. 2005;40:695–703.
87. Elting LS, Bodey GP. Septicemia due to *Xanthomonas* species and non-aeruginosa *Pseudomonas* species: increasing incidence of catheter-related infections. Medicine. 1990;69:196–206.
88. Hanna H, Afif C, Alakech B, et al. Central venous catheter-related bacteraemia due to Gram-negative bacilli: significance of catheter removal in preventing relapse. Infect Control Hosp Epidemiol. 2004;25:646–9.
89. Chee L, Brown M, Sasadeusz J, MacGregor L, Grigg AP. Gram-negative organisms predominate in Hickman line-related infections in non-neutropenic patients with hematological malignancies. J Infect. 2008;56:227–33.
90. Rodriguez-Creixems M, Alcala L, Munoz P, Cercenado E, Vicente T, Bouza E. Bloodstream infections: evolution and trends in the microbiology workload, incidence, and etiology, 1985–2006. Medicine (Baltimore). 2008;87:234–49.
91. Mermel LA, Farr BM, Sheretz RJ, Raad II, O'Grady N, Harris JAS, et al. Guidelines for the management of intravascular catheter-related infections. Clin Infect Dis. 2001;32:1249–72.
92. Strinden WD, Helgerson RB, Maki DG. Candida septic thrombosis of the great central veins associated with central catheters: clinical features and management. Ann Surg. 1985;202: 653–8.
93. Hanna H, Afif C, Alakech B, Boktour M, Tarrand J, Hachem R, et al. Central venous catheter-related bacteremia due to gram-negative bacilli: significance of catheter-removal in preventing relapse. Infect Control Hosp Epidemiol. 2004;25(8):646–9.
94. Nguyen MH, Peacock Jr JE, Tanner DC, et al. Therapeutic approaches in patients with candidemia: evaluation in a multicenter, prospective observational study. Arch Intern Med. 1995;155:2429–35.
95. Nucci M, Colombo AL, Silveira F, et al. Risk factors for death in patients with candidemia. Infect Control Hosp Epidemiol. 1998;19: 846–50.
96. Hung C-C, Chen Y-C, Chag S-C, Lu K-T, Hsieh W-C. Nosocomial candidemia in a university hospital in Taiwan. J Formas Med Assoc. 1996;95:19–28.
97. Rex JH, Bennett JE, Sugar AM, et al. Intravascular catheter-exchange and duration of candidemia. Clin Infect Dis. 1995;21:995–6.
98. Raad I, Hanna H, Boktour M, Girgawy E, Danawi H, Mardani M, et al. Management of central venous catheters in patients with cancer and candidemia. Clin Infect Dis. 2004;38:1119–27.
99. Mora-Duarte J, Betts R, Rotstein C, et al. Comparison of caspofungin and amphotericin B for invasive candidiasis. N Engl J Med. 2002;347:2020–9.
100. Oudiz RJ, Widlitz A, Beckman XJ, et al. Micrococcus-associated central venous catheter infection in patients with pulmonary arterial hypertension. Chest. 2004;126:90–4.
101. Dziekan G, Hahn A, Thune G, et al. Methicillin-resistant *Staphylococcus aureus* in a teaching hospital: investigation of nosocomial transmission using a matched case-control study. J Hosp Infect. 2000;46:263–70.
102. Raad I, Ramos E, Hachem R, et al. The crucial role of catéters in micrococcal bloodstream infections in cancer patients. Infect Control Hosp Epidemiol. 2009;30:83–5.
103. Chaftari AM, Kassis C, El Issa H, Al Wohoush I, Jiang Y, Rangaraj G, et al. Novel approach using antimicrobial catheters to improve the management of central line-associated bloodstream infections in cancer patients. Cancer. 2010 Dec 14. [Epub ahead of print]

Chapter 11
Intravascular Device-Related Infections: Catheter Salvage Strategies and Prevention of Device-Related Infection

Nasia Safdar and Dennis G. Maki

Abstract The use of intravascular devices for administration of chemotherapeutic drugs, fluids, blood products, and nutritional support is essential to the care of patients with cancer. Unfortunately, intravascular devices have great potential to produce iatrogenic disease, especially bloodstream infection originating from colonization of the device used for access or from contamination of the infusate administered through the device. Over two thirds of all healthcare-associated bacteremias originate from devices for vascular access. Probably, more than any other healthcare-associated infection, IVDR BSI is eminently preventable. The first step to preserve vascular access is a highly effective institutional program for the prevention of IVDR BSI. In recent years, high-quality research studies have delineated key measures for prevention, such as chlorhexidine (CHG) for cutaneous antisepsis, maximal barrier precautions, antiinfective-impregnated catheters, and the use of a CVC insertion "bundle," and IVDR BSI rates in the ICU have declined markedly in most hospitals. However, despite adherence to best practices, IVDR BSI continues to pose formidable challenges, especially in patients with cancer. Catheter salvage in the context of established IVDR BSI is particularly challenging, but recent advances such as antibiotic lock technique are now providing previously unavailable options.

Keywords Catheter infection • Bloodstream infection • Prevention • Treatment

Introduction

The use of intravascular devices for administration of chemotherapeutic drugs, fluids, blood products, and nutritional support is essential to the care of patients with cancer.

N. Safdar (✉)
Section of Infectious Diseases, Department of Medicine, University of Wisconsin Medical School, MFCB 5221, 1685 Highland Avenue, Madison, WI 53717, USA
e-mail: ns2@medicine.wisc.edu

Unfortunately, intravascular devices have great potential to produce iatrogenic disease, especially bloodstream infection (BSI) originating from colonization of the device used for access or from contamination of the infusate administered through the device [1–4]. Over two thirds of all healthcare-associated bacteremias originate from devices for vascular access [5].

Every year more than five million central venous catheters (CVC) are inserted in the United States [6]. More than 250,000 intravascular catheter-related blood stream infections (IVDR BSI) occur annually with an associated mortality of 12–25% [6]. A recent meta-analysis found mortality to be significantly increased in intensive care unit (ICU) patients who had IVDR BSI compared with those without IVDR BSI (OR, 1.96; 95% confidence interval [CI], 1.25–3.09) (Fig. 11.1) [7]. Each episode of IVDR BSI significantly increases hospital length of stay, and the added health-care costs range from $4,000 to $56,000 per episode [8–10].

Probably, more than any other healthcare-associated infection, IVDR BSI is eminently preventable [5, 11–14].

This chapter focuses on catheter salvage in IVDR BSI. The first step to preserve vascular access is a highly effective institutional program for the prevention of IVDR BSI. In recent years, high-quality research studies have delineated key measures for prevention, and IVDR BSI rates in the ICU have declined markedly in most hospitals [12, 15–26]. However, despite adherence to best practices, IVDR BSI continues to pose formidable challenges, especially in patients with cancer. Catheter salvage in the context of established IVDR BSI is particularly challenging, but recent advances are now providing previously unavailable options.

Pathogenesis of IVDR BSI

There are two major sources of IVD-related BSI: (1) colonization of the IVD, *device-related infection*, and (2) contamination of the fluid administered through the device, *infusate-related infection* [27]. Contaminated infusate is the cause of most *epidemic* intravascular device-related BSIs

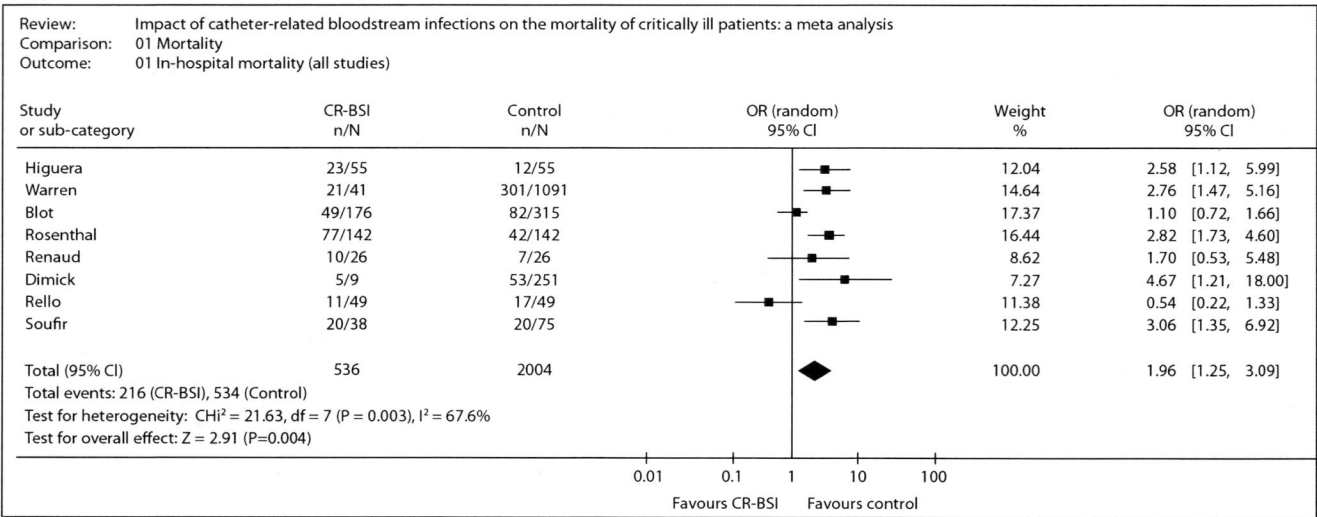

Fig. 11.1 Attributable mortality of IVDR BSI in critically ill patients. From Siempos et al. [7] with permission

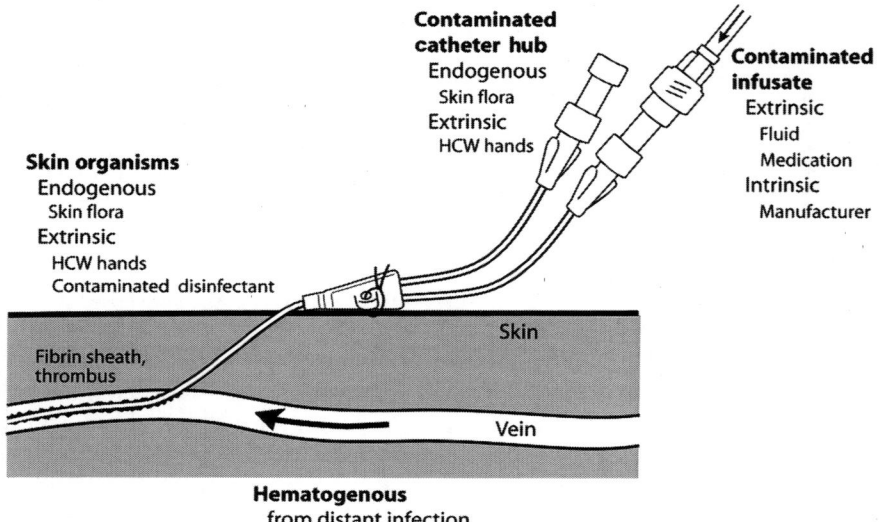

Fig. 11.2 Potential sources of infection of a percutaneous IVD: the contiguous skin flora, contamination of the catheter hub and lumen, contamination of infusate, and hematogenous colonization of the IVD from distant, unrelated sites of infection [174]

[4, 28]; by contrast, catheter-related infections are responsible for most *endemic* device-related BSIs. Understanding the pathogenesis of IVD-related BSIs is fundamental to devising effective strategies for the prevention and treatment of these infections; however, relatively few published studies have determined the mechanism of IVD-related colonization and infection using sophisticated molecular techniques to prove or disprove potential routes of infection [29–35].

In order for microorganisms to cause catheter-related infection, they must first gain access to the extraluminal or intraluminal surface of the device where they can adhere to and become incorporated into a biofilm that allows sustained colonization and ultimately hematogenous dissemination [36]. Microorganisms gain access to the implanted IVD by one of three mechanisms: skin organisms invade the percutaneous tract, probably facilitated by capillary action [37], at the time of insertion or in the days following; microorganisms contaminate the catheter hub (and lumen) when the catheter is inserted over a percutaneous guidewire or later manipulated [38]; or organisms are carried hematogenously to the implanted IVD from remote sources of local infection, such as a pneumonia [39] (Fig. 11.2).

With *short-term* IVDs (in place <14 days) – peripheral IV catheters, arterial catheters and noncuffed, nontunneled CVCs – most catheter-related BSIs are of cutaneous origin, from the insertion site, and gain access extraluminally or occasionally intraluminally [35, 40, 41]. For long-term catheters – tunneled, cuffed CVCs, totally implantable ports and PICCs – luminal colonization has been shown to be the major route of access leading to BSI [42, 43]. A characteristic pulsed-field gel electrophoresis image obtained from a short-term noncuffed CVC causing BSI is shown in Fig. 11.3 and a long-term catheter (PICC) in Fig. 11.4.

Microbiology

Antimicrobial resistance, now considered to be at global crisis levels, continues to loom large, and the organisms implicated in IVDR BSIs are no exception. In the past 2 decades, the proportion of IVDR BSIs caused by multidrug-resistant (MDR) organisms, such as methicillin-resistant *Staphylococcus aureus* (MRSA) and fluconazole-resistant *Candida* species, has risen inexorably [6, 44–46]. Overall, the organisms encountered most frequently in IVDR BSI are coagulase-negative staphylococci (CoNS) (31%), *S. aureus* (20%), Enterococci (9%), and *Candida* species (9%) [24–26, 44, 47].

In one large prospective surveillance study using data from SCOPE (Surveillance and Control of Pathogens of Epidemiological Importance), comprising 24,179 cases of nosocomial BSI reported over a 7-year period from 49 hospitals, rates of MRSA infection increased from 22% of all *S. aureus* BSIs in 1995 to 75% in 2001 ($P<0.001$), and resistance to vancomycin was found in 60% of *Enterococcus faecium* isolates [44].

Catheter Salvage in the Context of Prevention

In 2002, The Healthcare Infection Control Practices Advisory Committee (HICPAC) of the CDC published a comprehensive Guideline for the prevention of IVDR BSI, which is summarized in Table 11.1 [6]. This Guideline focuses on educating all healthcare workers on best practices for catheter insertion and care; choosing the optimal insertion site; practicing maximal antisepsis, including hand hygiene and barrier precautions; removing the device as soon as it is deemed unnecessary; and surveillance of catheter infection rates [5, 6]. Reviewed below are topics of importance in prevention as well as novel strategies not addressed in the guidelines (Table 11.2) [48–55]. The recommendations are rated based on the strength of evidence supporting them as follows. IA: strongly recommended for implementation and strongly supported by well-designed experimental, clinical, or epidemiologic studies; IB: strongly recommended for implementation and supported by some experimental, clinical or epidemiologic studies, and a strong theoretical rationale; IC: required by state or federal regulations, rules, or standards; II: suggested for implementation and supported by suggestive clinical or epidemiologic studies or a theoretical rationale [6].

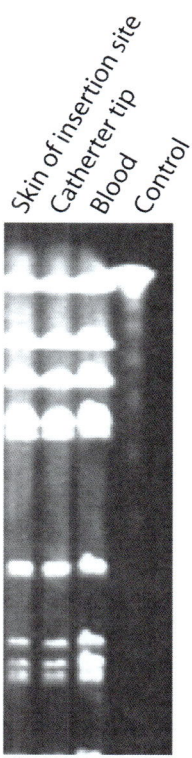

Fig. 11.3 Pulsed-field gel electrophoresis image showing the probable pathogenesis of a central venous catheter-related bacteremia with coagulase-negative Staphylococcus. The isolates from the catheter tip, blood, and skin of the insertion site were all concordant, indicating an extraluminal route of infection [35]

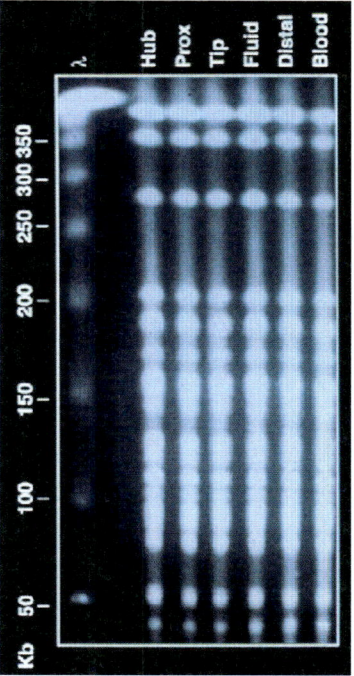

Fig. 11.4 Pulsed-field gel electrophoresis image showing the probable pathogenesis of a PICC-related bacteremia with *Serratia marcescens*. The isolates from the catheter tip, blood, hub, and fluid were all concordant, indicating an intraluminal route of infection

Table 11.1 Recommendations for prevention of IVDR BSI, 2002 CDC-HICPAC guideline [175]

Recommendation	Rating[a]
Education	
• Educate all relevant healthcare personnel regarding indications for IVC use, proper procedures for insertion and maintenance, and infection-control measures	IA
Surveillance	
• Conduct institutional surveillance for rates of IVDR BSI, monitor trends, identifying lapses in infection-control practices	IA
• Express ICU data as number of IVDR BSIs per 1,000 catheter days	IB
Antisepsis	
• Maximal sterile barrier precautions during catheter insertion: cap, mask, sterile gown, sterile gloves, and large sterile sheet	IA
• Hand hygiene: wash hands with antiseptic-containing soap and water or waterless alcohol-based product: before insertion or any manipulation of any IVC	IA
• Gloves: required for any manipulation of any IVC	IA
• Sterile gloves required for arterial and central catheters	
• Clean gloves acceptable for peripheral IVCs if site not touched after application of skin antiseptics	
• Cutaneous antisepsis: use before insertion and during dressing changes: 2% chlorhexidine is preferred, an iodophor or 70% alcohol are acceptable	IA
Insertion	
• When possible, use subclavian site when using a nontunneled CVC	IA
• Use designated personnel for insertion and maintenance of IVCs	IA
• Use sterile gauze or sterile, transparent semipermeable dressing	IA
• Do not give prophylactic antibiotics to prevent catheter colonization or BSI	IA
Maintenance	
• Change dressing at least weekly	II
• Monitor site visually or by palpation through intact dressing on regular basis and remove dressing for full exam if tender, fever without obvious source or other manifestations suggesting local or BSI	IB
• Do not routinely culture catheter tips	IB
• Do not use topical antibiotic ointments or creams (except with dialysis catheters)	IA
• Remove IVCs as soon as not necessary	IA
• Do not routinely replace CVCs, PICCs, HD catheters, or pulmonary artery catheters to prevent IVDR BSIs	IB
• Replace peripheral venous catheters at least every 72–96 h in adults	IB
• Replace administration sets no more frequently than at 72 h unless infection or unless infusing blood produces, or lipid emulsions	IB
• If after implementing a comprehensive strategy to reduce rates of IVDR BSIs and rates remain high, use antimicrobial or antiseptic-impregnated CVC in adults if CVC is expected to remain >5 days	IB
Novel strategies not addressed in current guidelines	
• Consider antimicrobial lock solutions for use in all long-term devices	IB
• Chlorhexidine-impregnated dressings (Biopatch®) should be used with all short-term catheters	IA
• A sutureless catheter securement device (StatLock®) is preferred to sutures	IB
• Adhere to the IHI bundle for CVCs	IA
• Chlorhexidine bathing in the ICU	IA

IVDR BSI catheter-related blood stream infection; *CVC* central venous catheter; *HD* hemodialysis; *IVC* intravenous catheter; *PICC* peripherally inserted central venous catheter

[a]CDC categories of evidence: *IA* strongly recommended for implementation and strongly supported by well-designed experimental, clinical, or epidemiologic studies; *IB* strongly recommended for implementation and supported by some experimental, clinical or epidemiologic studies, and a strong theoretical rationale; *IC* required by state or federal regulations, rules, or standards; *II* suggested for implementation and supported by suggestive clinical or epidemiologic studies or a theoretical rationale [6]

Cutaneous Antisepsis

Iodophors, such as 10% povidine-iodine, or 70% alcohol were the most widely used agents for cutaneous antisepsis of the insertion site in US centers [56, 57]. However, several studies, including a meta-analysis, have shown that 2% CHG is unequivocally superior for preventing IVDR BSI [54, 58] and is now recommended by the HICPAC Guideline as the agent of first choice (rating IA) [6, 56, 58].

Topical Antimicrobials

The HICPAC Guideline specifically recommends against the application of topical antimicrobial ointments or creams to the IVD insertion site, except in the case of hemodialysis catheters [6], to avoid promotion of fungal infection and antimicrobial resistance (rating IA). The Guideline also discourages the use of intranasal mupirocin for staphylococcal decolonization before IVD insertion or during the use of an IVD as a means to prevent colonization or IVDR BSI (rating IA) [6].

Table 11.2 Novel strategies for the prevention of intravascular device-related bloodstream infection

Strategy	References	Design	Technology	Outcome
Antimicrobial lock solutions	Safdar and Maki [48]	Meta-analysis	Vancomycin-containing locks vs. heparin	50% risk reduction (RR, 0.49; 95% CI, 0.26–0.95)
	Yahav et al. [52]	Systematic review and meta-analysis	Various antibiotics[a] Antibiotic plus antiseptic[b] Antiseptic[c]	Antibiotic solutions: RR, 0.44 (95% CI, 0.38–0.5) Nonantibiotic antiseptic solutions alone: RR, 0.9 (95% CI, 0.48–1.69) Nonantibiotic antiseptic solutions + other prevention methods[d]: RR, 0.25 (95% CI, 0.13–0.5)
	Sanders et al. [92]	Double-blind randomized trial	Ethanol-containing locks vs. heparin	OR, 0.18 (95% CI, 0.05–0.65)
Antimicrobial catheters	Veenstra et al. [51]	Meta-analysis	Antiseptic-impregnated CVCs[e]	OR, 0.56 (95% CI, 0.37–0.84)
	Ramritu et al. [50]	Systematic review	Antibiotic-impregnated CVCs[f]	RR, 0.39 (95% CI, 0.17–0.92)
	Crnich and Maki [174]	Meta-analysis	Silver-impregnated CVCs	RR, 0.40 (95% CI, 0.24–0.68)
	Ramritu et al. [50]	Systematic review	Antibiotic vs. first-generation antiseptic-impregnated CVCs	RR, 0.12 (95% CI 0.02–0.67)[g]
	Hockenhull et al. [176]	Meta-analysis	Antiinfective CVCs (all types)	OR, 0.49 (95% CI 0.37–0.64)[h]
Chlorhexidine dressings	Maki et al. [79]	RCT	Chlorhexidine-impregnated sponge dressing	IVDR BSI: RR 0.37 (0.17–0.80)
	Ho and Litton [49]	Meta-analysis	Chlorhexidine-impregnated dressing vs. placebo or povidone-iodine dressing	Catheter or exit site colonization: 14.3 vs. 27.2%; OR, 0.4 (95% CI, 0.26–0.61) IVDR BSIs: 2.2 vs. 3.8%; OR, 0.58 (95% CI, 0.29–1.14, $P=0.11$)
	Timsit et al. [80]	Randomized, controlled trial	Chlorhexidine-impregnated dressing vs. standard dressing	IVDR BSI: 0.4 vs. 1.3/1,000 catheter days; HR, 0.024 (95% CI, 0.09–0.65; $P=0.005$)
Cutaneous antisepsis	Chaiyakunapruk et al. [54]	Meta-analysis	Chlorhexidine vs. povidone-iodine	RR, 0.49 (95% CI, 0.28–0.88)[i]
	Maki et al. [58]	RCT	Chlorhexidine vs. alcohol vs. povidone-iodine	IVDR BSI RR 0.16, $P=0.04$
Mupirocin prophylaxis	Tacconelli et al. [55]	Meta-analysis	Mupirocin prophylaxis in dialysis patients[j]	Decrease in S. aureus bacteremia in hemodialysis patients by 78%; RR 0.22 (95% CI, 0.11–0.42)

CI confidence interval; *EDTA* ethylenediamine tetraacetic acid; *OR* odds ratio; *RR* relative risk
[a]Gentamicin; gentamicin+citrate; gentamicin+vancomycin; gentamicin+cefazolin; cefotaxime
[b]Minocycline with EDTA
[c]Citrate; citrate with taurolidine
[d]Nasal mupirocin and exit-site iodine dressing
[e]Chlorhexidine-silver sulfadiazine
[f]Minocycline and rifampin
[g]Reduced risk with antibiotic catheters
[h]Reduced risk with antiinfective catheters: all types combined, see text for subgroup analysis
[i]Reduced with chlorhexidine
[j]Six studies used intranasal mupirocin 2–3 times daily for 5–14 days with various maintenance schedules; 4 studies used mupirocin applied to catheter exit site

A meta-analysis of mupirocin prophylaxis to prevent *S. aureus* infections in patients undergoing dialysis showed a 63% reduction (95% CI), (50–73%) in the rate of overall *S. aureus* infections [55]. The study population included both hemodialysis and peritoneal dialysis patients. Of the ten studies, six used intranasal mupirocin 2–3 times daily for 5–14 days, with various maintenance schedules, and four used mupirocin applied to the catheter exit site. In patients undergoing hemodialysis, *S. aureus* bacteremias were reduced by 78% (relative risk [RR], 0.22; 95% CI, 0.11–0.42). However, the differences in site, frequency, and duration of mupirocin treatment in these studies and the resulting clinical heterogeneity make it difficult to offer robust recommendations [55].

A randomized, double-blind, placebo controlled trial evaluating mupirocin prophylaxis for nosocomial *S. aureus* infections in nonsurgical patients found that restricting the use of intranasal mupirocin to patients shown to be carriers on admission did not prevent nosocomial *S. aureus* infections [59]. Increasing reports of mupirocin resistance [60–65], call decolonization with mupirocin into question as a strategy to prevent IVDR BSI, even in hemodialysis centers, and we do not recommend topical or intranasal mupirocin for prevention of IVDR BSIs.

The early promise of mupirocin has suggested that other topical approaches to preventing IVDR BSIs bear study. One such agent is honey, which has long been known to have antibacterial properties. In a randomized, controlled trial (RCT) to compare the effect of thrice-weekly application of Medihoney (commercially available; pooled antibacterial honeys including *Leptospermum* species honey; Medihoney Pty Ltd, Brisbane, Australia) or mupirocin to the IVD exit site in 101 patients who were receiving hemodialysis through tunneled and cuffed CVCs, catheter-associated bacteremia rates in the two arms were similar (0.97 vs. 0.85 episodes per 1,000 catheter days; $P>0.05$) [66]. Although these results are promising, a larger trial powered to show equivalence or superiority and provide information on tolerance and effect of the topical agent on resistance patterns of infecting microorganisms is needed to establish the utility of Medihoney for the prevention of IVDR BSIs in patients receiving hemodialysis through cuffed and tunneled CVCs.

Maximal Barrier Precautions

The use of maximal barrier precautions, including cap, sterile gown, mask, large sterile drape, and sterile gloves, significantly reduce the rate of IVDR BSIs when used during catheter insertion [6, 67, 68]. In a RCT, Raad et al. compared maximal barrier precautions with limited precautions (e.g., sterile gloves and a small fenestrated drape) and found the CVC-related BSI rate to be 6.3 times higher in the control group ($P=0.06$) [67]. The HICPAC Guideline recommends that maximal barrier precautions be used for all central IVD insertions, including PICCs (rating IA) [6].

Insertion Site

According to the HICPAC Guideline, the preferred site for insertion of nontunneled CVCs in adult patients is the subclavian vein (rating 1A) [6]. The femoral site has been reported to be associated with higher rates of catheter colonization as well as increased risk of deep vein thrombosis compared to cephalad sites in adults [6, 40, 69–71]. In an RCT with uncuffed CVCs, comparing femoral and subclavian sites, catheters inserted in a femoral site were associated with a higher incidence of infectious complications (19.8 vs. 4.5%; $P<0.001$) [71].

The internal jugular vein site has also been associated with higher rates of IVDR BSI than the femoral or subclavian sites in several studies [6, 40, 72]. However, a recent RCT comparing the jugular and femoral sites found no difference in the risk for infection between the two sites (2.3 vs. 1.5, $P=0.42$) [73]. A prospective, observational study comparing the subclavian, internal jugular, and femoral insertion sites found colonization lowest at the subclavian site but no difference in rates of BSI between sites [74, 75].

Using real-time ultrasound guidance for catheter insertion significantly reduces mechanical complications deriving from catheter insertion and catheter infection [6, 76, 77]. In a recent randomized study, real-time ultrasound guidance vs. the landmark technique for catheter placement in the internal jugular vein resulted in significantly fewer complications, including fewer IVDR BSIs ($P<0.001$) [77]. A recent meta-analysis found that the use of ultrasound for insertion at internal jugular and subclavian vein sites reduced cannulation failure (RR, 0.32; 95% CI, 0.18–0.55), the need for multiple placement attempts (RR, 0.60; 95% CI, 0.45–0.79) and complications during catheter placement (RR, 0.22; 95% CI, 0.10–0.45), in comparison with insertions using anatomic landmarks [76].

Although no RCT to date has compared the three insertion sites, based on the available data, we recommend the subclavian site as the first preferred site for CVC insertion routinely employing real-time ultrasound to minimize mechanical complications.

Simulation-Based Training

A recent observational study, completed in an urban teaching hospital, evaluated the impact of a simulation-based educational intervention on the rates of IVDR BSI in a medical ICU [78]; third-year internal medicine and emergency medicine residents completed the educational program, which included a pretest, an informational video demonstrating proper CVC insertion technique, training with ultra-sound and hands-on practice using a simulator device, and a posttest with a required minimum score [78]. There were 3.2 infections per 1,000 catheter days in the 16 months prior to the educational intervention in this medical ICU and 4.9 infections per 1,000 catheter days in a comparator unit in the same hospital, the surgical ICU, during the preintervention period. The rate of IVDR BSIs in the medical ICU during the 16-month intervention period, when all of the second- and third-year residents had completed the training, decreased to 0.5/1,000 catheter days. The rate in the surgical ICU, where no rotating residents completed the simulation training, remained stable at 5.3/1,000 catheter days during the same 16-month time period [78]. This study affirms the value of cutting-edge programs for training healthcare personnel in proper CVC insertion techniques, addressing a priority recommendation in the CDC HICPAC Guideline for the Prevention of IVDR BSI [6].

Chlorhexidine-Impregnated Insertion Site Dressings

The application of a CHG-impregnated sponge dressing (BioPatch®, Johnson & Johnson Gateway) over the CVC insertion site has been shown to greatly reduce the incidence of IVDR BSI in several randomized trials [5, 56, 79–81]. A large, randomized, open, controlled trial compared this dressing to standard sterile dressings in 601 chemotherapy patients, with 9,731 catheterization days, recently showed a significant reduction in IVDR BSIs in the intervention group (6.4%, 19 of 300) compared to the control group (11.3%, 34 of 301; $P = 0.016$, RR, 0.54; 95% CI, 0.31–0.94) [81]. In ICU patients, the use of CHG-impregnated dressings led to significantly fewer IVDR BSIs when compared with standard sterile dressings, in a large, multicenter RCT ($P = 0.005$, HR 0.024, 95% CI, 0.09–0.65) [80].

The latest 2002 CDC Guideline makes no recommendations regarding the use of CHG-impregnated dressings. However, considerable emerging data indicate that CHG-impregnated dressings are effective in reducing IVDR BSIs, and we recommend their use (rating IA) [56, 79–81].

Chlorhexidine Bathing

Several before-after time-sequence trials have been undertaken to ascertain the impact of daily 4% CHG bathing to prevent healthcare-associated BSIs in critically ill ICU patients. Overall, CHG bathing, using either CHG-impregnated wipes or adding CHG to the bathwater, has been shown to have a positive outcome on CRBSIs [82–90]. However, patients with cancer who are not critically ill have not been studied. Daily CHG bathing is recommended if other, simpler measures for reducing CRBSI have been implemented, but rates of CRBSI continue to be high.

Antiinfective-Impregnated Catheters

The HIPAC Guideline recommends the use of antiinfective-coated CVCs if the catheter is expected to remain longer than 5 days and is used in combination with a comprehensive IVDR BSI reduction strategy (rating IB) [6]. However, the majority of the studies have focused on the use of antimicrobial-coated CVCs used as short-term devices, and few data have been published on their use as long-term devices [50, 56]. Several types of catheters are available: catheters coated either externally (first generation) or externally and internally (second generation) with chlorhexidine and sulfadiazine silver (CH-SS), catheters coated with minocycline or rifampin, and silver-impregnated catheters [5]. Silver-coated catheters include silver, platinum and carbon-coated catheters, and silver ion/alloy catheters [56].

A recent comprehensive meta-analysis of antiinfective-coated catheters included clinical trials comparing antimicrobial-coated CVCs with either a standard CVC or another antimicrobial-coated CVC [91]. The main outcomes were catheter colonization and catheter-related BSI. The first-generation chlorhexidine-silver sulfadiazine (CSS) CVCs were shown to reduce colonization (OR 0.51, 95% CI 0.42–0.60) and catheter-related BSI (OR 0.68, 95% CI 0.47–0.98). Minocycline-rifampin-coated CVCs also reduced catheter colonization (OR 0.39, 9%% CI 0.27–0.55) and catheter-related BSI (OR 0.29, 95% CI 0.16–0.52), and performed better than the CSS CVCs for reducing catheter colonization and BSI (OR 0.18, 95% CI 0.07–0.51).

The choice of which catheter to use is governed by many factors including efficacy, cost, cost-effectiveness, and risk of promoting drug resistance. A recent analysis (2008) found an estimated cost savings of £138.20 (approximately $227) for every antiinfective catheter inserted [10]. Antibiotic-resistance is a particular concern with antibiotic-impregnated catheters, although trials assessing the efficacy of minocycline-rifampin-coated catheters have not found evidence of emergence of drug resistance to date [50].

Antiinfective Lock Solutions

The major mechanism of IVDR BSI in long-term IVDs is intraluminal colonization. For this reason, antimicrobial lock solutions have been a logical step to prevent colonization of the intraluminal surfaces of long-term IVDs to prevent IVDR BSIs. A small volume of the antimicrobial solution is instilled into the lumen of the IVD and allowed to dwell for a proscribed period, after which it is either removed or flushed into the patient's bloodstream.

A meta-analysis of seven RCTs, involving mostly cancer patients, comparing a vancomycin-containing lock solution with sterile saline showed a significantly reduced risk of IVDR BSI (RR 0.49, 95% CI, 0.26–0.95) [48]. A recent systematic review and meta-analysis of RCTs in patients receiving maintenance hemodialysis of a variety of antiinfective lock solutions, including various antibiotic combinations, minocycline with ethylenediamine tetraacetic acid and nonantibiotic antiseptic solutions including citrate and citrate with taurolidine was recently reported [52]. All of the lock solutions reviewed showed significant benefit for prevention of IVDR BSI [52]. Ethanol has also recently been shown to be safe and effective as an antimicrobial lock solution [53, 56, 92]. A recently published prospective, double-blind, RCT comparing ethanol with heparinized saline in granulocytopenic hematology patients showed a fourfold reduction in the number of IVDR BSIs in the ethanol group compared to controls (OR 0.18, 95% CI, 0.05–0.65) [92]. While a number of new antibiotics show promise as lock solutions based on in vitro studies [93], further research of their efficacy in clinical trials is mandatory.

We recommend the use of antiinfective lock solutions for prevention of IVDR BSIs with long-term IVDs in patients at high risk for IVDR BSIs such as those receiving hemodialysis. In general, antiseptic lock solutions are preferable to antibiotic lock solutions because of their greater spectrum of activity and lesser risk of promoting antibiotic resistance.

Antiinfective Luer-Activated Devices

In addition to the above novel technology-based strategies for the prevention of IVDR BSI, an emerging role of needleless connectors in the pathogenesis of IVDR BSIs must be mentioned, with conjecture of possible preventive strategies.

Needleless connectors were developed in response to demands for enhanced safety for healthcare workers, to prevent needle-stick injuries, and are currently an integral component of infusion systems across North America. Although needleless connectors, when properly used, clearly reduce the risk for needle-stick injuries during access of an IVD or injection port [18, 94–97], a growing number of reports published over the past decade have raised concerns about the potential for an increased risk of iatrogenic IVDR-BSI associated with the use of luer-activated, valved connectors [40, 73, 98–101]. Most of these studies have been retrospective and uncontrolled, and suboptimal manipulation of the device, rather than the device itself, may have been responsible for some of the increased incidence of BSIs in some settings, however, many hospitals experienced sharp increases in primary BSI following introduction of a new luer-activated, valved connector and intensified infection control practices had no impact; only after removing the new connector from the hospital did the rates of CVC-associated BSI return to baseline levels [102]. Most notably, multiple commercial valved connectors have been implicated, indicating that these devices appear to have a generic risk of becoming contaminated during use and producing iatrogenic BSI.

Typically, healthcare personnel disinfect connectors with 70% (v/v) isopropyl alcohol before accessing them. Although needleless connectors appeared to reduce contamination in comparison with standard caps [103], a recent study by Menyhay and Maki found that conventional methods of disinfection of the membranous septum may not prevent microbial entry if the membrane of the luer-activated device (LAD) is heavily contaminated, which may account for the increased risk for CVC-associated BSIs seen in some centers [104].

The V-Link with VitalShield (Baxter Healthcare) is an LAD protected with an interior and exterior antimicrobial coating and was recently approved by the FDA. The V-Link with VitalShield is effective against 99.9% of pathogens known to cause IVDR BSIs in in vitro testing and was recently shown in a simulation study to prevent internal contamination, even with heavy contamination of the membranous septum [105].

Saralex-cl (Menyhay Healthcare Systems), another promising device, is an antimicrobial-barrier cap that threads onto the end of a needleless LAD system. A recent prospective in vitro study compared standard disinfection of common LADs using 70% isopropyl alcohol with the new antiseptic-barrier cap [106]. This new antiseptic cap, which bathes the connector septum with 0.25 mL of 2% CHG in 70% isopropyl alcohol, was almost totally effective in preventing transmission of pathogens across the membranes of precontaminated LADs when compared to standard disinfection with 70% alcohol (positive control, 100% transmission, standard disinfection with 70% alcohol, 20 transmissions in 30 trials, 67% transmission, Saralex-cl = 1 transmission in 60 trials, 1.6% transmission; $P<0.001$) [106]. Data on the clinical efficacy of antimicrobial-coated LADs and antimicrobial-barrier caps, based on an RCT, is needed.

Catheter Securement

Choices for securement of a percutaneous uncuffed CVC or PICC include sutures, tape, or novel catheter securement devices, such as StatLock® (Venetec International, CR Bard). Sutures are often painful for the patient, pose the risk of needle-stick injury to the provider placing them, and foster infection of the suture sites, potentially increasing the risk of catheter-related BSI. StatLock®, a sutureless catheter securement device, reduces catheter-related complications including IVDR BSIs [107–109]. A randomized trial comparing suture securement to the StatLock® with peripherally inserted central catheters, showed a significant reduction in the number of catheter-related BSIs in the StatLock® group (2 vs. 10; $P=0.032$) [108]. We recommend the use of a sutureless securement device for peripheral I.V. and extended-dwell catheters, such as noncuffed CVCs and PICCs.

Intensive Insulin Therapy

Glycemic control in critically ill ICU patients is essential for the prevention of IVDR BSI. However, the optimum level of glycemic control has been controversial. A large, RCT in 1,548 critically ill patients in a surgical ICU, the majority of whom were postsurgical patients, compared intensive insulin therapy – maintenance of blood glucose level between 80 and 110 mg/dL by using continuous infusions of insulin (insulin drips) with conventional insulin therapy – subcutaneous insulin given only if blood glucose levels exceeded 215 mg/dL, striving to maintain levels between 180 and 200 mg/dL [110]. The study found a markedly reduced ICU and hospital mortality with intensive glycemic control (8.0% with conventional treatment vs. 4.6% with intensive treatment; $P<0.04$); the greatest reduction in mortality was seen in patients with multi-organ failure due to a septic focus [110]. Most noteworthy, the incidence of nosocomial BSI was cut in half (8 vs. 4%). A similar study in medical ICU patients found no reduction in mortality or difference in bacteremia rates with intensive glycemic control [111].

A meta-analysis of 29 RCTs encompassing 8,432 patients found no difference in hospital mortality with tight glucose control vs. moderate control, glucose levels <150 mg/dL (21.6 vs. 23.3%; RR, 0.93; 95% CI, 0.85–1.03), and the results did not change when patients were stratified by type of ICU: surgical, medical, or medical-surgical. However, tight glucose control was associated with a reduced risk of septicemia (10.9 vs. 13.4%; RR, 0.76; 95% CI, 0.59–0.97) [112].

In the NICE SUGAR study, a large, randomized multicenter trial in 6,104 adult ICU patients, intensive glycemic control (goal 81–108 mg/dL) was associated with increased mortality compared to conventional control (goal ≤180 mg/dL) (OR, 1.14; 95% CI, 1.02–1.28; $P=0.02$) [113]. The study population included more medical than surgical ICU patients (intensive group: 36.9% surgical, 63.1% medical; conventional group: 37.2% surgical, 62.8% medical). Severe hypoglycemia (≤40 mg/dL) was significantly more common in the intensive control group (6.8 vs. 0.5%, $P<0.001$) [113].

A recent meta-analysis of 26 trials involving a total of 13,567 patients, including the data from the NICE SUGAR trial, found no mortality benefit to intensive insulin therapy in critically ill patients (pooled RR of death with intensive therapy using insulin drip as compared with moderate control using subcutaneous insulin (RR 0.93; 95% CI, 0.83–1.04)) [114]. However, when analyzed separately, surgical ICU patients experienced significant benefit (RR 0.63, 95% CI 0.44–0.91) while patients in nonsurgical ICUs did not.

Based on these studies, all hospitalized patients are likely to benefit from moderate glycemic control, and we recommend the use of intensive glycemic control with an insulin drip in surgical ICU patients to reduce the risk of healthcare-associated infections, particularly BSIs. However, stringent monitoring to avoid severe hypoglycemia is essential, and a glycemic target that can be achieved safely should be chosen, generally 120–150 mg/dL.

Achieving High-Level Compliance with Essential Control Measures Through Institutional Systems

A multifaceted approach with near-100% compliance is essential to consistently and maximally reduce the risk of IVDR BSI. The Institute for Healthcare Improvement (IHI) has promoted the concept of "bundles" to aid in risk reduction. A bundle, according to the IHI, is a structured way of improving the processes of care and patient outcomes using a set of practices, generally three to five, that when performed collectively and reliably, have been shown to improve patient outcomes [115]. The IHI-recommended evidence-based bundle for CVC care includes the following: (1) hand hygiene before IVD insertion; (2) maximal barrier precautions during the insertion procedure; (3) cutaneous antisepsis with CHG; (4) optimal catheter insertion site selection, with the subclavian vein the preferred site for CVCs, and (5) daily review of continued need for the, with immediate removal when no longer needed [115]. In an elegant time-sequence trial in 100 Michigan hospitals, Pronovost et al. showed that development of effective systems within the hospitals which assured a very high level of compliance with the bundle for every CVC insertion resulted in a striking reduction in IVDR BSI in the individual hospitals over 18 months, with a reduction from prestudy baseline of 0.62 (95% CI, 0.47–0.81) at 0–3 months and 0.34 (95% CI, 0.23–0.5) at 16–18 months [12]. These numbers represented an overall 66% reduction in rates of IVDR BSIs, which has now been maintained for 36 months [14].

Bhutta et al. undertook a prospective quasi-experimental study in a children's hospital, which included the stepwise introduction of interventions over a 5-year period [116]. The interventions included maximal barrier precautions, a transition to antibiotic-impregnated CVCs, annual hand washing campaigns, and the use of CHG in place of povidone-iodine. Significant decreases in rates of infection occurred over the intervention period and were sustained over a 3-year follow-up. Annual rates of CVC-associated BSI decreased from 9.7/1,000 days in 1997 to 3.0/1,000 days in 2005 (RR reduction, 0.75; 95% CI, 0.35–1.26). The investigators found that multifaceted interventions and development of systems to achieve uniformly high compliance reduce IVDR BSIs but require strong institutional support.

The recent implementation of a multifaceted approach in a pediatric cardiac intensive-care unit, which included CVC insertion and maintenance bundles, CHG-impregnated dressings, nurse and physician education, and the addition of a unit-based infection control nurse, resulted in a reduction in their rate of IVDR BSIs from 7.8 to 2.3 infections per 1,000 catheter days over a period of less than 2 years [117].

Pronovost et al. have outlined the essential steps to establishing an effective institutional system to achieve these recommended results [13].

Catheter Salvage in the Context of Treatment

The optimal management of IVDR BSI requires two basic clinical decisions: (1) the appropriate and timely administration of intravenous antiinfective therapy and (2) removal of the IVD or an attempt at catheter salvage (Fig. 11.5). A recent evidence-based Guideline from the Infectious Diseases Society of America is now available [118].

Systemic antiinfective therapy given intravenously should be selected based on the suspected or proven bloodstream pathogen(s) in accordance with published guidelines and resources [118]. It is extremely important to begin the therapy within 1 h of the encounter with clinical suspicion of IVDR BSI cite, as delays of 2 or more hours increase mortality by 30–40% [119].

The decision whether to remove the IVD is based on the clinical picture, the type of IVD being used and the organism in question. This decision becomes more complex when specific patient characteristics are considered, such as the type of device required (e.g., tunneled CVC or implanted port) and the ease of venous access.

First of all, we believe IVDs of all types should be promptly removed if the patient presents with septic shock and there is strong suspicion that IVDR BSI is the cause. The recent IDSA Guideline recommends removal of nontunneled catheters in all complicated infections (e.g., thrombosis, endocarditis, osteomyelitis) and in all infections caused by *S. aureus*, gram negative bacilli, Enterococcus, and *Candida* species [118]. In IVDR BSIs associated with tunneled or implantable devices, the catheters also require removal for all complicated infections (thrombosis, endocarditis, osteomyelitis), tunnel or pocket infections, and port abscesses, and for all infections caused by *S. aureus* and *Candida* spp.

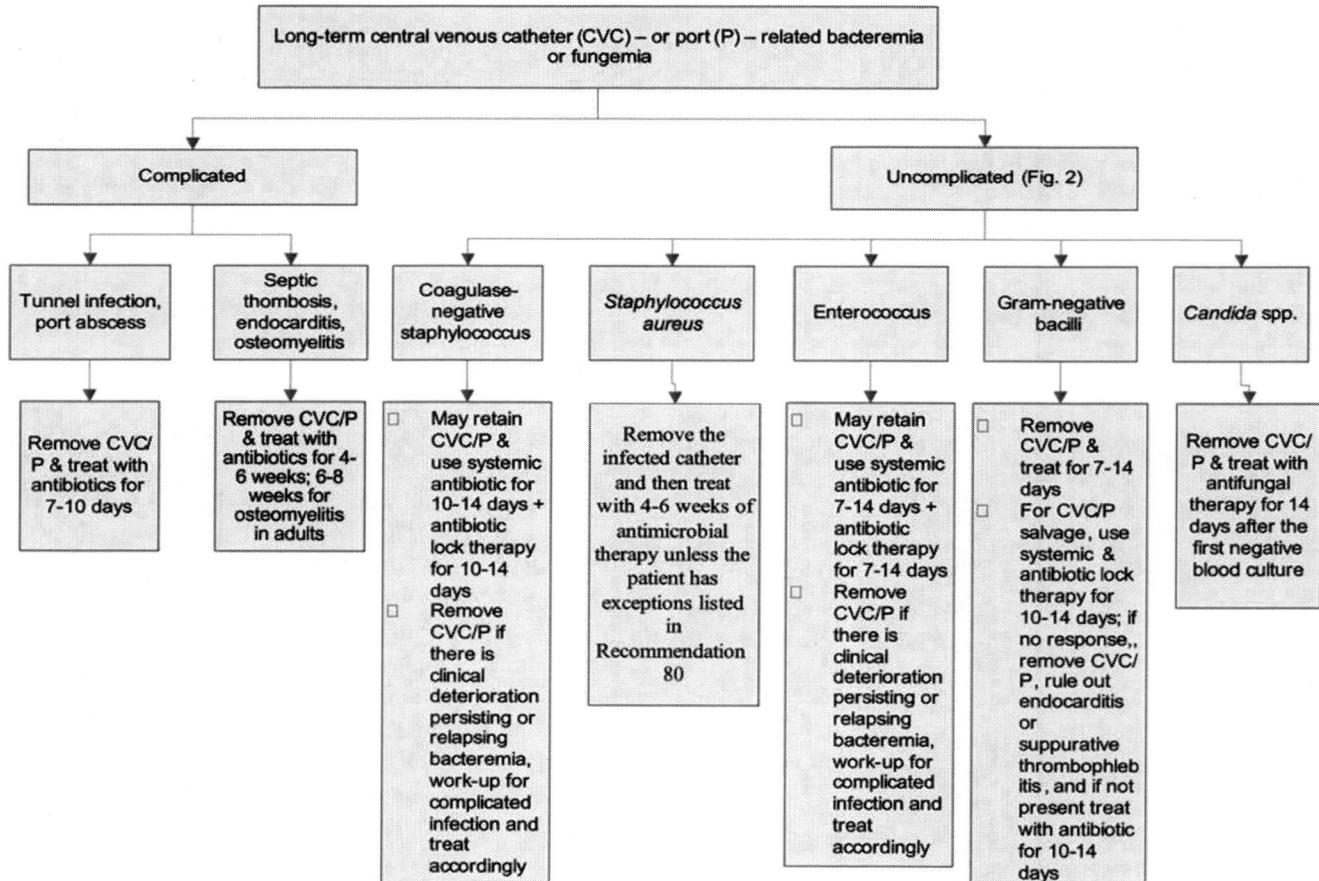

Fig. 11.5 Approach to the treatment of a patient with a long-term cuffed and tunneled central venous catheter (CVC) or a subcutaneous totally implanted port (P)-related bloodstream infection. From the IDSA guideline on management of IVDR BSI [168]

By the Guideline, catheter salvage regimens including the use of antibiotic lock therapy may be attempted, when necessary, for infections due to organisms *other* than *S. aureus*, fungi, *Pseudomonas aeruginosa*, *Bacillus* species, *Micrococcus* species, Propionibacteria, or mycobacteria [40, 118, 120].

Antiinfective Lock Therapy

The most frequently used implanted IVDs in patients with cancer are long-term cuffed and tunneled catheters, such as Hickman or Broviac catheters, and totally implanted subcutaneous central ports. Given that the major route of infection for these catheters is intraluminal contamination, a promising approach to the prevention of these infections has involved instilling an antiinfective solution into the device lumen or lumens to prevent colonization of the intraluminal surface by suspended planktonic-phase contaminants [121–123]. Antiinfective lock therapy (ALT) has also been applied, but much less rigorously studied for the *treatment* of IVDR BSI.

ALT for the treatment of IVDR BSI should always be used in conjunction with systemic antiinfective therapy when the goal is to successfully eradicate the BSI while retaining the device (Table 11.4). The likelihood of success of ALT varies with the infecting microorganism and the extent of infection. Recurrent bacteremia after parenteral therapy is more likely to occur if that therapy is administered through a retained catheter than if the catheter is removed. Several small cases series have shown ALT to be promising as adjunctive treatment when the original, presumably infected IVD is retained [121, 124–148]. In 21 open trials of ALT for IVDR BSI involving long-term catheters, with or without concomitant parenteral therapy, catheter salvage without relapse was achieved in 77% of episodes [135]. Table 11.3 summarizes the major studies that have examined lock therapy for adjunctive treatment of IVDR BSI with the goal of IVD salvage.

The only randomized trial of ALT to date compared a vancomycin or ceftazidime lock in addition to parenteral antibiotic therapy with parenteral antibiotic therapy plus a placebo lock [149]. The investigators found that in the analysis population of 44 patients (21 antibiotic lock arm and 23 in the placebo arm), by day 180, 33% of BSI in the antibiotic lock group had not been eradicated compared with 57% in the placebo arm (HR 0.55, $P=0.10$). Of note, only half of potentially eligible patients with an IVDR BSI met IDSA Guideline criteria for eligibility for this study. Frequent reasons for exclusion were the IVD was not available for >8–12 h/day for the antiinfective lock ($n=10$); yeast infection or mixed Gram-positive/negative infections ($n=13$); catheter removal preferred by the treating physician ($n=7$); and CRBSI <14 days after insertion, or pocket or/tunnel infection ($n=10$). Thus, barriers to the use of ALT are common and must be acknowledged when considering ALT as an option for adjunctive therapy of IVDR BSI.

To be practical in the acute care setting, the antiinfective lock regimen should exhibit efficacy over a sufficiently short dwell time to be practical in hospitalized patients with the need for extended "line time," for clinical use of the line. The minimum time recommended for exposure to the concentrated antiinfective lock solution is 60 min, if there is not a critical need for access, the dwell times should extend as long as possible [10]. Longer dwell times are possible in patients with hemodialysis catheters or implantable ports that are not routinely accessed on a daily basis.

The formation of a biofilm within the catheter lumen limits penetration of anti-infective solution and sterilization of the heavily colonized catheter. Bacteria within a biofilm require 100–1,000 times greater antiinfective concentrations to achieve killing as compared with the same organisms in the planktonic state [9]. Standard intravenous antimicrobial therapy does not reach sufficiently high concentrations to materially reduce the bacterial burden within a biofilm in the catheter lumen.

Stability and compatibility of the antiinfective lock solution with an accompanying anticoagulant must also be considered when ordering an antiinfective lock solution. Temperature, dwell time, addition of anticoagulant or other antiinfectives all

Table 11.3 Studies of antiinfective lock therapy as adjunctive treatment of intravascular device-related bloodstream infection

References	Type of lock therapy	Number of BSI receiving lock therapy	Salvage rate in lock group (%)	Relapses in lock group (%)	Catheter removals for failure in treatment group (%)
Messing et al. [145]	Antibiotic	22	20/22 (90)	NR	2/22 (9)
Dannenberg et al. [134]	Ethanol	24	23/24 (95)	0/24 (0)	1
Williams et al. [167]	Antibiotic	7	4/7 (57)	NR	2/7 (28)
Poole et al. [147]	Antibiotic	47	33/47 (70)	7/47 (15)	14/47 (30)
Rijnders et al. [149]	Antibiotic	22	14/21 (66)	3/21 (14)	3/21 (14)
Fortun et al. [139]	Antibiotic	19	16/19 (84)	2/19 (10)	1/19 (5)
Onder et al. [177]	Antibiotic	264	170/264 (64)	67/170 (39)	94/264 (36)
Aslam et al. [125]	N-acetylcysteine and tigecycline	18	15/18 (83)	NR	NR
Broom et al. [129]	Antibiotic and ethanol	17	15/17 (88)	0	2

NR not reported

Table 11.4 Final concentrations of antibiotic lock solution used for the treatment of intravascular device-related bloodstream infection

Antibiotic and dosage	Heparin or saline (IU/mL)
Vancomycin, 2.5 mg/mL	2,500 or 5,000
Vancomycin, 2.0 mg/mL	10
Vancomycin, 5.0 mg/mL	0 or 5,000
Ceftazidime, 0.5 mg/mL	100
Cefazolin, 5.0 mg/mL	2,500 or 5,000
Ciprofloxacin, 0.2 mg/mL	5,000
Gentamicin, 1.0 mg/mL	2,500
Ampicillin, 10.0 mg/mL	10 or 5,000
Ethanol, 70%	0

Adapted from the 2009 IDSA guidelines for management of IVDR BSI [168]

influence stability. In the case of ethanol lock solutions, the effect of ethanol on the mechanical and structural integrity of the catheter has been studied. These studies showed no change in the integrity of the catheter when exposed [27].

Although the duration of ALT has varied substantially among different studies (3–30 days), most studies have used a 2-week duration. Vancomycin, cefazolin, and ceftazidime remain stable in heparin solutions at 25 and 37°C for several days [178]. Not all antibiotic-heparin combinations can be used because precipitation can occur when some antibiotics are mixed with heparin, especially with high antibiotic concentrations [51, 150]. Ethanol is not compatible with heparin [151]. An ethanol lock should dwell for at least 60 min, then be removed and the VD flushed with *0.9% sodium chloride*. Heparin can then be instilled into the CVC/ID. Ethanol 50% is not a commercially available product. The compounded ethanol 50% (v/v) product is stable in syringes at room temperature for up to 28 days (unprotected from light) [35].

Table 11.4 lists antibiotic lock solutions that can be used without the risk of precipitation.

Exchange over a Guidewire

In patients with cancer who have long-term catheters and limited alternative sites for vascular access, catheter salvage is desirable, and another approach to salvage is to "exchange" the catheter (replace the infected catheter by a new uninfected catheter) over a guidewire. Current recommendations suggest that guidewire catheter exchange is acceptable in the management of suspected CVC-related BSI, although the catheter should be relocated to a new site if culture of the removed catheter confirms the diagnosis of CVC-related BSI. The evidence for this recommendation is, however, scant, and most studies have been undertaken in patients on hemodialysis [152, 153]. In patients with malignancy and thrombocytopenia, this procedure may be associated with an increased risk of bleeding.

The safety and efficacy of CVC exchange by guidewire after unsuccessful antimicrobial therapy were recently evaluated in a prospective quasi-experimental study of patients undergoing BMT or intensive chemotherapy [154]. CVC exchange was considered when fever and positive blood cultures persisted after 2 days of adequate antimicrobial therapy and no potential source of bacteremia other than CVC could be identified. The guidewire exchange was preceded and followed by a slow infusion of antimicrobial therapy. In 19 episodes of cryptogenic bacteremia during a 1-year period, 14 episodes (74%) were catheter-related and 71% of these were with CoNS. Guidewire replacement was accomplished uneventfully 4 (range 3–6) days after the development of bacteremia. In all cases, clinical signs of infection disappeared within 24 h after the exchange. Definitive catheter withdrawal was carried out a median of 16 days (range 3–42) after guidewire exchange; in all cases, the catheter culture was negative. The findings from this nonrandomized small study with no comparison group are intriguing, and this approach should be studied further, but at the present time, there is insufficient evidence to recommend its routine use.

Urokinase as Adjunctive Treatment for IVDR BSI

Catheter occlusion and thrombus formation can occur as part of an IVDR BSI. Dissolution of the infected thrombus using a thrombolytic agent such as urokinase may be a potential strategy to treat IVDR BSI in conjunction with antibiotics; however, this approach has not been adequately studied. In a prospective randomized trial in 63 children, 33 of whom received urokinase and antibiotics and 30 received antibiotics alone, the investigators found that treatment failures leading to catheter removal occurred in 9 of 33 in the experimental group and 9 of 30 in the control population ($P=NS$). Of note, all catheters in the study were shown to be free of thrombus by radiographic imaging prior to enrollment in the study. The role of urokinase as an adjuvant to antibiotics for the treatment of IVDR BSI is uncertain and is not recommended at the present time, but deserves further study.

IVDR BSI Pathogen-Specific Recommendations

Pathogen-specific recommendations are summarized in Tables 11.5 and 11.6 and described in more detail below.

Table 11.5 Recommendations for the use of antiinfective lock therapy for treatment of IVDR BSI

Recommendation	Strength of recommendation
Antibiotic lock is indicated for patients with IVDR BSI involving long-term catheters with no signs of exit site or tunnel infection for whom catheter salvage is the goal	B-II
For IVDR BSI, antibiotic lock should not be used alone; instead, it should be used in conjunction with systemic antimicrobial therapy, with both regimens administered for 7–14 days	B-II
Dwell times for antibiotic lock solutions should generally not exceed 48 h before reinstallation of lock solution; preferably, reinstallation should take place every 24 h for ambulatory patients with femoral catheters (B-II). However, for patients who are undergoing hemodialysis, the lock can be renewed after every dialysis session	B-II
Catheter removal is recommended for IVDR BSI due to *S. aureus* and *Candida* species, instead of treatment with antibiotic lock and catheter retention, unless there are unusual extenuating circumstances (e.g., no alternative catheter insertion site)	A-II
For patients with multiple positive catheter-drawn blood cultures that grow coagulase-negative staphylococci or gram-negative bacilli and concurrent negative peripheral blood cultures, antibiotic lock therapy can be given without systemic therapy for 10–14 days	B-III
For vancomycin, the concentration should be at least 1,000 times higher than the MIC (e.g., 5 mg/mL) of the microorganism involved	B-II
At this time, there are insufficient data to recommend an ethanol lock for the treatment of IVDR BSI	C-III

Adapted from the Infectious Diseases Society of America clinical practice guidelines for the diagnosis and management of intravascular catheter-related infection: 2009 update by the Infectious Diseases Society of America [168]

Table 11.6 Pathogen-specific recommendations regarding catheter salvage

Organism	Decision to remove CV or ID?	Decision to retain CVC/ID?	Salvage regimen	Salvage regimen failure?
S. aureus	Yes – always remove CVC/ID and treat with systemic antimicrobials	No – low success rate		
Coagulase-negative Staphylococcus	May retain – see salvage therapy	Yes – use salvage therapy	Systemic treatment plus ALT (antiinfectives and duration per infectious disease)	Remove CVC/ID if persistent or relapsing bacteremia or clinical deterioration
Gram-negative bacilli	If yes – remove CVC/ID and treat with systemic antiinfectives	If yes – use salvage therapy, only if not MDR GNB	Systemic treatment plus ALT (antiinfectives and duration per infectious disease)	If no response, remove CVC/ID and treat with systemic antiinfectives
Candida spp	Yes – remove CVC/ID and treat with systemic antifungal therapy	No – low success rate		

Candida spp.

The two major sources of candidemia are the CVC and translocation from the gastrointestinal tract in immunocompromised patients [155].

Candidemia deriving from IVDs is challenging to treat because of heavy biofilm formation on the surface of the catheter. In general, IVD removal is recommended for IVDR candidemia because of the risk of endophthalmitis, septic thrombophlebitis, and endocarditis if the candidemia is not quickly controlled, as conventional antifungal therapy will not effectively eradicate Candida organisms embedded in biofilm [156]. Preliminary studies, mainly in vitro, suggest that ethylene diamine tetra-acetic acid (EDTA) (an anticoagulant-chelating agent with antifungal as well as antibiofilm activity) might be useful as a lock agent. The utility of amphotericin B lipid complex (ABLC), with and without EDTA, was studied in an in vitro model of Candida biofilm. Clinical blood isolates from cancer patients infected with *Candida albicans* or *Candida parapsilosis* were used. ABLC+EDTA (30 mg/mL) was significantly more effective than ABLC alone, EDTA alone against *C. parapsilosis* at 6 h ($P \leq 0.01$) and against *C. albicans* at 8 h ($P \leq 0.04$) [157].

Staphylococcus aureus

The optimal duration of treatment for *S. aureus* bacteremia is unclear because of ever-present concern regarding complications such as endocarditis and hematogenous osteomyelitis. As many as a third of patients with *S. aureus* bacteremia will have metastatic infection [158]. In the past, prolonged treatment for 4–6 weeks for *S. aureus* bacteremia has been recommended.

Predictors of hematogenous metastatic infection include persistent bacteremia on therapy, evidence of cutaneous septic emboli, and community-acquired bacteremia [159].

In recent years, short-course therapy for *S. aureus* IVDR BSI has been extensively evaluated relying upon a transesophageal echocardiogram to rule out endocarditis cites. If the IVD is removed and there is no clinical evidence of metastatic infection, and the TEE shows no evidence of endocarditis, short-course parenteral antimicrobial therapy for 2 weeks in immunocompetent nonneutropenic patients is considered acceptable [62, 160, 179]. Of note, TEE is most sensitive for detecting endocarditis when performed 5–7 days after the onset of bacteremia [161].

Catheter salvage for S. aureus bacteremia is not recommended. Studies have shown that removal of vascular catheters infected with *S. aureus* is associated with more rapid clearance of the bacteremia and symptomatic improvement, with a higher cure rate, compared with catheter retention. Small series of patients in whom the catheter was retained and parenteral and ALT was employed have shown mixed results [147, 148, 162–167]. These studies suggest an unacceptably high failure rate for catheter salvage when *S. aureus* is the infecting pathogen. In extenuating circumstances, if the catheter is retained, the patient should receive systemic and ALT for at least 4 weeks (B-II). Catheter guide wire exchange should be done, if possible, and if done, an antimicrobial-impregnated catheter with an antiinfective intraluminal surface should be considered for the new catheter exchange (B-II).

For patients with catheters found to be colonized with *S. aureus* at removal who are not bacteremic, the recent IDSA management Guideline recommends a 5–7-day course of parenteral antibiotic therapy and close monitoring for signs of ongoing infection, with additional blood cultures, as indicated.

Coagulase-Negative Staphylococci

CoNS are the most frequent causative microorganisms in IVDR BSI. In the majority of patients, the clinical course is benign and complications are infrequent, with the exception of *Staphylococcus lugdenensis*, which produces invasive infection very similar to *S. aureus*. No randomized trials have been conducted on the optimal type and duration of antimicrobial treatment for IVDR BSI with CoNS. For uncomplicated infection by CoNS, treatment with ALT is considered acceptable if given in conjunction with systemic antimicrobial therapy for 10–14 days [168]. In an observational study of 188 patients with CoNS, Raad et al. found that patients in which the IVD was retained had a 6.6-fold (95% CI, 1.8–23.9) higher likelihood of having a recurrence than those patients whose IVD was removed or exchanged [169].

If the IVD is removed, antimicrobial treatment may be given for 5–7 days following device removal.

Gram-Negative Bacilli

Multiresistant (MDR) gram-negative bacilli are major pathogens in patients with cancer and the incidence of IVDR BSI caused by MDR gram-negative bacilli appears to be increasing [44]. Of particular concern is extended spectrum beta-lactamase producing gram-negative bacilli and the recent emergence of carbapenemase-producing *Klebsiella pneumoniae* [170]. Infections caused by these MDR bacteria are often associated with adverse clinical outcomes [171–173], in part because of a delay in initiating appropriate antimicrobial therapy. No randomized trials have been conducted to address optimal management of IVDR BSI with gram-negative bacilli. The IDSA Guideline recommends a 7–14-day course of antibiotic therapy tailored to the susceptibility of the infecting organism. ALT for catheter salvage may be considered for occasional patients with susceptible organisms and uncomplicated infection, but we do not recommend attempting catheter salvage for MDR gram-negative bacteremia deriving from an IVD.

References

1. Raad I, Hachem R, Hanna H, et al. Sources and outcome of bloodstream infections in cancer patients: the role of central venous catheters. Eur J Clin Microbiol Infect Dis. 2007;26(8):549–56.
2. Hachem R, Raad I. Prevention and management of long-term catheter related infections in cancer patients. Cancer Invest. 2002;20(7–8):1105–13.
3. Longuet P, Douard MC, Arlet G, Molina JM, Benoit C, Leport C. Venous access port-related bacteremia in patients with acquired immunodeficiency syndrome or cancer: the reservoir as a diagnostic and therapeutic tool. Clin Infect Dis. 2001;32(12):1776–83.
4. Safdar N, Maki DG. Antibiotic resistance and prevention of CVC-associated BSIs, catheter-associated urinary tract infection and clostridium difficile. In: Jarvis W, editor. Bennett and Brachman's hospital infections. Philadelphia: Lippincott, Williams and Wilkins; 2007. p. 395–416.
5. Raad I, Hanna H, Maki D. Intravascular catheter-related infections: advances in diagnosis, prevention, and management. Lancet Infect Dis. 2007;7(10):645–57.
6. O'Grady NP, Alexander M, Dellinger EP, et al. Guidelines for the prevention of intravascular catheter-related infections. Infect Control Hosp Epidemiol. 2002;23(12):759–69.
7. Siempos II, Kopterides P, Tsangaris I, Dimopoulou I, Armaganidis AE. Impact of catheter-related bloodstream infections on the mortality of critically ill patients: a meta-analysis. Crit Care Med. 2009;37(7):2283–9.
8. Pittet D, Tarara D, Wenzel RP. Nosocomial bloodstream infection in critically ill patients. Excess length of stay, extra costs, and attributable mortality. JAMA. 1994;271(20):1598–601.
9. Maki DG, Kluger DM, Crnich CJ. The risk of bloodstream infection in adults with different intravascular devices: a systematic review of 200 published prospective studies. Mayo Clin Proc. 2006;81(9):1159–71.
10. Hockenhull JC, Dwan K, Boland A, et al. The clinical effectiveness and cost-effectiveness of central venous catheters treated with

anti-infective agents in preventing bloodstream infections: a systematic review and economic evaluation. Health Technol Assess. 2008;12(12):1–154. Iii–iv, xi–xii.

11. Raad II. Commentary: zero tolerance for catheter-related bloodstream infections: the unnegotiable objective. Infect Control Hosp Epidemiol. 2008;29(10):951–3.

12. Pronovost P, Needham D, Berenholtz S, et al. An intervention to decrease catheter-related bloodstream infections in the ICU. N Engl J Med. 2006;355(26):2725–32.

13. McKee C, Berkowitz I, Cosgrove SE, et al. Reduction of catheter-associated bloodstream infections in pediatric patients: experimentation and reality. Pediatr Crit Care Med. 2008;9(1):40–6.

14. Pronovost PJ, Goeschel CA, Colantuoni E, et al. Sustaining reductions in catheter related bloodstream infections in Michigan intensive care units: observational study. BMJ. 2010;340:c309.

15. Centers for Disease Control. Reduction in central line-associated bloodstream infections among patients in intensive care units – Pennsylvania, April 2001–March 2005. MMWR Morb Mortal Wkly Rep. 2005;54(40):1013–6.

16. Frankel HL, Crede WB, Topal JE, Roumanis SA, Devlin MW, Foley AB. Use of corporate Six Sigma performance-improvement strategies to reduce incidence of catheter-related bloodstream infections in a surgical ICU. J Am Coll Surg. 2005;201(3): 349–58.

17. Gastmeier P, Geffers C. Prevention of catheter-related bloodstream infections: analysis of studies published between 2002 and 2005. J Hosp Infect. 2006;64(4):326–35.

18. Jeffries HE, Mason W, Brewer M, et al. Prevention of central venous catheter-associated bloodstream infections in pediatric intensive care units: a performance improvement collaborative. Infect Control Hosp Epidemiol. 2009;30(7):645–51.

19. Lobo RD, Levin AS, Oliveira MS, et al. Evaluation of interventions to reduce catheter-associated bloodstream infection: continuous tailored education versus one basic lecture. Am J Infect Control. 2010;38:440–8.

20. Miller RS, Norris PR, Jenkins JM, et al. Systems initiatives reduce healthcare-associated infections: a study of 22, 928 device days in a single trauma unit. J Trauma. 2010;68(1):23–31.

21. Render ML, Brungs S, Kotagal U, et al. Evidence-based practice to reduce central line infections. Jt Comm J Qual Patient Saf. 2006;32(5):253–60.

22. Rosenthal VD, Guzman S, Pezzotto SM, Crnich CJ. Effect of an infection control program using education and performance feedback on rates of intravascular device-associated bloodstream infections in intensive care units in Argentina. Am J Infect Control. 2003;31(7):405–9.

23. Zuschneid I, Schwab F, Geffers C, Ruden H, Gastmeier P. Reducing central venous catheter-associated primary bloodstream infections in intensive care units is possible: data from the German nosocomial infection surveillance system. Infect Control Hosp Epidemiol. 2003;24(7):501–5.

24. Edwards JR, Peterson KD, Andrus ML, Dudeck MA, Pollock DA, Horan TC. National Healthcare Safety Network (NHSN) report, data summary for 2006 through 2007, issued November 2008. Am J Infect Control. 2008;36(9):609–26.

25. Edwards JR, Peterson KD, Andrus ML, et al. National Healthcare Safety Network (NHSN) report, data summary for 2006, issued June 2007. Am J Infect Control. 2007;35(5):290–301.

26. Edwards JR, Peterson KD, Mu Y, et al. National Healthcare Safety Network (NHSN) report: data summary for 2006 through 2008, issued December 2009. Am J Infect Control. 2009;37(10): 783–805.

27. Maki DG, Goldman DA, Rhame FS. Infection control in intravenous therapy. Ann Intern Med. 1973;79(6):867–87.

28. Maki D, Mermel L. Infections due to infusion therapy. CINA-AGINCOURT. 1999;15:71–95.

29. Douard MC, Clementi E, Arlet G, et al. Negative catheter-tip culture and diagnosis of catheter-related bacteremia. Nutrition. 1994;10(5):397–404.

30. Nouwen JL, Wielenga JJ, van Overhagen H, et al. Hickman catheter-related infections in neutropenic patients: insertion in the operating theater versus insertion in the radiology suite. J Clin Oncol. 1999;17(4):1304.

31. Livesley MA, Tebbs SE, Moss HA, Faroqui MH, Lambert PA, Elliott TS. Use of pulsed field gel electrophoresis to determine the source of microbial contamination of central venous catheters. Eur J Clin Microbiol Infect Dis. 1998;17(2):108–12.

32. Darouiche RO, Raad II, Heard SO, et al. A comparison of two antimicrobial-impregnated central venous catheters. Catheter Study Group. N Engl J Med. 1999;340(1):1–8.

33. Maki DG, Stolz SM, Wheeler S, Mermel LA. Prevention of central venous catheter-related bloodstream infection by use of an antiseptic-impregnated catheter. A randomized, controlled trial. Ann Intern Med. 1997;127(4):257–66.

34. Garland JS, Alex CP, Sevallius JM, et al. Cohort study of the pathogenesis and molecular epidemiology of catheter-related bloodstream infection in neonates with peripherally inserted central venous catheters. Infect Control Hosp Epidemiol. 2008;29(3):243–9.

35. Safdar N, Maki DG. The pathogenesis of catheter-related bloodstream infection with noncuffed short-term central venous catheters. Intensive Care Med. 2004;30(1):62–7.

36. Marrie TJ, Costerton JW. Scanning and transmission electron microscopy of in situ bacterial colonization of intravenous and intraarterial catheters. J Clin Microbiol. 1984;19(5):687–93.

37. Cooper GL, Schiller AL, Hopkins CC. Possible role of capillary action in pathogenesis of experimental catheter-associated dermal tunnel infections. J Clin Microbiol. 1988;26(1):8–12.

38. Sitges-Serra A, Linares J, Garau J. Catheter sepsis: the clue is the hub. Surgery. 1985;97(3):355–7.

39. Maki DG, Jarrett F, Sarafin HW. A semiquantitative culture method for identification of catheter-related infection in the burn patient. J Surg Res. 1977;22(5):513–20.

40. Yokoe DS, Mermel LA, Anderson DJ, et al. A compendium of strategies to prevent healthcare-associated infections in acute care hospitals. Infect Control Hosp Epidemiol. 2008;29 Suppl 1:S12–21.

41. Bjornson HS, Colley R, Bower RH, Duty VP, Schwartz-Fulton JT, Fischer JE. Association between microorganism growth at the catheter insertion site and colonization of the catheter in patients receiving total parenteral nutrition. Surgery. 1982;92(4):720–7.

42. Sitges-Serra A, Puig P, Linares J, et al. Hub colonization as the initial step in an outbreak of catheter-related sepsis due to coagulase negative staphylococci during parenteral nutrition. JPEN J Parenter Enteral Nutr. 1984;8(6):668–72.

43. Raad I, Costerton W, Sabharwal U, Sacilowski M, Anaissie E, Bodey GP. Ultrastructural analysis of indwelling vascular catheters: a quantitative relationship between luminal colonization and duration of placement. J Infect Dis. 1993;168(2):400–7.

44. Wisplinghoff H, Bischoff T, Tallent SM, Seifert H, Wenzel RP, Edmond MB. Nosocomial bloodstream infections in US hospitals: analysis of 24,179 cases from a prospective nationwide surveillance study. Clin Infect Dis. 2004;39(3):309–17.

45. Trick WE, Fridkin SK, Edwards JR, Hajjeh RA, Gaynes RP. Secular trend of hospital-acquired candidemia among intensive care unit patients in the United States during 1989–1999. Clin Infect Dis. 2002;35(5):627–30.

46. Lorente L, Jimenez A, Santana M, et al. Microorganisms responsible for intravascular catheter-related bloodstream infection according to the catheter site. Crit Care Med. 2007;35(10):2424–7.

47. Sipsas NV, Lewis RE, Tarrand J, et al. Candidemia in patients with hematologic malignancies in the era of new antifungal agents

(2001–2007): stable incidence but changing epidemiology of a still frequently lethal infection. Cancer. 2009;115(20):4745–52.
48. Safdar N, Maki DG. Use of vancomycin-containing lock or flush solutions for prevention of bloodstream infection associated with central venous access devices: a meta-analysis of prospective, randomized trials. Clin Infect Dis. 2006;43(4):474–84.
49. Ho KM, Litton E. Use of chlorhexidine-impregnated dressing to prevent vascular and epidural catheter colonization and infection: a meta-analysis. J Antimicrob Chemother. 2006;58(2):281–7.
50. Ramritu P, Halton K, Collignon P, et al. A systematic review comparing the relative effectiveness of antimicrobial-coated catheters in intensive care units. Am J Infect Control. 2008;36(2):104–17.
51. Veenstra DL, Saint S, Saha S, Lumley T, Sullivan SD. Efficacy of antiseptic-impregnated central venous catheters in preventing catheter-related bloodstream infection: a meta-analysis. JAMA. 1999;281(3):261–7.
52. Yahav D, Rozen-Zvi B, Gafter-Gvili A, Leibovici L, Gafter U, Paul M. Antimicrobial lock solutions for the prevention of infections associated with intravascular catheters in patients undergoing hemodialysis: systematic review and meta-analysis of randomized, controlled trials. Clin Infect Dis. 2008;47(1):83–93.
53. Opilla MT, Kirby DF, Edmond MB. Use of ethanol lock therapy to reduce the incidence of catheter-related bloodstream infections in home parenteral nutrition patients. JPEN J Parenter Enteral Nutr. 2007;31(4):302–5.
54. Chaiyakunapruk N, Veenstra DL, Lipsky BA, Saint S. Chlorhexidine compared with povidone-iodine solution for vascular catheter-site care: a meta-analysis. Ann Intern Med. 2002;136(11):792–801.
55. Tacconelli E, Carmeli Y, Aizer A, Ferreira G, Foreman MG, D'Agata EM. Mupirocin prophylaxis to prevent *Staphylococcus aureus* infection in patients undergoing dialysis: a meta-analysis. Clin Infect Dis. 2003;37(12):1629–38.
56. Safdar N, Crnich CJ, Maki DG. The pathogenesis of ventilator-associated pneumonia: its relevance to developing effective strategies for prevention. Respir Care. 2005;50(6):725–39. discussion 739–41.
57. Clemence MA, Walker D, Farr BM. Central venous catheter practices: results of a survey. Am J Infect Control. 1995;23(1):5–12.
58. Maki DG, Ringer M, Alvarado CJ. Prospective randomised trial of povidone-iodine, alcohol, and chlorhexidine for prevention of infection associated with central venous and arterial catheters. Lancet. 1991;338(8763):339–43.
59. Wertheim HF, Vos MC, Ott A, et al. Mupirocin prophylaxis against nosocomial *Staphylococcus aureus* infections in nonsurgical patients: a randomized study. Ann Intern Med. 2004;140(6):419–25.
60. Babu T, Rekasius V, Parada JP, Schreckenberger P, Challapalli M. Mupirocin resistance among methicillin-resistant *Staphylococcus aureus*-colonized patients at admission to a tertiary care medical center. J Clin Microbiol. 2009;47(7):2279–80.
61. Orrett FA. The emergence of mupirocin resistance among clinical isolates of methicillin-resistant *Staphylococcus aureus* in Trinidad: a first report. Jpn J Infect Dis. 2008;61(2):107–10.
62. Perkins D, Hogue JS, Fairchok M, Braun L, Viscount HB. Mupirocin resistance screening of methicillin-resistant *Staphylococcus aureus* isolates at Madigan Army Medical Center. Mil Med. 2008;173(6):604–8.
63. Rossney A, O'Connell S. Emerging high-level mupirocin resistance among MRSA isolates in Ireland. Euro Surveill. 2008;13(14):8084.
64. Graber CJ, Schwartz BS. Failure of decolonization in patients with infections due to mupirocin-resistant strains of community-associated methicillin-resistant *Staphylococcus aureus*. Infect Control Hosp Epidemiol. 2008;29(3):284. author reply 284–5.
65. Cavdar C, Saglam F, Sifil A, et al. Effect of once-a-week vs thrice-a-week application of mupirocin on methicillin and mupirocin resistance in peritoneal dialysis patients: three years of experience. Ren Fail. 2008;30(4):417–22.
66. Tang Z, Mazabob J, Weavind L, Thomas E, Johnson TR. A time-motion study of registered nurses' workflow in intensive care unit remote monitoring. AMIA Annu Symp Proc. 2006:759–63.
67. Raad II, Hohn DC, Gilbreath BJ, et al. Prevention of central venous catheter-related infections by using maximal sterile barrier precautions during insertion. Infect Control Hosp Epidemiol. 1994;15(4 Pt 1):231–8.
68. Mermel LA, McCormick RD, Springman SR, Maki DG. The pathogenesis and epidemiology of catheter-related infection with pulmonary artery Swan-Ganz catheters: a prospective study utilizing molecular subtyping. Am J Med. 1991;91(3B):197S–205.
69. Goetz AM, Wagener MM, Miller JM, Muder RR. Risk of infection due to central venous catheters: effect of site of placement and catheter type. Infect Control Hosp Epidemiol. 1998;19(11): 842–5.
70. Joynt GM, Kew J, Gomersall CD, Leung VY, Liu EK. Deep venous thrombosis caused by femoral venous catheters in critically ill adult patients. Chest. 2000;117(1):178–83.
71. Merrer J, De Jonghe B, Golliot F, et al. Complications of femoral and subclavian venous catheterization in critically ill patients: a randomized controlled trial. JAMA. 2001;286(6):700–7.
72. Richet H, Hubert B, Nitemberg G, et al. Prospective multicenter study of vascular-catheter-related complications and risk factors for positive central-catheter cultures in intensive care unit patients. J Clin Microbiol. 1990;28(11):2520–5.
73. Do AN, Ray BJ, Banerjee SN, et al. Bloodstream infection associated with needleless device use and the importance of infection-control practices in the home health care setting. J Infect Dis. 1999;179(2):442–8.
74. Gowardman JR, Robertson IK, Parkes S, Rickard CM. Influence of insertion site on central venous catheter colonization and bloodstream infection rates. Intensive Care Med. 2008;34(6):1038–45.
75. Parienti JJ, Thirion M, Megarbane B, et al. Femoral vs jugular venous catheterization and risk of nosocomial events in adults requiring acute renal replacement therapy: a randomized controlled trial. JAMA. 2008;299(20):2413–22.
76. Randolph AG, Cook DJ, Gonzales CA, Pribble CG. Ultrasound guidance for placement of central venous catheters: a meta-analysis of the literature. Crit Care Med. 1996;24(12):2053–8.
77. Karakitsos D, Labropoulos N, De Groot E, et al. Real-time ultrasound-guided catheterisation of the internal jugular vein: a prospective comparison with the landmark technique in critical care patients. Crit Care. 2006;10(6):R162.
78. Barsuk JH, Cohen ER, Feinglass J, McGaghie WC, Wayne DB. Use of simulation-based education to reduce catheter-related bloodstream infections. Arch Intern Med. 2009;169(15):1420–3.
79. Maki DG, Mermel LA, Kluger D, Narans L, Knasinski V, Parenteau S, Covington P. The efficacy of a chlorhexidine impregnated sponge (Biopatch) for the prevention of intravascular catheter-related infection-a prospective randomized controlled multicenter study. 2000.
80. Timsit JF, Cheval C, Gachot B, et al. Usefulness of a strategy based on bronchoscopy with direct examination of bronchoalveolar lavage fluid in the initial antibiotic therapy of suspected ventilator-associated pneumonia. Intensive Care Med. 2001; 27(4):640–7.
81. Ruschulte H, Franke M, Gastmeier P, et al. Prevention of central venous catheter related infections with chlorhexidine gluconate impregnated wound dressings: a randomized controlled trial. Ann Hematol. 2009;88(3):267–72.
82. Bleasdale SC, Trick WE, Gonzalez IM, Lyles RD, Hayden MK, Weinstein RA. Effectiveness of chlorhexidine bathing to reduce catheter-associated bloodstream infections in medical intensive care unit patients. Arch Intern Med. 2007;167(19):2073–9.
83. Borer A, Gilad J, Porat N, et al. Impact of 4% chlorhexidine whole-body washing on multidrug-resistant Acinetobacter baumannii

skin colonisation among patients in a medical intensive care unit. J Hosp Infect. 2007;67(2):149–55.
84. Climo MW, Sepkowitz KA, Zuccotti G, et al. The effect of daily bathing with chlorhexidine on the acquisition of methicillin-resistant *Staphylococcus aureus*, vancomycin-resistant Enterococcus, and healthcare-associated bloodstream infections: results of a quasi-experimental multicenter trial. Crit Care Med. 2009;37(6): 1858–65.
85. Camus C, Bellissant E, Sebille V, et al. Prevention of acquired infections in intubated patients with the combination of two decontamination regimens. Crit Care Med. 2005;33:307–14.
86. Evans H, Dellit T, Chan J, Nathens A, Maier R, Cuschieri J. Effect of chlorhexidine whole-body bathing on hospital-acquired infections among trauma patients. Arch Surg. 2010;145(3):240.
87. Gould IM, MacKenzie FM, MacLennan G, Pacitti D, Watson EJ, Noble DW. Topical antimicrobials in combination with admission screening and barrier precautions to control endemic methicillin-resistant *Staphylococcus aureus* in an intensive care unit. Int J Antimicrob Agents. 2007;29(5):536–43.
88. Holder C, Zellinger M. Daily bathing with chlorhexidine in the ICU to prevent central line-associated bloodstream infections. JCOM. 2009;16(11):509–13.
89. Munoz Price L, Hota B, Stemer A, Weinstein R. Prevention of bloodstream infections by use of daily chlorhexidine baths for patients at a long term acute care hospital. Infect Control Hosp Epidemiol. 2009;30:1031–5.
90. Popovich KJ, Hota B, Hayes R, Weinstein RA, Hayden MK. Effectiveness of routine patient cleansing with chlorhexidine gluconate for infection prevention in the medical intensive care unit. Infect Control Hosp Epidemiol. 2009;30(10):959–63.
91. Casey AL, Mermel LA, Nightingale P, Elliott TS. Antimicrobial central venous catheters in adults: a systematic review and meta-analysis. Lancet Infect Dis. 2008;8(12):763–76.
92. Sanders J, Pithie A, Ganly P, et al. A prospective double-blind randomized trial comparing intraluminal ethanol with heparinized saline for the prevention of catheter-associated bloodstream infection in immunosuppressed haematology patients. J Antimicrob Chemother. 2008;62(4):809–15.
93. Bookstaver PB, Williamson JC, Tucker BK, Raad II, Sherertz RJ. Activity of novel antibiotic lock solutions in a model against isolates of catheter-related bloodstream infections. Ann Pharmacother. 2009;43(2):210–9.
94. Mendelson MH, Short LJ, Schechter CB, et al. Study of a needleless intermittent intravenous-access system for peripheral infusions: analysis of staff, patient, and institutional outcomes. Infect Control Hosp Epidemiol. 1998;19(6):401–6.
95. Skolnick R, LaRocca J, Barba D, Paicius L. Evaluation and implementation of a needleless intravenous system: making needlesticks a needless problem. Am J Infect Control. 1993;21(1):39–41.
96. Gartner K. Impact of a needleless intravenous system in a university hospital. J Healthc Mater Manage. 1993;11(8):44–6, 48–9.
97. Lawrence D. HAI – a high visibility problem: recent studies show that hospitals with low HAI rates rely heavily on IT, but the jury is still out on where a CIO should begin. Healthc Inform. 2008;25(12):22–24.
98. Cookson ST, Ihrig M, O'Mara EM, et al. Increased bloodstream infection rates in surgical patients associated with variation from recommended use and care following implementation of a needleless device. Infect Control Hosp Epidemiol. 1998;19(1):23–7.
99. McDonald LC, Banerjee SN, Jarvis WR. Line-associated bloodstream infections in pediatric intensive-care-unit patients associated with a needleless device and intermittent intravenous therapy. Infect Control Hosp Epidemiol. 1998;19(10):772–7.
100. Kellerman S, Shay DK, Howard J, et al. Bloodstream infections in home infusion patients: the influence of race and needleless intravascular access devices. J Pediatr. 1996;129(5):711–7.
101. Rupp ME, Sholtz LA, Jourdan DR, et al. Outbreak of bloodstream infection temporally associated with the use of an intravascular needleless valve. Clin Infect Dis. 2007;44(11):1408–14.
102. Maragakis LL, Bradley KL, Song X, et al. Increased catheter-related bloodstream infection rates after the introduction of a new mechanical valve intravenous access port. Infect Control Hosp Epidemiol. 2006;27(1):67–70.
103. Casey AL, Worthington T, Lambert PA, Quinn D, Faroqui MH, Elliott TS. A randomized, prospective clinical trial to assess the potential infection risk associated with the PosiFlow needleless connector. J Hosp Infect. 2003;54(4):288–93.
104. Menyhay SZ, Maki DG. Disinfection of needleless catheter connectors and access ports with alcohol may not prevent microbial entry: the promise of a novel antiseptic-barrier cap. Infect Control Hosp Epidemiol. 2006;27(1):23–7.
105. Maki DG. In vitro studies of a novel antimicrobial luer-activated needleless connector for prevention of catheter-related bloodstream infection. Clin Infect Dis. 2010;50(12):1580–7.
106. Menyhay SZ, Maki DG. Preventing central venous catheter-associated bloodstream infections: development of an antiseptic barrier cap for needleless connectors. Am J Infect Control. 2008;36(10):S174, e1–5.
107. Schears GJ. Summary of product trials for 10, 164 patients: comparing an intravenous stabilizing device to tape. J Infus Nurs. 2006;29(4):225–31.
108. Yamamoto AJ, Solomon JA, Soulen MC, et al. Sutureless securement device reduces complications of peripherally inserted central venous catheters. J Vasc Interv Radiol. 2002;13(1):77–81.
109. Frey AM, Schears GJ. Why are we stuck on tape and suture? A review of catheter securement devices. J Infus Nurs. 2006;29(1):34–8.
110. van den Berghe G, Wouters P, Weekers F, et al. Intensive insulin therapy in the critically ill patients. N Engl J Med. 2001;345(19):1359–67.
111. Van den Berghe G, Wilmer A, Hermans G, et al. Intensive insulin therapy in the medical ICU. N Engl J Med. 2006;354(5):449–61.
112. Wiener RS, Wiener DC, Larson RJ. Benefits and risks of tight glucose control in critically ill adults: a meta-analysis. JAMA. 2008;300(8):933–44.
113. Finfer S, Chittock DR, Su SY, et al. Intensive versus conventional glucose control in critically ill patients. N Engl J Med. 2009;360(13):1283–97.
114. Griesdale DE, de Souza RJ, van Dam RM, et al. Intensive insulin therapy and mortality among critically ill patients: a meta-analysis including NICE-SUGAR study data. CMAJ. 2009;180(8):821–7.
115. Haraden C. What is a bundle? 09/07/2006 ed: Institute for Healthcare Improvement. 2006.
116. Bhutta A, Gilliam C, Honeycutt M, et al. Reduction of bloodstream infections associated with catheters in paediatric intensive care unit: stepwise approach. BMJ. 2007;334(7589):362–5.
117. Costello JM, Morrow DF, Graham DA, Potter-Bynoe G, Sandora TJ, Laussen PC. Systematic intervention to reduce central line-associated bloodstream infection rates in a pediatric cardiac intensive care unit. Pediatrics. 2008;121(5):915–23.
118. Mermel LA, Farr BM, Sherertz RJ, et al. Guidelines for the management of intravascular catheter-related infections. J Intraven Nurs. 2001;24(3):180–205.
119. Heard SO, Wagle M, Vijayakumar E, et al. Influence of triple-lumen central venous catheters coated with chlorhexidine and silver sulfadiazine on the incidence of catheter-related bacteremia. Arch Intern Med. 1998;158(1):81–7.
120. Kassar R, Hachem R, Jiang Y, Chaftari AM, Raad I. Management of Bacillus bacteremia: the need for catheter removal. Medicine (Baltimore). 2009;88(5):279–83.
121. Bouza E, Burillo A, Munoz P. Catheter-related infections: diagnosis and intravascular treatment. J Chemother. 2001;13 Spec No 1(1):224–33.

122. Carratala J. Role of antibiotic prophylaxis for the prevention of intravascular catheter-related infection. Clin Microbiol Infect. 2001;7 Suppl 4:83–90.
123. Capdevila JA. Catheter-related infection: an update on diagnosis, treatment, and prevention. Int J Infect Dis. 1998;2(4):230–6.
124. Allon M. Saving infected catheters: why and how. Blood Purif. 2005;23(1):23–8.
125. Aslam S, Trautner BW, Ramanathan V, Darouiche RO. Pilot trial of N-acetylcysteine and tigecycline as a catheter-lock solution for treatment of hemodialysis catheter-associated bacteremia. Infect Control Hosp Epidemiol. 2008;29(9):894–7.
126. Battistella M, Walker S, Law S, Lok C. Antibiotic lock: in vitro stability of vancomycin and four percent sodium citrate stored in dialysis catheters at 37 degrees C. Hemodial Int. 2009;13(3):322–8.
127. Bestul MB, Vandenbussche HL. Antibiotic lock technique: review of the literature. Pharmacotherapy. 2005;25(2):211–27.
128. Bregenzer T, Widmer AF. Bloodstream infection from a Port-A-Cath: successful treatment with the antibiotic lock technique. Infect Control Hosp Epidemiol. 1996;17(12):772.
129. Broom J, Woods M, Allworth A, et al. Ethanol lock therapy to treat tunnelled central venous catheter-associated blood stream infections: results from a prospective trial. Scand J Infect Dis. 2008;40(5):399–406.
130. Buckler BS, Sams RN, Goei VL, et al. Treatment of central venous catheter fungal infection using liposomal amphotericin-B lock therapy. Pediatr Infect Dis J. 2008;27(8):762–4.
131. Carratala J. The antibiotic-lock technique for therapy of "highly needed" infected catheters. Clin Microbiol Infect. 2002;8(5):282–9.
132. Castagnola E, Moroni C, Gandullia P, et al. Catheter lock and systemic infusion of linezolid for treatment of persistent Broviac catheter-related staphylococcal bacteremia. Antimicrob Agents Chemother. 2006;50(3):1120–1.
133. Cuntz D, Michaud L, Guimber D, Husson MO, Gottrand F, Turck D. Local antibiotic lock for the treatment of infections related to central catheters in parenteral nutrition in children. JPEN J Parenter Enteral Nutr. 2002;26(2):104–8.
134. Dannenberg C, Bierbach U, Rothe A, Beer J, Korholz D. Ethanol-lock technique in the treatment of bloodstream infections in pediatric oncology patients with broviac catheter. J Pediatr Hematol Oncol. 2003;25(8):616–21.
135. del Pozo JL. Role of antibiotic lock therapy for the treatment of catheter-related bloodstream infections. Int J Artif Organs. 2009;32(9):678–88.
136. Del Pozo JL, Alonso M, Serrera A, Hernaez S, Aguinaga A, Leiva J. Effectiveness of the antibiotic lock therapy for the treatment of port-related enterococci, Gram-negative, or Gram-positive bacilli bloodstream infections. Diagn Microbiol Infect Dis. 2009;63(2):208–12.
137. Elwood RL, Spencer SE. Successful clearance of catheter-related bloodstream infection by antibiotic lock therapy using ampicillin. Ann Pharmacother. 2006;40(2):347–50.
138. Fernandez-Hidalgo N, Almirante B, Calleja R, et al. Antibiotic-lock therapy for long-term intravascular catheter-related bacteraemia: results of an open, non-comparative study. J Antimicrob Chemother. 2006;57(6):1172–80.
139. Fortun J, Grill F, Martin-Davila P, et al. Treatment of long-term intravascular catheter-related bacteraemia with antibiotic-lock therapy. J Antimicrob Chemother. 2006;58(4):816–21.
140. Kentos A, Struelens MJ, Thys JP. Antibiotic-lock technique for the treatment of central venous catheter infections. Clin Infect Dis. 1996;23(2):418–9.
141. Maya ID. Antibiotic lock for treatment of tunneled hemodialysis catheter bacteremia. Semin Dial. 2008;21(6):539–41.
142. Maya ID, Carlton D, Estrada E, Allon M. Treatment of dialysis catheter-related *Staphylococcus aureus* bacteremia with an antibiotic lock: a quality improvement report. Am J Kidney Dis. 2007;50(2):289–95.
143. Megged O, Shalit I, Yaniv I, Fisher S, Livni G, Levy I. Outcome of antibiotic lock technique for persistent central venous catheter-associated coagulase-negative Staphylococcus bacteremia in children. Eur J Clin Microbiol Infect Dis. 2010;29(2):157–61.
144. Messing B. Catheter-related sepsis during home parenteral nutrition. Clin Nutr. 1995;14 Suppl 1:46–51.
145. Messing B, Man F, Colimon R, Thuillier F, Beliah M. Antibiotic-lock technique is an effective treatment of bacterial catheter-related sepsis during parenteral nutrition. Clin Nutr. 1990;9(4):220–5.
146. Pagani JL, Eggimann P. Management of catheter-related infection. Expert Rev Anti Infect Ther. 2008;6(1):31–7.
147. Poole CV, Carlton D, Bimbo L, Allon M. Treatment of catheter-related bacteraemia with an antibiotic lock protocol: effect of bacterial pathogen. Nephrol Dial Transplant. 2004;19(5):1237–44.
148. Viale P, Pagani L, Petrosillo N, et al. Antibiotic lock-technique for the treatment of catheter-related bloodstream infections. J Chemother. 2003;15(2):152–6.
149. Rijnders BJ, Van Wijngaerden E, Vandecasteele SJ, Stas M, Peetermans WE. Treatment of long-term intravascular catheter-related bacteraemia with antibiotic lock: randomized, placebo-controlled trial. J Antimicrob Chemother. 2005;55(1):90–4.
150. Droste JC, Jeraj HA, MacDonald A, Farrington K. Stability and in vitro efficacy of antibiotic-heparin lock solutions potentially useful for treatment of central venous catheter-related sepsis. J Antimicrob Chemother. 2003;51(4):849–55.
151. Maiefski M, Rupp ME, Hermsen ED. Ethanol lock technique: review of the literature. Infect Control Hosp Epidemiol. 2009;30(11):1096–108.
152. Shaffer D. Catheter-related sepsis complicating long-term, tunnelled central venous dialysis catheters: management by guidewire exchange. Am J Kidney Dis. 1995;25(4):593–6.
153. Carlisle EJ, Blake P, McCarthy F, Vas S, Uldall R. Septicemia in long-term jugular hemodialysis catheters; eradicating infection by changing the catheter over a guidewire. Int J Artif Organs. 1991;14(3):150–3.
154. Martinez E, Mensa J, Rovira M, et al. Central venous catheter exchange by guidewire for treatment of catheter-related bacteraemia in patients undergoing BMT or intensive chemotherapy. Bone Marrow Transplant. 1999;23(1):41–4.
155. Raad I, Hanna H, Boktour M, et al. Management of central venous catheters in patients with cancer and candidemia. Clin Infect Dis. 2004;38(8):1119–27.
156. Shuford JA, Rouse MS, Piper KE, Steckelberg JM, Patel R. Evaluation of caspofungin and amphotericin B deoxycholate against *Candida albicans* biofilms in an experimental intravascular catheter infection model. J Infect Dis. 2006;194(5):710–3.
157. Bachmann SP, Ramage G, VandeWalle K, Patterson TF, Wickes BL, Lopez-Ribot JL. Antifungal combinations against *Candida albicans* biofilms in vitro. Antimicrob Agents Chemother. 2003;47(11):3657–9.
158. Ghanem GA, Boktour M, Warneke C, et al. Catheter-related *Staphylococcus aureus* bacteremia in cancer patients: high rate of complications with therapeutic implications. Medicine (Baltimore). 2007;86(1):54–60.
159. Nolan CM, Beaty HN. *Staphylococcus aureus* bacteremia. Current clinical patterns. Am J Med. 1976;60(4):495–500.
160. Rosen AB, Fowler Jr VG, Corey GR, et al. Cost-effectiveness of transesophageal echocardiography to determine the duration of therapy for intravascular catheter-associated *Staphylococcus aureus* bacteremia. Ann Intern Med. 1999;130(10):810–20.
161. Jacob S, Tong AT. Role of echocardiography in the diagnosis and management of infective endocarditis. Curr Opin Cardiol. 2002;17(5):478–85.

162. Rajpurkar M, Boldt-Macdonald K, McLenon R, et al. Ethanol lock therapy for the treatment of catheter-related infections in haemophilia patients. Haemophilia. 2009;15(6):1267–71.
163. Santarpia L, Pasanisi F, Alfonsi L, et al. Prevention and treatment of implanted central venous catheter (CVC)-related sepsis: a report after six years of home parenteral nutrition (HPN). Clin Nutr. 2002;21(3):207–11.
164. Saxena AK, Panhotra BR, Sundaram DS, Morsy MN, Al-Ghamdi AM. Enhancing the survival of tunneled haemodialysis catheters using an antibiotic lock in the elderly: a randomised, double-blind clinical trial. Nephrology (Carlton). 2006;11(4):299–305.
165. Simon A, Bode U, Beutel K. Diagnosis and treatment of catheter-related infections in paediatric oncology: an update. Clin Microbiol Infect. 2006;12(7):606–20.
166. Toltzis P. Antibiotic lock technique to reduce central venous catheter-related bacteremia. Pediatr Infect Dis J. 2006;25(5):449–50.
167. Williams N, Carlson GL, Scott NA, Irving MH. Incidence and management of catheter-related sepsis in patients receiving home parenteral nutrition. Br J Surg. 1994;81(3):392–4.
168. Mermel LA, Allon M, Bouza E, et al. Clinical practice guidelines for the diagnosis and management of intravascular catheter-related infection: 2009 update by the Infectious Diseases Society of America. Clin Infect Dis. 2009;49(1):1–45.
169. Raad I, Kassar R, Ghannam D, Chaftari AM, Hachem R, Jiang Y. Management of the catheter in documented catheter-related coagulase-negative staphylococcal bacteremia: remove or retain? Clin Infect Dis. 2009;49(8):1187–94.
170. Nadkarni AS, Schliep T, Khan L, Zeana CB. Cluster of bloodstream infections caused by KPC-2 carbapenemase-producing *Klebsiella pneumoniae* in Manhattan. Am J Infect Control. 2009;37(2):121–6.
171. Gasink LB, Fishman NO, Nachamkin I, Bilker WB, Lautenbach E. Risk factors for and impact of infection or colonization with aztreonam-resistant *Pseudomonas aeruginosa*. Infect Control Hosp Epidemiol. 2007;28(10):1175–80.
172. Lautenbach E, Patel JB, Bilker WB, Edelstein PH, Fishman NO. Extended-spectrum beta-lactamase-producing Escherichia coli and *Klebsiella pneumoniae*: risk factors for infection and impact of resistance on outcomes. Clin Infect Dis. 2001;32(8):1162–71.
173. Lautenbach E, Weiner MG, Nachamkin I, Bilker WB, Sheridan A, Fishman NO. Imipenem resistance among *Pseudomonas aeruginosa* isolates: risk factors for infection and impact of resistance on clinical and economic outcomes. Infect Control Hosp Epidemiol. 2006;27(9):893–900.
174. Crnich CJ, Maki DG. The promise of novel technology for the prevention of intravascular device-related bloodstream infection. II. Long-term devices. Clin Infect Dis. 2002;34(10):1362–8.
175. O'Grady NP, Alexander M, Dellinger EP, et al. Guidelines for the prevention of intravascular catheter-related infections. Centers for Disease Control and Prevention. MMWR Recomm Rep. 2002;51(RR-10):1–29.
176. Hockenhull JC, Dwan KM, Smith GW, et al. The clinical effectiveness of central venous catheters treated with anti-infective agents in preventing catheter-related bloodstream infections: a systematic review. Crit Care Med. 2009;37(2):702–12.
177. Onder AM, Chandar J, Billings AA, et al. Comparison of early versus late use of antibiotic locks in the treatment of catheter-related bacteremia. Clin J Am Soc Nephrol. 2008;3(4):1048–56.
178. Vaughan LM, Poon CY. Stability of ceftazidime and vancomycin alone and in combination in heparinized and nonheparinized peritoneal dialysis solution. Ann Pharmacother. 1994;28(5):572–6.
179. Fowler Jr VG, Li J, Corey GR, et al. Role of echocardiography in evaluation of patients with *Staphylococcus aureus* bacteremia: experience in 103 patients. J Am Coll Cardiol. 1997;30(4):1072–8.

Chapter 12
Pneumonia in the Cancer Patient

Scott E. Evans and Amar Safdar

Abstract Lower respiratory tract infections result in unacceptably high mortality among cancer patients. Pneumonias cause death in this population both directly through impairment of gas exchange and progression to system infection/sepsis, as well as indirectly by precluding delivery of necessary, antineoplastic therapies. Malignancy and treatment-related impairments of host immune responses and the emergence of multidrug-resistant organisms associated with recurrent exposures to hospital environments may not only enhance the risks of mortality, but also exacerbate the difficulty of diagnosing pneumonia in the cancer setting. As a consequence of disordered inflammatory responses, the typical clinical observations of pneumonia, including purulent respiratory secretions and early radiographic findings, may be inapparent or absent. A comprehensive review of etiology, clinical presentation, diagnosis, and management of pulmonary infections is presented in this chapter.

Keywords Pneumonia • MRSA • Fungal disease • CMV • Pneumococcus • Drug resistance • Immune defects

Lower respiratory tract infections result in unacceptably high mortality among cancer patients. Pneumonias cause death in this population both directly through impairment of gas exchange and progression to system infection/sepsis, as well as indirectly by precluding delivery of necessary, antineoplastic therapies [1–3]. Malignancy and treatment-related impairments of host immune responses and the emergence of multidrug-resistant (MDR) organisms associated with recurrent exposures to hospital environments may not only enhance the risks of mortality, but also exacerbate the difficulty of diagnosing pneumonia in the cancer setting. As a consequence of disordered inflammatory responses, the typical clinical observations of pneumonia, including purulent respiratory secretions and early radiographic findings, may be inapparent or absent. Adding to this diagnostic challenge is the frequent colonization of the upper airway with microorganisms that do not contribute to disease, rendering the diagnosis of pneumonia by conventional culture techniques difficult. Conversely, sterile respiratory tract cultures do not exclude an infectious etiology, particularly in the setting of recent exposure to broad-spectrum antibiotics.

Susceptibility to pneumonia in the cancer patient is not only conditioned by the type and degree of immune suppression, but also by its duration. Multiple immune defects may coexist among patients with cancer, which adds to the conundrum and spectrum of opportunistic infections. Immune defects, including compromised acellular and cellular (alveolar macrophages, mast cells, neutrophils) innate and/or altered adaptive immune function, leading to either inadequate immmunoglobulin or defective T-cell mediate defenses may promote the development of specific types of pneumonia. In addition, treatment-induced disruption of the respiratory mucosa and ciliary dysfunction may result in inadequate clearance of airway secretions, enhancing the likelihood of pneumonia. Hence, the individual patient's predilection for pneumonia in the cancer setting is best understood by examining the effect of malignancy and its treatment on specific host immune defenses (Table 12.1). Because the immune defect is often mixed, careful attention to clinical and radiographic features and recognition of nosocomial versus community-acquired sources of the infection are critical to making the diagnosis and guiding empiric antimicrobial therapy [4]. Delays in appropriate antimicrobial therapy increase the risk of secondary complications and infection-associated deaths, especially in severely immunosuppressed individuals. Therefore, it is common practice to initiate empiric and/or preemptive antimicrobial therapy in patients in whom the suspicion of infection is high. An approach to the diagnosis and treatment of cancer-related pneumonias based on the specific defects in the major arms of host immunity and broad categories of infection source is emphasized in

S.E. Evans (✉)
Department of Pulmonary Medicine, The University of Texas, M.D. Anderson Cancer Center, 1515 Holcombe Boulevard (Unit 1100), Houston, TX 77030, USA
e-mail: seevans@mdanderson.org

Table 12.1 Infections causing pneumonia in cancer patients based on the underlying immune defect

Immune defect	Bacteria	Fungi	Parasites	Viruses
Granulocytopenia	*Staphylococcus aureus*	*Aspergillus fumigatus*; non-*fumigatus Aspergillus*		Herpes simplex virus I and II
	Streptococcus pneumoniae	Non-*Aspergillus* hyalohyphomycosis such as *Pseudallescheria boydii*, *Fusarium solani*		Varicella-zoster virus
	Streptococcus species			
	Pseudomonas aeruginosa	*Mucorales* (zygomycoses)		
	Enterobacteriaceae	Dematiaceous (Black) fungi such as *Alternaria, Bipolaris, Curvularia, Scedosporium apiospermum, S. prolificans*		
	Escherichia coli			
	Klebsiella species			
	Stenotrophomonas maltophilia			
	Acinetobacter species			
Cell-mediated immune system Dysfunction	*Nocardia asteroides* complex	*Aspergillus* and non-*Aspergillus* filamentous molds	*Toxoplasma gondii*	Cytomegalovirus
	Salmonella species	*Pneumocystis jiroveci* (*P. carini*)	*Microsporidium* spp.	Respiratory viruses
	Rhodococcus equi	*Cryptococcus neoformans*	*Strongyloides stercoralis*	Influenza A and Influenza B
	R. bronchialis	Endemic mycoses due to *Histoplasma capsulatum, Coccidioides immitis, Blastomyces dermatitidis*		Parainfluenza type-3
	Listeria monocytogenes			Respiratory syncytial virus
	Mycobacterium tuberculous			Adenovirus
	Nontuberculous mycobacteria			Varicella-zoster virus
				HHV-6
				SARS-associated coronavirus
				Paramyxovirus
				Hantavirus
Humoral immune Dysfunction	*S. pneumoniae*			VZV
	Haemophilus influenzae			Echovirus
Splenctomy	*Neisseria meningitidis*			Enterovirus
	Capnocytophaga canimorsus			
	Campylobacter			
Mixed defects	*S. pneumoniae*	*P. jiroveci* (*P. carini*)	*T. gondii*	Respiratory viruses
	S. aureus	*Aspergillus* spp.	*S. stercoralis*	Influenza
	H. influenzae	*Candida* spp.		Parainfluenza
	K. pneumoniae	*C. neoformans*		Respiratory syncytial virus
	P. aeruginosa	*Mucorales* (zygomycoses)		Adenovirus
	Acinetobacter spp.	Endemic mycoses (severe systemic dissemination)		VZV
	Enterobacter spp.			
	S. maltophilia			
	N. asteroides complex			
	L. monocytogenes			
	Legionella spp.			

Note. Patients with mixed immune defects includes, recipients of allogeneic hematopoietic stem cell transplant; acute or chronic GVHD; myelodysplastic syndrome; adult T-cell leukemia lymphoma; antineoplastic agents like cyclophosphamide and fludarabine
VZV is rarely associated with systemic dissemination in patients with humoral immune defects, or even those with mixed immune dysfunctions
S. stercoralis may lead to serious, life-threatening hyperinfection syndrome in patients with marked cellular immune defects
HHV-6 Human herpesvirus-6

the early part of this section, followed by a more detailed discussion of selected pathogens that may cause fulminant infection in the cancer patient.

Specific Immune Defects

Disruption of local airway defense mechanisms often increases vulnerability to pneumonia among cancer patients. Breach of the respiratory epithelial barrier function and altered mucociliary clearance of secretions may occur as a result of cancer therapy, both through cell-specific injury and through generalized mucositis. Medical devices, such as nasogastric and endotracheal tubes, hinder coordinated glottic activities and mucociliary function and act as conduits for chronic colonization of pathogenic organisms [5]. Numerous defects of local innate defenses are also described following chemotherapy, including derangements of chemotaxis, phagocytosis, and killing by alveolar macrophages and resident mast cells. Respiratory epithelial cells tend to maintain their capacity for elaboration of inflammatory mediators following exposure to pathogens, despite cytotoxic chemotherapy [6, 7]. Yet, they are the primary interface with lower respiratory tract pathogens and are often susceptible to direct injury by MDR pathogens, due to the unique exposures of the cancer patients, as described further below. Further, concurrent alterations in systemic defense mechanisms, such as impairment of the circulating leukocytes of the innate immune system, are exceedingly common.

Neutrophils are exquisitely sensitive to the cytotoxic effects of chemotherapy, which may induce an agranulocytosis by direct myelotoxicity, as well as functional neutropenia by interfering with the phagocytic and chemotactic activity of these cells [8]. In addition, neutrophil dysfunction resulting from radiation therapy, corticosteroid administration and common cancer-related disorders, such as hypovolemia, prolonged hypoxemia, acidosis, and poorly controlled hyperglycemia, is a frequent problem. Severe neutropenia, defined as an absolute neutrophil count of ≤500 cells/μL, is associated with refractory lung infections caused by bacterial and fungal organisms [9]. In addition, the rapidity of onset of neutropenia and delay in neutrophil recovery play a role in the infection severity. More than 10% of patients with febrile neutropenia present with pulmonary infiltrates and infection remains the most frequent cause of radiographic abnormalities in these patients. The absence of consolidated infiltrates on chest radiographs does not exclude an evolving occult pneumonia, particularly in the setting of profound neutropenia (<100 cells/μL).

Severe pneumonias, including *de novo* infections and exacerbation of chronic lung infections, also arise in the setting of neutropenia. Gram-negative bacilli (GNB) including Enterobacteriaceae (*Klebsiella, Escherichia coli, Enterobacter, Citrobacter, Serretia*) and *Proteus* spp., [10] are the predominant source of pneumonias associated with neutropenic fever. MDR Gram-positive bacteria such as methicillin-resistant *Staphylococcus aureus* (MRSA) and extended spectrum beta-lactamase-producing Enterobacteriaceae are also frequently cultured in the setting of neutropenic pneumonia. The incidence of pulmonary infections caused by Gram-positive bacteria (*S. aureus, Streptococcus* spp., including *Streptococcus pneumoniae*) has decreased over the past three decades, while Gram-negative pneumonias, particularly those caused by *Pseudomonas* spp., have become an increasing source of life-threatening, necrotizing lung infection (Fig. 12.1) [11]. Other nonfermentative Gram-negative bacteria (NF-GNB) such as *Stenotrophomonas maltophilia* [12–15], *Achromobacter,* and *Alcaligenes* species have also increased in the recent years and often lead to difficult-to-treat infections [14, 16]. As is the case in almost all other populations, aspiration of infected material remains the predominant mechanism of entry for lower respiratory tract infection among cancer patients. However, hematogenous dissemination represents a uniquely common source of pneumonia among cancer patients, and bacteremia in febrile neutropenic patients may not present with an obvious primary site of origin. Initial antimicrobial therapy for febrile neutropenia in patients with pulmonary infiltrates should be broad in spectrum and provide antimicrobial activity against drug-resistant strains of *S. aureus* and *Pseudomonas aeruginosa*. Early deescalation therapy may be attempted in patients who have demonstrated prompt clinical response and in whom granulocyte recovery has occurred or is expected to occur in the near future, especially if a pathogen has been identified. Deescalation should be undertaken with caution in high-risk patients with poor clinical response to antimicrobial therapy;

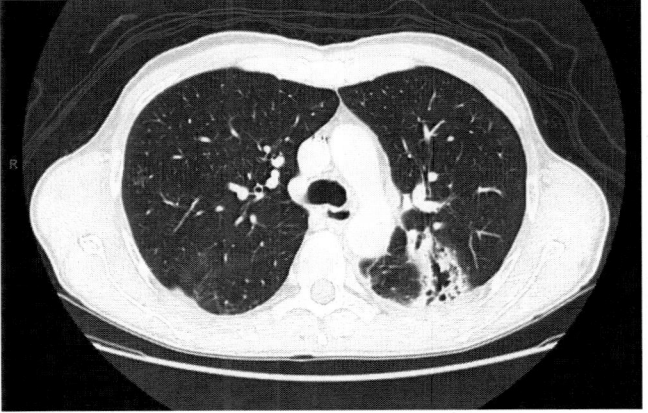

Fig. 12.1 *Pseudomonas* lung abscess in a patient with acute myelogenous leukemia awaiting bone marrow transplantation

persistent, severe, and/or long-standing granulocytopenia; or patients continuing on systemic immunosuppressive therapy.

In addition to neutropenia, cytotoxic antineoplastic therapies and hematologic malignancies may cause severe depression of humoral and cell-mediated adaptive immunity, resulting in inadequate immunoglobulin production and/or a variety of defective T and B cell-mediated defects. For example, immunoglobulin dyscrasias associated with hypogammaglobulinemia and defects in opsonization owing to asplenia are frequent among patients with certain types of lymphoreticular malignancies, such as multiple myeloma, chronic lymphocytic leukemia, and Waldenstom's macroglobulinemia. Hypocomplementemia associated with asplenia may lead to unchecked proliferation of encapsulated organisms that require opsonization with complement (C_3, C_5) for elimination. Furthermore, defects in antibody-dependent lymphocyte cytolytic activity may allow fulminant parasitic infections. Reduced T cell numbers and activity is a frequent finding among patients with Hodgkin's disease, hairy cell leukemia, adult T-cell leukemia, lymphocytic leukemia, and graft-versus-host disease (GVHD). In addition, viral illnesses, antineoplastic agents, and other immunosuppressive drugs (e.g., fludarabine, IL-2 inhibitors, antithymocyte globulins, calcinneurin inhibitors, tacrolimus, or glucocorticosteroids) may depress cellular immunity by inducing profound lymphopenia and/or interrupting activated T-cell inflammatory signal transduction pathways. Patients with cellular immune dysfunction are at increased risk of infection due to intracellular organisms such as *Listeria monocytogenes, Salmonella* spp., *Legionella* spp., *Pneumocystis jiroveci,* and *Toxoplasma gondii,* invasive pulmonary mycoses, and opportunistic viruses due to human cytomegalovirus, human herpesvirus-6 (HHV-6), and varicella-zoster virus. Thus, virtually every component of normal host immunity may be affected in an untoward manner by cancer or its treatment. The severe and oftentimes protracted immune suppression that follows encourages the development of unusual and intractable infections. Specific pathogens causing pneumonia that are commonly associated with depression of particular immune defects are listed in Table 12.1.

Community-Acquired Pneumonia (CAP). CAP, as defined by the Infectious Disease Society of America (IDSA) and the American Thoracic Society (ATS), refers to the radiographic and clinical development of pneumonia in patients who have not been hospitalized or resided in a nursing home for 14 or more days prior to the onset of symptoms and who do not meet criteria for HCAP [4]. The distinction of CAP from nosocomial pneumonia remains important, as it allows prediction of likely pathogens and permits prognostic estimations based on epidemiologic descriptions of the underlying cause. Consequently, this distinction provides a framework for decisions regarding the diagnostic evaluation and empiric antimicrobial therapy. Cancer patients are frequently exposed to the healthcare setting, both as inpatients and outpatients. Thus, pneumonia in the cancer patient is most often defined as hospital-acquired pneumonia (HAP) or healthcare-associated pneumonia (HCAP), rather than CAP.

The etiologic spectrum of bacterial pathogens causing CAP among those cancer patients with mild-to-moderate immunosuppression is similar to that of patients with no cancer history. However, a clinically insignificant microbial inoculum in the general population may cause severe infection among patients with underlying malignancy. *S. pneumoniae* remains the most commonly identified pathogen and the most frequent cause of lethal CAP [4]. Superinfection with MDR organisms is an emerging problem that complicates the management of CAP. *S. aureus*, nontypeable *Haemophilus influenzae*, *Pseudomonas* spp., and other GNB may also cause life-threatening CAP. Recently, other NF-GNB such as *Stenotrophomonas, Burkholderia, Chryseobacterium, Achromobacter,* and *Alcaligenes* species have been increasingly recognized as etiologic agents in both CAP and nosocomial infections [16, 17]. *S. pyogenes, Neisseria meningitidis,* and *Moraxella catarrhalis* also cause CAP less frequently. The incidence of CAP associated with the atypical pathogens such as *Mycoplasma pneumoniae, Chlamydia pneumoniae,* and *Legionella* spp. varies widely with patient age and geographic location. Viral pneumonias, most commonly influenza, parainfluenza, and adenoviral infections, are sources of CAP, which may cause severe pneumonias in the cancer setting.

The diagnosis of CAP is based on recovery of the likely pathogen from an otherwise sterile source (blood, urine, pleural fluid), isolation of a noncommensal organism in respiratory secretions, or positive results of selected serologic tests. Although the utility of Gram staining and culture of expectorated sputum in the diagnosis of pneumonia has been debated for years, carefully procured sputum specimens with cytologic confirmation of a lower respiratory source appear to be diagnostically useful, particularly if obtained before the initiation of antimicrobial therapy. Early and accurate diagnoses are critical to a successful outcome, although treatment should not be withheld while diagnostic interventions are undertaken. Antimicrobial selections are best based on knowledge of the infecting pathogen, if available, pneumonia severity, underlying immune status, and the presence of comorbid conditions [18, 19].

Hospital-Acquired Pneumonia. Lung infections that occur more than 48 h after hospital admission in patients without antecedent clinical symptoms or radiographic findings suggestive of pneumonia are referred to as HAP. HAP is a common complication in patients receiving treatment for cancer. Recently, the ATS and IDSA recognized HCAP as a distinct entity within the spectrum of HAP and ventilator-associated pneumonia (VAP) [20]. HCAP includes patients hospitalized in an acute care hospital for 2 or more days within 90 days of the current infection, patients treated in a hospital or hemodialysis clinic within 30 days of the pneumonia diagnosis, nursing home, or long-term care facility residents, and recipients of intravenous antibiotics, chemotherapy, or wound care within 30 days of the current infection. HAP, HCAP, and VAP comprise the majority of pneumonias in the cancer setting. The spectrum of pathogens in HCAP closely resembles late-onset HAP and VAP, particularly among elderly patients [21]. Thus, guidelines for the management of HCAP generally overlap with HAP and VAP. In the nonimmunosuppressed solid-organ cancer patient, HAP is most often seen in the intensive care units (ICUs). In fact, admission to the ICU increases the risk of pneumonia in these patients by nearly 20-fold. As many as 80% of ICU-related HAPs occur among patients receiving ventilatory support and the effect of VAP in ICU length of stay, ventilator days, and hospital length of stay is well documented [22].

The etiologic spectrum of microbial pathogens causing HAP among low-risk solid-organ cancer patients with no recent antibiotic exposure is similar as that seen in the general population. *H. influenzae, S. pneumoniae, S. aureus*, and Enterobacteriacea are frequently encountered. MRSA may cause refractory HAP, especially among patients with prior community-acquired MRSA colonization, antibiotic exposure, advanced age, and/or prolonged ventilatory support. Protracted mechanical ventilation and recent antibiotic administration are also associated with increased rates of HAP caused by *P. aeruginosa, Acinetobacter baumannii*-complex, *Enterobacter* spp., and emerging strains of MDR NF-GNB such as *S. maltophilia, Burkholderia cepacia complex*, and *Alcaligenes (Achromobacter)* species, which may be difficult to treat. Mortality rates associated with HAP due to MRSA or *P. aeruginosa* are disproportionately higher than those caused by other nosocomial bacterial pathogens [22].

Severe neutropenia remains an independent predictor of HAP due to NF-GNB. Invasive fungal disease in the severely neutropenic patients with absolute neutrophil counts of <150 cells/L are difficult to treat with antimicrobial therapy alone. Aerosolized antifungals and immune stimulants may also be considered in this context.

Polymicrobial isolates and MDR pathogens are more common among patients with HAP, particularly when it occurs as a late complication during hospitalization. Because of the frequency with which multiple organisms are identified on a single respiratory sample, recent evidence-based guidelines advocate the use of quantitative or semiquantitative lower respiratory tract cultures obtained either bronchoscopically or noninvasively as part of the initial evaluation of the patients with suspected HAP, VAP, or HCAP [20].

Empiric antibiotic selections for HAP that develop within 7 days of admission should target *S. pneumoniae, S. aureus (including MRSA), Streptococcus* spp., *H. influenzae*, and Enterobacteriaceae. Patients with late HAP (occurring >1 week after hospitalization) should receive empiric antimicrobial therapy that includes coverage for MDR-GNB. The scope of alternative antimicrobial choices in patients with refractory or slow-to-respond hospital- and/or ventilator-acquired pneumonia (VAP) should be based on institution-dependent susceptibility profiles.

Pneumonias Caused by Aspiration and Bronchial Obstruction. Aspiration of orogastric contents and mechanical obstruction of the airways may create a favorable milieu for pneumonia caused by microaerophilic or anaerobic bacteria (e.g., *Peptostreptococcus* spp.). A variety of factors, such as abnormal swallow function, altered cough reflex, impaired mucociliary clearance, altered mental status, use of sedating medications, chemotherapy-induced mucositis, supine positioning, gastroparesis, mechanical ventilation, and nasogastric tube feeding all contribute to the increased predilection for aspiration in the cancer setting. Pneumonia associated with large-volume aspiration of gastric contents typically occurs as a late finding. The acidic gastric contents act as a poor medium for bacterial growth. Thus, the initial clinical syndrome following aspiration of gastric contents arises from the direct caustic effect of the acidic aspirate on the cells of the alveolar-capillary interface (i.e., chemical pneumonitis). Pneumonia due to superimposed bacterial infection, if it occurs, presents as a later finding. ARDS, respiratory failure, and death may rapidly follow. Aspiration of oral contents, by contrast, results from inhalation of nonsterile oropharyngeal material. The clinical presentation is often insidious and the diagnosis is commonly inferred based on a compatible patient risk profile coupled with radiographic evidence of pneumonia. Chest radiographs may show areas of geographic abnormalities that correlate with the patient's position at the time of aspiration. For example, aspiration that occurs while the patient is in the upright position typically localizes to the basilar segments of the lower lobes, whereas the superior segments of the lower lobes and posterior segments of the upper lobes are more frequently affected following aspiration that occurs in the supine position. The major pathogens underlying nosocomial versus community-acquired aspiration pneumonias differ, and in a substantial portion of patients, a microbiologic diagnosis may not be established due to the limited yield of conventional anaerobic cultures. If necessary, such cultures may be best obtained bronchoscopically using a protected specimen brush or other protected strategy.

The management of patients with significant lung injury associated with the aspiration of gastric contents includes aggressive supportive care. Upper airway suctioning, pulmonary toilet, and if necessary, positive pressure ventilation comprise the mainstays of therapy. There is no clearly established role for corticosteroids in this setting, though the practice of prescribing moderate- to high-dose prednisolone is not uncommon. Early and aggressive antimicrobial therapy is recommended for patients with pneumonia secondary to aspiration of oropharyngeal contents. Antimicrobial selections should be tailored to the immune status of the patient and setting in which the aspiration occurred (community vs. nosocomial), but in general should be broad in spectrum and target Gram-negative organisms with or without anaerobic coverage. Anaerobic coverage should be considered for patients with periodontal disease, putrid sputum, or evidence of necrotizing pneumonia [23].

Solid tumors involving the lung may cause obstruction of the airways, atelectasis, and postobstructive pneumonia. Airway obstruction in this setting may be due to endobronchial tumor or an extraluminal mass that results in extrinsic compression of conducting airways. The associated pneumonias tend to be polymicrobial in nature (GNB, staphylococci, anaerobes) and may require relief of the obstruction to achieve adequate antimicrobial effects, even if appropriate antibiotics are selected. This is often most rapidly achieved through interventional bronchoscopic techniques such as tumor debulking by laser, electrocautery, or argon plasma coagulation with or without stent placement. Endobronchial brachytherapy or cryotherapy can be applied bronchoscopically as well, often with excellent results, but the time to effect is generally longer than with the formed strategies. Chemoradiation therapy can be similarly effective in relieving some obstructions, but the effect of these therapies is also delayed relative to bronchoscopic debulking.

Other Sources of Pneumonia. The lungs may also become infected via septic emboli arising from suppurative endovascular bacterial, and rarely, fungal infections. Infected intravascular septic deep venous thrombi are increasingly recognized as a potential source of infection in patients with cancer. The radiographic pattern in these patients is distinctive and includes multicentric, pleomorphic lung nodules, with asymmetric, relatively small, thick-walled cavities. In general, this appearance is distinct from the nonspecific infiltrates associated with hematogenous dissemination of distant site infections, as discussed previously.

Specific Pathogens

Nocardiosis. Nocardia asteroides complex, including *N. asteroids sensu stricto* and *N. farcinica*, accounts for nearly 90% of *Nocardia* infections, both in cancer patients and the general population. Risk factors for *Nocardia* pneumonia include profound deficiencies of cellular immunity, prolonged use of high-dose systemic corticosteroids, especially in the treatment of chronic lung diseases, [24] and the presence of GVHD. Although the latter two risk factors are often seen together (i.e., steroid treatment for GVHD), each appears to independently increase risk. Nodular pulmonary infiltrates are common radiographic findings, although reticulonodular or diffuse infiltrates are occasionally described. Solitary nodules associated with irregular, thick-walled cavities that mimic invasive pulmonary aspergillosis, histoplasmosis, necrotizing cancer, or chronic bacterial lung abscess have also been reported (Figs. 12.2 and 12.3). Indolent *Nocardia* pneumonia is clinically indistinguishable from other actinomycetes infections and from pneumonias caused by pulmonary eumycetes infections. Severely immunosuppressed cancer patients with refractory leukemia or allogenic hematopoetic stem cell transplant (HSCT) may

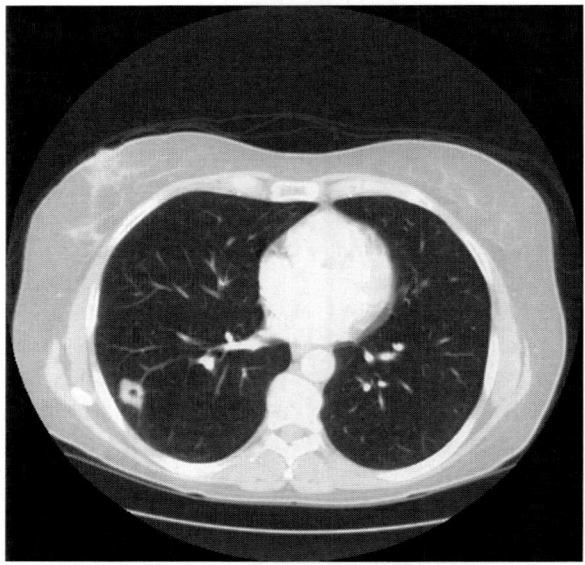

Fig. 12.2 Histoplasmosis in a patient with lung cancer

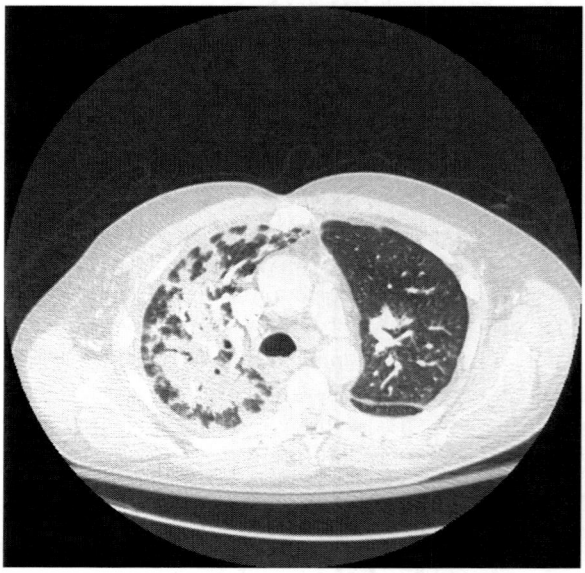

Fig. 12.3 *Nocardia abscessus* right lung infection in patient with lung cancer

present with pulmonary nocardiosis, a rapidly progressive, often multifocal form of *Norcardia*. Spontaneous pneumothorax and hemoptysis are widely reported presentations among immunocompromised patients (Fig. 12.3). Concomitant brain involvement is common, and preemptive evaluation is recommended to diagnose asymptomatic brain abscess in the setting of pulmonary disease. Trimethoprim-sulfamethoxazole (10–12 mg/kg daily) is effective against many *Nocardia* spp. Retrospective studies suggest improved outcomes when appropriate therapy is given for an extended period of time (6–12 months) [25]. Yet, despite antimicrobial therapy, pulmonary nocardiosis carries a high mortality in high-risk cancer patients [24]. Pulmonary actinomycosis typically presents in a very similar manner to nocardiasis, though sulfur granules are described more typically in samples from the former and infections classically cross tissue plans; pulmonary infection oftentimes involves the adjoining pleura and may erode through the chest wall. However, isolation of Actinomycetes from the respiratory tract should be evaluated critically, as in most patients their presence represents oropharyngeal contamination.

Tuberculous. *Mycobacterium tuberculous* is a rare cause of pulmonary infection in the developed world, but is still occasionally found in severely immunosuppressed cancer patients and in foreign-born individuals receiving cancer care in nonendemic regions of the world [26]. Patients with Hodgkin's disease and cancers of the head and neck, lung, and breast are considered at highest risk. Most pulmonary tuberculous infections in oncology centers in the United States are caused by reactivation of a remotely acquired latent infection. Pulmonary tuberculous may present as an insidious pneumonia that is difficult to distinguish from actinomycetes and eumycetes infection. Patients with impaired T-cell response may develop rapidly progressive tuberculous that follows a virulent bacterial infection. Systemic corticosteroid therapy is an independent predictor both of tuberculous reactivation and of a suboptimal response to combination antimicrobial therapy. Hence, once the diagnosis of tuberculous is established, every effort should be made to discontinue steroid therapy [26]. Just as observed in HIV-infected patients who initiate therapy with highly active antiretroviral therapy and demonstrate clinical worsening of their tuberculous pneumonia (i.e., immune reconstitution syndrome), tuberculous-related lung disease in cancer or stem cell transplant patients may infrequently worsen as patients' immune functions recover. Nonetheless, minimizing immune suppression is essential to clearing the mycobacteria.

Nontuberculous Mycobacteriosis (NTM). Pulmonary NTM is classically caused by *M. avium-intracellularae* complex and other slow-growing mycobacteria. These opportunistic pathogens can lead to chronic, indolent lung infections. In the United States, the rapidly growing mycobacteria (particularly *M. abscessus* and less frequently *M. fortuitum, M. smegmatis,* and *M. goodii*) have emerged as less frequent causes of NTM infections. The diagnosis of pulmonary NTM remains a challenge as identification of these mycobacteria in respiratory culture samples may result from colonization of the respiratory tract or environmental contamination. Causality is suggested by identification of NTM in sterile lower respiratory tract samples coupled with nonspecific clinical features, such as chronic nonproductive cough and exertional dyspnea. The cough may occasionally become productive, indicating underlying bronchiectasis. Fever, night sweats, weight loss, pleuritic chest pain, and pleural effusions are seldom seen. Radiographic features include upper lobe predominant nonspecific nodular lesions and small, thin-walled cavities. Chest CT findings demonstrating the characteristic "tree-in-bud" appearance may also be seen in patients with chronic infection. The so-called Lady Windermere syndrome, characterized by relapsing or refractory pulmonary NTM due to slow-growing mycobacteria, may be seen in patients with defects in endogenous interferon-gamma activity [27]. NTM pulmonary infections are usually insidious, although rapidly progressive disease has been seen in patients with profound defects in helper T-cells. Treatment should include at least two antimicrobial agents to which the *Mycobacterium* is susceptible, including rifampin, and should be given for 12–24 months. *M. kansasii* is antigenically similar to *M. tuberculous* and causes lung disease that is clinically and radiographically indistinguishable from pulmonary tuberculous. Endemic areas for *M. kansasii* infections in the US include the urban Southeast and Midwestern States. Due to associated architectural derangements and possibly because of impaired phagocytosis by alveolar macrophages, pneumoconioses are well-established predisposing conditions for NTM infection. Prolonged therapy (12–24 months) with rifampin plus one or two other susceptible antimicrobials is recommended.

Pneumocystis. *P. jiroveci* infections are primarily seen in patients with marked CD4 lymphocytopenia [28]. In most cancer patients, *Pneumocystis* pneumonia presents as a slowly progressive infection accompanied by nonproductive cough, exertional dyspnea, and hypoxemia, although an acute, rapidly progressive form that rapidly progresses to respiratory failure has been reported. CT evidence of perihilar infiltrates may be mistaken for pneumonitis caused by common acquired viral infections (RSV, influenza, parainfluenza type 3) or CMV during the early phase of the infection. Bronchoalveolar lavage typically has a high diagnostic yield, though lung biopsy is occasionally needed, as cancer patients typically have lower fungal burden than do HIV-infected patients. High-dose trimethoprim-sulfamethoxazole given for 21 days is the treatment of choice. Adjuvant systemic corticosteroids should be administered to most patients with severe hypoxemia. Oral atovaquone and parenteral pentamidine may be given to patients who are intolerant to sulfa-containing regimens.

Invasive Pulmonary Mycosis. Invasive pulmonary aspergillosis is the most common fungal pneumonia in cancer patients. Risk factors for invasive pulmonary aspergillosis include prolonged (>1 week) and severe (<100 cells/μL) neutropenia, refractory leukemia, allogeneic HSCT, GVHD immunosuppressive therapy, and high-dose systemic corticosteroid therapy [29, 30]. *Aspergillus fumigatus* is most prominent in this group, although amphotericin B-resistant *A. terreus* has recently emerged as the second most frequent *Aspergillus* spp. in cancer patients [31]. The near-exponential rise in pulmonary invasive fungal infections due to non-*Aspergillus* molds such as *Fusarium, Pseudallescheria boydii,* and *Scedosporium* spp. and the dematiaceous (black) molds that are often not susceptible to conventional antifungal agents poses a serious challenge in the selection of effective empiric and preemptive therapy. Fever, cough, and dyspnea, when present, suggest lung infection. Hemoptysis is not uncommon chest imaging studies are frequently nonspecific, though CT scans may reveal a highly suggestive "halo sign" or "crescent sign." In most cases of pulmonary mycosis, the only radiographic findings at the time of presentation are peripheral, pleural-based lung nodules, sometimes with thick-walled regular or irregular cavities (Fig. 12.4) [32]. Alveolar hemorrhage may occasionally herald an invasive pulmonary fungal infection.

A decline in the incidence of endemic mycoses, such as pulmonary histoplasmosis, blastomycosis, and coccidioidomycosis, as well as *Cryptococcus neoformans* infections, has been reported. This has largely been attributed to effective prophylaxis with fluconazole in immunosuppressed cancer patients. The incidence of Zygomycosis, on the other hand, has increased in recent years. This is likely related to the increased utilization of the recently available antifungal agent, voriconazole, with a concomitant decline in the use of amphotericin B. *Zygomycetes* organisms typically show a high level of susceptibility to amphotericin B. With the decreased utilization of this agent, rates of fungal infections at our institution caused by zygomycosis, invasive aspergillosis, and *Fusarium* species during the years 2002–2004 were 0.095/1,000, 0.302/1,000, and 0.073/1,000 patient-days, respectively [33].

The definitive diagnosis of pulmonary invasive fungal infection requires demonstration of fungal hyphae within the involved lung tissue. Therefore, the clinical diagnosis is often made by inference, as thrombocytopenia and coagulopathies often render biopsies unsafe. It is important to note that the isolation of molds in patients from peripheral or central venous blood samples may not indicate disseminated mycosis, even in severely immunosuppressed allogeneic HSCT recipients [34]. Similarly, isolation of fungi in respiratory samples may misrepresent the etiology of underlying pulmonary infiltrates. Therefore, the current consensus for invasive fungal infections diagnosis includes: (a) evaluation of host's predisposing factors such as prolonged granulocytopenia, high-risk HSCT, GVHD, immunosuppressive therapy; (b) clinical features (less often seen in cancer and stem cell transplant recipients); (c) radiographic features; and (d) isolation of pathogenic fungus from sterile respiratory sites. The measurement of fungal antigens such as serum galactomannan levels may be helpful in the detection of pulmonary mycosis. In a recent study of HSCT recipients, serum galactomannan levels were diagnostic in >85% of patients. The diagnostic utility of this test, however, was markedly compromised in the setting of antifungal therapy [35]. Newer diagnostic tests, including fungal DNA amplification in sterile samples, are currently under investigation and need clinical validation before routine use is recommended.

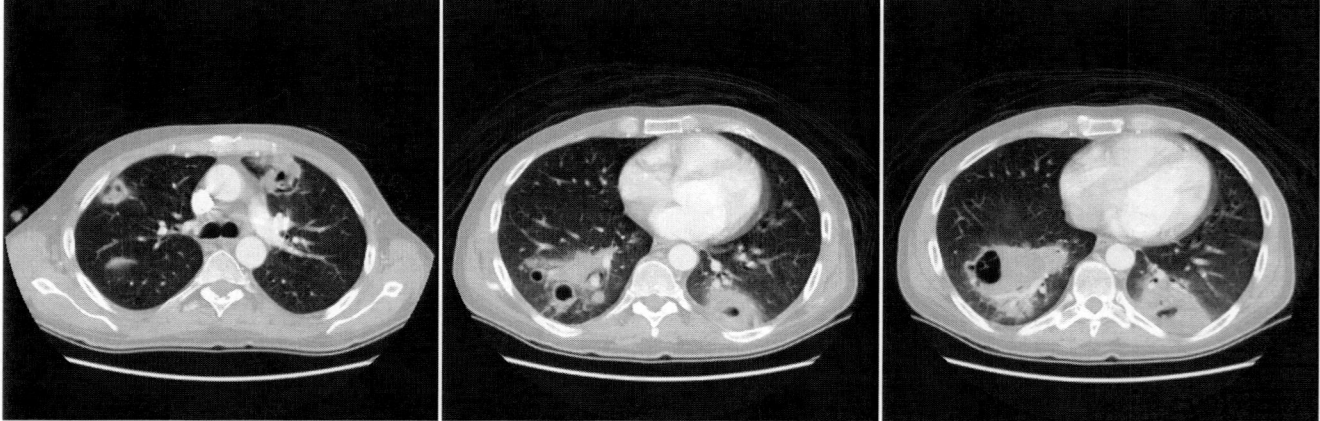

Fig. 12.4 Invasive *Aspergillus fumigatus* and *Rhizopus* multicentric cavitary pneumonia during graft-versus-host disease (GVHD) following donor lymphocyte infection in a patient with chronic lymphocytic leukemia and allogeneic hematopoietic stem cell transplantation; Postfungal pneumonia course was complicated by recurrent *Pseudomonas* and *Stenotrophomonas maltophilia* secondary lung infection

The treatment of pulmonary mycosis has improved considerably in the past ~10 years. The availability of voriconazole as primary therapy for invasive pulmonary aspergillosis [36] and caspofungin for salvage therapy of refractory invasive aspergillosis [37] is a promising addition to the antifungal armamentarium. Antifungal combinations may be prescribed for high-risk cancer patients and HSCT recipients with invasive mycosis. Due to the lack of prospective randomized trials, there is no consensus in recommending preferred antifungal combinations. A preliminary study using various antifungal combinations hinted modest superiority of caspofungin plus voriconazole in HSCT recipients with invasive fungal infections [38]. Reconstitution of the immune system, including recovery of severe granulocytopenia, remains the critical determinant in promoting resolution invasive fungal infections. Donor granulocyte transfusions and adjuvant recombinant T_H1 cytokines need prospective evaluation, although the results of preliminary observational studies among high-risk allogeneic HSCT recipients with disseminated mycosis appear promising [39].

Viruses. Human cytomegalovirus pneumonia is the most frequent cause of opportunistic viral complications in cancer patients with defective cellular immunity. Pulmonary Varicella-zoster virus and HHV-6 lung infections are difficult to distinguish from CMV pneumonitis. Seasonal respiratory viruses (RSV, Influenza A and B, Parainfluenza type 3, and Adenovirus) also cause serious lower respiratory tract infections in immunosuppressed cancer patients. Fever and nonproductive cough are prominent nonspecific features. In patients with extensive lung involvement, dyspnea may appear early in the course of infection. Viral antigen detection in nasal washes, tracheal aspirates, and bronchial specimens is most frequently used in determining active viral replication. Chest CT scans may show ground glass infiltrates, despite normal conventional chest radiographs. A normal chest CT scan in high-risk HSCT recipients with suspected viral pneumonitis excludes the possibility of infection in >95% of cases. The presence of CMV viremia is another helpful indicator in determining the etiology of a pulmonary process. The isolation of CMV antigen from lower respiratory tract secretions may not, however, necessarily indicate pulmonary infection, as patients with cellular immune defects may have intermittent low-level viral replication and shed virus without developing end-organ disease. Ganciclovir or foscarnet are commonly prescribed for systemic CMV and HHV-6 infections. Antiviral combinations with adjuvant immunoglobulin (IVIG) therapy are associated with variable results and presently not recommended for routine use. Human metapneumovirus (hMPV) has been recently recognized as a serious pulmonary pathogen. The spectrum of hMPV disease may range from mild upper respiratory tract infection to serious disseminated infection leading to respiratory failure and encephalitis. Ribavirin has been used successfully and intravenous ribavirin may be considered for patients with life-threatening hMPV disease [40].

Miscellaneous. Pulmonary *T. gondii* and *L. monocytogenes* infections can lead to serious, often life-threatening, complications in patients with profound cellular immune dysfunction and disease characteristics are described in detail elsewhere [41, 42].

References

1. Ahmed S, Siddiqui AK, Rossoff L, Sison CP, Rai KR. Pulmonary complications in chronic lymphocytic leukemia. Cancer. 2003;98(9):1912–7.
2. Safdar A, Armstrong D. Infectious morbidity in critically ill patients with cancer. Crit Care Clin. 2001;17(3):531–70, vii–viii.
3. Sculier J, Evans W, Feld R, et al. Superior vena caval obstruction syndrome in small cell lung cancer. Cancer. 1986;15:847–51.
4. Bartlett JG. Community-acquired pneumonia. Int J Clin Pract Suppl. 2000;54(115):18–22.
5. Ibrahim EH, Tracy L, Hill C, Fraser VJ, Kollef MH. The occurrence of ventilator-associated pneumonia in a community hospital: risk factors and clinical outcomes. Chest. 2001;120(2):555–61.
6. Agusti C, Rano A, Rovira M, et al. Inflammatory response associated with pulmonary complications in non-HIV immunocompromised patients. Thorax. 2004;59(12):1081–8.
7. Schleimer RP. Glucocorticoids suppress inflammation but spare innate immune responses in airway epithelium. Proc Am Thorac Soc. 2004;1(3):222–30.
8. Hubel K, Hegener K, Schnell R, et al. Suppressed neutrophil function as a risk factor for severe infection after cytotoxic chemotherapy in patients with acute nonlymphocytic leukemia. Ann Hematol. 1999;78(2):73–7.
9. Bodey GP, Buckley M, Sathe YS, Freireich EJ. Quantitative relationships between circulating leukocytes and infection in patients with acute leukemia. Ann Intern Med. 1966;64(2):328–40.
10. Yadegarynia D, Tarrand J, Raad I, Rolston K. Current spectrum of bacterial infections in patients with cancer. Clin Infect Dis. 2003;37(8):1144–5.
11. Chatzinikolaou I, Abi-Said D, Bodey GP, Rolston KV, Tarrand JJ, Samonis G. Recent experience with *Pseudomonas aeruginosa* bacteremia in patients with cancer: retrospective analysis of 245 episodes. Arch Intern Med. 2000;160(4):501–9.
12. Aisenberg G, Rolston KV, Dickey BF, Kontoyiannis DP, Raad II, Safdar A. *Stenotrophomonas maltophilia* pneumonia in cancer patients without traditional risk factors for infection, 1997-2004. Eur J Clin Microbiol Infect Dis. 2007;26(1):13–20.
13. Boktour M, Hanna H, Ansari S, et al. Central venous catheter and *Stenotrophomonas maltophilia* bacteremia in cancer patients. Cancer. 2006;106(9):1967–73.
14. Safdar A, Rodriguez GH, Balakrishnan M, Tarrand JJ, Rolston KV. Changing trends in etiology of bacteremia in patients with cancer. Eur J Clin Microbiol Infect Dis. 2006;25(8):522–6.
15. Safdar A, Rolston KV. *Stenotrophomonas maltophilia*: changing spectrum of a serious bacterial pathogen in patients with cancer. Clin Infect Dis. 2007;45(12):1602–9.
16. Aisenberg G, Rolston KV, Safdar A. Bacteremia caused by *Achromobacter* and *Alcaligenes* species in 46 patients with cancer (1989-2003). Cancer. 2004;101(9):2134–40.
17. Aisenberg G, Tarrand J, Rolston K, Kontoyiannis D, Raad I, Safdar A. *Stenotrophomonas maltophilia*: changing spectrum of bacterial pneumonia in cancer patients with low suspicion of *S. maltophilia* infection. Paper presented at: 15th European Congress of Clinical

Microbiology and Infectious Diseases (ECCMID); 2005; Copenhagen, Denmark.
18. Mandell LA, Bartlett JG, Dowell SF, File Jr TM, Musher DM, Whitney C. Update of practice guidelines for the management of community-acquired pneumonia in immunocompetent adults. Clin Infect Dis. 2003;37(11):1405–33.
19. Niederman MS, Mandell LA, Anzueto A, et al. Guidelines for the management of adults with community-acquired pneumonia. Diagnosis, assessment of severity, antimicrobial therapy, and prevention. Am J Respir Crit Care Med. 2001;163(7):1730–54.
20. American Thoracic Society; Infectious Diseases Society of America. Guidelines for the management of adults with hospital-acquired, ventilator-associated, and healthcare-associated pneumonia. Am J Respir Crit Care Med. 2005;171(4):388–416.
21. El-Solh A, Aquilina A, Dhillon R, Ramadan F, Nowak P, Davies J. Impact of invasive strategy on management of antimicrobial treatment failure in institutionalized older people with severe pneumonia. Am J Respir Crit Care Med. 2002;166:1038–43.
22. Rello J, Ollendorf DA, Oster G, et al. Epidemiology and outcomes of ventilator-associated pneumonia in a large US database. Chest. 2002;122(6):2115–21.
23. Marik PE. Aspiration pneumonitis and aspiration pneumonia. N Engl J Med. 2001;344(9):665–71.
24. Torres HA, Reddy BT, Raad II, et al. Nocardiosis in cancer patients. Medicine (Baltimore). 2002;81(5):388–97.
25. Uttamchandani RB, Daikos GL, Reyes RR, et al. Nocardiosis in 30 patients with advanced human immunodeficiency virus infection: clinical features and outcome. Clin Infect Dis. 1994;18(3):348–53.
26. De La Rosa GR, Jacobson KL, Rolston KV, Raad II, Kontoyiannis DP, Safdar A. *Mycobacterium tuberculosis* at a comprehensive cancer centre: active disease in patients with underlying malignancy during 1990-2000. Clin Microbiol Infect. 2004;10(8):749–52.
27. Safdar A, White DA, Stover D, Armstrong D, Murray HW. Profound interferon gamma deficiency in patients with chronic pulmonary nontuberculous mycobacteriosis. Am J Med. 2002;113(9):756–9.
28. Roblot F, Le Moal G, Godet C, et al. *Pneumocystis carinii* pneumonia in patients with hematologic malignancies: a descriptive study. J Infect. 2003;47(1):19–27.
29. Marr KA. Empirical antifungal therapy – new options, new tradeoffs. N Engl J Med. 2002;346(4):278–80.
30. Marr KA, Patterson T, Denning D. Aspergillosis. Pathogenesis, clinical manifestations, and therapy. Infect Dis Clin North Am. 2002;16(4):875–94, vi.
31. Hachem RY, Kontoyiannis DP, Boktour MR, et al. *Aspergillus terreus*: an emerging amphotericin B-resistant opportunistic mold in patients with hematologic malignancies. Cancer. 2004;101(7):1594–600.
32. Heussel CP, Kauczor HU, Heussel GE, et al. Pneumonia in febrile neutropenic patients and in bone marrow and blood stem-cell transplant recipients: use of high-resolution computed tomography. J Clin Oncol. 1999;17(3):796–805.
33. Kontoyiannis DP, Lionakis MS, Lewis RE, et al. Zygomycosis in a tertiary-care cancer center in the era of *Aspergillus*-active antifungal therapy: a case-control observational study of 27 recent cases. J Infect Dis. 2005;191(8):1350–60.
34. Safdar A, Bannister TW, Safdar Z. The predictors of outcome in immunocompetent patients with hematogenous candidiasis. Int J Infect Dis. 2004;8(3):180–6.
35. Marr KA, Balajee SA, McLaughlin L, Tabouret M, Bentsen C, Walsh TJ. Detection of galactomannan antigenemia by enzyme immunoassay for the diagnosis of invasive aspergillosis: variables that affect performance. J Infect Dis. 2004;190(3):641–9.
36. Herbrecht R, Denning DW, Patterson TF, et al. Voriconazole versus amphotericin B for primary therapy of invasive aspergillosis. N Engl J Med. 2002;347(6):408–15.
37. Maertens J, Raad I, Petrikkos G, et al. Efficacy and safety of caspofungin for treatment of invasive aspergillosis in patients refractory to or intolerant of conventional antifungal therapy. Clin Infect Dis. 2004;39(11):1563–71.
38. Marr K. Combination antifungal therapy: where are we now, and where are we going? Oncology (Williston Park). 2004;18(13 Suppl 7):24–9.
39. Safdar A, Rodriguez G, Ohmagari N, et al. The safety of interferon-gamma-1b therapy for invasive fungal infections after hematopoietic stem cell transplantation. Cancer. 2005;103(4):731–9.
40. Safdar A. Immune modulatory activity of ribavirin for serious human metapneumovirus disease: early i.v. therapy may improve outcomes in immunosuppressed SCT recipients. Bone Marrow Transplant. 2008;41(8):707–8.
41. Roemer E, Blau IW, Basara N, et al. Toxoplasmosis, a severe complication in allogeneic hematopoietic stem cell transplantation: successful treatment strategies during a 5-year single-center experience. Clin Infect Dis. 2001;32(1):E1–8.
42. Safdar A, Armstrong D. Listeriosis in patients at a comprehensive cancer center, 1955-1997. Clin Infect Dis. 2003;37(3):359–64.

Chapter 13
Noninfectious Lung Infiltrates That May Be Confused with Pneumonia in the Cancer Patient

Rana Kaplan, Lara Bashoura, Vickie R. Shannon, Burton F. Dickey, and Diane E. Stover

Abstract The clinical and radiographic presentation of noninfectious pulmonary disease can often mimic pneumonia in the cancer patient. This chapter provides an overview of some of the most commonly observed noninfectious entities which may be observed in the immunocompromised host with cancer. Hydrostatic and nonhydrostatic pulmonary edema, as well as transfusion-related acute lung injury, may cause bilateral airspace opacification that may be confused with an infectious process. Chemotherapy induced lung injury can occur with many classes of chemotherapeutic agents and requires a high index of clinical suspicion for diagnosis. It often results in distinct patterns of pathologic injury, which may present acutely, subacutely or chronically, and in some cases, up to years after initial administration of the chemotherapeutic agent. Radiation induced lung injury often causes a distinct pattern of radiographic abnormalities, which may occur many months after the initial radiation exposure. In hematopoietic stem cell transplant recipients, many pulmonary diagnoses, such as engraftment syndrome, idiopathic pneumonia syndrome and diffuse alveolar hemorrhage (occurring early) and cryptogenic organizing pneumonia (occurring late), can mimic infectious pneumonias. Small airway mucus impaction can present with tree-in-bud opacities on chest CT and mimics infectious bronchiolitis. It may resolve with only pulmonary hygiene maneuvers. A combined approach involving careful review of the patient's history, pattern of infiltrates on chest CT, and the use of bronchoscopy with bronchoalveolar lavage with or without transbronchial lung biopsy can often help provide clues to the noninfectious diagnosis.

Keywords Noninfectious • Lung infiltrates • Diffuse alveolar hemorrhage • Congestive heart failure • Drug toxicity • BOOP • Pulmonary alveolar proteinosis • Engraftment syndrome

R. Kaplan (✉)
Pulmonary Medicine Service, Memorial Sloan–Kettering Cancer Center, 1275 York Avenue, New York, NY 10065, USA
e-mail: kaplanr1@mskcc.org

Introduction

Pneumonia is the leading cause of death from infection among cancer patients and second most common cause of death after uncontrolled cancer itself. Therefore, the prevention, diagnosis, and treatment of pneumonia are critical to outcomes among cancer patients. During the workup of a symptom or sign, such as cough, fever, or chills, abnormalities in imaging studies of the lungs are commonly detected. Consideration of the differential diagnosis of a lung infiltrate in a cancer patient includes both infectious and several common noninfectious causes. Failure to accurately diagnose noninfectious causes of lung infiltrates can lead to unnecessary treatment with antibiotics, and more importantly, failure to address the underlying pathophysiologic process. This chapter is focused on the many clinical presentations that mimic infectious pneumonia.

Hydrostatic Pulmonary Edema (Congestive Heart Failure)

Cardiogenic (hydrostatic) pulmonary edema is frequently observed in cancer patients, probably due to the high prevalence of cardiac disease in this relatively elderly population, the large volumes of fluid administered with chemotherapy and antibiotics, chemotherapy-induced cardiotoxicity, and comorbidities (e.g., renal insufficiency) [1]. The classic presentation of cardiogenic pulmonary edema, consisting of acute, bilateral, symmetrical, perihilar infiltrates, an enlarged heart, and pleural effusions (see Fig. 13.1) in a patient with peripheral edema and bibasilar rales is easy to recognize. However, cardiogenic pulmonary edema may also be the cause of asymmetrical infiltrates in a patient with underlying lung disease, such as bullous emphysema, which precludes alveolar filling in localized regions (see Fig. 13.2). An enlarged heart may not be present on the radiograph if cardiac dysfunction is not long-standing, so that the heart has not had time to remodel (e.g., acute volume overload, or diastolic dysfunction secondary to acute ischemia).

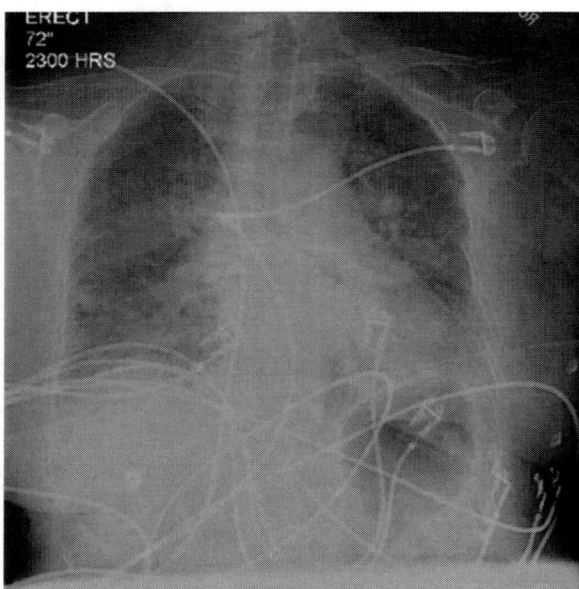

Fig. 13.1 Bilateral airspace opacities with a perihilar predominance and small bilateral pleural effusions are classic radiographic findings in *cardiogenic pulmonary edema*

Additional studies can be very helpful in establishing the diagnosis of cardiogenic pulmonary edema [2–4]. CT of the chest may show the diffuse nature of alveolar infiltrates and pleural effusions, less apparent on plain films, and may additionally reveal interstitial edema and cardiac chamber enlargement. Infiltrates may wax and wane in association with variations in patient weight, peripheral edema, or fluid administration. Echocardiography is very supportive when it reveals systolic dysfunction, but it is important to recognize that diastolic dysfunction is an equally prevalent cause of heart failure [5], potentially exacerbated by rhythm disturbances such as atrial fibrillation, valvular dysfunction, or transient ventricular wall stiffening due to ischemia. Brain natriuretic peptide (BNP) levels are quite specific and sensitive, but are less elevated in diastolic than in systolic dysfunction [5]. In the absence of heart failure, BNP levels can be elevated in patients with renal disease and obesity.

Nonhydrostatic Pulmonary Edema (Noncardiogenic Pulmonary Edema, Acute Lung Injury, and the Adult Respiratory Distress Syndrome)

Pulmonary edema due to increased permeability of the alveolo-capillary membrane can occur due to a wide variety of causes in cancer patients. Sepsis is the most common cause of permeability edema of the lungs in noncancer patients [6, 7] and can cause radiographic infiltrates in cancer patients. In addition, cancer patients are susceptible to lung injury from causes unique to this population, such as from chemotherapy or the effects of hematopoietic stem cell transplantation. Cancer patients are also frequently exposed to treatments associated with lung injury in the general hospital population, such as transfusion. These causes of permeability edema are addressed individually within the following sections.

Chemotherapy-Induced Lung Injury

Chemotherapy-induced lung injury (CILI) has been documented following administration of all categories of chemotherapeutic agents, including the newer molecular-targeted therapies. Lung toxicity from cancer chemotherapy results in a limited number of stereotypic histopathologic lung injury patterns that may involve the lung parenchyma, conducting airways, pleura, or pulmonary circulation (see Table 13.1 for types of chemotherapy-induced lung injury and associated chemotherapeutic agents).

Diagnoses that mimic CILI, such as pneumonia and cancer relapse, pose challenges for both pulmonary and infectious disease practitioners. There are no pathognomonic abnormalities for the diagnosis of CILI. A high index of suspicion, coupled with knowledge of risk factors, clinical presentation, radiologic manifestations, and histologic patterns is critical for early diagnosis and successful outcomes. The diagnosis is largely based on the association between drug exposure and the development of pulmonary illness, although, in some cases, lung injury can occur many years after the drug is discontinued. Chemotherapeutic agents, such as the nitrosoureas, for example, can cause pulmonary fibrosis up to 20 years after completion of therapy [8]. Evidence of rapid clinical and radiologic improvement following drug withdrawal supports the diagnosis; however, lung injury can progress despite withdrawal of certain drugs, such as bleomycin, busulfan, and BCNU.

CILI can present acutely, subacutely, or chronically and can be idiosyncratic, i.e., unrelated to dose or duration of therapy. Of the types of injury which could mimic infection, noncardiogenic pulmonary edema (NCPE), hypersensitivity pneumonitis (HP), and organizing pneumonia (OP) generally represent subacute processes that can occur days to weeks following drug administration. Chronic manifestations of drug toxicity, such as interstitial pneumonitis (i.e., nonspecific interstitial pneumonitis, or NSIP) and fibrosis (i.e., usual interstitial pneumonitis, or UIP), evolve insidiously over weeks to months and up to years after exposure (see Figs. 13.3a, b and 13.4a, b). The clinician should also be aware of drug synergisms causing diffuse alveolar damage (DAD)/NCPE following bleomycin/oxygen, gemcitabine/taxane, and vinca alkaloid/mitomycin combinations [9–11].

Low-grade fever, dyspnea, and nonproductive cough are the usual symptoms of subacute and chronic forms of drug

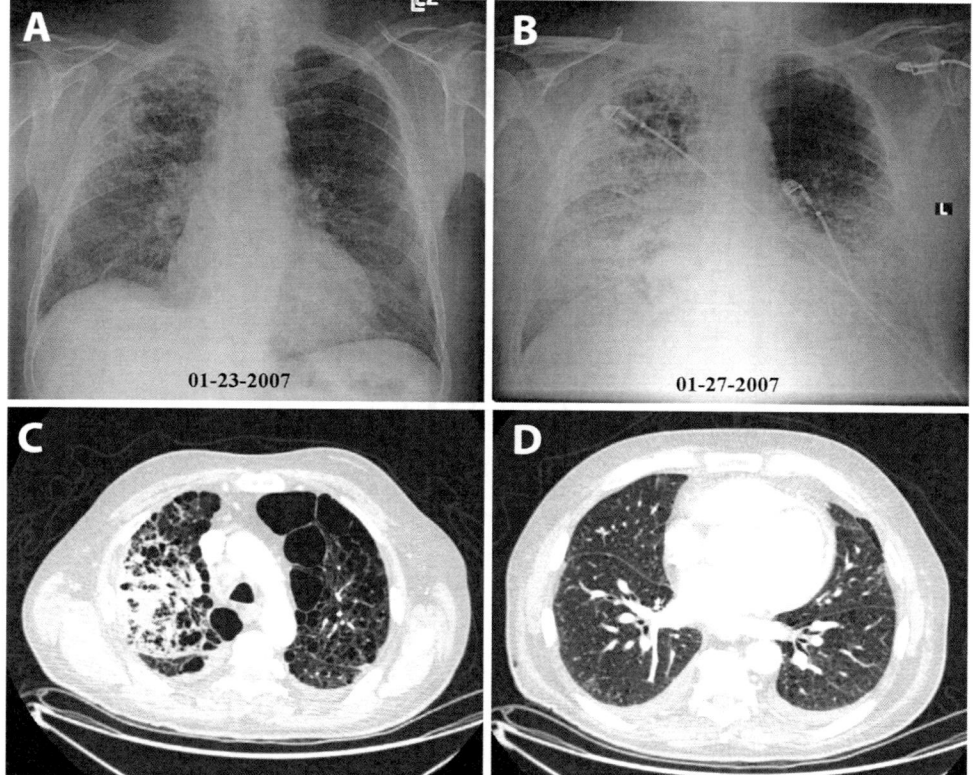

Fig. 13.2 *Atypical radiographic presentation of congestive heart failure.* A 68 year old male was receiving radiation therapy to a squamous cell carcinoma of the upper lobe of the right lung, because he was not felt to be a surgical candidate due to comorbidities, including coronary artery disease. He had received 19 of 37 planned fractions, when he was admitted because of increasing shortness of breath and cough thought to be due to pneumonia. (**A**) The PA radiograph on the upper left, taken one day prior to admission, shows the right upper lobe tumor with associated radiation pneumonitis. (**B**) The AP radiograph on the upper right, taken four days later, shows lung infiltrates that spare the left upper lobe. (**C**) However, CT angiogram on the lower panels, performed the day of admission, 01-24-2007, shows that the left upper chest is mostly occupied by emphysematous bullae, accounting for the sparing of the left upper lung field when pulmonary edema developed. (**D**) The remainder of the lung fields contain ground glass opacities, suggestive of *congestive heart failure*. The diagnosis of congestive heart failure was supported by the patient's history of prior episodes of pulmonary edema, bilateral 1+ ankle edema, a depressed left ventricular ejection fraction of 30–35%, moderate mitral regurgitation, elevated BNP of 1,043, transudative pleural effusion and improvement with diuresis

toxicity. Intractable respiratory impairment leading to respiratory failure and death may occur as the disease progresses.

Although radiographic changes in CILI are nonspecific, certain patterns are seen [12, 13]. Interstitial and mixed alveolar/interstitial abnormalities are commonly localized to the periphery of the lower lung zones and are the most frequent radiographic findings on chest CT in patients with chemotherapy-induced NSIP and UIP. DAD can present with pulmonary edema-like radiographs (see Fig. 13.5a), and OP often shows airspace consolidation mimicking bacterial pneumonia. Upper lobe predominate disease is characteristic of drug-induced hypersensitivity reactions (see Fig. 13.6a). CT scans and, occasionally, FDG-PET and gallium imaging may show abnormalities before chest radiographic changes and, in some cases, may precede clinical symptoms [14, 15].

Restrictive physiology and reduction in the diffusing capacity are commonly observed on lung function testing in CILI, with the latter often predating the onset of symptoms.

Histopathologic changes in CILI include endothelial swelling with exudation of fluid into the interstitium and intra-alveolar spaces. There is destruction of type I pneumocytes with proliferation of type II pneumocytes, which may appear large and "bizarre". Hyaline membranes may be seen in DAD (see Fig. 13.5b). Loosely formed granulomas are found in up to one third of lung biopsies in patients with methotrexate-induced lung injury, which is felt to represent a hypersensitivity reaction (see Fig. 13.6b).

Bronchoalveolar lavage (BAL) helps to exclude alternative pathologic processes, such as infection or malignancy [16]. A lymphocyte predominant alveolitis is most commonly observed in CILI. Transbronchial biopsy has limited utility in the diagnosis of CILI due to the inherent difficulty in extrapolating histopathologic patterns of lung involvement from small

Table 13.1 Types of chemotherapy-induced lung injury and some associated chemotherapeutic agents

LUNG INJURY	DRUG
UIP	bleomycin, busulfan, BCNU, melphalan, cyclophosphamide
NSIP	bleomycin, gemcitabine, mitomycin, docetaxel, dasatinib, nitrosureas
HP+	methotrexate, bleomycin, paclitaxel
OP+	bleomycin, interferon α or β*
DAD+	gefitinib, gemcitabine, cyclophosphamide
NCPE+	gemcitabine, cyclophosphamide, bleomycin, cytosine, arabinoside, docetaxel, fludarabine, mitomycin, vinca alkaloids, retinoic acid, methotrexate
LESS COMMON	
Diffuse alveolar hemorrhage	cytosine arabinoside, gemcitabine, mitomycin, retinoic acid, etoposide
Vascular changes	
Pulmonary hypertension	interferon α, mitomycin
Pulmonary veno-occlusive disease	bleomycin, busulfan, nitrosureas
Pleural effusion	dasatinib, docetaxel, methotrexate, busulfan
Pneumothorax	bleomycin, BCNU, retinoic acid
Mediastinal lymphadenopathy	methotrexate, bleomycin, interferon β
Bronchospasm	etoposide, interferon α and β, paclitaxel, vinca alkaloids

UIP = usual interstitial pneumonitis; **NSIP** = non-specific interstitial pneumonitis; **HP** = hypersensitivity pneumonitis; **OP** = organizing pneumonia; **DAD** = diffuse alveolar damage; **NCPE** = non-cardiogenic pulmonary edema
+In reporting histopathologic changes, there may be overlap between HP/EP, OP/EP and DAD/NCPE
*These cytokines have also been associated with granulomatous changes resembling sarcoidosis

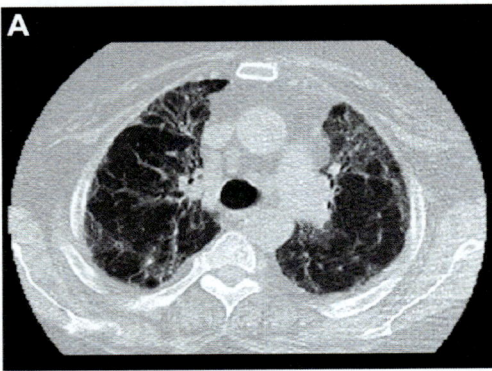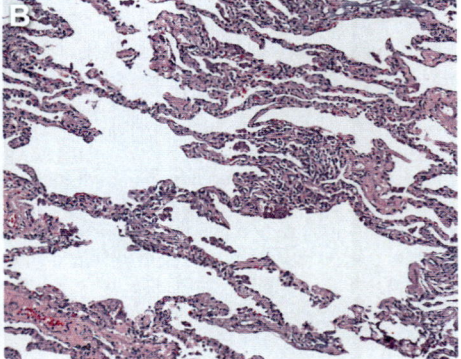

Fig. 13.3 *Pulmonary fibrosis* in a patient with a history of docetaxel use. (**A**) CT chest demonstrates a pattern of bilateral, symmetric, reticular infiltrates and ground glass opacities associated with traction bronchiectasis. (**B**) Histologic examination reveals *non-specific interstitial pneumonitis* (NSIP), characterized by uniform interstitial involvement of chronic inflammation, consisting mostly of lymphocytes and plasma cells, causing thickening of the alveolar walls

tissue samples and the lack of pathognomonic findings. Additionally, thrombocytopenia in the cancer treatment setting often precludes bronchoscopic biopsies. When safe, it should be performed along with BAL to help eliminate other diagnoses, such as infection or malignancy. Surgical lung biopsy should be considered, when fungal infection is an alternative diagnosis or when there is discordance between bronchoscopic biopsy and/or clinical or radiologic findings.

If pulmonary toxicity occurs, withdrawal of the offending agent is the mainstay of treatment. Although no controlled trials have explored the efficacy of corticosteroid therapy, a trial of systemic corticosteroid therapy is usually initiated in most cases. The optimal dose and duration of therapy are unknown; however, treatment with 1 mg/kg of prednisone daily is usually given, with a slow taper, as recurrence of symptoms has been reported in the setting of tapering. Given the increased incidence of *Pneumocystis jiroveci* pneumonia observed in non-HIV individuals with both hematologic malignancies and solid tumors on steroid therapy [17, 18], it is the authors' practice to routinely prescribe prophylactic trimethoprim–sulfamethoxazole

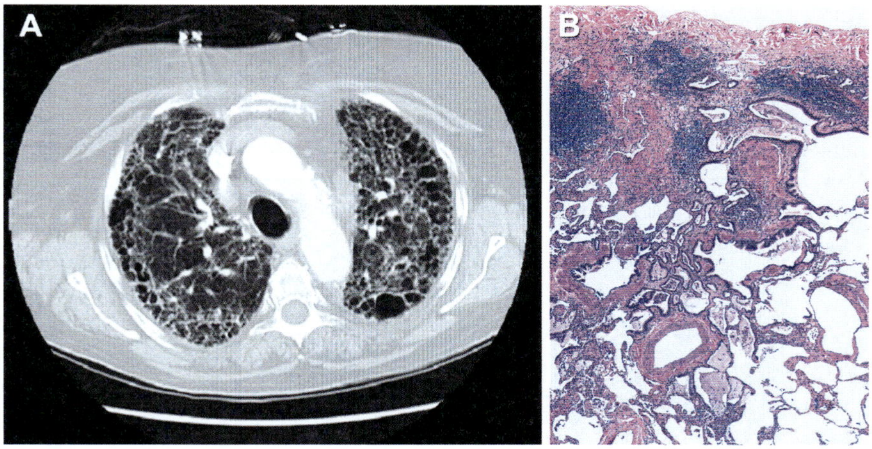

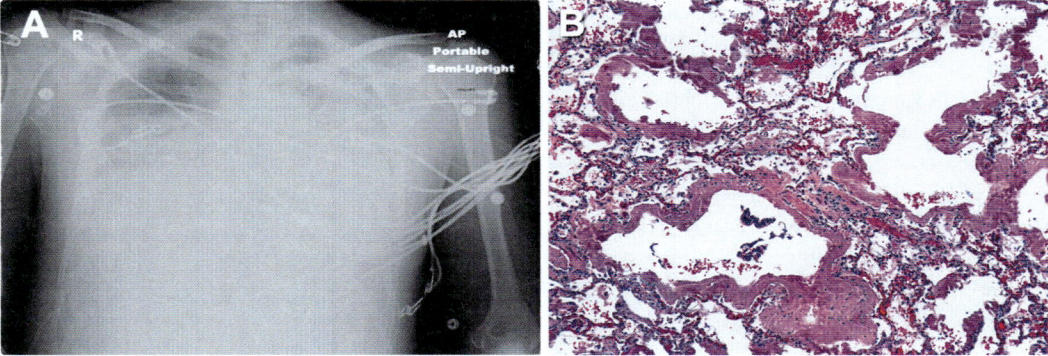

Fig. 13.4 *Idiopathic pulmonary fibrosis* (IPF). (**A**) Reticular infiltrates, associated with honeycombing and traction bronchiectasis in a basilar and peripheral predominance, are characteristic findings seen in CT imaging of IPF. (**B**) The histopathologic correlate of IPF is *usual interstitial pneumonia*, which is characterized by patchy, temporally heterogeneous subpleural fibrosis with honeycombing and the presence of fibroblastic foci

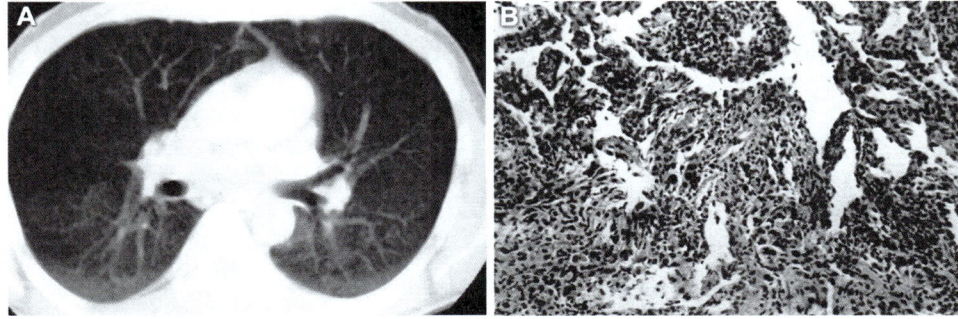

Fig. 13.5 *Diffuse alveolar damage.* (**A**) The chest radiograph demonstrates bilateral airspace opacities, characteristic of diffuse alveolar damage. (**B**) *Hyaline membranes* lining alveolar ducts are key features of acute diffuse alveolar damage on histopathologic examination; interstitial and alveolar edema may also be seen

Fig. 13.6 (**A**) CT chest findings in a patient with methotrexate-induced *hypersensitivity pneumonitis*. High resolution CT chest reveals poorly defined centrilobular nodules and diffuse ground glass attenuation. (**B**) Methotrexate can cause loosely formed non-necrotizing granulomas in a background of cellular interstitial inflammation

in conjunction with the high-dose steroid therapy. Reports exist of a negative rechallenge (i.e., no subsequent recurrence of pulmonary toxicity) with some chemotherapeutic agents, such as cyclophosphamide and methotrexate; rechallenging patients with drugs previously implicated in CILI is not recommended.

Radiation-Induced Lung Injury

The incidence and severity of radiation damage to the lungs are related principally to the volume of lung tissue irradiated, the total dose of radiation, the fraction into which the total dose is divided, and the quality of the radiation. Damage to the lung increases as the volume of the irradiated lung increases, and there is a threshold effect, such that irradiation of at least 10% of the lung is required to produce significant pulmonary toxicity. Radiation pneumonitis seldom occurs with fractionated doses of <20 Gy, but it is likely when doses exceed 60 Gy. The greater the number of fractions in which the radiation is given, the lower the damaging effect from the radiation. Certain chemotherapeutic agents, such as bleomycin and doxorubicin, are known to potentiate the damaging effects of radiation to the lung, especially when they are administered concomitantly.

Symptoms of acute radiation pneumonitis usually are seen 1½–3 months after the completion of radiation therapy [19]. The early onset of symptoms portends a more serious and protracted clinical course. Dyspnea is the more common symptom, followed by cough, which may be either nonproductive or productive of small amounts of pink sputum. Frank hemoptysis is rare early in the clinical course, though massive hemoptysis has been noted to occur as a late complication of pulmonary irradiation. Fever, if present, is usually low grade and transient.

The diagnosis of radiation pneumonitis can be made clinically on the basis of the timing of the onset of symptoms with the irradiation and the detection of typical radiographic abnormalities [20]. Early abnormalities include ground glass infiltrates, diffuse haziness, or indistinct pulmonary markings over the irradiated area. In both radiation pneumonitis and fibrosis, the abnormalities usually conform to the outlines of the field of radiation and may not adhere to anatomic borders (see Fig. 13.7). In "out of field" radiation pneumonitis, a rare complication thought to represent a hypersensitivity response, extensive radiographic changes are seen outside the radiation field, including the contralateral lung. Radiation-related bronchiolitis obliterans organizing pneumonia (BOOP) is a recently reported complication, seen predominantly in breast cancer patients. The infiltrates generally appear within an 18-month period from the time of radiation treatment, are always seen outside the irradiated lung (see Fig. 13.8), and can be bilateral [21, 22].

Carbon monoxide diffusing capacity is the parameter most predictive of impaired pulmonary function following

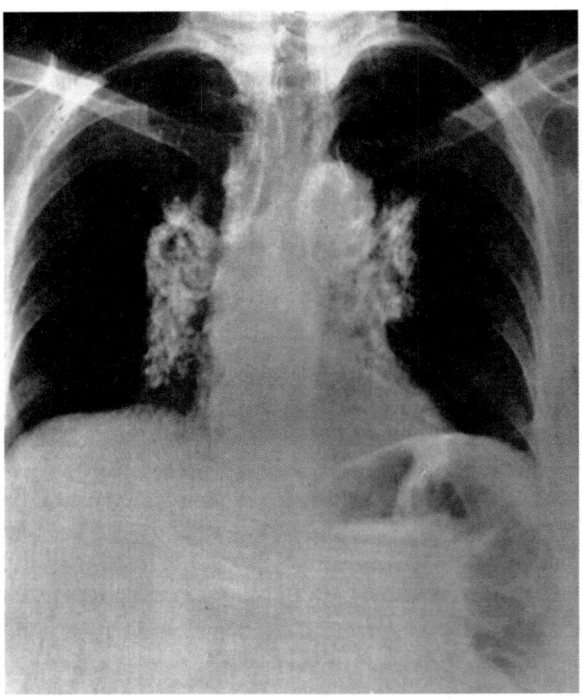

Fig. 13.7 Radiographic findings consistent with *radiation-induced pulmonary fibrosis* in a patient treated with mantle radiation for Hodgkin's lymphoma. Fibrosis and bronchiectasis are observed in a linear, geographic distribution corresponding to the field of radiation

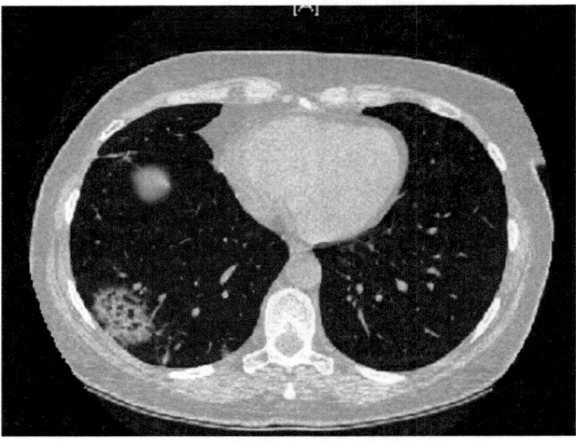

Fig. 13.8 *Radiation-induced BOOP*. CT chest findings characteristically show the location of these infiltrates outside of the portal of radiation, which, in this patient, was on the right chest wall

radiation therapy and may prognosticate a higher risk of ongoing pulmonary damage [23].

The histopathologic changes of radiation-induced pulmonary injury are not specific; vascular congestion, fibrin-rich exudate within alveoli, hyaline membranes, and hyperplasia of type II pneumocytes, with infiltration of fibroblasts and mast cells may be seen [24].

Although no controlled human clinical trials exist on the efficacy of steroid therapy, corticosteroids have resulted in an improvement in symptoms [25]. Common practice is to begin prednisone 1 mg/kg daily, in conjunction with trimethoprim–sulfamethoxazole for *Pneumocystis* prophylaxis, as soon as the diagnosis of symptomatic radiation pneumonitis is reasonably certain. The initial dose is maintained for several weeks and then reduced cautiously, based on symptom control. If steroids are tapered too rapidly, symptoms can be exacerbated, necessitating higher doses for longer periods. Most authors agree that steroids do not have a role in treatment in radiation-induced pulmonary fibrosis.

The clinical, histologic characteristics and response to steroids in radiation-induced BOOP are similar to that of cryptogenic organizing pneumonia (COP). A high relapse rate is seen with steroid tapers, and macrolides have been used with success in patients who are either intolerant to steroid therapy or in whom relapse of BOOP occurs with steroid taper [26].

Noninfectious Complications of Hematopoietic Stem Cell Transplantation

Hematopoietic stem cell transplantation (HSCT) is widely used in cancer therapy and is the only curative option for many patients with relapsed and high-risk malignancies. Despite advances in treatment regimens and supportive care, pulmonary complications still occur in up to 60% of HSCT recipients, accounting for significant morbidity and mortality [27]. Pulmonary complications are conveniently divided into those that occur "early" (during the first 100 days after transplantation) and those that occur "late" (see Table 13.2). These complications are mostly due to direct toxicities from conditioning regimens, delayed bone marrow recovery, prolonged immunosuppressive therapy, and graft-versus-host disease (GVHD). As the incidence of infectious pulmonary complications diminishing, largely due to effective prophylactic therapy, noninfectious pulmonary complications are emerging as a major cause of post-HSCT morbidity and mortality [28]. This section focuses on these noninfectious pulmonary complications and the many clinical presentations that often mimic infections.

Early-Onset Noninfectious Complications of HSCT

Pulmonary edema. Cardiogenic pulmonary edema is one of the most common early complications after HSCT. Common etiologies include cardiac dysfunction and/or an increase in hydrostatic capillary pressure, often from administration of large volumes of fluid. The clinical and radiographic manifestations are similar to those outlined in the section on hydrostatic pulmonary edema.

Engraftment syndrome. Engraftment syndrome (ES) is characterized by a constellation of symptoms and signs including fever, erythrodermatous skin rash, diarrhea, and NCPE with bilateral pulmonary infiltrates, which generally occur within 5 days of neutrophil engraftment following HSCT. In more severe cases, systemic involvement, i.e., renal failure, hepatic failure, encephalopathy, or seizures, may be observed. Seen most often following autologous HSCT, ES has also been described in those individuals who have undergone allogeneic HSCT with a nonmyeloablative preparative therapy. The pathophysiology of ES is not well understood. It is thought to result from endothelial injury, the production of cytokines and neutrophil degranulation, leading to capillary leak [29]. BAL may show a neutrophilic alveolitis. Surgical lung biopsies, when obtained, often reveal DAD. Treatment entails observation and supportive care (i.e., antibiotics, intravenous fluids) in mild cases. High-dose corticosteroid therapy is very effective, often resulting in rapid clinical improvement in those with progressive or symptomatic ES. Respiratory failure requiring mechanical ventilation has been observed, in up to one third of patients [30].

Idiopathic pneumonia syndrome (IPS). In 1993, a panel convened by the NIH proposed a broad working definition of IPS as widespread nonlobar radiographic infiltrates in the absence of congestive heart failure or evidence of lower respiratory tract infection [31]. IPS occurs in 10% of HSCT recipients, usually 14–90 days following transplantation. Mortality rates range from 50–70% [32]. Possible etiologies of IPS include direct toxic effects of the chemoradiation conditioning regimen, occult infection, and/or the release of inflammatory cytokines, secondary to some as yet unknown inciting stimuli. The association of IPS with the presence of

Table 13.2 Pulmonary complications following hematopoietic stem cell transplantation

Early (<100 days)	Late (>100 days)
Infectious pneumonia (e.g., bacterial, fungal)	Infectious pneumonia (e.g., viral, fungal, mycobacterial, bacterial)
Pulmonary edema	
Engraftment syndrome	Cryptogenic organizing pneumonia
Idiopathic pneumonia syndrome/Diffuse alveolar hemorrhage	Post-transplant lymphoproliferative disorder
Pulmonary veno-occlusive disease	Delayed pulmonary toxicity syndrome
Pulmonary alveolar proteinosis	Post-transplantation constrictive bronchiolitis

acute GVHD after allogeneic HSCT suggests that alloreactive T cells may be at least one of these stimuli [32].

The clinical presentation is nonspecific, with symptoms of dyspnea, cough, and fever associated with diffuse infiltrates on chest radiograph. The diagnosis of IPS largely relies on the exclusion of infection on lower respiratory samples obtained from a diagnostic procedure, e.g., BAL or lung biopsy. Common pathologic findings of NSIP and/or DAD may be seen. Although no randomized controlled trials of treatment for IPS are available, current standards include high-dose intravenous corticosteroids and supportive care, such as supplemental oxygen and broad-spectrum antibiotics. Recent data suggest a potential role for tumor necrosis factor-α (TNF-α) in the pathogenesis of IPS and there are ongoing clinical studies involving etanercept [33–36].

Diffuse alveolar hemorrhage (DAH). Posttransplantation DAH was initially described in autologous HSCT recipients as widespread lung injury manifested by diffuse radiographic infiltrates that occurred in the absence of identifiable infection [37]. DAH is now known to occur in both allogeneic and autologous transplant recipients and is seen in approximately 5% of all HSCT [38]. The etiology is unclear, but is not related to any specific coagulopathy or to thrombocytopenia [39]. Pretransplant high-dose chemotherapy, thoracic and/or total body irradiation, and undocumented infections are putative factors which may cause the initial injury, priming the lung for subsequent development of DAH. It can coincide with stem cell engraftment, but late onset (after the first 30 days) has been observed and is associated with a worse prognosis.

Symptoms include dyspnea, cough, and fever, with hemoptysis occurring in less than 20% of patients. Chest radiographs usually show diffuse alveolar and interstitial infiltrates in a central distribution. Bronchoscopic diagnostic criteria include progressively bloodier returns on BAL or the presence of 20% or more hemosiderin-laden macrophages on cytologic inspection of BAL fluid. However, these bronchoscopic criteria may be seen in association with diffuse lung injury from a wide variety of causes, including infections, congestive heart failure, and malignancy, often making a definitive diagnosis problematic. There are no prospective randomized trials addressing the treatment of DAH. Earlier retrospective studies demonstrated reduced need for mechanical ventilation and mortality in a cohort of patients receiving high-dose methylprednisolone. Although more recent observational studies found no survival benefit to high-dose corticosteroids [40, 41], they are routinely used in HSCT recipients with DAH.

Pulmonary veno-occlusive disease (PVOD). PVOD is a very rare complication of HSCT in which progressive occlusion of pulmonary veins and venules caused by intimal proliferation and fibrosis leads to pulmonary arterial hypertension (PAH) [42]. High-dose chemotherapy and infections are implicated as causes of PVOD. The onset is typically insidious, with progressive dyspnea and fatigue occurring 6–8 weeks after transplant [43]. Radiographic manifestations of PVOD include Kerley B lines, septal thickening, and poorly defined centrilobular ground glass opacities on CT scans. Right heart catheterization will reveal an elevated mean pulmonary artery pressure, but normal or low pulmonary capillary wedge pressure. The diagnosis of PAH secondary to PVOD is primarily one of exclusion and should be suspected in the HSCT patient, once alternative etiologies for PAH have been excluded; a definitive diagnosis is rendered only by surgical lung biopsy. No definitive treatment aside from lung transplantation is available for this condition. Some patients do tolerate arterial vasodilators, but fatal pulmonary edema has been described with the use of arterial vasodilators [44]. Although data from randomized, controlled trials for pharmacologic treatment of PAH secondary to PVOD do not exist, there are case reports documenting improvement in exercise capacity, dyspnea score, and hemodynamics in patients receiving treatment with either sildenafil alone, or sildenafil in conjunction with high-dose intravenous epoprostenol [45, 46].

Pulmonary alveolar proteinosis (PAP). PAP is another rare complication that may occur within the first 3 months after HSCT [47, 48]. Patients typically present with slowly progressive dyspnea and a nonproductive cough. Bilateral diffuse alveolar densities and diffuse ground glass attenuation with superimposed interlobular septal thickening and intralobular lines suggesting a "crazy paving" pattern on chest CT are nonspecific, but supportive, radiographic findings (see Fig. 13.9a). Bronchoscopic examination demonstrates copious, milky BAL effluent, which on cytologic examination contains foamy macrophages engorged with periodic acid-Schiff-positive intracellular inclusions and granular, acellular eosinophilic proteinaceous material (see Fig. 13.9b). Concentrically laminated phospholipid lamellar bodies may be seen on electron microscopy, which is occasionally necessary to confirm the diagnosis. Spontaneous reversal of PAP has been described after the resolution of neutropenia or an associated infection, when present. In patients with severe dyspnea and/or significant hypoxemia, whole lung lavage has been an effective form of treatment [49]. Preliminary data suggest that GM-CSF administered either subcutaneously or via nebulization improves lung function in some patients [50]. There is no role for corticosteroids, since they may increase mortality.

Late-Onset Noninfectious Complications of HSCT

Cryptogenic organizing pneumonitis (COP) [formerly, bronchiolitis obliterans organizing pneumonia (BOOP)]. COP occurs mostly in allogeneic HSCT recipients with GVHD or following CMV pneumonitis [51], with an onset usually between 1 and 13 months after transplantation. It is less common

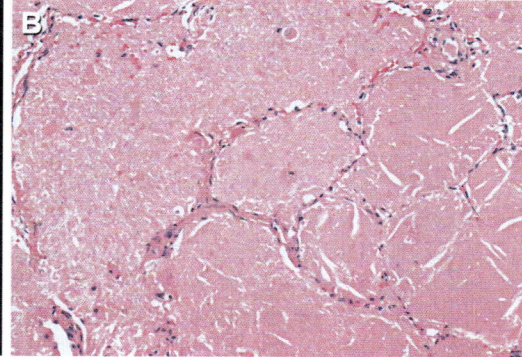

Fig. 13.9 *Pulmonary alveolar proteinosis* (PAP) in a patient with chronic myeloid leukemia. (**A**) CT chest demonstrates a "crazy paving" pattern, with a network of smoothly thickened reticular (i.e., septal) lines superimposed on ground glass opacities. (**B**) Histopathologic findings in PAP include the filling of alveolar spaces with eosinophilic proteinaceous material, which may stain periodic acid-Schiff-positive

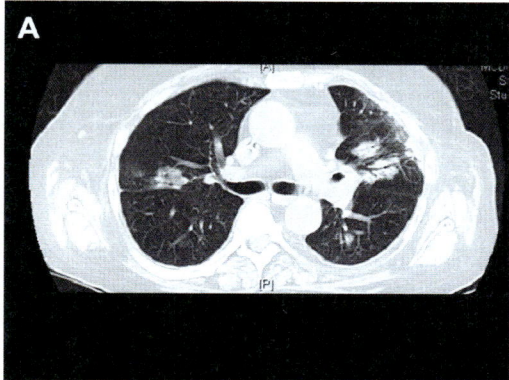
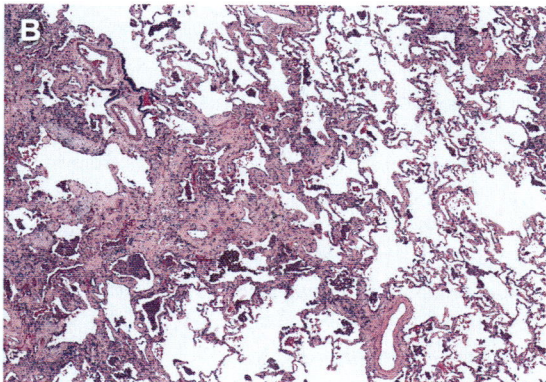

Fig. 13.10 *Organizing pneumonia* in a patient with a history of chronically waxing and waning pulmonary infiltrates. (**A**) Patchy airspace consolidation with air bronchograms, often in a subpleural location, is a characteristic radiographic presentation for organizing pneumonia. (**B**) On histopathologic examination, granulation tissue can be seen within the lumen of the distal air spaces, swirling into alveoli, associated with chronic inflammation in the surrounding alveoli

than posttransplantation constrictive bronchiolitis (PTCB) and should not be confused with it. Cough and fever are the most common symptoms on presentation; dyspnea, if present, is mild, and in some cases, patients are asymptomatic [52]. COP usually presents with patchy bilateral alveolar opacities which can be migratory on chest radiograph. The opacities have a lower lobe predominance and are peripheral in location. They may appear as ground glass opacities or consolidation with air bronchograms on high-resolution CT scans (see Fig. 13.10a). Occasionally, COP can present radiographically as a solitary nodule or mass mimicking a neoplasm or chronic nonresolving pneumonia. In one retrospective study of 43 cancer patients, 81% of patients with solid organ tumors had nodular or mass-like radiographic abnormalities and 19% presented with diffuse infiltrates [53]. In the same study, diffuse infiltrates were seen in the majority of patients with hematologic malignancies, including HSCT, and mimicked infection and drug-induced toxicity.

Pathologically, COP is characterized by the presence of granulation tissue within the lumen of the distal air spaces with or without bronchoalveolar involvement (see Fig. 13.10b). This pathologic picture can be seen with multiple other accompanying diagnoses, such as congestive heart failure, infections, and drug-induced toxicity; hence, in the HSCT recipient, other diagnoses should be excluded before a diagnosis of COP is made.

COP is highly responsive to corticosteroids. The minimal effective dose and duration of therapy are unknown; however, a prolonged steroid course with a slow taper is usually necessary due to high relapse rates. Macrolides have been used with success in some cases and might be considered in those individuals who are intolerant to steroid therapy or in whom relapse occurs [54]. Although the specific mechanism of action is not known, macrolides are thought to exert their beneficial effects through anti-inflammatory rather than antimicrobial activities.

Posttransplantation constrictive bronchiolitis (PTCB). PTCB is the most common pulmonary complication among long-term survivors of HSCT and is considered a manifestation of chronic GVHD. Contrary to COP, PTCB patients present with dyspnea without significant infiltrates on chest radiograph. While chest

CT imaging may show a mosaic pattern, it is often unremarkable even with advanced disease, presumably due to the uniformity of small airway obstruction. Since this disorder is not likely to be confused with pneumonia, it is not further considered here.

Posttransplantation lymphoproliferative disorder (PTLD). PTLD is an uncontrolled expansion of donor-derived EBV-infected B lymphocytes which develops in response to inadequate cytotoxic T-cell function [27, 55]. It occurs in approximately 1% of HSCT patients, usually within the first 4–12 months after transplant. The clinical constellation may include fever, lymphadenopathy, pharyngitis, hepatosplenomegaly, and neurologic symptoms. There appears to be a greater incidence of fulminant, disseminated PTLD in HSCT recipients as compared to solid organ transplant recipients, possibly accounting for the increased mortality associated with PTLD in this population [56]. The lung is involved only 20% of the time, usually as a component of disseminated disease, most commonly with ill-defined nodular infiltrates. It can also present as well-defined nodules, surrounded by a rim of ground glass density (halo sign), mimicking the features of invasive aspergillosis. Hilar and mediastinal adenopathy, and pleural effusions may also be seen. PTLD may be treated with anti-B-cell antibody therapy; rituximab (human–mouse chimeric monoclonal anti-CD20 antibody) is used for this purpose, with favorable response profiles and acceptable toxicity rates [57]. It has also been successfully treated with chemotherapy, as well as donor leukocytes.

Delayed pulmonary toxicity syndrome. This syndrome has been described in breast cancer patients undergoing autologous HSCT. Patients usually present around 10 weeks following transplantation with dry cough, dyspnea, and fever [58]. It is characterized by interstitial pneumonitis and fibrosis and is thought to be due to the toxic effects of high-dose chemotherapy, including cyclophosphamide, cisplatin, and BCNU. Pulmonary function testing reveals restrictive lung disease and a reduction in diffusing capacity. These patients respond favorably to steroid therapy, and the mortality rate is low.

Transfusion-Related Acute Lung Injury

Transfusion-related acute lung injury (TRALI) is defined as NCPE related to the transfusion of blood products. It is the leading cause of mortality from transfusions [59] and has been associated with all plasma-containing blood products, including immunoglobulins. The true incidence of TRALI is not known, but has been estimated at 0.02% per unit transfused and 0.16% per patient transfused [60]. Patients with TRALI commonly present with dyspnea, cough, fever, acute hypoxemia, and hypotension, generally within 1–6 h after the transfusion. Bilateral pulmonary infiltrates develop on chest radiograph. Transient leukopenia, due to pulmonary sequestration of the circulating pool of leukocytes, may be observed.

The mainstay of treatment for TRALI is to discontinue the transfusion, followed by supportive care, which includes administration of supplemental oxygen, resuscitation with intravenous fluids, and implementation of mechanical ventilatory support, when indicated. Although there has never been a randomized, controlled trial of glucocorticoid therapy, they have no demonstrated role in the treatment of TRALI and no effect on the 5–8% mortality. With supportive treatment, infiltrates resolve, usually within 96 h, and survivors have no long-term sequelae [61].

Small Airway Mucus Impaction

Peripheral lung linear and/or tree-in-bud opacities can be seen on chest CT in cancer patients due to impaction of small airways (bronchioles and distal bronchi) with mucus, accompanied to a variable extent by airway inflammation (see Fig. 13.11). These opacities often involve the right middle lobe and lingula, but can be seen in other lung regions. The differential diagnosis includes asthma, noninvasive fungal infection of the airway in a patient with or without a known asthmatic diathesis, recent viral infection, atypical mycobacterial infection, or impaired pathogen clearance due to immunosuppression. The importance of seeking a pathogen and the role of antibiotic treatment is not clear. We have found that physical measures directed at clearing impacted mucus from distal airways can be helpful. Aerosolization of 4 ml of 7% hypertonic saline solution twice daily has resulted in reduced cough, reduced sputum, and clearance of radiographic opacities in

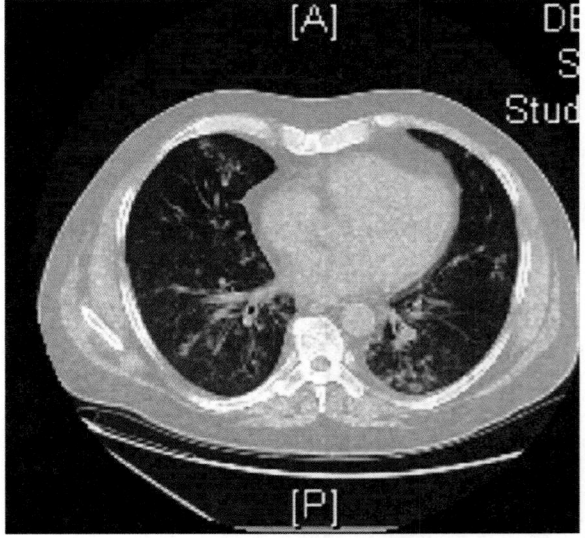

Fig. 13.11 Tree-in-bud infiltrates suggestive of *mucus impaction* in the small airways

some patients [62, 63]. An expiratory flutter valve may also be used to improve mucus clearance. In the case of mucus impaction following a viral respiratory infection, the virus has generally been cleared by the time radiographic abnormalities become evident. If an *Aspergillus* sp. is found in the airway lumen, antifungal agents are usually prescribed. It is debatable whether the morbidity imposed by use of multiple antibiotics to attempt to clear an atypical mycobacterial infection of the airways, in particular due to *M. avium* complex (MAC), is warranted, especially if minimal or no symptoms are present and radiographic and lung function changes are not progressive. In summary, there are no good studies to delineate the best treatment of this syndrome with or without MAC isolation.

Miscellaneous

Additional noninfectious causes of pulmonary infiltrates include pulmonary infarction from thromboembolic disease and metastatic or primary cancer. Venous thromboembolism is common in cancer patients [64] and may progress to lung infarction with radiographic infiltrates. If this diagnosis is suspected, a CT angiogram can be helpful in the differential diagnosis between pulmonary infarction and pneumonia. Infiltration of the lungs by cancer can also be mistaken for pneumonia. Rounded metastases to the lungs may resemble fungal or *Nocardia* infection, and localized lymphangitic spread can resemble viral or bacterial infection (see Fig. 13.12a, b). While

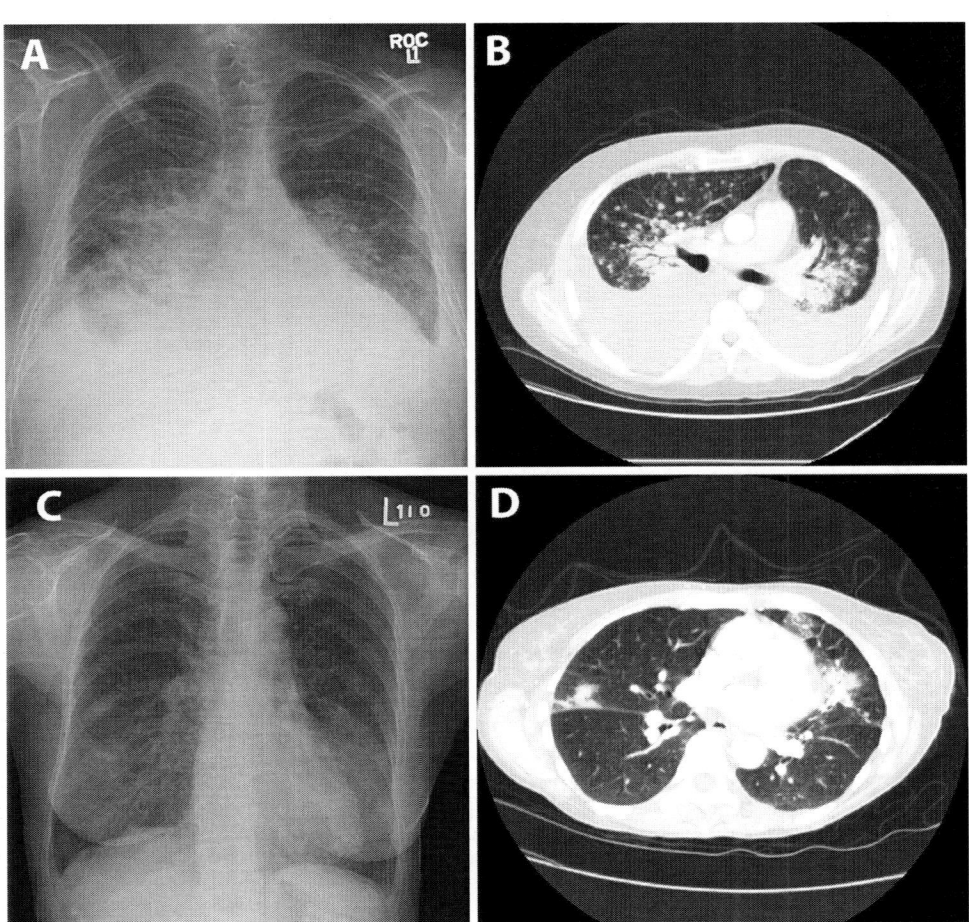

Fig. 13.12 *Tumor infiltration of lung tissue that can be confused with pneumonia. Top panel.* (**A**) On the left is an admission PA radiograph, of a 36 year old male with Hodgkin lymphoma diagnosed four years earlier. (**B**) On the right is a chest CT image the same day showing bilateral pleural effusions, hilar adenopathy, and perihilar consolidation, with multiple small nodules that are not contiguous with the consolidations. Despite extensive treatment with chemotherapy, there was progression of lung infiltrates. These were treated with multiple courses of antibiotics, despite the fact that video-assisted thoracoscopic biopsies of both lungs one year earlier, had all shown Hodgkin lymphoma. *Bottom panel.* The patient is a 68 year old female with chronic lymphocytic leukemia for seven years. On no treatment and routine follow-up, her white count had risen to 86,800 with an absolute lymphocyte count of 66,800, and she had developed a cough. (**C**) On the left, is an outpatient PA radiograph showing faint scattered lung infiltrates. (**D**) On the right, is a CT of the chest the same day showing new areas of consolidation. Transbronchial lung biopsy of the left lingula showed small lymphocytes with hyperchromatic nuclei, with the majority positive for both PAX-5 and CD5. The pathologic diagnosis was B-cell lymphocytic leukemia involving the lung parenchyma, with no evidence of acute pneumonia. Lymphoma and bronchoalveolar cancer are two malignancies that often mimic pneumonia, since they present with airspace consolidation, often with air bronchograms

infiltration of the lungs with malignant cells should be suspected in any patient with known cancer, atypical appearances due to prior treatment can complicate the presentation.

Summary

Multiple common noninfectious disorders in cancer patients are associated with radiographic lung infiltrates that can be confused with infectious pneumonia. Pneumonia is a serious complication in cancer patients and leads to an appropriately high index of suspicion, but accurate diagnosis of both infectious and noninfectious etiologies of lung infiltrates is essential to optimal treatment. The identification of noninfectious etiologies of lung infiltrates can sometimes be made on the basis of clinical findings and imaging studies, but invasive studies are sometimes necessary.

References

1. Yeh ET, Bickford C. Cardiovascular complications of cancer therapy: incidence, pathogenesis, diagnosis, and management. J Am Coll Cardiol. 2009;53(24):2231–47.
2. Hunt SA, Abraham WT, Chin MH, et al. 2009 Focused update incorporated into the ACC/AHA 2005 Guidelines for the Diagnosis and Management of Heart Failure in Adults: a report of the American College of Cardiology Foundation/American Heart Association Task Force on Practice Guidelines: developed in collaboration with the International Society for Heart and Lung Transplantation. Circulation. 2009;119(14):e391–479.
3. Wilson JF. In the Clinic. Heart failure. Ann Intern Med. 2007;147(11):ITC12-1-16.
4. Ware LB, Matthay MA. Clinical practice. Acute pulmonary edema. N Engl J Med. 2005;353(26):2788–96.
5. Maeder MT, Kaye DM. Heart failure with normal left ventricular ejection fraction. J Am Coll Cardiol. 2009;53(11):905–18.
6. Kollef MH, Schuster DP. The acute respiratory distress syndrome. N Engl J Med. 1995;332(1):27–37.
7. Piantadosi CA, Schwartz DA. The acute respiratory distress syndrome. Ann Intern Med. 2004;141(6):460–70.
8. Lohani S, O'Driscoll BR, Woodcock AA. 25-year study of lung fibrosis following carmustine therapy for brain tumor in childhood. Chest. 2004;126(3):1007.
9. Grande C, Villanueva MJ, Huidobro G, Casal J. Docetaxel-induced interstitial pneumonitis following non-small-cell lung cancer treatment. Clin Transl Oncol. 2007;9(9):578–81.
10. Sleijfer S. Bleomycin-induced pneumonitis. Chest. 2001;120(2):617–24.
11. Rivera MP, Kris MG, Gralla RJ, White DA. Syndrome of acute dyspnea related to combined mitomycin plus vinca alkaloid chemotherapy. Am J Clin Oncol. 1995;18(3):245–50.
12. Camus P, Bonniaud P, Fanton A, Camus C, Baudaun N, Foucher P. Drug-induced and iatrogenic infiltrative lung disease. Clin Chest Med. 2004;25(3):479–519, vi.
13. Copper Jr JA. Drug-induced lung disease. Adv Intern Med. 1997;42:231–68.
14. Erasmus JJ, McAdams HP, Rossi SE. High-resolution CT of drug-induced lung disease. Radiol Clin North Am. 2002;40(1):61–72.
15. Morikawa M, Demura Y, Mizuno S, Ameshima S, Ishizaki T, Okazawa H. FDG positron emission tomography imaging of drug-induced pneumonitis. Ann Nucl Med. 2008;22(4):335–8.
16. Costabel U, Guzman J, Bonella F, Oshimo S. Bronchoalveolar lavage in other interstitial lung diseases. Semin Respir Crit Care Med. 2007;28(5):514–24.
17. Yale SH, Limper AH. *Pneumocystis carinii* pneumonia in patients without acquired immunodeficiency syndrome: associated illness and prior corticosteroid therapy. Mayo Clin Proc. 1996;71(1):5–13.
18. Bollee G, Sarfati C, Thiery G, et al. Clinical picture of Pneumocystis jiroveci pneumonia in cancer patients. Chest. 2007;132(4):1305–10.
19. McDonald S, Rubin P, Phillips TL, Marks LB. Injury to the lung from cancer therapy: clinical syndromes, measurable endpoints, and potential scoring systems. Int J Radiat Oncol Biol Phys. 1995;31(5):1187–203.
20. De Jaeger K, Seppenwoolde Y, Boersma LJ, et al. Pulmonary function following high-dose radiotherapy of non-small-cell lung cancer. Int J Radiat Oncol Biol Phys. 2003;55(5):1331–40.
21. Abid SH, Malhotra V, Perry MC. Radiation-induced and chemotherapy-induced pulmonary injury. Curr Opin Oncol. 2001;13(4):242–8.
22. Arbetter KR, Prakash UB, Tazelaar HD, Douglas WW. Radiation-induced pneumonitis in the "nonirradiated" lung. Mayo Clin Proc. 1999;74(1):27–36.
23. Catane R, Schwade JG, Turrisi 3rd AT, Webber BL, Muggia FM. Pulmonary toxicity after radiation and bleomycin: a review. Int J Radiat Oncol Biol Phys. 1979;5(9):1513–8.
24. Gross N. Pulmonary effects of radiation therapy. Ann Intern Med. 1977;86:81–92.
25. Rubin P, Casarett GW. Clinical radiation pathology. Philadelphia: WB Saunders; 1968. p. 423–70.
26. Stover DE, Milite F, Zakowski M. A newly recognized syndrome: radiation-related bronchiolitis obliterans and organizing pneumonia. A case report and literature review. Respiration. 2001;68(5):540–4.
27. Kotloff RM, Ahya VN, Crawford SW. Pulmonary complications of solid organ and hematopoietic stem cell transplantation. Am J Respir Crit Care Med. 2004;170(1):22–48.
28. Limdo H, Lee J, Lee HG, et al. Pulmonary complications after hematopoietic stem cell transplantation. J Korean Med Sci. 2006;21(3):406–11.
29. Spitzer TR. Engraftment syndrome following hematopoietic stem cell transplantation. Bone Marrow Transplant. 2001;27(9):893–8.
30. Capizzi SA, Kumar S, Huneke NE, et al. Peri-engraftment respiratory distress syndrome during autologous hematopoietic stem cell transplantation. Bone Marrow Transplant. 2001;27(12):1299–303.
31. Clark JG, Hansen JA, Hertz MI, Parkman R, Jensen L, Peavy HH. NHLBI workshop summary. Idiopathic pneumonia syndrome after bone marrow transplantation. Am Rev Respir Dis. 1993;147(6 Pt 1):1601–6.
32. Watkins TR, Chien JW, Crawford SW. Graft versus host-associated pulmonary disease and other idiopathic pulmonary complications after hematopoietic stem cell transplant. Semin Respir Crit Care Med. 2005;26(5):482–9.
33. Yanik G, Hellerstedt B, Custer J, et al. Etanercept (Enbrel) administration for idiopathic pneumonia syndrome after allogeneic hematopoietic stem cell transplantation. Biol Blood Marrow Transplant. 2002;8(7):395–400.
34. Yanik GA, Ho VT, Levine JE, et al. The impact of soluble tumor necrosis factor receptor etanercept on the treatment of idiopathic pneumonia syndrome after allogeneic hematopoietic stem cell transplantation. Blood. 2008;112(8):3073–81.
35. Tun HW, Wallace KH, Grinton SF, Khoor A, Burger CD. Etanercept therapy for late-onset idiopathic pneumonia syndrome after nonmyeloablative allogeneic hematopoietic stem cell transplantation. Transplant Proc. 2005;37(10):4492–6.

36. Shukla M, Yang S, Milla C, Panoskaltsis-Mortari A, Blazar BR, Haddad IY. Absence of host tumor necrosis factor receptor 1 attenuates manifestations of idiopathic pneumonia syndrome. Am J Physiol Lung Cell Mol Physiol. 2005;288(5):L942–9.
37. Robbins RA, Linder J, Stahl MG, et al. Diffuse alveolar hemorrhage in autologous bone marrow transplant recipients. Am J Med. 1989;87(5):511–8.
38. Afessa B, Tefferi A, Litzow MR, Krowka MJ, Wylam ME, Peters SG. Diffuse alveolar hemorrhage in hematopoietic stem cell transplant recipients. Am J Respir Crit Care Med. 2002;166(5):641–5.
39. Jules-Elysee K, Stover DE, Yahalom J, White DA, Gulati SC. Pulmonary complications in lymphoma patients treated with high-dose therapy autologous bone marrow transplantation. Am Rev Respir Dis. 1992;146(2):485–91.
40. Majhail NS, Parks K, Defor TE, Weisdorf DJ. Diffuse alveolar hemorrhage and infection-associated alveolar hemorrhage following hematopoietic stem cell transplantation: related and high-risk clinical syndromes. Biol Blood Marrow Transplant. 2006;12(10):1038–46.
41. Lewis ID, DeFor T, Weisdorf DJ. Increasing incidence of diffuse alveolar hemorrhage following allogeneic bone marrow transplantation: cryptic etiology and uncertain therapy. Bone Marrow Transplant. 2000;26(5):539–43.
42. Salzman D, Adkins DR, Craig F, Freytes C, LeMaistre CF. Malignancy-associated pulmonary veno-occlusive disease: report of a case following autologous bone marrow transplantation and review. Bone Marrow Transplant. 1996;18(4):755–60.
43. Trobaugh-Lotrario AD, Greffe B, Deterding R, Deutsch G, Quinones R. Pulmonary veno-occlusive disease after autologous bone marrow transplant in a child with stage IV neuroblastoma: case report and literature review. J Pediatr Hematol Oncol. 2003;25(5):405–9.
44. Mandel J, Mark EJ, Hales CA. Pulmonary veno-occlusive disease. Am J Respir Crit Care Med. 2000;162(5):1964–73.
45. Kuroda T, Hirota H, Masaki M, et al. Sildenafil as adjunct therapy to high-dose epoprostenol in a patient with pulmonary veno-occlusive disease. Heart Lung Circ. 2006;15(2):139–42.
46. Barreto AC, Franchi SM, Castro CR, Lopes AA. One-year follow-up of the effects of sildenafil on pulmonary arterial hypertension and veno-occlusive disease. Braz J Med Biol Res. 2005;38(2):185–95.
47. Cordonnier C, Fleury-Feith J, Escudier E, Atassi K, Bernaudin JF. Secondary alveolar proteinosis is a reversible cause of respiratory failure in leukemic patients. Am J Respir Crit Care Med. 1994;149(3 Pt 1):788–94.
48. Tomonari A, Shirafuji N, Iseki T, et al. Acquired pulmonary alveolar proteinosis after umbilical cord blood transplantation for acute myeloid leukemia. Am J Hematol. 2002;70(2):154–7.
49. Beccaria M, Luisetti M, Rodi G, et al. Long-term durable benefit after whole lung lavage in pulmonary alveolar proteinosis. Eur Respir J. 2004;23(4):526–31.
50. Tazawa R, Hamano E, Arai T, et al. Granulocyte-macrophage colony-stimulating factor and lung immunity in pulmonary alveolar proteinosis. Am J Respir Crit Care Med. 2005;171(10):1142–9.
51. Afessa B, Litzow MR, Tefferi A. Bronchiolitis obliterans and other late onset non-infectious pulmonary complications in hematopoietic stem cell transplantation. Bone Marrow Transplant. 2001;28(5):425–34.
52. Maldonado F, Daniels CE, Hoffman EA, Yi ES, Ryu JH. Focal organizing pneumonia on surgical lung biopsy: causes, clinicoradiologic features, and outcomes. Chest. 2007;132(5):1579–83.
53. Mokhtari M, Bach PB, Tietjen PA, Stover DE. Bronchiolitis obliterans organizing pneumonia in cancer: a case series. Respir Med. 2002;96(4):280–6.
54. Stover DE, Mangino D. Macrolides: a treatment alternative for bronchiolitis obliterans organizing pneumonia? Chest. 2005;128(5):3611–7.
55. Papadopoulos EB, Ladanyi M, Emanuel D, et al. Infusions of donor leukocytes to treat Epstein–Barr virus-associated lymphoproliferative disorders after allogeneic bone marrow transplantation. N Engl J Med. 1994;330(17):1185–91.
56. Loren AW, Tsai DE. Post-transplant lymphoproliferative disorder. Clin Chest Med. 2005;26(4):631–45, vii.
57. Milpied N, Vasseur B, Parquet N, et al. Humanized anti-CD20 monoclonal antibody (Rituximab) in post transplant B-lymphoproliferative disorder: a retrospective analysis on 32 patients. Ann Oncol. 2000;11 Suppl 1:113–6.
58. Wilczynski SW, Erasmus JJ, Petros WP, Vredenburgh JJ, Folz RJ. Delayed pulmonary toxicity syndrome following high-dose chemotherapy and bone marrow transplantation for breast cancer. Am J Respir Crit Care Med. 1998;157(2):565–73.
59. Holness L, Knippen MA, Simmons L, Lachenbruch PA. Fatalities caused by TRALI. Transfus Med Rev. 2004;18(3):184–8.
60. Popovsky MA, Moore SB. Diagnostic and pathogenetic considerations in transfusion-related acute lung injury. Transfusion. 1985;25(6):573–7.
61. Looney MR, Gropper MA, Matthay MA. Transfusion-related acute lung injury: a review. Chest. 2004;126(1):249–58.
62. Donaldson SH, Bennett WD, Zeman KL, Knowles MR, Tarran R, Boucher RC. Mucus clearance and lung function in cystic fibrosis with hypertonic saline. N Engl J Med. 2006;354(3):241–50.
63. Elkins MR, Robinson M, Rose BR, et al. A controlled trial of long-term inhaled hypertonic saline in patients with cystic fibrosis. N Engl J Med. 2006;354(3):229–40.
64. Lee A. VTE in patients with cancer-diagnosis, prevention, and treatment. Thromb Res. 2008;123 Suppl 1:S50–4.

Chapter 14
Mucosal Barrier Injury and Infections

Nicole M.A. Blijlevens and J. Peter Donnelly

Abstract Neutropenia is well known as a risk factor for infectious complications of patients treated for hematological malignancies. Less is known about the impact of intensive chemotherapy on the epithelial innate immunity that protects us from infections due to opportunistic pathogens that reside on the mucosal surfaces. Injury to the mucosal barrier leads to barrier dysfunction, perturbed microbial signaling and inadequate host responses all of which increase the risk for life-threatening clinically- and microbilogically-defined infections. Greater awareness of mucosal barrier injury should help the physician to know better when and how to act when fever occurs during neutropenia.

Keywords Mucositis • Neutropenia • Infection • Cancer

Introduction

The number and variety of patients who are being treated for cancer with chemo-, radio- or targeted therapy continue to grow and more aggressive treatment modalities have resulted in a better overall survival, albeit often at the price of inducing profound damage to the host defences. Administration of potentially curative chemotherapy is relatively straightforward since internationally accepted treatment protocols dictate the dosages. Once the treatment has started, it becomes essential to monitor the patient as his natural host defence systems gradually disintegrate. Virtually, all cytotoxic therapy regimens, particularly the myeloablative regimens, deplete the pool of polymorphonuclear leucocytes, monocytes and lymphocytes and also attenuate the killing capacity of macrophages. As a result, the patient becomes further dependent on the vestiges of his innate immune system (e.g. complement, lysozyme, lectins), especially epithelial cells of the digestive tract and skin for protection against potentially lethal infectious complications. These epithelia form an anatomical and immunological barrier often referred to as the integument that serves as the front line against microbial invasion. Although these epithelia are highly organized and sophisticated structures, the barrier they create is not invincible to microorganisms, certainly not after it is damaged by anti-cancer therapy. Adequate supportive care is predicated by recognition of the disintegration of the primary host defence mechanisms aimed at early recognition and treatment of infection to improve survival.

Infections During Neutropenia

Over 50 years ago, Bodey et al. [1] showed a direct correlation between the severity and duration of neutropenia defined as an absolute neutrophil count of less than 0.5×10^9/L (500/mm^3) or a count less than 1.0×10^9/L (1,000/mm^3) expected to fall below 0.5×10^9/L (500/mm^3) and the risk of acquiring a life-threatening bacterial infection. Infections due to Gram-negative bacilli such as *Escherichia coli*, *Klebsiella pneumoniae* and *Pseudomonas aeruginosa* and Gram-positive cocci such as *Staphylococcus aureus* were notoriously lethal to patients who were undergoing treatment for acute leukaemia or lymphoma as these diseases intrinsically interfere directly with vital components of the immune system. Indeed, fever was often the first and the only sign of infection of these patients and potentially heralded a life-threatening infection which, if left untreated, might result in fulminant sepsis and even death. This led to the practice of starting therapy promptly at the onset of fever with antimicrobial agents that covered the most likely potential pathogens without waiting for the results of the blood cultures [2]. This was probably the single most important factor in saving life and became widely accepted as empirical therapy. Broad-spectrum synthetic penicillins and third- and fourth-generation cephalosporins, and carbapenems alone, or in various combinations as the

N.M.A. Blijlevens (✉)
Department of Haematology, Radboud University Nijmegen Medical Centre & Nijmegen University Centre for Infectious Diseaes,
P.O. Box 9101, 6500 HB Nijmegen, The Netherlands
e-mail: N.Blijlevens@hemat.umcn.nl

so-called double β-lactam combinations or together with an aminoglycoside were shown to be equally effective in large clinical trials that involved international cooperation [3]. However, in spite of changes in the spectrum of infectious agents, opportunistic pathogenic Gram-negative bacilli remain a threat because their virulence still accounts for serious morbidity and high early mortality rate [4]. Combination regimens of an anti-pseudomonal β-lactam, e.g. ceftazidime, and an aminoglycoside, e.g. amikacin covering *E. coli*, *P. aeruginosa*, *Klebsiella* species, other Enterobacteriaceae, and *S. aureus*, were not shown to be more effective than monotherapy [5]. These opportunistic pathogens are often part of the indigenous flora of the patient, but can be acquired during hospitalization. Whatever their origin, once they take up residence on the mucosal surfaces, they avail themselves of the opportunity to invade the body once the mucosal barrier is breached [6]. Modern anti-leukaemic therapy is inherently associated with breaches of the pulmonary and gastrointestinal mucosa, thereby allowing microorganisms originating from the damaged mucosal tracts ready access to the body [7]. Many centres therefore adopt prophylactic administration of anti-infective agents simultaneously with starting chemotherapy in an attempt to prevent these infections. A meta-analysis of 95 trials performed between 1973 and 2004 unequivocally showed a significant reduction in infection-related mortality, clinically defined and microbiologically defined infections (MDI) including bacteraemia, especially when fluoroquinolone was employed for patients treated for haematological malignancies [8]. Since these prophylactic agents were mainly targeted against the Enterobacteriaceae, a shift from Gram-negative to Gram-positive bacteria, including coagulase-negative staphylococci (CoNS) and the viridans streptococci, as the primary cause of bacteraemia in neutropenic patients was almost inevitable given their reduced susceptibility to the agents used for prophylaxis[9]. An epidemiological survey among hospitalized patients treated for haematological malignancies between 1995 and 2001 showed that approximately 70% (64% in 1995 and 76% in 2001) of all microbiologically confirmed febrile episodes were due to Gram-positive cocci and 18% (22% in 1995 and 14% in 2001) to Gram-negative bacilli [10]. Surprisingly, the use of vancomycin could be withheld empirically for treating persistent fever until the results of the cultures indicated otherwise [11]. Moreover, fever during neutropenia persisted in over 50% of 114 patients after treatment with broad-spectrum empirical therapy with or without teicoplanin [12]. A meta-analysis showed no negative impact of withholding glycopeptides on morbidity or mortality [13]. The use of leucocyte growth factors prevents febrile neutropenic episodes in patients treated for solid tumour or lymphoma only when the risk of febrile neutropenia is around 20%, but fails to do so in patients treated for leukaemia as most studies showed a shortening of duration of neutropenia, but no reduction in the incidence of febrile neutropenia or infections [14]. A recent meta-analysis could only show a slight reduction in MDI when growth factors were given to stem cell transplant (SCT) recipients after myeloablative conditioning [15]. The incidence of febrile neutropenia in those SCT recipients is almost 100%, but severe neutropenia is particularly short. These data indicate that duration of neutropenia is not necessarily the sole driver of the infection rate and many other factors play a role. Chemotherapeutic regimens designed to treat patients with acute lymphoblastic leukaemia incorporate high doses of corticosteroids rendering patients susceptible to infections typically related to impaired cellular immunity. The use of monoclonal antibodies further extends the suppression of B- and T-cell functions particularly when coinciding with prolonged, severe neutropenia.

Epithelial Innate Immunity

Only recently, it has become clear that the innate immune system not only specifically recognizes various classes of microorganisms, but also initiates and modulates the subsequent adaptive immune responses mediated by T cells and B cells through their interaction with antigen-presenting cells especially dendritic cells [16]. Epithelial cells as well as neutrophils and monocytes possess various pattern recognition receptors (PRRs) that sense conserved structures of the invading microorganisms, called pathogen-associated molecular patterns (PAMPs), and four major classes of PRRs have been identified; Toll-like receptors (TLR), C-type lectin receptors (LRs), NOD-like receptors (NLRs) and retinoic acid–inducible gene (RIG)-I-like receptors (RiG-I). The interaction of a PRR with a bacterial structure leads to activation of host response mechanisms, especially the release of cytokines and chemokines, responsible for elimination of the pathogen. For instance, human epithelial TLR4 directly protects the mucosa from *Candida* infection via a process involving cytokines and chemokines mediated by polymorphonuclear leukocytes. Infiltration of leukocytes of the mucosal tissues is not required [17]. Genetic variation, including single nucleotide polymorphisms (SNPs) in the non-HLA genes coding for PRRs, has been associated with increased susceptibility of SCT recipients to various bacterial and fungal infections [18]. For example, mannose-binding lectin (MBL2) is a PRR that activates complement independently of a specific antibody. MBL2 polymorphisms resulting in low MBL levels were associated with primary bacteraemia when there was mucosal damage following myeloablative TBI to prepare for an SCT [19].

A robust association between SNPs in NOD2/CARD15 and the outcome of allogeneic SCT has been reported by Holler et al. [20]. NOD2 is an intracytosolic PRR that senses the cell-wall component muramyl dipeptide (MDP) of certain bacteria and is expressed in Paneth cells, dendritic cells, neutrophils and monocytes [21]. Altered function due to NOD2 polymorphisms can result in uncontrolled inflammation of the gut mucosa, which plays a pathogenic role in Crohn's disease and acute GvHD [22]. Interestingly, this SNP effect was strongly reduced among SCT patients receiving oral intestinal decontamination with agents active mainly against Gram-positive bacteria. Finally, a wide array of cytokine gene polymorphisms has been studied in the context of SCT, including polymorphisms in IL10, TNF, IFNγ, IL6, IL1 and TGFβ1 [23]. The variety of SNPs influences the balance between activation of pro-inflammatory cytokines and the down-regulation of inflammation in mucosal tissues damaged by conditioning regimens. This inflammatory response is the first step in the development of acute GvHD after exposure to bacterial products (e.g. LPS) that cross the perturbed gastrointestinal barrier. The intact gastrointestinal epithelial barrier is capable in withstanding microbial invasion by expressing and secreting antimicrobial products including defensins, lipopolysaccharide-binding protein (LBP), lysozyme and cathelicidins, without any accompanying pro-inflammatory responses [24]. The intestinal tract is actually unique in this respect as it is constantly exposed to rich and varied commensal flora and infrequently to pathogenic bacteria. Most commensal microorganisms colonize the mucosal surfaces without gaining direct access to the epithelial barrier which is restricted to the strictly residential flora. Once the mucous layer recedes, attachment to the epithelial barrier can occur as first step in the process of translocation. Treatment with cytotoxic drugs places the epithelial defences under severe stress resulting in a process called mucosal barrier injury (MBI) [7].

Mucosal Barrier Injury

The pathobiology of cytotoxic therapy-induced mucositis was first described in 2004 and details are still being unravelled [25]. Briefly, the process begins as an inflammatory complication of anti-cancer treatment and occurs in five biological phases: (1) the initiation phase of free radical generation and induction of apoptotic cell death induced by both DNA and non-DNA damage, (2) the up-regulation and message generation phase where the master transcription factor, nuclear factor-κB (NF-κB), leads to the up-regulation of many genes resulting in the production of pro-inflammatory cytokines, (3) the amplification and signalling phase of these pro-inflammatory cytokines (TNF-α, IL1 and IL6), (4) Ulcerations, crypt hypoplasia, villous atrophy and cleavage of extracellular-matrix substrates such as collagen and fibronectin by activated matrix metalloproteinases are the net result. Microorganisms and their cell-wall products such as peptidoglycan and lipopolysacharide can breach the damaged physical barrier more easily and are able to activate tissue macrophages to produce more pro-inflammatory cytokines. The healing phase is the final stage in the process (5) when trefoil factors, secretory products of mucin-producing Goblet cells, in concert with matrix metalloproteinases down-regulate inflammation and restore the integrity of the mucosal barrier [26, 27]. Endogenous production of keratinocyte growth factor (KGF) is accelerated exclusively by mesenchymal cells, particularly fibroblasts. KGF is a paracrine mediator of mesenchymal-epithelial communication that plays a key role in maintaining the barrier function of epithelial tissues and the healing process after injury [28]. Mucositis of the entire alimentary tract is the clinical manifestation of the pathobiological process of MBI. Systemic drug exposure appears to be the key determinant of severe mucositis in a prospective audit of 197 patients with multiple myeloma (MM) or non-Hodgkin lymphoma (NHL) undergoing, respectively, high-dose melphalan (HDM) or BEAM chemotherapy and autologous stem cell transplantation [29]. Patients were 2.6 times more likely to develop severe mucositis when the dose of melphalan increased by 1 mg/kg of body weight. Dosing melphalan per kilogram bodyweight in either HDM or BEAM regimens tended to predict the risk of severe mucositis far better than dosing per body surface area [30, 31]. Furthermore, patients receiving a dose ≥70 mg/m² of melphalan had a 23-fold increased risk of developing mucositis ($p < 0.001$) compared with those receiving lower doses irrespective of depth of neutropenia [32]. Patients developing severe mucositis had a higher incidence of fever (68% vs. 47%, $p = 0.004$), more days of fever (4.2 vs. 3.0 days; $p = 0.033$) as well as a higher incidence of MDI (27% vs. 12%; $p = 0.013$) [33]. The length of hospital stay was increased by 2 days during chemotherapy cycles when both oral and gut mucositis were present [34]. The risk of mortality among SCT recipients suffering from severe oral mucositis was also increased [35]. Overall survival was significantly worse in patients with severe mucositis after high-dose chemotherapy regimen followed by autologous stem cell transplantation because of relapsed lymphoid malignancy [36].

Mucosal Barrier Injury and Infection

The median time to the onset of fever during neutropenia is around 12 days after starting myeloablative conditioning therapy when mucositis is at its worst and is independent of the nadir of neutropenia [37]. The inflammatory response measured by CRP and body temperature coincided with the occurrence of mucositis irrespective of the duration of neutropenia in 67 autologous SCT patients after HDM [38].

The systemic inflammatory response as measured by CRP, LPS-binding protein and IL8 of allogeneic SCT recipients after myeloablative conditioning was also predominantly related to the course of mucosal damage measured either by mucositis scoring scales, plasma citrulline levels or permeability tests [39]. The estimated surface area of the small intestine of adults is 200–300 m² and is roughly equivalent to the area of a soccer pitch. Damage of the epithelial lining of the small intestinal tract can be accurately documented by estimating the concentration of plasma citrulline which is almost exclusively produced by functional enterocytes [40]. The magnitude of the mucositis-related inflammatory response is not only boosted by bacteraemia, but often precedes it [41]. This is consistent with a study on rats exposed to chemotherapy in which the release of pro-inflammatory cytokines was associated with evolving mucositis and preceded microbial translocation [42]. Low citrulline levels reflecting intestinal MBI, rather than neutropenia per se, are associated with onset of bacteraemia [41]. In general, the risk of infection and use of antibiotics are significantly higher during chemotherapy cycles that are complicated by mucositis than during cycles without mucositis [34]. In particular, infections due to Gram-positive cocci tend to occur more frequently during cycles complicated by gut mucositis. Nowadays, Gram-positive cocci account for three of every four episodes of bacteraemia affecting patients treated for haematological malignancies (SCOPE project) [10]. CoNS are the most frequent isolates and, although CoNS bacteraemia is frequently associated with the use of central venous catheters, mucosal sites are also known to be an important portal of entry for these bacteria [43]. Indeed, plasmid pattern analysis of bacteraemic isolates of CoNS showed that the mucosa was the origin in 70% in haematology patients. CoNS bacteraemia mostly occurred within the first 2 weeks after transplant when gut integrity was markedly disturbed [44]. Bacteraemia due to oral viridans streptococci (OVS), mainly *Streptococcus mitis* and *S. oralis*, is clearly related to mucosal damage and can be associated with more serious complications such as sepsis and adult respiratory distress syndrome which carry a high mortality (80%) [45, 46]. Recipients of autologous SCT with oral ulcerative mucositis were found to be three times more likely to develop OVS bacteraemia than those without mucositis and the streptococci were isolated from blood cultures a median of 6 days (range 2–8 days) after transplant which is typically when the peak of mucositis occurs [47]. Drug-induced achlorhydria and the use of antimicrobial prophylaxis with fluoroquinolones contribute toward the development of OVS bacteraemia [48]. Significantly more patients develop infectious complications, including streptococcal bacteraemia, when the dose of cytarabine was increased from standard (200 mg/m²) to intermediate (1,000 mg/m²) [49]. Recently, a simple scoring system for predicting streptococcal infection was proposed, but unfortunately did not include mucositis [50]. Adding mucositis to the MASCC risk-index score used to assess low-risk febrile neutropenia patients might also further improve the tool [51]. *Candida* species normally reside on the mucosal surfaces of the digestive tract of many adults. Adherence to these surfaces appears to be a prerequisite for local infection and subsequent invasive disease since regular surveillance cultures of haematological patients have shown that colonization invariably precedes infection [52]. Patients treated for AML who developed invasive candidiasis had significantly lower serum D-xylose levels indicating malabsorption with the maximum difference noted at week 2 after start than patients without invasive disease [53]. SCT recipients prepared with regimens composed of TBI and patients treated with remission-induction regimens containing either high-dose cytarabine or an anthracycline have an increased risk of developing invasive *Candida* disease. The risk of candidaemia is also increased when patients suffer from a clinical picture designated as neutropenic enterocolitis or typhlitis [53]. The current term NE is used to describe an inflammatory process involving the colon, mainly caecum and adjacent parts of the small bowel in the context of chemotherapy-induced neutropenia and mucosal damage. NE is the example of MBI-related infection (Fig. 14.1). NE can potentially result in life-threatening complications such as ischemia, necrosis, haemorrhage, bacteraemia and perforation. There have only been a few prospective surveys published, but the incidence of NE is estimated to be 6.5% [54]. Mortality rates vary between 50 and 100% [55]. A systematic review of 21 studies (mainly case reports and reviews) reported a pooled incidence rate of 5.6% (84/1,489; 95% CI: 4.6–6.9%) in a subgroup of patients exclusively treated with intensive chemotherapy [56]. A similar analysis showed that 80% of patients with NE had been treated for haematological

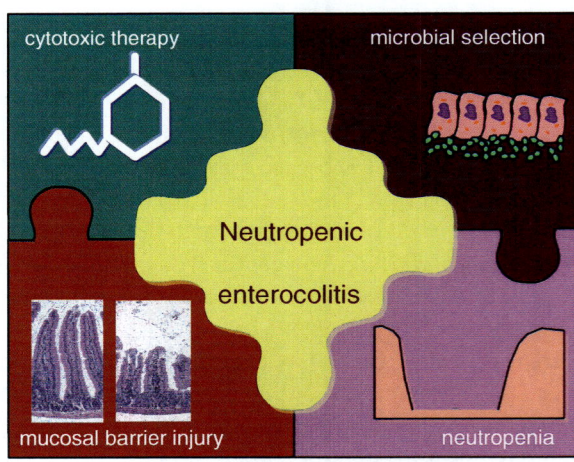

Fig. 14.1 Neutropenic enterocolitis – an example of mucosal barrier injury (MBI)-related infection

malignancies and that the overall mortality related to NE was 38% [57]. The common clinical manifestations of NE are fever, abdominal pain and diarrhoea [58]. These symptoms are not specific to NE and must be differentiated from other causes of abdominal complications such as appendicitis, pseudo-membranous colitis, ischemic colitis, obstruction and intussusceptions. NE occurs between 10 and 30 days after start of the cytotoxic treatment coinciding with MBI. Ultrasound sonography (US) or computer tomography (CT) proved to be more valuable in diagnosis and monitoring of clinical cases suspected of NE. The normal thickness of the bowel wall visualized by US is <2 mm and a thickening of >5 mm is considered abnormal and consistent with NE. Bowel wall thickening (BWT) between 2 and 5 mm is more difficult to interpret [59] and most reports adopt a threshold of >3 mm as being abnormal and supporting the diagnosis of NE. The typical five-layer morphology of ileum and colon seen by US and not CT scan is called the "gut-signature," suggesting that US is more accurate in measuring BWT [60]. However, the CT scan allows NE to be differentiated from other intestinal complications.

Summary

Recognizing MBI as an inflammatory complication of cytotoxic therapy should compel clinicians to change their approach in directing supportive therapy to those patients at greatest risk of developing infections during neutropenia (Table 14.1) Growth factors like recombinant human interleukin-11 which protect the integrity of the gut lowered the rate of bacteraemia in patients treated for acute leukaemia [61]. Moreover, the recombinant growth factor palifermin was able to significantly reduce the risk of febrile neutropenia and the rate of severe mucositis in patients undergoing SCT [62]. The possibility of treating or even preventing severe MBI will be an important step towards decreasing the infectious complications experienced by patients given intensive chemotherapy.

Table 14.1 MBI as a risk factor for infection

Why	The ulcerative phase of MBI allows translocation of residential microorganisms and their products from the alimentary tract into the bloodstream
Who	Intensive therapy for AML, MDS and HSCT recipients following myeloablative therapy
What	MBI as manifest by oral and gut mucositis
Where	Probably the gingival borders, soft tissues of the oral cavity, oesophagus, ileum, cecum and rectum
When	Second part of intensive chemotherapy, early (<14 days) after transplant, and during gut GVHD

References

1. Bodey GP, Buckley M, Sathe YS, Freireich EJ. Quantitative relationships between circulating leukocytes and infection in patients with acute leukemia. Ann Intern Med. 1966;64(2):328–40.
2. Schimpff SC, Satterlee W, Young VM, Serpick A. Empiric therapy with carbenicillin and gentamicin for febrile patients with cancer and granulocytopenia. N Engl J Med. 1971;284:1061–5.
3. De Pauw BE, Deresinski SC, Feld R, lane-Allman EF, Donnelly JP. Ceftazidime compared with piperacillin and trobramycin for the empiric treatment of fever in neutropenic patients with cancer – a multicenter randomized trial. Ann Intern Med. 1994;120:834–44.
4. Hughes WT, Armstrong D, Bodey GP, Bow EJ, Brown AE, Calandra T, et al. 2002 Guidelines for the use of antimicrobial agents in neutropic patients with cancer. Clin Infect Dis. 2002;34(6):730–51.
5. De Pauw BE, Raemaekers JM, Schattenberg A, Donnelly JP. Empirical and subsequent use of antibacterial agents in the febrile neutropenic patient. J Intern Med. 1997;242 Suppl 740:69–77.
6. Fainstein V, Rodriguez V, Turck M, Hermann G, Rosenbaum B, Bodey GP. Patterns of oropharyngeal and fecal flora in patients with adult leukemia. J Infect Dis. 1981;144:82–6.
7. Blijlevens NMA, Donnelly JP, De Pauw BE. Mucosal barrier injury: biology, pathology, clinical counterparts and consequences of intensive treatment for haematological malignancy: an overview. Bone Marrow Transplant. 2000;25:1269–78.
8. Gafter-Gvili A, Fraser A, Paul M, Leibovici L. Meta-analysis: antibiotic prophylaxis reduces mortality in neutropenic patients. Ann Intern Med. 2005;142(12 Pt 1):979–95.
9. Marchetti O, Calandra T. Infections in neutropenic cancer patients. Lancet. 2002;359(9308):723–5.
10. Wisplinghoff H, Seifert H, Wenzel RP, Edmond MB. Current trends in the epidemiology of nosocomial bloodstream infections in patients with hematological malignancies and solid neoplasms in hospitals in the United States. Clin Infect Dis. 2003;36:1103–10.
11. Vardakas KZ, Samonis G, Chrysanthopoulou SA, Bliziotis IA, Falagas ME. Role of glycopeptides as part of initial empirical treatment of febrile neutropenic patients: a meta-analysis of randomised controlled trials. Lancet Infect Dis. 2005;5(7):431–9.
12. Erjavec Z, De Vries-Hospers HG, Laseur M, Halie R, Daenen S. A prospective, randomized, double-blinded, placebo-controlled trial of empirical teicoplanin in febrile neutropenia with persistent fever after imipenem monotherapy. J Antimicrob Chemother. 2000;45:843–9.
13. Paul M, Borok S, Fraser A, Vidal L, Leibovici L. Empirical antibiotics against Gram-positive infections for febrile neutropenia: systematic review and meta-analysis of randomized controlled trials. J Antimicrob Chemother. 2005;55(4):436–44.
14. Smith TJ, Khatcheressian J, Lyman GH, Ozer H, Armitage JO, Balducci L, et al. 2006 Update of recommendations for the use of white blood cell growth factors: an evidence-based clinical practice guideline. J Clin Oncol. 2006;24(19):3187–205.
15. Dekker A, Bulley S, Beyene J, Dupuis LL, Doyle JJ, Sung L. Meta-analysis of randomized controlled trials of prophylactic granulocyte colony-stimulating factor and granulocyte-macrophage colony-stimulating factor after autologous and allogeneic stem cell transplantation. J Clin Oncol. 2006;24(33):5207–15.
16. Eckmann L. Innate immunity and mucosal bacterial interactions in the intestine. Curr Opin Gastroenterol. 2004;20(2):82–8.
17. Weindl G, Naglik JR, Kaesler S, Biedermann T, Hube B, Korting HC, et al. Human epithelial cells establish direct antifungal defense through TLR4-mediated signaling. J Clin Invest. 2007;117(12):3664–72.
18. Rocha V, Franco RF, Porcher R, Bittencourt H, Silva Jr WA, Latouche A, et al. Host defense and inflammatory gene polymorphisms are associated with outcomes after HLA-identical sibling bone marrow transplantation. Blood. 2002;100(12):3908–18.

19. Mullighan CG, Heatley SL, Danner S, Dean MM, Doherty K, Hahn U, et al. Mannose-binding lectin status is associated with risk of major infection following myeloablative sibling allogeneic hematopoietic stem cell transplantation. Blood. 2008;112(5):2120–8.
20. Holler E, Rogler G, Herfarth H, Brenmoehl J, Wild PJ, Hahn J, et al. Both donor and recipient NOD2/CARD15 mutations associate with transplant-related mortality and GvHD following allogeneic stem cell transplantation. Blood. 2004;104(3):889–94.
21. Strober W, Murray PJ, Kitani A, Watanabe T. Signalling pathways and molecular interactions of NOD1 and NOD2. Nat Rev Immunol. 2006;6(1):9–20.
22. Hugot JP, Chamaillard M, Zouali H, Lesage S, Cezard JP, Belaiche J, et al. Association of NOD2 leucine-rich repeat variants with susceptibility to Crohn's disease. Nature. 2001;411(6837):599–603.
23. Mullally A, Ritz J. Beyond HLA: the significance of genomic variation for allogeneic hematopoietic stem cell transplantation. Blood. 2007;109(4):1355–62.
24. Uehara A, Takada H. Synergism between TLRs and NOD1/2 in oral epithelial cells. J Dent Res. 2008;87(7):682–6.
25. Sonis ST. The pathobiology of mucositis. Nat Rev Cancer. 2004;4(4):277–84.
26. Beck PL, Wong JF, Li Y, Swaminathan S, Xavier RJ, Devaney KL, et al. Chemotherapy- and radiotherapy-induced intestinal damage is regulated by intestinal trefoil factor. Gastroenterology. 2004;126:796–808.
27. Parks WC, Wilson CL, Lopez-Boado YS. Matrix metalloproteinases as modulators of inflammation and innate immunity. Nat Rev Immunol. 2004;4:617–29.
28. Finch PW, Rubin JS. Keratinocyte growth factor/fibroblast growth factor 7, a homeostatic factor with therapeutic potential for epithelial protection and repair. Adv Cancer Res. 2004;91:69–136.
29. Blijlevens N, Schwenkglenks M, Bacon P, D'Addio A, Einsele H, Maertens J, et al. Prospective oral mucositis audit: oral mucositis in patients receiving high-dose melphalan or BEAM conditioning chemotherapy – European Blood and Marrow Transplantation Mucositis Advisory Group. J Clin Oncol. 2008;26(9):1519–25.
30. Grazziutti ML, Dong L, Miceli MH, Krishna SG, Kiwan E, Syed N, et al. Oral mucositis in myeloma patients undergoing melphalan-based autologous stem cell transplantation: incidence, risk factors and a severity predictive model. Bone Marrow Transplant. 2006;38(7):501–6.
31. Costa LJ, Micallef IN, Inwards DJ, Johnston PB, Porrata LF, Litzow MR, et al. Effect of the dose per body weight of conditioning chemotherapy on severity of mucositis and risk of relapse after autologous haematopoietic stem cell transplantation in relapsed diffuse large B cell lymphoma. Br J Haematol. 2008;143(2):268–73.
32. Kuhne A, Sezer O, Heider U, Meineke I, Muhlke S, Niere W, et al. Population pharmacokinetics of melphalan and glutathione S-transferase polymorphisms in relation to side effects. Clin Pharmacol Ther. 2008;83(5):749–57.
33. McCann S, Schwenkglenks M, Bacon P, Einsele H, D'Addio A, Maertens J, et al. The Prospective Oral Mucositis Audit: relationship of severe oral mucositis with clinical and medical resource use outcomes in patients receiving high-dose melphalan or BEAM-conditioning chemotherapy and autologous SCT. Bone Marrow Transplant. 2009;43(2):141–7.
34. Elting LS, Cooksley C, Chambers M, Cantor SB, Manzullo E, Rubenstein EB. The burdens of cancer therapy: clinical and economic outcomes of chemotherapy-induced mucositis. Cancer. 2003;98:1531–9.
35. Sonis ST, Oster G, Fuchs H, Bellm L, Bradford WZ, Edelsberg J, et al. Oral mucositis and the clinical and economic outcomes of hematopoietic stem-cell transplantation. J Clin Oncol. 2001;19(8):2201–5.
36. Fanning SR, Rybicki L, Kalaycio M, Andresen S, Kuczkowski E, Pohlman B, et al. Severe mucositis is associated with reduced survival after autologous stem cell transplantation for lymphoid malignancies. Br J Haematol. 2006;135(3):374–81.
37. Wardley AM, Jayson GC, Swindell R, Morgenstern GR, Chang J, Bloor R, et al. Prospective evaluation of oral mucositis in patients receiving myeloablative conditioning regimens and haematopoietic progenitor rescue. Br J Haematol. 2000;110(292):299.
38. van de Velden WJ, Blijlevens NM, Feuth T, Donnelly JP. Febrile mucositis in haematopoietic SCT recipients. Bone Marrow Transplant. 2009;43(1):55–60.
39. Blijlevens NM, Donnelly JP, DePauw BE. Inflammatory response to mucosal barrier injury after myeloablative therapy in allogeneic stem cell transplant recipients. Bone Marrow Transplant. 2005;36(8):703–7.
40. Wedlake L, McGough C, Hackett C, Thomas K, Blake P, Harrington K, et al. Can biological markers act as non-invasive, sensitive indicators of radiation-induced effects in the gastrointestinal mucosa? Aliment Pharmacol Ther. 2008;27(10):980–7.
41. Herbers AH, Blijlevens NM, Donnelly JP, de Witte TJ. Bacteraemia coincides with low citrulline concentrations after high-dose melphalan in autologous HSCT recipients. Bone Marrow Transplant. 2008;42(5):345–9.
42. Tsuji E, Hiki N, Nomura S, Fukushima R, Kojima J, Ogawa T, et al. Simultaneous onset of acute inflammatory response, sepsis-like symptoms and intestinal mucosal injury after cancer chemotherapy. Int J Cancer. 2003;107(2):303–8.
43. Costa SF, Miceli MH, Anaissie EJ. Mucosa or skin as source of coagulase-negative staphylococcal bacteraemia? Lancet Infect Dis. 2004;4(5):278–86.
44. Blijlevens NMA, van-'t Land B, Donnelly JP. Gram-positive bacteremia coincides with impaired gut integrity in HSCT recipients. Int J Infect Dis. 2002;6 Suppl 2:2S32–3.
45. Gassas A, Grant R, Richardson S, Dupuis LL, Doyle J, Allen U, et al. Predictors of viridans streptococcal shock syndrome in bacteremic children with cancer and stem-cell transplant recipients. J Clin Oncol. 2004;22(7):1222–7.
46. Vera-Llonch M, Oster G, Ford CM, Lu J, Sonis S. Oral mucositis and outcomes of allogeneic hematopoietic stem-cell transplantation in patients with hematologic malignancies. Support Care Cancer. 2007;15(5):491–6.
47. Ruescher TJ, Sodeifi A, Scrivani SJ, Kaban LB, Sonis ST. The impact of mucositis on alpha-hemolytic streptococcal infection in patients undergoing autologous bone marrow transplantation for hematologic malignancies. Cancer. 1998;82(11):2275–81.
48. Elting LS, Bodey GP, Keefe BH. Septicemia and shock syndrome due to viridans streptococci: a case-control study of predisposing factors. Clin Infect Dis. 1992;14(6):1201–7.
49. Deenik W, van der Holt B, Verhoef GE, Smit WM, Kersten MJ, Kluin-Nelemans HC, et al. Dose-finding study of imatinib in combination with intravenous cytarabine: feasibility in newly diagnosed patients with chronic myeloid leukemia. Blood. 2008;111(5):2581–8.
50. Cordonnier C, Buzyn A, Leverger G, Herbrecht R, Hunault M, Leclercq R, et al. Epidemiology and risk factors for Gram-Positive coccal infections in neutropenia: toward a more targeted antibiotic strategy. Clin Infect Dis. 2003;36:149–58.
51. de Souza V, Serufo JC, da Costa Rocha MO, Costa RN, Duarte RC. Performance of a modified MASCC index score for identifying low-risk febrile neutropenic cancer patients. Support Care Cancer. 2008;16(7):841–6.
52. Zollner-Schwetz I, Auner HW, Paulitsch A, Buzina W, Staber PB, Ofner-Kopeinig P, et al. Oral and intestinal *Candida* colonization in patients undergoing hematopoietic stem-cell transplantation. J Infect Dis. 2008;198(1):150–3.
53. Bow EJ, Loewen R, Cheang MS, Shore TB, Rubinger M, Schacter B. Cytotoxic therapy-induced D-xylose malabsorption and invasive

infection during remission-induction therapy for acute myeloid leukemia in adults. J Clin Oncol. 1997;15(6):2254–61.
54. Gorschluter M, Marklein G, Hofling K, Clarenbach R, Baumgartner S, Hah C, et al. Abdominal infections in patients with acute leukaemia: a prospective study applying ultrasonography and microbiology. Br J Haematol. 2002;117:351–8.
55. Gomez L, Martino R, Rolston KV. Neutropenic enterocolitis: spectrum of the disease and comparison of definite and possible cases. Clin Infect Dis. 1998;27:695–9.
56. Gorschluter M, Mey U, Strehl J, Ziske C, Schepke M, Schmidt-Wolf IG, et al. Neutropenic enterocolitis in adults: systematic analysis of evidence quality. Eur J Haematol. 2005;75(1):1–13.
57. Cardona AF, Ramos PL, Casasbuenas A. From case reports to systematic reviews in neutropenic enterocolitis. Eur J Haematol. 2005;75(5):445–6.
58. Sloas MM, Flynn PM, Kaste SC, Patrick CC. Typhlitis in children with cancer: a 30-year experience. Clin Infect Dis. 1993;17(3):484–90.
59. Dietrich CF, Hermann S, Klein S, Braden B. Sonographic signs of neutropenic enterocolitis. World J Gastroenterol. 2006;12(9):1397–402.
60. McCarville MB. Evaluation of typhlitis in children: CT versus US. Pediatr Radiol. 2006;36(8):890–1.
61. Ellis M, Zwaan F, Hedstrom U, Poynton CH, Kristensen J, Jumaa P, et al. Recombinant human interleukin 11 and bacterial infection in patients with haemological malignant disease undergoing chemotherapy: a double-blind placebo-controlled randomised trial. Lancet. 2003;361:275–80.
62. Spielberger R, Stiff P, Bensinger W, Gentile T, Weisdorf D, Kewalramani T, et al. Palifermin for oral mucositis after intensive therapy for hematologic cancers. N Engl J Med. 2004;351(25):2590–8.

Chapter 15
Bacterial Colonization and Host Immunity

Coralia N. Mihu, Karen J. Vigil, and Javier A. Adachi

Abstract The gastrointestinal (GI) tract is a highly evolved anatomical and functional structure that encounters a vast array of antigens, food particles, and microorganisms on a daily basis. The intestine has to perform the daunting function of absorbing nutrients essential for human life, while keeping us protected from luminal antigens, particles, and pathogens. The adult human intestine is home to an enormous number of microorganisms that is extraordinarily complex, collectively known as intestinal microbiota. Understanding our relationship with commensal flora has gained more depth in recent years; new data demonstrate that gastrointestinal microbiota plays an important role in defense against pathogenic organisms. Since it is only a thin monolayer of epithelial cells that separates us from the intestinal flora and pathogens, the intestine has acquired specialized cells organized in complex structures that have to perform the function of defending us against pathogens by initiating innate and adaptive immune responses. By constant signaling and communication, intestinal immune cells are organized in a vast and complex network that contributes to the maintenance of homeostasis.

Keywords Gastrointestinal tract • Immunity • Bacteria • Fungus • Colonization • Disease pathogenesis

Introduction

The gastrointestinal (GI) tract is one of the most complex and important organ systems. It performs two main functions: uptake of nutrients and digestion and maintaining immune homeostasis (mounting host immunological responses). Its extensive surface area – composed of a great diversity of cell types – as well as the vast amount of immune cells (the largest in the human body) and its resident microbiota makes it possible to develop these functions. Functional or genetic alteration of any of its three main components will result in the development of GI or systemic diseases.

The objective of this chapter is to provide a comprehensive review of the GI system architecture, its microbiome, the GI innate host immunity, and the complex interaction among these components.

Bacterial Colonization: Microbiota

The GI tract is the most heavily populated system by microbiota. In general, human beings have 10^{14} (100 trillion) microbes inhabiting their bodies of which 10^{12} organisms/g of fecal material are in the colon [1]. Initial culture-based studies report 400–500 distinct species in the gut microbiota, and it was estimated that >90% of them could be cultivated [2]. However, more recent 16S rRNA-based studies have shown that the gut microbiota was underestimated. The gut microbiome is diverse and includes eight phyla, with members of the Gram-negative Bacteroidetes and Gram-positive Firmicutes constituting between 60 and 80% of the total fecal community [3]. Additionally, although there is individual to individual variation, the community within an individual appears to be constant over time [4].

The GI microbiota has a mutualistic relationship with the host. Although it benefits receiving nutrients, the host takes advantage from some of its metabolic products. As an example, some bacteria from the Firmicutes division ferment nondigestible starch into short-chain fatty acids like butyrate that is not only the preferred energy source for colonocytes but also plays an important role in the maintenance of tissue homoeostasis and disease prevention [5].

Additionally, the microbiota drives some aspects of postnatal intestinal maturation. Colonization of germ-free mice with *Bacteroides thetaiotaomicron* – a component of the intestinal microflora of mice and humans – has been shown to allow the restoration of the fucosylation program in the small-intestinal epithelium that occurs during the time of

C.N. Mihu (✉)
Department of Infectious Diseases, Infection Control, and Employee Health, The University of Texas M.D. Anderson Cancer Center, 1515 Holcombe Boulevard (Unit 1460), Houston, TX 77030, USA
e-mail: CNMihu@mdanderson.org

weaning [6] and also to modulate the expression of genes involved in several important intestinal functions, including nutrient absorption, mucosal barrier fortification, xenobiotic metabolism, and angiogenesis [7].

Another microbiome–host interaction occurs in the host immune system. The microbiota provokes host immune responses. However it is still under investigation, the role of the host in the composition of the bacterial microbiota. Some studies have shown that secretory antibodies do not control its composition [8] while others have demonstrated that the host IgA is critical to its regulation of and the segmented filamentous bacteria antigens are strong stimuli of the mucosal immune system [9].

Therefore, we could say that the gut microbiota is part of a complex ecosystem along with the host mucosal epithelium and the host immunes system, and it plays a crucial role in homeostasis of the GI tract. Changes and disturbances in the GI microbiota play an important role in the pathogenesis of systemic and localized GI diseases either because of changes in the metabolic activity of an altered microbial community or because of the interaction between the microbiome and the host immune system. Perturbations of the normal microbiota have been linked to atopic dermatitis, eczema, food allergy, obesity, inflammatory bowel diseases, pouchitis, vaginitis, and infections such as antibiotic-associated diarrhea and *Clostridium difficile* infection.

In antibiotic-associated diarrhea, molecular phylogenetic analyses have shown temporal distinct changes in the diversity of fecal bacteria after antibiotic administration, including a marked decrease in the prevalence of butyrate-producing bacteria that resolved after the discontinuation of the antibiotic [10].

In *C. difficile* associated diarrhea, the fecal communities in patients with recurrent disease have been found to be highly variable in bacterial composition and characterized by markedly decreased diversity [11].

The microbial community in the human intestine may also play an important role in the pathogenesis of obesity. Collado et al. found that there is distinct composition of GI microbiota during pregnancy in overweight and normal-weight women. Bacteroides and *Staphylococcus* are significantly higher in the overweight state than in normal-weight women. Microbial counts have found to be higher in the third trimester of pregnancy, and high Bacteroides concentrations have been associated with excessive weight gain over pregnancy [12].

Finally, DNA-based techniques have demonstrated that patients with irritable bowel syndrome (IBS) have an increase number of total aerobes and great temporal instability of its microbiota [13]. Patients with different predominance of symptoms also have different microbiota. Diarrhea predominant IBS patients had lower numbers of *Lactobacilli* spp., while constipation predominant IBS patients had increased amounts of *Veillonella* spp [14].

Gastrointestinal Mucosa and Intestinal Immune Responses

The structure of GI mucosa varies from one site to another of the GI tract. It has three parts: a layer of specialized epithelial cells that line the lumen, the lamina propria (connective tissue with embedded vessels, nerves, and immune cells), and the muscularis mucosa. The GI tract surface has multiple invaginations called villi, which are lined with columnar epithelial cells. These cells have microvilli that help with the absorption of nutrients from digestion [15]. Interspersed in these structures are the gastrointestinal-associated lymphoid tissue (GALT) and the mesenteric lymph nodes (MLNs), which are the main tissues involved in GI immunity.

The intestinal immune system is the largest and most complex component of the immune system in general. In contrast to other parts of the body, it constantly encounters antigens and has to distinguish between harmful pathogens and commensal mucosal microbes that constitute microbiota. When pathogens are encountered, innate immune responses are generated immediately, producing a broad response directed mainly to decrease the pathogen load, while allowing for the highly specific adaptive immune response to succeed in clearing the pathogen.

The first line of defense between the external environment and the circulation is the intestinal epithelial cells themselves. Owing to their tight intercellular junctions, they provide a physical barrier that restricts access of pathogens to mucosal surfaces. Also, the brush border glycocalyx, the glycoproteins located in its border, prevents bacteria or large molecules to enter while allowing nutrients to cross [15]. Please review the previous Chap. 14 by Blijlvens and Donnelly for more information.

There are four different types of epithelial cells in the GI tract: columnar epithelial cells, goblet cells, enteroendocrine cells, and Paneth cells. Columnar epithelial cells can be found in the small intestine (enterocytes) or in the colon (colonocytes) and constitute 80% of the epithelial cell types. Goblet cells and enteroendocrine cells are located throughout the GI tract. Goblet cells are in charge of secreting mucin, while enteroendocrine cells integrate the GI system with the systemic nervous system. Paneth cells, initially described by Dr. Paneth in 1888, are found in the crypts of the small intestine and play an important role in innate immunity, mucosal inflammation, and absorption of fluids and nutrients [15, 16]. A more detailed review of the function of these cells is found later in this chapter.

In addition to being a mechanical barrier, intestinal epithelial cells are part of innate immune defense by secreting mucins, lysozymes, and defensins that prevent microbial adhesion and retain antimicrobial peptides and secretory antibodies inhibiting bacterial growth. Also, they transport luminal antigens for further presentation to underlying immune cells and secrete cytokines, such as interleukin (IL) 1-α, IL-1β, IL-6, IL-8, IL-10, IL-17, monocyte chemoattractant protein 1, granulocyte-macrophage colony-stimulating factor (GM-CSF), tumor necrosis factor α (TNF-α) and transforming growth factor β (TGF-β), chemokines, and eicosanoids that help in innate and adaptive responses [15].

Closely interspersed in the intestine and associated lymphoid tissue, there is a widespread network of bone marrow-derived innate immune cells, such as macrophages, mast cells, neutrophils, eosinophils, dendritic cells (DCs), and natural killer cells that each secrete a repertoire of cytokines and chemokines with functional profiles that partially overlap.

Antigen-presenting cells (APCs), comprising macrophages, conventional DCs, and plasmacytoid DCs, play a central role in initiating immune responses. In recent years, DCs have emerged as major players in shaping the immune responses in the gastrointestinal tract, by both maintaining tolerance toward microbiota and generating protection toward pathogens. This dual role can be explained by their unique structural and functional properties. There are several subpopulations of DCs located in the lymphoid structures of the intestine, such as Peyer's patches, isolated lymphoid follicles (ILF), and MLNs as well as in the lamina propria. Furthermore, the DCs population can be subdivided by the receptors expressed on their surface, which dictates the pattern of cytokine production and T-cell activation. For example, in the Peyer's patches CD11b+ subset of DCs produces IL-10 and Th2 priming, whereas CD11b-CD8α- and CD8α+ DCs produce IL-12 and later interferon-gamma (IFN-γ) by T cells [17].

As APCs DCs require antigen uptake by engulfing antigens already transported through the epithelial barrier by the microfold (M) cells, located at the dome of Peyer's patch, but also by expressing transepithelial projections of dendrites directly into the lumen in response to stimulation of epithelial cells Toll-like receptors (TLRs) by bacterial products [18, 19]. By constantly sampling the luminal antigens and microbiota, DCs continuously obtain immunological information about luminal commensals and pathogens.

Lamina propria DCs that have taken luminal antigens migrate to the draining MLN where they present antigen to T cells. This migration is constitutive and can occur in the absence of an infectious or inflammatory stimulus, although it can intensify in the presence of inflammatory stimuli. Chemokine receptor 7 (CCR7) appears critical for this migration [20]. These DCs are phenotypically mature, able to prime T cells. CCR7 receptors may be involved in promoting tolerance to mucosal antigens. Mice lacking CCR7 receptors have impaired ability to acquire tolerance to oral antigens [21]. Recent studies have shown that DCs from the lamina propria can promote generation of forkhead box P3 regulatory T cells (FOXP3+Treg), a process dependent on TGF-β and retinoic acid [22, 23]. Other mechanisms that can contribute to induction of tolerance are by induction of Th2 phenotype as well as promoting IgA secretion. It has been shown that DCs carrying commensal bacteria induce protective IgA [24].

In addition to promoting tolerance, DCs can induce adaptive immune responses that lead to generation of effector T cells directed toward clearance of intestinal pathogens. The mechanisms by which the DCs are able to promote tolerance vs. inflammation remain an area of active investigation. It has been suggested that the location and expression patterns of TLRs by intestinal epithelial cells may play a role. Alternatively, recruitment of DCs that have not been conditioned may be a factor. Another hypothesis that requires further investigation is uptake pathogenic species solely by DCs residing in MLNs [25].

Lastly, intestinal DCs play an important role in homing of recently activated T cells by promoting the expression of gut homing receptors (α4β7-integrin and CCR9) by both CD4+ and CD8+ T-cells subsets [26–28]. DCs are also involved in homing of IgA secreting B-cells [29].

Another important line of innate immune defense against pathogens is represented by antimicrobial peptides, a large group of peptides contained in the secretory granules of Paneth cells. Several members of this group have been the object of active investigation in the recent years, including α-defensins, angiogenins, and regIIIg.

Defensins are a family of evolutionary related peptides that have antimicrobial activity against bacteria and fungi. They are secreted by the Paneth cells into the crypt lumen by degranulation after stimulation by a variety of stimuli including gram positive, gram negative, and bacterial products such as lipopolysaccharide, lipoteichoic acid, lipid A, and muramyl dipeptide [30]. Recent studies performed in transgenic mice have shown that production of human defensin-5 protected mice against infection with *Salmonella typhimurium* [31]. It has been suggested that defensins may also play a role in antiparasitic immunity (*Giardia lamblia* and *Cryptosporidoim parvum*), but these findings need to be further confirmed [32, 33].

Angiogenin 4, produced by mouse Paneth cells, has antibacterial properties against *Enterococcus faecalis* and *Listeria monocytogenes*, two important gram positive pathogens, but does not affect other microorganisms such as *E. coli* or *Bacteroides thetaiotamicron*. Production of angiogenin 4 is stimulated by *B. thetaiotamicron*, suggesting that gut commensal microflora regulates the microbial environment and contributes to intestinal homeostasis through innate immune mechanisms [34].

More recently, a regenerating (Reg) family of proteins was described [35]. Structurally, C-type lectins, members of this family of proteins, are highly expressed at the level of the intestine. RegIIIg is found in mouse, with the counterpart in humans being HIP/PAP. RegIIIg binds to peptidoglycan expressed on the surface of the Gram-positive bacteria [36]. They appear to play an important role in the innate defense against *L. monocytogenes* and vancomycin-resistant *Enterococcus* [37, 38].

It has been observed that the repertoire of antimicrobial peptides changes along the small intestine; a subset of these molecules is upregulated in response to commensal flora, but not to enteric pathogens. This observation suggests that antimicrobial peptides produced by Paneth cells play a role in regulating commensal microbial homeostasis, in addition to protecting against infection [39].

In addition to secreting antimicrobial peptides, Paneth cells can express several inflammatory molecules, such as TNF, GM-CSF, and inducible NO synthase (iNOS) [40, 41]. Moreover, Paneth cells have a clear capacity to respond to inflammatory cytokines as shown in the induction of iNOS by TNF [42]. By releasing TNF, they are thought to be essential both in mucosal immunity against pathogens and in the development of Crohn's disease. IL-17 expression seems to play a role in systemic inflammation and shock induced by TNF [41], and recent studies have been showing its significant role in innate and adaptive immunity.

Innate immune mechanisms maintain rapid responses to mucosal pathogens but can lead to harmful inflammatory mucosal injury. The intrinsic control of these responses is comprised by a variety of down-regulatory pathways that are initiated by activation of the innate immune cells. These mechanisms are complex and partially overlap. A central role is played by interleukin 10 (IL-10), a potent anti-inflammatory cytokine which exerts its action on both innate and adaptive immunity. IL-10 prevents intestinal inflammation not only through T cells but also by reducing the antigen-presenting capacity of monocytes and DCs; it also exerts an inhibitory effect on the production of cytokines and chemokines by monocytes and macrophages while also inducing production of soluble inhibitory factors of proinflammatory cytokines (i.e., TNF-alpha) [43].

Adaptive immunity is a highly evolved mechanism of defense against pathogens. The most important characteristic of adaptive immunity is the presence of highly specific T- and B-cell receptors (TCRs and BCRs), which allow for an antigen-specific response. Another key characteristic is the presence of antigen-specific memory cells, which allow for a rapid, specific response upon rechallenge with the same antigen. T cells are characterized by the presence of CD4+ or CD8+ molecules, which are associated with the TCR and by the components of TCR (TCR$\alpha\beta$ or $\gamma\delta$). CD4+ and CD8+ cells recognize antigens presented by MHC class II molecules and class I respectively.

Several structural and functional characteristics singularize intestinal lymphoid edifice. It can be simplistically divided in the initiation compartment and the effector compartment.

Initiation compartment includes Peyer's patches, MLNs, as well as numerous ILFs. Mature Peyer's patches are found abundantly in distal ileum, but more recently have been described throughout the GI tract [44]. Structurally, Peyer's patches are similar to lymph nodes, containing large B-cell follicles with interspersed T-cell area; they are separated from the intestinal lumen by a single layer of epithelial cells named follicle-associated epithelium (FAE) and an area located immediately bellow the epithelium named subepithelial dome. The FAE contains microfold (M) cells, which are implicated in binding invasive pathogens as well as sampling particulate antigens. FAE also contains DCs, B and T cells, and macrophages. At this level, the initiation of the immune response occurs. M cells assist in antigen transport from the intestinal lumen, which is then passed on to the APCs, DCs playing an important role in this process, as outlined earlier in this chapter. APCs will subsequently move to the B-cell follicles and/or T-cell areas where they can interact and prime lymphocytes. The lymphocytes that are primed in the Payer's patches will migrate to the MLNs where they reside for an undefined period before migrating into the circulation and subsequently into the effector compartment. As previously mentioned, homing of primed T cells into the intestinal mucosa is facilitated by upregulation of certain receptors: $\alpha 4\beta 7$-integrin and CCR9, which are not expressed by T cells that are primed in peripheral lymphoid organs.

Different from other GALT tissues, MLNs can develop in the absence of growth factors. Interestingly, in germ-free mice MLNs are smaller but still functional due to a lack of stimulation from microbiota [45]. By contrast, ILFs which are found along the whole intestinal tract seem to develop under the stimulation of intestinal flora [46].

The effector compartment consists of lamina propria T cells and T cells interspersed in the intestinal epithelium, among the epithelial cells called intraepithelial lymphocytes (IELs). The phenotype and function of mucosal T cells remain an area of active investigation. Some populations of IELs are conventional CD4+ or CD8$\alpha\beta$+ T cells. Other populations are distinctively different from other lymphoid organs, such as CD8$\alpha\alpha$+$\gamma\delta$ TCR. Subsets of CD8+ T cells have cytotoxic activity. Other subset of T cells has effector/memory/regulatory/tissue repair functions [47]. Many studies in recent years have focused on regulatory T-cell subsets, which maintain intestinal homeostasis. The mechanisms underlying promotion of tolerance are very complex and partially redundant. Several subsets of T cells have been shown to have regulatory properties, among which CD4+Foxp3+ have a central role, but other CD4+ and CD8+ subsets also participate through IL-10 and transforming growth factor $\beta 1$ production and possibly other mechanisms [43].

B cells play an important role in intestinal immune responses by secreting IgA and cytokines. IgA production is a very important noninflammatory immune mechanism for the maintenance of intestinal homeostasis. IgA, one of the most abundant immunoglobulin isotypes produced in our body, is secreted as a dimmer by the intestinal B cells. Once secreted, it binds to a polymeric Ig receptor (pIgR), an antibody transporter located on the basolateral surface of the intestinal epithelial cells. Subsequently, it is transported to the surface of epithelial cells generating secretory IgA complexes. It can be produced in both intrafollicular and extrafollicular sites, in T-cell dependent and T-cell independent manner [24, 48]. Intestinal IgA performs multiple functions, including entrapment of dietary antigens and bacteria, interaction with local microbiota, maintenance of commensal bacterial flora (communities), and facilitation of antigen sampling by binding to M cells. Additionally, secretory IgA (sIgA) produced on mucosal surfaces promotes an anti-inflammatory environment [15]. Several factors such as IL-10 that promote tolerance also promote intestinal IgA production [49]. The mutualistic relationship is once again noted: IgA production is dependent on intestinal colonization and in turn it participates in immune exclusion by preventing the commensal bacteria to enter the intestinal surfaces [50].

Summary

The GI tract is a multifaceted anatomical and functional structure. There are intricate interactions between the immensely complex microbial populations comprising microbiota with the components of innate and adaptive immune system at the thin, fragile interface that separates the two worlds. Incessant signaling and communication between components is necessary to maintain homeostasis. Cancer and its therapies including chemotherapeutic agents but also antibiotics may disrupt this homeostasis and lead to unintended consequences. Although much progress has been made in recent years, understanding the ability of the GI tract to protect against pathogens while avoiding destructive inflammatory responses toward microbiota remains an area of active investigation.

References

1. Whitman WB, Coleman DC, Wiebe WJ. Prokaryotes: the unseen majority. Proc Natl Acad Sci. 1998;95:6578–83.
2. Moore WE, Holdeman LV. Human fecal flora: the normal flora of 20 Japanese-Hawaiians. Appl Microbiol. 1974;27:961–79.
3. Eckburg PB, Bik EM, Bernstein CN, et al. Diversity of the human intestinal microbial flora. Science. 2005;308:1635–8.
4. Delgado S, Ruas-Madiedo P, Suárez A, Mayo B. Interindividual differences in microbial counts and biochemical-associated variables in the feces of healthy Spanish adults. Dig Dis Sci. 2006;51:737–43.
5. Daly K, Cuff MA, Fung F, Shirazi-Beechey SP. The importance of colonic butyrate transport to the regulation of genes associated with colonic tissue homoeostasis. Biochem Soc Trans. 2005;33:733–5.
6. Bry L, Falk PG, Midtvedt T, Gordon JI. A model of host-microbial interactions in an open mammalian ecosystem. Science. 1996;273:1380–3.
7. Hooper LV, Wong MH, Thelin A, Hansson L, Falk PG, Gordon JI. Molecular analysis of commensal host-microbial relationships in the intestine. Science. 2001;291:881–4.
8. Sait L, Galic M, Strugnell RA, Janssen PH. Secretory antibodies do not affect the composition of the bacterial microbiota in the terminal ileum of 10-week-old mice. Appl Environ Microbiol. 2003;62:2100–9.
9. Suzuki K, Meek B, Doi Y, et al. Aberrant expansion of segmented filamentous bacteria in IgA-deficient gut. Proc Natl Acad Sci. 2004;101:1981–6.
10. Young VB, Schmidt TM. Antibiotic-associated diarrhea accompanied by large-scale alterations in the composition of the fecal microbiota. J Clin Microbiol. 2004;42:1203–6.
11. Chang JY, Antonopoulos DA, Kalra A, et al. Decreased diversity of the fecal Microbiome in recurrent *Clostridium difficile*-associated diarrhea. J Infect Dis. 2008;197:435–8.
12. Collado MC, Isolauri E, Laitinen K, Salminen S. Distinct composition of gut microbiota during pregnancy in overweight and normal-weight women. Am J Clin Nutr. 2008;88:894–9.
13. Matto J, Maunuksela L, Kajander K, et al. Composition and temporal stability of gastrointestinal microbiota in irritable bowel syndrome – a longitudinal study in IBS and control subjects. FEMS Immunol Med Microbiol. 2005;43:213–22.
14. Malinen E, Rinttila T, Kajander K, et al. Analysis of the fecal microbiota of irritable bowel syndrome patients and healthy controls with real-time PCR. Am J Gastroenterol. 2005;100:373–82.
15. McCracken VJ, Lorenz RG. The gastro-intestinal ecosystem: a precarious alliance among epithelium, immunity and microbiota. Cell Microbiol. 2001;3:1–11.
16. Porter EM, Bevins CL, Ghosh D, Ganz T. The multifaceted Paneth cell. Cell Mol Life Sci. 2002;59:156–70.
17. Coombes JL, Powrie F. Dendritic cells in intestinal immune regulation. Nat Rev Immunol. 2008;8:435–46.
18. Chieppa M, Rescigno M, Huang AY, Germain RN. Dynamic imaging of dendritic cell extension into the small bowel lumen in response to epithelial cell TLR engagement. J Exp Med. 2006;203:2841–52.
19. Niess JH, Brand S, Gu X, et al. CX3CR1-mediated dendritic cell access to the intestinal lumen and bacterial clearance. Science. 2005;307:254–8.
20. Jang MH, Sougawa N, Tanaka T, et al. CCR7 is critically important for migration of dendritic cells in intestinal lamina propria to mesenteric lymph nodes. J Immunol. 2006;176:803–10.
21. Worbs T, Bode U, Yan S, et al. Oral tolerance originates in the intestinal immune system and relies on antigen carriage by dendritic cells. J Exp Med. 2006;203:519–27.
22. Coombes JL, Siddiqui KR, Arancibia-Cárcamo CV, et al. A functionally specialized population of mucosal CD103+ DCs induces Foxp3+ regulatory T cells via a TGF-beta and retinoic acid-dependent mechanism. J Exp Med. 2007;204:1757–64.
23. Sun CM, Hall JA, Blank RB, et al. Small intestine lamina propria dendritic cells promote de novo generation of Foxp3 T reg cells via retinoic acid. J Exp Med. 2007;204:1775–85.
24. Macpherson AJ, Uhr T. Induction of protective IgA by intestinal dendritic cells carrying commensal bacteria. Science. 2004;303:1662–5.
25. Annacker O, Coombes JL, Malmstrom V, et al. Essential role for CD103 in the T cell-mediated regulation of experimental colitis. J Exp Med. 2005;202:1051–61.
26. Johansson-Lindbom B, Svensson M, Pabst O, et al. Functional specialization of gut CD103+ dendritic cells in the regulation of tissue-selective T cell homing. J Exp Med. 2005;202:1063–73.

27. Johansson-Lindbom B, Svensson M, Wurbel MA, Malissen B, Marquez G, Agace W. Selective generation of gut tropic T cells in gut-associated lymphoid tissue (GALT): requirement for GALT dendritic cells and adjuvant. J Exp Med. 2003;198: 963–9.
28. Stenstad H, Ericsson A, Johansson-Lindbom B, et al. Gut-associated lymphoid tissue-primed CD4+ T cells display CCR9-dependent and -independent homing to the small intestine. Blood. 2006;107: 3447–54.
29. Mora JR, Iwata M, Eksteen B, et al. Generation of gut-homing IgA-secreting B cells by intestinal dendritic cells. Science. 2006; 314:1157–60.
30. Ayabe T, Satchell DP, Wilson CL, Parks WC, Selsted ME, Ouellette AJ. Secretion of microbicidal alpha-defensins by intestinal Paneth cells in response to bacteria. Nat Immunol. 2000;1:113–8.
31. Porter EM, Liu L, Oren A, Anton PA, Ganz T. Localization of human intestinal defensin 5 in Paneth cell granules. Infect Immun. 1997;65:2389–95.
32. Aley SB, Zimmerman M, Hetsko M, Selsted ME, Gillin FD. Killing of *Giardia lamblia* by cryptdins and cationic neutrophil peptides. Infect Immun. 1994;62:5397–403.
33. Zaalouk TK, Bajaj-Elliott M, George JT, McDonald V. Differential regulation of beta-defensin gene expression during *Cryptosporidium parvum* infection. Infect Immun. 2004;72:2772–9.
34. Hooper LV, Stappenbeck TS, Hong CV, Gordon JI. Angiogenins: a new class of microbicidal proteins involved in innate immunity. Nat Immunol. 2003;4:269–73.
35. Cash HL, Whitham CV, Hooper LV. Refolding, purification, and characterization of human and murine RegIII proteins expressed in *Escherichia coli*. Protein Expr Purif. 2006;48:151–9.
36. Cash HL, Whitham CV, Behrendt CL, Hooper LV. Symbiotic bacteria direct expression of an intestinal bactericidal lectin. Science. 2006;313:1126–30.
37. Brandl K, Plitas G, Mihu CN, et al. Vancomycin-resistant enterococci exploit antibiotic-induced innate immune deficits. Nature. 2008;455:804–7.
38. Brandl K, Plitas G, Schnabl B, DeMatteo RP, Pamer EG. MyD88-mediated signals induce the bactericidal lectin RegIII gamma and protect mice against intestinal *Listeria monocytogenes* infection. J Exp Med. 2007;204:1891–900.
39. Karlsson J, Putsep K, Chu H, Kays RJ, Bevins CL, Andersson M. Regional variations in Paneth cell antimicrobial peptide expression along the mouse intestinal tract. BMC Immunol. 2008;9:37.
40. Ayabe T, Ashida T, Kohgo Y, Kono T. The role of Paneth cells and their antimicrobial peptides in innate host defense. Trends Microbiol. 2004;12:394–8.
41. Keshav S, Lawson L, Chung LP, Stein M, Perry VH, Gordon S. Tumor necrosis factor mRNA localized to Paneth cells of normal murine intestinal epithelium by in situ hybridization. J Exp Med. 1990;171:327–32.
42. Bultinck J, Sips P, Vakaet L, Brouckaert P, Cauwels A. Systemic NO production during (septic) shock depends on parenchymal and not on hematopoietic cells: in vivo iNOS expression pattern in (septic) shock. FASEB J. 2006;20:2363–5.
43. Izcue A, Coombes JL, Powrie F. Regulatory lymphocytes and intestinal inflammation. Annu Rev Immunol. 2009;27:313–38.
44. Hamada H, Hiroi T, Nishiyama Y, et al. Identification of multiple isolated lymphoid follicles on the antimesenteric wall of the mouse small intestine. J Immunol. 2002;168:57–64.
45. Gordon H, Pesti LG. The gnobiotic animal as a tools in the study of host-microbial relationships. Bacteriol Rev. 1971;35:390–429.
46. Lorenz RG, Chaplin DD, McDonald KG, McDonough JS, Newberry RD. Isolated lymphoid follicle formation is inducible and dependent upon lymphotoxin-sufficient B lymphocytes, lymphotoxin beta receptor, and TNF receptor I function. J Immunol. 2003;170:5475–82.
47. Cheroutre H, Madakamutil L. Acquired and natural memory T cells join forces at the mucosal front line. Nat Rev Immunol. 2004;4: 290–300.
48. Uematsu S, Fujimoto K, Jang MH, et al. Regulation of humoral and cellular gut immunity by lamina propria dendritic cells expressing Toll-like receptor 5. Nat Immunol. 2008;9:769–76.
49. Cerutti A. The regulation of IgA class switching. Nat Rev Immunol. 2008;8:421–34.
50. Macpherson AJ, McCoy KD, Johansen FE, Brandtzaeg P. The immune geography of IgA induction and function. Mucosal Immunol. 2008;1:11–22.

Chapter 16
Neutropenic Enterocolitis and *Clostridium difficile* Infections

Amar Safdar, Bruno P. Granwehr, Stephen A. Harold, and Herbert L. DuPont

Abstract Neutropenic enterocolitis is best defined as a clinical syndrome with features indistinguishable from other causes of bowel inflammation. Patients usually present with fever, abdominal pain, diarrhea, and have evidence of thickened bowel wall. This potentially fatal complication is not uncommon in neutropenic children, whereas in adults neutropenic enterocolitis is often seen in older patients with advanced cancer undergoing salvage chemotherapy for a hematologic malignancy. Patients with oro-intestinal mucosal damage following antineoplastic therapy are at an increased risk. The diagnosis is based on clinical features and evidence of diffuse or localized bowel wall thickening on CT scan; presence of air with in the bowel wall "pneumatosis intestinalis" indicates serious disease with an increased risk of perforation. Treatment is generally supportive with strict bowel rest, parenteral hydration, and nutritional support, along with broad spectrum antimicrobials. Myeloid growth factors promote early recovery form neutropenia. Surgery is reserved for patients with perforation of bowel with complicated peritonitis. In this chapter, a comprehensive discussion regarding *Clostridium difficile* (*C. diff*) is presented with emphasis on risk factors, clinical presentation, and antimicrobial therapy.

Keywords Neutropenia • Intestinal mucosal damage • Leukemia • Transplantation • Fever • Diarrhea • *Clostridium difficile*

Neutropenic Enterocolitis

Neutropenic enterocolitis (NEC) or typhlitis is a clinical syndrome characterized by fever, abdominal pain, and diarrhea [1–3]. Bowel wall thickening has been described, classically

A. Safdar (✉)
Department of Infectious Diseases, Infection Control, and Employee Health, The University of Texas M.D. Anderson Cancer Center, 1515 Holcombe Boulevard, Houston, TX 77030, USA
e-mail: amarsafdar@gmail.com

in the cecum; therefore, the term typhlitis from the Greek "typhlon" for cecum was used in earlier reports, this condition, however, involves all parts of postgastric intestinal tract [3, 4]. This potentially fatal complication of neutropenia is a form of colitis was originally described in patients undergoing chemotherapy for leukemia and solid organ cancer [1, 3–5]. The frequency may be as high as 26% based on autopsy findings in childhood leukemia cases [1, 4].

The diagnosis is difficult, most patients present with a nonspecific radiologic findings, and a differential diagnosis including appendicitis, ischemic colitis, pseudomembranous colitis, or antineoplastic drug or radiation toxicity [3, 5, 6]. Additionally, there is no internationally accepted standard for the diagnosis of NEC [3], with differences described between clinical presentation and diagnosis in children and adults [2, 3]. Given the challenge of accurate diagnosis, management becomes similarly difficult, involving supportive therapy with broad spectrum antimicrobials, strict bowel rest, and careful monitoring for complications that may require surgical intervention for perforated viscera [3, 5, 6].

In this chapter we present epidemiology, clinical presentation, and diagnosis and management of neutropenic colitis in adults and pediatric cancer patients.

Epidemiology

NEC has been described in association with chemotherapy, typically 10–14 days after cytotoxic chemotherapy, although cases have been described 30 days after chemotherapy [3, 5]. Patients with leukemia, aplastic anemia, and solid tumor undergoing high-dose chemotherapy are at an increased risk [3, 5]. Leukemia and other hematologic malignancies, as well as recipient of allogeneic stem cell transplantation with delayed engraftment or acute graft vs. host disease, account for approximately 75% of reported cases of NEC [2, 3].

Traditionally, cytotoxic drugs such as Ara-C and idarubicin are implicated [5]; whereas, recently a variety of other agents have been linked with NEC, including monoclonal antibody therapy with alemtuzumab [7], taxane-containing regimens [3, 8], cisplatin, and paclitaxel [3]. NEC may also be seen in noncancer population, recently a case was reported following unanticipated Chinese herbal drugs-induced neutropenia [9]. In children, similar agents have been associated with enterocolitis during neutropenia. A retrospective analysis from St. Jude's Children's hospital found a reduced risk of typhlitis in patients receiving Ara-C, methotrexate, and hydrocortisone along with trimethoprim-sulfamethoxazole [2]. By contrast, clinical trials with topotecan and irinotecan in children had to be terminated during the phase I due to high rates (45%) of typhlitis [10].

Neutropenia in patients with acute leukemia and those undergoing chemotherapy promotes translocation of microorganisms from host's intestinal lumen leading to tissue invasion and occasionally hematogenous dissemination. A retrospective study in pediatric cancer patients showed prolonged neutropenia and age >16 at cancer diagnosis were associated with a higher risk for typhlitis [2]. In a prospective study in adults, no specific risk factor for typhlitis was seen, and diagnosis was confirmed in 3.5% of cases [11]. An association with the presence of oropharyngeal mucositis and risk of NEC has been well described [4, 12].

NEC is a polymicrobial infection and organisms often associated with this disease entity include enteric Gram-negative bacteria (GNB) such as *Escherichia coli*, *Proteus* species, and nonfermentative gram-negatives in neutropenic patients like *Pseudomonas aeruginosa* and *Stenotrophomonas maltophilia* are of concern; among the Gram-positive bacteria, streptococci, enterococci including vancomycin-resistant *Enterococcus* (VRE), and coagulase negative staphylococcus species may be accompanied with *Candida* species [1, 5, 13, 14]. Cytomegalovirus or adenovirus enterocolitis may act as a trigger for a secondary NEC in some cases [5, 15].

Pathogenesis

The pathogenesis of necrotizing enterocolitis remains uncertain. In the earlier studies, association with leukemia prompted theories of bowel wall infiltration of tumor cells as the initial insult for development of colitis during neutropenia [15]. It was later proposed that chemotherapy neutropenia on its own promoting colitis [3, 5, 12] especially, in patients with enterotoxic chemotherapy-related bowel wall injury. Interestingly, in a large series of children with cancer, typhlitis was noted in 12% of patients in the absence of neutropenia [2], suggesting an important role for a primary process, such as cancer infiltration, chemotherapy-mediated damage, undiagnosed viral, or toxin-mediated enterocolic damage. Although, occurrence of this disease in patients with aplastic anemia [12] and noncancer patient with Chinese herb-induced neutropenia [9] suggests that severe neutropenic in certain individuals may lead to this clinical syndrome with no discernable prior damage to the intestinal tract.

Antimicrobial prophylaxis may influence the time of onset, etiology, and possibly incidence of NEC in patients undergoing cancer therapy. Antimicrobials are commonly used to prevent infections in high-risk patients with acute myelogenous leukemia, chronic lymphocytic leukemia, aplastic anemia, myelodysplastic syndrome, and those undergoing allogeneic stem cell transplantation. These antimicrobials have profound influence on microbial flora of the oro-intestinal tract, and may influence the potential organisms encountered with this syndrome [1, 5, 13, 14]. Increased use of high-dose chemotherapy and allogeneic stem cell transplantation in older patients may increase the rates of NEC. In a recent study, although in a small number of patients undergoing nonmyeloablative allogeneic stem cell transplant, the risk of typhlitis was only 6% [16].

Features on histopathologic examination of the involved bowel are diverse [3, 5]. These range from ischemic bowel in 12%, agranulocytic bowel in 19%, and pseudomembranous colitis in 69% [4]. Recent reports have shown findings indicative of mucosal damage and inflammation [4]. Some have reported leukemic infiltration of the bowel wall with no other significant findings [15, 17]. We suspect that NEC is a clinical syndrome of various primary causes, in most patients multiple factors appear to be responsible for this entity including severe neutropenia, young or advanced age, enteric insult due to cancer, drugs or bacterial toxins such as *Clostridium difficile*, subclinical viral disease, or unknown genetic polymorphisms that predispose some individuals to develop this disorder.

Diagnosis

In a retrospective study in adults, fever was present in 95%, 67% presented with abdominal pain which was often diffuse throughout the abdomen, and nearly all patients (95%) had diarrhea [5]. Presence of blood in the diarrheal stool indicated extensive intestinal wall damage and possibly herald bowel wall necrosis and perforation [5]. In a pediatric oncology study, 91% of patients exhibited abdominal pain, fever was present in 84%, and diarrhea in 72% of patients [2]. Distinguishing features for necrotizing enterocolitis in neutropenic patients are vague, and a high level of concern accompanied by frequent reevaluation remains central in the management for this potentially life-threatening complication in neutropenic cancer patients.

Fecal stool cultures provide limited information regarding the etiology of enterocolitis [18, 19]. Patients with concomitant bacteremia due to enteric organism(s) such as

Escherichia coli, enterococci, and streptococci give a partial spectrum of this polymicrobial disease, although sterile blood cultures do not exclude a low-grade, intermittent bacteremia and/or fungemia in the profoundly neutropenic susceptible patients [20]. Other common causes that may be mistaken for NEC include ischemic bowel injury, *C. difficile* colitis, appendicitis, or Ogilvie's syndrome [3]. To further complicate the diagnosis, there is a suggestion that the latter entities can coexist, with one small pediatric study suggesting that the combination of appendiceal thickening and enterocolitis may more likely to result in surgical intervention [21]. It was interesting to note that higher mortality was seen in children with NEC without evidence of appendicitis [21]. The frequency of NEC cases with concurrent or preceding *C. difficile* toxin-induced intestinal epithelia cell damage remains uncertain [22].

A comprehensive review of adult neutropenic patients with enterocolitis, appropriate diagnosis can be established by (1) >4 mm of bowel wall thickening on CT or ultrasonic abdominal scan combined with (2) clinical features such as fever, abdominal pain, and diarrhea (Fig. 16.1a) [3]. Several studies in pediatric and adults showed that a substantial proportion of neutropenic patients may not exhibit fever or abdominal pain during the early phase of the disease [2, 5, 11]. Therefore, a high level of suspicion in febrile neutropenic patients even in the absence of abdominal pain and/or distention with diarrhea or clinical or radiographic features of paralytic ileus should raise concerns for possible enterocolitis.

In older reports distal ileum and proximal colon were prominently involved in patients with this disease [23]. In recent reports, adult and pediatric neutropenic patients with clinical features of enterocolitis, mid and distal colon involvement is frequently appreciated and probably reflects frequently used sophisticated imaging scans [2, 3, 22]. As findings on abdominal ultrasounds and contrastenhanced CT scan are highly valuable [11], we recommend that bedside abdominal ultrasounds should be reserved for unstable patients in whom transport to the CT scan units is deferred, similarly, patients with other serious limitations for CT scan should than be evaluated with an abdominal X-rays and ultrasounds [2, 15].

The lack of an available gold standard for diagnosis of neutropenic colitis challenges the clinician to diagnose this syndrome. We suggest a combination of clinical symptoms such as abdominal pain, fever, or diarrhea in the setting of neutropenia and possibly cytotoxic chemotherapy combined with imaging studies (CT abdomen) that demonstrate bowel wall thickening (3–5 mm) and in severe case pneumatosis intestinalis may be used (Fig. 16.1b) [3, 11]. It is important to assess other potential treatable causes that may mimic these features such as ischemic colitis and *C. difficile* colitis. Some investigators have suggested that diagnosis of NEC should be reached after a thorough evaluation for other common etiologies [6].

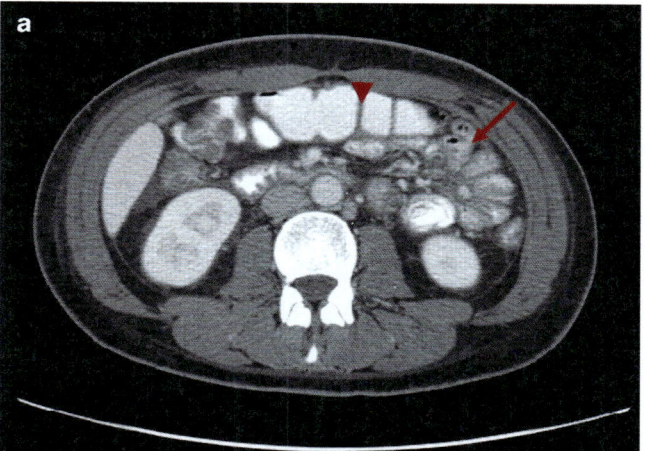

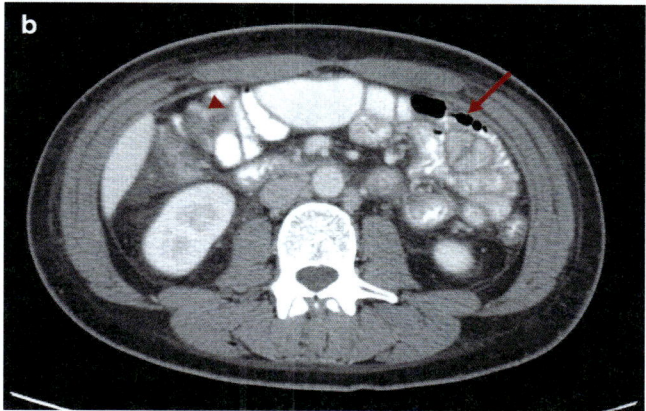

Fig. 16.1 CT scan findings show bowel wall thickening and areas of pneumatosis intestinalis in a patient with neutropenic enterocolitis. (**a**) Neutropenic colitis with thickening of the colon (*arrowhead*) and pneumatosis intestinalis (*arrow*), (**b**) Neutropenic colitis with thickening of the colon (*arrowhead*) and pneumatosis intestinalis (*arrow*)

Management

In patients with NEC, hastened recovery from neutropenia is important. Broad spectrum antimicrobial therapy is given for empiric coverage against enteric GNB, Gram-positive bacteria, and *Candida* species [3, 5, 13]. *Pseudomonas* species, other nonfermentative GNB, drug-resistant enteric GNB including extended spectrum beta-lactamases produces, and emergences of carbapenem-resistant enteric bacteria may further complicated empiric selection of appropriate antimicrobial choices. Similarly, vancomycin-resistant *Enterococcus*, multidrug-resistant staphylococci, and triazole-resistant yeast also play a role in the selection of appropriate therapy. In addition, there is a uniform recommendation to provide bowel rest, parenteral hydration, electrolyte, and nutritional support. Bowel decompression in patients with ileus with nasogastric intermittent suction may also be warranted in select patients [3, 5, 13]. Cases of prolonged neutropenia may benefit from recombinant myeloid growth factors such as G-CSF or GM-CSF and in select patients with refractory neutropenia, healthy donor-derived granulocyte transfusions may be considered [5, 6, 17].

Surgery should be deferred in neutropenic patients when possible. Patients with complicated peritonitis, surgical intervention considerably improved outcomes and survival (100%) compared with patients who were given conservative supportive care alone (9%) [14]. Surgery may also be considered in children who have radiographic evidence of appendicitis, as rupture of inflamed appendix may significantly complicate management of NEC [21]. Minimally invasive surgical procedures such as laparoscopic repair and removal of devitalized tissue when possible are desirable, and laparotomy for a two-stage hemicolectomy has also been done for patients with disease confined to the right colon [6, 12]. The timely institution of therapy is the most important predictor of outcomes in patients with NEC. Delay in diagnosis and institution of appropriate therapy herald a poor prognosis [4, 6].

Clostridium difficile Infection

C. difficile infection (CDI) is a debilitating complication in cancer patients undergoing antineoplastic therapy and/or hematopoietic stem cell transplantation [24, 25]. The recent increase in the frequency of these infections in hospitalized patients, especially due to a hypervirulent strain, has further accentuated concerns for serious inpatient potentially life-threatening complications among immunosuppressed oncology patients [26, 27]. Antibiotic prophylaxis with trimethoprim-sulfamethoxazole and fluoroquinolones has been widely used in leukemic patients with chemotherapy-induced neutropenia to prevent bacterial infections. These patients have a higher risk for infections not only due to resistant Gram-negative bacteria and fluoroquinolone-insensitive viridans streptococci but also due to antibiotic-associated CDI [28].

In an epidemiologic study among 248 patients, diagnosis of acute leukemia was significantly associated with carrier state of *C. diff* during an outbreak of clinical disease [15].

In neutropenic patients who are undergoing treatment for hematologic malignancies, the frequency of CDI was 7% among 875 courses of myelosuppressive chemotherapy [29]. In another study of 557 stool samples from 156 hospitalized cancer patients, *C. diff* or its toxin was identified in 35% of patients on oral antimicrobial prophylaxis, whereas *C. diff* was isolated in only 12% of other patients [30]. Therefore, CDI should be suspected in all hospitalized cancer patients with neutropenia who develop diarrheal illness, despite the fact that chemotherapy-induced oro-intestinal tract mucosal disruption may have indistinguishable clinical and radiologic features. Furthermore, in patients with leukemia, CDI has been associated with secondary systemic bacterial infections, such as vancomycin-resistant enterococcal intestinal colonization, and is at a significantly higher risk for VRE bacteremia following CDI [31].

Epidemiology and Risk Factors

The use of broad-spectrum antibiotics like fluoroquinolones has been identified as the most significant risk factor for CDI due to depletion of colonic aerobic flora. In addition, exposure to multiple antibiotics for the treatment of infections makes patients more vulnerable to this infection. Other precipitating factors that increase the risk for acquiring CDI include being elderly, immunosuppressed or with multiple comorbidities, receiving tube feedings, parenteral feedings, or undergoing gastrointestinal surgery, and cancer chemotherapy. Certain host-related factors like infection by human immunodeficiency virus, solid organ transplantation, or bone marrow transplantation render them particularly susceptible to CDI.

In a case-control study, treatment with low-dose chemotherapy, lack of parenteral use of vancomycin, and recent hospitalization were found to be independent predictors of CDI in oncology patients [32]. In an interesting study among children with cancer, no association was found between presence of toxigenic *C. diff* and receipt of antibiotics and/or administration of chemotherapy [33]. This absence of the classic risk factors seen in adults indicates that toxigenic strains of *C. diff* may in fact be part of the normal flora in young children [33]. However, outbreaks of CDI have been reported in pediatric oncology units [34]. On the other hand in adult oncology units, CDI outbreaks are more often seen in older individuals, those on antibiotics who are simultaneously treated with antineoplastic chemotherapy [35] or with chemotherapy alone [36]. Elderly patients are at a higher risk for developing serious CDI with an increased probability for recurrent CDI and secondary complications including prolonged bowel dysfunction, bowel perforation, and life-threatening toxic megacolon.

In another 2-year case-control study cancer patients compared with hospitalized patients without cancer were 22 times more likely to have received antibiotics during or 4 weeks prior to hospitalization. The trend for occurrence of CDI was higher in patients with exposure to an increased number of antibiotics [37]. Interestingly, the investigators noted a 7 times more likelihood of CDI in cancer patients treated with recombinant interleukine-2 [37]. In a case-control study in cancer patients with diarrhea, it was observed that patients with CDAD were 22 times more likely to have received any antibiotics and 7 times more likely to have received interleukin-2 during hospitalization or in the preceding month [37]. In patients with multiple myeloma or lymphoma, the risk of CDI is low although this risk increases following autologous stem cell transplantation to 15% [38, 39]. Fifteen percent of the patients who underwent autologous peripheral blood stem cell transplant experience CDI [38, 39]. Two thirds of these patients had multiple myeloma while 1/3 had lymphoma. However, this difference was not statistically significant. The risk factors associated with CDI in these patients were prior therapy with cephalosporins and intravenous vancomycin, On the other hand, patients treated with paclitaxel had a lower incidence of CDI when compared to those who were treated with hematopoietic growth factor as part of mobilization regimen [39]. Whereas inpatients undergoing allogeneic hematopoietic stem cell transplantation, nearly 50% of diarrheal episodes is due to acute graft-versus-host disease, while 15% is due to intestinal infections, and <5% is due to nosocomial CDI [40]. In another case-control study among outpatients at a cancer center, CDI was associated with prior antibiotic exposure and not unexpectedly, patients receiving clindamycin were nearly fourfold more likely to develop CDI; and for each additional day of clindamycin and oral cephalosporins, the patients were nearly twofold more likely to develop CDI [38].

Acute leukemia patients are exposed to higher risk of CDI while on chemotherapy due to probable intestinal track colonization and diarrheal disease [41–44]. 5-fluorouracil has been implicated in increasing the risk of CDI in patients with solid-organ cancer [45]; 5-fluorouracil-associated CDI was not seen in the older studies [46]. Treatment with mitoxantrone and etoposide has also been associated with CDI in patients with no antibiotic exposure for over 6 months [47]. Similarly, in patients with gynecologic malignancies, treatment with paclitaxel, carboplatin combination, or cisplatin-based has been noted to increase the risk for CDI [48–50]. In breast cancer patients undergoing autologous stem cell transplantation, the risk of CDI is nearly 10% [51]; whereas 16% of those receiving salvage therapy with ifosfamide, carboplatin, and etoposide for metastatic and refractory breast cancer experience grade 3–4 gastrointestinal toxicity, although the risk of CDI is only about 1% [52]. Others have observed that 45% of diarrheal episodes were due to *C. diff* in patients receiving intensive chemotherapy for disseminated germ cell cancer [53].

Pathogenesis

The surface layer proteins (SLPs) of *C. diff* play a significant role in activating the host immune response in CDI. SLPs are the outermost surface components of the bacterium that are responsible for their colonization and adhesion to the intestinal mucosa [54]. It has been proposed that SLPs attach to both the intestinal epithelial cells and some components of their extracellular matrix fibers, resulting in epithelial damage. In addition, the pathogenicity of CDI is attributed to the loss of the delicate balance between regulatory and inflammatory cytokines in the immune regulatory cells like monocytes and dendritic cells [55].

Although strains of *C. diff* are noninvasive, their toxins penetrate the mucosal barrier and initiate an immune response in the host [56]. Depending on the immune status of the individual, the latency period also varies from few days to 8 weeks and they clinically manifest with varying degrees of severity, from episodes of diarrhea to fatal toxic megacolon [57]. The ability of the host to produce specific antibodies against toxins and/or cellular antigens [58, 59] and to initiate the most appropriate cellular response [60] is a key factor accounting for the wide spectrum of the disease [61]. Low serum and/or intestinal antibody response to *C. diff* toxin A is associated with severe, prolonged, and recurrent *C. difficile* diarrhea [62]. This was not due to widespread humoral immune deficiency or of IgG subclass deficiency but due to selective reduction in IgG2 and IgG3 subclass responses [63]. Adequate antibody response to toxin A is therefore an important element in asymptomatic carriage of *C. diff* and in clinical recovery from CDI [61, 62].

Diagnosis

The diagnosis of CDI is based on both clinical as well as laboratory findings. Early diagnosis of CDI helps to initiate aggressive treatment and prevents complications like dehydration, electrolyte imbalance or depletion, and even hemorrhage. In patients presenting with diarrhea, diagnosis of CDI can be established by any of the following standard stool investigations: stool culture for *C. diff*, stool enzyme immunoassay for enterotoxin A and cytotoxin B, and tissue culture stool cytotoxicity test for toxin B. Colonoscopy or sigmoidoscopy can reveal Pseudomembranes, which are diagnostic of advanced CDI. At times they help diagnose CDI even before the stool results are available [64]. It is also important to consider a concurrent opportunistic infection in severely immunosuppressed neutropenic patients with CDAD. In patients with acute leukemia and in whom symptoms persist despite appropriate CDAD therapy, diagnostic assays for CMV reactivation, such as CMV antigenemia, serum fungal antigen like galactomannan, and if possible histological evaluation of tissue samples for special viral and fungal stains, may provide life-saving information.

Management

The mainstay of treatment is withdrawal or substitution of the offending antimicrobial agent and initiating specific treatment for CDI. Oral vancomycin 125 mg is given 4 times a day for 10 days and metronidazole 250 mg 4 times a day for 10 days is considered standard treatment. Administration of intravenous metronidazole can be used in patients unable to take oral drug. Although majority of the patients show significant symptomatic improvement within 2 days, the mean time ranges from 2 to 5 days. Recurrent CDI as well as reinfection of *C. diff* strains can be successfully treated with the same specific treatment regime. More severe cases of CDI should receive oral vancomycin as has been established in noncancer patients [65].

Other pharmaceutical agents that can be as effective as the vancomycin regime against CDI are teicoplanin 100 mg administered twice a day. Treatment with bacitracin and colestipol, an ion exchange resin though effective, produces response rates that are lower than with vancomycin [64].

Prevention and Control

Prevention of CDI should be given priority. Adopting barrier precaution using gloves can significantly reduce the spread of infection from patient to patient as well as from medical personnel. Hand washing using soap and water can protect hospital personnel from acquiring this infection. Isolation of patients with CDI, cleaning and disinfecting the rooms occupied by CDI patients with dilute clorox, and use of disposable rectal thermometers can reduce the incidence of CDI [66]. Restricted use of broad spectrum antibiotics has proved to reduce the incidence of CDI in hospitals. Administration of the probiotic *Saccharomyces boulardii* may have prophylactic value in reducing CDI in the setting of a hospital outbreak [64].

Summary

Neutropenic colitis was first described in the 1970s [67] as a clinical syndrome characterized by fever, abdominal pain, and diarrhea in the setting of neutropenia with bowel wall thickening. In the absence of large multicenter prospective trials in adults with this gastrointestinal complication management is based on anecdotal evidence. Patients with acute leukemia, aplastic anemia, or advanced solid organ malignancies treated with salvage high-dose cytotoxic chemotherapy are at increased risk [2, 3, 5, 13]. A high level of suspicion and evaluation for other frequently encountered conditions that mimic this syndrome is important. Most patients respond to a multifaceted approach including total bowel rest, parenteral hydration, electrolyte replacement, and nutritional support along with broad spectrum antimicrobial therapy [3, 5, 13]. Recombinant myeloid growth factors are important in the management of these patients and should be considered early in the course of therapy. Donor granulocyte transfusions are reserved for patients with refractory severe neutropenia and impending bowel perforation [5]. Finally, in patients with complicated peritonitis, surgical evaluation may be necessary [6, 14].

References

1. Katz JA, Wagner ML, Gresik MV, Mahoney Jr DH, Fernbach DJ. Typhlitis. An 18-year experience and postmortem review. Cancer. 1990;65:1041–7.
2. McCarville MB, Adelman CS, Li C, et al. Typhlitis in childhood cancer. Cancer. 2005;104:380–7.
3. Gorschluter M, Mey U, Strehl J, et al. Neutropenic enterocolitis in adults: systematic analysis of evidence quality. Eur J Haematol. 2005;75:1–13.
4. Dosik GM, Luna M, Valdivieso M, et al. Necrotizing colitis in patients with cancer. Am J Med. 1979;67:646–56.
5. Gomez L, Martino R, Rolston KV. Neutropenic enterocolitis: spectrum of the disease and comparison of definite and possible cases. Clin Infect Dis. 1998;27:695–9.
6. Wade DS, Nava HR, Douglass Jr HO. Neutropenic enterocolitis. Clinical diagnosis and treatment. Cancer. 1992;69:17–23.
7. Marie I, Robaday S, Kerleau JM, Jardin F, Levesque H. Typhlitis as a complication of alemtuzumab therapy. Haematologica. 2007;92:e62–3.
8. Oehadian A, Fadjari TH. Neutropenic enterocolitis in breast cancer patient after taxane-containing chemotherapy. Acta Med Indones. 2008;40:29–33.
9. Liou JM, Lin JT, Wu MS, Cheng TY, Shun CT, Wang HP. Typhlitis associated with *Candida albicans* and *Pseudomonas aeruginosa* infection in a patient with herbal drug-induced neutropenia. Ann Hematol. 2005;84:689–91.
10. Rodriguez-Galindo C, Crews KR, Stewart CF, et al. Phase I study of the combination of topotecan and irinotecan in children with refractory solid tumors. Cancer Chemother Pharmacol. 2006;57:15–24.
11. Aksoy DY, Tanriover MD, Uzun O, et al. Diarrhea in neutropenic patients: a prospective cohort study with emphasis on neutropenic enterocolitis. Ann Oncol. 2007;18:183–9.
12. Tokar B, Aydogdu S, Pasaoglu O, Ilhan H, Kasapoglu E. Neutropenic enterocolitis: is it possible to break vicious circle between neutropenia and the bowel wall inflammation by surgery? Int J Colorectal Dis. 2003;18:455–8.
13. Sloas MM, Flynn PM, Kaste SC, Patrick CC. Typhlitis in children with cancer: a 30-year experience. Clin Infect Dis. 1993;17:484–90.
14. Buyukasik Y, Ozcebe OI, Haznedaroglu IC, et al. Neutropenic enterocolitis in adult leukemias. Int J Hematol. 1997;66:47–55.
15. Gorschluter M, Marklein G, Hofling K, et al. Abdominal infections in patients with acute leukaemia: a prospective study applying ultrasonography and microbiology. Br J Haematol. 2002;117:351–8.
16. Shapira MY, Resnick IB, Bitan M, et al. Low transplant-related mortality with allogeneic stem cell transplantation in elderly patients. Bone Marrow Transpl. 2004;34:155–9.

17. Urbach DR, Rotstein OD. Typhlitis. Can J Surg. 1999;42:415–9.
18. Rolston KV, Bodey GP, Safdar A. Polymicrobial infection in patients with cancer: an underappreciated and underreported entity. Clin Infect Dis. 2007;45:228–33.
19. Davila ML. Neutropenic enterocolitis. Curr Opin Gastroenterol. 2006;22:44–7.
20. Pokorney BH, Jones JM, Shaikh BS, Aber RC. Typhlitis. A treatable cause of recurrent septicemia. JAMA. 1980;243:682–3.
21. McCarville MB, Thompson J, Li C, et al. Significance of appendiceal thickening in association with typhlitis in pediatric oncology patients. Pediatr Radiol. 2004;34:245–9.
22. Kirkpatrick ID, Greenberg HM. Gastrointestinal complications in the neutropenic patient: characterization and differentiation with abdominal CT. Radiology. 2003;226:668–74.
23. Thoeni RF, Cello JP. CT imaging of colitis. Radiology. 2006;240:623–38.
24. Leung S, Metzger BS, Currie BP. Incidence of *Clostridium difficile* infection in patients with acute leukemia and lymphoma after allogeneic hematopoietic stem cell transplantation. Infect Control Hosp Epidemiol. 2010;31:313–5.
25. Raza S, Baig MA, Russell H, Gourdet Y, Berger BJ. *Clostridium difficile* infection following chemotherapy. Recent Pat Antiinfect Drug Discov. 2010;5:1–9.
26. Hammond SP, Baden LR. Antibiotic prophylaxis during chemotherapy-induced neutropenia for patients with acute leukemia. Curr Hematol Malig Rep. 2007;2:97–103.
27. Nucci M, Anaissie E. Infections in patients with multiple myeloma in the era of high-dose therapy and novel agents. Clin Infect Dis. 2009;49:1211–25.
28. Heard SR, Wren B, Barnett MJ, Thomas JM, Tabaqchali S. *Clostridium difficile* infection in patients with haematological malignant disease. Risk factors, faecal toxins and pathogenic strains. Epidemiol Infect. 1988;100:63–72.
29. Gerard M, Defresne N, Daneau D, et al. Incidence and significance of *Clostridium difficile* in hospitalized cancer patients. Eur J Clin Microbiol Infect Dis. 1988;7:274–8.
30. Roghmann MC, McCarter Jr RJ, Brewrink J, Cross AS, Morris Jr JG. *Clostridium difficile* infection is a risk factor for bacteremia due to vancomycin-resistant enterococci (VRE) in VRE-colonized patients with acute leukemia. Clin Infect Dis. 1997;25:1056–9.
31. Hornbuckle K, Chak A, Lazarus HM, et al. Determination and validation of a predictive model for *Clostridium difficile* diarrhea in hospitalized oncology patients. Ann Oncol. 1998;9:307–11.
32. Burgner D, Siarakas S, Eagles G, McCarthy A, Bradbury R, Stevens M. A prospective study of *Clostridium difficile* infection and colonization in pediatric oncology patients. Pediatr Infect Dis J. 1997;16:1131–4.
33. Brunetto AL, Pearson AD, Craft AW, Pedler SJ. *Clostridium difficile* in an oncology unit. Arch Dis Child. 1988;63:979–81.
34. Blot E, Escande MC, Besson D, et al. Outbreak of *Clostridium difficile*-related diarrhoea in an adult oncology unit: risk factors and microbiological characteristics. J Hosp Infect. 2003;53:187–92.
35. Kamthan AG, Bruckner HW, Hirschman SZ, Agus SG. *Clostridium difficile* diarrhea induced by cancer chemotherapy. Arch Intern Med. 1992;152:1715–7.
36. Gifford AH, Kirkland KB. Risk factors for *Clostridium difficile*-associated diarrhea on an adult hematology-oncology ward. Eur J Clin Microbiol Infect Dis. 2006;25:751–5.
37. Arango JI, Restrepo A, Schneider DL, et al. Incidence of *Clostridium difficile*-associated diarrhea before and after autologous peripheral blood stem cell transplantation for lymphoma and multiple myeloma. Bone Marrow Transpl. 2006;37:517–21.
38. Cox GJ, Matsui SM, Lo RS, et al. Etiology and outcome of diarrhea after marrow transplantation: a prospective study. Gastroenterology. 1994;107:1398–407.
39. Palmore TN, Sohn S, Malak SF, Eagan J, Sepkowitz KA. Risk factors for acquisition of *Clostridium difficile*-associated diarrhea among outpatients at a cancer hospital. Infect Control Hosp Epidemiol. 2005;26:680–4.
40. Yolken RH, Bishop CA, Townsend TR, et al. Infectious gastroenteritis in bone-marrow-transplant recipients. N Engl J Med. 1982;306:1010–2.
41. Morales Chamorro R, Serrano Blanch R, Mendez Vidal MJ, et al. Pseudomembranous colitis associated with chemotherapy with 5-fluorouracil. Clin Transl Oncol. 2005;7:258–61.
42. Morris Jr JG, Jarvis WR, Nunez-Montiel OL, et al. *Clostridium difficile*. Colonization and toxin production in a cohort of patients with malignant hematologic disorders. Arch Intern Med. 1984;144:967–9.
43. Panichi G, Pantosti A, Gentile G, et al. *Clostridium difficile* colitis in leukemia patients. Eur J Cancer Clin Oncol. 1985;21:1159–63.
44. Rampling A, Warren RE, Bevan PC, Hoggarth CE, Swirsky D, Hayhoe FG. *Clostridium difficile* in haematological malignancy. J Clin Pathol. 1985;38:445–51.
45. Cascinu S, Catalano G. Have enteric infections a role in 5-fluorouracil-associated diarrhea? Support Care Cancer. 1995;3:322–3.
46. Jarvis B, Shevchuk YM. Recurrent *Clostridium difficile* diarrhea associated with mitoxantrone and etoposide: a case report and review. Pharmacotherapy. 1997;17:606–11.
47. Yamazawa K, Kanno H, Seki K, Kuzuta T, Matsui H, Sekiya S. Life-threatening *Clostridium difficile*-associated diarrhea induced by paclitaxel-carboplatin combination chemotherapy. Acta Obstet Gynecol Scand. 2001;80:768–9.
48. Barton T, Collis T, Stadtmauer E, Schuster M. Infectious complications the year after autologous bone marrow transplantation or peripheral stem cell transplantation for treatment of breast cancer. Clin Infect Dis. 2001;32:391–5.
49. Emoto M, Kawarabayashi T, Hachisuga MD, Eguchi F, Shirakawa K. *Clostridium difficile* colitis associated with cisplatin-based chemotherapy in ovarian cancer patients. Gynecol Oncol. 1996;61:369–72.
50. Resnik E, Lefevre CA. Fulminant *Clostridium difficile* colitis associated with paclitaxel and carboplatin chemotherapy. Int J Gynecol Cancer. 1999;9:512–4.
51. Chang AY, Hui L, Asbury R, Boros L, Garrow G, Rubins J. Ifosfamide, carboplatin and etoposide (ICE) in metastatic and refractory breast cancer. Cancer Chemother Pharmacol. 1999;44(Suppl):S26–8.
52. Nielsen H, Daugaard G, Tvede M, Bruun B. High prevalence of *Clostridium difficile* diarrhoea during intensive chemotherapy for disseminated germ cell cancer. Br J Cancer. 1992;66:666–7.
53. Martirosian G, Szczesny A, Cohen SH, Silva Jr J. Isolation of nontoxigenic strains of *Clostridium difficile* from cases of diarrhea among patients hospitalized in hematology/oncology ward. Pol J Microbiol. 2004;53:197–200.
54. Cerquetti M, Serafino A, Sebastianelli A, Mastrantonio P. Binding of *Clostridium difficile* to Caco-2 epithelial cell line and to extracellular matrix proteins. FEMS Immunol Med Microbiol. 2002;32:211–8.
55. Ausiello CM, Cerquetti M, Fedele G, et al. Surface layer proteins from *Clostridium difficile* induce inflammatory and regulatory cytokines in human monocytes and dendritic cells. Microbes Infect. 2006;8:2640–6.
56. Flegel WA, Muller F, Daubener W, Fischer HG, Hadding U, Northoff H. Cytokine response by human monocytes to *Clostridium difficile* toxin A and toxin B. Infect Immun. 1991;59:3659–66.
57. Castagliuolo I, LaMont JT. Pathophysiology, diagnosis and treatment of *Clostridium difficile* infection. Keio J Med. 1999;48:169–74.
58. Kyne L, Warny M, Qamar A, Kelly CP. Asymptomatic carriage of *Clostridium difficile* and serum levels of IgG antibody against toxin A. N Engl J Med. 2000;342:390–7.

59. Mulligan ME, Miller SD, McFarland LV, Fung HC, Kwok RY. Elevated levels of serum immunoglobulins in asymptomatic carriers of *Clostridium difficile*. Clin Infect Dis. 1993;16 Suppl 4:S239–44.
60. Johal SS, Lambert CP, Hammond J, James PD, Borriello SP, Mahida YR. Colonic IgA producing cells and macrophages are reduced in recurrent and non-recurrent *Clostridium difficile* associated diarrhoea. J Clin Pathol. 2004;57:973–9.
61. Sanchez-Hurtado K, Corretge M, Mutlu E, McIlhagger R, Starr JM, Poxton IR. Systemic antibody response to *Clostridium difficile* in colonized patients with and without symptoms and matched controls. J Med Microbiol. 2008;57:717–24.
62. Qamar A, Aboudola S, Warny M, et al. Saccharomyces boulardii stimulates intestinal immunoglobulin A immune response to *Clostridium difficile* toxin A in mice. Infect Immun. 2001;69:2762–5.
63. Katchar K, Taylor CP, Tummala S, Chen X, Sheikh J, Kelly CP. Association between IgG2 and IgG3 subclass responses to toxin A and recurrent *Clostridium difficile*-associated disease. Clin Gastroenterol Hepatol. 2007;5:707–13.
64. Gerding DN, Johnson S, Peterson LR, Mulligan ME, Silva Jr J. *Clostridium difficile*-associated diarrhea and colitis. Infect Control Hosp Epidemiol. 1995;16:459–77.
65. Zar FA, Bakkanagari SR, Moorthi KM, Davis MB. A comparison of vancomycin and metronidazole for the treatment of *Clostridium difficile*-associated diarrhea, stratified by disease severity. Clin Infect Dis. 2007;45:302–7.
66. Cohen SH, Gerding DN, Johnson S, et al. Clinical practice guidelines for *Clostridium difficile* infection in adults: 2010 update by the society for healthcare epidemiology of America (SHEA) and the infectious diseases society of America (IDSA). Infect Control Hosp Epidemiol. 2010;31:431–55.
67. Wagner ML, Rosenberg HS, Fernbach DJ, Singleton EB. Typhlitis: a complication of leukemia in childhood. Am J Roentgenol Radium Ther Nucl Med. 1970;109:341–50.

Chapter 17
Management of Reactivation of Hepatitis B and Hepatitis C During Antineoplastic Therapy

Marta Davila and Harrys A. Torres

Abstract Hepatitis viruses can cause serious illness in patient with cancer and those who have undergone stem cell transplantation (SCT). Patients with hematological malignancies chronically infected with either Hepatitis B virus (HBV) or Hepatitis C virus (HCV) are at risk for viral reactivation following chemotherapy. HBV reactivation is a common and serious complication but preventable. HCV has a lower reactivation rate following chemotherapy than HBV, but its presentation can be severe and nonpreventable. In this chapter, we review the management of reactivation of viral hepatitis during antineoplastic therapy affecting patients with cancer or SCT.

Keywords Hepatitis B • Hepatitis C • Reactivation

Introduction

Viral infections are common complications among cancer patients associated with significant morbidity and mortality; especially those with hematologic malignancies and those who have undergone stem cell transplantation (SCT). Hepatitis viruses can cause serious illness in these patient populations.

Patients with hematological malignancies chronically infected with either Hepatitis B virus (HBV) or Hepatitis C virus (HCV) showed a significantly higher incidence of severe liver dysfunction, after chemotherapy, compared with noninfected patients [1, 2]. In this chapter, we review the management of reactivation of viral hepatitis during antineoplastic therapy affecting patients with cancer or SCT recipients.

H.A. Torres (✉)
Department of Infectious Diseases, Infection Control, and Employee Health, The University of Texas M.D. Anderson Cancer Center, 1515 Holcombe, Unit 1460, Houston, TX 77030, USA
e-mail: htorres@mdanderson.org

Reactivation of Hepatitis B Virus

HBV reactivation is a well-recognized complication in cancer patients undergoing immunosuppressive therapy or hematopoietic SCT. Although it has been most reported in hepatitis B surface antigen (HBsAg) positive patients, it can also occur in those who are HBsAg negative but positive for the antibody to hepatitis B core antigen (anti-HBc) alone or with antibody to hepatitis B surface antigen (anti-HBs) [3, 4].

The reported frequency of HBV reactivation in HBV carriers undergoing chemotherapy ranges widely from 14 to 72% [3, 5]. The variation may be related to differences in patient populations, type of cancer (hematologic vs. solid), chemotherapy regimens, definition of HBV reactivation, and study designs.

Although there are no uniform diagnostic criteria available, most studies define HBV reactivation as an increase in serum HBV DNA level to more than 1 log higher than that of baseline, or an absolute increase exceeding 6 $\log_{10}$ copies/mL, or serum HBV DNA turning from negative to positive [6]. Hepatitis is commonly defined as a more than threefold increase of serum ALT on two consecutive determinations at least 5 days apart [6]. When evaluating patients with possible HBV reactivation, other causes of hepatitis should be excluded including superinfection with other viruses, drug toxicity, sino-occlusive disease, graft-versus-host disease, and liver involvement with tumor.

Pathogenesis and Clinical Manifestations

The typical course of reactivation starts with an increase in viral replication caused by the immune suppression of cytotoxic therapy [7, 8]. The degree of increase in viral replication can be demonstrated by a rise in HBV DNA in serum. During this time, there may be reappearance of HBeAg and HBsAg, with a decrease in anti-HBs titers. The second stage of reactivation occurs when chemotherapy is discontinued and the immune system is restored leading to the destruction of hepatocytes infected with HBV. Elevation in ALT levels and symptoms of hepatitis, including jaundice, may ensue. During this phase, HBV DNA levels may start to fall. The third phase of reactivation is recovery during which the clinical hepatitis resolves and HBV markers return to baseline levels [7]. Not all patients with HBV reactivation will go through all these phases. In some patients, HBV DNA remains high but there is no immune reconstitution; therefore, acute hepatitis does not develop. In others, the hepatitis phase is severe, leading to death. Yet, in other cases, the hepatitis phase persists and it may lead to the establishment of chronic hepatitis and deterioration of liver function [9].

HBV reactivation may be asymptomatic or may present with classic symptoms of hepatitis including fatigue, anorexia, jaundice, ascites, coagulopathy, and hepatic encephalopathy. Some patients may progress to liver failure and death. HBV reactivation may also result in significant delays or disruption in treatment and decreased overall survival [3, 10]. The mortality rate of HBV reactivation ranges from 5 to 40% [11, 12].

Risk Factors

Several risk factors are associated with an increased risk for HBV reactivation. Among them, a high serum HBV viral load has been consistently found to be one of the most important ones [13]. Other risk factors include a diagnosis of lymphoma or breast cancer, male gender, young age, use of steroids, and the use of certain chemotherapeutic agents (anthracyclines) [3, 14, 15]. Another viral factor that has been investigated is hepatitis B e antigen but the results are conflicting, and this is likely related to the presence of the precore/core promoter HBV mutants [3, 14, 16].

Monoclonal antibodies, such as rituximab (anti-CD20) and alemtuzumab (anti-CD52), have also been linked to HBV reactivation. Rituximab is effective in treating B-cell tumors and is used for the treatment of both low-grade and high-grade non-Hodgkin's lymphomas. The most frequent viral infection complicating rituximab therapy is HBV reactivation, and it accounts for 39% of the reported cases, with a 52% mortality rate due to liver failure [17].

Management of HBV Reactivation

Multiple studies have shown that prevention is superior to intervention at the time of reactivation. Preventative measures should start with screening for HBV markers before initiation of chemotherapy. Patients should be tested for HBsAg and anti-HBc and anti-HBs antibodies. Those who are HBsAg positive should be further tested for HBeAg, anti-HBe, and HBV DNA.

For HBsAg positive patients, prophylactic therapy for HBV should be started as soon as possible before initiation of chemotherapy or other immunosuppressive therapy [8, 10, 12]. Lamivudine, a nucleoside analog, has been commonly used in this setting with minimal toxicity. In a randomized controlled study, 30 HBsAg-positive lymphoma patients were randomized to receive lamivudine 100 mg daily 1 week prior to initiating chemotherapy or to have this treatment deferred until there was serologic evidence of HBV reactivation. None of the patients in the preemptive treatment group experienced reactivation, as opposed to eight patients (53%) in the deferred treatment group ($p=0.002$) [18]. In another randomized trial of 73 patients with hepatocellular carcinoma undergoing transarterial chemo-lipiodolization (TACL), patients were randomized to preemptive lamivudine 100 mg daily at the start of TACL vs. deferred treatment (control) until there was confirmation of HBV reactivation. Patients in the preemptive group were continued on lamivudine for 12 months after completion of TACL. Eleven patients (30%) in the control group and one patient (3%) in the preemptive treatment group developed HBV reactivation ($p=0.002$). In addition, there were significantly more episodes of overall hepatitis and severe grade of hepatitis in the control group [19]. A recent meta-analysis on the efficacy of preemptive lamivudine on HBV reactivation included 14 studies, with 275 patients in the treatment group and 475 control participants [20]. The relative risk (RR) in favor of preventive lamivudine vs. no prevention ranged from 0.00 to 0.21 for both HBV reactivation and HBV-related hepatitis. With one exception for an HBV-related death in one study, regardless of design, all studies reported beneficial effects of preventive lamivudine treatment [20].

The optimal time to start and discontinue anti-HBV treatment for the prevention of HBV reactivation remains uncertain. One concern is that the highest HBV reactivation rates have been observed in studies with the longest follow-ups after completion of chemotherapy [21]. Furthermore, reactivation rates after lamivudine withdrawal are significantly higher in patients with higher prechemotherapy HBV DNA levels and HepBeAg seropositivity [21]. For patients receiving conventional chemotherapy, lamivudine has been recommended for at least 6 months after discontinuation of all immunosuppression [7, 8, 12, 22]. Longer duration of treatment (12 months or more) may be necessary for patients receiving monoclonal antibody therapies or hematopoietic SCT [21, 23, 24]. Patients with high baseline HBV DNA (>2,000 IU/mL) should continue treatment until they reach treatment endpoints as in immunocompetent patients [22].

An area of concern with longer duration of lamivudine therapy is the development of resistant mutations [12].

There are newer nucleoside analogs approved for the treatment of patients with hepatitis B infection including adefovir, entecavir, telbivudine, and tenofovir. For those patients in need of prolonged anti-HBV therapy, it might be appropriate to use drugs with low-incidence of resistance (adefovir, entecavir, or tenofovir) as first-line preemptive therapy [22]. Interferons should not be used in patients undergoing cytotoxic therapy because of its bone marrow suppressive effects.

Patients who are HBsAg-negative and anti-HBc positive should be considered for antiviral prophylaxis, especially if prolonged immunosuppression or SCT is contemplated [7]. Prophylaxis should continue for at least 6 months after discontinuation of chemotherapy.

When managing a patient with the clinical diagnosis of HBV reactivation who has not received prophylactic anti-HBV therapy, all chemotherapy must be suspended and treatment with nucleoside analogs must be instituted. Experience with lamivudine indicates that this drug might be effective but mortality from hepatic failure may still be high [12, 23].

Reactivation of Hepatitis C Virus

The prevalence of HCV infection in cancer patients varies between 1.5 and 8.2% [1, 25, 26], and is more common than HBV infection even in endemic areas [1, 27]. On the other hand, although the prevalence of HCV infection in patients with cancer is high, patients with hematological malignancies and chronic HCV infection have a significantly lower incidence of severe liver dysfunction or viral reactivation following chemotherapy when compared to HBV-infected patients [1, 26]. The reason for this difference is unknown [1, 27]. Of interest, the mortality rate seems to be similar between HBV and HCV infected patients once severe hepatitis developed secondary to reactivation [28].

Currently, no uniform definition for HCV reactivation is available, but it has defined as a threefold or greater increase in serum alanine aminotransferase (ALT) level, in the absence of liver infiltration of cancer, hepatotoxic drugs, recent transfusion, and other systemic infections. Changes in liver enzymes should be accompanied by a sudden increase in serum HCV RNA level or reappearence of HCV RNA [27].

Pathogenesis and Clinical Manifestations

As reported for HBV infection [27, 29], reactivation of HCV occurs when chemotherapy depresses the immune system, leading to enhanced viral replication that exceeds largely the kinetics of the immune response and increased infected hepatocytes [30]. In addition, withdrawal of cytotoxic or immunosuppressive treatments may lead to an immunological rebound after a period of depressed cellular immunity with restoration of the host immune function and increase inflammatory activity in the liver, resulting in rapid destruction of the infected hepatocytes and liver injury [26, 30].

The possibility of HCV reactivation should be considered in patients with a history of chronic HCV infection developing liver dysfunction following chemotherapy. However, the timing of HCV reactivation may vary. It can occur during chemotherapy, but it is more frequently seen few weeks or months following withdrawal of chemotherapy and/or corticosteroids [26, 31–33]. In a series of 18 patients with hematologic malignancies who experienced acute exacerbation of chronic HCV infection, the increase in aminotransferase levels occurred at a mean of 19 days (range, 14–32 days) after withdrawal of chemotherapy, most commonly after the fourth or fifth cycle [32].

In the majority of cases, the acute elevation of ALT or HCV RNA is asymptomatic, with mild and transient elevation of the ALT levels. Some patients may have more severe flares with massive necrosis, liver failure, and death [34, 35]. In some of the fatal cases, HCV RNA levels increased dramatically during treatment, with a sharp decrease in HCV RNA and a marked increase in aminotransferase levels occurring on withdrawal of chemotherapy [35]. Of note, HCV viremia could be low in cases of severe hepatitis, probably because of massive liver cell necrosis and absence of suitable cells for viral replication [35]. Among patients who experienced severe hepatitis during chemotherapy, liver function tests return to normal within 2–3 weeks of discontinuation of the offending agent [32]. However, peak ALT levels above 6,000 IU/L with a delay recovery of about 7 weeks have been reported in cases of fulminant hepatitis [35].

In some cases of severe hepatitis due to HCV reactivation, chemotherapy needs to be discontinued [31, 32, 36]. Based on preliminary data from our institution, chemotherapy regimens in individuals with acute exacerbation of chronic HCV infection were discontinued in up to 22% of patients [25]. Chemotherapy can be restarted after the acute event when the liver function tests became normal.

In SCT recipients, severe hepatic dysfunction and fulminant hepatic failure can occur, with significantly increased HCV RNA levels during immunosuppressive therapy and fulminant hepatitis occurring after withdrawal of immunosuppressives, which most commonly included cyclosporine and/or prednisone [37–40].

HCV infection may be diagnosed using serological assays for antibodies and molecular tests for viral particles. Antibodies against HCV are detected by enzyme immunoassays that are very sensitive and very specific. However, cancer patients, especially those with hematologic malignancies, can have false-negative results [31, 41–43]. Even more, during chemotherapy and immunosuppressive therapy, HCV serology may be negative, thus making HCV RNA monitoring by polymerase chain reaction useful. Patients who are chronically infected with HCV, and are suspected to be having an HCV reactivation, should have HCV RNA levels measured for virologic confirmation [33].

Risk Factors

HCV reactivation in cancer patients appears to be more common in males, with underlying lymphoma (mainly non-Hodgkin's lymphoma), and prior exposure to corticosteroids [25, 26, 35]. Reactivation has also been reported in patients receiving chemotherapy for solid tumors [44], or SCT recipients [37, 40].

The presence of corticosteroids in the chemotherapy regimens is considered one of the most important risk factors for chemotherapy-induced HCV reactivation. These agents can induce the replication of HCV in vivo and in vitro [45]. Other chemotherapy or immunosuppressive drugs that have been linked to the reactivation of HCV include cyclophosphamide, doxorubicin, vincristine, cytarabine, bleomycin, etoposide, vinblastine, dacarbazine, busulfan, methotrexate, and cyclosporine [25, 35, 37, 40, 46], and the newer chemotherapy drugs rituximab and alemtuzumab [34, 46, 47]. However, it should be noted that many of these patients were treated simultaneously with corticosteroids [25, 34, 37, 46, 47]. The association between HCV reactivation and specifics HCV genotypes has not been clearly established.

Management of HCV Reactivation

The combination of pegylated interferon alfa and ribavirin can eradicate the HCV in more than 50% of patients. Combination therapy is more effective than monotherapy with either agent and has a higher rate of sustained virological response [48].

Unfortunately, the best strategy of managing HCV reactivation is not clear. Unlike HBV, there are no approved drugs for primary prophylaxis of HCV reactivation in chronically infected patients undergoing chemotherapy.

In HCV-infected cancer patients, the hematologic side effects of HCV drugs can exacerbate the side effects of chemotherapy, and fear for complications such as severe cytopenias and invasive infections has excluded the use of HCV therapy in patients undergoing intensive chemotherapy [36]. However, there is emerging data to suggest that antiviral treatment could be considered when liver dysfunction prohibits the administration of life-saving chemotherapy. Based on a recent small case series, combination therapy of standard interferon-alfa and ribavirin was given simultaneously to chemotherapy in three children with hematologic malignancies who presented with severe HCV exacerbation during intensive chemotherapy. The decision to initiate concomitant therapy was made when hepatic dysfunction led to complete inability to use chemotherapy. Patients were continued on antiviral treatment while they received intensive chemotherapy. Two children tolerated interferon plus ribavirin well, while the remaining patient developed severe febrile episodes, with prolonged neutropenia and depression [49]. Unfortunately, HCV therapy could be poorly tolerated and had to be discontinued due to severe hematologic toxicity in some adults in whom simultaneous use of antivirals and chemotherapy has been attempted [34]. In other study, ribavirin monotherapy administered during conditioning regimen and after transplant in HCV-infected patients requiring SCT appeared to be safe and effective in clearance of HCV RNA [50]. Large scale studies are needed to better define the cancer population that will benefit from this simultaneous therapeutic intervention.

Potential strategies to reduce the risk of HCV reactivation in cancer patients with chronic infection undergoing cytotoxic chemotherapy include the use of less aggressive and less immunosuppressive chemotherapy protocols in HCV-infected patients, and close monitoring of ALT throughout the course of chemotherapy, especially after immunosuppressive therapy is reduced or withdrawn, with early measurement of HCV RNA levels during episodes of potential viral reactivation.

To date, there is not enough information to recommend secondary antiviral prophylaxis for the population that has been exposed to HCV but are HCV negative.

Summary

HBV reactivation is a serious but preventable complication of immunosuppressive therapy. All patients at risk should be screened for HBV markers. Prophylactic anti-HBV therapy is effective. Lamivudine has been found to reduce the risk for HBV reactivation and HBV-associated morbidity and mortality. The use of newer nucleoside analogs is recommended for those who will require prolonged (>12 months) therapy. It seems that HCV have a lower reactivation rate following chemotherapy than HBV, but its presentation can be fatal. The best strategy of managing HCV reactivation is not clear.

References

1. Kawatani T, Suou T, Tajima F, et al. Incidence of hepatitis virus infection and severe liver dysfunction in patients receiving chemotherapy for hematologic malignancies. Eur J Haematol. 2001;67:45–50.
2. Kawatani T, Suou T, Tajima F, Ooi S, Kawasaki H. Hepatitis C virus infection in acute leukemia with liver dysfunction. Eur J Haematol. 1993;51:254–5.
3. Lok AS, Liang RH, Chiu EK, Wong KL, Chan TK, Todd D. Reactivation of hepatitis B virus replication in patients receiving cytotoxic therapy. Report of a prospective study. Gastroenterology. 1991;100:182–8.
4. Law JK, Ho JK, Hoskins PJ, Erb SR, Steinbrecher UP, Yoshida EM. Fatal reactivation of hepatitis B post-chemotherapy for lymphoma in a hepatitis B surface antigen-negative, hepatitis B core antibody-positive patient: potential implications for future prophylaxis recommendations. Leuk Lymphoma. 2005;46:1085–9.
5. Alexopoulos CG, Vaslamatzis M, Hatzidimitriou G. Prevalence of hepatitis B virus marker positivity and evolution of hepatitis B virus profile, during chemotherapy, in patients with solid tumours. Br J Cancer. 1999;81:69–74.
6. Lau GK. Hepatitis B reactivation after chemotherapy: two decades of clinical research. Hepatol Int. 2008;2:152–62.
7. Hoofnagle JH. Reactivation of hepatitis B. Hepatology. 2009;49:S156–65.
8. Mindikoglu AL, Regev A, Schiff ER. Hepatitis B virus reactivation after cytotoxic chemotherapy: the disease and its prevention. Clin Gastroenterol Hepatol. 2006;4:1076–81.
9. Su WP, Wen CC, Hsiung CA, et al. Long-term hepatic consequences of chemotherapy-related HBV reactivation in lymphoma patients. World J Gastroenterol. 2005;11:5283–8.
10. Yeo W, Chan PK, Ho WM, et al. Lamivudine for the prevention of hepatitis B virus reactivation in hepatitis B s-antigen seropositive cancer patients undergoing cytotoxic chemotherapy. J Clin Oncol. 2004;22:927–34.
11. Liang R, Lau GK, Kwong YL. Chemotherapy and bone marrow transplantation for cancer patients who are also chronic hepatitis B carriers: a review of the problem. J Clin Oncol. 1999;17:394–8.
12. Lalazar G, Rund D, Shouval D. Screening, prevention and treatment of viral hepatitis B reactivation in patients with haematological malignancies. Br J Haematol. 2007;136:699–712.
13. Lau GK, Leung YH, Fong DY, et al. High hepatitis B virus (HBV) DNA viral load as the most important risk factor for HBV reactivation in patients positive for HBV surface antigen undergoing autologous hematopoietic cell transplantation. Blood. 2002;99:2324–30.
14. Yeo W, Chan PK, Zhong S, et al. Frequency of hepatitis B virus reactivation in cancer patients undergoing cytotoxic chemotherapy: a prospective study of 626 patients with identification of risk factors. J Med Virol. 2000;62:299–307.
15. Yeo W, Zee B, Zhong S, et al. Comprehensive analysis of risk factors associating with Hepatitis B virus (HBV) reactivation in cancer patients undergoing cytotoxic chemotherapy. Br J Cancer. 2004;90:1306–11.
16. Jang JW, Choi JY, Bae SH, et al. Transarterial chemo-lipiodolization can reactivate hepatitis B virus replication in patients with hepatocellular carcinoma. J Hepatol. 2004;41:427–35.
17. Aksoy S, Harputluoglu H, Kilickap S, et al. Rituximab-related viral infections in lymphoma patients. Leuk Lymphoma. 2007;48:1307–12.
18. Lau GK, Yiu HH, Fong DY, et al. Early is superior to deferred preemptive lamivudine therapy for hepatitis B patients undergoing chemotherapy. Gastroenterology. 2003;125:1742–9.
19. Jang JW, Choi JY, Bae SH, et al. A randomized controlled study of preemptive lamivudine in patients receiving transarterial chemo-lipiodolization. Hepatology. 2006;43:233–40.
20. Loomba R, Rowley A, Wesley R, et al. Systematic review: the effect of preventive lamivudine on hepatitis B reactivation during chemotherapy. Ann Intern Med. 2008;148:519–28.
21. Hui CK, Cheung WW, Au WY, et al. Hepatitis B reactivation after withdrawal of pre-emptive lamivudine in patients with haematological malignancy on completion of cytotoxic chemotherapy. Gut. 2005;54:1597–603.
22. Lok AS, McMahon BJ. Chronic hepatitis B. Hepatology. 2007;45:507–39.
23. Yeo W, Johnson PJ. Diagnosis, prevention and management of hepatitis B virus reactivation during anticancer therapy. Hepatology. 2006;43:209–20.
24. Lau GK, He ML, Fong DY, et al. Preemptive use of lamivudine reduces hepatitis B exacerbation after allogeneic hematopoietic cell transplantation. Hepatology. 2002;36:702–9.
25. Torres HA, Mahale P, Davila M, Mulanovich V, Granwehr B, Kontoyiannis DP, Raad II. Hepatitis C virus infection in cancer patients: the story of a forgotten population. In: Abstracts of the 48th Annual Meeting of the Infectious Diseases Society of America; 21–24 Oct 2010. Canada: Vancouver; 2010.
26. Takai S, Tsurumi H, Ando K, et al. Prevalence of hepatitis B and C virus infection in haematological malignancies and liver injury following chemotherapy. Eur J Haematol. 2005;74:158–65.
27. Ozguroglu M, Bilici A, Turna H, Serdengecti S. Reactivation of hepatitis B virus infection with cytotoxic therapy in non-Hodgkin's lymphoma. Med Oncol. 2004;21:67–72.
28. Nakamura Y, Motokura T, Fujita A, Yamashita T, Ogata E. Severe hepatitis related to chemotherapy in hepatitis B virus carriers with hematologic malignancies. Survey in Japan, 1987–1991. Cancer. 1996;78:2210–5.
29. Keeffe EB. Hepatitis B virus reactivation with chemotherapy: diagnosis and prevention with antiviral prophylaxis. Rev Gastroenterol Disord. 2004;4:46–8.
30. Peffault de Latour R, Ribaud P, Robin M, et al. Allogeneic hematopoietic cell transplant in HCV-infected patients. J Hepatol. 2008;48:1008–17.
31. Gigliotti AR, Fioredda F, Giacchino R. Hepatitis B and C infection in children undergoing chemotherapy or bone marrow transplantation. J Pediatr Hematol Oncol. 2003;25:184–92.
32. Zuckerman E, Zuckerman T, Douer D, Qian D, Levine AM. Liver dysfunction in patients infected with hepatitis C virus undergoing chemotherapy for hematologic malignancies. Cancer. 1998;83:1224–30.
33. Mahale P, Davila M, Chemaly RF, Lewis RE, Hwang JP, Kontoyiannis DP, Torres HA. Acute exacerbation of chronic hepatitis C in cancer patients. In: Abstracts of the 48th Annual Meeting of the Infectious Diseases Society of America; 21–24 Oct 2010. Canada: Vancouver; 2010.
34. Anoop P, Wotherspoon A, Matutes E. Severe liver dysfunction from hepatitis C virus reactivation following alemtuzumab treatment for chronic lymphocytic leukaemia. Br J Haematol. 2010;148:484–6.
35. Vento S, Cainelli F, Mirandola F, et al. Fulminant hepatitis on withdrawal of chemotherapy in carriers of hepatitis C virus. Lancet. 1996;347:92–3.
36. Firpi RJ, Nelson DR. Management of viral hepatitis in hematologic malignancies. Blood Rev. 2008;22:117–26.
37. Kanamori H, Fukawa H, Maruta A, et al. Case report: fulminant hepatitis C viral infection after allogeneic bone marrow transplantation. Am J Med Sci. 1992;303:109–11.
38. Maruta A, Kanamori H, Fukawa H, et al. Liver function tests of recipients with hepatitis C virus infection after bone marrow transplantation. Bone Marrow Transplant. 1994;13:417–22.

39. Ljungman P, Johansson N, Aschan J, et al. Long-term effects of hepatitis C virus infection in allogeneic bone marrow transplant recipients. Blood. 1995;86:1614–8.
40. Fan FS, Tzeng CH, Hsiao KI, Hu ST, Liu WT, Chen PM. Withdrawal of immunosuppressive therapy in allogeneic bone marrow transplantation reactivates chronic viral hepatitis C. Bone Marrow Transplant. 1991;8:417–20.
41. Locasciulli A, Testa M, Pontisso P, et al. Prevalence and natural history of hepatitis C infection in patients cured of childhood leukemia. Blood. 1997;90:4628–33.
42. Poynard T, Yuen MF, Ratziu V, Lai CL. Viral hepatitis C. Lancet. 2003;362:2095–100.
43. Pawlotsky JM. Use and interpretation of virological tests for hepatitis C. Hepatology. 2002;36:S65–73.
44. Melisko ME, Fox R, Venook A. Reactivation of hepatitis C virus after chemotherapy for colon cancer. Clin Oncol (R Coll Radiol). 2004;16:204–5.
45. Magy N, Cribier B, Schmitt C, et al. Effects of corticosteroids on HCV infection. Int J Immunopharmacol. 1999;21:253–61.
46. Ennishi D, Terui Y, Yokoyama M, et al. Monitoring serum hepatitis C virus (HCV) RNA in patients with HCV-infected CD20-positive B-cell lymphoma undergoing rituximab combination chemotherapy. Am J Hematol. 2008;83:59–62.
47. Hsieh CY, Huang HH, Lin CY, et al. Rituximab-induced hepatitis C virus reactivation after spontaneous remission in diffuse large B-cell lymphoma. J Clin Oncol. 2008;26:2584–6.
48. Keating MR. Antiviral agents for non-human immunodeficiency virus infections. Mayo Clin Proc. 1999;74:1266–83.
49. Papaevangelou V, Varsami M, Papadakis V, et al. Hepatitis C treatment concomitant to chemotherapy as "salvage" therapy in children with hematologic malignancies. Pediatr Infect Dis J. 2010;29:277–80.
50. Ljungman P, Andersson J, Aschan J, et al. Oral ribavirin for prevention of severe liver disease caused by hepatitis C virus during allogeneic bone marrow transplantation. Clin Infect Dis. 1996;23:167–9.

Chapter 18
Management of Genitourinary Tract Infections

Amar Safdar and Maurie Markman

Abstract The risk of developing an infection in patients with genitourinary tract malignancy arise from a host of factors such as: (1) tumor encroachment and invasion of adjacent structures; (2) tumor necrosis; (3) complications arising from antineoplastic chemotherapy; (4) early and late effects of abdomiopelvic radiation therapy; (5) surgical tumor excision and removal of internal organs; (6) structural abnormalities resulting from surgical diversion procedures; and (7) other causes that disrupt protective barriers in urinary and female reproductive tract. The spectrum of causative organisms most frequently arise from patients' endogenous microflora. The vagina, lower urinary and intestinal tract colonization with bacteria and yeast serves as important sources for infection. The normal aerobic and anaerobic vaginal bacterial flora may be altered in patients undergoing antineoplastic therapy. Among factors that influence changes in colonization includes, hormonal dysfunction, frequent exposure to broad-spectrum antimicrobial agents, antineoplastic therapy, hospitalization, and instrumentization. Peritonitis, intraabdominal abscess, complicated urinary tract infection, surgical wound infection, skin and soft tissue infection such as cellulitis, necrotizing fasciitis, clostridial myonecrosis, and septic pelvic thrombophlebitis are important infectious complications encountered in patients with genitourinary tract malignancies.

Keywords Genitourinary tract • Cancer • Peritonitis • Intraabdominal abscess • Urinary tract infection • Surgical wound infection • Cellulitis • Necrotizing fasciitis • Clostridial myonecrosis • Septic pelvic thrombophlebitis

Introduction

The risk of developing an infection in patients with genitourinary tract malignancy arise from a number of factors such as: (1) tumor encroachment and invasion of adjacent structures; (2) tumor necrosis; (3) complications arising from antineoplastic chemotherapy; (4) early and late effects of abdomiopelvic radiation therapy; (5) surgical tumor excision and removal of internal organs; (6) structural abnormalities resulting from surgical diversion procedures; and (7) other causes that disrupt protective barriers in urinary and female reproductive tract [1, 2].

The spectrum of causative organisms most frequently arise from patients' endogenous microflora. The vagina, lower urinary, and intestinal tract colonization with bacteria and yeast serves as important sources for infection. The normal aerobic and anaerobic vaginal bacterial flora may be altered in patients undergoing antineoplastic therapy. Among factors that influence changes in colonization includes, hormonal dysfunction, frequent exposure to broad-spectrum antimicrobial agents, antineoplastic therapy, hospitalization, and instrumentization.

The female genital tract is rich in anaerobic microflora. Bacteria belonging to *Peptococcaceae* are the most prominent organisms in the normal vaginal flora. Quantitative vaginal cultures in recent studies showed that anaerobic bacteria outnumbered aerobic bacteria by nearly 10:1; these include peptococci, *Lactobacillus*, *Corynebacterium*, *Eubacterium*, and *Bacteroides* species which are common organisms isolated [3]. *Escherichia coli*, *Klebsiella* species, and *Enterobacter* species are the aerobic gram-negatives and streptococci, enterococci, and coagulase-negative staphylococcus are gram-positive bacteria isolated form of lower female genital tract. These organisms provide an important reference to local and invasive infections seen in patients undergoing treatment for gynecologic malignancy.

A. Safdar (✉)
Department of Infectious Diseases, Infection Control, and Employee Health, The University of Texas M.D. Anderson Cancer Center, 1515 Holcombe Boulevard, Houston, TX 77030, USA
e-mail: amarsafdar@gmail.com

Patient with Fever

In Table 18.1 factors that increase the risk for infection are shown. Awareness of specific cancer-therapy associated risks and host's underlying immune dysfunction may allow proper selection of empiric antibiotic therapy in critically ill patients prior to the results of microbiologic culture and radiographic studies becomes available. It is important to note that patients with gynecologic cancer may have a high risk of polymicrobial infections due to anatomic proximity to lower intestinal and urinary tracts [4]. In certain infections such as deep tissue abscess, cellulitis in patients with chronic fistula tract, presence of large necrotic tumor, history of multiple instrumentization probability of polymicrobial infection remains high [4]. Obstruction to pelvic venous and lymphatic flow in patients with advanced cancer with history of radiation therapy increases the risk for skin and soft tissue infection, deep pelvic infection, abscess formation, and septic thrombophlebitis. These may be difficult to distinguish from noninfectious tumor-related complications.

Table 18.1 Predisposing risk factors and infections in patients with gynecologic tumor

Tumor-related
Obstruction of gastrointestinal or urinary tract
Erosion into bowel, urinary tract, peritoneum or retroperitoneal
Necrosis of rapidly growing cancer promote abscess formation
Lymphatic obstruction
Surgery
Aspiration pneumonia
Hospital-acquired pneumonia, including ventilator-associated pneumonia
Wound infection, skin and skin structure infection
Tissue necrosis due to disruption of blood supply
Infected hematoma
Fistula tract communication between intestinal and urinary tracts
Complicated peritonitis
Septic deep thrombophlebitis
Fasciitis, myositis, and gas gangrene are rare complications
Chemotherapy
Febrile neutropenia
Pneumonia
Neutropenic enterocolitis
Radiation therapy
Enteritis
Urinary tract infection
Poor wound healing
Catheter and implantable devices
Device infection
Peritonitis
Bloodstream infection
Urinary tract infection

Tumor-Related

The tumor associated infections are dependent on the site and extent of tumor involvement. In patients with early stage of locally involved cancer such as stage I cervical cancer, most infections remain localized to vagina. Whereas, in patients with advanced cervical cancer infections may involve fallopian tubes, ovaries leading to tubo-ovarian abscess, uterine involvement may cause less frequently seen pyometra. Extension of these infections to adjacent structures such as urinary tract presents as ascending pyelonephritis; rectal abscess, and complicated peritonitis are serious and difficult-to-treat infections [5, 6]. It is also important to note that an infection may be the primary presentation of an undiagnosed malignancy involving female reproductive tract. In a study of postmenopausal women who presented with tubo-ovarian abscess, nearly half of these patients were subsequently diagnosed with a gynecologic malignancy [7]. Therefore, we recommend a thorough investigation for possible underlying cancer that should be considered in postmenopausal women or those with no risk factors for sexually transmitted diseases who present with tubo-ovarian abscess or pyometra.

The advances in improved outcomes for serious systemic bacterial and yeast infections are in most part due to availability of well-tolerated broad-spectrum antimicrobial agents. The recent emergence and spread of multidrug-resistant organisms, however, may mitigate these gains and even patients with solid-organ cancer with limited immune suppression may develop life-threatening septicemia and peritonitis as noted during 1970s [8].

Surgery-Related

Patient undergoing surgery for cervical cancer have higher rate of infectious complications while patients with endometrial cancer tolerate surgery better and have less infections during early and late postoperative period [9]. Pelvic exenteration is performed in patients with advanced and/or treatment refractory cervical and upper reproductive tract malignancy. Infections remain as serious morbidity following pelvic exenteration; early postsurgical wound infection and wound dehiscence are not uncommon [10]. Urinary tract infections are also frequently seen in patients with urinary fistula, and/or those who develop urethral obstruction. Studies show, greater than 40% of patients undergoing pelvic exenteration for gynecological and rectal cancer had urinary tract infection and wound dehiscence [11]. Late infections such as ascending pyelonephritis may be serious, as these infections are often recurrent and seen in patients with usually irreparable structural damage to the urinary reservoir, urethral stenosis, and anastomosis obstruction. Ureterointestinal fistula, stones in the urinary reservoir and stenosis all contribute to increase risk of infections and unless the anatomical abnormality are corrected, these patients remain at increased risk for recurrent urinary tract infections and complication arising from prolonged systemic antibiotic therapy and hospitalization.

Empiric therapy includes adequate coverage for possible polymicrobial infection, and choice should include drugs that provide adequate coverage for enteric coliforms, enterococci, including vancomycin-resistant *Enterococcus* species, especially in patient with known prior intestinal or genitourinary tract colonization due to these drug-resistant bacteria [12]. As most infections in this setting may also have an anaerobe as copathogen, even in patients with negative microbiologic evidence of anaerobic infection, antibiotic selection should entertain possibility of concurrent mixed anaerobic–aerobic infection. We recommend secondary suppressive antimicrobial therapy in patients with recurrent deep pelvic infection to reduced morbidity and subsequent hospitalization and surgeries. As it is critical to select high-risk patients judiciously, patients are not given prolonged courses of broad-spectrum antibiotics, inappropriately which is the single most important factor in promoting drug resistance in healthcare-associated infections.

Infections remain main concern in patients following radical vulvar resection and inguinal lymphadenectomy. Early postoperative cellulitis was noted in nearly one third of patients undergoing inguinal lymphadenectomy and in over 20%, early surgical wound breakdown also occurred [13]. Whereas, late cellulitis at surgical site was noted in patients with chronic lymphedema and in most patients surgical wound was not compromised [13].

Wound Infection

Infected surgical wound in patients following female genital tract surgery include *Staphylococcus aureus,* including multidrug-resistant strains (MRSA) obtained from healthcare microflora (healthcare-associated; HA) or community acquired (CA)-MRSA, which has now become the leading source of MRSA in the United States. *Streptococcus* species (group A, B, C and G) are also commonly pathogens in this population and nearly one third of infections, especially those with involvement of lower intestinal tract and urinary tract are less likely to be monomicrobial.

In patients treated with systemic corticosteroids for extended periods, patients with morbid obesity and those with diabetes mellitus have a higher risk of developing postoperative wound infections. Coagulase-negative staphylococcus, *Streptococcus* species, *S. aureus*, enteric gram-negative bacteria, and *Bacteroides* species are potential pathogens.

Patients who have a complicated hospital course following surgery may develop infections due to organisms acquired from the healthcare microenvironment. In critically ill patients, infections are treated empirically and spectrum of causative organism(s) may not be available at the time of medical decision making. Knowledge of regional and institutional prevalence of drug-resistant organisms is required in prescribing appropriate treatment regimen. The empiric therapy in patients with prolonged hospitalization, and anatomical abnormalities such as enterouretheral, entero-, rectovaginal or enterovesicular fistula increases probability of recurrent infection due to resistant HA-gram-negative bacteria such as *Pseudomonas* species, extended-spectrum beta-lactamases producing *Enterobacteriaceae*, including *E. coli*. Other nonfermentative gram-negative bacteria like *Acinetobacter* spp. and *Stenotrophomonas maltophilia* are often resistant to a wide spectrum of commonly used antibiotics and treatment for these multidrug-resistant (MDR) bacteria remains a daunting task [14, 15].

Intraabdominal and Pelvic Abscess

The secondary seeding of the intraperitoneal necrotic tumor mass in patients with bloodstream infection arising from a difference primary source such as urinary tract, or antineoplastic therapy-induced orointestinal mucositis may also occur. The spectrum of causative organism includes enteric bacteria such as *E. coli*, *Enterococcus*, *Staphylococcus* species, Bacteroides, and other anaerobes. *Candida* species infection is less frequent in nonneutropenic patients although patients with Candida species colonization at multiple sites in the body, exposure to prolonged broad-spectrum antibiotics, poorly controlled diabetes mellitus, systemic corticosteroid use, stay in critical care units, and presence of foreign devices may increase risk for invasive candidiasis.

Hematogenous or direct seeding of the retroperitoneal space may lead to paraspinal and psoas abscess, these infections escape early detection as patients may not have high-grade fever and de novo or sudden increase in chronic low back pain remain subject to interpretation. In the absence of a direct extension from intestinal or urinary tract, these retroperitoneal infections are usually monomicrobial, and diagnosis requires prompt aspiration of the infected collection. In tuberculous endemic regions, *Mycobacterium tuberculous* infection should be considered.

Pelvic abscesses that develop after instrumentization or following surgery are often polymicrobial and treatment is directed towards normal intestinal tract and cutaneous microflora.

Peritoneal infections following bowel perforation, anastomotic leaks, or fistula tracts may present with fever, abdominal pain and fistula drainage, and/or surgical wound dehiscence. Most infections, as expected are polymicrobial and *Enterobacteriaceae*, *S. aureus, Streptococcus* and *Enterococcus* species including vancomycin-resistant strains which are frequently encountered. *Bacteroides fragilis*, and *Clostridium* species are common anaerobes; *Fusobacterium*, *Peptostreptococcus,* and *Eubacterium* occur less frequently. Patients with peritoneal infections following surgery involving the nonsterile bowel and lower genitourinary tract may also have an increased risk for *Pseudomonas* species infection.

Chemotherapy and Radiation-Related

Patients with receiving chemotherapy may have increased risk of infection, neutropenia for less than a week increases risk for systemic bacterial infections due to *S. aureus* and *Pseudomonas* species. Patients who remain neutropenic for longer than 5 days are also at an increased risk for developing systemic *Candida* species infection [1, 2]. Disruption of orointestinal and genitourinary tract mucosa compromised an important barrier in prevention of bacterial and yeast invasion. In patients with severe treatment-induced mucositis, alpha hemolytic streptococcal and anaerobic septicemia may lead to devastating consequences [16].

Radiation therapy in patients with vulvar, vaginal, and cervical cancer causes microvascular damage to the tissue and may lead to difficult-to-treat intestinal, vaginal, and urologic complications.

Increased doses of radiation for gynecologic cancer have been associated with improved cancer-free survival [17]. Although with increase in radiation dose, the rate of complication has also risen [18]. Among noninfectious complications arising from high-dose radiotherapy include tissue and bone necrosis, fistula formation, enteritis, and fibrosis that may lead to vaginal, rectal, and ureteric stenosis and increased risk for secondary infection due to stagnation and inadequate tissue drainage [19]. Rarely, patients with radiation-induced necrosis of pelvic bones increase risk for secondary bone infection, these infection challenging and multifaceted treatment approach may be needed for implementing successful outcomes [20]. Patient with osteomyelitis in the setting of radiation-induced bone necrosis may need surgical debridement, appropriate selection of antibiotics given for a prolonged period. A high clinical suspicion remains critical in timely diagnosis of radiation-related infectious and noninfectious complication.

Bacteremia

In patients with solid-organ cancer, *E. coli* and coagulase-negative staphylococcus account for nearly 40% of bacteremia; whereas, *Pseudomonas*, *S. aureus,* and enterococcal bloodstream infection are 10% or less, each [21]. *Klebsiella* species, other *Enterobacteriaceae* and *S. maltophilia* are a serious concern and may become prominent bloodstream infection in certain geographic regions.

In cancer patients with bacteremia, who present with extensive tissue involvement/infection are significantly less likely to respond to antimicrobial therapy [22]. Other factors associated with poor prognosis in bacteremic patients with an underlying malignancy include shock, infection due to MDR bacteria, *Pseudomonas* and *Clostridium* species infection [22].

Bacteroides and *Clostridium* species are most frequent cause of anaerobic bacteremia, which are most frequently seen in patients with abdominal and pelvic malignancy [23]. Polymicrobial infections are more frequent in patients with anaerobic bacteremia compared with aerobic bacterial infections. In patients with anaerobic bacteremia concurrent candidemia is seldom noted. Over 90% of patients with nonsporulating anaerobic bacteremia may also have a deep tissue abscess [24]. Authors suggest that all patients with gynecologic malignancy who present with anaerobic bacteremia require thorough evaluation for an occult abdomiopelvic infected collection.

Clostridial bacteremia is often seen in patients with gastrointestinal, genitourinary cancer, and acute leukemia [25]. Nearly one third of patients with bacteremia with *Clostridium* species alone and nearly half with polymicrobial infection present with septic shock. *Clostridium perfringens* is common species, and *Clostridium septicum* is rare albeit, serious infection, and mostly seen in patients with an intraabdominal cancer [25]. Diffuse, rapidly spreading cellulitis involving the abdominal wall groin, and upper thigh area, gas gangrene, and acute intravascular hemolysis indicates possibility of clostridial infection [25]. Early appropriate therapy remains critical in improved response and outcome for patients with systemic anaerobic infection.

Febrile Neutropenia

During the first week of neutropenia, bacterial infections are prominent; if neutropenia extends, invasive candidiasis becomes a concern and in patients with greater than 2 weeks of profound neutropenia invasive mold infections such as aspergillosis may be occasionally encountered. [1, 2] However, in patients with gynecologic malignancy isolation of a mold even from a sterile body sites does not indicate invasive fungal disease; these patients with no predisposing factors [26], isolation of saprophytic molds represents colonization or a laboratory contamination.

Catheter-Related Bloodstream Infection

In patients with solid-organ cancer, nearly 70% of gram-positive bacteremia are associated with an infected catheter, similarly 60% of gram-negative bacteria are also related with an infected catheter whereas, only 19% of gram-negative bacteremia in patients with hematologic cancer are due to an infected catheter [27]. Coagulase-negative staphylococcus remains the most commonly isolated organisms in blood cultures drawn from an indwelling central venous catheter and frequently regarded as catheter-related infection. Similarly, S. aureus, including MRSA bacteremia may result from an infected indwelling catheter and successful therapy require selection of antimicrobial agents that penetrate the biofilm and are effective against the nonplanktonic, stationary phase of the bacteria [28].

Implantable Device Infections

Peritoneal, hepatic, and pleural implantable devices for delivering chemotherapy or drainage of recurring malignant effusions have successfully been used in the last decade. These devices are well tolerated, major complications including bowel perforation are uncommon and serious infections are seen in less than 5% of cases [29, 30]. Over all infections are seen in less than 20% of the cases, whereas serious infections including pocket infection are seldom noticed. When occur, pocket infection should be treated aggressively, requiring removal of the infected reservoir and appropriate systemic antimicrobial therapy [31]. Abdominal pain and chemotherapy-related discomfort remains the main problem with these chemotherapy infusion devices.

Urinary Tract Infection

Patients with gynecologic cancer have increased risk for urinary tract infection. The factors that promote infections are listed in (Table 18.2). Nearly one-third of patients while

Table 18.2 Factors promoting urinary tract infections

Tumor obstruction
Retrograde urine flow leading to ascending pyelonephritis
Stagnation in patients with outlet obstruction and abscess formation
Instrumentization
Cystoscopy-related introduction of pathogens
Dilatation of strictures
Foreign body
Urethral stent
Percutaneous nephrostomy tube placement/replacement[a]
Surgical drains for extended duration
Radiotherapy
Inflammation of bladder mucosa
Suppression of local innate cellular and acellular immune response
Surgery
Urinary diversions
Organ resection
lymph node dissection
Anastomotic leak
Chronic surgical wound breakdown
Chemotherapy
Neutropenia
Suppression of local immune surveillance and response to bacterial invasion
Mucosal damage and disruption

[a]Patients undergoing routine replacement of percutaneous nephrostomy tubes may develop transient into bacteremia in the event of prior colonization

undergoing pelvic radiotherapy for gynecologic cancer may have symptoms of urinary tract infection at the onset of therapy or develop infection during the course of radiation therapy [32]. Despite appropriate therapy, infections may recur and require several courses of antibiotic therapy [32]. Patients who have undergone pelvic exenteration remain at increased risk for ascending urinary tract infection; [10] recurrent pyelonephritis in these patients may lead to permanent renal damage. Older patients with advanced gynecological cancer are also being considered for pelvic exenteration surgery [33]. In these and other patients with lower renal reserves, a severe episode of pyelonephritis may further compromise renal function. We suggest in select group of high-risk patients preemptive antimicrobial therapy or even secondary antibiotic prophylaxis may be considered following recurrent episode of urinary tract infection.

Patients with urinary diversions including suprapubic cystostomy, neobladder/ileal pouch, and percutaneous nephrostomy tube placement increase the risk of recurrent and frequently difficult-to-treat infections. The management becomes further complicated due to presence of aberrant communications between the intestinal and urinary tract or genital and urinary tracts. Furthermore, patients given antimicrobial prophylaxis for prevention of secondary infections may develop breakthrough infections due to multidrug-resistant bacteria and yeasts.

Prevention of Surgical Infection

The overall postoperative infection rate has been as high as 46% and surgical site infection seen in nearly one fourth of patients [34]. The risk of postoperative infection is adversely effective by prolonged duration of surgery for >5 h, presence of remote infection at the time of surgery, and duration of hospitalization for longer than 3 weeks; in patients with all three risk factors the relative risk of infections increases to 7.3 compared to 3 in patients who have only one of these risk factors [34]. Risk factors that have been associated with an increased incidence of infection in patients undergoing surgery for reproductive tract carcinoma include lower socioeconomic status, preoperative colonization, failure to administer perioperative heparin, obesity, older patient age, a longer operative period, and a longer hospital stay before surgery. [35, 36] Extent of surgery plays a central role in predicting probability and severity of postoperative infections [9–11, 36]. However, these risk factors were not uniform among investigators' evaluations.

Guidelines for the administration of antibiotics to uninfected patients undergoing pelvic surgical procedures were first proposed by Ledger et al. [37]. There have been few studies evaluating prophylaxis for women undergoing radical pelvic surgery for gynecologic malignancies. Recently, cefazolin was showed to be inferior to cefotetan as a single-dose prophylaxis in women undergoing elective abdominal hysterectomy [38]. In a placebo-controlled trail using a broad-spectrum cephalosporin plus beta-lactamase inhibitor eliminated risk of major operation site infection up to 27% [39]. Interestingly, patients with preoperative cervical colonization did not increase postoperative complications including duration of hospitalization, operative time, or febrile episodes compared with patient in whom no cervical colonization was demonstrated [40]. Overall decrease in significant postoperative infections was reported in patients undergoing radical hysterectomy [41, 42]. The benefit however, was mostly reduced local surgical wound infection [43]. Prospective data have not resolved this issue. No significant difference in overall operative-site infection was observed after preoperative prophylaxis by research groups of Rosenshein et al. [44] or Marsden et al. [45], but significantly lower incidences of infection were reported by Sevin et al. [46] and Micha et al. [47]. Sevin et al. reported that a short course (three doses) of prophylaxis was as effective as a long course (12 doses) in preventing major infection after radical hysterectomy [48]. If separate operative-site data from prospective studies are combined, the overall incidence of pelvic infection and wound infection was significantly reduced by the administration of prophylactic antimicrobials.

A cost-benefit analysis of three doses of cefazolin antimicrobial prophylaxis showed 29% reduction in infectious morbidity following vaginal hysterectomy and an 18% reduction in postoperative infections in patients following abdominal hysterectomy [49].

One patient population that has a significant surgical incision breakdown is that of women undergoing radical vulvectomy. Anecdotal experience indicates the principle pathogens to be *S. aureus* and *S. epidermidis*. The administration of broad-spectrum medications, such as piperacillin or mezlocillin, did not significantly reduce the incidence of postoperative wound infection; 8 of 12 women undergoing radical vulvectomy for vulvar carcinoma who were given single-dose piperacillin or mezlocillin developed postoperative infections [50]. Drain sites fall into the same category. The foreign body undoubtedly contributes to the infections; local attention, rather than parenteral or oral antibiotics, is the appropriate preventive approach.

The first dose of an antibiotic should be given intravenously in the operating room. Combination regimens and prolonged administration did not appear to offer superior infection prevention when compared with that provided by a single agent given once. If the interval between the first dose and opening the vagina exceeds 2.5–3 h, a second intravenous dose should be given 15–30 min before the anticipated vaginal entry. This conclusion is based on data provided by Shapiro et al. [51]. This has not been clinically studied, but administration at longer fixed intervals has not enhanced protection at hysterectomy for benign indications. In patients who are expected to undergo prolonged surgical procedure (>4 h), and dose may be repeated after 4–6 h.

Bowel Preparation

Unobstructed Bowel

There are approximately 10^{11} bacteria in a gram of feces, making sepsis a major hazard if the colon is opened. It is desirable to reduce the patient's normal colonic microflora to diminish the postoperative infection rate in case it is necessary to perform colonic resection and reanastomosis. A recent multicenter, randomized trial has placed routine mechanical bowel preparation practice into serious question, as patients who underwent elective colorectal surgery, no difference in anastomotic leak, or other septic complications such as fascia dehiscence were noted in the group who had preoperative bowel preparation [52].

Clinical Syndromes

Peritonitis and Intraabdominal Abscess

The potential causes of infection include complications of the primary tumor, surgery, and radiation therapy. The tumor can compromise the integrity of the vaginal wall and allow seeding of endogenous vaginal flora into the pelvic and peritoneal cavities. Previous antibiotics, radiation therapy, and the tumor itself may alter the normal genital flora. The tumor can also erode into the bowel and allow entry of fecal material into the peritoneal cavity. Rare cases of several other syndromes arising from untreated pelvic tumor, including spontaneous clostridial gas gangrene and pneumoperitoneum, have been reported [53, 54]. Peritonitis, with or without abscess formation, may occur postoperatively after hysterectomy or with bowel injury. Radiation therapy to the pelvis can cause radiation enteritis, leading to a chronic diarrhea syndrome, which may develop years after radiation therapy is completed. These patients are also at higher risk for bowel adhesions and subsequent obstruction and subclinical perforation may present as late insidious intraabdominal or deep pelvic abscess.

Peritonitis may develop at any time, including at initial diagnosis due to tumor infiltration of bowel, immediately postoperatively, or days or weeks after surgery resulting from tumor infiltration, vascular insufficiency, or tissue necrosis following radiation therapy. The signs are generally dramatic and familiar: abdominal pain, fever, and signs of peritoneal irritation. However, among postoperative patients or patients who have received radiation or corticosteroid therapy, the physical findings may resemble those of a routine postoperative patient, making the diagnosis more difficult. To assure proper diagnosis, frequent examinations and close observation are required.

Abscess formation can also occur in several settings. In some patients, a subclinical microperforation of bowel is successfully walled off by the body's immune system, forming a pericolic or intraperitoneal abscess. This has been shown to occur 7–10 days after microperforation [55]. Fever or mechanical obstruction may be the only presenting signs. Subphrenic, psoas, or liver abscesses may present as a fever of unknown origin and may require a methodical, diligent evaluation for diagnosis. A fistula, usually caused by tumor but also occurring postoperatively, may form between any two organ systems, including the bladder, vagina, bowel, or skin. Persistent suppuration despite therapy or the presence of a feculent discharge from skin, bladder, or vagina may suggest the development of a fistula.

In patients who have clinical evidence of peritonitis but are unable to undergo surgery because of bulky tumor, multiple prior surgeries, or general debility, paracentesis with appropriate cultures may be useful in guiding antibiotic therapy. Blood cultures are only rarely positive. Radiologic investigation is generally required to diagnose an abscess. Regular plain X-ray films of the abdomen are seldom revealing. A contrast enhanced computed tomographic scan of the abdomen may show the collection. In a particularly confusing case in which abnormalities of scans can represent an abscess, metastatic tumor, or postoperative changes, a labeled leukocyte scan may be required to diagnose the abscess.

The diagnosis of a fistula requires demonstration of abnormal drainage from one organ system to another. This can be shown by intravenous or intravesical injection of dye for fistulae arising from the bladder, oral or rectal instillation of dye for those arising from the gastrointestinal tract, or a fistulogram for a fistula involving the skin.

In patients with unexplained bacteremia due to enteric gram-negative rods or anaerobes, with pelvic tumor, a radiologic evaluation is warranted for possible subclinical (micro) perforation or and aberrant communication with intestinal or lower urinary tract(s).

Acute, generalized peritonitis where gastrointestinal perforation is suspected requires urgent surgery to irrigate the peritoneum and repair perforation. Broad-spectrum antibiotic coverage with agents such as anti-pseudomonal penicillin, aminoglycosides, carbapenems, and coverage for coagulase-negative staphylococci and Enterococci are recommended for polymicrobial infections. Patients are also given empiric coverage for a possible Candida species infection. Effective treatment of an abscess requires drainage. Percutaneous drainage is adequate in most cases, but laparotomy may be needed, especially in patients with bulky tumor, extensive adhesion from prior surgeries, and/or radiation therapy. Large or persistent abscesses may require placement of a suction drain. Patients with fistulae generally require resection of the involved tissue. Patients who are inoperable can be treated, as suggested, with chronic suppressive antimicrobial therapy.

Wound Infections

There are important variables that influence the development of wound infection after surgery. These include hospital flora, patient flora, operative technique and variables, patient nutrition, and immunocompetency. Women being treated for reproductive tract cancer may be at risk because of specific problems with immunocompetency, possible prior chemotherapy or radiotherapy, poor nutritional status, hypoproteinemia, or low socioeconomic status. Additional risk factors for incisional infection include obesity and diabetes.

Surgical variables include operative procedures in excess of 4 h, breaks in surgical technique, excessive inoculum at the operative-site, excessive cautery, passive drains, shaving of the area in which the incision is made immediately before surgery, and placement and types of sutures. Infections may range from a mild cellulitis to a devastating fasciitis, deep infection with myonecrosis and mixed anaerobic–aerobic synergistic abdomiopelvic gangrene [56].

Cellulitis

Cellulitis is a relatively frequent occurrence. The presence of a foreign body in a wound is an unavoidable risk factor in many cases, but this variable should be removed or reduced as much as possible. Devitalized tissue, especially fat, can also act as a foreign body. Excess cautery causes thermal injury; the charred tissue may act as a foreign body. The presence of significant amounts of devitalized tissue usually produces a wound defect. A mechanical wound retractor placed for an extended duration can cause fat necrosis, and there appears to be only minimal ability to resorb these areas during wound healing. These areas should be carefully identified and excised before closing the wound. If drains are used, they should be closed, and drains should be vacuumed. Drains should not exit through the wound but rather through an adjacent puncture site, and they should be removed as early as possible. *S. aureus* is recovered from 50% or more of wound infections. If the operative procedure involves transection of the vagina, the infections may harbor other species of normal flora of the lower reproductive tract, such as gram-positive and gram-negative anaerobes and *Enterobacteriaceae*. Cellulitis of the leg occurs with increased frequency in patients after vulvectomy [57]. The affected leg is not always edematous. Group B beta-hemolytic streptococci are frequently recovered. Prophylactic therapy with oral penicillin may reduce recurrences in some patients [57].

The infected surgical incision should be explored. This can frequently be performed at the bedside. Opposing skin edges in such incisions are usually separated without difficulty and may expose underlying purulent material, seromas, hematomas, or any combination of these. The wound should be explored thoroughly, and, if the wound shows unusual features, aerobic and anaerobic cultures should be obtained. Foreign bodies such as sutures or drains should be removed, and obviously necrotic areas should be removed after the patient has been given parenteral pain medication. It is important to document deep fascial integrity. If this cannot be done at the bedside, it should be performed in the operating room.

The wound should be packed open with fine-mesh gauze approximated to the incisional margins. Gauze is used to fill the intervening spaces after each dressing change. The dressing is changed two to four times daily, with chemical and mechanical débridement of necrotic areas. In general, these débriding solutions should be removed from the wound with sterile normal saline before packing because they may impede healing. Except in unusual instances, it is unnecessary to administer parenteral antimicrobials. These incisions may be left open to heal by secondary intent, or they may be closed before discharge from the hospital after the margins are completely granulated. The optimal time for secondary closure is about the fourth day after institution of wound therapy. Studies have shown, normal wound healing was impaired in patients with anemia [58].

Necrotizing Fasciitis

Necrotizing fasciitis is a potentially life-threatening infection of the soft tissues above deep fascia that can involve the abdominal wall or vulva with extension to the proximal thighs and buttocks [59]. There are several descriptive names for this infection, such as beta-hemolytic streptococcal gangrene, hospital gangrene, gram-negative anaerobic cutaneous gangrene, nonclostridial gas gangrene, gangrenous erysipelas, or synergistic necrotizing cellulitis; but the name used by most is that coined by Wilson in 1952; that is, necrotizing fasciitis [60]. This significant infection has been reported in patients with endometrial cancer following irradiation and hysterectomy [61, 62]. It has also been found in endopelvic fascia, in a suprapubic catheter site during chemotherapy, in the vulva in diabetes, and after diagnostic laparoscopy [63].

Bacteria recovered from necrotizing fasciitis infectious sites include anaerobes, particularly *Peptostreptococcus*, *Prevotella*, and *Bacteroides* species, as well as *E. faecalis*, *S. aureus*, and *Enterobacteriaceae*. These bacteria produce large quantities of proteolytic and other enzymes and toxins that allow rapid spread to contiguous tissues. Superficial vessels are occluded, depriving the affected areas of oxygen, other nutrients, and antibiotics. This deprivation interferes with bacterial eradication. Patients at particularly high risk of developing this infection include women older than 50 years of age and those with arteriosclerotic heart disease, diabetes, or other chronic diseases.

The initial presentation of necrotizing fasciitis is of wound cellulitis, which fails to respond to standard antimicrobial therapy. The infection, however, seems to smolder, then rapidly progresses to involve the wound and to produce clinical sepsis. Mortality rates for this infection have been as high as 76%. The degree of disease evident on the skin is only a small fraction of the total amount of tissue that is involved because the skin is not the primary area of infection. Hallmarks of this infection include excessive pain, edema that is unusual for the apparently minimal degree of infection, and presence of superficial tissue crepitance. The skin overlying the affected area becomes blue or brown as the disease progresses, and there may be formation of bullae. Edema progresses, and there may be seepage of grayish fluid from the skin, which slips over underlying tissue and does not bleed if cut. Lack of familiarity with this infection and failure to recognize its signs may delay diagnosis. Even when recognized and treated early, there is a high mortality rate.

Diagnostic criteria as first outlined by Fisher et al. include [64]: (a) extensive necrosis of the superficial fascia with widespread undermining of surrounding tissue; (b) a moderate to severe systemic toxic reaction; (c) absence of muscle involvement; (d) failure to demonstrate *Clostridium* species in the wound or blood cultures; (e) absence of major vascular occlusion; and (f) histologic demonstration of intense leukocytic infiltration, focal necrosis of the superficial fascia and surrounding tissues, and microvascular thrombosis characterize this infection. Early diagnosis followed as soon as possible by appropriate treatment produces the highest cure rate. Radiologic evaluation, particularly with MRI, may confirm the diagnosis rapidly, and should be ordered whenever the disease is suspected. The average interval between diagnosis and initiation of treatment is approximately 5 days. If the interval is 4 days or less, survival rates are high, but an interval of 7 days or more is more likely to result in patient death because even intense antimicrobial therapy is rarely successful at this late stage. Broad-spectrum antimicrobial therapy is important, wide and often disfiguring surgical débridement is the treatment required for preservation of life. The excision must extend to viable tissue that bleeds. The areas of débridement should be treated as areas of burns. Adjunctive therapy with whirlpool baths and perhaps hyperbaric oxygen may be of use.

Clostridial Myonecrosis

Clostridial myonecrosis (gas gangrene) was described by Altmeier and Furste [65]. It is an infection that occurs in muscle and adjacent tissues beneath the deep fascia and is seen most commonly after trauma. However, it can be seen after intraabdominal surgery or surgery in an area that has been contaminated by feces. Mortality rates are about 25%, and poor prognosis factors are leukopenia, advanced age, renal failure, and intravascular hemolysis. *C. perfringens* (80–95%), *C. novyi* (10–40%), or *C. septicum* (5–20%) are common pathogens [66]. It is usually seen in association with gastrointestinal mucosal ulceration or perforation because *Clostridium* species are normal inhabitants of the gastrointestinal tract. *C. perfringens* may be isolated from as many as 20% of the women with nonsexually transmitted upper genital tract infections. The mere presence of *C. perfringens* in a wound does not mean that the patient will develop gas gangrene; it develops in only 1–2% of wounds in which that species can be isolated.

Early signs and symptoms of clostridial myonecrosis are tense edema in tissue that is extremely tender and pain that rapidly intensifies. If an incision is open, it is not uncommon to see a swollen, herniated muscle. There is frequently a serosanguinous, dirty discharge that has many gram-positive or gram-variable rods but few leukocytes. There may also be gas bubbles, and the secretions have a particularly sweet, offensive odor. The surrounding tissue frequently has crepitus. The skin becomes red to green-purple and then turns yellow before becoming a characteristic bronze color. The usual incubation period is about 2–3 days, but it can be as short as 6 h after the bacterial inoculation. With progression of the infection, the patient becomes obviously ill, pale, and sweaty, with increased pulse rate and decreased blood pressure. Temperature is usually elevated, but hypothermia may occur with shock. A positive wound culture may accompany the characteristic signs and symptoms of clostridial myonecrosis. X-ray or CT scan of the affected area frequently shows gas in deep tissues. Blood cultures grow clostridia in approximately 15% of the cases. It is common to find a decrease in hemoglobin and an increase in circulating leukocytes. Involved muscle is pale and edematous, with loss of elasticity, and it does not bleed or contract with stimulation. Histologic findings demonstrate coagulation necrosis of muscle fibers.

Clostridial myonecrosis is another infection that requires prompt and extensive débridement in the operating room. Cultures must be performed, and because clostridia may develop plasmid-mediated antibiotic-resistance, repeated cultures with sensitivity testing may be required if a patient is slow to respond. In addition to wide débridement, the treatment of choice is penicillin G at a dose of 1–2 million units every 2–3 h. Gram's stain also may indicate the presence of gram-negative bacteria, in which case coverage should be provided for those bacteria as well. Metronidazole, clindamycin, or carbapenems all of which have good in vitro activity against *C. perfringens* may be considered. Hyperbaric oxygen may be adjunctive, but its efficacy is uncertain.

Septic Pelvic Thrombophlebitis

Septic pelvic thrombophlebitis, also known as suppurative pelvic thrombophlebitis, is a disorder that has been diagnosed most frequently after antimicrobial therapy for pelvic infection after cesarean section or septic abortion, but it can be seen as a complication of infection after any type of pelvic surgery [67]. The mortality rate observed in 1917 was 52% after surgical therapy [68]. The use of antimicrobial prophylaxis and the enhanced antibacterial activity of current therapeutic regimens are presumed to be paramount in the disappearance of this potentially lethal infection. Septic pelvic thrombophlebitis is clot formation in the pelvic veins as a result of infection. It can be seen after hysterectomy, other pelvic operative procedures including brachytherapy, and in association with pelvic trauma or perirectal abscess. Classically, there is relative venous stasis before phlebitis that develops adjacent to pelvic infection. The intimal lining of the veins is invaded by bacteria, including Enterobacteriaceae, especially *E. coli*, aerobic and anaerobic streptococci, and *Bacteroides*. The veins involved may be the ovarian, hypogastric, or uterine, with essentially equal involvement in the right and left sides. If common iliac veins are involved, clot formation is more frequently seen on the left for unknown reasons. Infected clot may embolize to the lungs, kidneys, liver, brain, and spleen.

Presentation is essentially that of a fever of unknown cause, and the physician must rule out infections such as pyelonephritis, pneumonia, and pelvic or abdominal abscess. Persistent fever associated with tachycardia after clinical response to antimicrobial therapy for a pelvic infection is the most common presentation. In most cases clinical manifestation are not distinguishable; occasionally it may be possible to palpate tender cords in the vaginal fornices. In patients with bacteremia and septic emboli, chills are observed in two thirds of the patients, fever up to 41°C, and the variations in temperature may be quite hectic. Dyspnea, tachypnea, pleuritic pain, cough, hemoptysis, restlessness, anxiety, and perhaps angina may all be seen with septic embolization.

Compatible clinical presentation and CT or MRI scan are used for diagnosis [69]. Criteria for diagnosis of venous thrombosis using CT studies include enlargement of the involved vein(s), sharply defined vessel walls enhanced by contrast media, and a low-density intraluminal mass [70]. Diagnosis using MRI is based on intense intraluminal signals from clot in involved veins and a lack of signal with normal blood flow in uninvolved vessels; no contrast agent is needed. Blood culture should be performed if there is suspicion of septicemia. A ventilation-perfusion scan or contrast enhanced spiral CT scan should be performed if there is a suspicion for pulmonary embolization. A gallium scintiscan may be necessary to identify very small septic embolic foci in the lungs.

Early treatment of venous thrombosis was surgical [68]. The first to advocate the use of anticoagulants in addition to antibiotics were Schulman and Zatuchni [71].In some cases antibiotics alone may have been adequate and can be used in patients in whom anticoagulation can be detrimental [72]. In the largest published study of heparin therapy, the mean time to become afebrile was 2.5 days, and the average duration of heparin therapy was 8 days [73, 74]. It was unnecessary to initiate anticoagulation therapy in patients without evidence of emboli. Thromboembolism, during or after treatment with heparin has not been reported [75]. Antibiotic therapy must be continued. If there is significant improvement in the pulse rate and temperature pattern within 12–48 h after addition of heparin, reassessment is mandatory. Treatment with low molecular weight heparin has not been studied or standardized for this condition.

Noninfectious Causes of Fever

Not all patients with gynecologic malignancy and fever have an infection. Pulmonary embolus, drug-related fever, and tumor-related fever represent the main noninfectious sources of fever, but others, such as factitious fever and underlying collagen vascular disorder, must also be considered. The use of procalcitonin and neopterin levels have been suggested to help distinguish between infected and noninfected patients, although further studies are needed to validate these tests [76].

Pulmonary embolus should be considered in a bed-bound or postoperative patient with any combination of fever, chest pain, dyspnea, or an abnormal chest radiograph. Patients with bulky pelvic tumors are also at risk. A high level of suspicion is important and spiral chest CT scans or ventilation-perfusion scans may establish diagnosis; in rare instances a more definite pulmonary angiogram may be performed. Therapy remains anticoagulation with low molecular weight heparin. For patients who are unable to tolerate these drugs or who continue to have pulmonary emboli despite therapy, inferior vena caval filter are required.

Any antibiotic may cause fever [77]. Patients typically develop fever and a diffuse maculopapular rash after several days of therapy, although, eosinophilia is a helpful sign, when present. Mild elevations in liver function tests may be present though nonspecific. Atypical presentations of drug fever, including patients without rash or those who develop fever weeks into therapy or after completion of therapy, can also occur. The diagnosis is usually made by discontinuing the antibiotic and observing the patient. It is important to remember that some drug fevers may take as long as a week to resolve. Supportive measures, such as antipyretics and antipruritics, may decrease symptoms.

The diagnosis of tumor fever can be made only after systematic exclusion of all other potential causes of fever. Most patients with tumor fever have metastatic disease in the liver or lung. The fever may be as high as 40°C and patient often feels relatively well when afebrile. Patient suspected of having tumor fever, a clinical trial of broad-spectrum antibiotics is given. If the fever does not abate and no other clear infection source is evident, the likelihood of tumor fever increases.

Acknowledgement The authors are grateful to Drs. Donald Armstrong and Kent Sepkowitz of Memorial Sloan-Kettering Cancer Center for their contribution to this chapter.

References

1. Safdar A, Armstrong D. Infections in patients with neoplastic diseases. In: Grenvik M, Ayers SM, Holbrook PR, Shoemaker WC, editors. Textbook of critical care. 4th ed. Philadelphia: W.B. Saunders; 2000. p. 715–26.
2. Safdar A, Armstrong D. Infectious morbidity in critically ill patients with cancer. Crit Care Clin. 2001;17:531–70.
3. Evaldson G, Heimdahl A, Kager L, et al. The normal human anaerobic microflora. Scand J Infect Dis. 1982;35:9–15.
4. Rolston KVI, Bodey GP, Safdar A. Polymicrobial infection in patients with cancer: an underappreciated and underreported entity. Clin Infect Dis. 2007;45:228–33.
5. Barton DPJ, Fiorica JV, Hoffman MS, et al. Cervical cancer and tubo-ovarian abscesses: a report of three cases. J Reprod Med. 1993;38:561–4.

6. Imachi M, Tanaka S, Ishikawa S, et al. Spontaneous perforation of pyometra presenting as generalized peritonitis in a patient with cervical cancer. Gynecol Oncol. 1993;50:384–8.
7. Protopappas AG, Diakomanolis ES, Milingos SD, et al. Tubo-ovarian abscess in postmenopausal women: gynecological malignancy until proven otherwise. Eur J Obstet Gynecol Reprod Biol. 2004;114:203–9.
8. Inagaki J, Rodriguez V, Bodey GP. Causes of death in cancer patients. Cancer. 1974;33:568–73.
9. Iatrakis G, Sakellaropoulos G, Georgoulias N, et al. Gynecologic cancer and surgical infectious morbidity. Clin Exp Obstet Gynecol. 1998;25:36–7.
10. Chang HK, Lo KY, Chiang HS. Complications of urinary diversion after pelvic exenteration for gynecological malignancy. Int Urogynecol J. 2000;11:358–60.
11. Wydra D, Emerich J, Sawicki S, et al. Major complications following exenteration in cases of pelvic malignancies: a 10-year experience. World J Gastroenterol. 2006;12:1115–9.
12. Matar MJ, Safdar A, Rolston KV. Relationship of colonization with vancomycin-resistant enterococci and risk of systemic infection in patients with cancer. Clin Infect Dis. 2006;42:1506–7.
13. Gould N, Kamelle S, Tillmanns T, et al. Predictors of complications after inguinal lymphadenopathy. Gynecol Oncol. 2001;82:329–32.
14. Safdar A, Rolston KV. *Stenotrophomonas maltophilia*: changing spectrum of a serious bacterial pathogen in patients with cancer. Clin Infect Dis. 2007;45:1602–9.
15. Safdar A, Rodriguez GH, Balakrishnan M, et al. Changing trends in etiology of bacteremia in patients with cancer. Eur J Clin Microbiol Infect Dis. 2006;25:522–6.
16. Han XY, Kamana M, Rolston KV. Viridans streptococci isolated by culture from blood of cancer patients: clinical and microbiologic analysis of 50 cases. J Clin Microbiol. 2006;44:160–5.
17. Green JA, Kirwan JM, Tierney JF. Survival and recurrence after concomitant chemotherapy and radiotherapy for cancer of the uterine cervix. Lancet. 2001;385:781–6.
18. Yessaian A, Magistris A, Burger RA, et al. Radical hysterectomy followed by tailored postoperative therapy in the treatment of stage 1B2 cervical cancer: feasibility and indications for adjuvant therapy. Gynecol Oncol. 2004;94:61–6.
19. Jurado M, Martinez-Monge R, Garcia-Foncillas J, et al. Pilot study of concurrent cisplatin, 5-fluorouracil, and external beam radiotherapy prior to radical surgery +/− intraoperative electron beam radiotherapy in locally advanced cervical cancer. Gynecol Oncol. 1999;74:30–7.
20. Micha JP, Goldstein BH, Rettenmaier MA, et al. Pelvic radiation necrosis and osteomyelitis following chemoradiation for advanced stage vulvar and cervical carcinoma. Gynecol Oncol. 2006;101:349–52.
21. Anatoliotaki A, Valatas V, Mantadakis E, et al. Bloodstream infections in patients with solid tumors: associated factors, microbial spectrum and outcome. Infection. 2004;32:65–71.
22. Elting LS, Rubenstein EB, Rolston KV, et al. Outcomes of bacteremia in patients with cancer and neutropenia: observations from two decades of epidemiological and clinical trials. Clin Infect Dis. 1997;25:247–59.
23. Zahar JR, Farhat H, Chachaty E, et al. Incidence and clinical significance of anaerobic bacteremia in cancer patients: a 6-year retrospective study. Clin Microbiol Infect. 2005;11:724–9.
24. Fainstein V, Elting LS, Bodey GP. Bacteremia caused by non-sporulating anaerobes in cancer patients – a 12-year experience. Medicine (Baltimore). 1989;68:151–62.
25. Wynne JW, Armstrong D. Clostridial septicemia. Cancer. 1972;29:215–21.
26. Safdar A. Strategies to enhance immune function in hematopoietic transplantation recipients who have fungal infections. Bone Marrow Transplant. 2006;38:327–37.
27. Raad I, Hachem R, Hanna H, et al. Sources and outcome of bloodstream infections in cancer patients: the role of central venous catheters. Eur J Clin Microbiol Infect Dis. 2007;26:549–56.
28. Raad I, Hanna H, Jiang Y, et al. Comparative activities of daptomycin, linezolid, and tigecycline against catheter-related methicillin-resistant *Staphylococcus* bacteremic isolates embedded in biofilm. Antimicrob Agents Chemother. 2007;51:1656–60.
29. Strecker EP, Heber R, Boos I, et al. Preliminary experience with locoregional intraarterial chemotherapy of uterine cervical or endometrial cancer using the peripheral implantable port system (PIPS): a feasibility study. Cardiovasc Intervent Radiol. 2003;26:118–22.
30. Sakuragi N, Nakajima A, Nomura E, et al. Complications related to intraperitoneal administration of cisplatin or carboplatin for ovarian carcinoma. Gynecol Oncol. 2000;79:420–3.
31. Roybal JJ, Feliberti EC, Rouse L, et al. Pump removal in infected patients with hepatic chemotherapy pumps: when is it necessary? Am Surg. 2006;72:880–4.
32. Prasad KN, Pradhan S, Datta NR. Urinary tract infection in patients of gynecological malignancies undergoing external pelvic radiotherapy. Gynecol Oncol. 1995;57:380–2.
33. Roos EJ, Van Eijkeren MA, Boon TA, et al. Pelvic exenteration as treatment of recurrent or advanced gynecologic and urologic cancer. Int J Gynecol Cancer. 2005;15:624–9.
34. Velasco E, Thuler LC, Martins CA, et al. Risk factors for infectious complications after abdominal surgery for malignant disease. Am J Infect Control. 1996;24:1–6.
35. Brooker DC, Savage JE, Twiggs LB, et al. Infectious morbidity in gynecologic cancer. Am J Obstet Gynecol. 1987;156:513–20.
36. Morgan LS, Daly JW, Monif GR. Infectious morbidity associated with pelvic exenteration. Gynecol Oncol. 1980;10:318–28.
37. Ledger WJ, Gee C, Lewis WP. Guidelines for antibiotic prophylaxis in gynecology. Am J Obstet Gynecol. 1975;121:1038–45.
38. Hemsell DL, Johnson ER, Hemsell PG, et al. Cefazolin is inferior to cefotetan as single-dose prophylaxis for women undergoing elective total abdominal hysterectomy. Clin Infect Dis. 1995;20:677–84.
39. Hemsell DL, Bernstein SG, Bawdon RE, et al. Preventing major operative site infection after radical abdominal hysterectomy and pelvic lymphadenectomy. Gynecol Oncol. 1989;35:55–60.
40. Orr Jr JW, Shingleton HM, Hatch KD, et al. Correlation of perioperative morbidity and conization to radical hysterectomy interval. Obstet Gynecol. 1982;59:726–31.
41. Berkeley AS, Orr JW, Cavanagh D, et al. Comparative effectiveness and safety of cefotetan and cefoxitin as prophylactic agents in patients undergoing abdominal or vaginal hysterectomy. Am J Surg. 1988;155:81–5.
42. Mann Jr WJ, Orr JW, Shingleton HM, et al. Perioperative influences on infectious morbidity in radical hysterectomy. Gynecol Oncol. 1981;11:207–12.
43. Gussman D, Riva J, Carlson Jr JA. Prophylaxis for radical hysterectomy. Infect Surg. 1987;6:55.
44. Rosenshein NB, Ruth JC, Villar J, et al. A prospective randomized study of doxycycline as a prophylactic antibiotic in patients undergoing radical hysterectomy. Gynecol Oncol. 1983;15:201–6.
45. Marsden DE, Cavanagh D, Wisniewski BJ, et al. Factors affecting the incidence of infectious morbidity after radical hysterectomy. Am J Obstet Gynecol. 1985;152:817–21.
46. Sevin BU, Ramos R, Lichtinger M, et al. Antibiotic prevention of infections complicating radical abdominal hysterectomy. Obstet Gynecol. 1984;64:539–45.
47. Micha JP, Kucera PR, Birkett JP, et al. Prophylactic mezlocillin in radical hysterectomy. Obstet Gynecol. 1987;69:251–4.
48. Sevin BU, Ramos R, Gerhardt RT, et al. Comparative efficacy of short-term versus long-term cefoxitin prophylaxis against postoperative infection after radical hysterectomy: a prospective study. Obstet Gynecol. 1991;77:729–34.

49. Shapiro M, Schoenbaum SC, Tager IB, et al. Benefit-cost analysis of antimicrobial prophylaxis in abdominal and vaginal hysterectomy. JAMA. 1983;249:1290–4.
50. van Lindert AC, Giltaij AR, Derksen MD, et al. Single-dose prophylaxis with broad-spectrum penicillins (piperacillin and mezlocillin) in gynecologic oncological surgery, with observation on serum and tissue concentrations. Eur J Obstet Gynecol Reprod Biol. 1990;36:137–45.
51. Shapiro M, Munoz A, Tager IB, et al. Risk factors for infection at the operative site after abdominal or vaginal hysterectomy. N Engl J Med. 1982;307:1661–6.
52. Contant CM, Hop WC, van't Sant HP, et al. Mechanical bowel preparation for elective colorectal surgery: a multicenter randomized trial. Lancet. 2008;370:2112–7.
53. Braverman J, Adachi A, Lev-Gur M, et al. Spontaneous clostridia gas gangrene of uterus associated with endometrial malignancy. Am J Obstet Gynecol. 1987;156:1205–7.
54. Douvier S, Nabholtz JM, Friedman S, et al. Infectious pneumoperitoneum as an uncommon presentation of endometrial carcinoma: report of two cases. Gynecol Oncol. 1989;33:392–4.
55. Weinstein WM, Onderdonk AB, Bartlett JG, et al. Experimental intra-abdominal abscesses in rats: development of an experimental model. Infect Immun. 1974;10:1250–5.
56. Henderson W. Synergistic bacterial gangrene abdominal hysterectomy. Obstet Gynecol. 1977;49:24S.
57. Bouma J, Dankert J. Recurrent acute leg cellulitis in patients after radical vulvectomy. Gynecol Oncol. 1988;29:50–7.
58. Hunt TK, Rabkin J, von Smitten K. Effects of edema and anemia on wound healing and infection. Curr Stud Hematol Blood Transfus. 1986;53:101–13.
59. Bahary CM, Joel-Cohen SJ, Neri A. Necrotizing fasciitis. Obstet Gynecol. 1977;50:633–7.
60. Wilson B. Necrotizing fascitis. Am Surg. 1952;18:416.
61. Husseinzadeh N et al. Spontaneous occurrence of synergistic bacterial gangrene following external pelvic irradiation. Obstet Gynecol. 1984;63:859–62.
62. Hoffman MS, Turnquist D. Necrotizing fasciitis of the vulva during chemotherapy. Obstet Gynecol. 1989;74:483–4.
63. Roberts D. Necrotizing fasciitis of the vulva. Am J Obstet Gynecol. 1987;157:568.
64. Fisher JR, Conway MJ, Takeshita RT, et al. Necrotizing fasciitis. Importance of roentgenographic studies for soft-tissue gas. JAMA. 1979;241:803–6.
65. Altmeier WA. Gas gangrene. Surg Gynecol Obstet. 1947;84:504.
66. Pelletier JP, Plumbley JA, Rouse EA, Cina SJ. The role of *Clostridium septicum* in paraneoplastic sepsis. Arch Pathol Lab Med. 2000;124:353–6.
67. McNeeley Jr SG, Hopkins MP, Ehlerova B, et al. Infection on a gynecologic oncology service. Gynecol Oncol. 1990;37:183–7.
68. Miller C. Ligation or excision of the pelvic veins in the treatment of puerperal pyaemia. Surg Gynecol Obstet. 1917;25:431.
69. Twickler DM et al. Imaging of puerperal septic thrombophlebitis: prospective comparison of MR imaging, CT, and sonography. AJR Am J Roentgenol. 1997;169:1039–43.
70. Zerhouni EA, Barth KH, Siegelman SS. Demonstration of venous thrombosis by computed tomography. AJR Am J Roentgenol. 1980;134:753–8.
71. Schulman H, Zatuchni G. Pelvic thrombophlebitis in the puerperal and postoperative gynecology patient. Obscure fever as an indication for anticoagulant therapy. Am J Obstet Gynecol. 1964;90:1293.
72. Twickler DM, Setiawan AT, Evans RS, et al. Imaging of puerperal septic thrombophlebitis: prospective comparison of MR imaging, CT, and sonography. AJR Am J Roentgenol. 1997;169:1039–43.
73. Josey WE, Staggers Jr SR. Heparin therapy in septic pelvic thrombophlebitis: a study of 46 cases. Am J Obstet Gynecol. 1974;120:228–33.
74. Brown CE, Stettler RW, Twickler D, et al. Puerperal septic pelvic thrombophlebitis: incidence and response to heparin therapy. Am J Obstet Gynecol. 1999;181:143–8.
75. Lee AY et al. Low-molecular-weight heparin versus a coumarin for the prevention of recurrent venous thromboembolism in patients with cancer. N Engl J Med. 2003;349:146–53.
76. Ruokonen E et al. Procalcitonin and neopterin as indicators of infection in critically ill patients. Acta Anaesthesiol Scand. 2002;46:398–404.
77. Hirschmann JV. Fever of unknown origin in adults. Clin Infect Dis. 1997;24:291–300. Quiz 301–2.

Chapter 19
Central Nervous System Infections in Cancer Patients

Victor Mulanovich and Amar Safdar

Abstract Central nervous system (CNS) infections represent an important complication in cancer patients undergoing therapy. These infections are often difficult to diagnose, a high level of suspicion, prompt investigation, and institution of appropriate and early therapy remains critical for improved outcomes. A wide variety of viruses, bacteria, mycobacteria, fungi and parasitic meningeal, and brain disease makes empiric selection of antimicrobial therapy a daunting task. The factors that assist in the selection of initial therapy includes predisposing factors such as: (a) presence of prosthetic devices, (b) surgical manipulation, (c) host's immune defects either related to underlying malignancy, antineoplastic chemotherapy, or (d) complications arising from stem cell transplantation to name a few. For instance, patients with severe neutropenia have an increased risk for bacterial meningitis due to Gram-negative organisms, and fungal brain abscesses, where as patients with profound cellular immune defects are susceptible to *Listeria monocytogenes* infection, Cryptococcal meningitis and recrudescent herpesviruses, and toxoplasmosis. In evaluation of patients with CNS infections a knowledge of noninfectious causes that are clinically difficult to distinguish from an infection also need to be considered. In this regard, neoplastic meningitis, paraneoplastic syndrome, and recently described chemotherapy-induced reversible posterior leukoencephalopathy syndrome, are to name a few. Mental confusion and fever related to a drug is an important consideration in this population.

Keywords Encephalitis • Meningitis • Brain abscess • Shunt infection • Cancer • Transplantation • Noninfectious brain inflammation

V. Mulanovich (✉)
Infectious Diseases Department, The University of Texas,
M.D. Anderson Cancer Center, Houston, TX, USA
e-mail: vmulanov@mdanderson.org

Overview

Central nervous system (CNS) infections represent an important and difficult to diagnose complication of cancer and its therapy. Its presentation and differential diagnosis are affected by factors pertaining to the patient, the type of malignancy and its treatment. Patients may be at risk of CNS infection because of environmental exposure, such as mosquito bites transmitting viral encephalitis, or previous infections that may reactivate secondary to immunosuppressive treatments or stem cell transplantation (SCT). Hospitalizations increase the risk of colonization and infections with resistant bacteria. Cancer itself, such as hematologic malignancies, may cause immunocompromise. Treatment of malignancy often predisposes to CNS infection, in particular SCT, neurosurgical interventions, use of immunosuppressants, and chemotherapy-induced neutropenia.

The list of potential pathogens is large. A rational diagnostic approach has been presented in the past [1, 2]. We advocate following a methodical approach:

1. Identification of the clinical syndrome based on history, clinical exam, radiology, magnetic resonance imaging (MRI) if possible, although computed tomography (CT) of the brain may be used, and basic cerebrospinal fluid (CSF) results (if available). Four major neurologic syndromes, which may overlap to some degree, which will be discussed, are as follows: encephalitis, meningitis, brain abscess, or postsurgical infections.

2. Consideration of patient factors relevant to the particular syndrome, such as environmental exposures, age, type of malignancy, immunosuppression, history of neurosurgery. Noninfectious causes that may mimic infection should be entertained. Based on these factors, a list of potential pathogens that will be targeted with diagnostic tests and empiric treatment (steps 3 and 4) will be formulated.

3. Request of specific diagnostic tests, such as CSF cultures, polymerase chain reaction (PCR) testing for specific viruses and serology. Investigate extraneural sites of infection that may provide a diagnosis by means such as

blood cultures, sinus, or pulmonary imaging. Use stereotactic needle aspirate for diagnosis and treatment of a CNS abscess if indicated.
4. Empiric antimicrobial treatment while awaiting for an etiologic diagnosis.

The etiologic diagnosis may not be reached in a high percentage of patients. In this case the efficacy of empiric treatment has to be assessed by serial performance of clinical and radiologic exams and/or repeat CSF analysis. Disease progression may require performing brain biopsy in some cases.

We will discuss such an approach in the following pages.

Infectious Syndromes and Management

Encephalitis

Encephalitis is an inflammatory process in the brain parenchyma. Its hallmark is deterioration of cortical function, often referred to as encephalopathy. Other than infection, encephalopathy can be caused by autoimmune disease and/or vasculitis, neoplasias and paraneoplastic syndromes, metabolic derangements, hypoxia, trauma, drugs and toxins, vascular pathology (including hypertension, hemorrhage and ischemia), and nonconvulsive status epilepticus [3, 4].

In the United States there are ~19,000 hospitalizations each year with a diagnosis of encephalitis (An annual rate of 7.3 hospitalizations per 100,000 population) and 1,400 deaths. Although more than 100 different infectious agents have been identified as causative agents of encephalitis, the etiologic agent is not detected in the majority of cases. Khetsuriani et al. found no specific cause in 59.5% of encephalitis-associated hospitalizations from 1988 to 1997 [5]. The California Encephalitis Project identified the etiologic agent of only 29% of 1,570 prospectively identified immunocompetent patients with encephalitis between 1998 and 2005, despite extensive testing [4].

Infectious agents may cause encephalitis directly, when they invade the brain parenchyma or its supporting structures, or indirectly, when extraneural infection triggers it. These "parainfectious encephalitides" may be immune-mediated (e.g., acute disseminated encephalomyelitis (ADEM)) or occur when an infection-induced metabolic catastrophe leads to cerebral dysfunction, as in septic encephalopathy [3].

Clinical manifestations of encephalitis include fever, confusion, altered level of consciousness, and/or behavioral abnormalities. Fever may be absent or low grade, especially in the elderly and immunosuppressed. Altered mental status may range from mild lethargy to deep coma. The patient may be agitated, hallucinating, may have mood changes or frank psychosis. Generalized or focal seizures are frequent. Focal neurologic deficits such as aphasia, ataxia, or hemiparesis reflect the most affected brain regions. Meningeal inflammation is often present and, if significant, the term meningoencephalitis may be more appropriate [6].

The approach to the patient with infectious encephalitis takes into account his/her immune status, history of recent infectious syndrome such as fever and rash, diarrhea or upper respiratory infection, recent vaccination, and presence of sepsis or systemic inflammatory response syndrome. The following four groups are considered:

(a) *Encephalitis in an immunocompetent host who happens to have cancer*: The causative agent is often the same as encountered in noncancer patients. Epidemiologic data may help direct the investigation for an etiologic agent. Age, season of the year, geographic locale, diseases prevalent in the area, insect or animal contacts, travel, recreational or occupational activities may point towards a specific etiology and determine further diagnostic testing. The most common causes in the U.S. are herpes simplex virus (HSV), varicella zoster virus (VZV), and enteroviruses, which may also present as aseptic meningitis or as meningoencephalitis [4, 5]. Cases of Influenza encephalitis/encephalopathy have been reported since the 1918 pandemic (encephalitis lethargica) and with increased frequency in Japanese children. The onset of symptoms is within a few days of the first signs of infection; the mortality rate is 30% [7].

(b) *Encephalitis in an immunosuppressed host*: Reactivation of dormant infections, de novo infection with opportunistic pathogens and severe manifestations of less virulent ones occur in these patients. Herpesviruses cause persistent or latent infection in most humans and reactivate after solid organ or SCT or are transmitted from the donor to the transplant recipient. HSV remains an important consideration but is rare, maybe because the most immunocompromised patients receive prophylaxis. Human herpesvirus-6 (HHV-6) reactivates in ~50% of SCT patients 2–4 weeks posttransplant and may cause encephalitis, with predilection for the hippocampus, in a small number of patients, usually within the first 100 days posttransplant [8–10]. Preemptive therapy for HHV-6, triggered by high-level viremia, did not show advantage in preventing encephalitis in one Japanese study [11]. Cytomegalovirus (CMV) may affect the ependymal lining of the ventricles causing ventriculoencephalitis. Progression is rapid, MRI may show enhancement of the affected areas. CMV PCR may be positive in blood and/or CSF. High-level viremia, retinitis, or extraneural involvement may be present and provide a clue to the diagnosis [12]. VZV rarely causes CNS infection, cases of granulomatous cerebral angiitis following ophthalmic zoster [13, 14], clinically resembling a stroke, and progressive chronic encephalitis manifested in MRI as spherical white matter lesions without surrounding edema scattered throughout the white matter, have been reported in immunocompromised patients [15]. Epstein–Barr virus (EBV) can cause encephalitis and meningitis after primary infection or reactivation, in immunocompetent and immunocompromised hosts. Encephalitis is frequently accompanied by focal neurologic abnormalities. EBV-associated posttransplant lymphoproliferative disease (PTLD) presents usually within a year of transplantation and affects the CNS in 19% of cases [16–18].

West Nile virus (WNV) may be transmitted by mosquitoes, blood transfusion, or transplantation from a viremic donor, leading to meningoencephalitis after solid organ and hematopoietic SCT. Movement disorders and flaccid paralysis are often present. Patients receiving chemotherapy or otherwise immunosuppressed may also develop severe WNV disease [19–21].

Progressive multifocal leukoencephalopathy (PML) is caused by the polyomavirus JC. Eighty five percent of cases are associated with HIV infection. Immunosuppressive drugs such as corticosteroids, alkylating agents, purine analogs and some monoclonal antibodies (such as rituximab, natalizumab, etanercept, etc.), calcineurin inhibitors, and other drugs used mainly for the treatment of malignancies and in transplantation account for most of the rest. Cases have been described after SCT including autologous transplants. MRI findings include periventricular and subcortical white matter lesions that do not enhance and are not space occupying. PCR for JC virus in CSF has a sensitivity of 80% and specificity of 95%. Treatment is ineffective; cidofovir has been used with poor results. Withdrawal of immunosuppression is recommended [22–27].

Toxoplasma encephalitis occurs in SCT patients as subacute progressive or severe acute encephalitis. Altered mental status and focal neurological signs are common. Chorioretinitis, pneumonia, and multiorgan involvement are reported. Graft versus host disease (GVHD) is a predisposing factor. Diagnosis relies in finding multiple ring-enhancing lesions on MRI and *Toxoplasma* PCR in CSF or blood. Brain biopsy may be necessary [28–31]. CNS lymphoma, including PTLD, is the main differential diagnosis.

Acanthamoeba spp. and *Balamuthia mandrillaris* are free-living amebas that can rarely cause chronic granulomatous meningoencephalitis in patients with cancer and/or immunosuppression, including SCT. Diagnosis is difficult and requires culturing the organism from brain or skin lesion biopsies, so clinical suspicion is essential [32, 33].

Listeriosis, endemic mycoses, and *Mycobacterium tuberculous* are part of the differential diagnosis. Please refer to the appropriate chapters for a more detailed discussion.

(c) *Post-infectious or post-immunization encephalitis* is mediated by an immunologic response to an antigenic stimulus. ADEM accounts for the majority of cases. The usual latency is 4–21 days. Fever is present in 15% of adults and ~50% of children. Seizures occur in only 4% of adults and more frequently in children, often associated with fever. MRI usually reveals multifocal enhancing white matter lesions. The initial MRI may be normal, so repeat study it in 7–10 days is advised when the history of immunization and clinical presentation are suggestive [3].

(d) *Septic encephalopathy* is present in 50–70% of patients with sepsis [34]. It is defined as encephalopathy unexplained by lung, liver, kidney or cardiac dysfunction, or any of the previously discussed etiologies, in patients with an extraneural source of infection. It is a diagnosis of exclusion with no pathognomonic histopathology. It is most likely caused by mediators of inflammation that induce cerebral endothelial dysfunction and increased permeability of the blood-brain barrier. Ischemic changes are also found in patients dying from septic shock [3].

Diagnostic workup: Brain MRI is more sensitive and specific than CT in cases of suspected encephalitis [35]. Other conditions with similar presentation can be excluded. In ADEM, the MRI will show acute enhancing white matter lesions throughout the CNS [3]. CSF evaluation is essential. Viral encephalitis usually presents with mild mononuclear pleocytosis. Neutrophilic pleocytosis may be seen initially and may persist in WNV encephalitis. CSF protein is mild to moderately elevated. CSF eosinophilia suggests helminth infection, but is not specific. Low CSF glucose suggests bacterial infection (listeriosis, tuberculous), fungi or protozoa. Up to 10% of patients have normal CSF. Serology and PCR are the main diagnostic studies for viral agents. Viral cultures is of limited value; bacterial, fungal, and mycobacterial should be obtained [6].

Occasionally, the causative agent may be identified outside the CNS. Blood cultures may identify a bacterial pathogen (*Listeria*). Serum cryptococcal and CMV antigens and urine histoplasma antigen should be ordered if clinically indicated. In patients with respiratory symptoms, viral respiratory antigens or a PCR viral panel should be obtained from respiratory secretions. Diffuse pulmonary infiltrates may suggest *Mycoplasma* or viral infection; circumscribed infiltrates may be caused by infection with fungi, *Nocardia* or *M. tuberculous*.

Treatment recommendations: Since an etiologic diagnosis is not obtained in more than 70% of cases, empiric therapy directed at the most likely pathogens and treatable organisms is essential. Immunocompetent patients should be treated for HSV and VZV with intravenous acyclovir. Most patients are treated empirically for bacterial meningitis due to the clinical overlap (see next section). Listeriosis should be considered in pregnant, elderly, and immunocompromised patients,

Table 19.1 Causes of encephalitis, diagnostic method of choice, and recommended treatment in immunocompetent and immunocompromised patients. (1) Intraventricular γ-globulin for chronic or severe disease, (2) includes La Crosse, St. Louis encephalitis and Eastern, Western, and Venezuelan equine encephalitis viruses, (3) interferon-α-2b may be used for St. Louis encephalitis

Immunocompetent patients	Diagnosis	Treatment
Etiologic agent	Stool and throat cultures	Supportive 1
Enteroviruses	CSF RT-PCR	
HSV-1 and 2	CSF RT-PCR, MRI	Acyclovir
Varicella zoster virus	CSF PCR, MRI	Acyclovir
	DFA skin lesions	
Influenza A and B	Viral culture, antigen detection, PCR of respiratory secretions	Oseltamivir
West Nile virus	Serum + CSF IgM	Supportive
	CSF PCR	
Other mosquito-borne viruses 2	Serologic, CSF IgM	Supportive 3
HIV	HIV serology and RNA	HAART
Bartonella henselae (cat scratch disease)	Serology	Doxycycline or azithromycin (may add rifampin)
Rickettsia or *Ehrlichia*	Serology	Doxycycline
Immunocompromised patients		
Cytomegalovirus	CSF PCR, MRI	Gancyclovir + Foscarnet
Human herpesvirus 6	CSF PCR, MRI	Gancyclovir or Foscarnet
Epstein–Barr virus	CSF PCR, MRI	Supportive
JC virus	CSF PCR, MRI	Reverse immunosuppression
West Nile virus	Serum + CSF IgM	Supportive
	CSF PCR	
Listeria	Blood and CSF cultures	Ampicillin + gentamicin or trimethoprim/sulfamethoxazole
M. tuberculous	CSF AFB and culture	Four TB drugs per guidelines + Dexamethasone for meningitis
	CSF Gene-probe	
Coccidioides sp.	Serum + CSF antibodies and cultures	Azole or amphotericin per guidelines
Cryptococcus neoformans	Blood and CSF antigen and cultures	Amphotericin + flucytosine
Histoplasma capsulatum	Urine histoplasma antigen, CSF stains and culture	Liposomal amphotericin
Toxoplasmosis	Serum IgG (establish risk)	Pirimethamine + either sulfadiazine or clindamycin
	CSF PCR, MRI	
Postinfectious and postimmunization	MRI	Corticosteroids
		Plasma exchange
Septic encephalopathy	Diagnosis of exclusion	Treat underlying condition
		Supportive

and ampicillin added empirically. Rickettial and ehrlichial infections may present with fever, headache, and altered mental status in patients at risk for tick bites, doxycycline should be added in patients with probable exposure to ticks. Serologic tests for these pathogens are of limited value.

In moderate to severely immunocompromised patients herpesviruses and endemic fungi are the most important treatable agents and gancyclovir and/or foscarnet, plus voriconazole or liposomal amphotericin B are part of the empiric regimen. Meningitis again should also considered, including *Listeria*. Ten percent of toxoplasma encephalitis cases occur in HIV-negative patients, mostly after transplantation. Treatment with pyrimethamine plus sulfadiazine or clindamycin is standard. Trimethoprim/sulfamethoxazole has been used successfully to treat toxoplasmosis in AIDS patients [28–31].

Table 19.1 lists the most important pathogens in the first two groups and the diagnostic test of choice and general recommendations for therapy.

Meningitis

Signs of meningeal irritation and CSF pleocytosis are the hallmarks of this syndrome. Acute meningitis commonly presents in hours to days, chronic meningitis is defined as symptoms, signs, and/or CSF abnormalities for at least 4 weeks. Many infectious agents can cause encephalitis, meningitis, or both. It is not infrequent to have a mixed presentation, the term meningoencephalitis applies to those cases, nevertheless, separation is useful for diagnostic and therapeutic purposes.

The classic triad of fever, neck stiffness, and altered mental status is present in only 44% of cases of acute bacterial meningitis, however, 95% present with at least two of the following symptoms: headache, fever, neck stiffness, or altered mental status. In addition, 14% of patients are comatose and 33% have focal neurologic findings on admission [36]. Elderly patients tend to present less frequently with meningeal signs, headache, or fever and more with altered mental status, thus requiring a higher index of suspicion [37]. Symptoms tend to be less severe with viral meningitis, in which prodromal flu-like symptoms and characteristic rashes may be important diagnostic clues [38, 39].

When meningitis is suspected, blood cultures should be obtained and lumbar puncture performed immediately. If CSF can't be obtained promptly, appropriate empiric antibiotics should be started without delay. Criteria for obtaining a CT scan prior to lumbar puncture in adults have been published and are based in a prospective study of 301 patients by Hasbun et al., which showed that abnormal CT findings in patients with bacterial meningitis were associated with the following risk factors: age ≥60 years, history of CNS disease (e.g., mass lesion, stroke or focal infection), immunocompromised state, recent seizure (≤1 week), abnormal level of consciousness, or focal neurologic deficits [40, 41].

CSF analysis shows considerable overlap between bacterial and viral causes of meningitis. Gram stain using cytospin techniques has a yield of 50–90% for different bacterial pathogens, but decreases by >20% points with prior antimicrobial treatment. Only positive cultures or PCR for a specific pathogen are diagnostic. Latex agglutination has fallen out of favor but is still recommended for pretreated patients with a negative Gram stain. CSF lactate concentrations ≥4 mmol/L are predictive of bacterial infection in postoperative neurosurgical patients and a normal serum C-reactive protein has a high negative predictive value for the diagnosis of bacterial meningitis [40–45]. The approach to meningitis can be categorized as follows:

Acute bacterial meningitis is a neurologic emergency and therapy should be initiated as soon as possible after the diagnosis is considered to be likely [41]. Cancer patients can be classified in three groups according to risk of infection:

(a) *Community-acquired*: The predominant organisms are *Streptococcus pneumoniae* and *Neisseria meningitidis*. *Hemophilus influenzae* is now rare, thanks to vaccination. *Listeria monocytogenes* and aerobic Gram-negative bacilli must also be considered in adults over 50 years. Empiric antibiotic coverage with vancomycin plus ceftriaxone or cefotaxime is recommended, with the addition of ampicillin when listeriosis is suspected. The use of dexamethasone in patients with suspected or proven pneumococcal meningitis either immediately before or concomitant with the first dose of antibiotics is now recommended [41, 46], no specific data for cancer patients is available.

(b) *Neutropenic patients*: Acute bacterial meningitis is uncommon and associated with high morbidity and mortality. It affects predominantly patients with hematologic malignancies. Lukes et al. [47] reported Gram-negative organisms in 29 of 43 CNS infections in neutropenic adults in 1984. *Listeria* was the most common Gram-positive organism. More recently, Sommers and Hawkins reported Gram-positive predominance in neutropenic pediatric cancer patients, most of them had an underlying hematologic malignancy [48]. Staphylococci and Streptococci caused ten infections and *Klebsiella* and *Pseudomonas* one each. *Stomatococcus mucilaginosus*, a facultatively anaerobic Gram-positive coccus, causes sepsis in neutropenic patients with mucositis and caused meningitis in leukemic and SCT patients [49]. Viridans streptococci have emerged as a cause of bacteremia in severely neutropenic patients with the following risk factors: chemotherapy with high-dose Ara-C, use of quinolones or cotrimoxazole for prophylaxis and/or oropharyngeal mucositis. Penicillin resistance is common and cases of meningitis with or without sepsis have been reported [50, 51]. Other Gram-positive bacteria that may cause meningitis in neutropenic patients include *Staphylococcus aureus* [52] and *Corynebacterium jeikeium* [53]. Empiric therapy with vancomycin plus cefepime or ceftazidime is reasonable for neutropenic patients with hematologic malignancy. Again, ampicillin should be started if *Listeria* is suspected.

(c) *Nosocomial meningitis* occurs in patients with three distinct types of underlying conditions:

1. Patients with history of neurosurgery, neurosurgical device (discussed later) or CSF leakage.
2. Immunocompromised patients.
3. Patient with a distant focus of infection (pneumonia, sinusitis or otitis).

S. aureus and *S. pneumoniae* are the most common organisms. *Streptococcus epiderdimidis*, enteric Gram-negatives and *Pseudomonas aeruginosa* are also reported. Empiric treatment with vancomycin plus cefepime, ceftazidime, or meropenem is recommended [41, 54].

Patients with nasopharyngeal carcinoma have anatomic changes in the upper respiratory tract that predispose them to sinusitis and otitis; they often receive radiotherapy and may develop osteoradionecrosis of the skull base, and therefore have an increased risk of bacterial meningitis, brain abscess, or cavernous sinus thrombosis [55].

Viral (aseptic) meningitis: Aseptic meningitis is defined by the absence of a bacterial pathogen. Viruses are the main cause. Age and immune status influence the severity of presentation. More than 90% of all viral meningitis is caused by enteroviruses, which are transmitted primarily by fecal–oral contamination and less commonly by respiratory secretions. In temperate climates, most cases occur in summer and early fall. Gastrointestinal symptoms and rash are common. Enterovirus 71 presents with vesicular hand-foot-and-mouth disease [39]. HSV-1 and 2 can cause meningitis with or without genital or oral lesions. Recurrent episodes of aseptic meningitis (Mollaret's meningitis) have been linked to HSV-2 reactivation. VZV may also present as meningitis, the occurrence of herpes zoster may herald it [39].

WNV infection often presents as meningitis, which has lower mortality and less complications than WNV encephalitis. Additionally, acute flaccid paralysis similar to paralytic poliomyelitis was described in up to 10% of patients, and only half of them had concomitant meningitis or encephalitis [56]. Other viruses more commonly associated with encephalitis, such as St. Louis and La Crosse viruses, may present with meningeal signs and symptoms (Table 19.1). As with viral encephalitis, diagnosis of viral meningitis depends on epidemiologic clues, blood and CSF serology, and CSF PCR. Treatment, other than acyclovir for HSV and VZV, is supportive.

Other infectious causes of meningitis: Cryptococcal meningitis is a disease of patients with cellular immune deficiencies. Please refer to chapter 26 for a more detailed discussion. Infrequently, cases are described in "immunocompetent" patients and in patients with leukemia or SCT [57–59].

In the appropriate setting and with the right risk factors, Spirochetes (Lyme borreliosis, syphilis and *Leptospira spp.*), endemic fungi (*Histoplasma, Coccidioides, Blastomyces*), and *M. tuberculous* must be considered in the differential diagnosis. The presentation is usually subacute and sometimes chronic. Molds are extremely rare causes of meningitis in patients with hematologic malignancy. Few cases of *Aspergillus* and other molds have been described [60, 61].

Candida meningitis is a rare entity mostly limited to neonates and neurosurgical patients. McCullers et al. reported 12 patients with leukemia and *Candida* meningitis, eight had positive blood cultures and only one had an Ommaya reservoir. Autopsies on seven of eight revealed disseminated multiorgan disease. All had prolonged neutropenia and one had SCT [62]. The routine use of antifungal prophylaxis in high-risk patients with prolonged neutropenia has made this entity rare.

Non-infectious causes of meningitis: Connective tissue disease, malignancy, and drugs such as nonsteroidal anti-inflammatories and intravenous immunoglobulin [39, 63] may cause a meningitis syndrome.

Chronic meningitis: Defined as meningitis persisting for >4 weeks, is caused mainly by *M. tuberculous* and endemic fungi, especially *Cryptococcus*. *Histoplasma* causes chronic meningitis in children and individuals with impaired T-cell immunity and has been described in association with AML [64]. Lyme disease presented as lymphocytic meningitis in a patient with CLL [65], syphilis, and brucellosis can be considered if there are risk factors. Patients with hypo- or agammaglobulinemia can develop enterovirus chronic meningitis or meningoencephalitis, often fatal [66]. Enterovirus meningoencephalitis has been reported after rituximab therapy. Enterovirus PCR in CSF may provide the diagnosis. Response to high-dose intravenous immunoglobulin and the antiviral pleconaril has been reported [67, 68]. Parvovirus B19 caused chronic meningitis in a patient with ALL [69]. Noninfectious causes include neoplastic meningitis, sarcoidosis, lupus erythematous, vasculitides, and drug toxicity or reactions [70].

Brain Abscess

Brain abscess is a focal infection that begins as a localized area of cerebritis that develops a necrotic center. Well-vascularized (ring-enhancing on CT) tissue surrounds the area leading to the formation of a capsule that walls off the abscess. The process takes >14 days in experimental animal models [71].

The epidemiology, diagnosis, and management of brain abscesses changed radically with antibiotic and surgical treatment of dental, otic and sinus infections, the advent of CT scans and MRI, the introduction of stereotactic brain biopsies, and the increased incidence among very immunosuppressed patients, especially with hematologic malignancies and SCT.

Etiology and risk factors: Infection may spread from adjacent structures such as the paranasal sinuses, middle ear, and teeth, either directly or indirectly through venous drainage. Early antibiotic and surgical treatment of these infections has diminished its importance as a cause of brain abscess. Direct seeding in the case of postoperative infections will be discussed in the next section. Hematogenous spread from distant sources, especially endocarditis, line infection and pneumonia may also occur. The source of infection is not found in 20–30% of cases. Bacteria are by far the most common cause in immunocompetent patients. Table 19.2 shows the most frequent etiologic agents for each of the above mentioned categories [71–73].

Cancer patients are often immunocompromised, and the etiology of brain abscess is quite different. Patients most frequently affected are those with hematologic malignancies, SCT, and primary CNS tumors or brain metastases taking high doses of corticosteroids, often in association with temozolamide [74, 75]. A case series of 12 pediatric cancer patients with brain abscesses found 11 cases due to fungi, seven of them *Aspergillus*, two *Candida*, and one case of *L. monocytogenes*. Eight patients had leukemia (two had allogeneic transplants) and four had CNS tumors [76]. Three

Table 19.2 Brain abscess: risk factors and etiologic agents

Risk factor	Frequent etiologic agents
Contiguous source (Sinusitis, otic or odontogenic infection)	Aerobic and anaerobic streptococci
	Haemophilus sp.
	Anaerobes (*Bacteroides, Fusobacterium, Actinomyces*)
	Pseudomonas, Enterobacteriaceae (otogenic)
Hematogenous spread (Endocarditis, pulmonary, GI or urinary sources)	*Staphylococcus aureus* and streptococci
	Listeria monocytogenes
	Anaerobes (from lung of GI tract)
	Pseudomonas, Enterobacteriaceae (from lungs or urinary tract)
Postoperative infections	*S. aureus* and streptococci
	Pseudomonas, Enterobacteriaceae
Penetrating trauma	*S. aureus* and *S. epiderdimidis*
	Clostridium sp.
	Enterobacteriaceae
Immunocompromised host (Hematopoietic malignancy, stem cell transplant, high dose corticosteroids/other immunosuppressive agents)	Molds (mainly *Aspergillus*)
	Candida sp.
	Nocardia
	Toxoplasma gondii
	L. monocytogenes
	Other: *Trypanosoma, Mycobacteria*, bacteria (see above)

out of 13 patients with solid tumors with invasive aspergillosis had brain invasion [75]. The incidence of brain abscess is highest among SCT recipients, with reports of 2–5% [77–79]. Fungal pathogens accounted for 92% of cases. *Aspergillus* and *Candida* are the most common [76, 78]. The lungs, sinuses, and skin are frequently the source of CNS mold infections, while candidemia accompanies two thirds of *Candida* brain abscesses. Bacteria, especially Gram-negatives, and *Toxoplasma gondii* are seen with less frequency [78]. *Nocardia* sp. may also cause brain abscess, often originating in the lungs or skin. In patients from endemic areas of the Americas, *Trypanosoma cruzi* may reactivate and present as an area of localized encephalitis termed "chagoma." Donors infected with *T. cruzi* may transmit infection to transplant recipients [80, 81].

The classic clinical presentation includes dull, nonspecific headache, fever (seen in 50–80% of cases), focal neurological findings (30–60%), and seizures (20–30%). SCT patients have fever (83%) and altered mental status (50%) more commonly, with or without neurologic deficits [71, 73, 78]. Acute deterioration with meningismus may be due to abscess rupture into the ventricular space. Signs of increased intracranial pressure (altered mental status, nausea and vomiting) may herald herniation. Coma at presentation is an independent risk factor for mortality [71].

Diagnosis depends on imaging. Brain CT scan shows cerebritis as a focal hypodensity (edema) that enhances with contrast. The classic ring-enhancing lesion is associated with a mature brain abscess. MRI shows hypointense lesions with ring-enhancement following gadolinium administration in T1-weighted sequences. In T2-weighted images a hyperintense central area of pus is surrounded by a well-defined hypointense capsule and surrounding edema. Stereotactic brain biopsy allows for confirmation and identification of the causal organism. Positive blood cultures or identification of an extraneural source of infection (such as *Aspergillus* or *Nocardia* pneumonia, bacterial or fungal sinusitis or otitis) will help when biopsy or surgery is not an option. Lumbar puncture is infrequently done because of the risk of herniation and frequent negative results, unless there is associated meningitis.

In patients with cancer, differentiating between brain tumor (new or recurrent) and abscess is often difficult. Pus produces hyperintense signals on MRI diffusion-weighted sequences while necrotic tumor centers produce iso- or hypointense signals. Brain metastases and glioblastomas occasionally display hyperintense signals and may be confused with abscess. Intratumor hemorrhage may also limit the interpretation. CNS toxoplasmosis is difficult to differentiate from lymphoma and PTLD in SCT patients since both may present as single or multiple nodular or ring-enhancing lesions. Tuberculomas, histoplasmomas, cryptococcomas, aspergillomas, nocardiosis and, even more rarely, neurocysticercosis, schistosomiasis, and cerebral syphilitic gummas can be confused with a brain tumor or metastatic disease [82–84].

Antibiotic management of bacterial brain abscess is best directed by microbiologic diagnosis. Empiric therapy may be selected based on the likely bacterial etiology as listed in Table 19.2, however, since patients are often very ill and cancer patients may be at higher risk of resistant bacterial infections, broad-spectrum coverage with vancomycin 15 mg/kg every 8 h plus either meropenem 2 g every 8 h or the combination of metronidazole plus cefepime or ceftazidime are reasonable initial therapies while awaiting culture results.

Fungal brain abscess has shown poor response to traditional antifungals with or without surgery. Amphotericin B and liposomal amphotericin B were the most frequently used treatments [76–79]. The use of voriconazole has been reported to improve outcomes with complete or partial response in 28 (35%) of 81 patients. SCT patients had the worst response (15%) [85].

Stereotactic needle aspiration provides therapeutic drainage and specimens for culture and other studies [71]. Prior antibiotic therapy decreases culture positivity by 50% [73]. Open craniotomy is now rarely performed. Response to therapy is monitored with CT or MRI and duration of therapy is determined in part by radiologic resolution of inflammatory signs. Traditionally, 6–8 weeks of parenteral antibiotics have been recommended. Shorter intravenous courses followed by oral antibiotics have been used successfully even in patients who either could not have or refused aspiration or surgery [71, 86].

Postoperative Infections

CSF shunt infections: CSF shunts are used in the management of hydrocephalus, and have a proximal portion that enters the CSF space and a distal portion that may either drain internally to the peritoneal or pleural cavity or a blood vessel, or externally as in external ventricular drains (EVDs), used for temporary drainage. They may have reservoirs for intermittent percutaneous access [87].

EVD infection is defined as one positive CSF culture, except when skin flora is recovered, in which case a repeat positive culture or abnormal CSF and/or clinical findings consistent with infection are required. An average incidence of these infections is 10% although infectious complications have been seen in up to 27% in some series. Risk factors include the presence of subarachnoid or intraventricular hemorrhage, duration of catheter placement for >5 days, frequent manipulation of the EVD system, and repeat shunting [87–90]. Use of antibiotics for the duration of EVD placement to prevent infection is controversial, with some studies showing decreased incidence of infections while others show no change in incidence and selection of more resistant organisms [88, 91, 92]. Etiologic agents include skin flora such as coagulase-negative staphylococci and *S. aureus*, *Propionibacterium acnes* as well as resistant Gram-negatives commonly seen in ICU, including *Pseudomononas* sp., *Acinetobacter* sp. [93], and Enterobacteriaceae. *Candida* infections are infrequent and occur in patients with risk factors for candidemia and patients treated for bacterial CSF infections [94].

Internal shunt infections often mimic shunt malfunction, presenting with headache, drowsiness, and vomiting. Fever and CSF abnormalities are common. Only one third of patients develop meningeal irritation since most infections remain contained in the ventricles and are caused by low-virulence organisms, mostly skin flora (*Staphylococci*, *P. acnes*), and less commonly by Gram-negatives. Most infections present early after shunt placement or revision. CSF cultures obtained from the valve or ventricles have a higher yield than lumbar puncture. CT or MRI imaging may rarely show a brain abscess. Infection of the distal shunt portion may manifest as peritonitis or bacteremia depending on whether it drains in the peritoneum or the vascular system [87, 95].

Treatment of CSF shunt infections includes removal of its components, a new temporary EVD and intravenous antibiotics. Empiric coverage includes vancomycin plus either cefepime, ceftazidime, or meropenem. The timing of internal shunt reimplantation depends on the infecting organism and negativization of CSF cultures. Specific indications for use of the intraventricular route for antibiotic administration are not well established. They may be beneficial [41, 96]. Conservative treatment with antibiotics alone or "one stage" shunt replacement has a higher risk of relapse [41, 95, 96].

The Infectious Diseases Society of America has published treatment recommendations [41].

Postcraniotomy infections occur in <1 to >8% of intracranial surgical procedures [97] and may be superficial, such as scalp infections and bone flap osteitis, or deep, including meningitis-ventriculitis, brain abscess, and empyema. Most scheduled craniotomies are considered clean surgeries. Entry through the paranasal sinuses or mastoid is considered clean-contaminated, and open fractures from trauma are considered contaminated [98]. Antibiotic prophylaxis decreases the incidence of superficial but not deep infections and may select for more resistant organisms in the later [98, 99]. *S. aureus* is the most frequent pathogen followed by other Gram-positive bacteria, and, less commonly, hospital-acquired Gram-negatives. The risk of infection is higher in those with a preceding craniotomy, operative time >4 h, emergency or trauma surgery, external CSF leakage or early subsequent operation. In patients recovering from surgery for malignant glioma, it is difficult to differentiate clinically or by imaging between early recurrence of tumor, postoperative hyperperfusion, and intracranial infection. Fever and local signs of wound infection may be present. Infections tend to occur early, 70% in the first month and 85% within 2 months, while tumor recurrence usually occurs after 6 months, rarely before 3 months [100]. Surgical debridement and antibiotics are the treatment of choice. Empiric therapy is similar to CSF shunt infections.

Postoperative meningitis may be bacterial or aseptic, the later is likely a reaction to heme breakdown products, and posterior fossa surgery is a known predisposing factor. Empiric therapy followed by discontinuation if CSF cultures are negative after 3 days, provided the sample was taken before antibiotics were administered, was found prospectively to be an effective strategy in one study [101].

Noninfectious Problems that May Mimic Infection

1. Neoplastic meningitis is most commonly seen in patients with disseminated progressive cancer (60–70%), but in 5–10% of cases it may be the initial manifestation of cancer. The incidence varies according to tumor type, and is highest with some lymphomas and leukemias. The most common solid tumors include breast cancer (3%) and small-cell lung cancer (6%). Symptoms are varied, depending on the CNS territory invaded by the tumor. Headache, altered mental status, and ataxia are the most common (50%). Cranial nerve compromise (40%) and spinal symptoms (60%) are frequently reported. MRI shows leptomeningeal enhancement and tumor nodules in less than 60% and communicating hydrocephalus in

8–10%. CSF analysis may show pleocytosis (63%), elevated protein (80%), and decreased glucose (55%). Malignant cells are found in 50% on the first CSF sample and 25% more in the second one. Autopsy data shows up to 40% of patients with neoplastic meningitis lack positive CSF cytology. Thus, it may be difficult to differentiate from subacute or chronic meningitis and chemical meningitis [102].

2. Paraneoplastic neurological syndromes (PNS) may affect any part of the central and peripheral nervous system, the neuromuscular junction or muscle. In 50% of cases onconeural antibodies are found, suggesting an immune-mediated disorder. PNS are rapidly progressive and may cause severe disability. They are rare (less than 0.01% of cancer patients) and antedate the diagnosis of cancer in almost 80% of patients. Some may be confused with infection. Paraneoplastic encephalomyelitis is characterized by neuronal loss and inflammatory infiltrates in multiple areas of the CNS. Seventy five percent of patients have underlying small-cell lung cancer. Limbic encephalitis has a subacute onset with confusion and short-term memory loss, sometimes after a prodrome of fevers and headache. Seizures, hallucinations, and sleep disturbances may follow. Small-cell lung cancer, testicular tumors, and breast cancer are the most frequent underlying cancers. Treatment is directed at the tumor and immune modulation may be beneficial in select cases [103, 104].

3. Reversible posterior leukoencephalopathy syndrome (RPLS) was described by Hinchey et al. in 1996 in seven patients receiving cyclosporine or tacrolimus after transplantation or for aplastic anemia, one receiving interferon alpha for metastatic melanoma and seven more with either eclampsia (three patients) or acute hypertensive encephalopathy (four patients) [105]. RPLS presents subacutely with headaches (53%), visual symptoms (39%), seizures (87%), and altered mental status/encephalopathy (92%) [105, 106]. Blood pressure elevations can be severe or, more often, mild to moderate. The syndrome can be confused with acute encephalitis. Since the clinical presentation is nonspecific, diagnosis relies on MRI, which shows bilateral white matter abnormalities suggestive of edema in the posterior regions of the cerebral hemispheres. Other areas may be involved [105, 107]. Capillary leak caused by drugs that affect the endothelium or increase blood pressure or blood volume and secondarily tax endothelial function is the proposed mechanism. The posterior part of the brain has decreased sympathetic innervation and is thus believed to be more vulnerable [105–108]. RPLS is usually reversible within 2 weeks. Treatment includes discontinuation of the offending drug, control of hypertension, and supportive treatment. In a large series, malignancy was present in 32% and transplantation in 24% of cases of RPLS [106]. Reports of chemotherapeutic agents linked to RPLS continue to enlarge the list, now including platinum analogs (cisplatin, carboplatin), antimetabolites (gemcitabine), folate antagonists, anthracyclines, and vinca alkaloids. Growth factors, high-dose corticosteroids and antiangiogenic-targeted therapies such as Bevacizumab and sorafenib have been implicated. Many of this drugs cause hypertension and have the potential to cause endothelial damage. RPLS has been reported as soon as hours after drug administration and as late as 1 month later [108].

4. GVHD neurological involvement commonly manifests as neuromuscular problems. Angiitis of the CNS is a rare complication of allogeneic SCT. Patients present with acute or subacute focal neurological deficits, encephalopathy, or neuropsychological impairment approximately 2 years after transplantation. Gray and white matter ischemia and cerebral hemorrhages are found in autopsy. Most patients had history of acute and chronic GVHD [109–111]. Two cases of GVHD presenting solely as encephalitis in similar patients have been reported [112, 113].

References

1. Pruitt AA. Nervous system infections in patients with cancer. Neurol Clin. 2003;21(1):193–219.
2. Pruitt AA. Central nervous system infections in cancer patients. Semin Neurol. 2004;24(4):435–52.
3. Davies NW, Sharief MK, Howard RS. Infection-associated encephalopathies: their investigation, diagnosis, and treatment. J Neurol. 2006;253(7):833–45.
4. Glaser CA, Honarmand S, Anderson LJ, et al. Beyond viruses: clinical profiles and etiologies associated with encephalitis. Clin Infect Dis. 2006;43(12):1565–77.
5. Khetsuriani N, Holman RC, Anderson LJ. Burden of encephalitis-associated hospitalizations in the United States, 1988–1997. Clin Infect Dis. 2002;35(2):175–82.
6. Tunkel AR, Glaser CA, Bloch KC, et al. The management of encephalitis: clinical practice guidelines by the Infectious Diseases Society of America. Clin Infect Dis. 2008;47(3):303–27.
7. Studahl M. Influenza virus and CNS manifestations. J Clin Virol. 2003;28(3):225–32.
8. Drobyski WR, Knox KK, Majewski D, Carrigan DR. Brief report: fatal encephalitis due to variant B human herpesvirus-6 infection in a bone marrow-transplant recipient. N Engl J Med. 1994;330(19):1356–60.
9. Fotheringham J, Akhyani N, Vortmeyer A, et al. Detection of active human herpesvirus-6 infection in the brain: correlation with polymerase chain reaction detection in cerebrospinal fluid. J Infect Dis. 2007;195(3):450–4.
10. Yoshida H, Matsunaga K, Ueda T, et al. Human herpesvirus 6 meningoencephalitis successfully treated with ganciclovir in a patient who underwent allogeneic bone marrow transplantation from an HLA-identical sibling. Int J Hematol. 2002;75(4):421–5.
11. Ogata M, Satou T, Kawano R, et al. Plasma HHV-6 viral load-guided preemptive therapy against HHV-6 encephalopathy after allogeneic stem cell transplantation: a prospective evaluation. Bone Marrow Transplant. 2008;41(3):279–85.

12. Miller GG, Boivin G, Dummer JS, et al. Cytomegalovirus ventriculoencephalitis in a peripheral blood stem cell transplant recipient. Clin Infect Dis. 2006;42(4):e26–9.
13. Fukumoto S, Kinjo M, Hokamura K, Tanaka K. Subarachnoid hemorrhage and granulomatous angiitis of the basilar artery: demonstration of the varicella-zoster-virus in the basilar artery lesions. Stroke. 1986;17(5):1024–8.
14. Verghese A, Sugar AM. Herpes zoster ophthalmicus and granulomatous angiitis. An ill-appreciated cause of stroke. J Am Geriatr Soc. 1986;34(4):309–12.
15. Weaver S, Rosenblum MK, DeAngelis LM. Herpes varicella zoster encephalitis in immunocompromised patients. Neurology. 1999;52(1):193–5.
16. Garamendi I, Montejo M, Cancelo L, et al. Encephalitis caused by Epstein–Barr virus in a renal transplant recipient. Clin Infect Dis. 2002;34(2):287–8.
17. Phowthongkum P, Phantumchinda K, Jutivorakool K, Suankratay C. Basal ganglia and brainstem encephalitis, optic neuritis, and radiculomyelitis in Epstein–Barr virus infection. J Infect. 2007;54(3):e141–4.
18. Volpi A. Epstein–Barr virus and human herpesvirus type 8 infections of the central nervous system. Herpes. 2004;11 Suppl 2:120A–7.
19. Brenner W, Storch G, Buller R, Vij R, Devine S, DiPersio J. West Nile virus encephalopathy in an allogeneic stem cell transplant recipient: use of quantitative PCR for diagnosis and assessment of viral clearance. Bone Marrow Transplant. 2005;36(4):369–70.
20. Hong DS, Jacobson KL, Raad II, et al. West Nile encephalitis in 2 hematopoietic stem cell transplant recipients: case series and literature review. Clin Infect Dis. 2003;37(8):1044–9.
21. Kleinschmidt-DeMasters BK, Marder BA, Levi ME, et al. Naturally acquired West Nile virus encephalomyelitis in transplant recipients: clinical, laboratory, diagnostic, and neuropathological features. Arch Neurol. 2004;61(8):1210–20.
22. Hopfinger G, Plessl A, Grisold W, et al. Progressive multifocal leukoencephalopathy after rituximab in a patient with relapsed follicular lymphoma and low IgG levels and a low CD4+ lymphocyte count. Leuk Lymphoma. 2008;49(12):2367–9.
23. Kiewe P, Seyfert S, Korper S, Rieger K, Thiel E, Knauf W. Progressive multifocal leukoencephalopathy with detection of JC virus in a patient with chronic lymphocytic leukemia parallel to onset of fludarabine therapy. Leuk Lymphoma. 2003;44(10):1815–8.
24. Osorio S, de la Camara R, Golbano N, et al. Progressive multifocal leukoencephalopathy after stem cell transplantation, unsuccessfully treated with cidofovir. Bone Marrow Transplant. 2002;30(12): 963–6.
25. Pelosini M, Focosi D, Rita F, et al. Progressive multifocal leukoencephalopathy: report of three cases in HIV-negative hematological patients and review of literature. Ann Hematol. 2008;87(5):405–12.
26. Reddy N, Abel TW, Jagasia M, Morgan D, Weaver K, Greer J. Progressive multifocal leukoencephalopathy in a patient with follicular lymphoma treated with multiple courses of rituximab. Leuk Lymphoma. 2009;50(3):460–2.
27. Weber T. Progressive multifocal leukoencephalopathy. Neurol Clin. 2008;26(3):833–54, x–xi.
28. Aoun M, Georgala A, Mboumi K, et al. Changing the outcome of toxoplasmosis in bone marrow transplant recipients. Int J Antimicrob Agents. 2006;27(6):570–2.
29. De Medeiros BC, De Medeiros CR, Werner B, Loddo G, Pasquini R, Bleggi-Torres LF. Disseminated toxoplasmosis after bone marrow transplantation: report of 9 cases. Transpl Infect Dis. 2001;3(1):24–8.
30. Montoya JG, Liesenfeld O. Toxoplasmosis. Lancet. 2004;363(9425):1965–76.
31. Pagano L, Trape G, Putzulu R, et al. *Toxoplasma gondii* infection in patients with hematological malignancies. Ann Hematol. 2004;83(9):592–5.
32. Anderlini P, Przepiorka D, Luna M, et al. Acanthamoeba meningoencephalitis after bone marrow transplantation. Bone Marrow Transplant. 1994;14(3):459–61.
33. Deetz TR, Sawyer MH, Billman G, Schuster FL, Visvesvara GS. Successful treatment of Balamuthia amoebic encephalitis: presentation of 2 cases. Clin Infect Dis. 2003;37(10):1304–12.
34. Eidelman LA, Putterman D, Putterman C, Sprung CL. The spectrum of septic encephalopathy. Definitions, etiologies, and mortalities. JAMA. 1996;275(6):470–3.
35. Maschke M, Kastrup O, Forsting M, Diener HC. Update on neuroimaging in infectious central nervous system disease. Curr Opin Neurol. 2004;17(4):475–80.
36. van de Beek D, de Gans J, Spanjaard L, Weisfelt M, Reitsma JB, Vermeulen M. Clinical features and prognostic factors in adults with bacterial meningitis. N Engl J Med. 2004;351(18):1849–59.
37. Cabellos C, Verdaguer R, Olmo M, et al. Community-acquired bacterial meningitis in elderly patients: experience over 30 years. Medicine (Baltimore). 2009;88(2):115–9.
38. Ihekwaba UK, Kudesia G, McKendrick MW. Clinical features of viral meningitis in adults: significant differences in cerebrospinal fluid findings among herpes simplex virus, varicella zoster virus, and enterovirus infections. Clin Infect Dis. 2008;47(6):783–9.
39. Irani DN. Aseptic meningitis and viral myelitis. Neurol Clin. 2008;26(3):635–55, vii–viii.
40. Hasbun R, Abrahams J, Jekel J, Quagliarello VJ. Computed tomography of the head before lumbar puncture in adults with suspected meningitis. N Engl J Med. 2001;345(24):1727–33.
41. Tunkel AR, Hartman BJ, Kaplan SL, et al. Practice guidelines for the management of bacterial meningitis. Clin Infect Dis. 2004;39(9):1267–84.
42. Cunha BA. Distinguishing bacterial from viral meningitis: the critical importance of the CSF lactic acid levels. Intensive Care Med. 2006;32(8):1272–3; author reply 4.
43. Gerdes LU, Jorgensen PE, Nexo E, Wang P. C-reactive protein and bacterial meningitis: a meta-analysis. Scand J Clin Lab Invest. 1998;58(5):383–93.
44. Leib SL, Boscacci R, Gratzl O, Zimmerli W. Predictive value of cerebrospinal fluid (CSF) lactate level versus CSF/blood glucose ratio for the diagnosis of bacterial meningitis following neurosurgery. Clin Infect Dis. 1999;29(1):69–74.
45. Sormunen P, Kallio MJ, Kilpi T, Peltola H. C-reactive protein is useful in distinguishing Gram stain-negative bacterial meningitis from viral meningitis in children. J Pediatr. 1999;134(6):725–9.
46. van de Beek D, de Gans J, Tunkel AR, Wijdicks EF. Community-acquired bacterial meningitis in adults. N Engl J Med. 2006;354(1):44–53.
47. Lukes SA, Posner JB, Nielsen S, Armstrong D. Bacterial infections of the CNS in neutropenic patients. Neurology. 1984;34(3):269–75.
48. Sommers LM, Hawkins DS. Meningitis in pediatric cancer patients: a review of forty cases from a single institution. Pediatr Infect Dis J. 1999;18(10):902–7.
49. Abraham J, Bilgrami S, Dorsky D, et al. *Stomatococcus mucilaginosus* meningitis in a patient with multiple myeloma following autologous stem cell transplantation. Bone Marrow Transplant. 1997;19(6):639–41.
50. Balkundi DR, Murray DL, Patterson MJ, Gera R, Scott-Emuakpor A, Kulkarni R. Penicillin-resistant *Streptococcus mitis* as a cause of septicemia with meningitis in febrile neutropenic children. J Pediatr Hematol Oncol. 1997;19(1):82–5.
51. Tokuda K, Nishi J, Yoshinaga M, et al. Sepsis and meningitis due to penicillin-resistant viridans streptococci in neutropenic children. Pediatr Int. 2000;42(2):174–7.
52. Matsubara H, Makimoto A, Higa T, et al. Successful treatment of meningoencephalitis caused by methicillin-resistant *Staphylococcus aureus* with intrathecal vancomycin in an allogeneic peripheral

blood stem cell transplant recipient. Bone Marrow Transplant. 2003;31(1):65–7.
53. Johnson A, Hulse P, Oppenheim BA. *Corynebacterium jeikeium* meningitis and transverse myelitis in a neutropenic patient. Eur J Clin Microbiol Infect Dis. 1992;11(5):473–4.
54. Weisfelt M, van de Beek D, Spanjaard L, de Gans J. Nosocomial bacterial meningitis in adults: a prospective series of 50 cases. J Hosp Infect. 2007;66(1):71–8.
55. Liang KL, Jiang RS, Lin JC, et al. Central nervous system infection in patients with postirradiated nasopharyngeal carcinoma: a case-controlled study. Am J Rhinol Allergy. 2009;23(4):417–21.
56. Kramer LD, Li J, Shi PY. West Nile virus. Lancet Neurol. 2007;6(2):171–81.
57. Mavinkurve-Groothuis AM, Bokkerink JP, Verweij PE, Veerman AJ, Hoogerbrugge PM. Cryptococcal meningitis in a child with acute lymphoblastic leukemia. Pediatr Infect Dis J. 2003;22(6):576.
58. Mendpara SD, Ustun C, Kallab AM, Mazzella FM, Bilodeau PA, Jillella AP. Cryptococcal meningitis following autologous stem cell transplantation in a patient with multiple myeloma. Bone Marrow Transplant. 2002;30(4):259–60.
59. Urbini B, Castellini C, Rondelli R, Prete A, Pierinelli S, Pession A. Cryptococcal meningitis during front-line chemotherapy for acute lymphoblastic leukemia. Haematologica. 2000;85(10): 1103–4.
60. Madrigal V, Alonso J, Bureo E, Figols FJ, Salesa R. Fatal meningoencephalitis caused by Scedosporium inflatum (*Scedosporium prolificans*) in a child with lymphoblastic leukemia. Eur J Clin Microbiol Infect Dis. 1995;14(7):601–3.
61. Saitoh T, Matsushima T, Shimizu H, et al. Successful treatment with voriconazole of Aspergillus meningitis in a patient with acute myeloid leukemia. Ann Hematol. 2007;86(9):697–8.
62. McCullers JA, Vargas SL, Flynn PM, Razzouk BI, Shenep JL. Candidal meningitis in children with cancer. Clin Infect Dis. 2000;31(2):451–7.
63. Scribner CL, Kapit RM, Phillips ET, Rickles NM. Aseptic meningitis and intravenous immunoglobulin therapy. Ann Intern Med. 1994;121(4):305–6.
64. Pereira GH, Padua SS, Park MV, Muller RP, Passos RM, Menezes Y. Chronic meningitis by histoplasmosis: report of a child with acute myeloid leukemia. Braz J Infect Dis. 2008;12(6):555–7.
65. Schweighofer CD, Fatkenheuer G, Staib P, Hallek M, Reiser M. Lyme disease in a patient with chronic lymphocytic leukemia mimics leukemic meningeosis. Onkologie. 2007;30(11):564–6.
66. McKinney Jr RE, Katz SL, Wilfert CM. Chronic enteroviral meningoencephalitis in agammaglobulinemic patients. Rev Infect Dis. 1987;9(2):334–56.
67. Ganjoo KN, Raman R, Sobel RA, Pinto HA. Opportunistic enteroviral meningoencephalitis: an unusual treatable complication of rituximab therapy. Leuk Lymphoma. 2009;50(4):673–5.
68. Kiani-Alikhan S, Skoulidis F, Barroso A, et al. Enterovirus infection of neuronal cells post-Rituximab. Br J Haematol. 2009;146(3):333–5.
69. Sinclair JP, Croxson MC, Thomas SM, Teague LR, Mauger DC. Chronic parvovirus B19 meningitis in a child with acute lymphocytic leukemia. Pediatr Infect Dis J. 1999;18(4):395–6.
70. Hildebrand J, Aoun M. Chronic meningitis: still a diagnostic challenge. J Neurol. 2003;250(6):653–60.
71. Mathisen GE, Johnson JP. Brain abscess. Clin Infect Dis. 1997;25(4):763–79; quiz 80–1.
72. Tattevin P, Bruneel F, Clair B, et al. Bacterial brain abscesses: a retrospective study of 94 patients admitted to an intensive care unit (1980 to 1999). Am J Med. 2003;115(2):143–6.
73. Tonon E, Scotton PG, Gallucci M, Vaglia A. Brain abscess: clinical aspects of 100 patients. Int J Infect Dis. 2006;10(2):103–9.
74. Damek DM, Lillehei KO, Kleinschmidt-DeMasters BK. Aspergillus terreus brain abscess mimicking tumor progression in a patient with treated glioblastoma multiforme. Clin Neuropathol. 2008;27(6):400–7.
75. Ohmagari N, Raad II, Hachem R, Kontoyiannis DP. Invasive aspergillosis in patients with solid tumors. Cancer. 2004;101(10):2300–2.
76. Antunes NL, Hiriharan S, DeAngelis LM. Brain abscesses in children with cancer. Med Pediatr Oncol. 1998;31(1):19–21.
77. Baddley JW, Salzman D, Pappas PG. Fungal brain abscess in transplant recipients: epidemiologic, microbiologic, and clinical features. Clin Transplant. 2002;16(6):419–24.
78. Hagensee ME, Bauwens JE, Kjos B, Bowden RA. Brain abscess following marrow transplantation: experience at the Fred Hutchinson Cancer Research Center, 1984–1992. Clin Infect Dis. 1994;19(3):402–8.
79. Jantunen E, Volin L, Salonen O, et al. Central nervous system aspergillosis in allogeneic stem cell transplant recipients. Bone Marrow Transplant. 2003;31(3):191–6.
80. Di Lorenzo GA, Pagano MA, Taratuto AL, Garau ML, Meli FJ, Pomsztein MD. Chagasic granulomatous encephalitis in immunosuppressed patients. Computed tomography and magnetic resonance imaging findings. J Neuroimaging. 1996;6(2):94–7.
81. Marchiori PE, Alexandre PL, Britto N, et al. Late reactivation of Chagas disease presenting in a recipient as an expansive mass lesion in the brain after heart transplantation of chagasic myocardiopathy. J Heart Lung Transplant. 2007;26(11):1091–6.
82. Omuro AM, Leite CC, Mokhtari K, Delattre JY. Pitfalls in the diagnosis of brain tumours. Lancet Neurol. 2006;5(11):937–48.
83. Lambertucci JR, Souza-Pereira SR, Carvalho TA. Simultaneous occurrence of brain tumor and myeloradiculopathy in *Schistosomiasis mansoni*: case report. Rev Soc Bras Med Trop. 2009;42(3):338–41.
84. Rettenmaier NB, Epstein HD, Oi S, Robinson PA, Goldstein BH. Cerebral nocardia masquerading as metastatic CNS disease in an endometrial cancer patient. Eur J Gynaecol Oncol. 2009;30(1): 90–2.
85. Schwartz S, Ruhnke M, Ribaud P, et al. Improved outcome in central nervous system aspergillosis, using voriconazole treatment. Blood. 2005;106(8):2641–5.
86. Skoutelis AT, Gogos CA, Maraziotis TE, Bassaris HP. Management of brain abscesses with sequential intravenous/oral antibiotic therapy. Eur J Clin Microbiol Infect Dis. 2000;19(5):332–5.
87. Zunt JR. Iatrogenic infections of the central nervous system. In: Sheld WM, Whitley RJ, Marra CM, editors. Infection of the central nervous system. Philadelphia: Lippincott Williams & Wilkins; 2004.
88. Arabi Y, Memish ZA, Balkhy HH, et al. Ventriculostomy-associated infections: incidence and risk factors. Am J Infect Control. 2005;33(3):137–43.
89. Hoefnagel D, Dammers R, Ter Laak-Poort MP, Avezaat CJ. Risk factors for infections related to external ventricular drainage. Acta Neurochir (Wien). 2008;150(3):209–14; discussion 14.
90. Mayhall CG, Archer NH, Lamb VA, et al. Ventriculostomy-related infections. A prospective epidemiologic study. N Engl J Med. 1984;310(9):553–9.
91. Alleyne CH, Jr., Hassan M, Zabramski JM. The efficacy and cost of prophylactic and periprocedural antibiotics in patients with external ventricular drains. Neurosurgery. 2000;47(5):1124–7; discussion 7–9.
92. Poon WS, Ng S, Wai S. CSF antibiotic prophylaxis for neurosurgical patients with ventriculostomy: a randomised study. Acta Neurochir Suppl. 1998;71:146–8.
93. Kralinsky K, Krcmeryova T, Tuharsky J, Krcmery V. Nosocomial Acinetobacter meningitis. Pediatr Infect Dis J. 2000;19(3):270–1.
94. Montero A, Romero J, Vargas JA, et al. Candida infection of cerebrospinal fluid shunt devices: report of two cases and review of the literature. Acta Neurochir (Wien). 2000;142(1):67–74.

95. Conen A, Walti LN, Merlo A, Fluckiger U, Battegay M, Trampuz A. Characteristics and treatment outcome of cerebrospinal fluid shunt-associated infections in adults: a retrospective analysis over an 11-year period. Clin Infect Dis. 2008;47(1):73–82.
96. Arnell K, Enblad P, Wester T, Sjolin J. Treatment of cerebrospinal fluid shunt infections in children using systemic and intraventricular antibiotic therapy in combination with externalization of the ventricular catheter: efficacy in 34 consecutively treated infections. J Neurosurg. 2007;107(3 Suppl):213–9.
97. McClelland 3rd S, Hall WA. Postoperative central nervous system infection: incidence and associated factors in 2111 neurosurgical procedures. Clin Infect Dis. 2007;45(1):55–9.
98. Korinek AM. Risk factors for neurosurgical site infections after craniotomy: a prospective multicenter study of 2944 patients. The French Study Group of Neurosurgical Infections, the SEHP, and the C-CLIN Paris-Nord. Service epidemiologie hygiene et prevention. Neurosurgery. 1997;41(5):1073–9; discussion 9–81.
99. Korinek AM, Baugnon T, Golmard JL, van Effenterre R, Coriat P, Puybasset L. Risk factors for adult nosocomial meningitis after craniotomy: role of antibiotic prophylaxis. Neurosurgery. 2006;59(1):126–33; discussion 33.
100. Vogelsang JP, Wehe A, Markakis E. Postoperative intracranial abscess–clinical aspects in the differential diagnosis to early recurrence of malignant glioma. Clin Neurol Neurosurg. 1998;100(1):11–4.
101. Zarrouk V, Vassor I, Bert F, et al. Evaluation of the management of postoperative aseptic meningitis. Clin Infect Dis. 2007;44(12):1555–9.
102. Gleissner B, Chamberlain MC. Neoplastic meningitis. Lancet Neurol. 2006;5(5):443–52.
103. Graus F, Dalmau J. Paraneoplastic neurological syndromes: diagnosis and treatment. Curr Opin Neurol. 2007;20(6):732–7.
104. Honnorat J, Antoine JC. Paraneoplastic neurological syndromes. Orphanet J Rare Dis. 2007;2:22.
105. Hinchey J, Chaves C, Appignani B, et al. A reversible posterior leukoencephalopathy syndrome. N Engl J Med. 1996;334(8):494–500.
106. Lee VH, Wijdicks EFM, Manno EM, Rabinstein AA. Clinical spectrum of reversible posterior leukoencephalopathy syndrome. Arch Neurol. 2008;65(2):205–10.
107. Hinchey JA. Reversible posterior leukoencephalopathy syndrome: what have we learned in the last 10 years? Arch Neurol. 2008;65(2):175–6.
108. Vaughn C, Zhang L, Schiff D. Reversible posterior leukoencephalopathy syndrome in cancer. Curr Oncol Rep. 2008;10(1):86–91.
109. Campbell JN, Morris PP. Cerebral vasculitis in graft-versus-host disease: a case report. AJNR Am J Neuroradiol. 2005;26(3):654–6.
110. Ma M, Barnes G, Pulliam J, Jezek D, Baumann RJ, Berger JR. CNS angiitis in graft vs host disease. Neurology. 2002;59(12):1994–7.
111. Padovan CS, Bise K, Hahn J, et al. Angiitis of the central nervous system after allogeneic bone marrow transplantation? Stroke. 1999;30(8):1651–6.
112. Iwasaki Y, Sako K, Ohara Y, et al. Subacute panencephalitis associated with chronic graft-versus-host disease. Acta Neuropathol. 1993;85(5):566–72.
113. Marosi C, Budka H, Grimm G, et al. Fatal encephalitis in a patient with chronic graft-versus-host disease. Bone Marrow Transplant. 1990;6(1):53–7.

Chapter 20
Endocarditis in Oncology Patients

Sara E. Cosgrove and Aruna Subramanian

Abstract Although relatively uncommon in the general population with an incidence of 2–7 cases per 100,000 person-years, infective endocarditis (IE) is associated with significant morbidity and mortality. Recent studies suggest that the incidence of IE in oncology patients overall has increased and that it is reasonable to maintain a baseline suspicion in patients who present with the appropriate clinical scenario. An in-depth review of epidemiology, risk factors, clinical presentation, diagnosis, and medical and surgical management of IE in oncology patients is presented in this chapter.

Keywords Infective endocarditis • Antibiotic therapy • Diagnosis • Surgical intervention

Epidemiology

Although relatively uncommon in the general population with an incidence of 2–7 cases per 100,000 person years, infective endocarditis (IE) is associated with significant morbidity and mortality [1]. The incidence of IE in oncology patients has not been defined and traditionally is thought to be low. Some have hypothesized that because many oncology patients, particularly those with leukemia, have low platelet counts because of their disease or therapy, they are unable to effectively form the essential lesion of endocarditis – a mass of platelets and fibrin adherent to the endothelial surface of the heart within which circulating microorganisms have enmeshed. Indeed, in a study of the hearts at autopsy of 420 patients with acute leukemia between 1954 and 1964, none had endocarditis, although 7% had myocardial abscesses generally associated with disseminated infection [2].

However, recent studies suggest that the incidence of IE in oncology patients overall has increased and that it is reasonable to maintain a baseline suspicion in patients who present with the appropriate clinical scenario. In a study evaluating a large international cohort of patients with IE, 230 (8%) of 2,772 patients had cancer [3]. Interestingly, in this same cohort, similar numbers of patients were on hemodialysis (8%), a recognized risk for IE due to long-term catheter use and frequent access of the vascular system, events that also often occur in oncology patients undergoing therapy. An additional analysis of this cohort specifically evaluated patients with both nosocomial and nonnosocomial healthcare-associated IE, which made up 34% of the cohort of patients with noninjecting drug use-associated IE. Of these patients, 16% had cancer and 15% were on immunosuppressive therapy. *Staphylococcus aureus* was the most common cause of infection, occurring in about 45% of patients, about half of whom had methicillin-resistant strains.

Very few studies specifically investigate IE in oncology patients (Table 20.1). Early case series focused on an association between long-term central venous access and risk of coagulase-negative staphylococcal bacteremia and subsequent endocarditis, predominantly involving the right side of the heart in patients with hematologic malignancy [4–6]. Indeed, this pathogen and *S. aureus* appeared to be the predominant causes of IE in the oncology population, while streptococci were reported infrequently. This more closely mirrored the distribution of pathogens in healthcare-associated IE and stood in contrast to the usual distribution of pathogens among patients with community-acquired native-valve endocarditis who were not injecting drug users in which one third to one half of cases were caused by streptococci [1, 3, 7]. Interestingly, the incidence of native-valve coagulase-negative staphylococcal IE might be even higher in the oncology population than had been described among patients with healthcare-associated IE, perhaps because of the frequency and duration of central venous catheterization in the former group. Also of interest in these series was the finding that IE developed despite the presence of thrombocytopenia in many cases.

S.E. Cosgrove (✉)
Division of Infectious Diseases, Johns Hopkins University School of Medicine, 600 N. Wolfe Street, Baltimore, MD 21287, USA
e-mail: scosgro1@jhmi.edu

Table 20.1 Studies of IE in oncology populations

Author	Year	Population	Number	Incidence	Type of malignancy	Predominant organisms	Notes
Liepman [4]	1980–1981	Adult leukemia patients	3	Not stated	AML (100%)	S. epidermidis (66%)	All with indwelling catheters and thrombocytopenia
Quinn [6]	1982–1983	Oncology center, adult allogeneic bone marrow transplant patients	3	3/246 (1.2%) patients undergoing BMT	Leukemia undergoing BMT	Coagulase-negative staph (100%)	All with Hickman catheters; all right-sided IE
Martino [5]	1986–1987	Adult allogeneic and autologous bone marrow transplant patients	7	7/141 (5%) patients undergoing BMT	Leukemia undergoing BMT (100%)	S. epidermidis (57%)	All with Hickman catheters; all right-sided; 5/7 with thrombocytopenia
Yusef [8]	1994–2004	Oncology center, adult patients	26	26/654 (4%) patients with echo requested to rule out IE	About half with hematologic malignancy and half with solid organ cancer	S. aureus (35%) Coagulase-negative staph (23%) Enterococcus spp. (11%) E. coli (8%)	45 patients with vegetations by echo; 19 with negative blood cultures – the authors speculate that most of these cases were NBTE; 69% of patients with IE had a central venous catheter; 31% had thrombocytopenia; 21 had left-sided involvement

In a larger series of patients identified at a large oncology center between 1994 and 2004 which included patients with both hematologic (51%) and solid organ malignancy, S. aureus, coagulase-negative staphylococci, and Enterococcus species accounted for over two thirds of cases of IE in patients with positive blood cultures [8]. In contrast to previous series and although most patients with culture positive IE had central lines (69%), 21 (81%) of 26 patients had involvement of the mitral or aortic valves with only three patients having right-sided IE. Consequently, the risk of peripheral embolic events was high, occurring in 15 (58%) patients.

Risk Factors for IE

Risk factors for development of IE include both preexisting valvular abnormalities, such as rheumatic valve disease, degenerative heart disease, mitral valve prolapse, congenital heart disease, hypertrophic cardiomyopathy, and the presence of a prosthetic valve, and host conditions, such as intravenous drug abuse and the presence of an indwelling central venous catheter or cardiac device. Prosthetic-valve endocarditis accounts for about 15–20% of patients with IE in recent studies [9, 10]. The risk of PVE is greatest in the first 6 months following valve replacement, but continues indefinitely. Most cases seen within the first year are caused by S. aureus and methicillin-resistant coagulase-negative staphylococci. After this time, the causative pathogens of PVE are similar to those of NVE, although the relative incidence of staphylococcal infections remains greater.

Clinical Presentation

Patients with IE have traditionally been divided into those with subacute presentations and those with acute presentations. The former is characterized by a more indolent illness that develops over weeks with low-grade fevers and minimal cardiac dysfunction in patients with underlying valvular disease and is usually caused by organisms with lower virulence such as α-hemolytic streptococci (viridans streptococci). The later is characterized by an acute syndrome of systemic toxicity and rapid progression with intracardiac and extracardiac complications, is usually caused by *S. aureus,* and can occur on normal valves.

The majority of patients (~80–90%) present with fever, although it may be absent in patients either of advanced age, with chronic renal failure or who have received prior antibiotics. Other nonspecific symptoms include chills, anorexia, weight loss, myalgia, cough, and back pain. About 85% of patients with native-valve IE have heart murmurs, although this is usually related to the predisposing valvular lesion; only 10–40% of patients have a new or changed murmur. The classically described peripheral signs of IE are rarely seen in the modern era because patients are diagnosed before these sequelae of long-standing disease develop. These include petechiae which often involve the conjunctiva or distal extremities; splinter hemorrhages; Osler nodes which are painful nodules on the finger and toe pads; and retinal lesions known as Roth spots. However, clinical manifestations of embolic events are often seen because emboli occur in about 40% of patients. These include renal emboli that may present as flank pain or hematuria; splenic emboli that can manifest as left shoulder or left upper quadrant pain; septic pulmonary emboli indicated by pleuritic chest pain or back pain; emboli to the extremities which, if small, can cause capillary occlusion and painful spots on the fingers and toes, and if large, can involve arteries and lead to limb ischemia; and cerebral emboli which most commonly involve the middle cerebral artery. Neurologic events are common in IE, occurring in up to 25% of patients and also include hemorrhage, transient ischemic attack, meningitis, and mycotic aneurysm [11]. Any new neurologic signs, including persistent headache, should be evaluated by MRI and MRA or angiography.

Diagnosis and Investigation

The "modified Duke criteria" are the most commonly used algorithm for diagnosing IE (Fig. 20.1) [12, 13]. These criteria combine clinical, laboratory, and imaging data to estimate the likelihood of IE. While IE is unlikely if these criteria are not met, it is important to recognize that the original intent was to create a standardized definition for research purposes. Thus, if these criteria are not met, but there is a strong clinical suspicion for IE, additional patient evaluation and treatment, if appropriate, should ensue.

Adequate numbers of appropriately obtained blood cultures are crucial in diagnosing IE. The majority of patients with IE will have positive blood cultures – upwards of 90–95%. The most likely reason for negative blood cultures is prior receipt of antibiotics; thus, every effort should be made to obtain three sets of blood cultures with a minimum of 10 ml of blood in each bottle prior to the initiation of antibiotics. If a patient has a central venous catheter, no more than one set should be drawn from the line. In a patient with a subacute presentation who has received antibiotics and has no evidence of sepsis, progressive valvular dysfunction, or heart failure, antibiotics should be withheld for 2–3 days and blood cultures obtained off antibiotics. Unfortunately, this is often not possible in the oncology population, where patients are more likely to have infection with organisms that present acutely, such as *S. aureus*, or may be neutropenic or otherwise significantly immunosuppressed.

Follow-up blood cultures should be obtained to document clearance of bacteremia and again a few days after initial clearance. In addition, additional blood cultures should be drawn if a patient has a persistent fever or develops new fevers or other concerning symptoms while on therapy. Fever beyond 7 days may indicate failure of antimicrobial therapy or the presence of a myocardial abscess, focal extracardiac infection, emboli, or hypersensitivity to an antimicrobial agent.

Finally, if infection with an unusual or fastidious organism is suspected, discussion with the microbiology laboratory should occur regarding additional approaches to evaluation of blood cultures. In addition, serologic tests for infection with *Brucella* spp., *Legionella* spp., *C. burnetii, Chlamydia* spp., and *Bartonella* spp. can be obtained, usually in consultation with infectious diseases.

All patients with suspected IE should undergo echocardiography to assess for the size and location of vegetations, the presence of valve ring abscess, and any evidence of valvular or ventricular dysfunction. While the specificity of transthoracic echocardiography (TTE) for detecting vegetations is high (91–98%), the sensitivity is in the range of 45–60%, particularly when vegetations are less than 1 cm in size [14, 15]. In addition, TTE is a poor modality for evaluating prosthetic valves or assessing the presence of perivalvular abscess or leaflet perforation. When evaluating an echocardiogram result, it is important to know how the quality of the exam was graded by the cardiologist. A negative TTE of good quality can rule out most cases of IE when the likelihood of disease is felt to be low. However, if the quality of the exam is low or the patient is at intermediate to high risk of IE, a transesophageal echocardiogram (TEE) should be obtained. TEE has a sensitivity of ~90% for identifying vegetations and offers improved imaging of the pulmonic valves, prosthetic valves, and intracardiac complications due to IE [16].

Fig. 20.1 Modified Duke clinical criteria for diagnosis of infective endocarditis

Major criteria

Positive blood culture
- Two separate blood cultures yielding organisms that typically cause infective endocarditis (viridans streptococci, *Streptococcus bovis*, HACEK[a], *Staphylococcus aureus* or community-acquired enterococci without a primary focus)
- Persistently positive blood cultures (defined as positive blood cultures drawn more than 12 hours apart *or* all of three or a majority of four or more separate positive blood cultures, the first and last drawn at least 1 hour apart)
- Single positive blood culture for *Coxiella burnetii* or antiphase I IgG antibody titer > 1:800

Evidence of endocardial involvement
- Echocardiography positive for infective endocarditis[b]
  Oscillating intracardiac mass on a valve or supporting structure in the path of regurgitant jets or on implanted material in the absence of an alternative anatomical explanation
  Abscess
  New partial dehiscence of a prosthetic valve
- New valvular regurgitation (change in pre-existing murmur is not adequate)

Minor criteria
- *Predisposing heart condition or intravenous drug use*
- *Fever (≥ 38.0°C)*
- *Vascular phenomenon* (major arterial emboli, septic pulmonary infarcts, mycotic aneurysm, intracranial haemorrhage, conjunctival hemorrhages or Janeway lesions)
- *Immunological phenomenon* (glomerulonephritis, Osler nodes, Roth spots or rheumatoid factor)
- *Microbiological evidence* (positive blood culture, but less than major criterion,[c] *or* serological evidence of active infection with an organism consistent with infective endocarditis)

[a]*Haemophilus* spp., *Actinobacillus actinomycetemcomitans*, *Cardiobacterium hominis*, *Eikenella corrodens* and *Kingella kingae*
[b]TEE recommended in patients with prosthetic valves, complicated endocarditis, and who have possible endocarditis
[c]Excludes a single positive culture for coagulase-negative staphylococci or organisms that do not cause infective endocarditis

Source: Durack *et al. Am J Med* 1994; **96**: 200-9 and

Li JS et al. Clin Infect Dis 2000; *30-633-8.*

Management

In addition to the aforementioned blood cultures and echocardiography, all patients should undergo a detailed history and physical examination, laboratory work, chest X-ray, and an ECG. A prolonged PR interval or intraventricular conduction disturbance on ECG can indicate a valve ring abscess, particularly in aortic valve infective endocarditis. New conduction abnormalities are highly specific for paravalvular infection, but are not sensitive [17].

Risk factors for relevant organisms should be taken into consideration when selecting empiric therapy for oncology patients with IE. Based on the epidemiology of IE in this population, coverage directed against *S. aureus*, including methicillin-resistant strains, and coagulase-negative staphylococci (CoNS) is recommended, usually with vancomycin.

Given that infections caused by Gram-negative bacilli, yeast, or fastidious organisms are rare causes of IE in oncology patients, initial coverage directed at these pathogens is unnecessary in most cases, unless there is a specific reason to have concern that they may be involved. The American Heart Association has issued guidelines for organism-specific antimicrobial therapy and treatment for the most common organisms in oncology patients is summarized in Table 20.2 and discussed in the organism-specific sections below [18].

The strongest indication for valve replacement in a patient with IE is development of congestive heart failure as delaying surgery in these patients has been associated with increased mortality [19, 20]. Other situations in which surgery should be strongly considered include myocardial invasion such as valve ring abscess or fistula formation, large

Table 20.2 Infective endocarditis treatment regimens

Infecting Organism	Antibiotic	Dose	Duration	Comments
Viridans streptococcal and *Streptococcus bovis* native-valve endocarditis				
1. Fully sensitive to Penicillin (MIC ≤ 0.12 mcg/ml)	Penicillin G	3 million units IV Q4H	4 weeks	
	OR			
	Ceftriaxone	2 g IV Q24H	4 weeks	
	OR			
	[Penicillin G or Ceftriaxone]	3 million units IV Q4H 2 g IV Q24H	2 weeks 2 weeks	Use 2 week regimen for uncomplicated cases only
	PLUS			
	Gentamicin	3 mg/kg IV Q24H	2 weeks	
	OR			
	Vancomycin	15 mg/kg IV Q12H	4 weeks	Use for severe Penicillin allergy only Goal Vancomycin trough 15–20 mcg/ml
2. Relatively resistant to Penicillin (MIC > 0.12 mcg/ml and ≤ 0.5 mcg/ml)	[Penicillin G or Ceftriaxone]	4 million units IV Q4H 2 g IV Q24H	4 weeks 4 weeks	
	PLUS			
	Gentamicin	3 mg/kg IV Q24H	2 weeks	
	OR			
	Vancomycin	15 mg/kg IV Q12H		Use for severe Penicillin allergy only Goal Vancomycin trough 15–20 mcg/ml
3. Penicillin MIC > 0.5 mcg/ml or nutritionally variant streptococci	Treat as Enterococcal endocarditis			
Viridans streptococcal and *Streptococcus bovis* prosthetic-valve endocarditis				
1. Fully sensitive to Penicillin (MIC ≤ 0.12 mcg/ml)	[Penicillin G or Ceftriaxone]	4 million units IV Q4H 2 g IV Q24H	6 weeks 2 weeks	
	+/-			
	Gentamicin	3 mg/kg IV Q24H	2 weeks	
	OR			
	Vancomycin	15 mg/kg IV Q12H	6 weeks	Use only for Penicillin resistance or severe Penicillin allergy (consider desensitization to Ampicillin or Penicillin) Goal Vancomycin trough 15–20
2. Relatively or fully resistant to Penicillin (MIC > 0.12 mcg/ml)	[Penicillin G or Ceftriaxone]	4 million units IV Q4H 2 g IV Q24H	6 weeks 6 weeks	
	+/-			
	Gentamicin	3 mg/kg IV Q24H	2 weeks	
	OR			
	Vancomycin	15 mg/kg IV Q12H		Goal Vancomycin trough 15–20 mcg/ml
Enterococcal endocarditis				
1. Low-level resistance to Gentamicin	[Ampicillin or Penicillin G]	2 g IV Q4H 3–5 million units IV Q4H	4–6 weeks	4 weeks of therapy in most cases 6 weeks for those with symptoms > 3 months or prosthetic valve
	PLUS			
	Gentamicin	1 mg/kg IV Q8H	4–6 weeks	Goal Gentamicin peak = 3–4 mcg/ml and trough <1 mcg/ml
	OR			
	Vancomycin	15 mg/kg IV Q12H	6 weeks	Use only for Penicillin resistance or severe PCN allergy (consider desensitization to Ampicillin or Penicillin) Goal Vancomycin trough 15–20 mcg/ml Goal Gentamicin peak = 3–4 mcg/ml and trough < 10 mcg/ml
	PLUS			
	Gentamicin	1 mg/kg IV Q8H	6 weeks	
2. High level resistance to Gentamicin but low-level resistance to Streptomycin	Replace Gentamicin with Streptomycin in above regimens	7.5 mg/kg IV Q12H		Goal Streptomycin peak = 20–35 mcg/ml and trough <10 mcg/ml

(continued)

Table 20.2 (continued)

Infecting Organism	Antibiotic	Dose	Duration	Comments
Staphylococcal native-valve endocarditis				
1. Methicillin susceptible	Oxacillin OR Nafcillin	2 g IV Q4H 2 g IV Q4H	Uncomplicated: 4 weeks Complicated: 6 weeks	Drugs of choice for MSSA. Addition of Gentamicin 1 mg/kg IV Q8H optional. Goal Gentamicin peak = 3–4 mcg/ml and trough <1 mcg/ml
2. Methicillin susceptible and non-severe PCN allergy	Cefazolin	2 g IV Q8H	Uncomplicated: 4 weeks Complicated: 6 weeks	Addition of Gentamicin 1 mg/kg IV Q8H optional. Goal Gentamicin peak = 3–4 mcg/ml and trough <1 mcg/ml
3. Methicillin resistant or Penicillin allergy	Vancomycin	15 mg/kg IV Q12H	6 weeks	Use only for Methicillin resistance or severe Penicillin allergy (consider desensitization to Oxacillin or Nafcillin). Goal Vancomycin trough 15–20 mcg/ml
	OR Daptomycin	6–12 mg/hg IV Q24H	6 weeks	Use only for Methicillin resistance or severe Penicillin allergy (consider desensitization to Oxacillin or Nafcillin)
Staphylococcal prosthetic-valve endocarditis				
1. Methicillin sensitive	Oxacillin PLUS	2 g IV Q4H	6 weeks	
	Gentamicin AND	1 mg/kg IV Q8H	2 weeks	Goal Gentamicin peak = 3–4 mcg/ml and trough <1 mcg/ml
	Rifampin	300 mg PO Q8H	6 weeks after blood cultures have cleared	
2. Methicillin resistant or Penicillin allergy	Vancomycin PLUS	15 mg/kg IV Q12H	6 weeks	Consider desensitization to Oxacillin or Nafcillin if severe Penicillin allergy.
	Gentamicin AND	1 mg/kg IV Q8H	2 weeks	Goal Vancomycin trough 15–20 mcg/ml. Goal Gentamicin peak = 3–4 mcg/ml and trough <1 mcg/ml
	Rifampin	300 mg PO Q8H	6 weeks after blood cultures have cleared	

vegetation >1 cm with large embolization or vegetation >1.5 cm even without vegetation, most cases of PVE caused by *S. aureus*, and failure to respond to antimicrobial therapy, including cases with infection with highly resistant organisms or yeast and mold [19, 21]. These patients should be evaluated early in the clinical course by a cardiovascular surgeon in case urgent intervention is required. In general, if a patient has a strong indication for surgery, it should not be delayed to wait for clearance of blood cultures as reinfection of implanted valves occurs relatively infrequently provided that the patient is on appropriate therapy at the time of the operation [19, 22]. Surgery should be delayed in patients whose course is complicated by neurologic events given the risk of intracerebral hemorrhage on cardiopulmonary bypass. In general, waiting 2–4 weeks after a large embolic infarct (>2 cm) and 4 weeks after intracerebral hemorrhage is recommended; shorter waiting periods may be possible with smaller lesions [23]. With regard to duration of antimicrobial therapy postoperatively, patients with negative blood and valve cultures should complete the already planned course of therapy. For patient with positive valve cultures and most patients with PVE, a full course of therapy postoperatively should be given.

Etiologic Agents

Below the etiologic agents of IE most relevant to oncology patients are reviewed. IE caused by Gram-negative organisms, HACEK organisms, and causes of culture-negative IE are not further discussed.

Staphylococcus aureus

Bacteremia with *S. aureus* is relatively common in oncology patients, likely due to the high frequency of central venous catheter use in this population. In the general population, about one third of patients with *S. aureus* bacteremia will develop metastatic complications resulting either from hematogenous seeding of a distant site or from local extension of infection [24–26]. These sites include bone and joints, especially when prosthetic material is present; the epidural space and intervertebral discs; intra-abdominal organs such as the kidneys and spleen; and heart valves, including previously normal valves.

Interestingly, in the oncology population, there may be a difference in the rate of the occurrence of metastatic spread of *S. aureus* depending on the presence of neutropenia. Nonneutropenic oncology patients appear to be at significant risk for seeding other sites in the setting of *S. aureus* bacteremia. In one study of 52 nonneutropenic patients in which the source of infection was device-related in 42%, tissue-infection related in 44%, and unknown in 13%, 17 (33%) patients developed metastatic infections, including eight cases of IE, six cases of bone and joint infection, and three cases of renal infection [27]. In a study that evaluated outcomes of 91 patients with catheter-related *S. aureus* bacteremia of whom 63% had solid tumors and 81% were not neutropenic at the time of bacteremia, 36 (40%) had at least one complication [28]. Patients with solid tumors had significant risk for intravascular complications which included 3 cases of IE and 15 cases of septic thrombosis. Of note, rates of receipt of TTE and TEE were low in the cohort – 35% and 12%, respectively – and only 22% of patients had a venous flow study to evaluate for venous thrombosis. Thus, the true incidence of IE and other endovascular infection in the setting of *S. aureus* bacteremia is likely underestimated.

In studies that have evaluated neutropenic hematologic malignancy patients, IE associated with *S. aureus* bacteremia has been observed in very few patients (range 0–0.5%) [29–33]. Rates of other metastatic complications were also low in these studies, although osteomyelitis, septic pulmonary emboli, and meningitis were observed rarely [30, 31, 34]. Hypotheses for these findings include early initiation of antistaphylococcal therapy because of empiric treatment of neutropenic fever and inability of prolonged survival of *S. aureus* organisms within neutrophils due to their absence [35].

An important caveat in interpreting these results is that the studies were all retrospective and did not comment on whether patients had aggressive evaluations for spread of *S. aureus* infection with TTE, TEE or other symptom-based imaging (e.g., magnetic resonance imaging of the spine to rule out an epidural abscess or osteomyelitis in a patient with significant back pain). Thus, the suggestion made by one author that shorter courses of therapy be considered in these patients should not be undertaken without a complete evaluation for metastatic seeding of *S. aureus*. It is also important to note that although these studies did not find a high rate of metastatic spread, many did find that *S. aureus* bacteremia among neutropenic patients was associated with an increased risk of septic shock and death relative to nonneutropenic patients [28–31].

Because the presence of *S. aureus* bacteremia is a significant risk factor for IE, all patients with *S. aureus* bacteremia should undergo echocardiography to rule out vegetations. Many experts recommend use of TEE based on its superior sensitivity for detection of IE as well as intracardiac abcesses and valvular perforation in patients with *S. aureus* bacteremia [36–38]. At a minimum, TEE should be performed if a patient has a prosthetic valve, permanent cardiac device, prolonged bacteremia (>48 h) or fever (>72 h), or cardiac conduction abnormalities OR if short-course, 2-week therapy is planned. Of note, while a TEE of native valves that does not identify evidence of endocarditis makes the diagnosis of endocarditis unlikely, other criteria, such as the absence of other metastatic foci, must be met before the decision is made to give a short course of therapy [39].

Every effort should be made to identify and drain abscesses and remove infected devices to maximize therapeutic response. Antimicrobial therapy of *S. aureus* IE is based on the organism's susceptibility to methicillin. Methicillin susceptible isolates should be treated with antistaphylococcal penicillins whenever possible, given their superior efficacy relative to vancomycin [40]. Cefazolin is an alternative in patients with nonsevere penicillin allergies and desensitization to an antistaphylococcal penicillin should be considered in patients with type 1 allergies to penicillin. Guidelines from the American Heart Association note that the addition of initial (first 3–5 days), low-dose, synergistic gentamicin (1 mg/kg IV Q8H) is optional in the treatment of IE caused by MSSA [18]. This practice has not been shown to improve patient outcomes, although it appears to reduce the duration of bacteremia by about a day in patients with MSSA native-valve endocarditis [41]. However, this minimal benefit is likely outweighed by the potential for nephrotoxicity, which was seen in 24% of patients in a recent clinical trial [42].

Treatment of methicillin-resistant *S. aureus* IE can be challenging. Vancomycin is generally considered the drug of first choice as it has been used to cure many patients over the past 40 years. However, vancomycin is slowly bactericidal and has been associated with prolonged duration of bacteremia and occasionally clinical failure. This failure has been seen in patients without evidence of vancomycin resistance using conventional microbiologic testing. Some patients are infected with heteroresistant MRSA where subpopulations of organisms have minimum inhibitory concentrations (MICs) of vancomycin indicative of reduced susceptibility (4–32 µg/ml) [43]. In addition, patients with MRSA with vancomycin MICs of 2 µg/ml may be at increased risk for clinical failure [44, 45]. Although the use of higher doses of vancomycin to improve response has not been well studied, current guidelines recommend vancomycin troughs of 15–20 µg/ml for treatment of serious MRSA infections including IE [46].

An alternative to vancomycin is daptomycin, a bactericidal lipopeptide that is FDA-approved at a dose of 6 mg/kg daily for the treatment of *S. aureus* bacteremia and right-sided endocarditis based on a trial showing that it was as effective as standard therapy, consisting of initial low-dose gentamicin plus either vancomycin or an antistaphylococcal penicillin [47]. Because six patients in the trial had emergence of reduced susceptibility to daptomycin during the study, it has been suggested that higher doses of daptomycin (8–12 mg/kg daily) be used in seriously ill patients or those with left-sided IE [48, 49, 99].

Prosthetic-valve IE caused by *S. aureus* should be treated with three agents to avoid emergence of resistance. These include either an antistaphylococcal penicillin or vancomycin based on susceptibilities of the organisms plus low-dose gentamicin and rifampin. Rifampin should be started after blood cultures clear to minimize emergence of rifampin resistance and care should be given to assess for drug interactions [50]. Most patients with *S. aureus* PVE will require repeat valve replacement to optimize outcomes; therefore, cardiac surgeons should be involved in the patient's care from the time of presentation [21].

Coagulase-Negative Staphylococci

While CoNS have long been frequent pathogens in prosthetic-valve IE, they were the cause of 7.8% of cases of native-valve IE in a recent multicenter study [51]. In addition, they were the second commonest cause of IE in oncology patients in a study assessing endocarditis in this population [8]. Most CoNS IE is caused by *S. epidermidis*, although other species have been implicated such as *S. lugdinensis*, *S. hominis*, *S. saprophyticus*, and *S. haemolyticus*. The epidemiology of native-valve CoNS IE appears similar to that of native-valve *S. aureus* IE in that it is often healthcare-acquired and associated with indwelling catheters, hemodialysis access, and recent invasive procedures [51]. However, patients tend to have a longer duration of symptoms before the IE is detected, both because the organism can be more indolent and possibly because CoNS in blood cultures is often a contaminant and does not attract clinical attention. Indeed, it can be challenging to assess whether CoNS growing in blood cultures represents contamination or infection. In general, patients with true infection will have more than one set of blood cultures taken from different sites growing CoNS, particularly in the setting of endovascular infection. If such infection is suspected, blood cultures should be obtained peripherally; repeated blood cultures growing CoNS that are drawn from central lines may represent colonization of the catheter and not infection. It is relevant to note that although most of the reported cases of CoNS IE in oncology patients have been associated with a central catheter, some may have the mucosa as a source, particularly in those with neutropenia [4–6, 52].

CoNS isolates from patients with suspected or proven IE should be speciated to rule out infection caused by *S. lugdunensis*, a species of CoNS known for its increased virulence manifested by valvular destruction and myocardial abscess formation [53]. In contrast to *S. epidermidis*, this organism is usually susceptible to antistaphylococcal penicillins which should be used preferentially for treatment. Because of high rates of resistance to antistaphylococcal penicillins among *S. epidermidis* isolates, vancomycin is generally the agent of choice for most cases of CoNS IE. Regimens for PV IE due to CoNS are the same as those for *S. aureus* and include a three-drug regimen and evaluation by a cardiothoracic surgeon.

Streptococci

Although streptococci have traditionally been considered the most common cause of IE in the community setting, they appear to be less common among patients with healthcare-associated IE, including oncology patients. Most streptococcal IE is caused by α-hemolytic streptococci, also known as viridans group streptococci. Within this group, the majority of cases are caused by *Streptococcus sanguis*, *Streptococcus mitis*, and *Streptococcus mutans* [54–56].

Interestingly, despite the infrequency of streptococcal IE, bacteremia due to viridans streptococci is relatively common in neutropenic patients with cancer, accounting for 15–30% of all bacteremias in this population [57]. Streptococcal bacteremia in neutropenic patients is associated with oropharyngeal mucositis, receipt of high doses of cytosine arabinoside, and recent chemotherapy while receipt of penicillin for prophylaxis and early receipt of antibiotics for neutropenic fever appear to be protective [57, 58]. The organisms most commonly isolated in this population are similar to those that cause IE, *S. sanguis*, *S. mitis*, and *S. oralis* [57, 58]. However, few cases of IE following viridans streptococcal bacteremia have been noted. Two cases (8%) of IE were reported in one study to have developed following viridans streptococcal bacteremia; one of the two patients had previous valvular abnormalities [57]. Nevertheless, if an oncology patient presents with multiple blood cultures growing viridans streptococci, IE should be ruled out with echocardiography, particularly if the patient has a history of underlying valvular disease. It should also be suspected in patients presenting with low-grade fevers and malaise over a period of weeks.

Treatment recommendations are based on the minimal inhibitory concentration (MIC) of penicillin and are described in Table 20.2; it is important to request for the MIC of penicillin if it is not reported by the microbiology laboratory. The frequency of penicillin nonsusceptible viridans streptococci has increased among oncology patients, a finding likely related to the use of penicillin and ampicillin for prophylaxis [59–61]. Thus, empiric therapy for viridans streptococci bacteremia before the MIC of penicillin is known should be with vancomycin in the oncology population at most institutions. There is some controversy regarding the optimal therapy for penicillin-resistant viridans streptococcal IE; recommendations include high-dose penicillin plus low-dose gentamicin, ceftriaxone plus low-dose gentamicin, or vancomycin [62, 63].

Among other streptococcal species that cause IE, *Streptococcus bovis* deserves particular mention because of its association both with IE and with colonic neoplasm. There are two biotypes of S. bovis: biotype I is now termed *S. galloyticus* subspecies *gallolyticus,* biotype II is further characterized into strain 1, *S. gallolyticus* subspecies *S. lutetiensis,* and strain 2, *S. gallolyticus* subspecies *pasteurianus* [64]. When biotype I is isolated in blood cultures, IE is also present in 60–94% of cases, and underlying malignant or premalignant colonic lesions can be detected in 40–100% of cases [64–67]. Bacteremia with biotype 2 is associated with hepatobiliary disease and much less commonly IE or colonic neoplasm. As most microbiology labs do not distinguish between the two biotypes when reporting culture results, any patient with *S. bovis* bacteremia should undergo echocardiography as well as colonoscopy. *S. bovis* IE is treated in the same manner as viridans streptococcal IE.

Other streptococcal types include the *Streptococcus milleri* group (*S. anginosus*, *S. constellatus*, and *S. intermedius*) and the nutritionally deficient streptococci (*Abiotrophia defectiva, Granulicatella adiacens, Granulicatella para-adiacens, Granulicatella balaenopterae,* and *Granulicatella elegans*). Of the former group, *S. anginosus* is most likely to cause IE, but overall this occurs uncommonly. The nutritionally deficient streptococci are often tolerant to penicillin; thus combination therapy is often needed for cure [68].

Enterococci

Historically, enterococci are the etiology in ~6–10% of cases of IE, although this percentage appears to be higher among patients with healthcare-associated IE [1, 3, 7]. In addition, a recent multicenter study found that patients with enterococcus IE were more likely to have cancer than patients with IE caused by other organisms (21% vs. 8%) [69]. *E. faecalis* IE is significantly more common than *E. faecium* IE, and the most frequent sources are infection of the urinary tract, particularly in the setting of instrumentation, followed by infections involving the GI tract and central catheters [70]. Between 8 and 32% of patients with enterococcal bacteremia, either have or will develop IE and this risk is significantly increased if the isolate is *E. faecalis* or the patient has a prosthetic valve [71].

Oncology patients with enterococcal bacteremia should be assessed carefully for the possibility of IE, particularly if blood cultures are persistently positive or in the setting of a prosthetic valve. It is particularly important to establish the diagnosis because treatment for enterococcal IE may be different than treatment for a less severe enterococcal infection. Combination therapy with a cell wall-active agent (penicillin, ampicillin, or vancomycin) plus an aminoglycoside with enterococcal activity (gentamicin or streptomycin) is required to eradicate enterococci in IE because enterococci are inhibited but not killed by penicillin, ampicillin, and vancomycin alone. Enterococci with high-level resistance to gentamicin (MIC $500 \geq$ mg/l) should be tested for high-level resistance to streptomycin (MIC $\geq 2,000$ mg/l); streptomycin can be used if high-level resistance is not present. Neither gentamicin nor streptomycin should be used when there is high-level resistance to both. A possible alternative to aminoglycosides in the treatment of *E. faecalis* is the addition of ceftriaxone to ampicillin, which has been associated with clinical cure rates in 67.4% of patients [72]. Although uncommon, IE caused by vancomycin-resistant enterococcus has been reported and is associated with poor outcomes [73].

Fungi

Although infections caused by *Candida* and *Aspergillus* are common in patients with malignancy, IE due to these organisms is rare in this and in the overall population. Reviews of the published literature between 1965 and 2005 revealed 237 cases of *Candida* IE, 94 cases of *Aspergillus* IE, and significantly smaller numbers of IE caused by other yeast and molds [74, 75]. Only 33 of 2,760 (1.2%) patients in a multinational database of prospective cases of IE had infection caused by *Candida* (11 patients had other fungal organisms that were not defined further) [76]. In this cohort, the majority of organisms were *C. albicans* (48%), followed by *C. parapsilosis* (21%), *C. glabrata* (15%), and *C. tropicalis* (9%). Risk factors for candida IE included having a prosthetic valve, a short-term indwelling catheter, or recent coronary artery bypass grafting, but not malignancy. In a report evaluating 168 oncology patients with candidiasis studied at necropsy, 17 (10%) were found to have cardiac involvement, although none of these patients had a past history of cardiac disease [77]. Sixteen of the patients had leukemia or lymphoma. While all patients had abscesses in the myocardium and eight had mural endocardial involvement, no patients had valvular involvement. All patients with cardiac involvement had evidence of disseminated infection and the majority had *Candida* growing in blood cultures. *Candida* IE should be considered in oncology patients who have risk factors for IE (prosthetic valve, other valvular abnormalities, indwelling catheters), blood cultures with growth of *Candida* that is usually persistent, and evidence of peripheral embolization, as large vegetations and associated embolic events occur commonly in this disease.

Combination of surgical and medical management is generally recommended for *Candida* IE. Amphotericin B is considered the drug of choice, largely based on more extensive clinical experience with this agent, although treatment with echinocandins has been successful in some reports [78]. Valve replacement surgery followed by 6–8 weeks of antifungal therapy is recommended. For patients who are unable to undergo surgery, long-term suppressive therapy with fluconazole is recommended and has been associated with cure in some patients.

Cardiac infection due to *Aspergillus* species is uncommon in oncology patients and generally manifests as myocardial abscesses, rather than IE, in hematologic malignancy patients with other evidence of disseminated fungal disease [2]. The majority of cases of *Aspergillus* IE reported in the literature occur in patients following cardiac surgery with prosthetic valves [79]. In the few reports of *Aspergillus* IE in oncology patients, patients develop initial *Aspergillus* infection during the time of severe myelosuppression and go on to develop vegetative lesions after recovery of their cell counts [80]. Premortem diagnosis can be difficult as patients generally do not have blood cultures that grow the organism, either because of intermittent fungemia or challenges with isolation of the organisms in routine blood culture media [81]. *Aspergillus* vegetations are often large and are frequently associated with embolization; in one series, the diagnosis was initially established in 7 of 35 patients when fungal forms were found in arterial emboli that had been removed [79]. *Aspergillus* IE has also been associated with macroangiopathic hemolytic anemia in patients with hematologic malignancies, and the appearance of this clinical syndrome should prompt echocardiography [80, 81]. In addition, a patient with persistent unexplained fever and known disseminated Aspergillosis should undergo echocardiography.

Aspergillus IE in oncology patients is associated with significant, almost universal, mortality, both because patients usually have disseminated disease at the time of presentation and because treatment is challenging. A combination of medical and surgical therapy is required. Resection of the vegetation and infected valve and removal of other areas of mural involvement should be undertaken. Traditionally, Amphotericin B has been used for therapy; however, there are emerging reports of use of voriconazole alone or in combination for treatment and recent guidelines suggest that voriconazole be considered as first-line therapy [34, 82, 83].

Prolonged suppressive therapy with voriconazole is indicated in most cases.

Nonbacterial Thrombotic Endocarditis in Oncology Patients

Nonbacterial thrombotic endocarditis (NBTE), previously called marantic endocarditis, results from the deposition of masses of fibrin and platelets that do not contain microorganisms or inflammatory cells on often-normal heart valves. Consequently, blood cultures do not grow organisms. Although the exact pathogenesis is not fully understood, the condition has been associated with both increased levels of circulating cytokines that may lead to endothelial damage and a hypercoagulable state with enhanced activation of platelets and the coagulation cascade [84, 85]. In addition, there appears to be an association between NBTE and the presence of disseminated intravascular coagulation. In one autopsy study, 71% of patients had both conditions [86].

The incidence of NBTE appears to be relatively high in oncology patients. In one study, TTE was performed on 200 ambulatory patients with solid tumors and 100 control patients without overt heart disease or known malignancy. Cardiac vegetations were detected in 19% of the solid tumor patients compared to only 2% of the control group [87]. Other studies have reported a lower incidence of NBTE in cancer patients (0.96–1.3%); however, these have been autopsy studies and some authors have suggested that, by the time autopsy occurs, many patients who may have had NBTE no longer have evidence of cardiac vegetation because of peripheral embolization [86, 88].

NBTE is most frequently associated with solid tumors, most commonly adenocarcinoma of the lung and pancreas. However, it has been described in patients with almost all malignancies, including those involving the gastrointestinal tract, breast, and prostate; melanoma; lymphoma; and multiple myeloma [87–91]. Most oncology patients with NBTE have disseminated metastatic disease, although occasionally NBTE is seen with localized tumors.

NBTE is characterized by small multiverrucous vegetations that are found in areas of high blood flow such as the line of valve closure of the mitral and aortic valves. Right-sided valvular involvement is uncommon. Because of the lack of inflammation, the vegetations do not strongly adhere to the valves, and consequently, while they rarely cause valvular damage, they tend to embolize easily. Embolism rates range from 14 to 91% with an average of 42% and clinically important sites of embolism include the cerebral, coronary, splenic, renal and mesenteric vessels and, more rarely, major peripheral vessels [89].

The most common and most morbid clinical presentation of NBTE is an acute neurologic event. In one autopsy study, cerebral embolic infarction was noted in 42 (49%) of 86 patients with NBTE; 32 (76%) patients were symptomatic with about half having a focal neurologic deficit only and half presenting with diffuse encephalopathy [92]. Most patients had widespread metastatic disease at the time of presentation and half died from cerebral or other infarcts. Patients with NBTE-related embolic strokes appear to have a particular stroke pattern on diffusion-weighted magnetic resonance imaging consisting of multiple, widely distributed small and large strokes [93].

In addition to neurologic complications, cardiac dysfunction caused by embolism to the coronary vessels can complicate NBTE; intramyocardial arterial thrombosis occurs in one quarter to one third of patients with 6.7–9% developing clinical significant myocardial infarction [94]. Embolism to the kidneys may result in hematuria, while embolism to the spleen may manifest as left upper quadrant pain.

The diagnosis of NBTE should be considered in any oncology patient with evidence of arterial or venous embolism or disseminated intravascular coagulation. An initial evaluation should include a careful physical exam to assess for other embolic lesions followed by relevant imaging studies to evaluate abnormal findings, several sets of blood cultures to rule out infective endocarditis, laboratory investigations to assess for the presence of disseminated intravascular coagulation, and TTE. If suspicion for NBTE is high and TTE does not show a vegetation, TEE should be considered as it appears to have a higher diagnostic yield in NBTE [95].

One of the main challenges in diagnosing NBTE is distinguishing it from infective endocarditis, particularly because many oncology patients are on antibiotics which can cause blood cultures to not grow organisms in the setting of infective endocarditis. Some differences between IE and NBTE are noted in Table 20.3. Specifically, patients with NBTE are less likely to have fever, leukocytosis, blood cultures growing organisms, and valvular destruction and its sequelae and are more likely to have associated disseminated intravascular coagulation and CNS and coronary emboli than patients with IE.

Treatment of patients with NBTE includes both systemic anticoagulation and treatment of the underlying malignancy. The latter is often difficult as many patients have advanced metastatic cancer, but surgical resection or shrinkage of tumors with chemotherapy or radiation may lead to resolution of NBTE [96]. Although there are limited clinical data regarding the efficacy of heparin in curbing embolic events associated with NBTE, it is considered the first-choice agent for anticoagulation. Traditionally, therapy has been with unfractionated heparin, although low-molecular-weight heparin may also be effective. Cessation of heparin has been associated with occurrence of additional embolic events and is not recommended unless the malignancy can be controlled. Despite the high frequency of subclinical and clinical cerebral embolism in NBTE, treatment with heparin does not appear to promote brain hemorrhage [97].

The role of cardiac surgery to treat NBTE is not well studied. It could be considered in patients with reasonable functional status who have severe valvular dysfunction that cannot be medically managed or recurrent embolic events despite anticoagulation [98]. Vegectomy rather than valve replacement may be possible in some cases if the valve structure remains intact. Subsequent risk of recurrent NBTE after these procedures has not been studied.

Table 20.3 Comparison of infective endocarditis and nonbacterial thrombotic endocarditis

Characteristic	Infective endocarditis	Nonbacterial thrombotic endocarditis
Fever	~90% of patients	Uncommon
New murmur	~10–40%	~15%
Leukocytosis	Common	Uncommon
Positive blood cultures	~90%	Uncommon
Involved valves	Left- and right-sided involvement	Right-sided involvement rare
Valvular function	Often impaired due to valvular invasion	Often unaffected
Frequency of emboli	15–40%	14–91%
Common sites of embolization	Renal > splenic > coronary > cerebral	Cerebral > coronary > renal > splenic
Pattern of cerebral embolism	Solitary lesion, territorial infarction, or multiple punctate lesions	Multiple, widely distributed, small and large strokes
Concomitant disseminated intravascular coagulation	Rare	Common

References

1. Tleyjeh IM, Steckelberg JM, Murad HS, et al. Temporal trends in infective endocarditis: a population-based study in Olmsted County, Minnesota. JAMA. 2005;293:3022–8.
2. Roberts WC, Bodey GP, Wertlake PT. The heart in acute leukemia. A study of 420 autopsy cases. Am J Cardiol. 1968;21:388–412.
3. Murdoch DR, Corey GR, Hoen B, et al. Clinical presentation, etiology, and outcome of infective endocarditis in the 21st century: the International Collaboration on Endocarditis-Prospective Cohort Study. Arch Intern Med. 2009;169:463–73.
4. Liepman MK, Jones PG, Kauffman CA. Endocarditis as a complication of indwelling right atrial catheters in leukemic patients. Cancer. 1984;54:804–7.
5. Martino P, Micozzi A, Venditti M, et al. Catheter-related right-sided endocarditis in bone marrow transplant recipients. Rev Infect Dis. 1990;12:250–7.
6. Quinn JP, Counts GW, Meyers JD. Intracardiac infections due to coagulase-negative *Staphylococcus* associated with Hickman catheters. Cancer. 1986;57:1079–82.
7. Benito N, Miro JM, de Lazzari E, et al. Health care-associated native valve endocarditis: importance of non-nosocomial acquisition. Ann Intern Med. 2009;150:586–94.
8. Yusuf SW, Ali SS, Swafford J, et al. Culture-positive and culture-negative endocarditis in patients with cancer: a retrospective observational study, 1994–2004. Medicine. 2006;85:86–94.
9. Hoen B, Alla F, Selton-Suty C, et al. Changing profile of infective endocarditis: results of a 1-year survey in France. JAMA. 2002;288:75–81.
10. Wang A, Athan E, Pappas PA, et al. Contemporary clinical profile and outcome of prosthetic valve endocarditis. JAMA. 2007;297:1354–61.
11. Heiro M, Nikoskelainen J, Engblom E, Kotilainen E, Marttila R, Kotilainen P. Neurologic manifestations of infective endocarditis: a 17-year experience in a teaching hospital in Finland. Arch Intern Med. 2000;160:2781–7.
12. Durack DT, Lukes AS, Bright DK. New criteria for diagnosis of infective endocarditis: utilization of specific echocardiographic findings. Duke Endocarditis Service. Am J Med. 1994;96:200–9.
13. Li JS, Sexton DJ, Mick N, et al. Proposed modifications to the Duke criteria for the diagnosis of infective endocarditis. Clin Infect Dis. 2000;30:633–8.
14. Evangelista A, Gonzalez-Alujas MT. Echocardiography in infective endocarditis. Heart. 2004;90:614–7.
15. Reynolds HR, Jagen MA, Tunick PA, Kronzon I. Sensitivity of transthoracic versus transesophageal echocardiography for the detection of native valve vegetations in the modern era. J Am Soc Echocardiogr. 2003;16:67–70.
16. Mugge A, Daniel WG, Frank G, Lichtlen PR. Echocardiography in infective endocarditis: reassessment of prognostic implications of vegetation size determined by the transthoracic and the transesophageal approach. J Am Coll Cardiol. 1989;14:631–8.
17. Meine TJ, Nettles RE, Anderson DJ, et al. Cardiac conduction abnormalities in endocarditis defined by the Duke criteria. Am Heart J. 2001;142:280–5.
18. Baddour LM, Wilson WR, Bayer AS, et al. Infective endocarditis: diagnosis, antimicrobial therapy, and management of complications: a statement for healthcare professionals from the Committee on Rheumatic Fever, Endocarditis, and Kawasaki Disease, Council on Cardiovascular Disease in the Young, and the Councils on Clinical Cardiology, Stroke, and Cardiovascular Surgery and Anesthesia, American Heart Association: endorsed by the Infectious Diseases Society of America. Circulation. 2005;111:e394–434.
19. Olaison L, Pettersson G. Current best practices and guidelines indications for surgical intervention in infective endocarditis. Infect Dis Clin North Am. 2002;16:453–75. xi.
20. Vikram HR, Buenconsejo J, Hasbun R, Quagliarello VJ. Impact of valve surgery on 6-month mortality in adults with complicated, left-sided native valve endocarditis: a propensity analysis. JAMA. 2003;290:3207–14.
21. John MD, Hibberd PL, Karchmer AW, Sleeper LA, Calderwood SB. Staphylococcus aureus prosthetic valve endocarditis: optimal management and risk factors for death. Clin Infect Dis. 1998;26:1302–9.
22. Alexiou C, Langley SM, Stafford H, Lowes JA, Livesey SA, Monro JL. Surgery for active culture-positive endocarditis: determinants of early and late outcome. Ann Thorac Surg. 2000;69:1448–54.
23. Derex L, Bonnefoy E, Delahaye F. Impact of stroke on therapeutic decision making in infective endocarditis. J Neurol. 2009;257:315–21.
24. Fowler Jr VG, Olsen MK, Corey GR, et al. Clinical identifiers of complicated *Staphylococcus aureus* bacteremia. Arch Intern Med. 2003;163:2066–72.
25. Lautenschlager S, Herzog C, Zimmerli W. Course and outcome of bacteremia due to *Staphylococcus aureus*: evaluation of different clinical case definitions. Clin Infect Dis. 1993;16:567–73.
26. Ringberg H, Thoren A, Lilja B. Metastatic complications of *Staphylococcus aureus* septicemia. To seek is to find. Infection. 2000;28:132–6.
27. Gopal AK, Fowler Jr VG, Shah M, et al. Prospective analysis of *Staphylococcus aureus* bacteremia in nonneutropenic adults with malignancy. J Clin Oncol. 2000;18:1110–5.
28. Ghanem GA, Boktour M, Warneke C, et al. Catheter-related *Staphylococcus aureus* bacteremia in cancer patients: high rate of complications with therapeutic implications. Medicine (Baltimore). 2007;86:54–60.
29. Espersen F, Frimodt-Moller N, Rosdahl VT, Jessen O, Faber V, Rosendal K. *Staphylococcus aureus* bacteremia in patients with hematological malignancies and/or agranulocytosis. Acta Med Scand. 1987;222:465–70.
30. Gonzalez-Barca E, Carratala J, Mykietiuk A, Fernandez-Sevilla A, Gudiol F. Predisposing factors and outcome of *Staphylococcus aureus* bacteremia in neutropenic patients with cancer. Eur J Clin Microbiol Infect Dis. 2001;20:117–9.
31. Skov R, Gottschau A, Skinhoj P, Frimodt-Moller N, Rosdahl VT, Espersen F. *Staphylococcus aureus* bacteremia: a 14-year nationwide study in hematological patients with malignant disease or agranulocytosis. Scand J Infect Dis. 1995;27:563–8.
32. Sotman SB, Schimpff SC, Young VM. *Staphylococcus aureus* bacteremia in patients with acute leukemia. Am J Med. 1980;69:814–8.
33. Venditti M, Falcone M, Micozzi A, et al. *Staphylococcus aureus* bacteremia in patients with hematologic malignancies: a retrospective case-control study. Haematologica. 2003;88:923–30.
34. Walsh TJ, Anaissie EJ, Denning DW, et al. Treatment of aspergillosis: clinical practice guidelines of the Infectious Diseases Society of America. Clin Infect Dis. 2008;46:327–60.
35. Gresham HD, Lowrance JH, Caver TE, Wilson BS, Cheung AL, Lindberg FP. Survival of *Staphylococcus aureus* inside neutrophils contributes to infection. J Immunol. 2000;164:3713–22.
36. Abraham J, Mansour C, Veledar E, Khan B, Lerakis S. *Staphylococcus aureus* bacteremia and endocarditis: the Grady Memorial Hospital experience with methicillin-sensitive *S. aureus* and methicillin-resistant *S. aureus* bacteremia. Am Heart J. 2004;147:536–9.
37. Fowler Jr VG, Li J, Corey GR, et al. Role of echocardiography in evaluation of patients with *Staphylococcus aureus* bacteremia: experience in 103 patients. J Am Coll Cardiol. 1997;30:1072–8.
38. Sullenberger AL, Avedissian LS, Kent SM. Importance of transesophageal echocardiography in the evaluation of *Staphylococcus aureus* bacteremia. J Heart Valve Dis. 2005;14:23–8.

39. Cosgrove SE, Fowler Jr VG. Management of methicillin-resistant *Staphylococcus aureus* bacteremia. Clin Infect Dis. 2008;46 Suppl 5:S386–93.
40. Chang FY, Peacock Jr JE, Musher DM, et al. *Staphylococcus aureus* bacteremia: recurrence and the impact of antibiotic treatment in a prospective multicenter study. Medicine (Baltimore). 2003;82:333–9.
41. Korzeniowski O, Sande MA. Combination antimicrobial therapy for *Staphylococcus aureus* endocarditis in patients addicted to parenteral drugs and in nonaddicts: a prospective study. Ann Intern Med. 1982;97:496–503.
42. Cosgrove SE, Vigliani GA, Fowler Jr VG, et al. Initial low-dose gentamicin for *Staphylococcus aureus* bacteremia and endocarditis is nephrotoxic. Clin Infect Dis. 2009;48:713–21.
43. Khosrovaneh A, Riederer K, Saeed S, et al. Frequency of reduced vancomycin susceptibility and heterogeneous subpopulation in persistent or recurrent methicillin-resistant *Staphylococcus aureus* bacteremia. Clin Infect Dis. 2004;38:1328–30.
44. Lodise TP, Graves J, Evans A, et al. Relationship between vancomycin MIC and failure among patients with methicillin-resistant *Staphylococcus aureus* bacteremia treated with vancomycin. Antimicrob Agents Chemother. 2008;52:3315–20.
45. Soriano A, Marco F, Martinez JA, et al. Influence of vancomycin minimum inhibitory concentration on the treatment of methicillin-resistant *Staphylococcus aureus* bacteremia. Clin Infect Dis. 2008;46:193–200.
46. Rybak MJ, Lomaestro BM, Rotschafer JC, et al. Therapeutic monitoring of vancomycin in adults summary of consensus recommendations from the American Society of health-system pharmacists, the infectious diseases society of America, and the society of infectious diseases pharmacists. Pharmacotherapy. 2009;29:1275–9.
47. Fowler Jr VG, Boucher HW, Corey GR, et al. Daptomycin versus standard therapy for bacteremia and endocarditis caused by *Staphylococcus aureus*. N Engl J Med. 2006;355:653–65.
48. Cunha BA, Eisenstein LE, Hamid NS. Pacemaker-induced *Staphylococcus aureus* mitral valve acute bacterial endocarditis complicated by persistent bacteremia from a coronary stent: cure with prolonged/high-dose daptomycin without toxicity. Heart Lung. 2006;35:207–11.
49. Figueroa DA, Mangini E, Amodio-Groton M, et al. Safety of high-dose intravenous daptomycin treatment: three-year cumulative experience in a clinical program. Clin Infect Dis. 2009;49:177–80.
50. Riedel DJ, Weekes E, Forrest GN. Addition of rifampin to standard therapy for treatment of native valve infective endocarditis caused by *Staphylococcus aureus*. Antimicrob Agents Chemother. 2008;52:2463–7.
51. Chu VH, Woods CW, Miro JM, et al. Emergence of coagulase-negative staphylococci as a cause of native valve endocarditis. Clin Infect Dis. 2008;46:232–42.
52. Costa SF, Miceli MH, Anaissie EJ. Mucosa or skin as source of coagulase-negative staphylococcal bacteraemia? Lancet Infect Dis. 2004;4:278–86.
53. Patel R, Piper KE, Rouse MS, Uhl JR, Cockerill 3rd FR, Steckelberg JM. Frequency of isolation of *Staphylococcus lugdunensis* among staphylococcal isolates causing endocarditis: a 20-year experience. J Clin Microbiol. 2000;38:4262–3.
54. Mylonakis E, Calderwood SB. Infective endocarditis in adults. N Engl J Med. 2001;345:1318–30.
55. Parker MT, Ball LC. Streptococci and aerococci associated with systemic infection in man. J Med Microbiol. 1976;9:275–302.
56. Roberts RB, Krieger AG, Schiller NL, Gross KC. Viridans streptococcal endocarditis: the role of various species, including pyridoxal-dependent streptococci. Rev Infect Dis. 1979;1:955–66.
57. Bochud PY, Eggiman P, Calandra T, Vanmelle G, Saghafi L, Francioli P. Bacteremia due to viridans *Streptococcus* in neutropenic patients with cancer – clinical spectrum and risk-factors. Clin Infect Dis. 1994;18:25–31.
58. Richard P, Amador Del Valle G, Moreau P, et al. Viridans streptococcal bacteraemia in patients with neutropenia. Lancet. 1995;345:1607–9.
59. Reinert RR, von Eiff C, Kresken M, et al. Nationwide German multicenter study on the prevalence of antibiotic resistance in streptococcal blood isolates from neutropenic patients and comparative in vitro activities of quinupristin-dalfopristin and eight other antimicrobials. J Clin Microbiol. 2001;39:1928–31.
60. Tunkel AR, Sepkowitz KA. Infections caused by viridans streptococci in patients with neutropenia. Clin Infect Dis. 2002;34:1524–9.
61. Wisplinghoff H, Reinert RR, Cornely O, Seifert H. Molecular relationships and antimicrobial susceptibilities of viridans group streptococci isolated from blood of neutropenic cancer patients. J Clin Microbiol. 1999;37:1876–80.
62. Fujitani S, Rowlinson MC, George WL. Penicillin G-resistant viridans group streptococcal endocarditis and interpretation of the American Heart Association's Guidelines for the Treatment of Infective Endocarditis. Clin Infect Dis. 2008;46:1064–6.
63. Levy CS, Kogulan P, Gill VJ, Croxton MB, Kane JG, Lucey DR. Endocarditis caused by penicillin-resistant viridans streptococci: 2 cases and controversies in therapy. Clin Infect Dis. 2001;33:577–9.
64. Vaska VL, Faoagali JL. *Streptococcus bovis* bacteraemia: identification within organism complex and association with endocarditis and colonic malignancy. Pathology. 2009;41:183–6.
65. Corredoira J, Alonso MP, Coira A, et al. Characteristics of *Streptococcus bovis* endocarditis and its differences with *Streptococcus viridans* endocarditis. Eur J Clin Microbiol Infect Dis. 2008;27:285–91.
66. Ruoff KL, Miller SI, Garner CV, Ferraro MJ, Calderwood SB. Bacteremia with *Streptococcus bovis* and *Streptococcus salivarius*: clinical correlates of more accurate identification of isolates. J Clin Microbiol. 1989;27:305–8.
67. Tripodi MF, Fortunato R, Utili R, Triassi M, Zarrilli R. Molecular epidemiology of *Streptococcus bovis* causing endocarditis and bacteraemia in Italian patients. Clin Microbiol Infect. 2005;11:814–9.
68. Liao CH, Teng LJ, Hsueh PR, et al. Nutritionally variant streptococcal infections at a University Hospital in Taiwan: disease emergence and high prevalence of beta-lactam and macrolide resistance. Clin Infect Dis. 2004;38:452–5.
69. McDonald JR, Olaison L, Anderson DJ, et al. Enterococcal endocarditis: 107 cases from the international collaboration on endocarditis merged database. Am J Med. 2005;118:759–66.
70. Fernandez Guerrero ML, Goyenechea A, Verdejo C, Roblas RF, de Gorgolas M. Enterococcal endocarditis on native and prosthetic valves: a review of clinical and prognostic factors with emphasis on hospital-acquired infections as a major determinant of outcome. Medicine (Baltimore). 2007;86:363–77.
71. Anderson DJ, Murdoch DR, Sexton DJ, et al. Risk factors for infective endocarditis in patients with enterococcal bacteremia: a case-control study. Infection. 2004;32:72–7.
72. Gavalda J, Len O, Miro JM, et al. Brief communication: treatment of *Enterococcus faecalis* endocarditis with ampicillin plus ceftriaxone. Ann Intern Med. 2007;146:574–9.
73. Stevens MP, Edmond MB. Endocarditis due to vancomycin-resistant enterococci: case report and review of the literature. Clin Infect Dis. 2005;41:1134–42.
74. Ellis ME, Al-Abdely H, Sandridge A, Greer W, Ventura W. Fungal endocarditis: evidence in the world literature, 1965–1995. Clin Infect Dis. 2001;32:50–62.
75. Pierrotti LC, Baddour LM. Fungal endocarditis, 1995–2000. Chest. 2002;122:302–10.
76. Baddley JW, Benjamin Jr DK, Patel M, et al. Candida infective endocarditis. Eur J Clin Microbiol Infect Dis. 2008;27:519–29.
77. Ihde DC, Roberts WC, Marr KC, et al. Cardiac candidiasis in cancer patients. Cancer. 1978;41:2364–71.

78. Pappas PG, Kauffman CA, Andes D, et al. Clinical practice guidelines for the management of candidiasis: 2009 update by the Infectious Diseases Society of America. Clin Infect Dis. 2009;48:503–35.
79. Carrizosa J, Levison ME, Lawrence T, Kaye D. Cure of *Aspergillus ustus* endocarditis on a prosthetic valve. Arch Intern Med. 1974;133:486–90.
80. Nishiura T, Miyazaki Y, Oritani K, et al. Aspergillus vegetative endocarditis complicated with schizocytic hemolytic anemia in a patient with acute lymphocytic leukemia. Acta Haematol. 1986;76:60–2.
81. Chim CS, Ho PL, Yuen ST, Yuen KY. Fungal endocarditis in bone marrow transplantation: case report and review of literature. J Infect. 1998;37:287–91.
82. Reis LJ, Barton TD, Pochettino A, et al. Successful treatment of Aspergillus prosthetic valve endocarditis with oral voriconazole. Clin Infect Dis. 2005;41:752–3.
83. Vassiloyanakopoulos A, Falagas ME, Allamani M, Michalopoulos A. *Aspergillus fumigatus* tricuspid native valve endocarditis in a non-intravenous drug user. J Med Microbiol. 2006;55:635–8.
84. Asopa S, Patel A, Khan OA, Sharma R, Ohri SK. Non-bacterial thrombotic endocarditis. Eur J Cardiothorac Surg. 2007;32:696–701.
85. el-Shami K, Griffiths E, Streiff M. Nonbacterial thrombotic endocarditis in cancer patients: pathogenesis, diagnosis, and treatment. Oncologist. 2007;12:518–23.
86. Bedikian A, Valdivieso M, Luna M, Bodey GP. Nonbacterial thrombotic endocarditis in cancer patients: comparison of characteristics of patients with and without concomitant disseminated intravascular coagulation. Med Pediatr Oncol. 1978;4:149–57.
87. Edoute Y, Haim N, Rinkevich D, Brenner B, Reisner SA. Cardiac valvular vegetations in cancer patients: a prospective echocardiographic study of 200 patients. Am J Med. 1997;102:252–8.
88. Rosen P, Armstrong D. Nonbacterial thrombotic endocarditis in patients with malignant neoplastic diseases. Am J Med. 1973;54:23–9.
89. Deppisch LM, Fayemi AO. Non-bacterial thrombotic endocarditis: clinicopathologic correlations. Am Heart J. 1976;92:723–9.
90. Gonzalez Quintela A, Candela MJ, Vidal C, Roman J, Aramburo P. Non-bacterial thrombotic endocarditis in cancer patients. Acta Cardiol. 1991;46:1–9.
91. Kalangos A, Pretre R, Girardet C, Ricou E, Faidutti B. An atypical aortic valve non-bacterial thrombotic endocarditis in the course of multiple myeloma. Eur Heart J. 1997;18:351–2.
92. Graus F, Rogers LR, Posner JB. Cerebrovascular complications in patients with cancer. Medicine (Baltimore). 1985;64:16–35.
93. Singhal AB, Topcuoglu MA, Buonanno FS. Acute ischemic stroke patterns in infective and nonbacterial thrombotic endocarditis: a diffusion-weighted magnetic resonance imaging study. Stroke. 2002;33:1267–73.
94. Kuramoto K, Matsushita S, Yamanouchi H. Nonbacterial thrombotic endocarditis as a cause of cerebral and myocardial infarction. Jpn Circ J. 1984;48:1000–6.
95. Dutta T, Karas MG, Segal AZ, Kizer JR. Yield of transesophageal echocardiography for nonbacterial thrombotic endocarditis and other cardiac sources of embolism in cancer patients with cerebral ischemia. Am J Cardiol. 2006;97:894–8.
96. Cockburn M, Swafford J, Mazur W, Walsh GL, Vauthey JN. Resolution of nonbacterial endocarditis after surgical resection of a malignant liver tumor. Circulation. 2000;102:2671–2.
97. Rogers LR, Cho ES, Kempin S, Posner JB. Cerebral infarction from non-bacterial thrombotic endocarditis. Clinical and pathological study including the effects of anticoagulation. Am J Med. 1987;83:746–56.
98. Rabinstein AA, Giovanelli C, Romano JG, Koch S, Forteza AM, Ricci M. Surgical treatment of nonbacterial thrombotic endocarditis presenting with stroke. J Neurol. 2005;252:352–5.
99. Liu C, Bayer A, Cosgrove SE, Daum RS, Friakin SK, Gorwitz RJ, Kaplan SL, Karchmer AW, Levine DP, Murray BE, Rybak MJ, Talan DA, Chambers HF. Clinical practice guidelines by the Infections Diseases Society of America for the treatment of methicillin – resistant. *Staphylococcus aureus* infections in adults and children. Clin Infect Dis. 2011;52:e18–55.

Chapter 21
Skin Disorders Difficult to Distinguish from Infection

Sharon Hymes, Susan Chon, and Ana Ciurea

Abstract Dermatologists and infectious disease specialists are often called upon to evaluate skin lesions in cancer patients, especially when an infectious etiology is suspected. Many different organisms can affect the skin, and these are comprehensively reviewed in other chapters. This section will review some of the noninfectious skin eruptions that mimic cutaneous infections. These noninfectious diagnoses may be suspected after review of the patient history, and are often confirmed by skin evaluation and biopsy as indicated. The morphology of the primary skin lesion, the one that has not been manipulated or otherwise treated, often provides important diagnostic clues.

This chapter is intended to help the clinician generate a differential diagnosis when evaluating cutaneous lesions in cancer patients. Using the morphology of the primary lesion as a starting point, we then list the noninfectious diagnosis that could be considered and the infectious process it mimics.

Keywords Skin disorder • Mimic infection • Vesiculobullous lesions • Pustular lesions • Reactive neutrophilic dermatoses

Vesiculobullous Lesions

A vesicle is a sharply circumscribed fluid-filled blister measuring 0.5 cm or less, while a bulla is usually greater than 0.5 cm. The configuration may be solitary, grouped or annular, and the distribution may be localized or widespread. From an infectious disease point of view, vesicles and bullae are most often associated with viral eruptions, and these are frequently herpetic. Vesicles and bullae are also produced when an infectious pathogen produces necrosis of the overlying skin. Isolated bullae, especially when on a background of erythema, may look like impetigo or cellulitis. However, many vesiculobullous eruptions in cancer patients are noninfectious, and alternative etiologies are reviewed.

Acute Dermatitis

Differential Diagnosis: Viral Exanthem or Cellulitis

Acute dermatitis is characterized by vesicles and bullae, often precipitated by allergic or irritant reactions caused by an exogenous agent contacting the skin. In the oncology setting, this is often seen under dressings or after the application of topical antibiotics (Fig. 21.1). When corresponding to the outline of the bandages, the bullae may be linear but not dermatomal, helping to distinguish this from herpes zoster. When the diagnosis is uncertain, a skin biopsy demonstrates the hallmark changes of spongiosis, characterized by inter- and intracellular edema in the epidermis, rather than the multinucleated giant cells characteristic of herpes infections. Although acute dermatitis is not in itself contagious, it is not uncommon for the lesions to become secondarily infected. On occasion, eczematous vesicles and bullae develop in a generalized and distant distribution from the original contact, a phenomenon known as autosensitization dermatitis. This should be distinguished from disseminated herpetic disease.

Mechanical Blisters

Differential Diagnosis: Viral Exanthem or Ecthyma

Mechanical blisters occur in areas subject to friction (Fig. 21.2), pressure, burns, or extravasations of toxic substances, including some types of parenteral chemotherapy. Chemotherapeutic agents may be irritants, which produce inflammation or phlebitis but not tissues necrosis, or they may be vesicants which

S. Hymes (✉)
Department of Dermatology, The University of Texas,
M.D. Anderson Cancer Center, 1515 Holcombe Blvd.
(Unit 1452), Houston, TX 77030-4009, USA
e-mail: srhymes@mdanderson.org

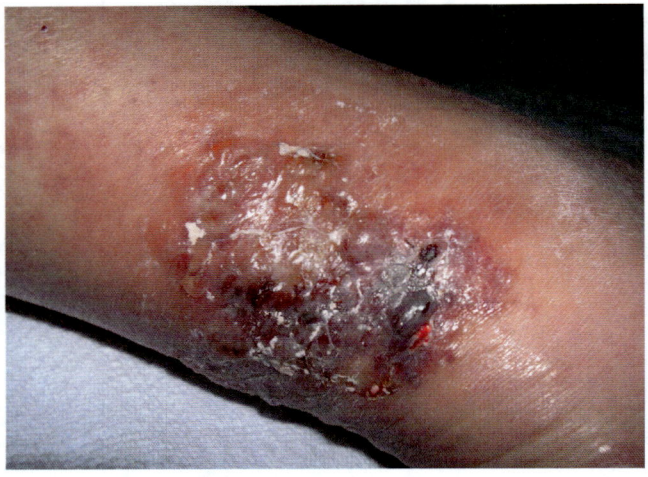

Fig. 21.1 Acute dermatitis. There are prominent blisters, erythema, and crusting after the application topical Neomycin

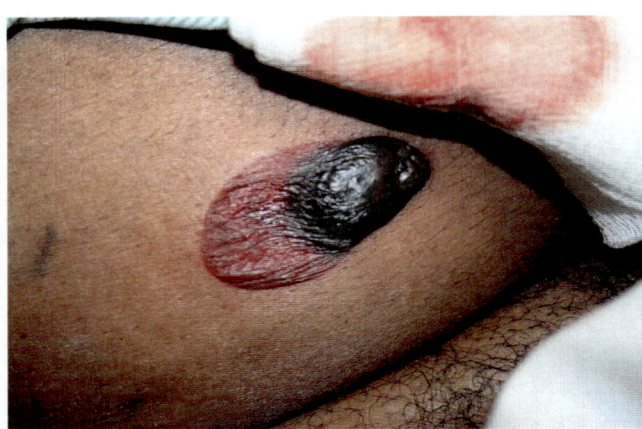

Fig. 21.3 Purpura from injections in a patient with thrombocytopenia

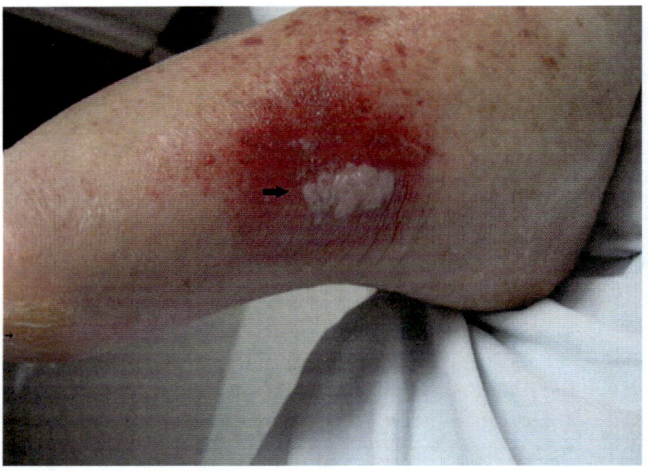

Fig. 21.2 Friction blister. This larger blister marked by an *arrow* is secondary to rubbing from an ill-fitting shoe. The smaller blister on the left is from edema

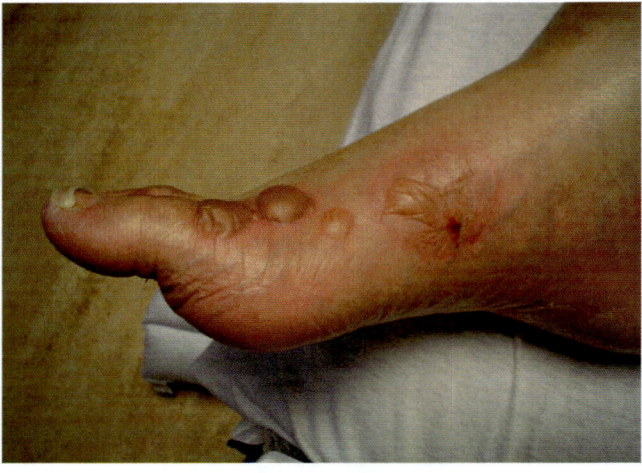

Fig. 21.4 Coma bullae after a barbiturate overdose

are more tissue destructive [1]. Hemorrhagic bullae may occur at the site of subcutaneous injections, or at phlebotomy sites in thrombocytopenic patients. In these cases, the history will likely confirm the diagnosis (Fig. 21.3).

Coma Bullae

Differential Diagnosis: Viral Exanthem, Cellulitis, or Ecthyma

Also called barbiturate or neurologic blisters, coma bullae usually appear over sites of pressure and are sometimes associated with macular erythema or violaceous plaques. The etiology is multifactorial, but in some cases, a direct toxic drug effect has been implicated. Many drugs are excreted through the eccrine glands and presumably produce eccrine gland necrosis resulting in blister formation. Barbiturates are the most frequently reported causative agent [2, 3], but similar findings have been noted in association with other medications, as well as coma and central nervous system disorders [4]. These bullae have been reported in up to 4–5% in patients hospitalized for drug-induced coma, and although they typically occur in pressure areas on the extremities and trunk after several hours or days, the bullae occasionally appear as early as 1 hour after acute intoxication. In addition, areas not typically prone to pressure may be involved (Fig. 21.4) [5].

Edema and Lymphedema Bullae

Differential Diagnosis: Cellulitis

Large bullae may develop in the setting of acute exacerbation of edema or of anasarca, often on the distal lower extremities. Early on, they are tense and clear, and biopsy demonstrates spongiosis (inter and intracellular epidermal edema) with dilated dermal vessels. In the cancer patient, lymphedema bullae are a difficult management problem produced by extensive lymph node dissection, ionizing radiation therapy, or tumor obstruction. Chronic lymphedema produces characteristic skin changes including verrucous hyperkeratosis, fibrosis, and hyperkeratosis, which may become superinfected.

Diabetic Blisters

Differential Diagnosis: Cellulitis

The term bullosis diabeticorum was first introduced in 1967 [6] and refers to the development of spontaneous bullous lesions in patients with diabetes mellitus. The pathogenesis may be related to angiopathy or trauma, and the bullae tend to be clear and tense. This needs to be differentiated from infectious cellulitis.

Bullous Insect Bite Reaction

Differential Diagnosis: Ecthyma, Viral Exanthem, Cellulitis

This is an exaggerated response to insect bites resulting in papulovesicles, bullae, and occasionally necrotic lesions. This phenomenon has been reported primarily in the setting of chronic lymphocytic leukemia (CLL), but may also occur with other hematoproliferative disorders like mantle cell lymphoma, and human immunodeficiency virus infection [7, 8]. Prominent eosinophil infiltration and degranulation within these lesions likely contribute to the severity of symptoms [9]. Many patients have no recollection of the bite.

Bullous Graft-Versus-Host-Disease (GVHD)

Differential Diagnosis: Cellulitis

Acute and chronic GVHD may be vesicular or bullous [10]. In severe acute disease, there is damage at the epidermal–dermal junction that may be severe enough to allow the epidermis to separate completely from the dermis when traction or pressure is applied; this has been termed the Nikolsky sign (Fig. 21.5). Chronic sclerodermoid GVHD, like idiopathic scleroderma, may also exhibit bullae. Although the pathogenesis is unknown, biopsy shows typical fibrotic changes and dermal edema [11, 12]. As the bullae resolve, the slowly healing erosions and ulcerations should be monitored for secondary bacterial superinfection.

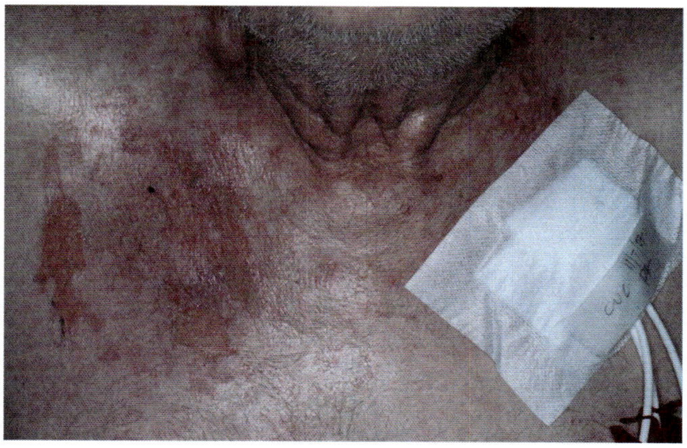

Fig. 21.5 Graft-versus-host disease with positive Nikolsky sign and epidermal detachment

Bullous Drug Eruptions

Differential Diagnosis: Viral Infection

Bullous drug eruptions may be localized or widespread (Fig. 21.6). When localized, they are referred to as fixed drug eruptions, and are characterized by recurrence at same location following drug reexposure. This eruption, occurring 1–2 weeks after the first exposure and within 24 hours of reexposure, is characterized by a localized area of erythema and bullae which resolve with a "slate gray" color (Fig. 21.7).

A variety of medications may also produce autoimmune blistering, sometimes characterized by the deposition of linear IgA at the dermal–epidermal junction. This is of particular interest to infectious disease specialists as it has been reported with multiple antibiotics including vancomycin, beta-lactam antibiotics, trimethoprim-sulfamethoxazole, penicillin, metronidazole, and rifampicin [13]. It has also been reported after interferon [14], lithium carbonate, diclofenac, and glibenclamide [15–18]. Linear IgA deposition in the skin has also been associated with malignancy [19] including that of the esophagus [20], colon [21], and pancreas [22].

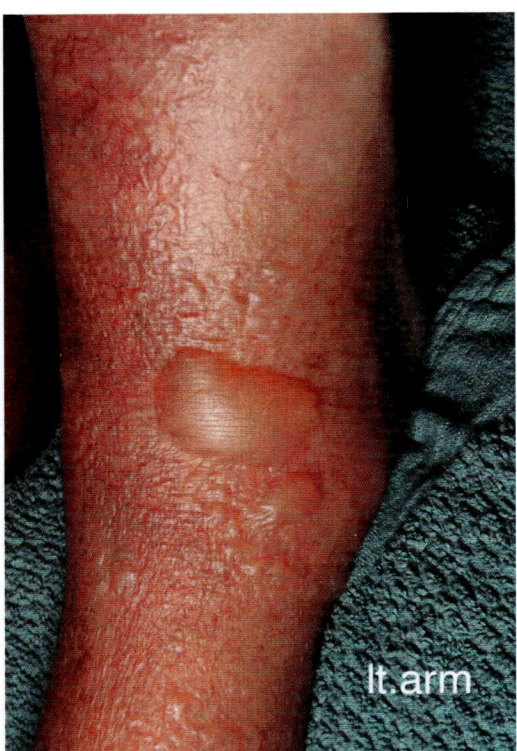

Fig. 21.6 Bullous drug eruption on background of erythema secondary to cytarabine

Autoimmune Bullous Dermatoses

Differential Diagnosis: Viral Infection, Scabies

Dermatitis herpetiformis is associated with thyroid disease, particularly Hashimoto thyroiditis [24], as well as enteropathy-associated T-cell lymphoma. Clinically, these very pruritic tiny vesicles may be suggestive of scabies infestation or herpes. The biopsy shows characteristic neutrophils in the dermal papillae and direct immunofluorescence shows granular deposits of IgA. Conversely, the incidence of non-Hodgkin's lymphoma is significantly increased in patients with dermatitis herpetiformis [25–27].

Pemphigus is an autoimmune blistering disease that affects skin and mucous membranes, with characteristic flaccid bullae and a positive Nikolsky sign (Fig. 21.8). Multiple drugs have been associated with the development of pemphigus. Drugs of interest to the infectious disease specialist include thiol drugs like ampicillin, drugs with an active amide group such as penicillins, nonthiol, nonamide drugs containing a phenol group such as cefadroxil and rifampicin [13, 28]. Other culprits include penicillamine, captopril, beta blockers, progesterone, heroin, and pyrazole compounds [15]. The eruption occurs a few weeks after starting the medication, and the diagnosis is made by histology which shows an intraepidermal vesicle with acantholysis, and direct immunofluorescence of perilesional skin which demonstrates IgG and/or C3 binding to the intercellular cement substance or keratinocyte cell surface [15].

Paraneoplastic pemphigus, also called paraneoplastic autoimmune multiorgan syndrome [29], was described by Anhalt et al. in 1990 as a mucocutaneous disease invariably associated with neoplasia [30, 31] including lymphomas,

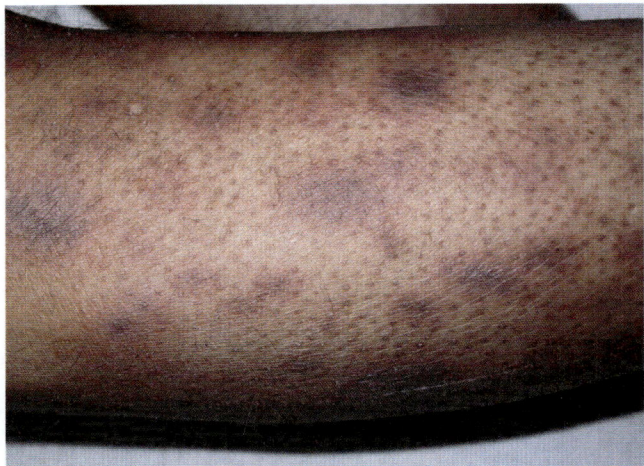

Fig. 21.7 Fixed drug eruption characterized by well-demarcated erythematous to slate gray plaques, in this case secondary to naproxen

Phototoxic drug eruptions may also be bullous, with the characteristic finding of involvement in UV exposed areas. This has been described recently with paclitaxel [23].

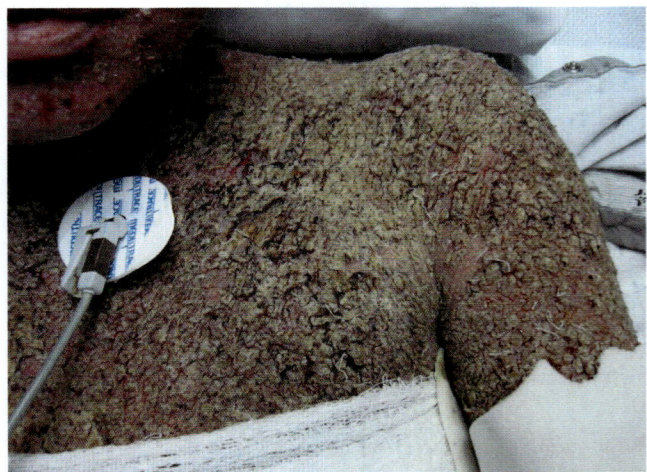

Fig. 21.8 Pemphigus produces superficial blistering with crusts

CLL, Castleman disease [32], Waldenstrom macroglobulinemia, thymoma, retroperitoneal sarcoma, bronchogenic carcinoma [15], and mastocytosis [33]. The lesions are heterogeneous, but the patients classically develop severe mucosal erosions, stomatitis, and skin eruptions that may resemble other autoimmune bullous disorders, drug eruptions, lichen planus, or erythema multiforme [15](Fig. 21.9). The patients may develop bronchiolitis obliterans and pulmonary infiltrates. Immunoprecipitation demonstrates the presence of antibodies against the plakin family [15]. Antibodies to desmoglein 1 and 3, similar to those found in classic pemphigus, may play a role [34, 35].

Bullous pemphigoid presents with tense skin blisters and, less commonly, mucosal involvement (Fig. 21.10). It is characterized by autoantibodies located in the hemidesmosomal complex of the skin basement membrane zone. It may occur de novo, associated with other autoimmune disease or with systemic malignancy. Some antibiotics, including amoxicillin [36], cephalexin [37], and ciprofloxacin [38] have been reported to cause drug-induced disease. Bullous pemphigoid and mucosal scarring cicatricial (scarring) pemphigoid may occur as manifestation of immune dysregulation after stem cell transplantation [39, 40]. It is diagnosed by its histologic features, as well as positive direct and indirect immunofluorescence microscopy.

Porphyria Cutanea Tarda (PCT) and Pseudoporphyria Cutanea Tarda

Differential Diagnosis: Viral Infection, Bacterial Infection

PCT is caused by decreased catalytic activity of uroporphyrinogen decarboxylase. There are acquired and hereditary variants associated with a clinical spectrum of vesiculobullae, skin fragility, erosions, crusts, scarring dyspigmentation, hypertrichosis, photosensitivity, and occasional scleromoid changes (Fig. 21.11). This may be associated with hepatitis C [41], HIV [42], hepatoma [43], estrogen, alcohol abuse, and iron overloading, especially in cancer patients who have received multiple transfusions [44].

Pseudoporphyria is a rare photosensitive disorder that clinically resembles PCT but lacks the biochemical derangements in porphyrin metabolism. It is often drug induced and has been associated with nalidixic acid, tetracycline, chlorthalidone, pyridoxine, naproxen, furosemide, etretinate, cyclosporine, intravenous 5-fluorouracil, imatinib [45], and voriconazole [46, 47]. It has also been associated with end-stage renal failure [48] (Fig. 21.12).

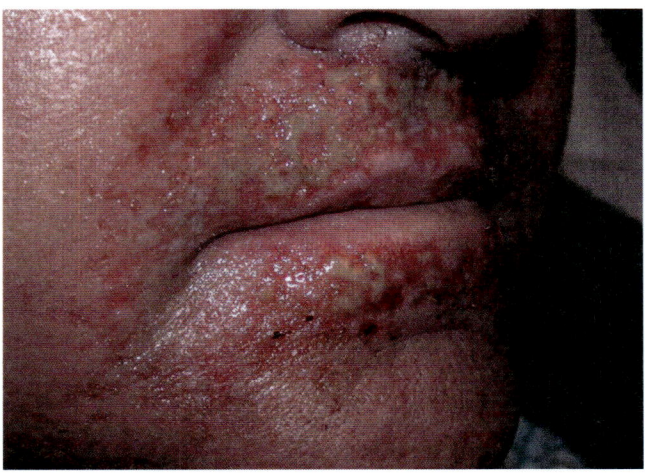

Fig. 21.9 Paraneoplastic pemphigus with epidermal denudation. This patient also had severe stomatitis

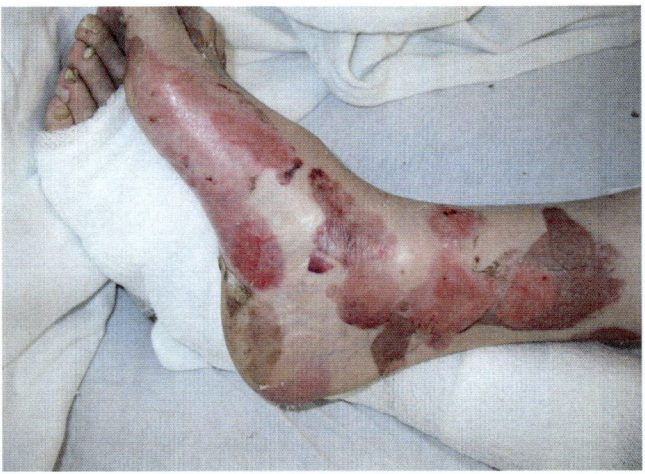

Fig. 21.10 Bullous pemphigoid produces tense and ruptured bullae on the legs of this patient

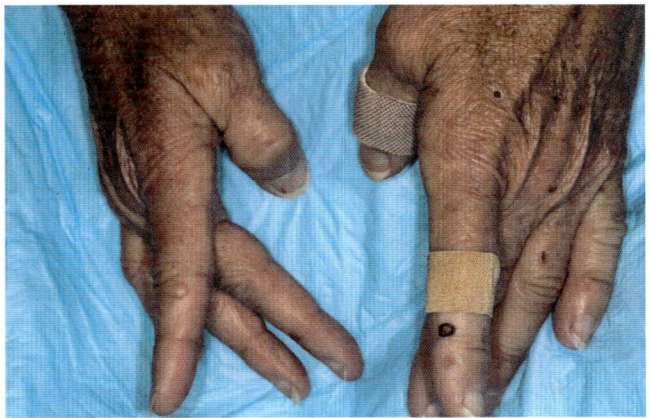

Fig. 21.11 Porphyria cutanea tarda is characterized by skin fragility especially on the sun-exposed hands leading to erosions and bullae

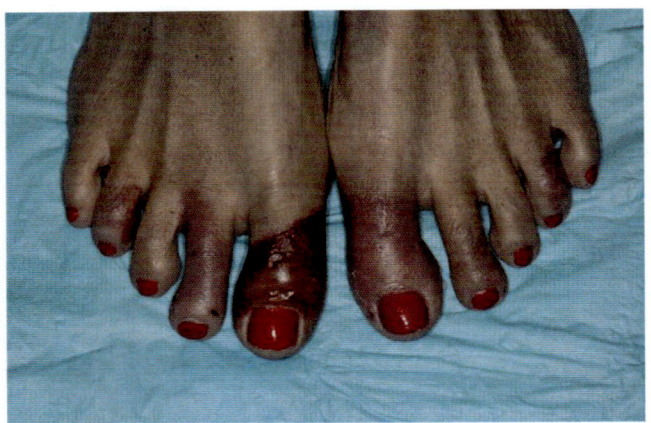

Fig. 21.12 Pseudoporphyria characterized by subepidermal bullae in a patient with renal failure

Miliaria Crystallina

Differential Diagnosis: Herpes Viral Infection

Also known as sudamina, miliaria crystallina is characterized by a diffuse eruption of 1–2 mm superficial asymptomatic vesicles on a noninflamed base, sometimes appearing as "drops of water" (Fig. 21.13). These vesicles appear in crops, typically on the trunk. This eruption is often mistaken for disseminated herpes, but the onset is related to heat and humidity or the profuse sweating accompanying persistent febrile illness. The individual vesicles are extremely fragile, rupturing spontaneously or with slight friction, and resolve with a superficial desquamation. Therapy is generally not required because the eruption is self-limited.

Pustular Lesions

Sterile pustular lesions may be seen as solitary or over most of the body surface. They may be mistaken for bacterial, fungal, or superinfected herpetic infections.

Acute Generalized Exanthematous Pustulosis (AGEP)

Differential Diagnosis: Bacterial, Fungal or Viral Infections

AGEP is also known as a pustular drug eruption as 90% of cases are related to medication administration (Fig. 21.14). The eruption is of sudden onset and appears on average of 5 days after the medication is started; in 50% of cases it starts within first 24 h. Initially, there is a diffuse exanthematous erythema followed by eruption of multiple monoform nonfollicular pustules less than 5 mm in diameter. Widespread superficial desquamation occurs after a few days and fever is common along with systemic neutrophilia and eosinophilia. Once the inciting agent is discontinued, the eruption resolves within 15 days without sequelae [49]. In up to 80% of cases, pustular drug eruptions are secondary to antibiotics including beta-lactam antibiotics, macrolides [49], and cephalosporins [50, 51]. Pustular eruptions may also occur after imatinib [52].

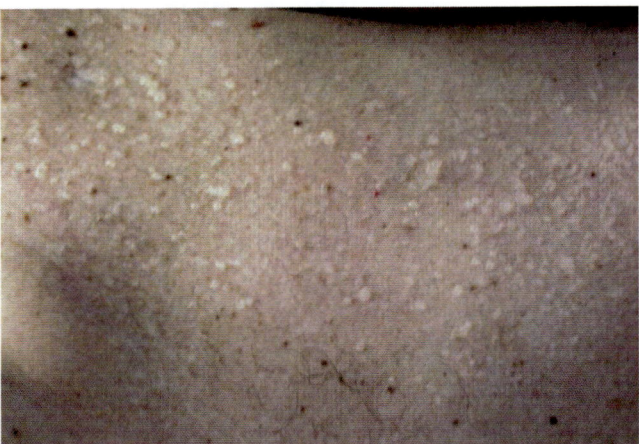

Fig. 21.13 Miliaria crystallina is characterized by translucent, fragile vesicles secondary to sweat duct obstruction. This may be confused with herpetic infections

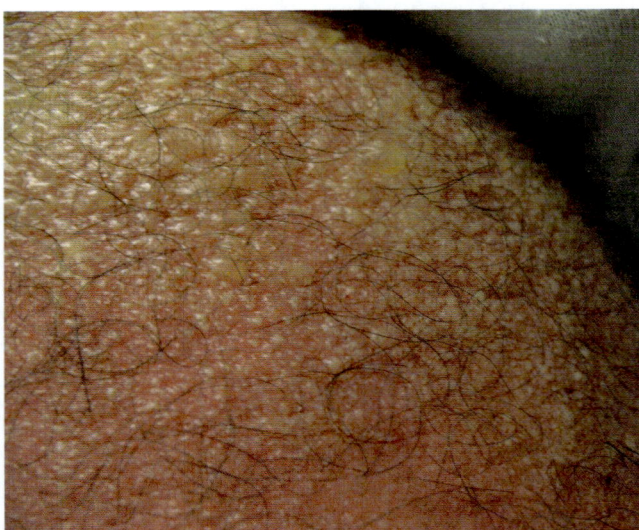

Fig. 21.14 Acute generalized exanthematous pustulosis produces large and small sterile, nonfollicular pustules, sometimes on an erythematous base

Reactive Neutrophilic Dermatoses

Differential Diagnosis: Bacterial, Fungal or Viral Infections

These are a spectrum of dermatoses that are mediated by neutrophils. They frequently have systemic manifestations and associations with underlying diseases, such as inflammatory bowel disease and internal malignancies. The management of these disorders with systemic corticosteroids and nonsteroidal immunosuppressive or immunomodulatory agents is common [53]. Sweet syndrome, pyoderma gangrenosum, Bechet disease, and bowel-associated dermatosis-arthritis syndrome are examples of these dermatoses.

Sweet syndrome and pyoderma gangrenosum may look like ecthyma, erysipelas, cellulitis, viral, fungal, and mycobacterial infections. These are neutrophilic disorders that often start with erythematous papules and plaques; they may resemble cellulitis or erysipelas [54]. In the case of Sweet syndrome, also called febrile neutrophilic dermatosis, these may become pustular or bullous (Fig. 21.15). The patients often develop an associated fever and peripheral leukocytosis, all of which resolve promptly with glucocorticoid therapy [55]. It is thought to be a hypersensitivity reaction of unknown cause characterized by infiltration of polymorpholeukocytes in the skin. The majority of cases of Sweet syndrome follow a febrile upper respiratory tract infection and therefore acute and self-limited. Other infectious agents that have been associated include Yersinia, Toxoplasma, Salmonella, and Mycobacterium. It has also been reported with inflammatory bowel disease, Behcet syndrome and drugs like trimetoprim-sulfamethoxazole and the granulocyte-colony stimulating factor [56]. Hematologic malignancies or solid tumors are present in about 10–15% of cases [55, 57]. The most common associated malignancy is AML but it can also be seen in association with CML [58], lymphomas, anemias, or polycythemias [55]. The lesions may precede the diagnosis of leukemia. Associated solid tumors are of any type, but most commonly genitourinary, breast, and gastrointestinal [53].

Patients with pyoderma gangrenosum develop ulcers with a purple overhanging edge and prominent pathergy. It is also associated with rheumatologic disorders, malignancy, and inflammatory bowel disease (Fig. 21.16).

Behçet disease (BD) was named in 1937 after the Turkish dermatologist Hulusi Behçet, who first described the triple-symptom complex of recurrent oral apthous ulcers, genital ulcers, and uveitis [59]. This chronic mucocutaneous disorder is diagnosed by means of clinical criteria, defined by oral and genital apthae, pustular vasculitic cutaneous lesions, ocular, gastrointestinal, and vascular manifestations [60] (Fig. 21.17). Although more prevalent in the Middle East, Behcet disease has been reported all over the world. The skin lesions are pyoderma and furunculosis [60]. The ulcers in Behcet disease present as superficial gray erosions and deeply punched out erosions that affects the lips, gums, cheeks, and tongue. The apthous lesions, whether on the mouth or genitalia, begin as vesicles or pustules and tend to heal with scar formation [60].

Bowel-associated dermatosis-arthritis syndrome is a well-recognized complication in patients who have had jejunoileal bypass for morbid obesity. It consists of an influenza-like illness with increased temperature, chills, polyarthralgia, myalgia, and inflammatory papules and pustules that are 2–4 mm in diameter and that usually appear on the

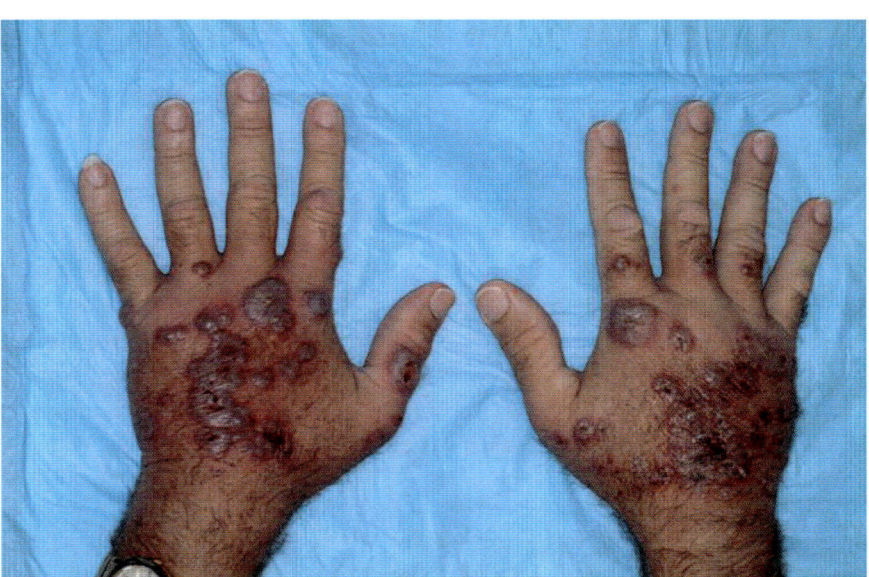

Fig. 21.15 Acute febrile neutrophilic dermatosis (Sweet syndrome) with red nodules, plaques, and blisters on the hands. Pathology often confirms the diagnosis

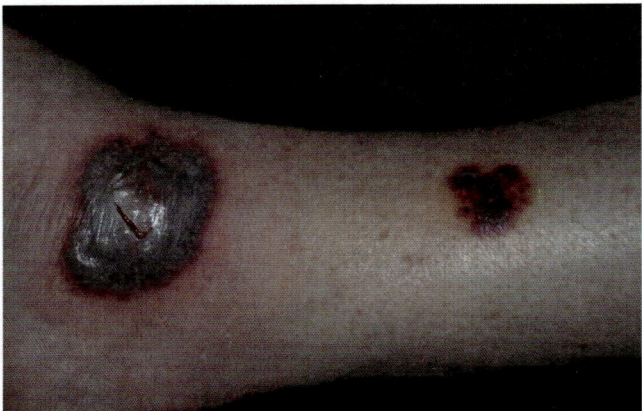

Fig. 21.16 Pyoderma gangrenosum. The lesion on the left shows an erosion with a purple overhanging border and central necrotic bulla. The lesion on the right is earlier and hemorrhagic

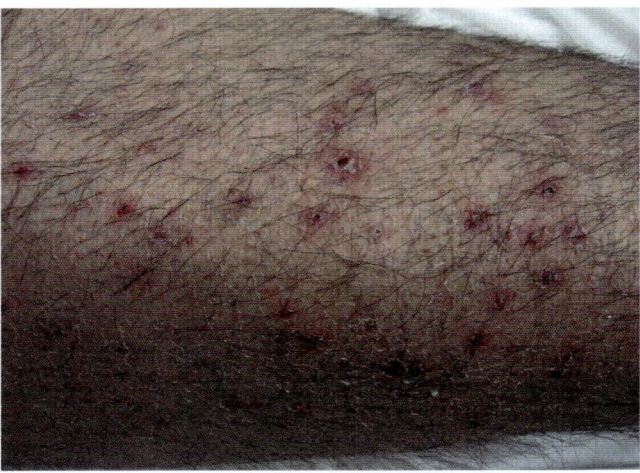

Fig. 21.18 EGFR-induced acneiform pustulosis. Monoform papulopustules are present on the extremities secondary to epidermal growth factor receptor inhibitor in patient with colon cancer

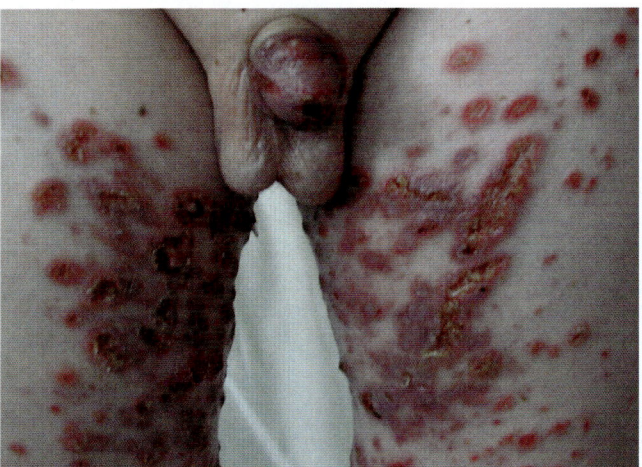

Fig. 21.17 Behcet disease showing recurrent ulcerations on the skin and genital mucosa in a patient with iridocyclitis and apthae of the oral mucous membranes

extremities and the upper part of the trunk. It involves bacterial overgrowth causing complement activation with subsequent deposition of antibody complexes in skin and synovium [61]. Histology shows a perivascular lymphocytic infiltrate and a leukocytoclastic vasculitis of dermal capillaries. Pustular pyoderma gangrenosum and infections should be considered in the differential diagnosis.

Acneiform Eruptions

Differential Diagnosis: Bacterial or Fungal Folliculitis

Acne is a follicular disease characterized by abnormal keratinization, inflammation, presence of Propionibacterium acnes in sebum, and increased sebum production, under hormonal control. Precursor lesions are noninflammatory (comedo and microcomedo) and inflammatory (papules, pustules and nodules) on face and upper trunk. The inflammation is triggered by follicular wall rupture and subsequent immune responses that promote follicular plugging and microcomedo formation [62]. Drug-induced acne is usually abrupt in onset and monomorphous. In cancer patient on systemic corticosteroids, an acneiform eruption is not uncommon, but comedones are rarely seen. Antibiotics such as tetracyclines and isoniazid, as well as chemotherapeutic agents such as azathioprine, cyclosporin, and sirolimus may produce acneiform drug eruptions [13]. Patients on epidermal growth factor receptor inhibitors, EGFRI, often have characteristic pustular eruptions, frequently associated with paronychia that is severe enough to significantly impact their lives [52, 63]. Rather than the diffuse pustulosis seen with AGEP, this eruption commonly found in an acneiform distribution on the face, scalp, chest, and back is characterized by a perifollicular lymphocytic infiltrate or suppurative neutrophilic folliculitis [1, 64] (Fig. 21.18).

Eosinophilic Folliculitis

Differential Diagnosis: Bacterial or Fungal Folliculitis

This presents as erythematous pruritic papules and pustules, some edematous, on face, trunk, extremities, and scalp. It has a male predominance with increased incidence in Japan. Typically, it has an abrupt onset that resolves in 1 week then reoccurs in crops several weeks later. It has been associated with HIV disease with CD4 counts <300.

Grover Disease

Differential Diagnosis: Bacterial or Fungal Folliculitis

Also know as transient acantholytic dermatosis, this disease is characterized by a sparse eruption, often of limited extent in persons over 50 years of age. The lesions are red papules and fragile vesicles that erode into scaly papules and plaques limited to the chest, shoulder girdle area, and upper abdomen. It is exacerbated by heat and often confused with bacterial folliculitis (Fig. 21.19).

Miliaria Rubra

Differential Diagnosis: Bacterial, Fungal, or Viral Folliculitis

Obstruction of the eccrine sweat duct may create small non-follicular red macules and papules topped by a vesicle or pustule, commonly called "prickly heat." This is not uncommonly seen at sites of occlusion, especially on the back of febrile immobile patients.

Neutrophilic Eccrine Hidradenitis

Differential Diagnosis: Cellulitis

This has also been termed chemotherapy-associated eccrine hidradenitis and appears at a mean of 8 days after infusion. It is characterized by painful erythematous papules and plaques, usually on the trunk [3]. Alkylating agents, anthracyclines, antimetabolites, platinum compounds, taxanes, vinca alkaloids, mitotic inhibitors, and G-CSF and GM-CSF may induce this disorder [1, 65–67] (Fig. 21.20).

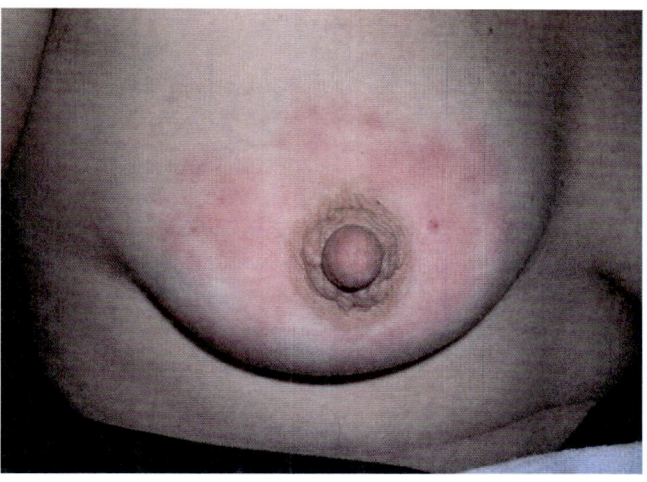

Fig. 21.20 Neutrophilic eccrine hidradenitis. These painful, erythematous plaques on the breast may be confused with cellulitis

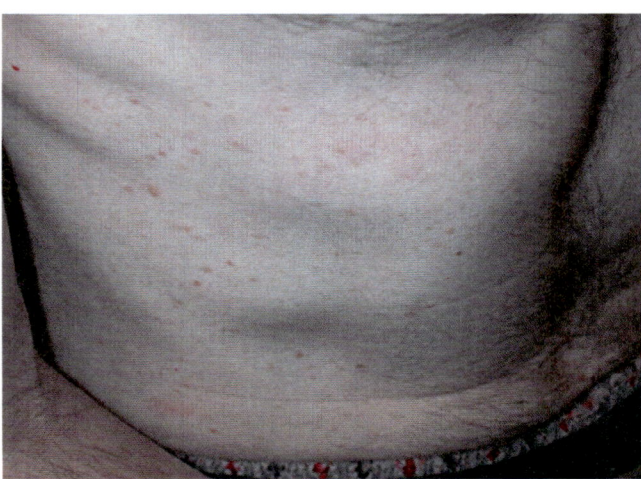

Fig. 21.19 Grover disease (transient acantholytic dermatosis) is characterized by pruritic red–brown keratotic papules on the chest that may be confused with infectious folliculitis

Papulosquamous Lesions

A papule is a raised growth less than 1 cm; a plaque is a raised growth greater than 1 cm. Squamous lesions have characteristic epidermal changes such as scale. The distribution of the lesions helps to further refine diagnostic possibilities.

Dermatitis

Differential Diagnosis: Cellulitis or Superficial Fungal Infection

Also known as eczema, this skin condition has a variety of etiologies, usually described by the preceding adjective, i.e. atopic, contact or irritant dermatitis (Fig. 21.21). The classic skin findings are erythematous, often itchy, scaly patches, and plaques. Due to the chronicity and pruritic nature of this condition, long-standing lesions often become secondarily infected and 90% will be culture positive for *Staphylococcus aureus* leading to impetigo [68].

Pityriasis alba is a variant of atopic dermatitis characterized by hypopigmented patches that are associated with fine, sometimes powdery scale. The most common areas of involvement are the face especially the forehead and

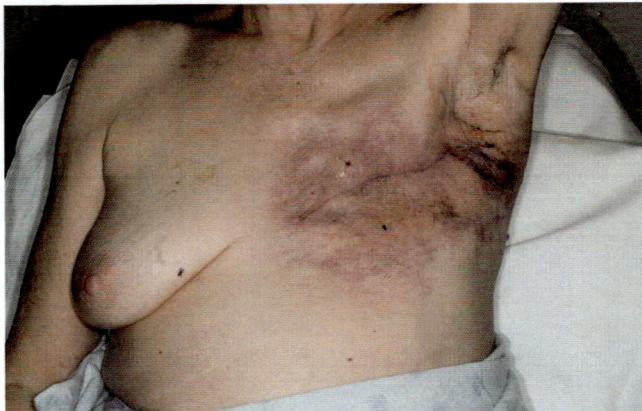

Fig. 21.21 Irritant dermatitis from a breast prosthesis. This needs to be distinguished from cellulitis

cheeks, but can also be seen on the trunk and extremities. The eruption can be preceded by mild asymptomatic erythema. The lesions are usually self-limited and do not require treatment. The hypopigmentation is due to a decreased number of melanocytes and decreased pigment production [69]. Potassium hydroxide examination of a superficial skin scraping can rule out cutaneous dermatophyte infections.

Stasis dermatitis often causes patchy or confluent erythema which must be differentiated from cellulitis. Excoriations or minimal trauma may precipitate erosions and ulcers which may become secondarily superinfected. When chronic venous insufficiency is present, examination of the lower extremities show various combinations of varicosities, dyspigmentation with hemosiderin deposition, or even fibrotic changes termed lipodermatosclerosis. Ulcers often occur around the medial malleolus. Both extremities may be affected with patches of dermatitis. Pruritis is more likely a feature of dermatitis, and pain more likely with cellulitis.

Dermatitis after ionizing radiation often produces persistent tender or edematous erythema which may be mistaken for cellulitis (Fig. 21.22). It is important to identify any superinfection, especially with organisms like *Staphylococcus aureus*, which may act as a superantigen and increase the inflammation [70, 71].

Drug eruptions may be papulosquamous, and when present in intertriginous areas are confused with dermatophyte or yeast infections. This has been reported with chemotherapeutic agents like gefitinib [72] and busulfan. Symmetrical drug-related intertriginous and flexural exanthema may also be seen is association with antibiotic therapy [73].

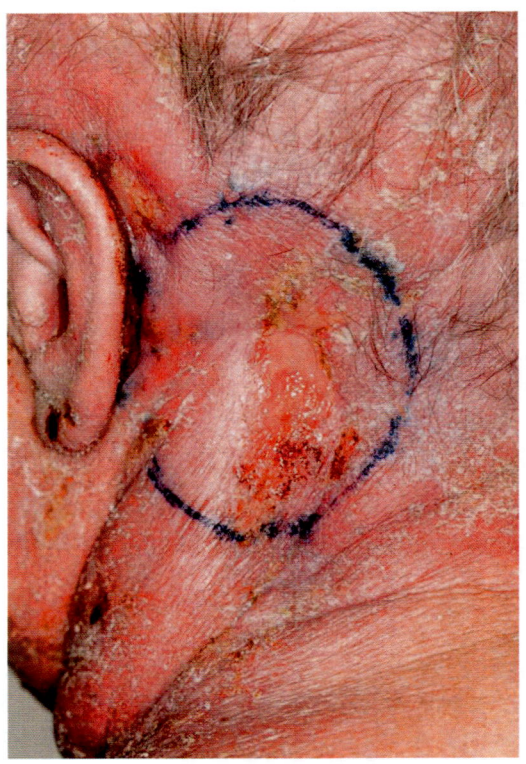

Fig. 21.22 Radiation dermatitis with erythema that may be mistaken for infection

Psoriasis

Differential Diagnosis: Superficial Fungal Infection

Psoriatic plaques may be mistaken for cutaneous fungal infections due to their similar clinical appearance. This skin disease is a common affliction affecting over 2% of the general population, with a bimodal peak at the 3rd and 6th decade of life. The well-demarcated papules and annular plaques often are covered in a thick silvery scale and can be distributed all over the body with a predilection for the scalp, elbows, and knees (Fig. 21.23). When the morphology is annular or ring shaped, the lesions can mimic cutaneous fungal infections. Psoriasis of the hands and feet demonstrates erythema with diffuse scaling and thickened nails reminiscent of onychomycosis. Pustular eruptions of the hands and feet may also represent a form of psoriasis that can be indistinguishable from tinea and dyshidrotic dermatitis. Cancer patients who are placed on systemic corticosteroids and chemotherapy often find that their psoriasis improves, only to flare with pustular lesions when these drugs are withdrawn [74].

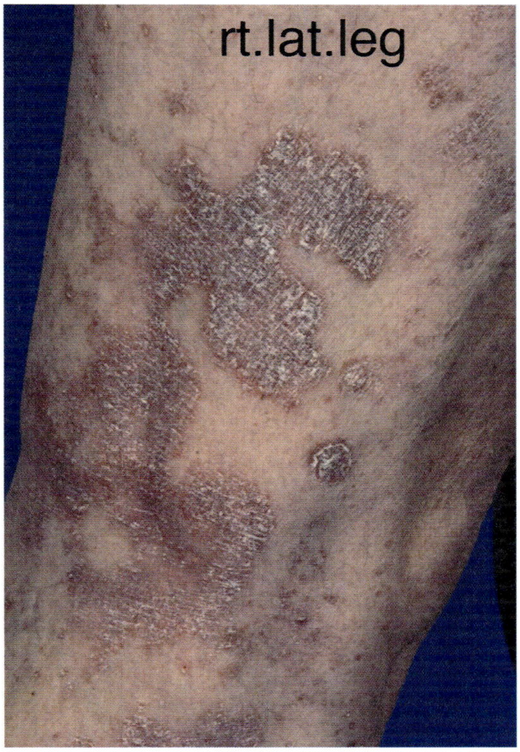

Fig. 21.23 Psoriasis vulgaris. Psoriasis produces an erythematous plaque covered with white or silvery scale which can be confused with fungal infection

Pityriasis Rubra Pilaris

Differential Diagnosis: Superficial Fungal Infection

This eruption often starts with erythema and scaling of the scalp and face and thickening of the palms and soles. Scaly, salmon-colored plaques and hyperkeratotic follicular- based papules are seen on the trunk and extremities. A characteristic finding is "islands of sparing" within the involved areas. Skin biopsy is helpful to distinguish this from psoriasis and fungal infection and a search for occult malignancy should be considered if the presentation is atypical, or in older patients.

Pityriasis Rosea

Differential Diagnosis: Superficial Fungal or Spirochete Infection

This is a two-phase inflammatory skin condition. The onset begins with a herald patch, which is a solitary erythematous papule or plaque, either oval or round, with a collarette of scale. At this stage, it can easily be misinterpreted as a fungal infection. Within 2 weeks, a diffuse truncal rash appears with similar lesions. Pityriasis rosea is postulated to be due to a viral infection although this is not proven [75]. A higher incidence of pityriasis rosea in the fall and winter has been observed. The disease is self-limited and resolves often with 6–8 weeks.

Mycosis Fungoides and Cutaneous T-Cell Lymphoma

Differential Diagnosis: Superficial Fungal Infection

There are many clinical variants, but the classic subtype begins with erythematous patches that may evolve into scaly erythematous plaques. The evolution of this condition can vary from asymptomatic, stable, and indolent or progressing to more serious disease with tumors, erythroderma, and blood involvement (Sezary syndrome). The subtle erythematous patches are nonspecific, and may resemble superficial fungal infection. The diagnosis of mycosis fungoides can be elusive and multiple biopsies with T-cell receptor gene rearrangement studies may also be necessary.

Purpuric and Petechial Lesions

Purpura or hemorrhage into the skin may be a sign of more serious disease in immunocompromised patients. Cancer patients are especially susceptible to polymicrobial opportunistic infections that present this way. When not infectious, vasculitis, the inflammation of the blood vessel walls, often precedes the purpura and can be caused by medications, neoplasms, or other systemic diseases, leading to significant morbidity and mortality. The most common purpuric dermatoses that can mimic underlying infections will be reviewed.

Leukocytoclastic Vasculitis

Differential Diagnosis: Bacterial or Fungal Infection

Leukocytoclastic vasculitis, an inflammation of the small dermal blood vessel walls often presents as macular or palpable nonblanchable purpura usually on the lower extremities or in areas of localized pressure (Fig. 21.24). The

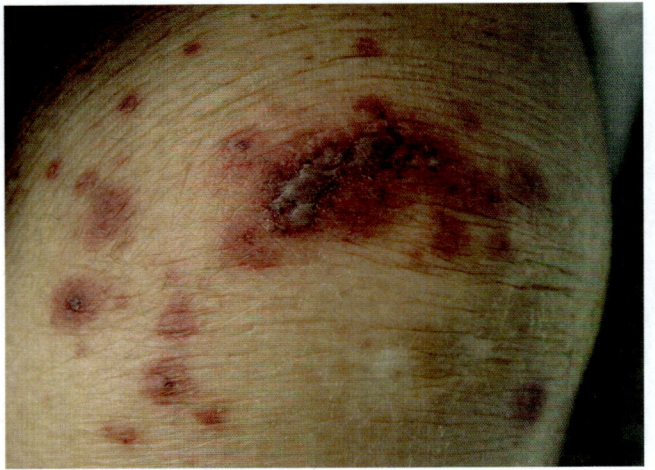

Fig. 21.24 Leukocytoclastic vasculitis is characterized by purpuric confluent papulovesicles on the legs in this patient

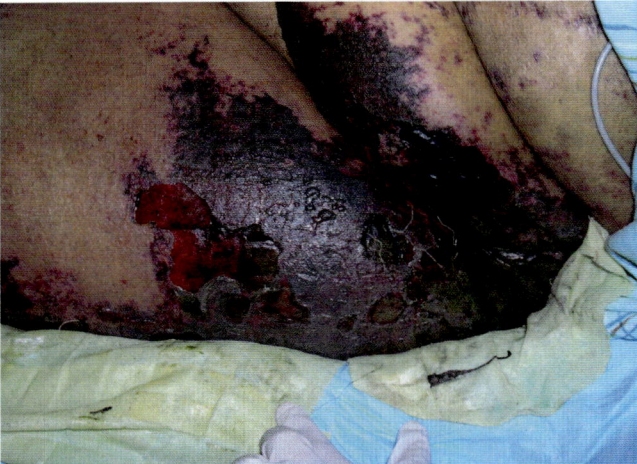

Fig. 21.25 Disseminated intravascular coagulation. Purpura and tissue necrosis involving the abdomen, buttocks, and legs

diagnosis can be made clinically and confirmed by skin biopsy that shows inflammation of the small vessels with neutrophils, extravasated erythrocytes, and fibrinoid necrosis in the blood vessel walls.

Superficial Thrombophlebitis

Differential Diagnosis: Cellulitis

Characterized by inflammation and thrombosis in the superficial venous system, this condition results in erythema, swelling, and tenderness in the extremity.

This is to be distinguished from cellulitis, which is an infection of the underlying deeper dermis and subcutaneous tissue.

Disseminated Intravascular Coagulation (DIC)

Differential Diagnosis: Fungal or Bacterial Sepsis

This disorder of coagulation causes a consumption of clotting factors and the production of fibrin split products. Patients will have signs of blood loss as well as end-organ damage due to thrombosis of large and small vessels. Cutaneous findings include petechiae, purpura, bleeding from mucocutaneous orifices and wounds, soft tissue hematomas, acral cyanosis with possible ischemia, and necrosis (Fig. 21.25). The most common associated conditions are underlying infection, sepsis, trauma, malignancy, and transfusion reactions. Therefore, a thorough investigation of all possible underlying causes is warranted in these cases [76].

Calciphylaxis

Differential Diagnosis: Ecthyma, Cellulitis, Deep Fungal, or Bacterial Infection

Calciphylaxis produces vascular calcification leading to ischemia of the skin and soft tissues (Fig. 21.26). It is most commonly seen in patients with chronic renal disease and hyperparathyroidism. Clinically, the involved areas develop reticulate, violaceous patches which are painful and may progress to necrosis. The exact etiology of calciphylaxis is unknown. Various theories propose either protein C dysfunction or exposure to sensitizing agents that then cause deposition of calcium in tissues [77, 78].

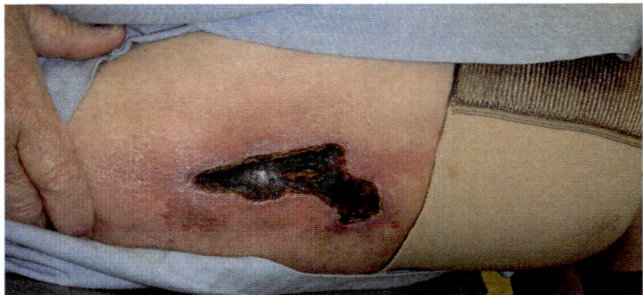

Fig. 21.26 Calciphylaxis characterized by stellate ulceration and hemorrhagic crusts can be confused with ecthyma

Petechiae

Differential Diagnosis: Rickettsial, Bacterial, or Fungal Infection

Petechiae are pinpoint nonblanchable erythematous macules due to leaking of blood into the skin. They occur in the setting of thrombocytopenia, abnormal platelet function, localized pressure or trauma, increase in intravascular venous pressure, or vitamin C deficiency. However, some Rickettsial infections can often start with small erythematous macules on the wrists and ankles with petechiae.

Lesions of the Adipose Tissue

Differential Diagnosis: Cellulitis, Deep Fungal, or Mycobacterial Infection

Panniculitis refers to diseases in which the major abnormality is an inflammation of the subcutaneous fat presenting as subcutaneous nodules. The clinical lesions are red-to-violaceous nodules and plaques that have a predilection for the legs. The nodules may be tender and ulcerated or they may remain asymptomatic and intact. Fat necrosis is usually present and associated with vascular changes. Histopathologically, the inflammatory processes may show considerable overlap. From the practical standpoint of diagnosis and management, patients with panniculitis can be placed into the following groups:

Cold Panniculitis

This is an acute, nodular, erythematous eruption with livedo mottling usually limited to areas exposed to the cold. It is commonly seen in children and women, and systemic diseases are not associated with this group of patients.

Pancreatic Panniculitis

Circulating lipases from pancreatic carcinoma and acute pancreatitis can produce fat necrosis that results in tender subcutaneous nodules that simulate erythema nodosum. Fever, eosinophilia, and arthralgia may accompany the disease (Fig. 21.27).

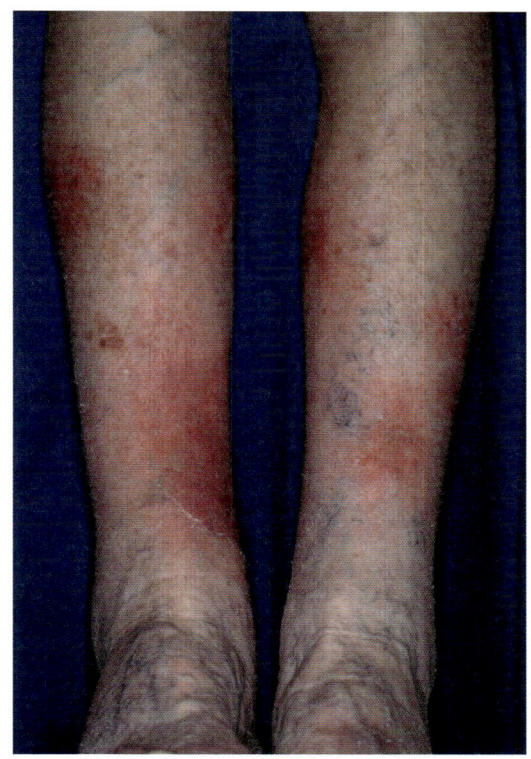

Fig. 21.27 Pancreatic panniculitis. Painless subcutaneous nodules of pancreatic fat necrosis

Nodular Vasculitis

This presents as tender, subcutaneous nodules of the calves of middle-aged women. The lesions are bilateral, often ulcerate, and recur over years. It has long been considered as a cutaneous hypersensitivity reaction to Mycobacterium tuberculous, but has also been associated with HIV [79] and hepatitis C [80] and drugs including dasatinib [81] and imatinib [82] (Fig. 21.28).

Septal panniculitis (Erythema nodosum, EN)

The most common form of inflammatory panniculitis with most cases occurring in young adult women. The eruption consists of bilateral, symmetrical, deep tender nodules 1–10 cm in diameter located pretibially. The onset is acute, frequently associated with malaise, arthralgias, arthritis, and leg edema. The nodules last a few days to weeks, appearing in crops, and then slowly involute.

EN is a reactive process, commonly associated with streptococcal, beta-hemolytic infection, usually within 3 weeks from the onset of the disease. Other associations

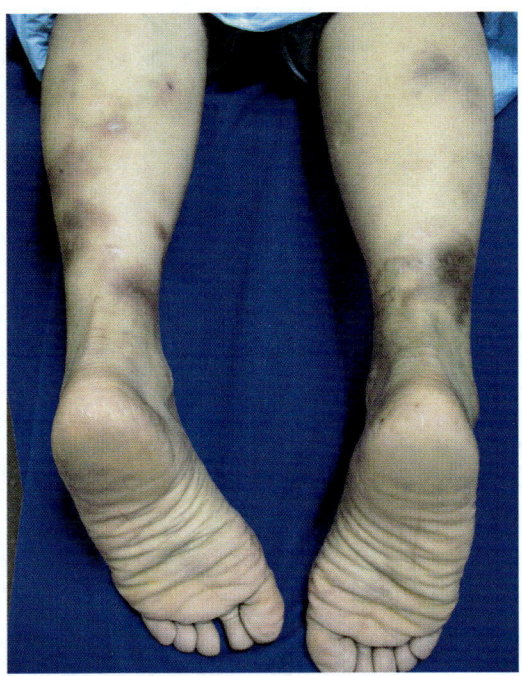

Fig. 21.28 Nodular vasculitis. Tender subcutaneous nodules on the calves of a middle-aged woman

include primary tuberculous, intestinal infection with Yersinia, Salmonella, or Shigella and in endemic areas, systemic fungal infections (coccidiomycosis, histoplasmosis, sporotrichosis, and blastomycosis) should be considered. Other noninfectious causes of EN include sarcoidosis, inflammatory bowel diseases, hematologic malignancies, pregnancy, and medications including oral contraceptives. Spontaneous resolution usually occurs within 3–6 weeks without scarring.

Sclerosing Panniculitis (Lipodermatosclerosis)

This occurs primarily on the medial lower legs of obese women older than age 40. However, this may occur in the setting of chronic lower extremity edema in the cancer patient. There is marked woody induration in a stocking distribution as a result of fibrosis of subcutaneous fat.

Traumatic panniculitis

Most commonly occurs on the trunk and breast in women. Lesions present as firm subcutaneous masses of variable tenderness, and may mimic mastitis.

Erythematous Lesions

The term erythema means redness (hyperemia) of the skin and most of the skin conditions in this category are blanchable. A number of skin conditions are referred as reactive erythemas: urticaria and angioedema, erythema multiforme, Stevens–Johnson syndrome (SJS), toxic epidermal necrolysis (TEN), eosinophilic dermatosis, and gyrate erythemas. Confluent erythema may be mistaken for cellulitis, and the gyrate erythemas which are annular or polycyclic, may be confused with superficial fungal infections. These entities represent the cutaneous reaction to an underlying systemic process which may be infectious, malignant, or drug related. The primary lesions are erythematous plaques that are annular or arcuate, transient or fixed.

Urticaria and Angioedema

Differential Diagnosis: Cellulitis, Superficial Fungal Infection

Acute urticaria is a common, acute, self-limited eruption of smooth, pruritic erythematous papules and plaques produced by localized edema. They change in size and shape with time and are usually present for a few hours and less than 2 days. Chronic urticaria is defined as urticaria lasting longer than 6 weeks. Although urticaria results from transient dermal edema, angioedema results from deep swelling within subcutaneous sites. The etiology of an acute episode of urticaria can sometimes be determined, but chronic urticaria is often idiopathic. When the lesions are annular, it may be mistaken for tinea, and angioedema must be distinguished from cellulitis.

Erythema Multiforme (EM)/Stevens–Johnson Syndrome (SJS) and Toxic Epidermal Necrolysis (TEN)

Differential Diagnosis: Disseminated Viral, Bacterial, or Fungal Infections

The lesions of EM may be macular, urticarial, and vesiculobullous (Fig. 21.29). The eruption has a predilection for the back of the hands, palms, soles, and the extensor surfaces of the limbs. They may spread to the rest of the body, or be generalized from the start. The macular lesions are bright red and well circumscribed and they frequently become urticarial within a few hours. Iris or target lesions are urticarial

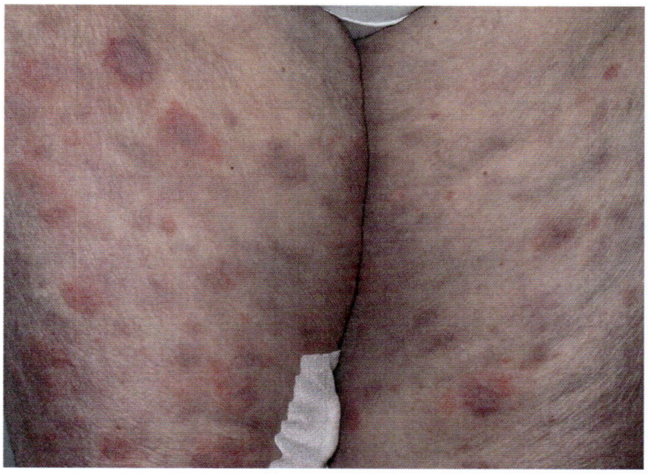

Fig. 21.29 Erythema multiforme characterized by target lesions

patches with dusky centers and bright red active borders. Mucosal involvement begins with bullae that break very soon after formation and leave denuded areas that undergo a variety of changes. Healing of mucosal lesions takes place without scarring, unless there has been secondary bacterial infection. In the case of SJS, the lips, buccal mucosa, palate, conjunctivae, urethra, and vagina are frequently involved. It is often defined as severe erythema multiforme with mucosal involvement, visceral involvement, or both. These diseases are part of a continuum of immunologically mediated mucocutaneous diseases of varying degrees of severity. When the lesions become bullous, pustular, or necrotic, the differential diagnosis may include disseminated herpes, bacterial or fungal infection.

TEN is a severe reaction characterized by confluent blisters resulting in detachment of the epidermis from the dermis, leading to denudation of greater than 30% of the body surface area (Fig. 21.30). The differential diagnosis includes staphylococcal scalded skin syndrome (SSSS), which causes more superficial epidermal blisters that can be readily distinguished by skin biopsy.

EM, SJS, and TEN have multiple etiologies. Infectious diseases are the important causes of EM in children and young adults [83], whereas drug reactions [84–86] and malignancy [86] are more important factors in adults. Herpes simplex infection may be followed 7–10 days later by EM. The diagnosis may be established by biopsy, culture, or direct antigen immunofluorescence. Other etiologic infectious agents are Mycoplasma pneumoniae, Coxsackie B-5, influenza type A and echo viruses [87].

Erythema Annulare Centrifugum

Differential Diagnosis: Superficial Fungal, Bacterial, or Rickettsial Infection

The most common gyrate erythema is characterized by polycyclic, erythematous plaques, sometimes with trailing scale, that grow eccentrically and slowly (2–3 mm/day). The lesions disappear over several weeks and are replaced by new ones that follow a similar course, usually on the trunk, buttocks, and inner thighs (Fig. 21.31). Some cases are associated with dermatophyte infection elsewhere, but the lesions themselves do not contain fungus. It is rarely associated with internal malignancy such as Hodgkin's lymphoma [88], Mantle B-cell non-Hodgkin's lymphoma [89], breast carcinoma [90], CLL [91], myeloma [92], and tumors of the gastrointestinal tract [93]. The clinical presentation can mimic secondary syphilis, tinea corporis and cruris, Hansen disease, and Lyme disease.

Erythema Gyratum Repens

Differential Diagnosis: Superficial Fungal Infection

This uncommon, morphologically distinctive eruption is an indicator of serious disease, usually internal malignancy. Lesions consist of undulating wavy bands of slightly elevated

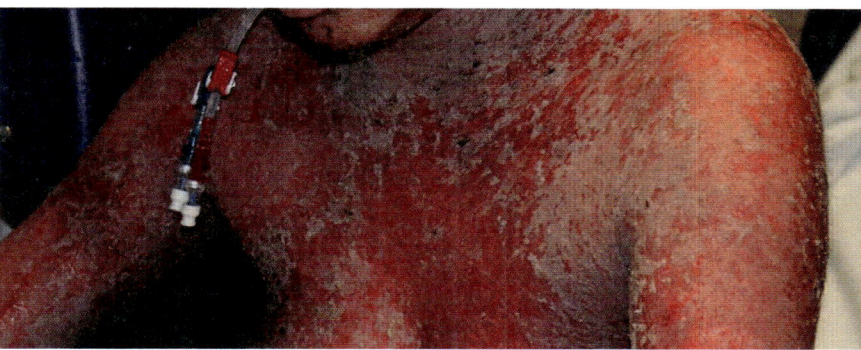

Fig. 21.30 Toxic epidermal necrolysis. Erythroderma and detachment of the epidermis and erosions affecting more than 30% body surface

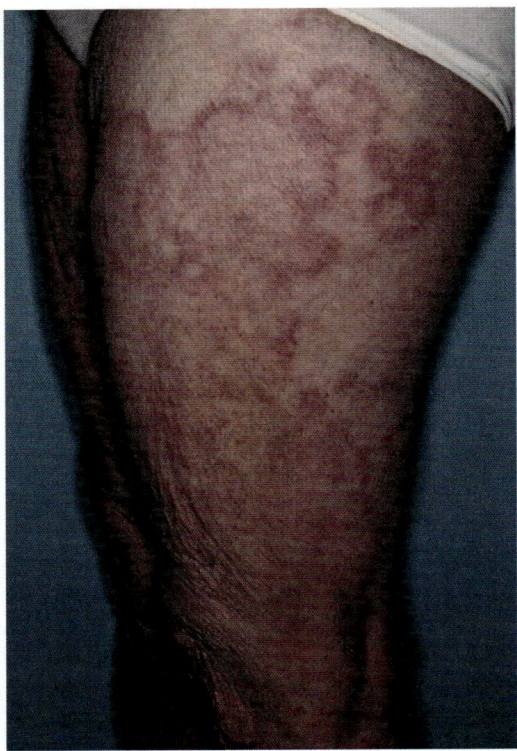

Fig. 21.31 Erythema annulare centrifugum characterized by annular and polycyclic plaques with delicate scaling on the inner margin of the advancing edge on the legs

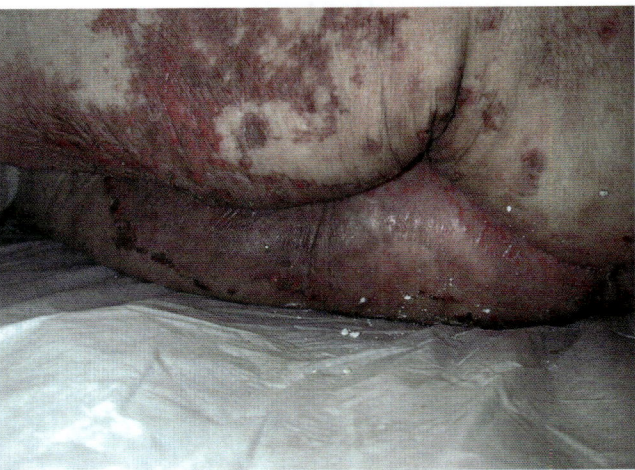

Fig. 21.32 Necrolytic migratory erythema with erythematous patches that blister centrally, erode, and heal with hyperpigmentation on the perineum

scaly erythema over the entire body. Lesions migrate rapidly (up to 1 cm/day) and are characteristically concentric, giving the skin a "wood grain" appearance. This distinctive migratory eruption has been mostly associated with lung cancer, esophageal, and breast cancer. With adequate control of the cancer the dermatitis usually abates, however this may not be possible in cases of metastatic disease at diagnosis [94].

Necrolytic Migratory Erythema

Differential Diagnosis: Mucocutaneous Candidiasis

This rare syndrome is associated with glucagon-secreting tumors of the pancreas that occurs in periorificial, flexural, and acral areas and closely resembles the lesions associated with zinc deficiency. There are active erythematous, gyrate, or circinate borders with confluence [94, 95] (Fig. 21.32). Most patients have diabetes or glucose intolerance, and hyperglucagonemia, in addition to the rash. Other common manifestations include anemia, weight loss, diarrhea, atrophic glossitis, and angular cheilitis. Additional laboratory findings are low serum zinc level and hypoaminoacidemia. The eruption may resemble chronic mucocutaneous candidiasis, severe seborrheic dermatitis, and acrodermatitis enteropathica [94, 95]. Removal of the pancreatic tumor leads to resolution; however, in half of the cases, metastases have occurred at the time of diagnosis. Necrolytic acral erythema produces similar erythematous or gyrate lesions on the acral surface has been reported in association with hepatitis C [96].

Chemotherapy-Induced Acral Blisters and Erythema (Palmoplantar Erythrodysesthesia Syndrome, Hand–Foot Syndrome)

Differential Diagnosis: Cellulitis, Viral Infection

This reactive and usually painful erythema of the hands and feet may be seen following chemotherapy with a variety of agents including cytarabine, doxorubicin, capecitabine, taxanes and 5-fluorouracil, and methotrexate [52, 97]. More recently it has been associated with some of the multikinase inhibitors, including sorafenib and sunitinib [52, 98]. Erythema is followed by blistering and superficial desquamation, associated with the dose and duration of infusion [1].

Granuloma Annulare

Differential Diagnosis: Superficial Fungal Infection

This is a granulomatous process which presents with annular and serpiginous plaques usually on the extremities (Fig. 21.33). They occur most often on the dorsum of

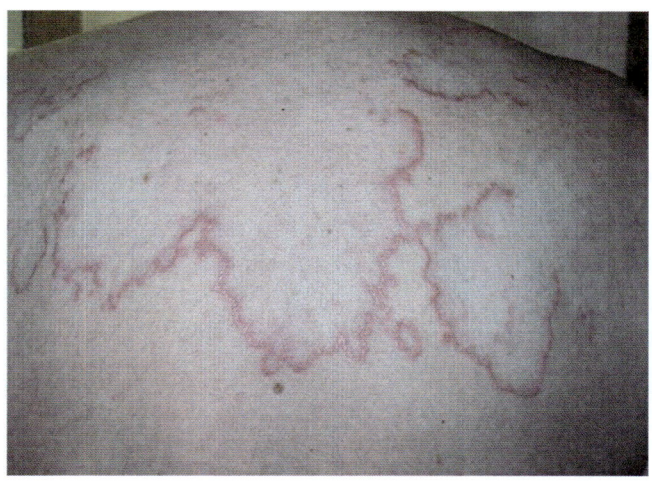

Fig. 21.33 Granuloma annulare producing annular plaques that can be confused with fungal infection erythema migrans associated with Lyme disease

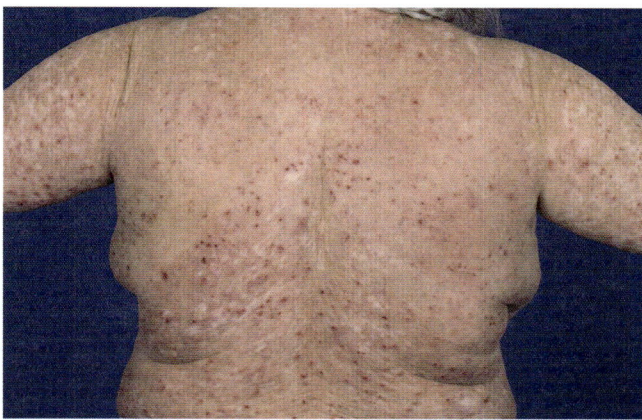

Fig. 21.34 Hypereosinophilic syndrome with diffuse dermatitis and excoriations which may be confused with scabies

the hands and arms, then legs and feet. There is usually no significant scale. Biopsy of the indurated borders reveals a granulomatous dermatitis with histiocytic infiltration, degeneration of collagen and elastic fibers, and mucin deposition. The lesions are self-limited and must be distinguished from a fungal infection.

Eosinophilic Dermatoses

Differential Diagnosis: Bacterial, Fungal, Mycobacterial Infections

The eosinophilic dermatoses are a heterogenous group in which the histopathologic findings are characterized by many eosinophils in the inflammatory infiltrate. The most common causes include arthropod bites, drug eruptions, allergic contact dermatitis, and atopic dermatitis.

Granuloma faciale (GF) is a distinct disease characterized by a single or multiple red–brown plaques on the face. Although the clinical appearance is usually quite distinctive, it can be mistaken for syphilis and leprosy, and is resistant to therapy [99].

Eosinophilic cellulitis (Wells syndrome) presents as recurrent painful or pruritic erythematous indurated plaques, persistent urticaria, and eosinophilia, both peripheral and in the bone marrow. The pathogenesis of Wells syndrome is unknown, but so-called triggers have been described in some cases, including myeloproliferative diseases, insect bites, and drugs [100]. Toxocara canis and other parasitic disorders can present with clinical and pathological findings similar to Wells syndrome [101]. Wells syndrome often has a striking clinical presentation resembling bacterial cellulitis and erysipelas, and usually improves dramatically after administration of systemic corticosteroids.

Hypereosinophilic syndrome is often a myeloproliferative disease defined as peripheral eosinophilia for more than 6 months, more than 1,500/µl absolute eosinophil count, lack of evidence of parasitic, allergic, or other known cause of eosinophilia, and signs and symptoms of multiorgan involvement, including the heart, central nervous system (CNS), skin, and respiratory tract [102, 103] (Fig. 21.34). Thromboembolic disease is not infrequent. Cutaneous lesions occur in more than half of all cases and range from pruritic macules, papules, and nodules to urticaria and angioedema. Ulcerated or nonulcerated nodules, erythroderma, and mucosal ulcerations are less common cutaneous manifestations. The differential diagnosis includes Churg–Strauss syndrome, parasitic infections (toxocariasis, strongylodiasis), and lymphoproliferative diseases [102, 103].

Ulcerative Lesions and Skin Tumors

Differential Diagnosis: Bacterial, Fungal, Mycobacterial, Parasitic Infections

An infectious etiology should always be considered when a skin ulcer develops in a cancer patient, especially when they are immunosuppressed. Noninfectious causes may be considered after this is excluded. Skin fibrosis and poor wound healing is frequently seen in the context of radiation fibrosis [70] or sclerodermoid GVHD [104] (Fig. 21.35). Mal perforans or neuropathic ulcers are associated with altered skin sensation resulting in the inability to detect and avoid skin trauma, and may be a consequence of chemotherapy-induced sensory neuropathy. Neurotic excoriations may produce factitial changes that result in erosions and ulcers. Chronic nonhealing ulcers should be biopsied to rule out tumor, which may be primary or metastatic. At the same time, a tissue culture biopsy may be performed for fungal, mycobacterial, and bacterial culture. Primary and metastatic skin tumors may mimic infections or cellulitis, especially when the lymphatic system is involved (Fig. 21.36). Solitary tumors may resemble ecthyma or septic emboli (Fig. 21.37).

Hair and Scalp Lesions

Differential Diagnosis: Fungal and bacterial Infections

Alopecias may be divided into scaring and nonscarring forms. The scarring or cicatricial forms may present with sterile pustules and are often mistaken for infectious folliculitis, secondary to bacteria or dermatophytes (Fig. 21.38). In these neutrophilic dermatoses, follicular hyperkeratosis rather than infection is thought to play a role, although *Staphylococcus aureus* is commonly found [105]. Dissecting folliculitis may respond better to oral retinoids rather than to antibiotics [106]. Conversely, a rather bland, scaly alopecia is occasionally associated with the infiltration of neoplastic cells, which destroys hair follicles by inducing fibroplasia via inflammatory mediators. The most common neoplasm is metastatic breast carcinoma. Other causes include squamous and basal cell carcinomas, angiosarcoma, gastric carcinoma, placental site trophoblastic tumor, and mycosis fungoides [107].

Summary

A wide variety of cutaneous infections have been described in cancer patients. As clinicians, we know that these patients are often prone to commonplace skin problems which may be more difficult to recognize because of confounding factors

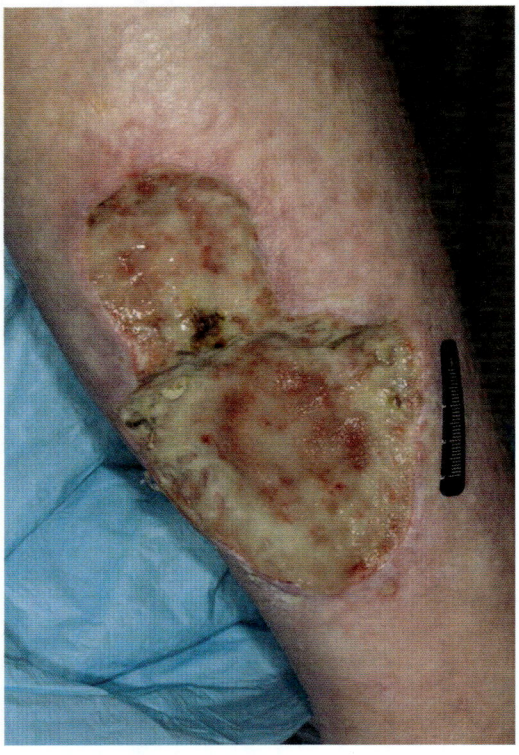

Fig. 21.35 Chronic leg ulcers developing in patient with poor wound healing from sclerodermoid GVHD

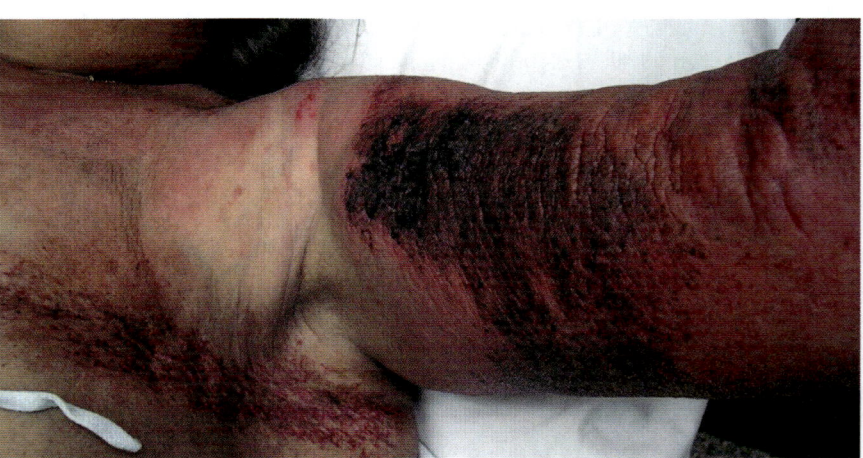

Fig. 21.36 Metastatic breast carcinoma mimicking cellulitis

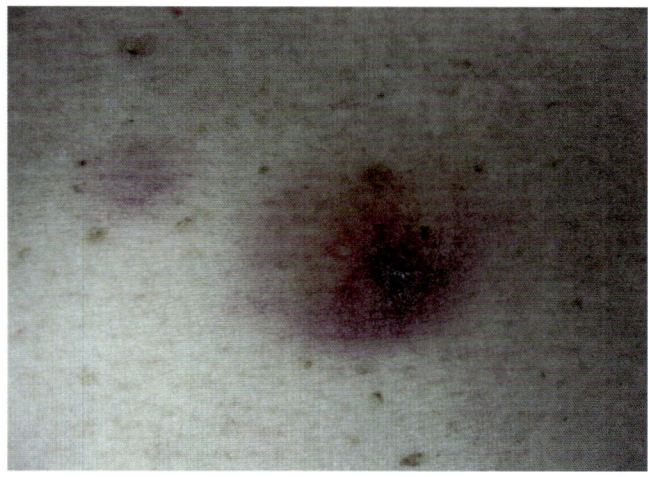

Fig. 21.37 Leukemia cutis mimicking ecthyma or septic emboli

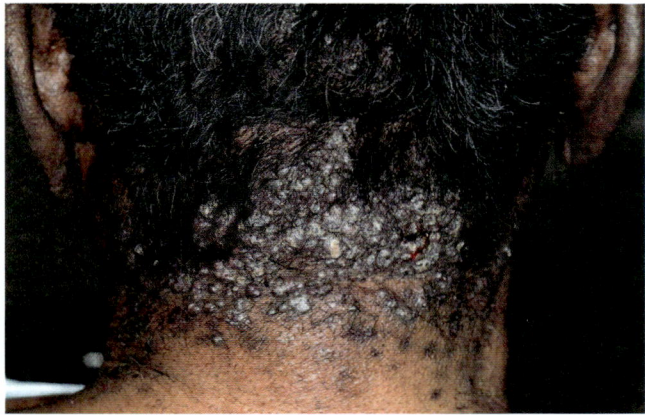

Fig. 21.38 Acne keloidalis mimicking a bacterial or fungal infection

like immunosuppression and pancytopenia. Unusual noninfectious skin lesions and paraneoplastic eruptions also occur in this setting. Teamwork between the infectious disease specialist, dermatologist, and pathologist is critical in distinguishing infectious lesions from dermatologic eruptions that mimic infectious disorders.

References

1. Sanborn RE, Sauer DA. Cutaneous reactions to chemotherapy: commonly seen, less described, little understood. Dermatol Clin. 2008;26:103–19, ix.
2. Groschel D, Gerstein AR, Rosenbaum JM. Skin lesions as a diagnostic aid in barbiturate poisoning. N Engl J Med. 1970;283:409–10.
3. Wenzel FG, Horn TD. Nonneoplastic disorders of the eccrine glands. J Am Acad Dermatol. 1998;38:1–17; quiz 8–20.
4. Judge TG, Nisbet NH. Trophoneurotic blisters in elderly hemiplegics. Lancet. 1967;1:811–2.
5. Holten C. Cutaneous phenomena in acute barbiturate poisoning. Acta Derm Venereol Suppl (Stockh). 1952;32:162–8.
6. Cantwell Jr AR, Martz W. Idiopathic bullae in diabetics. Bullosis diabeticorum. Arch Dermatol. 1967;96:42–4.
7. Rosen LB, Frank BL, Rywlin AM. A characteristic vesiculobullous eruption in patients with chronic lymphocytic leukemia. J Am Acad Dermatol. 1986;15:943–50.
8. Barzilai A, Shpiro D, Goldberg I, et al. Insect bite-like reaction in patients with hematologic malignant neoplasms. Arch Dermatol. 1999;135:1503–7.
9. Davis MD, Perniciaro C, Dahl PR, Randle HW, McEvoy MT, Leiferman KM. Exaggerated arthropod-bite lesions in patients with chronic lymphocytic leukemia: a clinical, histopathologic, and immunopathologic study of eight patients. J Am Acad Dermatol. 1998;39:27–35.
10. Schauder CS, Hymes SR, Rapini RP, Zipf TF. Vesicular graft-versus-host disease. Int J Dermatol. 1992;31:509–10.
11. Moreno JC, Valverde F, Martinez F, et al. Bullous scleroderma-like changes in chronic graft-versus-host disease. J Eur Acad Dermatol Venereol. 2003;17:200–3.
12. Hymes SR, Farmer ER, Burns WH, et al. Bullous sclerodermalike changes in chronic graft-vs-host disease. Arch Dermatol. 1985;121:1189–92.
13. Ramdial PK, Naidoo DK. Drug-induced cutaneous pathology. J Clin Pathol. 2009;62:493–504.
14. Kocyigit P, Akay BN, Karaosmanoglu N. Linear IgA bullous dermatosis induced by interferon-alpha 2a. Clin Exp Dermatol. 2009;34:e123–4.
15. Yeh SW, Ahmed B, Sami N, Razzaque Ahmed A. Blistering disorders: diagnosis and treatment. Dermatol Ther. 2003;16:214–23.
16. Scott JE, Ahmed AR. The blistering diseases. Med Clin North Am. 1998;82:1239–83.
17. Wojnarowska F. What's new in linear IgA disease? J Eur Acad Dermatol Venereol. 2000;14:441–3.
18. Richards SS, Hall S, Yokel B, Whitmore SE. A bullous eruption in an elderly woman. Vancomycin-associated linear IgA dermatosis (LAD). Arch Dermatol. 1995;131(1447–8):50–1.
19. Nassar D, Gabillot-Carre M, Ortonne N, et al. Atypical linear IgA dermatosis revealing angioimmunoblastic T-cell lymphoma. Arch Dermatol. 2009;145:342–3.
20. Green ST, Natarajan S. Linear IgA disease and oesophageal carcinoma. J R Soc Med. 1987;80:48–9.
21. Lai-Cheong JE, Groves RW, Banerjee P. Linear IgA bullous dermatosis associated with adenocarcinoma of the ascending colon. J Eur Acad Dermatol Venereol. 2007;21:978–9.
22. Adamic M, Potocnik M, Pavlovic MD. Linear IgA bullous dermatosis in a patient with advanced pancreatic carcinoma. Clin Exp Dermatol. 2008;33:503–5.
23. Cohen PR. Photodistributed erythema multiforme: paclitaxel-related, photosensitive conditions in patients with cancer. J Drugs Dermatol. 2009;8:61–4.
24. Cunningham MJ, Zone JJ. Thyroid abnormalities in dermatitis herpetiformis. Prevalence of clinical thyroid disease and thyroid autoantibodies. Ann Intern Med. 1985;102:194–6.
25. Collin P, Pukkala E, Reunala T. Malignancy and survival in dermatitis herpetiformis: a comparison with coeliac disease. Gut. 1996;38:528–30.
26. Sigurgeirsson B, Agnarsson BA, Lindelof B. Risk of lymphoma in patients with dermatitis herpetiformis. BMJ. 1994;308:13–5.
27. Leonard JN, Tucker WF, Fry JS, et al. Increased incidence of malignancy in dermatitis herpetiformis. Br Med J (Clin Res Ed). 1983;286:16–8.
28. Brenner S, Bialy-Golan V, Ruocco A. Drug-induced pemphigus. Clin Dermatol. 1998;16:393–7.

29. Nguyen VT, Ndoye A, Bassler KD, et al. Classification, clinical manifestations, and immunopathological mechanisms of the epithelial variant of paraneoplastic autoimmune multiorgan syndrome: a reappraisal of paraneoplastic pemphigus. Arch Dermatol. 2001;137:193–206.
30. Anhalt GJ. Paraneoplastic pemphigus: the role of tumours and drugs. Br J Dermatol. 2001;144:1102–4.
31. Anhalt GJ, Kim SC, Stanley JR, et al. Paraneoplastic pemphigus. An autoimmune mucocutaneous disease associated with neoplasia. N Engl J Med. 1990;323:1729–35.
32. Chorzelski T, Hashimoto T, Maciejewska B, Amagai M, Anhalt GJ, Jablonska S. Paraneoplastic pemphigus associated with Castleman tumor, myasthenia gravis and bronchiolitis obliterans. J Am Acad Dermatol. 1999;41:393–400.
33. Eccersley LR, Hoffbrand AV, Rustin MH, McNamara CJ. Paraneoplastic pemphigus associated with systemic mastocytosis. Am J Hematol. 2009;84:847–8.
34. Wang L, Bu D, Yang Y, Chen X, Zhu X. Castleman's tumours and production of autoantibody in paraneoplastic pemphigus. Lancet. 2004;363:525–31.
35. Aho S, Mahoney MG, Uitto J. Plectin serves as an autoantigen in paraneoplastic pemphigus. J Invest Dermatol. 1999;113:422–3.
36. Alcalay J, David M, Ingber A, Hazaz B, Sandbank M. Bullous pemphigoid mimicking bullous erythema multiforme: an untoward side effect of penicillins. J Am Acad Dermatol. 1988;18:345–9.
37. Czechowicz RT, Reid CM, Warren LJ, Weightman W, Whitehead FJ. Bullous pemphigoid induced by cephalexin. Australas J Dermatol. 2001;42:132–5.
38. Kimyai-Asadi A, Usman A, Nousari HC. Ciprofloxacin-induced bullous pemphigoid. J Am Acad Dermatol. 2000;42:847.
39. Szabolcs P, Reese M, Yancey KB, Hall RP, Kurtzberg J. Combination treatment of bullous pemphigoid with anti-CD20 and anti-CD25 antibodies in a patient with chronic graft-versus-host disease. Bone Marrow Transplant. 2002;30:327–9.
40. Aisa Y, Mori T, Nakazato T, et al. Cicatricial pemphigoid of the oropharynx after allogeneic stem cell transplantation for relapsed follicular lymphoma. Int J Hematol. 2005;82:266–9.
41. Daoud MS, Gibson LE, Daoud S, el-Azhary RA. Chronic hepatitis C and skin diseases: a review. Mayo Clin Proc. 1995;70:559–64.
42. Hogan D, Card RT, Ghadially R, McSheffrey JB, Lane P. Human immunodeficiency virus infection and porphyria cutanea tarda. J Am Acad Dermatol. 1989;20:17–20.
43. Salata H, Cortes JM, de Enriquez Salamanca R, et al. Porphyria cutanea tarda and hepatocellular carcinoma. Frequency of occurrence and related factors. J Hepatol. 1985;1:477–87.
44. McLaren GD, Muir WA, Kellermeyer RW. Iron overload disorders: natural history, pathogenesis, diagnosis, and therapy. Crit Rev Clin Lab Sci. 1983;19:205–66.
45. Timmer-de Mik L, Kardaun SH, Kramer MH, Hayes DP, Bousema MT. Imatinib-induced pseudoporphyria. Clin Exp Dermatol. 2009;34:705–7.
46. Kwong WT, Hsu S. Pseudoporphyria associated with voriconazole. J Drugs Dermatol. 2007;6:1042–4.
47. Sharp MT, Horn TD. Pseudoporphyria induced by voriconazole. J Am Acad Dermatol. 2005;53:341–5.
48. Green JJ, Manders SM. Pseudoporphyria. J Am Acad Dermatol. 2001;44:100–8.
49. Roujeau JC, Bioulac-Sage P, Bourseau C, et al. Acute generalized exanthematous pustulosis. Analysis of 63 cases. Arch Dermatol. 1991;127:1333–8.
50. Jackson H, Vion B, Levy PM. Generalized eruptive pustular drug rash due to cephalexin. Dermatologica. 1988;177:292–4.
51. Fayol J, Bernard P, Bonnetblanc JM. Pustular eruption following administration of cefazolin: a second case report. J Am Acad Dermatol. 1988;19:571.
52. Heidary N, Naik H, Burgin S. Chemotherapeutic agents and the skin: an update. J Am Acad Dermatol. 2008;58:545–70.
53. Callen JP. Neutrophilic dermatoses. Dermatol Clin. 2002;20:409–19.
54. Dompmartin A, Troussard X, Lorier E, et al. Sweet syndrome associated with acute myelogenous leukemia. Atypical form simulating facial erysipelas. Int J Dermatol. 1991;30:644–7.
55. Cohen PR. Sweet's syndrome–a comprehensive review of an acute febrile neutrophilic dermatosis. Orphanet J Rare Dis. 2007;2:34.
56. Park JW, Mehrotra B, Barnett BO, Baron AD, Venook AP. The Sweet syndrome during therapy with granulocyte colony-stimulating factor. Ann Intern Med. 1992;116:996–8.
57. Cohen PR, Kurzrock R. Sweet's syndrome and malignancy. Am J Med. 1987;82:1220–6.
58. Cohen PR, Kurzrock R. Chronic myelogenous leukemia and Sweet syndrome. Am J Hematol. 1989;32:134–7.
59. Behcet H. Uber rezidivierende, aphthose, durchein Virus verursachte Geschwure am Mund, am Auge und anden Genitalien. Dermatol Wochenschr. 1937;36:1152–7.
60. Ghate JV, Jorizzo JL. Behcet's disease and complex aphthosis. J Am Acad Dermatol. 1999;40:1–18; quiz 9–20.
61. Jorizzo JL, Schmalstieg FC, Dinehart SM, et al. Bowel-associated dermatosis-arthritis syndrome. Immune complex-mediated vessel damage and increased neutrophil migration. Arch Intern Med. 1984;144:738–40.
62. James WD. Clinical practice. Acne. N Engl J Med. 2005;352:1463–72.
63. Osio A, Mateus C, Soria JC, et al. Cutaneous side-effects in patients on long-term treatment with epidermal growth factor receptor inhibitors. Br J Dermatol. 2009;161:515–21.
64. Busam KJ, Capodieci P, Motzer R, Kiehn T, Phelan D, Halpern AC. Cutaneous side-effects in cancer patients treated with the anti-epidermal growth factor receptor antibody C225. Br J Dermatol. 2001;144:1169–76.
65. Susser WS, Whitaker-Worth DL, Grant-Kels JM. Mucocutaneous reactions to chemotherapy. J Am Acad Dermatol. 1999;40:367–98; quiz 99–400.
66. Alley E, Green R, Schuchter L. Cutaneous toxicities of cancer therapy. Curr Opin Oncol. 2002;14:212–6.
67. Baack BR, Burgdorf WH. Chemotherapy-induced acral erythema. J Am Acad Dermatol. 1991;24:457–61.
68. Leyden JJ, Marples RR, Kligman AM. Staphylococcus aureus in the lesions of atopic dermatitis. Br J Dermatol. 1974;90:525–30.
69. Zaynoun ST, Aftimos BG, Tenekjian KK, Bahuth N, Kurban AK. Extensive pityriasis alba: a histological histochemical and ultrastructural study. Br J Dermatol. 1983;108:83–90.
70. Hymes SR, Strom EA, Fife C. Radiation dermatitis: clinical presentation, pathophysiology, and treatment 2006. J Am Acad Dermatol. 2006;54:28–46.
71. Hill A, Hanson M, Bogle MA, Duvic M. Severe radiation dermatitis is related to Staphylococcus aureus. Am J Clin Oncol. 2004;27:361–3.
72. Lin SS, Tsai TH, Yang HH. Rare cutaneous side-effect of gefitinib masquerading as superficial dermatophytosis. Clin Exp Dermatol. 2009;34:528–30.
73. Wolf R, Orion E, Matz H. The baboon syndrome or intertriginous drug eruption: a report of eleven cases and a second look at its pathomechanism. Dermatol Online J. 2003;9:2.
74. Tsankov N, Angelova I, Kazandjieva J. Drug-induced psoriasis. Recognition and management. Am J Clin Dermatol. 2000;1:159–65.
75. Prantsidis A, Rigopoulos D, Papatheodorou G, et al. Detection of human herpesvirus 8 in the skin of patients with pityriasis rosea. Acta Derm Venereol. 2009;89:604–6.
76. Levi M, Toh CH, Thachil J, Watson HG. Guidelines for the diagnosis and management of disseminated intravascular coagulation.

British Committee for Standards in Haematology. Br J Haematol. 2009;145:24–33.
77. Weenig RH, Sewell LD, Davis MD, McCarthy JT, Pittelkow MR. Calciphylaxis: natural history, risk factor analysis, and outcome. J Am Acad Dermatol. 2007;56:569–79.
78. Goldsmith DJ. Calciphylaxis, thrombotic diathesis and defects in coagulation regulation. Nephrol Dial Transplant. 1997;12: 1082–3.
79. Friedman PC, Husain S, Grossman ME. Nodular tuberculid in a patient with HIV. J Am Acad Dermatol. 2005;53:S154–6.
80. Fernandes SS, Carvalho J, Leite S, et al. Erythema induratum and chronic hepatitis C infection. J Clin Virol. 2009;44:333–6.
81. Assouline S, Laneuville P, Gambacorti-Passerini C. Panniculitis during dasatinib therapy for imatinib-resistant chronic myelogenous leukemia. N Engl J Med. 2006;354:2623–4.
82. Ugurel S, Lahaye T, Hildenbrand R, et al. Panniculitis in a patient with chronic myelogenous leukaemia treated with imatinib. Br J Dermatol. 2003;149:678–9.
83. Choy AC, Yarnold PR, Brown JE, Kayaloglou GT, Greenberger PA, Patterson R. Virus induced erythema multiforme and Stevens-Johnson syndrome. Allergy Proc. 1995;16:157–61.
84. Hazin R, Ibrahimi OA, Hazin MI, Kimyai-Asadi A. Stevens-Johnson syndrome: pathogenesis, diagnosis, and management. Ann Med. 2008;40:129–38.
85. MacGregor JL, Silvers DN, Grossman ME, Sherman WH. Sorafenib-induced erythema multiforme. J Am Acad Dermatol. 2007;56:527–8.
86. Auquier-Dunant A, Mockenhaupt M, Naldi L, Correia O, Schroder W, Roujeau JC. Correlations between clinical patterns and causes of erythema multiforme majus, Stevens-Johnson syndrome, and toxic epidermal necrolysis: results of an international prospective study. Arch Dermatol. 2002;138:1019–24.
87. French LE, Prins C. Erythema multiforme, Stevens-Johnson syndrome and toxic epidermal necrolysis. In: Bolognia J, Rapini R, editors. Dermatology. Spain: Mosby, Elsevier; 2008. p. 288.
88. Leimert JT, Corder MP, Skibba CA, Gingrich RD. Erythema annulare centrifugum and Hodgkin's disease: association with disease activity. Arch Intern Med. 1979;139:486–7.
89. Carlesimo M, Fidanza L, Mari E, et al. Erythema annulare centrifugum associated with mantle b-cell non-Hodgkin's lymphoma. Acta Derm Venereol. 2009;89:319–20.
90. Panasiti V, Devirgiliis V, Curzio M, et al. Erythema annulare centrifugum as the presenting sign of breast carcinoma. J Eur Acad Dermatol Venereol. 2009;23:318–20.
91. Helbling I, Walewska R, Dyer MJ, Bamford M, Harman KE. Erythema annulare centrifugum associated with chronic lymphocytic leukaemia. Br J Dermatol. 2007;157:1044–5.
92. Krrok G, Waldenstrom JG. Relapsing annular erythema and myeloma successfully treated with cyclophosphamide. Acta Med Scand. 1978;203:289–92.
93. Ravic-Nikolic A, Milicic V, Jovovic-Dagovic B, Ristic G. Gyrate erythema associated with metastatic tumor of gastrointestinal tract. Dermatol Online J. 2006;12:11.
94. Stone SP, Buescher LS. Life-threatening paraneoplastic cutaneous syndromes. Clin Dermatol. 2005;23:301–6.
95. Gantcheva ML, Broshtilova VK, Lalova AI. Necrolytic migratory erythema: the outermost marker for glucagonoma syndrome. Arch Dermatol. 2007;143:1221–2.
96. Geria AN, Holcomb KZ, Scheinfeld NS. Necrolytic acral erythema: a review of the literature. Cutis. 2009;83:309–14.
97. Millot F, Auriol F, Brecheteau P, Guilhot F. Acral erythema in children receiving high-dose methotrexate. Pediatr Dermatol. 1999;16:398–400.
98. Lipworth AD, Robert C, Zhu AX. Hand-foot syndrome (hand-foot skin reaction, palmar-plantar erythrodysesthesia): focus on sorafenib and sunitinib. Oncology. 2009;77:257–71.
99. Marcoval J, Moreno A, Peyr J. Granuloma faciale: a clinicopathological study of 11 cases. J Am Acad Dermatol. 2004;51:269–73.
100. Afsahi V, Kassabian C. Wells syndrome. Cutis 2003;72:209–12; quiz 8.
101. Hurni MA, Gerbig AW, Braathen LR, Hunziker T. Toxocariasis and Wells' syndrome: a causal relationship? Dermatology. 1997;195:325–8.
102. Gleich GJ, Leiferman KM. The hypereosinophilic syndromes: current concepts and treatments. Br J Haematol. 2009;145:271–85.
103. Ogbogu PU, Bochner BS, Butterfield JH, et al. Hypereosinophilic syndrome: a multicenter, retrospective analysis of clinical characteristics and response to therapy. J Allergy Clin Immunol. 2009;124:1319–25.e3.
104. Hymes SR, Turner ML, Champlin RE, Couriel DR. Cutaneous manifestations of chronic graft-versus-host disease. Biol Blood Marrow Transplant. 2006;12:1101–13.
105. Otberg N, Kang H, Alzolibani AA, Shapiro J. Folliculitis decalvans. Dermatol Ther. 2008;21:238–44.
106. Scerri L, Williams HC, Allen BR. Dissecting cellulitis of the scalp: response to isotretinoin. Br J Dermatol. 1996;134:1105–8.
107. Scheinfeld N. Review of scalp alopecia due to a clinically unapparent or minimally apparent neoplasm (SACUMAN). Acta Derm Venereol. 2006;86:387–92.

Part III
Major Etiologic Agents

Chapter 22
Overview of Invasive Fungal Disease in Oncology Patients

Amar Safdar

Abstract The spectrum of invasive fungal disease has changed considerably in the past 2 decade. Since early 1990s, triazole prophylaxis has resulted in a significant decline in cases of invasive candidiasis among patients undergoing hematopoietic stem cell transplantation and those with acute leukemia. Recently, reduced rates of invasive mold disease following echinocandin and antimold triazoles use during the high-risk periods have ushered optimism. This trend in effective drug-mediated prevention has not been without setbacks including unexpected toxicity due to drug–drug interaction, and difficult-to-treat breakthrough fungal disease due to previously uncommon yeasts and filamentous fungi. The rise in virulent non-*albicans Candida* species and non-*Aspergillus* molds has, to some extent, compromised the recent advances in early diagnosis and effective antifungal therapy. As the understanding of hosts' genetic (polymorphisms) vulnerability to fungal disease improves, next generation of diagnostic assays (DNA proliferation, microarray and other technologies) gain clinical validation, approach toward mitigating underlying immune defects with recombinant cytokines, strategies to restore innate and adaptive immune dysfunction become feasible, and target-specific effective antineoplastic therapy is introduced in the cancer fighting armamentarium; these accomplishments in a new era for improved outcomes in cancer patients who are susceptible to invasive fungal disease.

Keywords Fungal infections • Aspergillosis • Candidiasis • Cancer • Leukemia • Bone marrow transplantation

The spectrum of invasive fungal disease has changed considerably in the past 2 decade. Since early 1990s, triazole prophylaxis has resulted in a significant decline in cases of invasive candidiasis among patients undergoing hematopoietic stem cell transplantation and those with high-risk hematologic malignancies [1]. An increase in non-*albicans Candida* breakthrough infections in patients given fluconazole prophylaxis [2, 3] appears to be a small setback as in a recent registry of over 2,000 cases of invasive candidiasis only 3% of these infections were seen in patients following stem cell transplantation whereas, 17% had solid-organ cancer, a group in whom antifungal prophylaxis is not given routinely [4]. Similarly, a significant decline in invasive mold disease has also been shown in randomized trials in patients given micafungin or posaconazole prophylaxis [5, 6]. These drugs have also not been without disadvantages such as unexpected drug–drug interaction and toxicity, problems arising from unpredictable bioavailability of the newer antifungal agents, and difficult-to-treat breakthrough fungal disease due to previously less common yeasts and filamentous fungi [7, 8].

Introduction of echinocandin drugs was an important addition in the existing choices for candidiasis therapy. The agents in this class such as caspofungin and micafungin have shown promising results in neutropenic patients with persistent fever, or for patients with invasive *Candida* species infections including fungemia, acute disseminated candidiasis, intra-abdominal infections, and *Candida* abscesses [9–11]. A similar benefit has been seen in randomized trials for the treatment of invasive aspergillosis in cancer and transplant population. Voriconazole had a significant impact on the overall survival in immunosuppressed patients with IA compared with the old standard of therapy [12]. As these agents have become widely used in susceptible cancer and transplant population, it was not unexpected to find improved outcomes among cancer patients with invasive mold infection. In a recent registry-based analysis of 234 HSCT recipients with fungal disease, the short-term mortality among patients with IA was comparable or less than the crude mortality noted in patients with invasive candidiasis (36 vs. 49%, respectively) [13]. This improved survival has been echoed in several recent reports of invasive aspergillosis in patients with hematologic malignancies and stem cell transplantation [14–16].

The research in understanding the immunopathogenesis of invasive fungal diseases has recently uncovered the central

A. Safdar (✉)
Department of Infectious Diseases, Infection Control, and Employee Health, The University of Texas M.D. Anderson Cancer Center, 1515 Holcombe Boulevard, Houston, TX 77030, USA
e-mail: amarsafdar@gmail.com

role of innate immune defense pathways such as pattern recognition receptors (PRR) in preventing fungal colonization and fungal tissue invasion [17, 18]. These and other similar important advances in elucidating the complex host–pathogen interaction and the role of various facets of immune defenses that come in to play at different stages in fungal infection have opened the door for asking the very basic question; why certain patients with similar risk factors and exposure develop IFD and other do not? The association in hosts' genetic polymorphism and fungal colonization, invasive fungal disease and more importantly predictor of response to antifungal therapy, and disease recurrence remains in the early phase of exploration. There have been certain interesting observations, such as polymorphisms in genes encoding for Dectin-1 may increase the risk for colonization due to *Candida* species [19]. Individuals with Dectin-1 gene polymorphism along with other immune pathways such as TLR-4, IL-10, TNF receptor-2, and plasminogen may also have an increased susceptibility for invasive aspergillosis [20–25]. However, much work needs to be done to understand clinical impact of these apparently random single gene or gene-cluster polymorphisms on susceptibility for fungal disease, disease progression, response to antifungal therapy, and in what group of patients it is suitable to consider immunotherapy.

The immunotherapy for fungal infection is also gaining traction; this field has received a boost from the recent developments on understanding the host–pathogen immune interaction and role of various components of innate and more importantly adaptive cellular immune effector pathways in the development of invasive fungal disease [26–28]. Since the use of donor granulocyte transfusion in the early twentieth century, and awaking in the 1960s, and reawaking in the past decade, little progress was made in this field [29, 30]. This changed with the development of recombinant myeloid growth factors such as G-CSF and GM-CSF, furthermore, Th1 cytokines like interferon gamma that favorably influenced the natural course of invasive fungal disease in animal experiments and in nonrandomized clinical studies [31–33]. The field of adaptive immunotherapy for fungal disease is also gaining momentum in the recent years [34, 35] and future prospects look promising.

In conclusion, this section focuses on all clinically relevant aspects of invasive fungal disease in the immunosuppressed cancer and stem cell transplant patients. These include epidemiology, immunopathogenesis, clinical presentation, and diagnosis. The discussion on antifungal therapy is supplemented with chapters relating to issues regarding molecular and clinical bases for drug resistance, pharmacokinetic and pharmacodynamics of the antifungal drugs in the special host. The topic of current and future strategies for restoring innate and adaptive immune dysfunction is also presented. The recent accomplishments ushers an era for improved outcomes in cancer patients susceptible to and being treated for invasive fungal disease.

References

1. Goodman JL, Winston DJ, Greenfield RA, Chandrasekar PH, Fox B, Kaizer H, et al. A controlled trial of fluconazole to prevent fungal infections in patients undergoing bone marrow transplantation. N Engl J Med. 1992;326:845–51.
2. Wingard JR, Merz WG, Rinaldi MG, Johnson TR, Karp JE, Saral R. Increase in *Candida krusei* infection among patients with bone marrow transplantation and neutropenia treated prophylactically with fluconazole. N Engl J Med. 1991;325:1274–7.
3. Safdar A, van Rhee F, Henslee-Downey JP, Singhal S, Mehta J. *Candida glabrata* and *Candida krusei* fungemia after high-risk allogeneic marrow transplantation: no adverse effect of low-dose fluconazole prophylaxis on incidence and outcome. Bone Marrow Transplant. 2001;28:873–8.
4. Horn DL, Neofytos D, Anaissie EJ, et al. Epidemiology and outcomes of candidemia in 2019 patients: data from the prospective antifungal therapy alliance registry. Clin Infect Dis. 2009;48:1695–703.
5. van Burik JA, Ratanatharathorn V, Stepan DE, Miller CB, Lipton JH, Vesole DH, et al. Micafungin versus fluconazole for prophylaxis against invasive fungal infections during neutropenia in patients undergoing hematopoietic stem cell transplantation. Clin Infect Dis. 2004;39:1407–16.
6. Cornely OA, Maertens J, Winston DJ, Perfect J, Ullmann AJ, Walsh TJ, et al. Posaconazole vs. fluconazole or itraconazole prophylaxis in patients with neutropenia. N Engl J Med. 2007;356:348–59.
7. Marty FM, Cosimi LA, Baden LR. Breakthrough zygomycosis after voriconazole treatment in recipients of hematopoietic stem-cell transplants. N Engl J Med. 2004;350:950–2.
8. Kontoyiannis DP, Lionakis MS, Lewis RE, Chamilos G, Healy M, Perego C, et al. Zygomycosis in a tertiary-care cancer center in the era of Aspergillus-active antifungal therapy: a case-control observational study of 27 recent cases. J Infect Dis. 2005;191:1350–60.
9. Walsh TJ, Teppler H, Donowitz GR, Maertens JA, Baden LR, Dmoszynska A, et al. Caspofungin versus liposomal amphotericin B for empirical antifungal therapy in patients with persistent fever and neutropenia. N Engl J Med. 2004;351:1391–402.
10. Mora-Duarte J, Betts R, Rotstein C, Colombo AL, Thompson-Moya L, Smietana J, et al. Comparison of caspofungin and amphotericin B for invasive candidiasis. N Engl J Med. 2002;347:2020–9.
11. Pappas PG, Rotstein CM, Betts RF, Nucci M, Talwar D, De Waele JJ, et al. Micafungin versus caspofungin for treatment of candidemia and other forms of invasive candidiasis. Clin Infect Dis. 2007;45:883–93.
12. Herbrecht R, Denning DW, Patterson TF, Bennett JE, Greene RE, Oestmann JW, et al. Voriconazole versus amphotericin B for primary therapy of invasive aspergillosis. N Engl J Med. 2002;347:408–15.
13. Neofytos D, Horn D, Anaissie E, et al. Epidemiology and outcome of invasive fungal infection in adult hematopoietic stem cell transplant recipients: analysis of Multicenter Prospective Antifungal Therapy (PATH) Alliance registry. Clin Infect Dis. 2009;48:265–73.
14. Upton A, Kirby KA, Carpenter P, et al. Invasive aspergillosis following hematopoietic cell transplantation: outcomes and prognostic factors associated with mortality. Clin Infect Dis. 2007;44:531–40.
15. Nivoix Y, Velten M, Letscher-Bru V, et al. Factors associated with overall and attributable mortality in invasive aspergillosis. Clin Infect Dis. 2008;47:1176–84.
16. Cordonnier C, Ribaud P, Herbrecht R, et al. Prognostic factors for death due to invasive aspergillosis after hematopoietic stem cell transplantation: a 1-year retrospective study of consecutive patients at French transplantation centers. Clin Infect Dis. 2006;42:955–63.
17. Lamaris GA, Lewis RE, Chamilos G, et al. Caspofungin mediated b-glucan unmasking and enhancement of human polymorphonuclear neutrophil activity against Aspergillus and non-Aspergillus hypae. J Infect Dis. 2008;198:186–92.

18. Hohl TM, Feldmesser M, Perlin DS, Pamer EG. Caspofungin modulates inflammatory responses to Aspergillus fumigatus through stage-specific effects on fungal b-glucan exposure. J Infect Dis. 2008;198:176–85.
19. Plantinga TS, van der Velden WJ, Ferwerda B, et al. Early stop polymorphism in human DECTIN-1 is associated with increased candida colonization in hematopoietic stem cell transplant recipients. Clin Infect Dis. 2009;49:724–32.
20. Bochud PY, Chien JW, Marr KA, et al. Toll-like receptor 4 polymorphisms and aspergillosis in stem-cell transplantation. N Engl J Med. 2008;359:1766–77.
21. Carvalho A, Cunha C, Carotti A, et al. Polymorphisms in Toll-like receptor genes and susceptibility to infections in allogeneic stem cell transplantation. Exp Hematol. 2009;37:1022–9.
22. Ferwerda B, McCall MB, Alonso S, et al. TLR4 polymorphisms, infectious diseases, and evolutionary pressure during migration of modern humans. Proc Natl Acad Sci USA. 2007;104:16645–50.
23. Seo KW, Kim DH, Sohn SK, et al. Protective role of interleukin-10 promoter gene polymorphism in the pathogenesis of invasive pulmonary aspergillosis after allogeneic stem cell transplantation. Bone Marrow Transplant. 2005;36:1089–95.
24. Sainz J, Perez E, Hassan L, et al. Variable number of tandem repeats of TNF receptor type 2 promoter as genetic biomarker of susceptibility to develop invasive pulmonary aspergillosis. Hum Immunol. 2007;68:41–50.
25. Zaas AK, Liao G, Chien JW, et al. Plasminogen alleles influence susceptibility to invasive aspergillosis. PLoS Genet. 2008;4:e1000101.
26. Safdar A. Difficulties with fungal infections in acute myelogenous leukemia patients: immune enhancement strategies. Oncologist. 2007;12 Suppl 2:2–6.
27. Safdar A. Strategies to enhance immune function in hematopoietic transplantation recipients who have fungal infections. Bone Marrow Transplant. 2006;38(5):327–37.
28. Safdar A. Immunomodulation therapy for invasive aspergillosis – discussion on myeloid growth factors, recombinant cytokines and antifungal drug immune modulation. Curr Fungal Infect Rep. 2010;4:1–7.
29. Freireich EJ, Levin RH, Whang J, Carbone PP, Bronson W, Morse EE. The function and face of transfused leukocytes from donors with chronic myelocytic leukemia in leukopenic recipients. Ann NY Acad Sci. 1964;113:1081–90.
30. Seidel MG, Peters C, Wacker A, Northoff H, Moog R, Boehme A, et al. Randomized phase III study of granulocyte transfusions in neutropenic patients. Bone Marrow Transplant. 2008;42(10): 679–84.
31. Safdar A, Rodriguez G, Ohmagari N, Kontoyiannis DP, Rolston KV, Raad II, et al. The safety of interferon-gamma-1b therapy for invasive fungal infections after hematopoietic stem cell transplantation. Cancer. 2005;103:731–9.
32. Gil-Lamaignere C, Winn RM, Simitsopoulou M, Maloukou A, Walsh TJ, Roilides E. Inteferon gamma and granulocyte-macrophage colony-stimulating factor augment the antifungal activity of human polymorphonuclear leukocytes against Scedosporium spp.: comparison with Aspergillus spp. Med Mycol. 2005;43:253–60.
33. Dignani MC, Rex JH, Chan KW, Dow G, deMagalhaes-Silverman M, Maddox A, et al. Immunomodulation with interferon-gamma and colony-stimulating factors for refractory fungal infections in patients with leukemia. Cancer. 2005;104:199–204.
34. Tramsen L, Beck O, Schuster FR, et al. Generation and characterization of anti-Candida T cells as potential immunotherapy in patients with Candida infection after allogeneic hematopoietic stem-cell transplantation. J Infect Dis. 2007;196:485–92.
35. Tramsen L, Koehl U, Tonn T, et al. Clinical-scale generation of human anti-Aspergillus T cells for adoptive immunotherapy. Bone Marrow Transplant. 2009;43:13–9.

Chapter 23
Diagnosis of Invasive Fungal Disease

Dionissios Neofytos and Kieren Marr

Abstract The diagnosis of invasive fungal infections (IFI) relies on the critical assessment of clinical presentation, associated risk factors, and careful interpretation of the appropriate diagnostic tests. Frequently, clinicians have to initiate antifungal therapy based on their clinical suspicion and without having made a definitive diagnosis, particularly in cancer or other critically ill patients. To complicate diagnosis, isolation of fungal organisms does not imply pathogenicity, especially from nonsterile sites, and may not necessitate treatment. Hence, making the diagnosis of an IFI in clinical practice requires suspicion of disease, mostly on the acuity and severity of clinical signs and symptoms, and necessitates careful consideration of findings. In this chapter we will review the traditional diagnostic modalities (culture, histopathology, and imaging) and recently developed diagnostic tools (BG, PCR, and GM EIA) for the diagnosis of IFIs. This review will focus on the diagnosis of the most commonly identified IFIs in cancer patients, specifically invasive candidiasis (IC), invasive aspergillosis (IA), and zygomycosis.

Keywords Invasive fungal infection • PCR • Galactomannan assay • Fungal antigen assays • CT scan • Beta glucan • Candidiasis • Aspergillosis • Zygomycosis

Introduction

The diagnosis of invasive fungal infections (IFI) relies on the critical assessment of clinical presentation, associated risk factors, and careful interpretation of the appropriate diagnostic tests. Frequently, clinicians have to initiate antifungal therapy based on their clinical suspicion and without having made a definitive diagnosis, particularly in cancer or other critically ill patients. To complicate diagnosis, isolation of fungal organisms does not imply pathogenicity, especially from nonsterile sites, and may not necessitate treatment. Hence, making the diagnosis of an IFI in clinical practice requires suspicion of disease, depends mostly on the acuity and severity of clinical signs and symptoms, and necessitates careful consideration of findings.

The identification of a yeast or mold in the mycology laboratory has – historically – been based on their appearance under the microscope and growth in culture. Isolation varies by the media used, the experience of the mycology laboratory personnel, and the occasional slow and cumbersome growth of certain fungi. In addition, blood cultures, considered the reference diagnostic test for the diagnosis of candidemia, have been associated with a sensitivity ranging from 50 to 70% [1–7]. Similarly, the sensitivity of tissue and bronchoalveolar lavage (BAL) cultures for *Aspergillus* spp. has ranged between 30–52 and 0–67%, respectively [8–21]. The need for faster and more sensitive diagnostic tests has led to the recent development and implementation of multiple tests to augment detection of microbial components, including the β-D-glucan (BG), fungal polymerase chain reaction (PCR), and the double-sandwich galactomannan enzyme immunoassay (GM EIA). However, the study of diagnostic tests for IFIs is limited mainly due to the absence of a reference standard other than histopathologic confirmation of diagnosis and insensitivity of this "gold standard." In this chapter we will review the traditional diagnostic modalities (culture, histopathology, and imaging) and recently developed diagnostic tools (BG, PCR, and GM EIA) for the diagnosis of IFIs. This review will focus on the diagnosis of the most commonly identified IFIs in cancer patients, specifically invasive candidiasis (IC), invasive aspergillosis (IA), and zygomycosis. The diagnostics of other yeasts and molds and endemic fungi, rarely encountered in cancer patients, will not be reviewed.

D. Neofytos (✉)
Division of Infectious Diseases, The Johns Hopkins Hospital,
600 N. Wolfe Street, Baltimore, MD 21287, USA
e-mail: dneofyt1@jhmi.edu

Invasive Candidiasis

Clinical Syndromes

Two major clinical syndromes of IC among cancer patients will be discussed in this section: candidemia and hepatosplenic candidiasis. Cancer patients share multiple risk factors for candidemia by virtue of their underlying disease and therapies administered. Most commonly candidemia results from translocation of *Candida* spp. through the gastrointestinal tract due to mucositis caused by chemotherapy. In addition, most cancer patients have a central intravenous catheter, presenting additional risks for candidemia. Candidemia may be sustained despite administration of appropriate therapy, present as sepsis, and rapidly disseminate to involve other organs (e.g., endophthalmitis, osteomyelitis). A diffuse maculopapular skin rash may occasionally be observed among neutropenic patients with IC (Fig. 23.1). Patients with hematologic malignancies may also develop hepatosplenic candidiasis due to invasion of the portal venous system and subsequent spread of *Candida* spp. into the liver or/and spleen (see Sect. III). Hepatosplenic candidiasis may present with persistent fever, severe right-sided abdominal pain, abnormal liver function tests, and multiple liver, spleen, and/or kidney micronodular lesions on imaging tests.

Diagnosis of Candidemia

Microbiology and Culture

Although widely considered the "gold standard," blood cultures for the diagnosis of candidemia have been associated with a sensitivity historically ranging from 21.3 to 54% [1–7, 22]. The advent of lysis centrifugation has increased the diagnostic yield of blood cultures for the diagnosis of candidemia, albeit with limitations including higher rates of contamination and additional cost and required personnel [23]. For instance, a retrospective review of 41 confirmed cases of IC among 803 autopsies showed that blood cultures with lysis centrifugation were positive in 28 and 58% of patients with single-organ and disseminated IC, respectively [1]. Notably, the majority of patients with disseminated disease had a hematologic malignancy. The automated continuous monitoring blood culture systems and use of special fungal media have been used to increase our ability to identify *Candida* species [24]. Diagnosis has been reported to be better and faster when using the Mycosis IC/F medium, particularly for patients with *C. glabrata* candidemia [24]. Although special "fungal" blood cultures are not widely utilized, it appears that blood cultures in special media may increase the diagnostic yield. Prospective studies in specific patient populations are required before definitive conclusions can be drawn.

Candida speciation: The identification of *Candida* spp. may provide significant information about the source of candidemia (e.g., association between *C. parapsilosis* and intravenous central catheters) and the selection of the appropriate antifungal agent. The latter can be based on specific *Candida* spp. susceptibility patterns (e.g., *C. krusei* – resistance to fluconazole, *C. lusitaniae* – resistance to polyenes) or/and susceptibility testing, particularly important for *C. glabrata* (against the azoles) and *C. parapsilosis* (against the echinocandins). Historically, a germ tube test is performed for the differentiation of *C. albicans* (or/and *C. dubliniensis*) from other *Candida* species. Results can be available within 1–2 h, but the test requires sufficient growth of *Candida* that may further delay the diagnosis for 1–3 days. More recently,

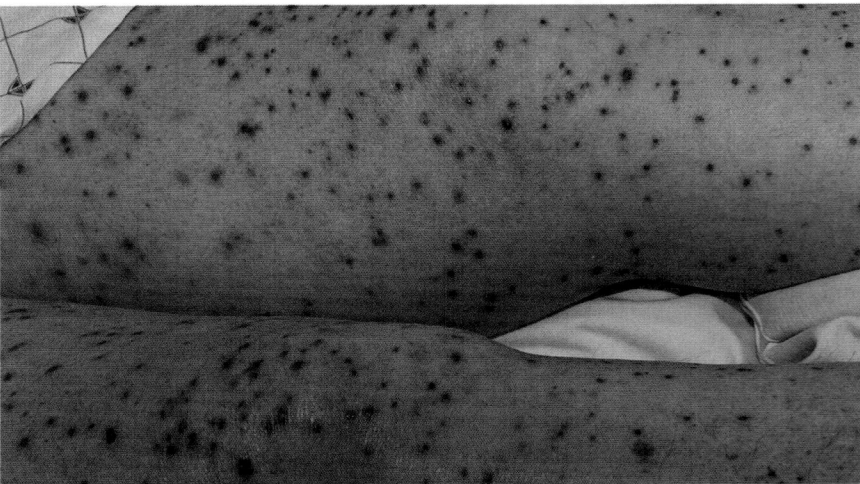

Fig. 23.1 Disseminated maculopapular skin rash in a neutropenic patient with acute myelogenous leukemia with *C. tropicalis* candidemia

the germ tube test has been applied directly on positive blood cultures with a sensitivity and specificity of 87.1 and 100%, respectively, for the identification of *C. albicans* when compared to the results obtained from fungal colonies [25]. In clinical practice, the identification of germ tube-positive yeasts would imply the presence of *C. albicans,* usually susceptible to fluconazole. Germ tube-negative yeasts may include *C. krusei* which is inherently resistant to fluconazole and *C. glabrata* which may be or become resistant to fluconazole and other azoles. Notably, not all germ tube-negative *Candida* spp. are azole-resistant, as *C. tropicalis* and *C. parapsilosis* remain highly susceptible to fluconazole and *C. krusei* is susceptible to voriconazole.

The Peptide Nucleic Acid Fluorescent In Situ Hybridization (PNA-FISH) test has been studied and recently introduced in clinical practice for the rapid identification of *Candida* species. The PNA-FISH for *C. albicans* has had a sensitivity, specificity, positive, and negative predictive value of 99, 100, 100, and 99.3%, respectively [26]. More recently, a multicenter study evaluated the performance of a rapid two-color PNA-FISH assay for detection of *C. albicans* and *C. glabrata* directly from positive blood culture bottles [25]. Among 197 routine blood cultures positive for yeast by Gram stain, PNA-FISH test detected *C. albicans* and *C. glabrata* with a sensitivity of 98.7 and 100%, respectively, and a specificity of 100% for both. More data are required for the use of PNA-FISH test for the diagnosis of IC due to other *Candida* species.

Beta-D-Glucan Assay

Nonculture diagnostic tests, such as the BG assay, may be useful adjuncts for the diagnosis of candidemia. BG is a cell wall component of a wide variety of fungi and can be detected by its ability to activate factor G of the horseshoe crab coagulation cascade [27]. There are two different assays for the detection of BG: the Fungitec-G glucan (Seikagaku) and the Glucatell (or Fungitell) test (Associates of Cape Cod). The reagents used in these two tests are derived from different species of horseshoe crabs: the amebocyte enzymes from *Tachypleus tridentatus* for the Fungitec assay and the enzymes from *Limulus polyphemus* amebocytes for the Glucatell assay [27]. The former test has been extensively studied and used in Japan, whereas the latter has been cleared by the United States Food and Drug Administration (FDA) for the diagnosis of IFIs.

In one of the preliminary studies, BG was studied in serum samples from 283 patients with newly diagnosed acute myelogenous leukemia or myelodysplastic syndrome [27]. Twenty patients developed a proven or probable IFI; 11 of these IFIs were IC. Using a predefined cutoff value of 60 pg/mL, the sensitivity and specificity of a single positive specimen was 100 and 90%, respectively. The positive and negative predictive value of the test was 43 and 100%, respectively. Notably, BG was positive at a median of 10 days before the clinical diagnosis of a proven or probable IFI was made. In another case-control study including patients from six different clinical sites in the US, a single blood sample was drawn from each subject within 72 h of the diagnosis of an IFI [28]. In that study, only a minority of patients had an underlying malignancy (28.8%) and IC was the most common diagnosis: 111 cases of proven ($n=107$) and probable ($n=4$) IC. Using a BG cutoff of 60 pg/mL, the assay had a sensitivity of 82.6% for IC. Notably, sensitivity differed among *Candida* spp., with the assay performing worse for *C. parapsilosis* (sensitivity: 72.2%).

Based on the above, the BG appears to be a promising tool for the diagnosis of candidemia in patients with hematologic malignancies, albeit with certain limitations. The optimal frequency of testing has not been established as yet. False positive results have been reported in patients requiring hemodialysis with cellulose membranes, use of cotton gauze and surgical sponges, administration of immunoglobulin products or antitumor polysaccharides (e.g., lentina, polysaccharide K, schizophyllan) [28–32]. There have also been reports of false positive GM results associated with bacterial infections (e.g., *P. aeruginosa, S. pneumoniae*), perhaps due to production of BG or similar molecules [33, 34]. Other limitations of the test include the variable performance among different *Candida* spp. (e.g., *C. parapsilosis*) and relative lack of specificity (other fungi, e.g., *Aspergillus* spp., *Pneumocystis* spp. produce this antigen). Finally, one needs to be considerate of the relatively low positive predictive value when applied on patient populations with a low prevalence of candidemia; hence, careful targeting of the assay to high-risk populations is necessary [35–37].

Polymerase Chain Reaction

There are few data to support the use of a PCR assay for the diagnosis of candidemia in cancer patients. In a study of 72 patients with a hematologic malignancy and neutropenic fever from Italy, the sensitivity and specificity of PCR for the diagnosis of IC were 92.9 and 97.6%, respectively [38]. Another group from Brazil evaluated the efficacy of a PCR assay for the diagnosis of candidemia in 225 patients with high risks [39]. With the minority of study subjects being cancer patients, the reported sensitivity, specificity, positive and negative predictive value were 72.1, 91.2, 65.9, and 93.2%, respectively. Similar observations come from studies on nonneutropenic intensive care unit patients [40]. Considering the relatively low sensitivity of blood cultures, PCR may prove to be a significant adjunct for the diagnosis of candidemia particularly in high risk patients, such as cancer patients. However, a major limitation of most PCR assays is their relative lack of specificity, mostly due to high rates of contamination. The test may not be applicable to smaller institutions or resource-poor countries due to requirements for highly trained personnel, special equipment, and higher costs. The above will likely result in running PCR assays for the diagnosis of candidemia in batches rather than on a daily (or even more frequent) basis, thus minimally affecting time to diagnosis compared to more traditional diagnostic tests. Widespread use awaits standardization, commercialization, and further study.

Diagnosis of Hepatosplenic Candidiasis

Hepatosplenic candidiasis develops typically after *Candida* spp. invade the portal vasculature, disseminating to the liver and/or spleen. Clinical manifestations typically coincide with inflammation developed after resolution of neutropenia. Definitive diagnosis requires biopsy of hepatic lesions that may reveal hyphal forms consistent with *Candida* species. The diagnosis is suggested by the presence of multiple lesions of the liver and spleen, occasionally described as "bull's eye" appearing on abdominal CT scan or magnetic resonance imaging (MRI) (Fig. 23.2) [41]. Frequency of candidemia among patients with hepatosplenic candidiasis has historically ranged between 8 and 19% [41, 42]. While the constellation of fever, abdominal pain, elevated alkaline phosphatase, and liver lesions is suggestive of hepatosplenic candidiasis, multiple organisms, including bacterial and filamentous fungi, can cause a similar syndrome. Clinicians should also be aware that lesions (and symptoms) can get worse with progressive inflammation, despite appropriate antifungal therapy.

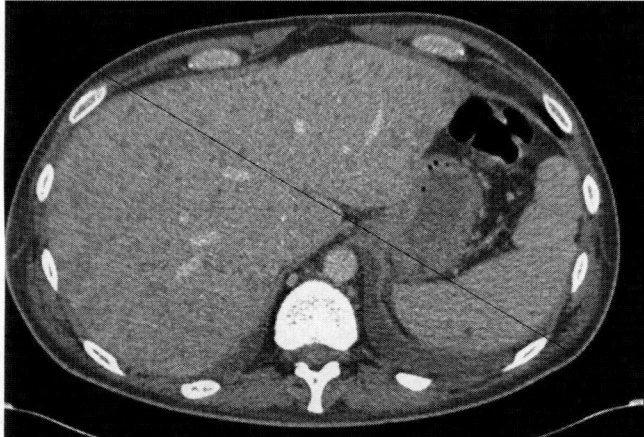

Fig. 23.2 Thirty nine-year old male patient with a history of acute myelogenous leukemia presenting with neutropenic fever, abdominal pain, elevated liver function tests and liver and spleen lesions on abdominal CT, consistent with hepatospenic candidiasis

Invasive Mold Infections

Clinical Syndromes

Invasive mold infections among immunocompromised hosts may present with local invasion (e.g., sinusitis, pulmonary involvement) or disseminate to involve multiple sites. Local invasion of the sinuses and lungs follows mold inhalation, and skin involvement most frequently occurs through direct inoculation. Spread of the organisms to other sites may happen contiguously (e.g., sinus to orbit and brain) or hematogenously (e.g., brain, skin, liver). Pulmonary invasive disease is the most commonly observed clinical syndrome due to molds among cancer patients. Multiple molds may cause disease, including *Aspergillus* spp., the Zygomycetes, and *Fusarium* species. Few clinical clues are typical with presentation. One classic finding is the presence of multiple maculopapular to ulcerated skin lesions, which, especially in the presence of positive blood cultures, is highly suggestive of fusariosis (Fig. 23.3) [43]. However, most other molds, including *Aspergillus* and the Zygomycetes may disseminate to involve the skin.

Diagnosis of Invasive Mold Infections

Imaging

Invasive mold infections affecting the lungs may present with different patterns on a chest CT, including small or large nodules, patchy, segmental, or wedge-shaped consolidations, peribronchial infiltrates with a tree-in-bud distribution, and cavitation [44, 45]. Systematic use of chest CT for the diagnosis of pulmonary IA can significantly decrease the time to diagnosis of IA among neutropenic patients [46, 47]. Improved outcomes based on early diagnosis of pulmonary IA with the use of the halo sign were observed in a study that analyzed the radiographic findings from 235 patients with pulmonary IA who participated in the Global Comparative Aspergillosis Study [48, 49]. Patients with a halo sign were more likely to survive by 12 weeks (71 vs. 53%, $p<0.01$) and respond to the administered treatment (52 vs. 29%, $p<0.001$), regardless of neutropenic status or underlying condition [48]. This may be, in part, due to the earlier recognition of IA and prompt initiation of antifungal treatment at an earlier stage leading to improved outcomes.

Two CT patterns have been associated with early and late pulmonary IA: the "halo" and the "crescent" sign, respectively (Fig. 23.4). Kuhlman et al. first described the significance of the halo sign on a chest CT for the diagnosis of IA in patients with acute leukemia [50]. This refers to a nodular

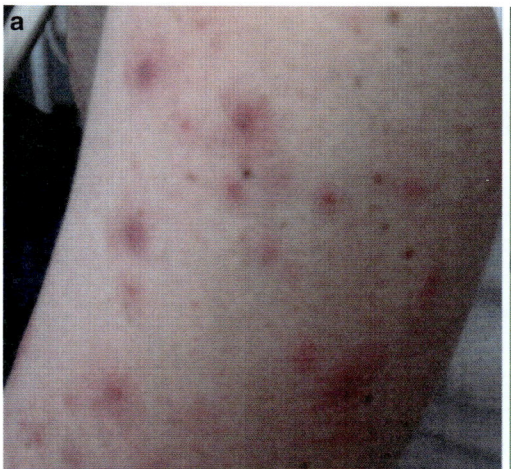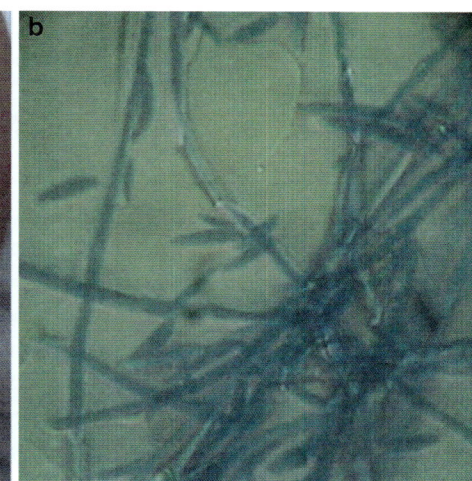

Fig. 23.3 Nineteen-year old male patient with relapsed acute myelogenous leukemia presenting 5 days after a mismatched related allogeneic HSCT with fever and multiple maculopapular skin lesions (**a**). His skin biopsy and blood cultures were positive for *Fusarium* species (**b**)

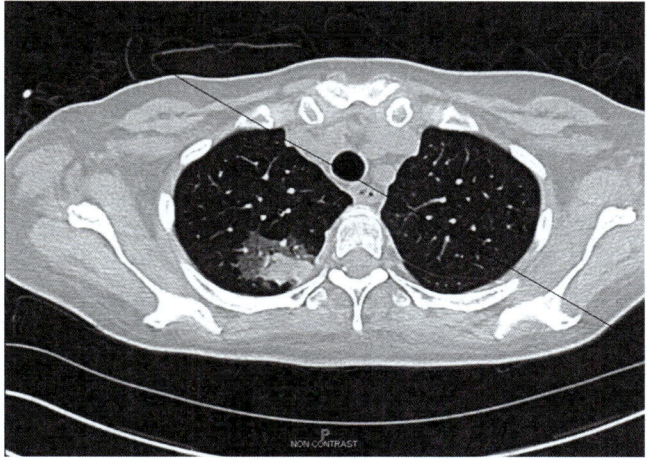

Fig. 23.4 Thirty nine-year old female patient with relapsed acute myelogenous leukemia presenting 3 months after a matched unrelated allogeneic HSCT recipient with cough, fever, and mild dyspnea. The patient was being treated with high dose corticosteroids for severe skin graft versus host disease. She was diagnosed with pulmonary invasive aspergillosis based on the halo sign shown on her chest CT and the presence of *A. fumigatus* in her bronchoalveolar lavage

lesion or mass surrounded by a halo of alveolar hemorrhage, showing as ground-glass attenuation on CT [50–53]. The halo sign may appear in 60–93% of neutropenic patients with pulmonary IA [3, 44–46, 48, 54]. Although the halo sign has been most frequently associated with pulmonary IA, other infections can present similarly, including other filamentous fungi (e.g., zygomycosis) and bacterial infections (e.g., *Pseudomonas* spp.) [53, 55, 56].

Historically, zygomycosis has been associated with sizable nodular, occasionally cavitary, lung lesions [57–59]. However, the majority of old studies have included mixed patient populations, with diabetic patients representing a significant proportion [57–59]. In addition, most lesions described were based on chest XRs rather than CT scans [57–59]. More recent data suggest that presence of multiple (>10) lung nodular lesions (OR: 19.8; $p=0.012$) or a pleural effusion (OR: 5.07; $p=0.042$) may be more suggestive of pulmonary zygomycosis vs. IA among patients with an underlying hematologic malignancy [60]. Notably, the presence of the halo or crescent signs, cavity, or mass was not found to be a predictor of pulmonary zygomycosis. Although the above findings need to be further validated, they could – potentially – be useful in the differential diagnosis of hematologic patients with a suspected pulmonary invasive mold infection on imaging.

It is important to remember that these classic findings – halo and cavitation – are common in neutropenic patients. However, more recent studies are emphasizing that nonneutropenic patients with high risks, such as allogeneic HSCT recipients postengraftment with graft-versus-host-disease (GVHD), may present with variable radiographic findings. For instance, it has been reported that bronchopneumonias or focal infiltrates may be more common compared to isolated nodules in nonneutropenic allogeneic HSCT recipients with documented IA [61].

Histopathology and Microbiology

Histopathologic confirmation of sterile tissue invasion remains the "gold standard" to establish a proven diagnosis of an invasive mold infection [62]. The presence of septate narrow hyphal forms with acute angle branching is suggestive of *Aspergillus* spp., but other filamentous fungi (e.g., *Fusarium* spp., *Penicillium* spp., *Scedosporium* spp.) may look similar under the microscope. The Zygomycetes appear with characteristic broad, nonseptate hyphae with right-angle branching when specimens are stained with calcofluor white or methenamine silver stains. Although suggestive, histopathologic findings do not definitively identify the pathogen. Microbiologic identification of the fungal genus and species should be pursued if feasible, as it may have important implications in the management of cancer patients with fungal infections.

However, culture of filamentous fungi is not easy. Sensitivity rates of sputum cultures for the diagnosis of pulmonary IA have ranged between 15 and 69%. Similarly, the sensitivity of tissue and BAL cultures for *Aspergillus* spp. has ranged between 30–52 and 0–67%, respectively [8–21]. Sensitivity rates of sputum and BAL cultures for the diagnosis of zygomycosis have been in the range of 25% [63]. Hence, cultures may be negative despite presence of disease. In addition, performing an invasive procedure (e.g., bronchoscopy) or obtaining tissue for a biopsy may not always be feasible. To further complicate the diagnostic process, isolation of a fungal organism does not necessarily imply pathogenicity. Fungal pathogens (e.g., *A. niger*) may represent mere colonization of the airway and incidentally growth in a sputum or BAL culture. Hence, interpretation of culture results necessitates careful consideration of the host and clinical presentation.

Galactomannan Antigen

Reiss and Lechmann were the first to report the detection of *Aspergillus* antigens for the diagnosis of IA [64]. Since then, significant progress has been made, eventually leading to the availability of commercial assays. Galactomannan is a polysaccharide present in the cell wall of *Aspergillus*, which is released during the growth of *Aspergillus* hyphae. Currently, the Platelia sandwich enzyme-linked immunosorbent assay (ELISA; BioRad, Marnes-La-Coquette, France) is the assay that has been most extensively studied and used. Positive and negative controls are included in each assay as well as a standardized serum specimen with 1 ng/mL of GM. The process may take up to 3–4 h and the assays are run in batches in most institutions. The optical density index (ODI) of each sample is used to define positivity, calculated by dividing the OD of each sample with that of the threshold control. ODI cutoffs have ranged between 0.5 and 1.5 in different studies, with an ODI of 0.5 suggested as the cutoff by the FDA. The Platelia GM EIA has been approved by the FDA for use only on serum samples; approval of the test on BAL is under evaluation.

The performance of the serum GM EIA has varied among studies, depending on the patient population and age, number of serum samples required to define positivity, certainty of diagnosis, administration of concomitant antibacterial and antifungal agents, and the ODI cutoff used [49, 65–71]. Sensitivity and specificity have differed based on the ODI cutoff ranging from 64–78 to 81–95% for ODI of 1.5 and 0.5 ng/mL, respectively [72] In a meta-analysis of 27 studies with a total of 4,000 patients, the overall sensitivity and specificity of the GM EIA for the diagnosis of IA (proven and probable) were 61% (95% CI 59–63%) and 93% (95% CI 92–94%), respectively [73]. The assay appeared to perform better in patients with an underlying hematological malignancy or among HSCT vs. solid organ transplant (SOT) recipients [73]. The latter may, in part, be due to the low prevalence of IA among most SOT recipients and the small number of SOT recipients included in these studies. The use of GM EIA may significantly quicken the diagnosis of pulmonary IA and affect the costs associated the management of this infection [66, 74].

Administration of piperacillin-tazobactam or amoxicillin-clavulanate has been associated with false positive results [47, 75–78]. In fact, in one study piperacillin-tazobactam was the only factor significantly associated with false positive GM EIA results in 38 of 42 (90.5%) patients with positive GM EIAs; the GM EIA was positive in 3 of 4 batches of piperacillin-tazobactam in this study [77]. The presence of organisms that share cross-reacting antigens (e.g., *Penicillium* spp., *Paecilomyces* spp., *Alternaria* spp., *Cladosporium herbarum*, *Acremonium* spp., *Alternaria alternata*, *Fusarium oxysporum*, *Wangiella dermatitidis*, and *Rhodotorula rubra*) may also decrease the specificity of the test [65, 79]. Severe mucositis and gastrointestinal GHVD following HSCT can occasionally lead to false positive results, likely due to translocation of GM across the intestinal mucosa during periods of reduced mucosal integrity. Younger age has been associated with lower specificity rates, predominantly attributed to the high concentration of GM in children's food (e.g., cereals) [49]. Recent data suggest that the performance of the GM EIA may be variable for the different *Aspergillus* spp. with sensitivity being lower among patients with IA due to *A. fumigatus* (13%) compared to non-*fumigatus Aspergillus* spp. (49%; $p<0.0001$) [80]. Finally, based on animal and human data, the performance of serum GM appears – in part – to depend on the fungal burden [66, 81–87]. In fact, administration of antifungal agents with mold activity has been found to decrease the sensitivity of GM EIA [67, 80].

GM EIA in other than blood specimens: GM is a water-soluble carbohydrate, and thus can be detected in fluids other than blood, including urine, BAL, cerebrospinal fluid (CSF), and pleural fluid. Sensitivity of the GM EIA in BAL has ranged between 60 and 100%, depending on the patient population studied, ODI cutoff used, certainty of diagnosis, and bronchoscopy performance [88–95]. False positive assays can occur when BAL is contaminated with galactomannan in the setting of airway colonization. Despite, specificity has been reported to be as high as 95% among HSCT and lung transplant recipients [89, 93]. In a case-control study among HSCT recipients, Musher et al. reported a sensitivity and specificity of 76 and 94%, respectively, for the diagnosis of IA using the GM EIA on BAL samples at an ODI cutoff of 0.5 [89]. Notably, among 22 culture-negative BAL specimens from patients with IA, the sensitivity of the GM EIA was 59%, suggesting that more than half of HSCT recipients with a negative culture on their BAL could be diagnosed with this assay. In fact, 25 additional procedures were performed among 18 HSCT recipients with negative BAL cultures; the authors estimated that 8 of 12 additional bronchoscopies and 8 of 13 lung biopsies might have been avoided if the GM EIA was applied on the initial BAL [89]. The combination of GM EIA and early chest CT may result in earlier diagnosis of IA [82, 83]. Many institutions have started using the GM EIA on BAL specimens pending the clearance of the assay by the FDA.

The performance of GM testing in the urine has varied based on the patient population and method used for the detection of GM [96–101]. The sensitivity and specificity of antigenuria using the latex agglutination test among HSCT recipients with autopsy-proven IA were 57 and 53%, respectively, compared to 43 and 53% for antigenemia [96]. It has been suggested that the diagnostic yield of the urine GM EIA may increase if urine is concentrated by tenfold [100]. False positive results of urine GM have ranged between 8 and 47%, attributed to a variety of factors, including urine contamination with *Aspergillus* spp. [96, 98, 99]. GM can also be detected in the CSF of patients with central nervous system or pleural fluid of patients with lung disease, although most results come from case reports/series and more prospective data are required to make further conclusions [102–104].

Beta-D-Glucan Assay

The BG is a cell wall component of a variety of fungi, including *Aspergillus* species. It is being evaluated as a diagnostic aid for numerous IFIs, given its lack of specificity, with reasonable reported sensitivities. The sensitivity of the serum BG assay for the diagnosis of IA has ranged between 55 and 87.5% [28, 105–107]. For instance, in a retrospective review of 456 autopsies, 54 (11.8%) cases of proven IFIs were identified, 41 of which had a BG test performed within 2 weeks prior to death [35]. With the vast majority of IFIs (70%) being IA, the sensitivity and specificity of the BG assay at a cutoff of 60 pg/mL were 85.4 and 95.2%, respectively.

Polymerase Chain Reaction

The use of PCR for the diagnosis of IA in cancer patients has been studied using different blood products (e.g., whole blood, plasma, serum), BAL, and CSF [95, 103, 107–128]. Sensitivity and specificity of blood PCR for the diagnosis of IA have ranged between 64–100 and 63.5–100%, respectively [129]. PCR for the diagnosis of IA has been limited due to, in part, lack of standardization and commercially available assays [129]. Results have varied based on the specimen used (e.g., whole blood, plasma, serum, BAL), PCR technique (e.g., real-time vs. nested), DNA extraction methods, target genes (e.g., 18S vs. 28S rRNA vs. mtDNA), patient population studied (e.g., hematologic malignancy vs. other), or the number of samples tested [128]. For instance, testing serum may be less sensitive (55–70%) than whole blood (57–100%), perhaps as a result of the partial loss of fungal particles during processing [71, 111, 114, 122, 126, 130–132]. Sample volume may also affect the sensitivity of the test, with large serum volumes yielding higher sensitivity (100%) compared to smaller serum volumes (76.5%) [133].

A major limitation of the test is its relative lack of specificity due to – among others – potential contamination of the specimens during processing. The specificity of blood PCR for the diagnosis of IA in patients with a hematologic malignancy may increase from 37 to 89% when two consecutive positive samples are required to establish the diagnosis [108, 111]. The occasional homology of probes used with the DNA of other filamentous fungi may further increase the false positive rates observed in PCR assay results. Caution should be called here, as a "false positive" result may represent subclinical or early infection (early true positive) which might have affected the performance of the PCR assays in previous studies [116, 128].

PCR has been successfully applied to identify fungi in tissues and to further identify organisms to the species level. For instance, PCR and restriction fragment-length polymorphism analysis have been used retrospectively for the identification of the Zygomycetes in tissue [134, 135]. Moreover, two seminested PCR assays identifying *Aspergillus* spp. and the Zygomycetes were prospectively studied on respiratory tract biopsy samples from 56 immunocompromised hosts with suspected invasive mold infections [136]. Among 27 (48%) patients with histopathologically confirmed mold infections, 18 (66.7%), 6 (22.2%), and 3 (11.1%) were found to have IA, zygomycosis, and another mold infection, respectively. PCR was found to be significantly better compared to traditional cultures in detecting an invasive mold infection (26 of 27 vs. 17 of 27, respectively; $p = 0.006$).

Diagnosis of Invasive Fungal Sinus Disease

Sinus disease presents with fever, facial numbness or tenderness, and necrotic areas appearing as dark colored eschars in the nares or oral cavity. Concomitant neutropenia may result in a subtle clinical presentation of sinus disease and hence lead to late diagnosis and worse outcomes. Clinical suspicion among patients at risk should prompt aggressive diagnostic work-up, including sinus CT scan or magnetic resonance (MRI) and sinus biopsy, if feasible [137, 138]. Necrotic lesions are not necessary to establish diagnosis. Invasive fungal sinusitis among cancer patients may also present as severe soft tissue edema and mucoperiosteal thickening on a CT scan [138]. Lesions are frequently unilateral and contiguous bone erosion may occur [138]. As imaging tests are not as sensitive for the diagnosis of invasive fungal sinusitis, diagnosis relies on biopsy and culture of the affected tissue. The absence of distinct lesions upon direct visualization of the sinuses should not exclude tissue biopsy. Concomitant sinus and lung disease may be suggestive of zygomycocis, although *Aspergillus* spp. and other molds, including the dematiaceous molds, may have similar presentations [60, 139–141].

Summary

Establishing the diagnosis of IFIs first depends on having an early and accurate suspicion of disease, depending on the knowledge of host risks and local epidemiology. In the past several years, availability of nonculture based assays to detect fungal antigens and nucleic acids have opened up new pathways to increase sensitivity of detecting fungi in tissues, although much needs to be learned about how to best utilize them in clinical practice.

References

1. Berenguer J, Buck M, Witebsky F, Stock F, Pizzo PA, Walsh TJ. Lysis-centrifugation blood cultures in the detection of tissue-proven invasive candidiasis disseminated versus single-organ infection. Diagn Microbiol Infect Dis. 1993;17(2):103–9.
2. Bodey GP. Fungal infections complicating acute leukemia. J Chronic Dis. 1966;19(6):667–87.
3. Kami M, Machida U, Okuzumi K, et al. Effect of fluconazole prophylaxis on fungal blood cultures: an autopsy-based study involving 720 patients with haematological malignancy. Br J Haematol. 2002;117(1):40–6.
4. Louria DB, Kaminski T. The effects of four antimicrobial drug regimens on sputum superinfection in hospitalized patients. Am Rev Respir Dis. 1962;85:649–65.
5. Myerowitz RL, Pazin GJ, Allen CM. Disseminated candidiasis. Changes in incidence, underlying diseases, and pathology. Am J Clin Pathol. 1977;68(1):29–38.
6. Taschdjian CL, Kozinn PJ, Fink H, Cuesta MB, Caroline L, Kantrowitz AB. Post mortem studies of systemic candidiasis: I. Diagnostic validity of precipitin reaction and probable origin of sensitization to cytoplasmic candidal antigens. Sabouraudia. 1969;7(2):110–7.
7. Gaines JD, Remington JS. Diagnosis of deep infection with *Candida*. A study of *Candida* precipitins. Arch Intern Med. 1973;132(5):699–702.
8. Bodey G, Bueltmann B, Duguid W, et al. Fungal infections in cancer patients: an international autopsy survey. Eur J Clin Microbiol Infect Dis. 1992;11(2):99–109.
9. Albelda SM, Talbot GH, Gerson SL, Miller WT, Cassileth PA. Role of fiberoptic bronchoscopy in the diagnosis of invasive pulmonary aspergillosis in patients with acute leukemia. Am J Med. 1984;76(6):1027–34.
10. Caillot D, Casasnovas O, Bernard A, et al. Improved management of invasive pulmonary aspergillosis in neutropenic patients using early thoracic computed tomographic scan and surgery. J Clin Oncol. 1997;15(1):139–47.
11. Horvath JA, Dummer S. The use of respiratory-tract cultures in the diagnosis of invasive pulmonary aspergillosis. Am J Med. 1996;100(2):171–8.
12. Kahn FW, Jones JM, England DM. The role of bronchoalveolar lavage in the diagnosis of invasive pulmonary aspergillosis. Am J Clin Pathol. 1986;86(4):518–23.
13. Levy H, Horak DA, Tegtmeier BR, Yokota SB, Forman SJ. The value of bronchoalveolar lavage and bronchial washings in the diagnosis of invasive pulmonary aspergillosis. Respir Med. 1992;86(3):243–8.
14. McWhinney PH, Kibbler CC, Hamon MD, et al. Progress in the diagnosis and management of aspergillosis in bone marrow transplantation: 13 years' experience. Clin Infect Dis. 1993;17(3):397–404.
15. Tarrand JJ, Lichterfeld M, Warraich I, et al. Diagnosis of invasive septate mold infections. A correlation of microbiological culture and histologic or cytologic examination. Am J Clin Pathol. 2003;119(6):854–8.
16. Treger TR, Visscher DW, Bartlett MS, Smith JW. Diagnosis of pulmonary infection caused by *Aspergillus*: usefulness of respiratory cultures. J Infect Dis. 1985;152(3):572–6.
17. von Eiff M, Roos N, Schulten R, Hesse M, Zuhlsdorf M, van de Loo J. Pulmonary aspergillosis: early diagnosis improves survival. Respiration. 1995;62(6):341–7.
18. Young RC, Bennett JE, Vogel CL, Carbone PP, DeVita VT. Aspergillosis. The spectrum of the disease in 98 patients. Medicine (Baltimore). 1970;49(2):147–73.
19. Reichenberger F, Habicht J, Matt P, et al. Diagnostic yield of bronchoscopy in histologically proven invasive pulmonary aspergillosis. Bone Marrow Transplant. 1999;24(11):1195–9.
20. Saito H, Anaissie EJ, Morice RC, Dekmezian R, Bodey GP. Bronchoalveolar lavage in the diagnosis of pulmonary infiltrates in patients with acute leukemia. Chest. 1988;94(4):745–9.
21. Baron O, Guillaume B, Moreau P, et al. Aggressive surgical management in localized pulmonary mycotic and nonmycotic infections for neutropenic patients with acute leukemia: report of eighteen cases. J Thorac Cardiovasc Surg. 1998;115(1):63–8; discussion 68–9.
22. Hart PD, Russell Jr E, Remington JS. The compromised host and infection. II. Deep fungal infection. J Infect Dis. 1969;120(2):169–91.
23. Creger RJ, Weeman KE, Jacobs MR, et al. Lack of utility of the lysis-centrifugation blood culture method for detection of fungemia in immunocompromised cancer patients. J Clin Microbiol. 1998;36(1):290–3.
24. Meyer MH, Letscher-Bru V, Jaulhac B, Waller J, Candolfi E. Comparison of mycosis IC/F and plus Aerobic/F media for diagnosis of fungemia by the bactec 9240 system. J Clin Microbiol. 2004;42(2):773–7.
25. Sheppard DC, Locas MC, Restieri C, Laverdiere M. Utility of the germ tube test for direct identification of *Candida albicans* from positive blood culture bottles. J Clin Microbiol. 2008;46(10):3508–9.

26. Wilson DA, Joyce MJ, Hall LS, et al. Multicenter evaluation of a *Candida albicans* peptide nucleic acid fluorescent in situ hybridization probe for characterization of yeast isolates from blood cultures. J Clin Microbiol. 2005;43(6):2909–12.
27. Odabasi Z, Mattiuzzi G, Estey E, et al. Beta-D-glucan as a diagnostic adjunct for invasive fungal infections: validation, cutoff development, and performance in patients with acute myelogenous leukemia and myelodysplastic syndrome. Clin Infect Dis. 2004;39(2):199–205.
28. Ostrosky-Zeichner L, Alexander BD, Kett DH, et al. Multicenter clinical evaluation of the (1–3) beta-D-glucan assay as an aid to diagnosis of fungal infections in humans. Clin Infect Dis. 2005;41(5):654–9.
29. Pickering JW, Sant HW, Bowles CA, Roberts WL, Woods GL. Evaluation of a (1->3)-beta-D-glucan assay for diagnosis of invasive fungal infections. J Clin Microbiol. 2005;43(12):5957–62.
30. Nakao A, Yasui M, Kawagoe T, Tamura H, Tanaka S, Takagi H. False-positive endotoxemia derives from gauze glucan after hepatectomy for hepatocellular carcinoma with cirrhosis. Hepatogastroenterology. 1997;44(17):1413–8.
31. Kato A, Takita T, Furuhashi M, Takahashi T, Maruyama Y, Hishida A. Elevation of blood (1->3)-beta-D-glucan concentrations in hemodialysis patients. Nephron. 2001;89(1):15–9.
32. Ikemura K, Ikegami K, Shimazu T, Yoshioka T, Sugimoto T. False-positive result in limulus test caused by limulus amebocyte lysate-reactive material in immunoglobulin products. J Clin Microbiol. 1989;27(9):1965–8.
33. Mennink-Kersten MA, Donnelly JP, Verweij PE. Detection of circulating galactomannan for the diagnosis and management of invasive aspergillosis. Lancet Infect Dis. 2004;4(6):349–57.
34. Mennink-Kersten MA, Ruegebrink D, Verweij PE. Pseudomonas aeruginosa as a cause of 1, 3-beta-D-glucan assay reactivity. Clin Infect Dis. 2008;46(12):1930–1.
35. Obayashi T, Negishi K, Suzuki T, Funata N. Reappraisal of the serum (1–3)-beta-D-glucan assay for the diagnosis of invasive fungal infections–a study based on autopsy cases from 6 years. Clin Infect Dis. 2008;46(12):1864–70.
36. Upton A, Leisenring W, Marr KA. (1-->3) beta-D-glucan assay in the diagnosis of invasive fungal infections. Clin Infect Dis. 2006;42(7):1054–6; author reply 1056.
37. Herbrecht R, Berceanu A. Beta-D-glucan detection test: a step toward preemptive therapy for fungal infections in leukemic patients? Clin Infect Dis. 2008;46(6):886–9.
38. Morace G, Pagano L, Sanguinetti M, et al. PCR-restriction enzyme analysis for detection of *Candida* DNA in blood from febrile patients with hematological malignancies. J Clin Microbiol. 1999;37(6):1871–5.
39. Moreira-Oliveira MS, Mikami Y, Miyaji M, Imai T, Schreiber AZ, Moretti ML. Diagnosis of candidemia by polymerase chain reaction and blood culture: prospective study in a high-risk population and identification of variables associated with development of candidemia. Eur J Clin Microbiol Infect Dis. 2005;24(11):721–6.
40. McMullan R, Metwally L, Coyle PV, et al. A prospective clinical trial of a real-time polymerase chain reaction assay for the diagnosis of candidemia in nonneutropenic, critically ill adults. Clin Infect Dis. 2008;46(6):890–6.
41. Thaler M, Pastakia B, Shawker TH, O'Leary T, Pizzo PA. Hepatic candidiasis in cancer patients: the evolving picture of the syndrome. Ann Intern Med. 1988;108(1):88–100.
42. Anttila VJ, Ruutu P, Bondestam S, et al. Hepatosplenic yeast infection in patients with acute leukemia: a diagnostic problem. Clin Infect Dis. 1994;18(6):979–81.
43. Nucci M, Marr KA, Queiroz-Telles F, et al. *Fusarium* infection in hematopoietic stem cell transplant recipients. Clin Infect Dis. 2004;38(9):1237–42.
44. Kami M, Kishi Y, Hamaki T, et al. The value of the chest computed tomography halo sign in the diagnosis of invasive pulmonary aspergillosis. An autopsy-based retrospective study of 48 patients. Mycoses. 2002;45(8):287–94.
45. Horger M, Hebart H, Einsele H, et al. Initial CT manifestations of invasive pulmonary aspergillosis in 45 non-HIV immunocompromised patients: association with patient outcome? Eur J Radiol. 2005;55(3):437–44.
46. Caillot D, Couaillier JF, Bernard A, et al. Increasing volume and changing characteristics of invasive pulmonary aspergillosis on sequential thoracic computed tomography scans in patients with neutropenia. J Clin Oncol. 2001;19(1):253–9.
47. Weisser M, Rausch C, Droll A, et al. Galactomannan does not precede major signs on a pulmonary computerized tomographic scan suggestive of invasive aspergillosis in patients with hematological malignancies. Clin Infect Dis. 2005;41(8):1143–9.
48. Greene RE, Schlamm HT, Oestmann JW, et al. Imaging findings in acute invasive pulmonary aspergillosis: clinical significance of the halo sign. Clin Infect Dis. 2007;44(3):373–9.
49. Herbrecht R, Letscher-Bru V, Oprea C, et al. *Aspergillus* galactomannan detection in the diagnosis of invasive aspergillosis in cancer patients. J Clin Oncol. 2002;20(7):1898–906.
50. Kuhlman JE, Fishman EK, Siegelman SS. Invasive pulmonary aspergillosis in acute leukemia: characteristic findings on CT, the CT halo sign, and the role of CT in early diagnosis. Radiology. 1985;157(3):611–4.
51. Mori M, Galvin JR, Barloon TJ, Gingrich RD, Stanford W. Fungal pulmonary infections after bone marrow transplantation: evaluation with radiography and CT. Radiology. 1991;178(3):721–6.
52. Potente G. Computed tomography in invasive pulmonary aspergillosis. Acta Radiol. 1989;30(6):587–90.
53. Greene R. The radiological spectrum of pulmonary aspergillosis. Med Mycol. 2005;43 Suppl 1:S147–54.
54. Ribaud P, Chastang C, Latge JP, et al. Survival and prognostic factors of invasive aspergillosis after allogeneic bone marrow transplantation. Clin Infect Dis. 1999;28(2):322–30.
55. Primack SL, Hartman TE, Lee KS, Muller NL. Pulmonary nodules and the CT halo sign. Radiology. 1994;190(2):513–5.
56. Lee YR, Choi YW, Lee KJ, Jeon SC, Park CK, Heo JN. CT halo sign: the spectrum of pulmonary diseases. Br J Radiol. 2005;78(933):862–5.
57. McAdams HP, Rosado de Christenson M, Strollo DC, Patz EF Jr. Pulmonary mucormycosis: radiologic findings in 32 cases. AJR Am J Roentgenol. 1997;168(6):1541–8.
58. Lee FY, Mossad SB, Adal KA. Pulmonary mucormycosis: the last 30 years. Arch Intern Med. 1999;159(12):1301–9.
59. Dykhuizen RS, Kerr KN, Soutar RL. Air crescent sign and fatal haemoptysis in pulmonary mucormycosis. Scand J Infect Dis. 1994;26(4):498–501.
60. Chamilos G, Marom EM, Lewis RE, Lionakis MS, Kontoyiannis DP. Predictors of pulmonary zygomycosis versus invasive pulmonary aspergillosis in patients with cancer. Clin Infect Dis. 2005;41(1):60–6.
61. Kojima R, Tateishi U, Kami M, et al. Chest computed tomography of late invasive aspergillosis after allogeneic hematopoietic stem cell transplantation. Biol Blood Marrow Transplant. 2005;11(7):506–11.
62. De Pauw B, Walsh TJ, Donnelly JP, et al. Revised definitions of invasive fungal disease from the european organization for research and treatment of Cancer/Invasive fungal infections cooperative group and the national institute of allergy and infectious diseases mycoses study group (EORTC/MSG) consensus group. Clin Infect Dis. 2008;46(12):1813–21.
63. Kontoyiannis DP, Wessel VC, Bodey GP, Rolston KV. Zygomycosis in the 1990s in a tertiary-care cancer center. Clin Infect Dis. 2000;30(6):851–6.

64. Reiss E, Lehmann PF. Galactomannan antigenemia in invasive aspergillosis. Infect Immun. 1979;25(1):357–65.
65. Swanink CM, Meis JF, Rijs AJ, Donnelly JP, Verweij PE. Specificity of a sandwich enzyme-linked immunosorbent assay for detecting *Aspergillus* galactomannan. J Clin Microbiol. 1997;35(1):257–60.
66. Marr KA, Balajee SA, McLaughlin L, Tabouret M, Bentsen C, Walsh TJ. Detection of galactomannan antigenemia by enzyme immunoassay for the diagnosis of invasive aspergillosis: variables that affect performance. J Infect Dis. 2004;190(3):641–9.
67. Marr KA, Laverdiere M, Gugel A, Leisenring W. Antifungal therapy decreases sensitivity of the *Aspergillus* galactomannan enzyme immunoassay. Clin Infect Dis. 2005;40(12):1762–9.
68. Maertens J, Verhaegen J, Demuynck H, et al. Autopsy-controlled prospective evaluation of serial screening for circulating galactomannan by a sandwich enzyme-linked immunosorbent assay for hematological patients at risk for invasive aspergillosis. J Clin Microbiol. 1999;37(10):3223–8.
69. Machetti M, Feasi M, Mordini N, et al. Comparison of an enzyme immunoassay and a latex agglutination system for the diagnosis of invasive aspergillosis in bone marrow transplant recipients. Bone Marrow Transplant. 1998;21(9):917–21.
70. Bretagne S, Marmorat-Khuong A, Kuentz M, Latge JP, Bart-Delabesse E, Cordonnier C. Serum *Aspergillus* galactomannan antigen testing by sandwich ELISA: practical use in neutropenic patients. J Infect. 1997;35(1):7–15.
71. Bretagne S, Costa JM, Bart-Delabesse E, Dhedin N, Rieux C, Cordonnier C. Comparison of serum galactomannan antigen detection and competitive polymerase chain reaction for diagnosing invasive aspergillosis. Clin Infect Dis. 1998;26(6):1407–12.
72. Leeflang MM, Debets-Ossenkopp YJ, Visser CE, et al. Galactomannan detection for invasive aspergillosis in immunocompromized patients. Cochrane Database Syst Rev. 2008;(4): CD007394.
73. Pfeiffer CD, Fine JP, Safdar N. Diagnosis of invasive aspergillosis using a galactomannan assay: a meta-analysis. Clin Infect Dis. 2006;42(10):1417–27.
74. Maertens J, Theunissen K, Verhoef G, et al. Galactomannan and computed tomography-based preemptive antifungal therapy in neutropenic patients at high risk for invasive fungal infection: a prospective feasibility study. Clin Infect Dis. 2005;41(9): 1242–50.
75. Sulahian A, Touratier S, Ribaud P. False positive test for *Aspergillus* antigenemia related to concomitant administration of piperacillin and tazobactam. N Engl J Med. 2003;349(24):2366–7.
76. Walsh TJ, Shoham S, Petraitiene R, et al. Detection of galactomannan antigenemia in patients receiving piperacillin-tazobactam and correlations between in vitro, in vivo, and clinical properties of the drug-antigen interaction. J Clin Microbiol. 2004;42(10): 4744–8.
77. Adam O, Auperin A, Wilquin F, Bourhis JH, Gachot B, Chachaty E. Treatment with piperacillin-tazobactam and false-positive *Aspergillus* galactomannan antigen test results for patients with hematological malignancies. Clin Infect Dis. 2004;38(6):917–20.
78. Aubry A, Porcher R, Bottero J, et al. Occurrence and kinetics of false-positive *Aspergillus* galactomannan test results following treatment with beta-lactam antibiotics in patients with hematological disorders. J Clin Microbiol. 2006;44(2):389–94.
79. Kappe R, Schulze-Berge A. New cause for false-positive results with the pastorex *Aspergillus* antigen latex agglutination test. J Clin Microbiol. 1993;31(9):2489–90.
80. Hachem RY, Kontoyiannis DP, Chemaly RF, Jiang Y, Reitzel R, Raad I. Utility of galactomannan enzyme immunoassay and (1, 3) beta-D-glucan in diagnosis of invasive fungal infections: low sensitivity for *Aspergillus* fumigatus infection in hematologic malignancy patients. J Clin Microbiol. 2009;47(1):129–33.
81. Francis P, Lee JW, Hoffman A, et al. Efficacy of unilamellar liposomal amphotericin B in treatment of pulmonary aspergillosis in persistently granulocytopenic rabbits: the potential role of bronchoalveolar D-mannitol and serum galactomannan as markers of infection. J Infect Dis. 1994;169(2):356–68.
82. Becker MJ, de Marie S, Fens MH, Verbrugh HA, Bakker-Woudenberg IA. Effect of amphotericin B treatment on kinetics of cytokines and parameters of fungal load in neutropenic rats with invasive pulmonary aspergillosis. J Antimicrob Chemother. 2003;52(3):428–34.
83. Becker MJ, Lugtenburg EJ, Cornelissen JJ, Van Der Schee C, Hoogsteden HC, De Marie S. Galactomannan detection in computerized tomography-based broncho-alveolar lavage fluid and serum in haematological patients at risk for invasive pulmonary aspergillosis. Br J Haematol. 2003;121(3):448–57.
84. Berenguer J, Allende MC, Lee JW, et al. Pathogenesis of pulmonary aspergillosis. Granulocytopenia versus cyclosporine and methylprednisolone-induced immunosuppression. Am J Respir Crit Care Med. 1995;152(3):1079–86.
85. Petraitis V, Petraitiene R, Sarafandi AA, et al. Combination therapy in treatment of experimental pulmonary aspergillosis: synergistic interaction between an antifungal triazole and an echinocandin. J Infect Dis. 2003;187(12):1834–43.
86. Petraitiene R, Petraitis V, Groll AH, et al. Antifungal efficacy of caspofungin (MK-0991) in experimental pulmonary aspergillosis in persistently neutropenic rabbits: pharmacokinetics, drug disposition, and relationship to galactomannan antigenemia. Antimicrob Agents Chemother. 2002;46(1):12–23.
87. Sulahian A, Boutboul F, Ribaud P, Leblanc T, Lacroix C, Derouin F. Value of antigen detection using an enzyme immunoassay in the diagnosis and prediction of invasive aspergillosis in two adult and pediatric hematology units during a 4-year prospective study. Cancer. 2001;91(2):311–8.
88. Verweij PE, Latge JP, Rijs AJ, et al. Comparison of antigen detection and PCR assay using bronchoalveolar lavage fluid for diagnosing invasive pulmonary aspergillosis in patients receiving treatment for hematological malignancies. J Clin Microbiol. 1995;33(12):3150–3.
89. Musher B, Fredricks D, Leisenring W, Balajee SA, Smith C, Marr KA. *Aspergillus* galactomannan enzyme immunoassay and quantitative PCR for diagnosis of invasive aspergillosis with bronchoalveolar lavage fluid. J Clin Microbiol. 2004;42(12):5517–22.
90. Nguyen MH, Jaber R, Leather HL, et al. Use of bronchoalveolar lavage to detect galactomannan for diagnosis of pulmonary aspergillosis among nonimmunocompromised hosts. J Clin Microbiol. 2007;45(9):2787–92.
91. Meersseman W, Lagrou K, Maertens J, Van Wijngaerden E. Invasive aspergillosis in the intensive care unit. Clin Infect Dis. 2007;45(2):205–16.
92. Meersseman W, Lagrou K, Maertens J, et al. Galactomannan in bronchoalveolar lavage fluid: a tool for diagnosing aspergillosis in intensive care unit patients. Am J Respir Crit Care Med. 2008;177(1):27–34.
93. Husain S, Paterson DL, Studer SM, et al. *Aspergillus* galactomannan antigen in the bronchoalveolar lavage fluid for the diagnosis of invasive aspergillosis in lung transplant recipients. Transplantation. 2007;83(10):1330–6.
94. Clancy CJ, Jaber RA, Leather HL, et al. Bronchoalveolar lavage galactomannan in diagnosis of invasive pulmonary aspergillosis among solid-organ transplant recipients. J Clin Microbiol. 2007;45(6):1759–65.
95. Frealle E, Decrucq K, Botterel F, et al. Diagnosis of invasive aspergillosis using bronchoalveolar lavage in haematology patients: influence of bronchoalveolar lavage human DNA content on real-time PCR performance. Eur J Clin Microbiol Infect Dis. 2009; 28(3):223–32.

96. Ansorg R, Heintschel von Heinegg E, Rath PM. *Aspergillus* antigenuria compared to antigenemia in bone marrow transplant recipients. Eur J Clin Microbiol Infect Dis. 1994;13(7):582–9.
97. Dupont B, Huber M, Kim SJ, Bennett JE. Galactomannan antigenemia and antigenuria in aspergillosis: studies in patients and experimentally infected rabbits. J Infect Dis. 1987;155(1):1–11.
98. Haynes K, Rogers TR. Retrospective evaluation of a latex agglutination test for diagnosis of invasive aspergillosis in immunocompromised patients. Eur J Clin Microbiol Infect Dis. 1994;13(8):670–4.
99. Rogers TR, Haynes KA, Barnes RA. Value of antigen detection in predicting invasive pulmonary aspergillosis. Lancet. 1990;336(8725):1210–3.
100. Salonen J, Lehtonen OP, Terasjarvi MR, Nikoskelainen J. *Aspergillus* antigen in serum, urine and bronchoalveolar lavage specimens of neutropenic patients in relation to clinical outcome. Scand J Infect Dis. 2000;32(5):485–90.
101. Stynen D, Goris A, Sarfati J, Latge JP. A new sensitive sandwich enzyme-linked immunosorbent assay to detect galactofuran in patients with invasive aspergillosis. J Clin Microbiol. 1995;33(2):497–500.
102. Ray P, Chakrabarti A, Jatana M, Sharma BS, Pathak A. Western blot analysis of cerebrospinal fluid for detection of *Aspergillus* antigens. Mycopathologia. 1995;131(2):103–6.
103. Kami M, Shirouzu I, Mitani K, et al. Early diagnosis of central nervous system aspergillosis with combination use of cerebral diffusion-weighted echo-planar magnetic resonance image and polymerase chain reaction of cerebrospinal fluid. Intern Med. 1999;38(1):45–8.
104. Weiner MH, Talbot GH, Gerson SL, Filice G, Cassileth PA. Antigen detection in the diagnosis of invasive aspergillosis. utility in controlled, blinded trials. Ann Intern Med. 1983;99(6):777–82.
105. Senn L, Robinson JO, Schmidt S, et al. 1, 3-beta-D-glucan antigenemia for early diagnosis of invasive fungal infections in neutropenic patients with acute leukemia. Clin Infect Dis. 2008;46(6):878–85.
106. Pazos C, Ponton J, Del Palacio A. Contribution of (1->3)-beta-D-glucan chromogenic assay to diagnosis and therapeutic monitoring of invasive aspergillosis in neutropenic adult patients: a comparison with serial screening for circulating galactomannan. J Clin Microbiol. 2005;43(1):299–305.
107. Kawazu M, Kanda Y, Nannya Y, et al. Prospective comparison of the diagnostic potential of real-time PCR, double-sandwich enzyme-linked immunosorbent assay for galactomannan, and a (1->3)-beta-D-glucan test in weekly screening for invasive aspergillosis in patients with hematological disorders. J Clin Microbiol. 2004;42(6):2733–41.
108. Cesaro S, Stenghele C, Calore E, et al. Assessment of the lightcycler PCR assay for diagnosis of invasive aspergillosis in paediatric patients with onco-haematological diseases. Mycoses. 2008;51(6):497–504.
109. Buchheidt D, Baust C, Skladny H, Baldus M, Brauninger S, Hehlmann R. Clinical evaluation of a polymerase chain reaction assay to detect *Aspergillus* species in bronchoalveolar lavage samples of neutropenic patients. Br J Haematol. 2002;116(4):803–11.
110. El-Mahallawy HA, Shaker HH, Ali Helmy H, Mostafa T, Razak Abo-Sedah A. Evaluation of pan-fungal PCR assay and *Aspergillus* antigen detection in the diagnosis of invasive fungal infections in high risk paediatric cancer patients. Med Mycol. 2006;44(8):733–9.
111. Florent M, Katsahian S, Vekhoff A, et al. Prospective evaluation of a polymerase chain reaction-ELISA targeted to *Aspergillus fumigatus* and *Aspergillus flavus* for the early diagnosis of invasive aspergillosis in patients with hematological malignancies. J Infect Dis. 2006;193(5):741–7.
112. Ferns RB, Fletcher H, Bradley S, Mackinnon S, Hunt C, Tedder RS. The prospective evaluation of a nested polymerase chain reaction assay for the early detection of *Aspergillus* infection in patients with leukaemia or undergoing allograft treatment. Br J Haematol. 2002;119(3):720–5.
113. Halliday C, Hoile R, Sorrell T, et al. Role of prospective screening of blood for invasive aspergillosis by polymerase chain reaction in febrile neutropenic recipients of haematopoietic stem cell transplants and patients with acute leukaemia. Br J Haematol. 2006;132(4):478–86.
114. Hebart H, Loffler J, Meisner C, et al. Early detection of *Aspergillus* infection after allogeneic stem cell transplantation by polymerase chain reaction screening. J Infect Dis. 2000;181(5):1713–9.
115. Hebart H, Loffler J, Reitze H, et al. Prospective screening by a panfungal polymerase chain reaction assay in patients at risk for fungal infections: implications for the management of febrile neutropenia. Br J Haematol. 2000;111(2):635–40.
116. Jordanides NE, Allan EK, McLintock LA, et al. A prospective study of real-time panfungal PCR for the early diagnosis of invasive fungal infection in haemato-oncology patients. Bone Marrow Transplant. 2005;35(4):389–95.
117. Khot PD, Ko DL, Hackman RC, Fredricks DN. Development and optimization of quantitative PCR for the diagnosis of invasive aspergillosis with bronchoalveolar lavage fluid. BMC Infect Dis. 2008;8:73.
118. Komatsu H, Fujisawa T, Inui A, et al. Molecular diagnosis of cerebral aspergillosis by sequence analysis with panfungal polymerase chain reaction. J Pediatr Hematol Oncol. 2004;26(1):40–4.
119. Lass-Florl C, Gunsilius E, Gastl G, et al. Diagnosing invasive aspergillosis during antifungal therapy by PCR analysis of blood samples. J Clin Microbiol. 2004;42(9):4154–7.
120. Hummel M, Spiess B, Kentouche K, et al. Detection of *Aspergillus* DNA in cerebrospinal fluid from patients with cerebral aspergillosis by a nested PCR assay. J Clin Microbiol. 2006;44(11):3989–93.
121. Hummel M, Spiess B, Roder J, et al. Detection of *Aspergillus* DNA by a nested PCR assay is able to improve the diagnosis of invasive aspergillosis in paediatric patients. J Med Microbiol. 2009;58(Pt 10):1291–7.
122. Raad I, Hanna H, Sumoza D, Albitar M. Polymerase chain reaction on blood for the diagnosis of invasive pulmonary aspergillosis in cancer patients. Cancer. 2002;94(4):1032–6.
123. Raad I, Hanna H, Huaringa A, Sumoza D, Hachem R, Albitar M. Diagnosis of invasive pulmonary aspergillosis using polymerase chain reaction-based detection of *Aspergillus* in BAL. Chest. 2002;121(4):1171–6.
124. Scotter JM, Campbell P, Anderson TP, Murdoch DR, Chambers ST, Patton WN. Comparison of PCR-ELISA and galactomannan detection for the diagnosis of invasive aspergillosis. Pathology. 2005;37(3):246–53.
125. Sanguinetti M, Posteraro B, Pagano L, et al. Comparison of real-time PCR, conventional PCR, and galactomannan antigen detection by enzyme-linked immunosorbent assay using bronchoalveolar lavage fluid samples from hematology patients for diagnosis of invasive pulmonary aspergillosis. J Clin Microbiol. 2003;41(8):3922–5.
126. Skladny H, Buchheidt D, Baust C, et al. Specific detection of *Aspergillus* species in blood and bronchoalveolar lavage samples of immunocompromised patients by two-step PCR. J Clin Microbiol. 1999;37(12):3865–71.
127. Williamson EC, Leeming JP, Palmer HM, et al. Diagnosis of invasive aspergillosis in bone marrow transplant recipients by polymerase chain reaction. Br J Haematol. 2000;108(1):132–9.
128. White PL, Linton CJ, Perry MD, Johnson EM, Barnes RA. The evolution and evaluation of a whole blood polymerase chain reaction assay for the detection of invasive aspergillosis in hematology patients in a routine clinical setting. Clin Infect Dis. 2006;42(4):479–86.

129. Donnelly JP. Polymerase chain reaction for diagnosing invasive aspergillosis: getting closer but still a ways to go. Clin Infect Dis. 2006;42(4):487–9.
130. Yamakami Y, Hashimoto A, Tokimatsu I, Nasu M. PCR detection of DNA specific for *Aspergillus* species in serum of patients with invasive aspergillosis. J Clin Microbiol. 1996;34(10):2464–8.
131. Van Burik JA, Myerson D, Schreckhise RW, Bowden RA. Panfungal PCR assay for detection of fungal infection in human blood specimens. J Clin Microbiol. 1998;36(5):1169–75.
132. Einsele H, Hebart H, Roller G, et al. Detection and identification of fungal pathogens in blood by using molecular probes. J Clin Microbiol. 1997;35(6):1353–60.
133. Suarez F, Lortholary O, Buland S, et al. Detection of circulating *Aspergillus fumigatus* DNA by real-time PCR assay of large serum volumes improves early diagnosis of invasive aspergillosis in high-risk adult patients under hematologic surveillance. J Clin Microbiol. 2008;46(11):3772–7.
134. Larche J, Machouart M, Burton K, et al. Diagnosis of cutaneous mucormycosis due to Rhizopus microsporus by an innovative PCR-restriction fragment-length polymorphism method. Clin Infect Dis. 2005;41(9):1362–5.
135. Machouart M, Larche J, Burton K, et al. Genetic identification of the main opportunistic Mucorales by PCR-restriction fragment length polymorphism. J Clin Microbiol. 2006;44(3):805–10.
136. Rickerts V, Mousset S, Lambrecht E, et al. Comparison of histopathological analysis, culture, and polymerase chain reaction assays to detect invasive mold infections from biopsy specimens. Clin Infect Dis. 2007;44(8):1078–83.
137. Roithmann R, Shankar L, Hawke M, Chapnik J, Kassel E, Noyek A. Diagnostic imaging of fungal sinusitis: eleven new cases and literature review. Rhinology. 1995;33(2):104–10.
138. DelGaudio JM, Swain Jr RE, Kingdom TT, Muller S, Hudgins PA. Computed tomographic findings in patients with invasive fungal sinusitis. Arch Otolaryngol Head Neck Surg. 2003;129(2):236–40.
139. Waitzman AA, Birt BD. Fungal sinusitis. J Otolaryngol. 1994;23(4):244–9.
140. deShazo RD, Chapin K, Swain RE. Fungal sinusitis. N Engl J Med. 1997;337(4):254–9.
141. Drakos PE, Nagler A, Or R, et al. Invasive fungal sinusitis in patients undergoing bone marrow transplantation. Bone Marrow Transplant. 1993;12(3):203–8.

Chapter 24
Invasive Candidiasis in Management of Infections in Cancer Patients

Matteo Bassetti, Malgorzata Mikulska, Juan Gea-Banacloche, and Claudio Viscoli

Abstract *Candida* infections are increasing. Nonalbicans *Candida* are now the most commonly isolated species in immunocompromised patients. The determination of serum beta-D-glucan may allow early diagnosis, but the best implementation of this new technology as screening or diagnostic test remains to be determined. From the therapeutic standpoint, the echinocandins have changed the management of invasive candidiasis due to their effectiveness and excellent safety and drug interaction profile.

Keywords *Candida* • Beta-D-glucan • Echinocandin • Neutropenia

Introduction

Candida is the yeast responsible for most human fungal infections, ranging in severity from mucocutaneous disease to multisystemic invasive disease. The incidence of systemic *Candida* infections, particularly candidemia, has increased significantly in recent years, being the fourth most common pathogen isolated in blood cultures [1]. Apart from *Candida albicans*, other species (nonalbicans) are being isolated more frequently and currently account for the majority of episodes of candidemia in many groups of immunocompromised patients [2, 3].

The diagnostic and therapeutic challenges presented by *Candida* infections are being met by advances in serologic markers and drug development. From the diagnostic standpoint, although blood cultures may be negative in invasive candidiasis [4], the use of beta-D-glucan offers the possibility of early diagnosis [5, 6]. From the therapeutic standpoint, even if widespread use of antifungal prophylaxis predisposes to infections due to species with intrinsic or acquired resistance to some antifungal agents, the echinocandins offer an excellent therapeutic alternative with low toxicity and few interactions in cancer patients [7].

Candida colonization, the presence of the yeast on mucocutaneous surfaces without any sign of invasion, must be distinguished from infection, where there is a clinically evident pathological process with mucosal damage and inflammation. A culture of oropharyngeal, intestinal, or genital material that grows *Candida* species is clinically insignificant unless there are signs or symptoms of infection, as it is part of the normal flora.

Candidemia, the presence of *Candida* species in the blood, may be a manifestation of disseminated disease or it may sometimes reflect only a colonization of an indwelling intravenous catheter [8]. Nonetheless, all the cases of candidemia require treatment with an antifungal agent [9, 10]; it should never be assumed that removal of a catheter alone is an adequate therapy for candidemia.

Mortality rate in case on invasive candidiasis, particularly candidemia, remains high, but can be decreased by rapidly administered antifungal therapy [3, 11–14]. Cancer patients at highest risk for *Candida* infection may be potential candidates for prophylaxis or empirical or preemptive therapy [15].

Epidemiology

Invasive candidiasis is an increasingly important nosocomial infection, particularly in patients who are malnourished, long time hospitalized, and immunocompromised [1, 3, 8, 16, 17].

In Europe, an autopsy-based study showed an increase of invasive fungal disease over the last 10 years [18]. *Candida* infections affect patients with disrupted mechanical barriers (such as skin and mucous membranes, including the presence of central venous catheter) and with deficits in phagocytosis (e.g., neutropenia). Candidemia is now the fourth most common type of nosocomial bloodstream infection, accounting for 9% of cases in a national survey of United States hospitals from 1995 to 2002 [1], and *Candida* species are increasingly isolated from surgical site and urinary tract

C. Viscoli (✉)
Division of Infectious Diseases, San Martino Hospital
and University of Genoa, Genoa, Italy
e-mail: viscoli@unige.it

Table 24.1 Resistance patterns among different *Candida* species

	Fluconazole	Itraconazole	Voriconazole	Posaconazole	Amphotericin B	Echinocandins
C. albicans	S	S	S	S	S	S
C. glabrata	S-DD or R	S-DD or R	S-DD or R	S-DD or R	S to I	S
C. krusei	R	S-DD or R	S	S	S to I	S
C. lusitaniae	S	S	S	S	S to R	S
C. parapsilosis	S	S	S	S	S	S or rarely R
C. tropicalis	S	S	S	S	S	S

I intermediate; *S* susceptible; *S-DD* susceptible dose-dependent; *R* resistant

infections [19]. Moreover, there has also been an increase in bloodstream infections due to nonalbicans species of *Candida* [12, 13, 20], surpassing *C. albicans* in some series [2, 3]. *Candida glabrata*, *Candida parapsilosis*, *Candida tropicalis*, and *Candida krusei* seem to be more common in immunocompromised patients [12, 21], perhaps related to the selective pressure caused by antifungal prophylaxis with fluconazole [21–26]. However, other factors such as geography, age, and concomitant therapies may contribute as well [27–30]. Table 24.1 reports susceptibility of selected species to the most commonly used antifungals. Given that *C. krusei* is intrinsically resistant to fluconazole and *C. glabrata* is either resistant or exhibits a dose-dependent susceptibility, these are the species more common in case of fluconazole administration. Moreover, *C. glabrata* can cause also a breakthrough infection in case of prophylaxis with other triazoles, namely itraconazole [31]. Nosocomial *C. parapsilosis* infection is frequently related to indwelling catheter and parenteral nutrition by CVC has been reported [32].

The mortality in candidemia remains high with most recent randomized controlled trials reporting mortality in the 20–40% range [33–36], even if the attributable mortality is only 10–15% [33].

Pathogenesis

C. albicans is a part of the normal endogenous flora and is present in the gastrointestinal tract of 40–50% of individuals. Colonization is a mandatory first step in developing invasive candidiasis. Changes in endogenous flora which promote increased fungal growth on mucosal surfaces, together with damage of intestinal mucosa, can predispose patients to invasive infections. The loss of integrity of the gastrointestinal tract, as a result of either the disease or the cytotoxic chemotherapy, can create a portal by which *Candida* passes from the gastrointestinal tract into the bloodstream [37]. However, in the case of *Candida* catheter-related infections, including septic thrombophlebitis, the skin at the site of vascular catheter entry, rather than the gastrointestinal tract, is the most likely portal of entry [38].

Although the infecting strain is most often part of the host's endogenous flora, nosocomial acquisition of *Candida* species has been described [19, 39, 40]. The organism has spread via contaminated solutions in some cases [39], whereas the hands of healthcare workers have been the probable source in others [40].

Table 24.2 Patients who are at increased risk of invasive candidiasis

Congenital deficit of cellular immunity
Deficit of cellular immunity secondary to infection (HIV)
Recipients of solid organ transplant
Recipients of hematopoietic stem cell transplant
Low birth weight infants

Table 24.3 Risk factors for invasive candidiasis in cancer patients

Neutropenia, secondary to chemotherapy or aplasia
Treatment with immunosuppressive agents (including glucocorticosteroids, chemotherapeutic agents, and immunomodulators)
Colonization with yeasts
Central venous catheter
Parenteral nutrition, particularly with high-concentration carbohydrate solutions
Prolonged broad-spectrum antibiotic therapy
High APACHE II scores
Acute renal failure, particularly if requiring hemodialysis
Prior surgery, particularly abdominal
Gastrointestinal tract perforations and anastomotic leaks
Bacteremia with enteric organisms
Severe mucositis
Total body irradiation
Graft versus host diseases with mucosal damage
Long-term hospitalization, with changes in endogenous flora

Risk Factors

Patients who are at increased risk of *Candida* infection and numerous risk factors for invasive candidiasis, which are particularly frequent in cancer patients during hospital stay, have been described and are outlined in Tables 24.2 and 24.3 [11–13, 20, 22, 41, 42]. Patients who are immunocompromised or admitted to intensive care units (ICU) have the highest risk of developing candidemia. In the case of cancer patients, next to granulocytopenia, the use of pharmacological doses of corticosteroids and indwelling catheters is the most important factor facilitating the development of candidiasis. Additionally, chemotherapeutic agents associated with extensive gastrointestinal mucosal damage or abdominal surgical procedures further predispose to yeast infections.

Diagnosis

A positive blood culture remains a cornerstone for the diagnosis of invasive candidiasis. Cultures of nonsterile materials, such as pharyngeal swab, bronco-alveolar lavage, and urine, which grow *Candida,* should be carefully examined in consideration of clinical signs and risk factors for candidiasis in order to discriminate between a colonization and an infection.

Definitions

As for other invasive mycoses, the definitions of invasive candidiasis have been developed and modified [43, 44]. Proven invasive fungal disease due to *Candida* species requires a positive result of a histopathologic, cytopathologic, or direct microscopic examination of a sterile material from a normally sterile site (other than mucous membranes) showing pseudohyphae or true hyphae of *Candida.* Positive blood cultures also constitute a proven invasive fungal disease, if there are clinical signs or symptoms of infection or if predisposing host factors (especially neutropenia) are present.

Candidiasis is considered disseminated when after an episode of candidemia within the previous 2 weeks, there is visceral or ophthalmic involvement. These are indicated by the presence of small, target-like abscesses (bull's-eye lesions) in liver or spleen, or progressive retinal exudates on ophthalmologic examination. The signs and symptoms consistent with sepsis syndrome indicate acute disseminated candidiasis, whereas their absence denotes chronic disseminated disease.

Urinary infection due to *Candida* can be diagnosed in case of two positive results of culture of urine samples for yeasts in absence of urinary catheter or if there are *Candida* casts in urine in absence of urinary catheter.

Chronic disseminated candidiasis can be diagnosed as probable in the presence of characteristic target-like radiological lesions, demonstrated by CT, MRI, or ultrasound, as well as elevated serum alkaline phosphatase level, even if no microbiological confirmation is found.

Blood Cultures

Unfortunately, blood culture techniques are relatively insensitive. Moreover, studies from several decades ago showed that blood cultures were positive in only approximately 50% of patients who were found to have disseminated candidiasis at autopsy [4]. Since then, improved, more sensitive microbiological detection systems were developed. However, blood cultures are still often negative in patients with disseminated candidiasis and the diagnosis is often made on clinical grounds. Moreover, blood cultures require from 1 to 4 days to become positive, and in seriously ill patients, more rapid and sensitive diagnostic techniques are warranted. Thus, a number of noninvasive rapid diagnostic tests have been explored.

Nonculture-Based Methods

Noninvasive techniques, such as presence of *Candida* antigens, their metabolites, or antibodies in serum (mannan, enolase, antimannan antibodies), have been developed. However, their clinical utility is limited due to high rate of false positive and false negative results. The colonization with *Candida* can decrease the specificity of antibody assay, while the fact that immunocompromised hosts may be unable to produce antibodies can decrease test's sensitivity. Detection of circulating *Candida* antigens or metabolites seemed promising, but was proved to be insufficiently sensitive for clinical purposes [45, 46].

The newest indirect diagnostic test is based on the detection of beta-D-glucan, which is present in the cell wall of many fungi, including *Candida, Aspergillus, Fusariumm, Trichosporon, Saccharomyces,* and *Acremonium* infection [5, 47]. Serum beta-D-glucan was included among mycological criteria in new definitions of invasive fungal diseases [44], and several studies have reported its high sensitivity and specificity [5, 6]. It has been used as a screening test obtained twice a week in neutropenic patients [5] as well systematically twice weekly and then more frequently in the presence of fever during neutropenia [48]. Although the test seems useful, it remains unclear what the best screening or diagnostic strategy with beta-D-glucan can be in terms of efficacy and cost for the management of candidiasis in daily clinical practice. We have had cases of documented candidemia where a positive beta-D-glucan preceded the positive blood cultures by several days. The availability (or lack thereof) of results in real time is an important consideration that may make the implementation of the test difficult.

Molecular diagnosis with polymerase chain reaction (PCR) seems promising; however, it is time-consuming and lacks intralaboratory standardization. Therefore, it remains useful for clinical studies and is not routinely recommended [43, 44].

Radiological Signs

Chronic disseminated candidiasis (hepatosplenic candidiasis) is characterized by peripheral, target-like abscesses (bull's-eye lesions) in liver or spleen. These lesions may be documented by ultrasound, computed tomography, and magnetic resonance [49]. Serial studies are often required, as the microabscesses may be undetectable during neutropenia, but manifest at the time of neutrophil recovery [50]. The radiological signs and symptoms can be strongly suggestive of invasive mycosis, but occasionally lymphoma, other fungal infections, and tuberculous or other disseminated mycobacterial disease may present a similar pattern.

Clinical Presentation

There are numerous clinical manifestations of diseases caused by Candida, which can be divided into mucocutaneous and deep organ involvement. Mucous membrane infections include oral candidiasis (thrush), acute atrophic candidiasis of the tongue, chronic atrophic candidiasis ("denture sore mouth"), angular cheilitis, and Candida leukoplakia. Candida esophagitis is an invasive infection of the esophageal mucosa. Other manifestations of mucocutaneous Candida infections are vaginitis, balanitis, paronychia, onychomycosis, and chronic mucocutaneous candidiasis.

The clinical forms particularly important in cancer patients will be reviewed in detail.

Esophagitis

Esophageal disease was believed to be initiated by direct spread from oral disease; however, it may occur frequently without thrush. It is frequent in patients with AIDS, cancer, particularly hematological malignancies, and in transplant recipients. According to an autopsy study from a cancer hospital, esophagus and stomach were the sites most frequently involved in gastrointerstinal candidiasis in these patients [51].

The most common symptoms include painful swallowing, a feeling of obstruction on swallowing, and retrosternal chest pain. Nausea and vomiting may also occur. Among the complications, hemorrhage and dissemination should be mentioned, particularly with involvement of the whole gastrointestinal tract in cancer patients.

The diagnosis is made definitively by biopsy during endoscopy; however, endoscopic appearance of ulceration and white patches (pseudomembranes) can be strongly suggestive.

Candidemia

The clinical manifestations of candidemia vary from mild fever to a full-blown sepsis syndrome (fever, chills, hypotension), indistinguishable from severe bacterial infection. Of note, in cancer patients receiving corticosteroid therapy, fever might be absent, thus an episode of candidemia may be initially asymptomatic. Clinical signs of hematogenous spread of Candida include predominantly characteristic eye lesions (chorioretinitis, endophthalmitis) or skin lesions, both described further below. Rarely, muscle abscesses can form. Additionally, signs of multiorgan system failure may be present due to involvement of the organs like kidneys, heart, liver, spleen, lungs, eyes, and brain.

Skin Lesions in Disseminated Candidiasis

In case of disseminated candidiasis, different types of lesions have been described [52]. The most frequent ones are painless, nodular, small (0.5–1 cm in diameter), and pink to red. They may be either single or numerous, distributed over the entire body [53]. Most patients with these lesions are neutropenic and affected by disseminated candidiasis. Other possible lesions may resemble ecthyma gangrenosum [54] or purpura fulminans [55]. A punch biopsy and histological examination is the most accurate diagnostic method.

Chronic Disseminated Candidiasis (Hepatosplenic Candidiasis)

The clinical sign and symptoms of hepatosplenic candidiasis include fever, abdominal pain, hepatosplenomegaly, and an increase in markers of cholestasis, particularly alkaline phosphatase. Radiological imagining reveals the aforementioned characteristic target-like lesions. Most of these infections have occurred in severely immunocompromised patients and become manifest during their recovery from neutropenia.

Ocular Infection

The incidence of ophthalmologic lesions in case of candidemia ranges from 2 to 26%. The most common are endophthalmitis and chorioretinitis. Endophthalmitis can become evident up to 2 weeks after the diagnosis of candidemia and is correlated with the dissemination of fungal infection to other internal organs.

Clinical signs and symptoms include visual disturbances, such as blurring or floating scotomas, eye pain, and even blindness. However, cases of asymptomatic Candida endophthalmitis have been reported, thus a fundoscopic exam is mandatory in case of blood cultures positive for

Candida. Importantly, patients in the ICU may be too ill to report any symptoms.

Usually, on fundoscopic exam, the lesions are white, cotton ball-like, chorioretinal in origin, and can rapidly progress to involve the vitreous. Diagnosis can be made by the characteristic picture plus, in half of the cases, an episode of known candidemia. Unlike vitrectomy, aspiration of the anterior chamber is rarely diagnostic.

Diagnosis of ocular lesions is particularly important because they can cause permanent blindness and they may indicate underlying dissemination to other internal organs.

Endocarditis

Cardiac *Candida* infections are almost exclusively diagnosed in patients fitted with a central venous catheters or a prosthetic valve, in those undergoing cardiac surgery, and in drug addicts. Large vegetations are characteristic and, peripheral embolization phenomena are frequent. *Candida* endocarditis usually requires valve replacement and prolonged antifungal treatment [56], although a few case reports and case series show that medical management alone may be successful when there are contraindications to surgery [57–61].

Trombophlebitis

The infection of vascular prostheses or anastomoses is possible in patients undergoing vascular surgery with implementation of large prosthetic materials. Management usually requires catheter removal and drainage or resection of the vein, or intravenous treatment with echinocandin or AmB followed by fluconazole.

Intra-abdominal Infections

They are usually secondary to perforations of gastrointestinal tract or to abdominal surgeries, particularly when liver or biliary vessels are involved.

Urinary Tract Candidiasis

The clinical importance of candiduria remains unclear. Urinary catheters are frequently colonized with *Candida*, and catheter replacement can successfully resolve the presence of fungi in the urine. In case of asymptomatic candiduria, therapy is usually not indicated, with the exception of patients at high risk for disseminated candidiasis, such as neonates, neutropenic adults, or those undergoing urologic procedures. Cancer patients often belong to one or more of these categories, and the possibility of disseminated candidiasis should be considered and ruled out. Imaging of the kidneys and collecting system may be indicated. Symptomatic cystitis, when *Candida* is the only pathogen growing in urine culture, may require antifungal therapy. Fluconazole is generally the treatment of choice (and the only azole that achieves high enough concentration in the urine), but AmB may be necessary if the isolate is *C. glabrata*.

Prophylaxis and Treatment of *Candida* Infection

Systemic antifungal agents with activity against *Candida* include amphotericin B (AmB, both deoxycholate (AmB-d) [34, 62] and lipid formulations (L-AmB) [33], triazoles (fluconazole [63], itraconazole [64], voriconazole [65, 66], and posaconazole [67]), and echinocandins (micafungin, caspofungin, and anidulafungin) are presented in Table 24.4 [33, 34, 36]. Not all agents have been compared in all the different *Candida* infections and settings, so recommendations are based both on evidence and reasonable extrapolations [9].

Prophylaxis

Knowing which patients are at increased risk for candidiasis allows for selective use of antifungal prophylaxis. The main indications in cancer patients are prolonged neutropenia and hematopoietic stem cell transplantation. Randomized controlled trials have confirmed the efficacy of fluconazole (400 mg [6 mg/kg] daily) [68, 69], itraconazole [70, 71], posaconazole (200 mg 3 times daily) [72], voriconazole [73], and micafungin (50 mg daily) [74]. All these agents have shown to effectively prevent invasive candidiasis, but the clinical trials have been performed in different patient populations. In prolonged neutropenia (mainly acute leukemia), posaconazole 200 mg every 8 h was superior to fluconazole or itraconazole and was associated with improved survival [72]. Studies in stem cell transplantation have not shown superiority of any antifungal prophylaxis, although agents with activity against mold have the added advantage of resulting in less *Aspergillus* infections.

Treatment

The *Candida* infections most important in Oncology are mucocutaneous (thrush and esophageal), acute disseminated

Table 24.4 Systemic agents with activity against *Candida* spp.

Antifungal agent	Adult dose for systemic candidiasis/candidemia	Described resistant species	Evidence-supported usage
Azoles	Inhibit ergosterol synthesis. Inhibit to various degrees some cytochrome P-450 isoenzymes, with decreased clearance of several drugs important in oncology, including vinca alkaloids, cyclophosphamide, calcineurin inhibitors, and sirolimus		
Fluconazole	800 mg loading, then 400 mg/day	*C. krusei, C. glabrata*	Prophylaxis during neutropenia and oropharyngeal and esophageal candidiasis therapy of invasive candidiasis
			Urinary tract *Candida* infection
Itraconazole	Avoid initiating an oral agent in cases of systemic candidiasis	*C. glabrata* may exhibit or develop decreased susceptibility	Prophylaxis during neutropenia and stem cell transplantation, esophageal candidiasis
Posaconazole			Prophylaxis during neutropenia and oropharyngeal and esophageal candidiasis
Voriconazole	400 mg (6 mg/kg) d12h for 2 doses, then 4 mg/kg/12 h		Candidemia, oropharyngeal and esophageal candidiasis, invasive candidiasis. Prophylaxis during neutropenia
Echinocandins	Inhibit synthesis of beta-glucan, a constituent of the cell wall. Only available for intravenous administration. Few toxicities. Few significant interactions (possible interaction cyclosporine A-caspofungin). Equivalent efficacy against *Candida* spp. J-shaped in vitro growth curve inhibition for some yeasts has unknown clinical significance. All are approved for use in candidemia as well as oropharyngeal and esophageal candidiasis, invasive candidiasis		
	Prophylaxis during neutropenia in stem cell transplant		
Caspofungin	70 mg loading, followed by 50 mg daily	*C. parapsilosis* sensu strictu may be resistant	Candidemia (equivalent to AmB-d)
Micafungin	100 mg daily		Candidemia (equivalent to L-AB)
			Prophylaxis during neutropenia in stem cell transplant
Anidulafungin	200 mg loading, then 100 mg daily		Invasive candidiasis (superior to fluconazole)
Amphotericin B	Binds to ergosterol and disrupts the osmotic integrity of the fungal cell wall. Lipid formulations seem to be equally effective, less toxic		
Amphotericin B deoxycholate lipid formulations	0.5–1 mg/kg/day	*C. lusitaniae* is resistant; *C. glabrata* may exhibit decreased susceptibility	
Amphotericin B lipid formulations	3–5 mg/kg/day		

candidiasis (candidemia), and chronic disseminated candidiasis (hepatosplenic candidiasis).

Mucocutaneous Candidiasis

For mild cases of mucocutaneous candidiasis, clotrimazole troches (10 mg 5 times daily) or nystatin suspension or pastilles may be used. For moderate-to-severe disease, fluconazole (100–200 mg daily) is usually the first-line agent. Fluconazole failures can usually be successfully treated with itraconazole or posaconazole. Voriconazole and amphotericin suspension may be used when the other regimens fail. For refractory cases, echinocandins (there is no evidence that there are significant differences in terms of efficacy between the three currently available) may used, but they may also be used as first-line agents if there are contraindications (e.g., drug interactions) for the use of the other agents. Amphotericin B deoxycholate (AmB-d) 0.3 mg/kg/day is also effective.

Candidemia and Acute Disseminated Candidiasis

Only a few multicenter randomized controlled trials have compared different treatment options for acute invasive candidiasis [34, 35, 62, 63, 75–77]. The IDSA guidelines appropriately distinguish between the treatment of suspected candidiasis and the treatment of documented candidemia and further separate neutropenic from nonneutropenic patients [9], based on the fact that most controlled trials of echinocandins have included only a few neutropenic patients.

In cases of suspected candidiasis in neutropenic patients, the options include caspofungin or another echinocandin or AmB (either deoxycholate 1 mg/kg or a lipid formulation (L-AmB) 3–5 mg/kg). In patients with hypotension, severe sepsis, or septic shock, many experts would still prefer AmB. Voriconazole or fluconazole IV should be considered only if the patient was not receiving azole prophylaxis. In nonneutropenic patients, the IDSA recommends (as expert opinion only, not evidence-based) an echinocandin of fluconazole as first-line therapy,

In documented candidemia, the choice will be influenced by the prior use of azole prophylaxis as well as the particular species of *Candida*. An echinocandin, AmB, or fluconazole may all be reasonable options depending on the circumstances. Patients who were on azole prophylaxis should receive an echinocandin or AmB. Regarding species-specific recommendation, for *C. glabrata* and *C. krusei* most experts would choose an echinocandin; *C. parapsilosis* is less susceptible in vitro to echinocandins, and in some trials, a disproportionate amount of the echinocandin failures were caused by this species.

The need to remove the intravenous catheter in neutropenic patients with candidemia has been questioned, based on the fact that the catheter may not be the portal of entry (as opposed to ICU-acquired candidemia, in which the catheter is usually to blame and should routinely be removed) [10]. However, in cases of candidemia, we usually remove and replace intravascular catheters when feasible [78].

Chronic Disseminated Candidiasis

Most successful experience in chronic disseminated candidiasis has been with AmB [79, 80] or fluconazole [81, 82]. Echinocandins have also reported to be successful [83, 84]. Accordingly, all these are endorsed by the IDSA as acceptable options for the treatment of this disease. The emphasis is on the prolonged duration of treatment (until resolution of the lesions, usually weeks) and the need for continued treatment during subsequent episodes of immunosuppression or neutropenia [9].

References

1. Wisplinghoff H, Bischoff T, Tallent SM, Seifert H, Wenzel RP, Edmond MB. Nosocomial bloodstream infections in US hospitals: analysis of 24, 179 cases from a prospective nationwide surveillance study. Clin Infect Dis. 2004;39:309–17.
2. Hachem R, Hanna H, Kontoyiannis D, Jiang Y, Raad I. The changing epidemiology of invasive candidiasis: *Candida glabrata* and *Candida krusei* as the leading causes of candidemia in hematologic malignancy. Cancer. 2008;112:2493–9.
3. Horn DL, Neofytos D, Anaissie EJ, et al. Epidemiology and outcomes of candidemia in 2019 patients: data from the prospective antifungal therapy alliance registry. Clin Infect Dis. 2009;48:1695–703.
4. Berenguer J, Buck M, Witebsky F, Stock F, Pizzo PA, Walsh TJ. Lysis-centrifugation blood cultures in the detection of tissue-proven invasive candidiasis. Disseminated versus single-organ infection. Diagn Microbiol Infect Dis. 1993;17:103–9.
5. Odabasi Z, Mattiuzzi G, Estey E, et al. Beta-D-glucan as a diagnostic adjunct for invasive fungal infections: validation, cutoff development, and performance in patients with acute myelogenous leukemia and myelodysplastic syndrome. Clin Infect Dis. 2004;39:199–205. Epub 2004 Jun 28.
6. Ostrosky-Zeichner L, Alexander BD, Kett DH, et al. Multicenter clinical evaluation of the (1–>3) beta-D-glucan assay as an aid to diagnosis of fungal infections in humans. Clin Infect Dis. 2005;41:654–9.
7. Tamura K, Urabe A, Yoshida M, et al. Efficacy and safety of micafungin, an echinocandin antifungal agent, on invasive fungal infections in patients with hematological disorders. Leuk Lymphoma. 2009;50:92–100.
8. Fridkin SK. The changing face of fungal infections in health care settings. Clin Infect Dis. 2005;41:1455–60.
9. Pappas PG, Kauffman CA, Andes D, et al. Clinical practice guidelines for the management of candidiasis: 2009 update by the Infectious Diseases Society of America. Clin Infect Dis. 2009;48:503–35.
10. Mermel LA, Allon M, Bouza E, et al. Clinical practice guidelines for the diagnosis and management of intravascular catheter-related infection: 2009 Update by the Infectious Diseases Society of America. Clin Infect Dis. 2009;49:1–45.
11. Fraser VJ, Jones M, Dunkel J, Storfer S, Medoff G, Dunagan WC. Candidemia in a tertiary care hospital: epidemiology, risk factors, and predictors of mortality. Clin Infect Dis. 1992;15:414–21.
12. Nguyen MH, Peacock Jr JE, Tanner DC, et al. Therapeutic approaches in patients with candidemia. Evaluation in a multicenter, prospective, observational study. Arch Intern Med. 1995;155:2429–35.
13. Nucci M, Colombo AL, Silveira F, et al. Risk factors for death in patients with candidemia. Infect Control Hosp Epidemiol. 1998;19:846–50.
14. Blot SI, Vandewoude KH, Hoste EA, Colardyn FA. Effects of nosocomial candidemia on outcomes of critically ill patients. Am J Med. 2002;113:480–5.
15. Almyroudis NG, Segal BH. Prevention and treatment of invasive fungal diseases in neutropenic patients. Curr Opin Infect Dis. 2009;22:385–93.
16. Pappas PG, Rex JH, Lee J, et al. A prospective observational study of candidemia: epidemiology, therapy, and influences on mortality in hospitalized adult and pediatric patients. Clin Infect Dis. 2003;37:634–43.
17. Tortorano AM, Peman J, Bernhardt H, et al. Epidemiology of candidaemia in Europe: results of 28-month European Confederation of Medical Mycology (ECMM) hospital-based surveillance study. Eur J Clin Microbiol Infect Dis. 2004;23:317–22.
18. Schwesinger G, Junghans D, Schroder G, Bernhardt H, Knoke M. Candidosis and aspergillosis as autopsy findings from 1994 to 2003. Mycoses. 2005;48:176–80.
19. Jarvis WR. Epidemiology of nosocomial fungal infections, with emphasis on *Candida* species. Clin Infect Dis. 1995;20:1526–30.
20. Viscoli C, Girmenia C, Marinus A, et al. Candidemia in cancer patients: a prospective, multicenter surveillance study by the Invasive Fungal Infection Group (IFIG) of the European Organization for Research and Treatment of Cancer (EORTC). Clin Infect Dis. 1999;28:1071–9.
21. Bassetti M, Righi E, Costa A, et al. Epidemiological trends in nosocomial candidemia in intensive care. BMC Infect Dis. 2006;6:21.
22. Abi-Said D, Anaissie E, Uzun O, Raad I, Pinzcowski H, Vartivarian S. The epidemiology of hematogenous candidiasis caused by different *Candida* species. Clin Infect Dis. 1997;24:1122–8.
23. Girmenia C, Martino P. Fluconazole and the changing epidemiology of candidemia. Clin Infect Dis. 1998;27:232–4.
24. Abbas J, Bodey GP, Hanna HA, et al. *Candida krusei* fungemia. An escalating serious infection in immunocompromised patients. Arch Intern Med. 2000;160:2659–64.
25. Bodey GP, Mardani M, Hanna HA, et al. The epidemiology of *Candida glabrata* and *Candida albicans* fungemia in immunocompromised patients with cancer. Am J Med. 2002;112:380–5.
26. Malani PN, Bradley SF, Little RS, Kauffman CA. Trends in species causing fungaemia in a tertiary care medical centre over 12 years. Mycoses. 2001;44:446–9.

27. Garbino J, Kolarova L, Rohner P, Lew D, Pichna P, Pittet D. Secular trends of candidemia over 12 years in adult patients at a tertiary care hospital. Medicine. 2002;81:425–33.
28. Cuenca-Estrella M, Rodriguez D, Almirante B, et al. In vitro susceptibilities of bloodstream isolates of *Candida* species to six antifungal agents: results from a population-based active surveillance programme, Barcelona, Spain, 2002-2003. J Antimicrob Chemother. 2005;55:194–9.
29. Diekema DJ, Messer SA, Brueggemann AB, et al. Epidemiology of candidemia: 3-year results from the emerging infections and the epidemiology of Iowa organisms study. J Clin Microbiol. 2002;40:1298–302.
30. Lin MY, Carmeli Y, Zumsteg J, et al. Prior antimicrobial therapy and risk for hospital-acquired *Candida glabrata* and *Candida krusei* fungemia: a case-case-control study. Antimicrob Agents Chemother. 2005;49:4555–60.
31. Paterson PJ, McWhinney PH, Potter M, Kibbler CC, Prentice HG. The combination of oral amphotericin B with azoles prevents the emergence of resistant *Candida* species in neutropenic patients. Br J Haematol. 2001;112:175–80.
32. Almirante B, Rodriguez D, Cuenca-Estrella M, et al. Epidemiology, risk factors, and prognosis of *Candida parapsilosis* bloodstream infections: case-control population-based surveillance study of patients in Barcelona, Spain, from 2002 to 2003. J Clin Microbiol. 2006;44:1681–5.
33. Kuse ER, Chetchotisakd P, da Cunha CA, et al. Micafungin versus liposomal amphotericin B for candidaemia and invasive candidosis: a phase III randomised double-blind trial. Lancet. 2007;369:1519–27.
34. Mora-Duarte J, Betts R, Rotstein C, et al. Comparison of caspofungin and amphotericin B for invasive candidiasis. N Engl J Med. 2002;347:2020–9.
35. Pappas PG, Rotstein CM, Betts RF, et al. Micafungin versus caspofungin for treatment of candidemia and other forms of invasive candidiasis. Clin Infect Dis. 2007;45:883–93.
36. Reboli AC, Rotstein C, Pappas PG, et al. Anidulafungin versus fluconazole for invasive candidiasis. N Engl J Med. 2007;356:2472–82.
37. Cole GT, Halawa AA, Anaissie EJ. The role of the gastrointestinal tract in hematogenous candidiasis: from the laboratory to the bedside. Clin Infect Dis. 1996;22 Suppl 2:S73–88.
38. Benoit D, Decruyenaere J, Vandewoude K, et al. Management of candidal thrombophlebitis of the central veins: case report and review. Clin Infect Dis. 1998;26:393–7.
39. Pfaller MA. Nosocomial candidiasis: emerging species, reservoirs, and modes of transmission. Clin Infect Dis. 1996;22 Suppl 2:S89–94.
40. Vazquez JA, Sanchez V, Dmuchowski C, Dembry LM, Sobel JD, Zervos MJ. Nosocomial acquisition of *Candida albicans*: an epidemiologic study. J Infect Dis. 1993;168:195–201.
41. Blumberg HM, Jarvis WR, Soucie JM, et al. Risk factors for candidal bloodstream infections in surgical intensive care unit patients: the NEMIS prospective multicenter study. The National Epidemiology of Mycosis Survey. Clin Infect Dis. 2001;33:177–86.
42. Chow JK, Golan Y, Ruthazer R, et al. Risk factors for albicans and non-albicans candidemia in the intensive care unit. Crit Care Med. 2008;36:1993–8.
43. Ascioglu S, Rex JH, de Pauw B, et al. Defining opportunistic invasive fungal infections in immunocompromised patients with cancer and hematopoietic stem cell transplants: an international consensus. Clin Infect Dis. 2002;34:7–14.
44. De Pauw B, Walsh TJ, Donnelly JP, et al. Revised definitions of invasive fungal disease from the European Organization for Research and Treatment of Cancer/Invasive Fungal Infections Cooperative Group and the National Institute of Allergy and Infectious Diseases Mycoses Study Group (EORTC/MSG) Consensus Group. Clin Infect Dis. 2008;46:1813–21.
45. Reiss E, Morrison CJ. Nonculture methods for diagnosis of disseminated candidiasis. Clin Microbiol Rev. 1993;6:311–23.
46. Walsh TJ, Hathorn JW, Sobel JD, et al. Detection of circulating *Candida* enolase by immunoassay in patients with cancer and invasive candidiasis. N Engl J Med. 1991;324:1026–31.
47. Yoshida M, Obayashi T, Iwama A, et al. Detection of plasma (1 –> 3)-beta-D-glucan in patients with *Fusarium*, *Trichosporon*, *Saccharomyces* and *Acremonium* fungaemias. J Med Vet Mycol. 1997;35:371–4.
48. Senn L, Robinson JO, Schmidt S, et al. 1, 3-Beta-D-glucan antigenemia for early diagnosis of invasive fungal infections in neutropenic patients with acute leukemia. Clin Infect Dis. 2008;46:878–85.
49. Masood A, Sallah S. Chronic disseminated candidiasis in patients with acute leukemia: emphasis on diagnostic definition and treatment. Leuk Res. 2005;29:493–501.
50. Karthaus M, Ganser A. Hepatosplenic candidiasis in patients with acute leukaemia. Br J Haematol. 2000;109:672.
51. Eras P, Goldstein MJ, Sherlock P. *Candida* infection of the gastrointestinal tract. Medicine. 1972;51:367–79.
52. Lindblad R, al-Obaidy A, Mobacken H, Rodjer S. Diagnostically usable skin lesions in *Candida* septicaemia. Mycoses. 1989;32:416–20.
53. Bodey GP, Luna M. Skin lesions associated with disseminated candidiasis. JAMA. 1974;229:1466–8.
54. Suster S, Rosen LB. Intradermal bullous dermatitis due to candidiasis in an immunocompromised patient. JAMA. 1987;258:2106–7.
55. Silverman RA, Rhodes AR, Dennehy PH. Disseminated intravascular coagulation and purpura fulminans in a patient with *Candida* sepsis. Biopsy of purpura fulminans as an aid to diagnosis of systemic *Candida* infection. Am J Med. 1986;80:679–84.
56. Steinbach WJ, Perfect JR, Cabell CH, et al. A meta-analysis of medical versus surgical therapy for *Candida* endocarditis. J Infect. 2005;51:230–47.
57. Aaron L, Therby A, Viard JP, Lahoulou R, Dupont B. Successful medical treatment of *Candida albicans* in mechanical prosthetic valve endocarditis. Scand J Infect Dis. 2003;35:351–2.
58. Lopez-Ciudad V, Castro-Orjales MJ, Leon C, et al. Successful treatment of *Candida parapsilosis* mural endocarditis with combined caspofungin and voriconazole. BMC Infect Dis. 2006;6:73.
59. Melamed R, Leibovitz E, Abramson O, Levitas A, Zucker N, Gorodisher R. Successful non-surgical treatment of *Candida tropicalis* endocarditis with liposomal amphotericin-B (AmBisome). Scand J Infect Dis. 2000;32:86–9.
60. Stripeli F, Tsolia M, Trapali C, et al. Successful medical treatment of *Candida* endocarditis with liposomal amphotericin B without surgical intervention. Eur J Pediatr. 2008;167:469–70.
61. Westling K, Thalme A, Julander I. *Candida albicans* tricuspid valve endocarditis in an intravenous drug addict: successful treatment with fluconazole. Scand J Infect Dis. 2005;37:310–1.
62. Rex JH, Bennett JE, Sugar AM, et al. A randomized trial comparing fluconazole with amphotericin B for the treatment of candidemia in patients without neutropenia. Candidemia Study Group and the National Institute. N Engl J Med. 1994;331:1325–30.
63. Rex JH, Pappas PG, Karchmer AW, et al. A randomized and blinded multicenter trial of high-dose fluconazole plus placebo versus fluconazole plus amphotericin B as therapy for candidemia and its consequences in nonneutropenic subjects. Clin Infect Dis. 2003;36:1221–8.
64. Graybill JR, Vazquez J, Darouiche RO, et al. Randomized trial of itraconazole oral solution for oropharyngeal candidiasis in HIV/AIDS patients. Am J Med. 1998;104:33–9.
65. Kullberg BJ, Sobel JD, Ruhnke M, et al. Voriconazole versus a regimen of amphotericin B followed by fluconazole for candidaemia in non-neutropenic patients: a randomised non-inferiority trial. Lancet. 2005;366:1435–42.
66. Ally R, Schurmann D, Kreisel W, et al. A randomized, double-blind, double-dummy, multicenter trial of voriconazole and fluconazole in

the treatment of esophageal candidiasis in immunocompromised patients. Clin Infect Dis. 2001;33:1447–54.
67. Vazquez JA, Skiest DJ, Nieto L, et al. A multicenter randomized trial evaluating posaconazole versus fluconazole for the treatment of oropharyngeal candidiasis in subjects with HIV/AIDS. Clin Infect Dis. 2006;42:1179–86.
68. Goodman JL, Winston DJ, Greenfield RA, et al. A controlled trial of fluconazole to prevent fungal infections in patients undergoing bone marrow transplantation [see comments]. N Engl J Med. 1992;326:845–51.
69. Slavin MA, Osborne B, Adams R, et al. Efficacy and safety of fluconazole prophylaxis for fungal infections after marrow transplantation–a prospective, randomized, double-blind study. J Infect Dis. 1995;171:1545–52.
70. Marr KA, Crippa F, Leisenring W, et al. Itraconazole versus fluconazole for prevention of fungal infections in patients receiving allogeneic stem cell transplants. Blood. 2004;103:1527–33.
71. Winston DJ, Maziarz RT, Chandrasekar PH, et al. Intravenous and oral itraconazole versus intravenous and oral fluconazole for long-term antifungal prophylaxis in allogeneic hematopoietic stem-cell transplant recipients. A multicenter, randomized trial. Ann Intern Med. 2003;138:705–13.
72. Cornely OA, Maertens J, Winston DJ, et al. Posaconazole vs. fluconazole or itraconazole prophylaxis in patients with neutropenia. N Engl J Med. 2007;356:348–59.
73. Wingard JR, Carter SL, Walsh TJ, Kurtzberg J, Small TN, Gersten ID, et al. Results of a randomized, double-blind trial of fluconazole vs. voriconazole for the prevention of invasive fungal infections in 600 allogeneic blood and marrow transplant patients. Blood. 2007;110:55a.
74. van Burik JA, Ratanatharathorn V, Stepan DE, et al. Micafungin versus fluconazole for prophylaxis against invasive fungal infections during neutropenia in patients undergoing hematopoietic stem cell transplantation. Clin Infect Dis. 2004;39:1407–16.
75. Phillips P, Shafran S, Garber G, et al. Multicenter randomized trial of fluconazole versus amphotericin B for treatment of candidemia in non-neutropenic patients. Canadian Candidemia Study Group. Eur J Clin Microbiol Infect Dis. 1997;16:337–45.
76. Reboli A, Rotstein C, Pappas P, Schranz J, Krause D, Walsh T. Anidulafungin vs. fluconazole for treatment of candidemia and invasive candidiasis (C/IC). 45th annual Interscience Conference on Antimicrobial Agents and Chemotherapy, Washington (abstract M-718); 2005.
77. Betts RF, Nucci M, Talwar D, et al. A Multicenter, double-blind trial of a high-dose caspofungin treatment regimen versus a standard caspofungin treatment regimen for adult patients with invasive candidiasis. Clin Infect Dis. 2009;48:1676–84.
78. Walsh TJ, Rex JH. All catheter-related candidemia is not the same: assessment of the balance between the risks and benefits of removal of vascular catheters. Clin Infect Dis. 2002;34:600–2.
79. Walsh TJ, Whitcomb PO, Revankar SG, Pizzo PA. Successful treatment of hepatosplenic candidiasis through repeated cycles of chemotherapy and neutropenia. Cancer. 1995;76:2357–62.
80. Walsh TJ, Whitcomb P, Piscitelli S, et al. Safety, tolerance, and pharmacokinetics of amphotericin B lipid complex in children with hepatosplenic candidiasis. Antimicrob Agents Chemother. 1997;41:1944–8.
81. Anaissie E, Bodey GP, Kantarjian H, et al. Fluconazole therapy for chronic disseminated candidiasis in patients with leukemia and prior amphotericin B therapy. Am J Med. 1991;91:142–50.
82. Kauffman CA, Bradley SF, Ross SC, Weber DR. Hepatosplenic candidiasis: successful treatment with fluconazole. Am J Med. 1991;91:137–41.
83. Altintas A, Ayyildiz O, Isikdogan A, Atay E, Kaplan MA. Successful initial treatment with caspofungin alone for hepatosplenic candidiasis in a patient with acute myeloblastic leukemia. Saudi Med J. 2006;27:1423–4.
84. Sora F, Chiusolo P, Piccirillo N, et al. Successful treatment with caspofungin of hepatosplenic candidiasis resistant to liposomal amphotericin B. Clin Infect Dis. 2002;35:1135–6.

Chapter 25
Management of Aspergillosis, Zygomycosis, and Other Clinically Relevant Mold Infections

Konstantinos Leventakos and Dimitrios P. Kontoyiannis

Abstract Invasive mold infections (IMIs) are a major cause of morbidity and mortality in severely immunocompromised hematologic malignancy patients and hematopoietic stem cell transplantations recipients. Invasive aspergillosis caused by *Aspergillus fumigatus* is the most common cause of IMI, but recent advances in the pharmacotherapy of fungal infections and an increase in the number of patients at risk have caused an epidemiologic shift towards infections with resistant non-*fumigatus Aspergillus* species and non-*Aspergillus* molds such as Zygomycetes. Patient outcome is a function of immune function recovery, early diagnosis, and multiple interventions, such as with broad-spectrum antifungal therapy and adjunct immunotherapy and surgery in select patients. In this chapter, we review the utility of new diagnostic modalities such as the galactomannan test, the 1,3-beta-D-glucan test, and fungal DNA tests in diagnosing IMIs early. We focus on modern antifungal agents (the lipid formulations of amphotericin B, the broad-spectrum azoles, and the echinocandins) and evaluate them in the context of evolving prophylactic, preemptive, and targeted therapies for IMIs.

Keywords Aspergillosis • Zygomycosis • Invasive mold infections • Prophylaxis • Prevention • Treatment

Brief Review of the Evolving Epidemiology of Invasive Mold Infections

Recent advances in oncology and transplantation have led to prolonged survival in critically ill and severely immunocompromised cancer patients. However, these patients' pleiotropic and profound immune defects (Table 25.1) have led to the emergence of invasive fungal infections (IFIs) and specifically invasive mold infections (IMIs) [1, 2].

Since the 1990s, the widespread use of fluconazole for antifungal prophylaxis has decreased the incidence of candidiasis, but increased the incidence of IMIs, especially aspergillosis. Invasive aspergillosis (IA) remains a leading cause of death in leukemia patients and stem cell transplantation (SCT) recipients, although recent reports have documented a decreasing mortality rate, perhaps reflecting earlier diagnosis and the use of voriconazole-based regimens [3, 4]. An alarming swift in the epidemiology of IA is the increasing incidence of non-*fumigatus Aspergillus* spp. that are resistant to antifungals like *A. terreus* and *A. ustus* [5, 6]. In addition, there is an increase in the incidence of uncommon and difficult-to-treat opportunistic molds such as Zygomycetes, *Fusarium* spp., *Scedosporium* spp., and phaeohyphomycetes [7, 8]. Zygomycosis in particular has emerged as a superinfection in patients on voriconazole, a broad-spectrum triazole that has no activity against Zygomycetes [9]. Voriconazole is the preferred agent for treatment or perhaps prophylaxis against IA in many hematology centers. This opportunistic mycosis poses a great challenge as it manifests clinical similarly to IA, there is no reliable method of early diagnosis, and delayed treatment that has activity against Zygomycetes is associated with a dire clinical outcome [10]. The decreasing autopsy rates in hematology units – at our center, current rates approach 7% in the leukemia and SCT units (K. Leventakos and D.P. Kontoyiannis, unpublished data) – disguise the true incidence of IFIs and IMIs. In addition, this vanishing "gold standard" makes it difficult to reliably assess the true utility of new diagnostics and therapies.

Diagnostic Criteria and Novel Diagnostics

Substantial delays in diagnosing IMIs remain a major impediment to their successful treatment. Recently, the European Organization for Research and Treatment of Cancer/Invasive Fungal Infections Cooperative Group and the National

---

D.P. Kontoyiannis (✉)
Department of Infectious Diseases, Infection Control, and Employee Health, Unit 402, The University of Texas M.D. Anderson Cancer Center, 1515 Holcombe Boulevard, Houston, TX 77030, USA
e-mail: dkontoyi@mdanderson.org

Table 25.1 Risk factors for IFIs in HSCT recipients.

- History of IFI, especially IA or chronic systemic candidiasis, prior to transplantation
- History of ongoing steroid therapy or steroid therapy prior to BMT
- Underlying hematologic malignancy (AML, malignancy not in remission)
- Allogeneic transplantation (with unrelated cord blood recipients at highest risk)
- Duration of neutropenia >20 days
- Age >40 years
- History of cytomegalovirus disease or cytomegalovirus reactivation
- Colonized with fungi such as *Aspergillus* spp., *Fusarium* spp., zygomycetes, *Scedosporium* spp., and *Candida tropicalis*
- GvHD grade III or IV

Institute of Allergy and Infectious Diseases Mycoses Study Group revised their definitions of invasive fungal disease [11]. The revised definitions retain the original classifications of "proven," "probable," and "possible" IMIs. For most conditions, proven infections require proof of hyphal elements in diseased tissue. To characterize a case as probable, a host factor, clinical features, and a mycologic or nonculture-based surrogate marker (e.g., galactomannan, beta-glucan, or as determined by polymerase chain reaction [PCR]) must be present. Possible invasive fungal disease is more strictly defined to include patients with the appropriate host factors and sufficient clinical evidence of invasive fungal disease, but no mycologic evidence. For rare molds, the isolation of fungus in respiratory secretions, skin, and blood is not synonymous with invasive disease. Most such cases represent contamination or colonization, even among high-risk patients [8, 12]. For example, in our recent experience with the significance of the isolation of black molds at MD Anderson Cancer center, most of the cases did not represent infections [8].

In clinical practice, conventional diagnostic methods based on histologic evaluation and culture remain the cornerstones for diagnosing IMIs [13]. Cultures allow for speciation and susceptibility testing, which may provide useful treatment information. Invasive procedures such as biopsy may be required, but they may not be feasible in patients who are clinically unstable or severely hypoxic (in the case of bronchoscopy) or who have low platelet counts. Even when biopsy is feasible, it may not provide a specific diagnosis when culture remains negative as occurs in almost 50% of cases [14]. In addition, *Fusarium*, *Scedosporium*, and *Acremonium* spp. have histologic characteristics that cannot be distinguished from those of IA. In situ hybridization directed against ribosomal 18S RNA sequences can rapidly and accurately distinguish between these species [15]. Recent efforts have been oriented towards identifying a nonculture-based marker for rapid, reliable diagnosis. Thus, the identification of fungal antigens, metabolites, and DNA has enhanced current diagnostic modalities.

The galactomannan assay is the most studied of new diagnostic tests. Galactomannan is a heat-stable heteropolysaccharide that is released from the cell wall during hyphae growth in tissues. A double-sandwich enzyme-linked immunosorbent galactomannan assay (galactomannan detection threshold at concentrations as low as 0.5 ng/mL) has been approved by the U.S. Food and Drug Administration for use with serum samples [16]. False-positive results have been described in patients receiving beta-lactam antibiotics. Variables that reduce the fungal load and consequently reduce the levels of circulating galactomannan, such as antifungal prophylaxis and treatment, can alter the results [17, 18]. Galactomannan can be detected in bronchoalveolar fluid, urine, and cerebrospinal fluid, but these approaches have not been standardized.

1,3-beta-D-glucan is an integral cell-wall component in a number of pathogenic yeasts and filamentous fungi (exceptions include Zygomycetes, *Cryptococcus* spp., and *Trichosporon* spp.). A sensitive (1 pg/mL) colorimetric beta-glucan detection assay is now commercially available. The presence of beta-glucan in serum indicates the presence of fungal invasion, but it is not species-specific [19, 20]. False-positive results can occur in dialysis patients, immunoglobulin recipients, those exposed to glucan-containing gauge, and those treated with certain antimicrobials. It has been reported that the combination of galactomannan and beta-glucan improves the specificity (to 100%) and sensitivity (to 100%) of each test in high-risk hematologic patients by identifying false-positive reactions [20].

PCR – usually by amplifying ribosomal fungal DNA – has been regarded as a promising method of early detection of IA. One of the advantages of PCR is the capability of rapid detection and molecular identification of opportunistic molds besides *Aspergillus* [21]. However, these diagnostic platforms have not been standardized; thus they remain investigational.

Radiologic methods play a pivotal role in diagnosing IMIs [22]. Computed tomography (CT) findings – the most important being the "halo sign" and "air crescent sign" – have facilitated the diagnosis of pulmonary IMIs. The halo sign is highly specific for acute IA in severely neutropenic patients, but its sensitivity is low; it is also transient: 75% of initial halo signs disappear within a week [22, 23]. It has been reported that a positive halo sign may be associated with a better outcome in IA as it is a marker for early suspicion of and early therapy of IA [24, 25]. The radiologic distinction between IA and zygomycosis in high-risk leukemia or SCT patients is important because of the lack of reliable serologic methods for diagnosing zygomycosis. Single-institution retrospective studies have shown that the "reverse halo sign" and the presence of sinusitis, pleural effusion, ten or more lung nodules or reverse halo sign on chest CT are suggestive of zygomycosis [26, 27].

Current Systemic Antifungals with Mold Activity

Amphotericin B and its Lipid Formulations

Amphotericin B (AMB) is a broad-spectrum fungicidal polyene that has in vitro activity against most molds (the rare exceptions include *A. terreus*, *Fusarium solani*, and *Scedosporium* spp.). The common dose-limiting renal and infusion-related toxicities of D-AMB, an agent that has been in use for over 50 years, led to the introduction of three lipid formulations of AMB (LF-AMB): AMB lipid complex (ABLC), AMB colloidal dispersion, and liposomal AMB (L-AMB). All LF-AMBs have reduced nephrotoxicity compared with D-AMB because they functionally spare the kidneys [28]. IMI patients typically require prolonged therapy; these agents are preferred for systemic AMB-based therapy in high-risk cancer patients. Although no comparative trials between the lipid formulations of AMB and D-AMB in IMIs have been conducted, LF-AMBs appear to be equally efficacious and they are clearly less toxic than D-AMB.

An even more controversial issue is whether there are clinically meaningful differences between the various LF-AMB as there are, based mostly on preclinical data, differences with respect to the rate and extent of drug delivery to the respiratory tract, the most common site of involvement in IMIs. Specifically, ABLC results in substantially higher drug concentrations in lung tissue when compared with L-AMB; therefore, ABLC may result in more rapid and complete *Aspergillus* killing [29]. The current role of the LFABs in the treatment of IMIs remains significant because of their broad tissue distribution and spectrum that makes them favorable for preemptive strategies and for targeted therapies in a variety of documented IMIs progressing on a triazole or echinocandin-based therapy [30].

Second-Generation Triazoles

Voriconazole is an orally and intravenously available azole with high bioavailability (over 90%) and broad tissue distribution [31]. Voriconazole inhibits cytochrome P-450 14a-demethylase, which is an enzyme of the sterol biosynthesis pathway; it has a broad spectrum of activity against a variety of pathogenic molds, with the notable exceptions of Zygomycetes and *Scedosporium prolificans*. The drug is metabolized in the liver by CYP540; CYP540-inhibiting and -inducing agents and pharmacogenetic differences (e.g., idiosyncratic variations due to CYP2C19 polymorphisms) may dramatically change the drug's pharmacokinetics. Because of voriconazole's complex metabolism, dose-related toxicities, and narrow therapeutic range, researchers have investigated the utility of therapeutic drug monitoring of voriconazole [32]. Even though the current data cannot establish a therapeutic range of voriconazole, a low level in a patient who does not respond to voriconazole therapy should lead to an increase of the regimen [33]. Common side effects of voriconazole include transaminase elevation and visual disturbances [34]. The latter is a rather unique side effect of voriconazole and is reversible upon discontinuation of the drug.

Posaconazole, an orally available analog of itraconazole, has the same mechanism of action as other azoles. On the basis of data from preclinical and salvage studies, posaconazole has an impressive spectrum of activity against molds, including Zygomycetes [35]. Its availability only as an oral formulation (it cannot be used in severely ill patients in the intensive care unit or in patients with gastrointestinal dysfunction) and poor absorption in undernourished patients or patients with mucositis are major limitations of its use. When posaconazole is administered after a high-fat meal, its bioavailability increases by 400%; thus, patients are strongly advised to take posaconazole after a good meal [36]. It is well tolerated and has few side effects, and it has a narrower drug interaction profile than voriconazole because it only inhibits CYP3A4 [37]. Limited data reveal an association between low posaconazole serum levels and suboptimal treatment outcome; that and posaconazole's unpredictable absorption support the use of routine therapeutic drug monitoring in some patients.

Validated assays have been developed for the new generation of triazoles and the results of several clinical trials suggest that therapeutic antifungal drug monitoring can be useful for reducing drug toxicity and optimizing efficacy. Further studies are needed to determine optimal timing of monitoring, to refine concentration goals, and to better delineate targeted monitoring for specific patient populations and clinical scenarios [38].

Echinocandins

The echinocandins inhibit (1,3)-beta-D-glucan synthase, which is the key enzyme for the production of beta-glucan, a critical component of the cell wall of many medically important fungi [39]. This inhibition results in disruption of the growing cell wall and the death of susceptible cells [40]. Laboratory ex vivo data support the immunopharmacologic mode of echinocandin action that enhances phagocytosis of fungal hyphae by means of beta-glucan unmasking [41]. All three Food and Drug Administration-approved echinocandins (caspofungin, micafungin, and anidulafungin) are water-soluble and are only available intravenously. They have linear pharmacokinetics, and because they are not CYP450 substrates or inhibitors, they have no drug–drug interactions, unlike members of the azole family [42–44]. This class of antifungals is extremely well tolerated, which is consistent with their unique, fungus-specific mechanism of action. All three echinocandins have a limited spectrum of activity in vitro against non-*Aspergillus* molds.

IMI Prevention and Prophylaxis

Reports on nosocomial outbreaks of IMIs have linked cases to hospital construction, the absence of appropriate barriers between patients and the environment, and the presence of fungal spores in room air samples [45, 46]. A meta-analysis of 16 controlled trials found that HEPA filtration had no effect on mortality in neutropenic patients with hematologic malignancies and SCT recipients. Protected environments appeared to be beneficial, but there were insufficient data to support definite conclusions [47]. The Centers for Disease Control recommends the use of HEPA filters in allogeneic SCT recipient patients' rooms [48].

The optimal antifungal prophylactic has been an evolving issue, perhaps reflecting the introduction of several new agents in the clinical practice (Table 25.2). The emergence of IA in the last two decades necessitates the use of mold-active prophylaxis or fluconazole prophylaxis combined with effective surveillance (e.g., based on periodic galactomannan measurements and/or chest CT) to detect IA early [49]. Which of these two strategies is the most effective in specific patient subgroups is unknown. In addition, we do not know which antifungal agents and delivery methods (oral, inhaled, or intermittent intravenous) are the most effective. In a multicenter, randomized, nonblinded study, an echinocandin (micafungin) was found to be more effective than fluconazole [50]. In this study which has been questioned about the choice of study population and the prophylactic period length, micafungin was found to have superior efficacy. The lack of large comparative studies, the IV-only formulation of echinocandins, and reports for breakthrough mold infections makes echinocandins' role in prophylaxis needing more research [51].

Lipid formulations of AMB as prophylaxis have been tried either as daily administration, weekly, or twice weekly schedules. These agents' "depot" pharmacokinetic characteristics and long elimination times make them attractive for intermittent prophylaxis, avoiding the unreliability of azole-based oral prophylaxis in selected patients. The need for definite conclusions regarding safety and efficacy, since all current data come from noncomparative studies, can be answered by a well-developed randomized trial [52]. A recent study evaluated the effectiveness of aerosolized L-AMB in patients who at the same time were on fluconazole [53]. Fewer patients in the aerosolized prophylaxis arm developed IA; the most common reason for treatment discontinuation was cough. Further research is needed on the safety and efficacy of aerosolized polyenes.

In one study, prophylactic posaconazole was similar to fluconazole for prophylaxis against fungal infections among patients with graft-versus-host disease (GvHD) in overall mortality. Posaconazole was superior in preventing IA and reducing the rate of deaths related to fungal infections [54]. In a substudy of posaconazole pharmacokinetics in the GvHD population, patients with symptomatic diarrhea during acute GvHD had lower serum drug levels and tended to be more prone to infections due to their lower levels [55]. In another study of patients undergoing chemotherapy for acute myelogenous leukemia or myelodysplastic syndrome, posaconazole prevented IFIs more effectively than did either fluconazole or/and itraconazole and improved overall survival [56]. These two studies' results are reflected in the most recent Infectious Diseases Society of America (IDSA) recommendations on prophylaxis in these patient groups [13]. According to these guidelines, antifungal prophylaxis with posaconazole can be recommended in HSCT recipients with GvHD who are at high risk for IA aspergillosis and in patients with acute myelogenous leukemia or myelodysplastic syndrome who are at high risk for IA. Prophylactic voriconazole was also compared with fluconazole and galactomannan monitoring in a large randomized trial in allogeneic SCT recipients. Both agents were administered for at least 100 days after allogeneic SCT [56, 57]. Fewer IFIs, especially IAs, were found in the voriconazole arm of this study, although

Table 25.2 Options for prophylactic use of antifungal drugs in HSCT recipients

No risk factors for IMIs
- *Autologous HSCT*: fluconazole (200–400 mg/day) starting at day 0 until the resolution of neutropenia and mucositis
- *Allogeneic HSCT*: fluconazole (400 mg/day) starting at day 0 for 75 days in myeloablative and nonmyeloablative allograft recipients

Risk factors for IMIs (only for allogeneic HSCT)
- *Voriconazole*: patients in whom *Aspergillus* (and *Candida* and other rare fungi) but not Zygomycetes is a major consideration, such as lack of iron overload, lack of concomitant diabetes, lack of infliximab for GvHD, and lack of prolonged prior exposure to voriconazole, but who have a history of cytomegalovirus reactivation or aspergillosis
- *Posaconazole*: patients in whom *Aspergillus* and Zygomycetes (and *Candida* and other rare fungi) are major considerations, such as iron overload, concomitant diabetes, chronic corticosteroids or infliximab for GvHD, recent cytomegalovirus reactivation, and prior prolonged exposure to voriconazole. Ambulatory patients with severe liver dysfunction or who experience intolerance to or prohibitory drug interactions with voriconazole (e.g., severe rash)
- *Echinocandins* (e.g., 50 mg/day of caspofungin intravenously): hospitalized or ambulatory patients in whom Zygomycetes is not a major consideration and who have severe liver dysfunction or experience intolerance to or prohibitory drug interactions with voriconazole or posaconazole
- *L-AMB* (2 or 3 times a week): patients who cannot take oral mold-active azoles or intravenous echinocandins and have normal renal function

IFI rates were generally low because the population was at low or intermediate risk. Furthermore, the total mortality rates did not differ between the two arms of the study.

The use of second-generation azole as mold prophylaxis in high-risk patients is gaining acceptance, even though these drugs are more complicated to administer than is fluconazole. Issues that arise and need to be answered by future prospective studies are the need of therapeutic drug monitoring of these drugs and the changing validity of blood-based diagnostic assays because mold-active prophylaxis reduces their sensitivity [18]. In the current era of mold-active prophylaxis, it is needed to define which patients need to be covered with mold-active prophylaxis (and for how long) and which patients have less risk so that fluconazole is adequate as prophylaxis. Nevertheless, close evaluation for breakthrough infections is warranted for these patients. Finally, the increased survival of IMI patients in the setting of continuous immunosuppression necessitates secondary prevention strategies. For example, experience and data on the best treatment for relapsing IA are lacking. The high mortality rate of patients with relapsing IA shows that aggressive approaches (e.g., rapid tapering of immunosuppression, using a low threshold for switching to investigational antifungals, and antifungal therapy plus immune restoration strategies) are needed [58].

Empiric and Preemptive Therapy

The effectiveness of empiric antifungal treatment of neutropenic fever was documented in prospective randomized trials. L-AMB, voriconazole, and caspofungin were effective treatments in high- and low-risk patients with persistent febrile neutropenia [59–61]. A comprehensive strategy for this use of antifungal drugs is shown in Fig. 25.1. It is unclear whether the indiscriminate empiric use of antifungals or a measured approach that includes risk stratification, early use of chest CT, and nonculture serologic diagnostic (e.g., galactomannan assay or PCR) is the most efficacious, least toxic, and most cost-effective. The available options for the usage of antifungal drugs for preemptive therapy are shown in Table 25.3. A large randomized, nonblinded, European study (PREVERT trial) [62] did not show that preemptive approach is clinically more useful and more cost-effective compared to the traditional empiric approach. Future studies are needed that stratify patients by risk and use more sensitive methods for early diagnosis. There is no question that early antifungal therapy triggered by the detection of halo sign, an early radiologic marker of IA, is associated with better outcomes [24, 63, 64]. In addition, a single-institution retrospective study showed that a 1-week treatment delay of effective treatment compared with early treatment doubled the mortality rate in a case series of 35 patients with zygomycosis [10].

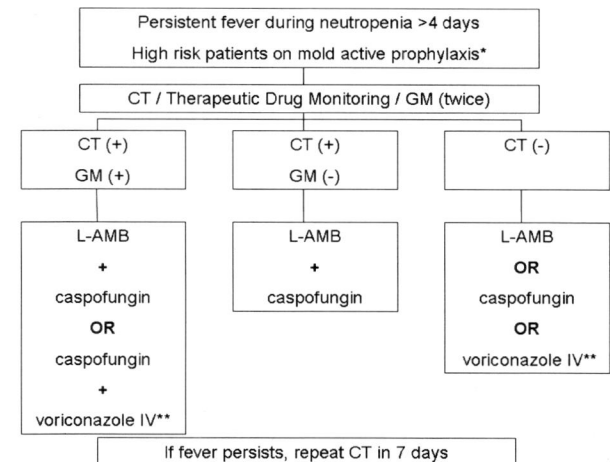

Fig. 25.1 Empiric management of fever in neutropenic SCT patients: use of antifungal drugs

Table 25.3 Options for preemptive therapy of IFIs

For suspected pulmonary mold infections	Voriconazole because *Aspergillus* is the most common mold infection, unless there are contraindications or a suspicion of voriconazole-resistant mycosis (e.g., zygomycetes infection) • 5 mg/kg/day of LF-AMB • Appropriate clinical and radiographic follow-up (including bronchoalveolar lavage or biopsy) coordinated with the infectious disease and pulmonary teams
Febrile BMT patients with twice-positive galactomannan assay results and no other signs or symptoms of infection	Trial of antifungal therapy (voriconazole, caspofungin LF-AMB) with an infectious disease consult
Patients on high-dose steroids for diffuse alveolar hemorrhage or idiopathic pulmonary syndrome[a]	Mold-active azoles such as voriconazole or itraconazole

[a]Rationale: patients with diffuse infiltrates early after transplantation who are negative for infection (on bronchoalveolar lavage or biopsy) are at high risk for subsequent mold infections because they are often treated with high doses of corticosteroids (4 mg/kg/day)

Targeted Therapy for Selected IMIs

Aspergillosis

Voriconazole has emerged as the preferred therapy for IA on the basis of results from a pivotal, large randomized nonblinded study comparing voriconazole with AMB-D (1–1.5 mg/kg/day) in 144 patients with documented IA [64].

This recommendation has been endorsed by several organizations, including the IDSA [13]. L-AMB was also endorsed as an effective alternative primary therapy on the basis of the results of a recent double-blind prospective trial that randomly assigned neutropenic leukemia patients to 3 or 10 mg/kg/day for 14 days, followed by 3 mg/kg/day (AmBiLoad trial) [63]. No statistically significant differences in the overall treatment response were found between the standard and high-dose regimens, but nephrotoxicity and hypokalemia were more common in the high-dose group.

The interest in combination antifungal therapy as primary therapy for IA developed from the observation that the preferred first-line drug, voriconazole, has failure rates approaching 70% in high-risk patients such as SCT recipients [64]. Therefore, it seems that there is much room for improvement, and the early administration of combined antifungal drugs may become an important treatment for IA [65]. A large randomized study is underway evaluating voriconazole plus placebo to anidulafungin plus voriconazole in patients with documented IA. This study hopefully will shed light on the true benefit of combined azole-echinocandin-based primary therapy.

Meanwhile, there are two points of special interest that should be noted in relevance to voriconazole-based combinations as primary therapy. Because voriconazole is used as front-line therapy for IA, it cannot be assumed that the combination of caspofungin and voriconazole will be effective in patients who do not experience a response to voriconazole. In addition, given the emergence of breakthrough Zygomycetes infections in patients undergoing voriconazole prophylaxis or empirical treatment, specific diagnoses are particularly important in high-risk patients because zygomycosis has a similar manifestation to that of IA. Similarly, the combination of an echinocandin and LF-AMB is unclear in IA. The results of small single-institution retrospective studies suggest that LF-AMB and caspofungin are effective against IA, especially as primary therapy [66]. A small prospective, randomized study comparing high-dose L-AMB (10 mg/kg/day) with low-dose L-AMB (3 mg/kg/day) and caspofungin in 30 IA patients (24 probable and six proven) (Combistrat trial) showed that combination therapy was associated with a better (but not statistically significant) response [67]. However, no firm conclusions could be drawn because of the small sample size and the undocumented status of most cases. In addition, it is unclear whether the combination of LF-AMB and echinocandin is beneficial in patients with IA that is refractory to LF-AMB given as monotherapy. Similar results were obtained in our retrospective study [68] and a recent observational prospective study of micafungin plus L-AMB in SCT patients with refractory IA [69]. It can be concluded that combination therapy for IA cannot be widely recommended; therefore, physicians should consider it on a case-by-case basis, accounting for clinical and laboratory evidence.

The effectiveness of salvage antifungal therapy is not known in patients with IA that is refractory or intolerant to voriconazole. Single-institution retrospective salvage studies have evaluated the combination of voriconazole and caspofungin [70]. A multicenter observational study assessed the effectiveness of caspofungin combined with other antifungal drugs in 53 patients with IA that was intolerant or refractory to front-line therapy. The combination of caspofungin and voriconazole resulted in a successful outcome in 54% of patients [71]. The complexities and biases in salvage therapy trials preclude firm recommendations. Combination antifungal therapy or immunotherapy with an LF-AMB, caspofungin, or posaconazole can be used [13].

Zygomycosis

Early diagnosis of zygomycosis is crucial because delayed AMB-based therapy results in poor clinical outcomes [10]. Posaconazole salvage therapy is promising. In a retrospective study that included 91 patients with zygomycosis, the rate of success (i.e., either complete or partial response) at 12 weeks after treatment initiation was 60% [72]. In a nonrandomized, multicenter, compassionate trial that evaluated oral posaconazole as salvage therapy for zygomycosis, the overall survival rate was 79%; survival was also associated with surgical resection of affected tissue and stabilization or improvement of the underlying illness [73]. In a recent study of diabetic patients with rhino-orbital-cerebral mucormycosis treated with combination polyene-caspofungin therapy, patients treated with ABLC and caspofungin had superior success [74]. Advances in our understanding of iron metabolism's role in zygomycosis pathogenesis have led us to use nondeferoxamine iron chelators, such as deferasirox, in combination treatment [75–77]. An open label trial of deferasirox and L-AMB is currently underway to assess their safety and tolerability (DEFEAT Study).

Fusariosis, Phaehyphomycosis, and Scedosporiosis

The rarity and opportunistic nature of fusariosis, phaeohyphomycosis, and scedosporiosis prevent us from determining the optimal treatment regimen and precludes an organized experience for the treatment. Azole-based therapy (voriconazole and posaconazole) provides the best chance for survival, with or without LF-AMB, reduced immunosuppression, and adjunct immunotherapy (e.g., donor white blood cell transfusions [78]).

Summary

We have witnessed important advances in the treatment of IMIs during the last decades. The population at risk is continuously increasing, and the spectrum of emerging pathogens is endlessly expanding. Fortunately, our antifungal armamentarium includes newer antifungal drugs, and we have entered an era in which more sophisticated prophylactic and preemptive strategies and combination therapies can be tailored for patients on the basis of their unique epidemiologic characteristics and risk factors. Indeed, these new therapies will be tested in clinical trials that will establish evidence-based standards of care for patients with IMIs.

References

1. Kontoyiannis DP, Bodey GP. Invasive aspergillosis in 2002: an update. Eur J Clin Microbiol Infect Dis. 2002;21:161–72.
2. Chamilos G, Luna M, Lewis RE, et al. Invasive fungal infections in patients with hematologic malignancies in a tertiary care cancer center: an autopsy study over a 15-year period (1989–2003). Haematologica. 2006;91:986–9.
3. Neofytos D, Horn D, Anaissie E, et al. Epidemiology and outcome of invasive fungal infection in adult hematopoietic stem cell transplant recipients: analysis of Multicenter Prospective Antifungal Therapy (PATH) Alliance registry. Clin Infect Dis. 2009;48:265–73.
4. Wingard JR, Ribaud P, Schlamm HT, Herbrecht R. Changes in causes of death over time after treatment for invasive aspergillosis. Cancer. 2008;112:2309–12.
5. Balajee SA, Weaver M, Imhof A, Gribskov J, Marr KA. *Aspergillus fumigatus* variant with decreased susceptibility to multiple antifungals. Antimicrob Agents Chemother. 2004;48:1197–203.
6. Steinbach WJ, Benjamin Jr DK, Kontoyiannis DP, et al. Infections due to *Aspergillus terreus*: a multicenter retrospective analysis of 83 cases. Clin Infect Dis. 2004;39:192–8.
7. Nucci M, Marr KA. Emerging fungal diseases. Clin Infect Dis. 2005;41:521–6.
8. Ben-Ami R, Lewis RE, Raad II, Kontoyiannis DP. Phaeohyphomycosis in a tertiary care cancer center. Clin Infect Dis. 2009;48:1033–41.
9. Kontoyiannis DP, Lionakis MS, Lewis RE, et al. Zygomycosis in a tertiary-care cancer center in the era of *Aspergillus*-active antifungal therapy: a case-control observational study of 27 recent cases. J Infect Dis. 2005;191:1350–60.
10. Chamilos G, Lewis RE, Kontoyiannis DP. Delaying amphotericin B-based frontline therapy significantly increases mortality among patients with hematologic malignancy who have zygomycosis. Clin Infect Dis. 2008;47:503–9.
11. De Pauw B, Walsh TJ, Donnelly JP, et al. Revised definitions of invasive fungal disease from the European Organization for Research and Treatment of Cancer/Invasive Fungal Infections Cooperative Group and the National Institute of Allergy and Infectious Diseases Mycoses Study Group (EORTC/MSG) Consensus Group. Clin Infect Dis. 2008;46:1813–21.
12. Lionakis MS, Kontoyiannis DP. The significance of isolation of saprophytic molds from the lower respiratory tract in patients with cancer. Cancer. 2004;100:165–72.
13. Walsh TJ, Anaissie EJ, Denning DW, et al. Treatment of aspergillosis: clinical practice guidelines of the Infectious Diseases Society of America. Clin Infect Dis. 2008;46:327–60.
14. Tarrand JJ, Lichterfeld M, Warraich I, et al. Diagnosis of invasive septate mold infections. A correlation of microbiological culture and histologic or cytologic examination. Am J Clin Pathol. 2003;119:854–8.
15. Hayden RT, Isotalo PA, Parrett T, et al. In situ hybridization for the differentiation of *Aspergillus, Fusarium,* and *Pseudallescheria* species in tissue section. Diagn Mol Pathol. 2003;12:21–6.
16. Mennink-Kersten MA, Donnelly JP, Verweij PE. Detection of circulating galactomannan for the diagnosis and management of invasive aspergillosis. Lancet Infect Dis. 2004;4:349–57.
17. Marr KA, Balajee SA, McLaughlin L, Tabouret M, Bentsen C, Walsh TJ. Detection of galactomannan antigenemia by enzyme immunoassay for the diagnosis of invasive aspergillosis: variables that affect performance. J Infect Dis. 2004;190:641–9.
18. Marr KA, Laverdiere M, Gugel A, Leisenring W. Antifungal therapy decreases sensitivity of the *Aspergillus* galactomannan enzyme immunoassay. Clin Infect Dis. 2005;40:1762–9.
19. Pickering JW, Sant HW, Bowles CA, Roberts WL, Woods GL. Evaluation of a (1->3)-beta-D-glucan assay for diagnosis of invasive fungal infections. J Clin Microbiol. 2005;43:5957–62.
20. Pazos C, Ponton J, Del Palacio A. Contribution of (1->3)-beta-D-glucan chromogenic assay to diagnosis and therapeutic monitoring of invasive aspergillosis in neutropenic adult patients: a comparison with serial screening for circulating galactomannan. J Clin Microbiol. 2005;43:299–305.
21. Donnelly JP. Polymerase chain reaction for diagnosing invasive aspergillosis: getting closer but still a ways to go. Clin Infect Dis. 2006;42:487–9.
22. Caillot D, Mannone L, Cuisenier B, Couaillier JF. Role of early diagnosis and aggressive surgery in the management of invasive pulmonary aspergillosis in neutropenic patients. Clin Microbiol Infect. 2001;7 Suppl 2:54–61.
23. Caillot D, Couaillier JF, Bernard A, et al. Increasing volume and changing characteristics of invasive pulmonary aspergillosis on sequential thoracic computed tomography scans in patients with neutropenia. J Clin Oncol. 2001;19:253–9.
24. Greene RE, Schlamm HT, Oestmann JW, et al. Imaging findings in acute invasive pulmonary aspergillosis: clinical significance of the halo sign. Clin Infect Dis. 2007;44:373–9.
25. Caillot D, Casasnovas O, Bernard A, et al. Improved management of invasive pulmonary aspergillosis in neutropenic patients using early thoracic computed tomographic scan and surgery. J Clin Oncol. 1997;15:139–47.
26. Chamilos G, Marom EM, Lewis RE, Lionakis MS, Kontoyiannis DP. Predictors of pulmonary zygomycosis versus invasive pulmonary aspergillosis in patients with cancer. Clin Infect Dis. 2005;41:60–6.
27. Wahba H, Truong MT, Lei X, Kontoyiannis DP, Marom EM. Reversed halo sign in invasive pulmonary fungal infections. Clin Infect Dis. 2008;46:1733–7.
28. Dupont B. Overview of the lipid formulations of amphotericin B. J Antimicrob Chemother. 2002;49 Suppl 1:31–6.
29. Lewis RE, Liao G, Hou J, Chamilos G, Prince RA, Kontoyiannis DP. Comparative analysis of amphotericin B lipid complex and liposomal amphotericin B kinetics of lung accumulation and fungal clearance in a murine model of acute invasive pulmonary aspergillosis. Antimicrob Agents Chemother. 2007;51:1253–8.
30. Lanternier F, Lortholary O. Liposomal amphotericin B: what is its role in 2008? Clin Microbiol Infect. 2008;14 Suppl 4:71–83.
31. Theuretzbacher U, Ihle F, Derendorf H. Pharmacokinetic/pharmacodynamic profile of voriconazole. Clin Pharmacokinet. 2006;45:649–63.
32. Pascual A, Calandra T, Bolay S, Buclin T, Bille J, Marchetti O. Voriconazole therapeutic drug monitoring in patients with invasive mycoses improves efficacy and safety outcomes. Clin Infect Dis. 2008;46:201–11.
33. Lewis RE. What is the "therapeutic range" for voriconazole? Clin Infect Dis. 2008;46:212–4.

34. Johnson LB, Kauffman CA. Voriconazole: a new triazole antifungal agent. Clin Infect Dis. 2003;36:630–7.
35. Gonzalez GM, Fothergill AW, Sutton DA, Rinaldi MG, Loebenberg D. In vitro activities of new and established triazoles against opportunistic filamentous and dimorphic fungi. Med Mycol. 2005;43:281–4.
36. Courtney R, Radwanski E, Lim J, Laughlin M. Pharmacokinetics of posaconazole coadministered with antacid in fasting or nonfasting healthy men. Antimicrob Agents Chemother. 2004;48:804–8.
37. Raad II, Graybill JR, Bustamante AB, et al. Safety of long-term oral posaconazole use in the treatment of refractory invasive fungal infections. Clin Infect Dis. 2006;42:1726–34.
38. Andes D, Pascual A, Marchetti O. Antifungal therapeutic drug monitoring: established and emerging indications. Antimicrob Agents Chemother. 2009;53:24–34.
39. Denning DW. Echinocandin antifungal drugs. Lancet. 2003;362:1142–51.
40. Bowman JC, Hicks PS, Kurtz MB, et al. The antifungal echinocandin caspofungin acetate kills growing cells of *Aspergillus fumigatus* in vitro. Antimicrob Agents Chemother. 2002;46:3001–12.
41. Lamaris GA, Lewis RE, Chamilos G, et al. Caspofungin-mediated beta-glucan unmasking and enhancement of human polymorphonuclear neutrophil activity against *Aspergillus* and non-*Aspergillus* hyphae. J Infect Dis. 2008;198:186–92.
42. Vazquez JA, Sobel JD. Anidulafungin: a novel echinocandin. Clin Infect Dis. 2006;43:215–22.
43. Chandrasekar PH, Sobel JD. Micafungin: a new echinocandin. Clin Infect Dis. 2006;42:1171–8.
44. Walsh TJ, Raad I, Patterson TF, et al. Treatment of invasive aspergillosis with posaconazole in patients who are refractory to or intolerant of conventional therapy: an externally controlled trial. Clin Infect Dis. 2007;44:2–12.
45. Boyce JM, Pittet D. Guideline for Hand Hygiene in Health-Care Settings. Recommendations of the Healthcare Infection Control Practices Advisory Committee and the HICPAC/SHEA/APIC/IDSA Hand Hygiene Task Force. Society for Healthcare Epidemiology of America/Association for Professionals in Infection Control/Infectious Diseases Society of America. MMWR Recomm Rep. 2002;51:1–45; quiz CE1–4.
46. Thio CL, Smith D, Merz WG, et al. Refinements of environmental assessment during an outbreak investigation of invasive aspergillosis in a leukemia and bone marrow transplant unit. Infect Control Hosp Epidemiol. 2000;21:18–23.
47. Eckmanns T, Ruden H, Gastmeier P. The influence of high-efficiency particulate air filtration on mortality and fungal infection among highly immunosuppressed patients: a systematic review. J Infect Dis. 2006;193:1408–18.
48. Guidelines for preventing opportunistic infections among hematopoietic stem cell transplant recipients. MMWR Recomm Rep. 2000;49:1–125; CE1–7.
49. Slavin MA, Osborne B, Adams R, et al. Efficacy and safety of fluconazole prophylaxis for fungal infections after marrow transplantation–a prospective, randomized, double-blind study. J Infect Dis. 1995;171:1545–52.
50. van Burik JA, Ratanatharathorn V, Stepan DE, et al. Micafungin versus fluconazole for prophylaxis against invasive fungal infections during neutropenia in patients undergoing hematopoietic stem cell transplantation. Clin Infect Dis. 2004;39:1407–16.
51. Chou LS, Lewis RE, Ippoliti C, Champlin RE, Kontoyiannis DP. Caspofungin as primary antifungal prophylaxis in stem cell transplant recipients. Pharmacotherapy. 2007;27:1644–50.
52. Marr KA. Primary antifungal prophylaxis in hematopoietic stem cell transplant recipients: clinical implications of recent studies. Curr Opin Infect Dis. 2008;21:409–14.
53. Rijnders BJ, Cornelissen JJ, Slobbe L, et al. Aerosolized liposomal amphotericin B for the prevention of invasive pulmonary aspergillosis during prolonged neutropenia: a randomized, placebo-controlled trial. Clin Infect Dis. 2008;46:1401–8.
54. Ullmann AJ, Lipton JH, Vesole DH, et al. Posaconazole or fluconazole for prophylaxis in severe graft-versus-host disease. N Engl J Med. 2007;356:335–47.
55. Krishna G, Martinho M, Chandrasekar P, Ullmann AJ, Patino H. Pharmacokinetics of oral posaconazole in allogeneic hematopoietic stem cell transplant recipients with graft-versus-host disease. Pharmacotherapy. 2007;27:1627–36.
56. Cornely OA, Maertens J, Winston DJ, et al. Posaconazole vs. fluconazole or itraconazole prophylaxis in patients with neutropenia. N Engl J Med. 2007;356:348–59.
57. Siwek GT, Pfaller MA, Polgreen PM, et al. Incidence of invasive aspergillosis among allogeneic hematopoietic stem cell transplant patients receiving voriconazole prophylaxis. Diagn Microbiol Infect Dis. 2006;55:209–12.
58. Sipsas NV, Kontoyiannis DP. Clinical issues regarding relapsing aspergillosis and the efficacy of secondary antifungal prophylaxis in patients with hematological malignancies. Clin Infect Dis. 2006;42:1584–91.
59. Walsh TJ, Finberg RW, Arndt C, et al. Liposomal amphotericin B for empirical therapy in patients with persistent fever and neutropenia. National Institute of Allergy and Infectious Diseases Mycoses Study Group. N Engl J Med. 1999;340:764–71.
60. Walsh TJ, Pappas P, Winston DJ, et al. Voriconazole compared with liposomal amphotericin B for empirical antifungal therapy in patients with neutropenia and persistent fever. N Engl J Med. 2002;346:225–34.
61. Walsh TJ, Teppler H, Donowitz GR, et al. Caspofungin versus liposomal amphotericin B for empirical antifungal therapy in patients with persistent fever and neutropenia. N Engl J Med. 2004;351:1391–402.
62. Cordonnier C, Pautas C, Maury S, et al. Empirical versus preemptive antifungal therapy for high-risk, febrile, neutropenic patients: a randomized, controlled trial. Clin Infect Dis. 2009;48:1042–51.
63. Cornely OA, Maertens J, Bresnik M, et al. Liposomal amphotericin B as initial therapy for invasive mold infection: a randomized trial comparing a high-loading dose regimen with standard dosing (AmBiLoad trial). Clin Infect Dis. 2007;44:1289–97.
64. Herbrecht R, Denning DW, Patterson TF, et al. Voriconazole versus amphotericin B for primary therapy of invasive aspergillosis. N Engl J Med. 2002;347:408–15.
65. Chamilos G, Kontoyiannis DP. The rationale of combination antifungal therapy in severely immunocompromised patients: empiricism versus evidence-based medicine. Curr Opin Infect Dis. 2006;19:380–5.
66. Aliff TB, Maslak PG, Jurcic JG, et al. Refractory Aspergillus pneumonia in patients with acute leukemia: successful therapy with combination caspofungin and liposomal amphotericin. Cancer. 2003;97:1025–32.
67. Caillot D, Thiebaut A, Herbrecht R, et al. Liposomal amphotericin B in combination with caspofungin for invasive aspergillosis in patients with hematologic malignancies: a randomized pilot study (Combistrat trial). Cancer. 2007;110:2740–6.
68. Kontoyiannis DP, Hachem R, Lewis RE, et al. Efficacy and toxicity of caspofungin in combination with liposomal amphotericin B as primary or salvage treatment of invasive aspergillosis in patients with hematologic malignancies. Cancer. 2003;98:292–9.
69. Kontoyiannis DP, Ratanatharathorn V, Young JA, et al. Micafungin alone or in combination with other systemic antifungal therapies in hematopoietic stem cell transplant recipients with invasive aspergillosis. Transpl Infect Dis. 2009;11:89–93.
70. Marr KA, Boeckh M, Carter RA, Kim HW, Corey L. Combination antifungal therapy for invasive aspergillosis. Clin Infect Dis. 2004;39:797–802.
71. Maertens J, Glasmacher A, Herbrecht R, et al. Multicenter, noncomparative study of caspofungin in combination with other

antifungals as salvage therapy in adults with invasive aspergillosis. Cancer. 2006;107:2888–97.
72. van Burik JA, Hare RS, Solomon HF, Corrado ML, Kontoyiannis DP. Posaconazole is effective as salvage therapy in zygomycosis: a retrospective summary of 91 cases. Clin Infect Dis. 2006;42:e61–5.
73. Greenberg RN, Mullane K, van Burik JA, et al. Posaconazole as salvage therapy for zygomycosis. Antimicrob Agents Chemother. 2006;50:126–33.
74. Reed C, Bryant R, Ibrahim AS, et al. Combination polyene-caspofungin treatment of rhino-orbital-cerebral mucormycosis. Clin Infect Dis. 2008;47:364–71.
75. Walsh TJ, Kontoyiannis DP. Editorial commentary: what is the role of combination therapy in management of zygomycosis? Clin Infect Dis. 2008;47:372–4.
76. Ibrahim AS, Gebermariam T, Fu Y, et al. The iron chelator deferasirox protects mice from mucormycosis through iron starvation. J Clin Invest. 2007;117:2649–57.
77. Reed C, Ibrahim A, Edwards Jr JE, Walot I, Spellberg B. Deferasirox, an iron-chelating agent, as salvage therapy for rhinocerebral mucormycosis. Antimicrob Agents Chemother. 2006;50:3968–9.
78. Safdar A. Antifungal immunity and adjuvant cytokine immune enhancement in cancer patients with invasive fungal infections. Clin Microbiol Infect. 2007;13:1–4.

Chapter 26
Cryptococcal Disease and Endemic Mycosis

Johan A. Maertens and Hélène Schoemans

Abstract *Cryptococcus* and the endemic fungi (*Histoplasma, Blastomyces,* and *Coccidioides*) can cause severe, even life-threatening, pulmonary and extrapulmonary disease in immunocompromised patients, including cancer patients and transplant recipients. This chapter describes the epidemiology, clinical manifestations, diagnosis, and treatment of these infections in patients with prolonged immunodeficiency.

Keywords Cryptococcus • Cancer • Immune suppression • Histoplasmosis • Blastomycosis • Coccidioidomycosis

Cryptococcal Disease

Cryptococcosis, a potentially life-threatening invasive fungal disease caused by the encapsulated, nonmycelial budding yeast, *Cryptococcus neoformans*, is a common opportunistic infection in acquired immunodeficiency syndrome (AIDS) patients and solid organ transplant recipients, but remains a relatively uncommon disease in patients with malignancy [1, 2]. This fungus is widely distributed worldwide and is particularly abundant in soil contaminated by pigeon droppings. In general, incidence rates below 2% have been found at autopsy surveys in cancer patients [3]. This low incidence can be partially due to the widespread use of azole prophylaxis (in particular fluconazole) and the routine empirical use of antifungals in many cancer patients at risk for cryptococcosis. As a consequence, most (retrospective) studies consist of case reports or small case series only. Hence, many aspects of the epidemiology and clinical features of cryptococcosis in cancer patients remain poorly documented.

The majority of *Cryptococcus* infections in immunocompromised patients are caused by *C. neoformans* var. *grubii* (serotype A) or var. *neoformans* (serotype D). *Cryptococcus gattii* (previously *C. neoformans* serotypes B and C) is responsible for a smaller proportion of cases, often in otherwise healthy immunocompetent patients in distinct geographic locations (northern Australia and Papua New Guinea and more recently Vancouver Island) [4]. Exposure to this ubiquitous environmental fungus is common, with the majority of people being exposed by the age of 5 years. Inhalation of basidospores is thought to be the primary portal of entry. Person-to-person transmission does not occur. Upon inhalation, these pathogens may be cleared, may be retained as dormant living yeast within pulmonary lymph nodes (similar to that of tuberculous), or may disseminate, depending on host immune response, virulence of the organism, and size of the inoculum. Cell-mediated immunity plays a critical role in the host defense and protective pulmonary inflammatory responses are dependent on interferon-gamma and tumor necrosis factor-α, leading to a Th1-weighted immunity [5].

Prior to the AIDS epidemic, only approximately 300 cases of cryptococcosis had been reported in the medical literature. Historically, cryptococcosis has typically been described in cancer patients with impaired T-cell immunity (e.g., patients with Hodgkin's disease) or in patients who received high doses of corticosteroids or purine analogs. As a result, patients with hematological malignancies, especially lymphoma and chronic leukemia, were predominant in older series [6, 7]. More recently, novel immunosuppressive monoclonal antibody therapies have been reported as emerging risk factors, including the use of infliximab, efalizumab, adalimumab (an anti-TNF-α monoclonal), and alemtuzumab, an anti-CD52 monoclonal that causes profound CD4 lymphopenia and that is used in the treatment of chronic B-cell malignancies, T-cell malignancies and solid organ transplants, and the use of antithymocyte globulin (ATG) [8, 9].

Clinical findings in cryptococcosis are generally caused by pulmonary and neurologic abnormalities, although the fungus can disseminate to virtually all organs of the body, including prostate and eye [10]. In addition, underlying immunodeficiencies (e.g., use of steroids) may attenuate the clinical signs and symptoms of cryptococcosis [10]. The onset of symptoms in immunocompromised patients is generally subacute, but rapidly progressive disease may occur [10, 11].

J.A. Maertens (✉)
Department of Hematology, Acute Leukemia and Stem Cell Transplantation Unit, University Hospitals Leuven,
Campus Gasthuisberg, Herestraat 49, 3000, Leuven, Belgium
e-mail: johan.maertens@uzleuven.be

Meningitis or meningoencephalitis and pulmonary cryptococcosis are the predominant manifestations in cancer patients [10].

Central nervous system cryptococcosis commonly results from dissemination from the lungs and usually presents as subacute meningitis with prominent neurological symptoms and defects. Patients frequently complain of unbearable headache, with or without fever. Other features include seizures, vomiting, visual disturbances, altered sensorium, hemiparesis, hemisensory signs, and cranial neuropathies [12]. These findings should always raise suspicion of cryptococcosis and need to be differentiated from other causes of meningitis, including tuberculous meningitis and carcinomatous or lymphomatous meningitis. Diagnosis of cryptococcosis with CNS involvement is based on positive *Cryptococcus* antigen titer, culture, or visualizing the organism by India ink staining of cerebrospinal fluid (CSF) [12]. *Cryptococcus* antigen testing (by latex agglutination test or ELISA) is almost always positive, except very early in the course of the disease (low fungal burden) and in certain patients with cryptococcomas [13]. However, a positive CSF culture remains the gold standard. Routine antifungal susceptibility testing is of little value because primary resistance is rare and cut-offs for susceptibility remain ill-defined. Neuro-imaging, computed tomographic (CT) scan, or preferably magnetic resonance imaging (MRI) of the brain with contrast should be carried out in all patients with cryptococcal meningitis to rule out space-occupying lesions [14]. A lumbar puncture with manometry is also highly recommended [15].

Cryptococcosis is an emerging respiratory mycosis and many HIV-negative patients infected with *Cryptococcus* will present with signs of pulmonary involvement [5]. However, the nonspecific constellation of symptoms of pulmonary disease, including fever, (dry) cough, chest pain, weight loss, dyspnea, night sweats, and hemoptysis, makes a differential diagnosis with other pulmonary conditions (e.g., tuberculous or lung metastasis) in cancer patients difficult. In some cases, pulmonary cryptococcosis may result in respiratory failure. The radiographic features of pulmonary cryptococcosis are clearly influenced by the underlying immune status of the patient [5]. Findings are nonspecific and can broadly be categorized into (1) solitary or multiple smooth or spiculated pulmonary nodules; (2) focal or multifocal consolidations; and (3) diffuse interstitial infiltrates. Lymphadenopathy and pleural effusions have also been reported. Diagnosis of pulmonary cryptococcosis requires culture and identification of the organism from a pulmonary specimen, and ideally, histopathologic evidence of tissue invasion. Sputum samples are the most readily obtainable samples, but are limited by decreased sensitivity. Invasive diagnostic procedures such as bronchoscopy with bronchoalveolar lavage (BAL), transbronchial biopsy, or percutaneous or open-lung biopsy will result in a higher diagnostic yield. *C. neoformans* will grow on most bacterial and fungal culture media within 2–7 days [16]. Earlier studies have demonstrated that cryptococcal antigen testing of BAL samples (titer >1:8) was a very effective tool for diagnosing cryptococcal pneumonia [17].

Cryptococcus species are not considered normal respiratory flora in humans. Hence, especially among immunocompromised cancer patients, isolation from a respiratory sample must be considered significant. In these cases, a thorough search for dissemination and an accurate evaluation of fungal burden should be started, including serum cryptococcal antigen testing, fungal blood and urine cultures, and examination of CSF. Serum cryptococcal antigen detection (a titer of ≥1:4) is very accurate for diagnosing disseminated disease. In patients with cryptococcal meningitis, antigen positivity will be found in more than 90% of the tested CSF samples and in more than 80% of the tested serum samples. However, the diagnostic utility of the serum test is limited in patients with isolated pulmonary disease.

More unusual presentations of cryptococcosis include cryptococcemia, mimicking candidemia, and cryptococcal cellulitis, mimicking nonspecific panniculitis.

All infected immunocompromised patients, HIV-positive and HIV-negative, should receive antifungal therapy, even if they are asymptomatic. In addition, all these patients should have serum antigen titers obtained and a lumbar puncture performed with CSF cultures and antigen titers to determine CNS involvement. The goal of antifungal treatment in cryptococcal disease is to prevent dissemination, to sterilize infected tissue, and to prevent recurrence. Clearly, successfully achieving these goals will be closely related to the host immunity; therefore, different approaches have been recommended for immunocompromised and immunocompetent patients.

Recommendations for antifungal therapy of cryptococcosis in non-HIV-infected cancer patients are hampered by the paucity of data. However, given the high risk of fungal dissemination in all immunocompromised patients (albeit predominantly studied in HIV-positive patients), we still recommend an induction course of antifungal therapy, followed by consolidation and maintenance treatment [18]. Amphotericin B deoxycholate (0.7–1.0 mg/kg/day) plus flucytosine for 2 weeks remains the mainstay of induction therapy in most immunocompromised patients. A recent randomized controlled trial showed that high-dose amphotericin B deoxycholate (1 mg/kg/day) was significantly more rapidly fungicidal than standard-dose amphotericin B (0.7 mg/kg) in HIV-patients with meningitis [19]. In the context of preexisting renal impairment or concomitant use of nephrotoxic drugs (e.g., calcineurin inhibitors), substitution with liposomal amphotericin B (3–4 mg/kg) or amphotericin B lipid complex (5 mg/kg) is preferable. In addition, flucytosine, given at a dose of 100 mg/kg (orally or intravenously), remains the agent of choice for use in combination with amphotericin B. Although many hemato-oncologists are hesitant to use flucytosine in cancer patients, particularly given its myelosuppressive properties, lack of flucytosine in the induction phase was independently associated with mycological failure at 2 weeks in a large prospective study in France in HIV-positive and HIV-negative patients [20]. Furthermore, less than 14 days of flucytosine therapy was independently associated with treatment failure at 90 days [21]. Although fluconazole (400 mg/day) is recommended as initial therapy for nonsevere, nonmeningeal disease [18], we still recommend initial therapy with amphotericin B and flucytosine for all cancer patients, especially in view of the poor outcomes seen in patients with initial dissemination. This combination induction therapy is then followed by consolidation with oral fluconazole 400–800 mg/day for a minimum of 8 weeks. Finally, in HIV-positive patients, fluconazole maintenance therapy (200 mg/day) is usually given for 6–12 months, depending on the CD4 cell count. The need for prolonged maintenance prophylaxis in HIV-negative patients is less clear-cut; the decision to discontinue should be based on host immune recovery and improvement in clinico-radiological findings. For instance, in a series from the MDACC, most patients did not receive more than 4 months of therapy [1]. The newer triazoles, voriconazole and posaconazole, have a role in the salvage setting. Echinocandins are not effective against cryptococcosis and therefore should not be used.

More recently, clinical research is focusing on the use of adjunctive immunotherapies, in particular the use of recombinant interferon-gamma, and on the use of heat shock protein 90 antibodies. Another important part of the integrated approach is the management of raised CSF pressure associated with cryptococcal meningitis, often requiring serial lumbar punctures or the (temporary) placement of shunts. Finally, cryptococcal immune reconstitution syndrome (IRIS) has also been reported in HIV-negative patients, including solid organ transplant recipients following tapering of immunosuppressive drugs and following T-cell recovery after alemtuzumab therapy. If IRIS patients deteriorate despite maintained antifungal therapy and controlled CSF drainage and if no alternative diagnoses have been found, a short course with corticosteroids may proof useful [18].

The outcome of cancer patients with cryptococcosis is ill-defined. A study from MSKCC found a significantly worse outcome for cancer patients than for HIV-infected patients [22] and a French study found underlying cancer to be the strongest predictor of fatal cryptococcosis among HIV-negative individuals [23]. However, a more recent case series from MDACC reported much better outcomes in cancer patients [1]. In this latter study, all patients who died of cryptococcosis had either lymphopenia or concurrent infections, a regular finding in these patients. According to a multivariate analysis in HIV-negative patients, age above 60 years, hematological malignancy, and organ failure were independent predictors of mortality [10]. Of note, cryptococcal infection does not preclude subsequent transplantation procedures, provided secondary prophylaxis is given. In the future, it is hoped that vaccines or boosting of the immunity will prevent or eliminate the disease.

Endemic Mycosis

Coccidioidomycosis

Although the exact incidence remains unknown, infection with *Coccidiodes immitis* is a very rare event in cancer patients, even in areas endemic for coccidioidomycosis (also known as valley fever). This finding may in part be explained by the frequent empirical use of antifungals in febrile cancer patients without a specific diagnosis, the low index of suspicion, and the lack of autopsy data.

In healthy individuals, this infection, which is endemic in the desert regions of the southwestern United States, in adjacent regions of Mexico, and in other areas of Central and South America, usually presents as a self-limiting, often asymptomatic pulmonary infection [24]. However, patients who have suppressed cellular immunity, including cancer patients, are at increased risk of developing extrapulmonary and disseminated disease. In a case series of 55 immunocompromised patients, dissemination was found in more than 20%, far exceeding the observed rate of 1 or 2% in immunocompetent individuals [25].

Most of the reports are hampered by small numbers of cases, but it seems that these infections are more frequent in patients with non-Hodgkin's lymphoma and chronic lymphocytic leukemia, underscoring again the importance of deficiencies in T-cell immunity. Of note, these infections can be diagnosed months or years after the initial diagnosis of a hematological malignancy, either as primary infection or as reactivation of a previous episode [25]. More recently, an increased risk for coccidioidomycosis has also been reported following anti-TNF-α monoclonal antibody therapy [26]. Finally, in endemic regions, around 5% of solid organ transplant recipients have evidence of disease and, although prior coccidioidomycosis does not contraindicate transplantation, early identification and treatment or prophylaxis seems prudent [27].

Unifocal or multifocal pulmonary disease is present in 95% of the cases; dissemination may occur to skin, central nervous system, or other single organs. Only very few patients will present with disseminated disease without evidence of pulmonary involvement. In cancer patients, coccidioidomycosis carries a mortality up to 50%, albeit greatly increased by steroid treatment or cytotoxic therapy [25].

Rapid diagnosis is possible based on microscopic examination of respiratory specimens or tissues [28]. Cultures will be infrequently positive and are time-consuming. Detection of circulating antibodies (serological assays), although frequently used, yields questionable sensitivity and specificity [29]. More recently, a specific *Coccidiodes* enzyme immunoassay has been developed, detecting urinary antigen in 71% of immunosuppressed patients with moderately severe-to-severe disease. Specificity was high, but cross-reactivity occurred in 10% of patients infected with other endemic mycosis [30]. Recently, several smaller studies have demonstrated the usefulness of in-house-developed polymerase chain reaction assays in establishing the diagnosis.

Azole antifungals have clearly become the standard therapy for coccidioidomycosis [24]. Based on the Landmark study of Galgiani et al., itraconazole capsules 200 mg twice daily are preferred above fluconazole [31]. Posaconazole, structurally related to itraconazole, can be used in case of itraconazole failure. Amphotericin B deoxycholate or a lipid-based formulation can be used in patients unable to tolerate azole therapy or in patients with rapidly progressive disease. Although clinical efficacy with echinocandins has been seen in scattered case reports, their use cannot be recommended in the absence of clinical studies.

Blastomycosis

Infection with *Blastomyces dermatitidis* is endemic in the southeastern and south central states of the United States and the Great Lakes region, as well as in locations near the Missouri, Mississippi, and Ohio Rivers [32]. Although formerly thought to be more prominent in men in the fourth through sixth decade of life, recent data from the Nationwide Inpatient Sample Database fail to confirm this finding [33].

Systemic infection with *B. dermatitidis* usually follows an inhalation exposure. Alveolar macrophages then play a critical role in inhibiting transformation of the mold into the yeast phase and T-cells are the chief mediators of immunity to *B. dermatitidis*. Specifically, a Th-1 response is primarily responsible for effective immunologic control of infection [32].

The range of clinical symptoms associated with blastomycosis is broad. Almost any organ system can be involved, with severity ranging from mild-to-rapidly fatal, depending on the underlying immune status [34, 35]. The most common presentation is acute or chronic pulmonary infection. Patients with acute pneumonia present with mild-to-moderate flu-like symptoms with nonproductive cough, or more symptomatically with sputum, fever, and pleuritic chest pain. Chronic pneumonia is far more common and is characterized by nonspecific findings, such as low-grade fever, constitutional symptoms, and chronic productive cough. Chest radiographic features are nonspecific as well, demonstrating nodular or lobar infiltrates, often with cavitation. Skin and subcutaneous involvement is the second most frequent manifestation of blastomycosis [35].

Although the published experience is (very) small, recognition of blastomycosis in the expanding population of immunocompromised hosts is a real clinical problem. Indeed, blastomycosis affects less than 1% of solid organ transplant recipients in endemic regions, but causes ARDS or miliary disease in 15% of the infected patients [36]. This manifestation is associated with a 50–90% mortality rate, despite appropriate therapy. Also, stem cell transplant recipients and patients receiving chemotherapy are at risk [37]. The exact incidence rate remains unknown, but up to 40% of these infected patients will develop ARDS and miliary disease, resulting in a rapidly fatal outcome. HIV-infected patients are another population of interest; again, disease manifestations tend to be very severe with disease-related mortality rates approaching 40% within the first weeks [38].

Diagnosis, which is often delayed due to unawareness of clinicians of this possibility, rests heavily on culture and histopathology. However, the organism may take weeks to be isolated in culture and histopathologic examination requires a dedicated and well-trained pathologist. Given the low-to-very low sensitivities (complement fixation 9%, immune-diffusion 28%, ELISA 77%), most experts do not recommend using the currently available serological tests for diagnosis [39]. However, antigen can be detected in urine, serum, and bronchial lavage fluid using the routinely available *Blastomyces* enzyme immunoassay (MiraVista Diagnostics, Indianapolis, Indiana) [40]. High sensitivity and specificity of 93 and 98%, respectively, was noted in one study, comparing favorably against serological testing. In addition, serial testing may be a method to monitor disease progression [41]. However, the assay is somewhat limited by significant cross-reactivity with *Histoplasma capsulatum*.

Even in the absence of comparative clinical trial data, patients with moderately severe-to-severe forms of blastomycosis (such as most cancer patients) should receive initial therapy with amphotericin B, either deoxycholate (0.7–1.0 mg/kg) or lipid-based (3–5 mg/kg) for 1 or 2 weeks, followed by a consolidation therapy with itraconazole (200 mg bid, following a loading dose of 200 mg 3 times per day for 3 days) for at least 12 months (or lifelong in case of continued immunosuppression) [42]. Of note, given the erratic absorption of itraconazole, monitoring of serum itraconazole concentrations is strongly recommended. However, target serum levels and dose-adjustment protocols for itraconazole have not been established. Patients with central nervous system involvement should receive initial therapy with a lipid-based formulation of amphotericin B. The drug of choice for continued oral maintenance therapy in these particular cases is unclear, but voriconazole looks promising, provided therapeutic drug monitoring is performed. Finally, patients presenting with ARDS due to blastomycosis may benefit from adjunctive therapy with corticosteroids and may suffer from infection-related adrenal insufficiency, underscoring the need for a multidisciplinary approach.

Histoplasmosis

Histoplasmosis, caused by *H. capsulatum*, is the most common endemic mycosis reported in immunocompromised patients, most likely because it is the most common endemic mycosis overall. The dimorphic fungus *H. capsulatum* is endemic in the Ohio and Mississippi River valleys and in Central and South America. In these areas, skin tests surveys demonstrate that over half of the population acquired histoplasmosis during infancy. Smaller foci of histoplasmosis also exist in southeastern Asia, Africa, and the south of Europe [43]. In general, healthcare providers in these areas are familiar with the recognition, diagnosis, and therapy of histoplasmosis. However, nowadays, an increasing number of cases are recognized in nonendemic areas, especially in immunocompromised patients with prior exposure to endemic areas, either through travel or residence [44]. In some of these cases, histoplasmosis occurs months to years later following low-inoculum exposure, making the diagnosis more difficult.

This fungus is abundantly present in soil contaminated by droppings from birds and bats, in old buildings, and in caves. Again, infection follows an inhalation exposure. Aerosolized microconidia are inhaled and phagocytized by alveolar macrophages. Upon phagocytosis, the organism converts to its yeast phase and disseminates throughout the reticuloendothelial system [45]. Once specific cell-mediated immunity develops, T cells will activate the macrophages, enabling them to kill the organism. However, in case of defective cell-mediated immunity, viable organisms will remain within these macrophages and cause progressive disease. Obviously, the severity of disease will depend on the burden of inhaled conidia and the host immune response. In severely immunosuppressed patients, even a small inoculum can cause severe pulmonary infection of disseminated histoplasmosis. Patients at increased risk include AIDS patients with low CD4 counts, those receiving corticosteroids and other immunosuppressive drugs, patients suffering from hematological malignancies and, more recently, patient receiving anti-TNF-α monoclonal antibodies; the risk for solid organ transplant recipients and stem cell transplantation recipients appears to be low, even in endemic areas. Of note, since *H. capsulatum* is a viable intracellular organism, it can be transmitted with donated organs. When diagnosis is made timely and adequate therapy is installed, mortality tends to be low, even in immunosuppressed patients. However, too often diagnosis is not established until late in the course, especially in nonendemic regions.

Patients who are immunosuppressed usually develop clinical picture of severe pneumonia or that of disseminated disease [46]. They appear ill, present with chills, high fever, dyspnea, dry cough, and chest pain, and can progress rapidly to acute respiratory distress syndrome. In case of dissemination, they manifest with severe signs of sepsis or organ failure: shock with ARDS, adrenal insufficiency, disseminated intravascular coagulation, central nervous system involvement, mucosal and skin lesions, pancytopenia, and markedly elevated liver enzymes. Hemophagocytic syndrome (with extremely high serum ferritin levels) has been reported occasionally as a detrimental complication of histoplasmosis.

Culture of the organism from involved tissue provides a definite diagnostic test, but is limited by delayed positivity for up to 4–6 weeks [43, 44]. Histopathology can provide a more rapid result (within days), but requires a pathologist skilled in recognition of fungal pathogens [29]. Hence, in acutely ill patients suspected for disseminated histoplasmosis, a tissue biopsy (e.g., bone marrow, liver, skin, etc.) for histopathologic evaluation should be performed without any delay [43]. In patients with pulmonary infiltrates, BAL with or without biopsies should be performed as soon as possible. Serological tests, although useful for diagnosis of histoplasmosis, lack sensitivity in disseminated disease, probably because of underlying immunosuppression. In addition, following acute infection, antibodies may persist for several years, incorrectly suggesting active disease in patients with other diagnoses, or (false) positive assays may result from cross-reactivity in patients with other endemic mycoses [29, 44].

The *Histoplasma* antigen sandwich enzyme immunoassay (offered by MiraVista Diagnostics, Indianapolis, Indiana) is very useful for the rapid diagnosis of disseminated histoplasmosis in HIV-positive patients [47, 48]. When available, antigen can be found within 24–48 h in approximately 90% of these patients with disseminated disease and in up to 75% of cases of acute pulmonary histoplasmosis. Urine specimens yield the highest sensitivity, but antigen can also be detected in other body fluids, including serum, CSF, and BAL fluid specimens. False-positive results have been reported in blastomycosis, paracoccidioidomycosis, penicilliosis, and occasionally in aspergillosis. However, one should realize that few data are available on the usefulness of this assay in HIV-negative immunosuppressed patients. Of note is that histoplasmosis may be a cause of false-positive results in the Platelia *Aspergillus* antigen assay (Bio-Rad Laboratories, Marnes-la-Coquette, France and Hercules, California); patients with invasive aspergillosis, however, do not exhibit false-positive *Histoplasma* antigen tests. Again, serial testing may be used to monitor antifungal therapy [49].

Antifungal therapy with amphotericin B (1–2 weeks) is indicated for all patients presenting with moderately severe-to-severe acute pulmonary histoplasmosis and severe progressive disseminated disease [50]. In a randomized trial in HIV-infected patients with severe disseminated histoplasmosis, liposomal amphotericin B (3 mg/kg daily) resulted in improved survival when compared with amphotericin B deoxycholate [51]. As the condition improves, a step-down therapy with itraconazole (200 mg twice daily following a loading dose of 200 mg 3 times daily for 3 days) can be initiated and continued for at least 12 months (or longer in case of persistent immunodeficiency) and until clinical findings have resolved [50]. Preferably, antigenuria should resolve before discontinuation of antifungal therapy. A short course of methylprednisolone (0.5–1 mg/kg/day) may be beneficial in patients with respiratory complications and ARDS. Less severe cases of pulmonary or disseminated histoplasmosis can be treated with oral itraconazole only. In every case, it is recommended to monitor serum itraconazole levels to ensure adequate absorption; a serum concentration above 1 µg/mL is recommended.

Patients with central nervous system histoplasmosis require special attention. They should be treated with higher-dose (5 mg/kg) liposomal amphotericin B, for at least 4–6 weeks, followed by prolonged oral maintenance therapy (at least 12 months) with an azole. The azole of choice in this particular setting remains unknown. Both fluconazole and itraconazole have been used, but also voriconazole and posaconazole have been used anecdotally. All echinocandins lack activity against *H. capsulatum*; they should not be used. Prophylaxis with itraconazole may be appropriate in specific circumstances in HIV-negative immunosuppressed patients. However, the best way of preventing histoplasmosis in immunocompromised patients might be via reduction of environmental exposure (specific recommendations are available from the National Institute for Occupational Safety and Health) [52].

References

1. Kontoyiannis DP, Peitsch WK, Reddy BT, Whimbey EE, Han XY, Bodey GP, et al. Cryptococcosis in patients with cancer. Clin Infect Dis. 2001;32:e145–50.
2. Pagano L, Fianchi L, Caramatti C, D'Antonio D, Melillo L, Caira M, et al. Cryptococcosis in patients with hematologic malignancies. A report from GIMEMA-infection program. Haematologica. 2004;89:852–6.
3. Kume H, Yamazaki T, Abe M, Tanuma H, Okudaira M, Okayasu I. Increase in aspergillosis and severe mycotic infection in patients with leukemia and MDS: comparison of the data from the Annual of the Pathological Autopsy Cases in Japan in 1989, 1993 and 1997. Pathol Int. 2003;53:744–50.
4. Jarvis JN, Harrison TS. HIV-associated cryptococcal meningitis. AIDS. 2007;21:2119–29.
5. Jarvis JN, Harrison TS. Pulmonary cryptococcosis. Semin Respir Crit Care Med. 2008;29:141–50.
6. Kaplan MH, Rosen PP, Armstrong D. Cryptococcosis in a cancer hospital: clinical and pathological correlates in forty-six patients. Cancer. 1977;39:2265–74.
7. Sepkowitz KA. Opportunistic infections in patients with and without acquired immunodeficiency syndrome. Clin Infect Dis. 2002;34:1098–107.
8. Jarvis JN, Dromer F, Harrison TS, Lortholary O. Managing cryptococcosis in the immunocompromised host. Curr Opin Infect Dis. 2008;21:596–603.
9. Wu G, Vilchez RA, Eidelman B, Fung J, Kormos R, Kusne S. Cryptococcal meningitis: an analysis among 5, 521 consecutive organ transplant recipients. Transpl Infect Dis. 2002;4:183–8.
10. Pappas PG, Perfect JR, Cloud GA, Larsen RA, Pankey GA, Lancaster DJ, et al. Cryptococcosis in human immunodeficiency virus-negative patients in the era of effective azole therapy. Clin Infect Dis. 2001;33:690–9.
11. Baddley JW, Perfect JR, Oster RA, Larsen RA, Pankey GA, Henderson H, et al. Pulmonary cryptococcosis in patients without HIV infection: factors associated with disseminated disease. Eur J Clin Microbiol Infect Dis. 2008;27:937–43.
12. Satishchandra P, Mathew T, Gadre G, Nagarathna S, Chandramukhi A, Mahadevan A, et al. Cryptococcal meningitis: clinical, diagnostic and therapeutic overviews. Neurol India. 2007;55:226–32.
13. Stamm AM, Polt SS. False-negative cryptococcal antigen test. JAMA. 1980;244:1359.
14. Smith AB, Smirniotopoulos JG, Rushing EJ. From the archives of the AFIP: central nervous system infections associated with human immunodeficiency virus infection: radiologic-pathologic correlation. Radiographics. 2008;28:2033–58.
15. Pappas PG. Managing cryptococcal meningitis is about handling the pressure. Clin Infect Dis. 2005;40:480–2.
16. Shirley RM, Baddley JW. Cryptococcal lung disease. Curr Opin Pulm Med. 2009;15:254–60.
17. Baughman RP, Rhodes JC, Dohn MN, Henderson H, Frame PT. Detection of cryptococcal antigen in bronchoalveolar lavage fluid: a prospective study of diagnostic utility. Am Rev Respir Dis. 1992;145:1226–9.
18. Perfect JR, Dismukes WE, Dromer F, Goldman DL, Graybill JR, Hamill RJ, et al. Clinical practice guidelines for the management of cryptococcal disease: 2010 update by the Infectious Diseases Society of America. Clin Infect Dis. 2010;50:291–322.
19. Bicanic T, Wood R, Meintjes G, Rebe K, Brouwer A, Loyse A, et al. High-dose amphotericin B with flucytosine for the treatment of cryptococcal meningitis in HIV-infected patients. Clin Infect Dis. 2008;47:123–30.
20. Dromer F, Mathoulin-Pélissier S, Launay O, Lortholary O; French Cryptococcosis Study Group. Determinants of disease presentation and outcome during cryptococcosis: the CryptoA/D study. PLoS Med. 2007;4:e21.
21. Dromer F, Bernede-Bauduin C, Guillemot D, Lortholary O. Major role for amphotericin B-flucytosine combination in severe cryptococcosis. PLoS Med. 2008;3:e2870.
22. White M, Cirrincione C, Blevins A, Armstrong D. Cryptococcal meningitis: outcome in patients with AIDS and patients with neoplastic disease. J Infect Dis. 1992;165:960–3.
23. Dromer F, Mathoulin S, Dupont B, Brugiere O, Letenneur L. Comparison of the efficacy of amphotericin B and fluconazole in the treatment of cryptococcosis in human immunodeficiency virus-negative patients: retrospective analysis of 83 cases. French Cryptococcosis Study Group. Clin Infect Dis. 1996;22:S154–60.
24. Galgiani JN, Ampel NM, Blair JE, Catanzaro A, Johnson RH, Stevens DA, et al. Coccidioidomycosis. Clin Infect Dis. 2005;41:1217–23.
25. Blair JE, Smilack JD, Caples SM. Coccidioidomycosis in patients with hematologic malignancies. Arch Intern Med. 2005;165:113–7.

26. Bergstrom L, Yocum DE, Ampel NM, Villanueva I, Lisse J, Gluck O, et al. Increased risk of coccidioidomycosis in patients treated with tumor necrosis factor alpha antagonists. Arthritis Rheum. 2004;50:1959–66.
27. Blair JE. Approach to the solid organ transplant patient with latent infection and disease caused by Coccidioides species. Curr Opin Infect Dis. 2008;21:415–20.
28. Saubolle MA, McKellar PP, Sussland D. Epidemiological, clinical, and diagnostic aspects of coccidioidomycosis. J Clin Microbiol. 2007;45:26–30.
29. Wheat JL. Approach to the diagnosis of endemic mycoses. Clin Chest Med. 2009;30:379–89.
30. Durkin M, Connolly P, Kuberski T, Myers R, Kubak BM, Bruckner D, et al. Diagnosis of coccidioidomycosis with use of the Coccidioides antigen enzyme immunoassay. Clin Infect Dis. 2008;47:e69–73.
31. Galgiani JN, Catanzaro A, Cloud GA, Johnson RH, Williams PL, Mirels LF, et al. Comparison of oral fluconazole and itraconazole for progressive, nonmeningeal coccidioidomycosis. A randomized, double-blind trial. Mycoses Study Group. Ann Intern Med. 2000;133:676–86.
32. McKinnell JA, Pappas PG. Blastomycosis: new insights into diagnosis, prevention, and treatment. Clin Chest Med. 2009;30:227–39.
33. Chu JH, Feudtner C, Heydon K, Walsh TJ, Zaoutis TE. Hospitalizations for endemic mycoses: a population-based national study. Clin Infect Dis. 2006;42:822–5.
34. Bradsher RW, Chapman SW, Pappas PG. Blastomycosis. Infect Dis Clin North Am. 2003;17:21–40.
35. Lemos LB, Baliga M, Guo M. Blastomycosis. Ann Diagn Pathol. 2002;6:194–203.
36. Gauthier GM, Safdar N, Klein BS, Andes DR. Blastomycosis in solid organ transplant recipients. Transpl Infect Dis. 2007;9:310–7.
37. Kauffman CA. Endemic mycoses in patients with hematologic malignancies. Semin Respir Infect. 2002;17:106–12.
38. Pappas PG, Pottage JC, Powderly WG, Fraser VJ, Stratton CW, McKenzie S, et al. Blastomycosis in patients with the acquired immunodeficiency syndrome. Ann Intern Med. 1992;116:847–53.
39. Kauffman CA. Endemic mycoses: blastomycosis, histoplasmosis, and sporotrichosis. Infect Dis Clin North Am. 2006;20:645–62.
40. Durkin M, Witt J, Lemonte A, Wheat B, Connolly P. Antigen assay with the potential to aid in diagnosis of blastomycosis. J Clin Microbiol. 2004;42:4873–5.
41. Mongkolrattanothai K, Peev M, Wheat LJ, Marcinak J. Urine antigen detection of blastomycosis in pediatric patients. Pediatr Infect Dis J. 2006;25:1076–8.
42. Chapman SW, Dismukes WE, Proia LA, Bradsher RW, Pappas PG, Threlkeld MG, et al. Clinical practice guidelines for the management of blastomycosis: 2008 update by the Infectious Diseases Society of America. Clin Infect Dis. 2008;46:1801–12.
43. Kauffman CA. Diagnosis of histoplasmosis in immunosuppressed patients. Curr Opin Infect Dis. 2008;21:421–5.
44. Wheat LJ. Histoplasmosis: a review for clinicians from non-endemic areas. Mycoses. 2006;49:274–82.
45. Kauffman CA. Histoplasmosis. Clin Chest Med. 2009;30:217–25.
46. Kauffman CA. Histoplasmosis: a clinical and laboratory update. Clin Microbiol Rev. 2007;20:115–32.
47. Connolly PA, Durkin MM, Lemonte AM, Hackett EJ, Wheat LJ. Detection of histoplasma antigen by quantitative enzyme immunoassay. Clin Vaccine Immunol. 2007;14:1587–91.
48. Gutierrez ME, Canton A, Connolly P, Zarnowski R, Wheat LJ. Detection of Histoplasma capsulatum antigen in Panamanian patients with disseminated histoplasmosis and AIDS. Clin Vaccine Immunol. 2008;15:681–3.
49. Wheat LJ. Improvements in diagnosis of histoplasmosis. Expert Opin Biol Ther. 2006;6:1207–21.
50. Wheat LJ, Freifeld AG, Kleiman MB, Baddley JW, McKinsey DS, Loyd JE, et al. Clinical practice guidelines for the management of histoplasmosis: 2007 update by the Infectious Diseases Society of America. Clin Infect Dis. 2007;45:807–25.
51. Johnson PC, Wheat LJ, Cloud GA, Goldman M, Lancaster D, Bamberger DM, et al. Safety and efficacy of liposomal amphotericin B compared with conventional amphotericin B for induction therapy of histoplasmosis in patients with AIDS. Ann Intern Med. 2002;137:105–9.
52. Lenhart SW, Schafer MP, Singal M. Histoplasmosis: protecting workers at risk. DHHS Publication No. 97–146, 1997.

Chapter 27
Current Controversies in the Treatment of Fungal Infections

Christopher D. Pfeiffer, John R. Perfect, and Barbara D. Alexander

Abstract With improved laboratory techniques and the availability of new antifungal agents, complexity in the treatment of invasive fungal disease has rapidly increased over the past decade, stimulating a debate on the best management strategies. In this chapter, we address four important areas of current uncertainty, including (1) the role of therapeutic drug monitoring for voriconazole and posaconazole, (2) the utility of in vitro antifungal susceptibility testing of yeasts and moulds, (3) the optimal treatment of zygomycosis, and (4) the value of combination therapy for invasive aspergillosis. For each topic, we examine the available evidence surrounding the ambiguity and then offer data-driven recommendations on how to proceed with management.

Keywords Voriconazole • Posaconazole • Drug level • Monitoring • Antifungal susceptibility testing • Combination antifungal therapy

Role of Therapeutic Drug Monitoring for Voriconazole and Posaconazole

The utility of therapeutic drug monitoring (TDM) hinges on certain attributes of a medication. These important qualities include (1) an unpredictable blood or tissue drug level, (2) evidence that the drug level correlates with either toxicity or efficacy, and (3) the availability of an accurate drug assay [1]. Drug levels are often influenced by several factors including absorption, metabolism, and drug interactions. As experience has increased with the newer extended-spectrum azoles, mounting evidence suggests that TDM may be necessary for these drugs. The following sections address the evidence for and against voriconazole and posaconazole TDM and are summarized in Table 27.1.

C.D. Pfeiffer (✉)
Department of Medicine, Division of Infectious Diseases and International Health, Duke University Medical Center, 116G Carl Bldg. Research Dr, Durham, NC 27710, USA
e-mail: christopher.pfeiffer@duke.edu

Voriconazole

Despite excellent oral bioavailability, voriconazole drug levels are variable in healthy volunteers and patients [2–5]. Studies have demonstrated both metabolism and drug interactions to be important sources of this unpredictability.

The major mechanism of voriconazole elimination is hepatic metabolism through the cytochrome P450 system, including isoenzymes CYP2C9, CPY2C29, CYP3A4, and CYP2C19 [6]. The affinity of voriconazole appears to be highest for CYP2C19, and polymorphisms in this gene can result in variable rates of metabolism of the drug. Those with the wild-type allele ("extensive metabolizers") have up to fourfold decreased plasma concentration of voriconazole as compared to those homozygous for the "poor metabolizer" phenotype [7, 8]. Importantly, the estimated frequency of CYP2C19 polymorphisms is different among ethnic groups: 20% of Asians compared with 2–5% of Caucasians and African-Americans are poor metabolizers of the drug [1, 6, 8, 9].

Further, voriconazole interacts with many coadministered drugs as it is an inhibitor of several isoenzymes in the cytochrome P450 system (CYP2C19, CYP2C9, and CYP3A4) (see Table 27.2). The type of interaction depends on whether the coadministered drug acts as a substrate, inducer, or inhibitor of one of the noted P450 isoenzymes. Inducers or inhibitors of these enzymes may decrease or increase voriconazole plasma concentrations, respectively. For example, coadministration of efavirenz, an isoenzyme inhibitor, results in increased levels of voriconazole while rifampin, a potent isoenzyme inducer, reduces the mean area under the curve (AUC) and mean maximum concentration (C_{max}) of voriconazole by up to 95% [10, 11]. In some cases, the impact of voriconazole coadministration with another drug is hard to predict particularly when the two drugs have competing effects on the same isoenzyme [10].

Initially, based on data from six clinical trials ($n = 280$), no concrete relationship between voriconazole concentration and efficacy could be established [10]. However, more recent reports have correlated low voriconazole levels with poor outcome [12–15]. One study of 52 patients revealed

Table 27.1 Relevant voriconazole and posaconazole therapeutic drug monitoring (TDM) parameters

Drug	Predictable serum levels	Serum level correlated to efficacy	Serum level correlated to toxicity	Accurate assay available	TDM indicated	TDM targets
Voriconazole	No	More certain	Yes	Yes	Yes	Trough level between 1.0 and 5.5 µg/ml
Posaconazole	No	Less certain	No	Maybe	For specific scenarios	Steady-state level >0.5–0.7 µg/ml

Table 27.2 Major voriconazole and posaconazole drug interactions (% change in C_{max}, if available)

Voriconazole			Posaconazole	
Effects of other drugs on voriconazole	Effects of voriconazole on other drugs	2-Way interactions (levels of each drug affected)	Effects of other drugs on posaconazole	Effects of posaconazole on other drugs
Rifampin (↓93%)[a]	Sirolimus (↑700%)[a]	Rifabutin[a]	Rifabutin (↓43%)	Sirolimus (↑572%)[a]
Ritonavir (↓66–82%)[a]	QT prolongators[a,b]	Efavirenz[c]	Phenyoin (↓41%)	QT prolongators[a,b]
St. John's Wort (↓59%)[a]	Ergot alkaloids[a]	Other NNRTIs	Cimetidine (↓39%)	Ergot alkaloinds[a]
Barbiturates (↓)[a]	Cyclosporin (↑)[d]	Protease inhibitors	Efavirenz (↓45%)	Cyclosporine (↑)[d]
Cimetidine (→18%)	Tacrolimus (↑100%)[e]	Phenytoin	Boost	Tacrolimus (↑121%)[e]
Isoniazid (→)	Methadone (↑31–65%)	Omeprazole		Rifabutin (↑31%)
Amiodarone	Warfarin	Fluoxetine		Midazolam (↑30–126%)
	Statins	Oral contraceptives		Phenytoin (↑16%)
	Benzodiazepines			Ritonavir (↑49%)
	Calcium-channel blockers			Atazanavir (↑155%)
	Sulfonylureas			Vinca alkaloids
	Vinca alkaloids			Statins
	Other PPIs			Calcium-channel blockers
	Other SSRIs			Digoxin
	NSAIDS			Amiodarone

References [10, 28, 138]
PPI proton pump inhibitor; *SSRI* selective serotonin reuptake inhibitor; *NNRTI* nonnucleoside reverse transcriptase inhibitor
[a] Coadministration of the two medications is contraindicated
[b] QT prolongators/CYP3A4 substrates include terfenadine, astemizole, pimozide, cisapride, quinidine, and halofantrine among others
[c] Suggested dosing when coadministered is efavirenz 300 mg daily (decreased) and voriconazole 400 mg BID (increased)
[d] Cyclosporine dose should be reduced 50% with voriconazole and 25% with posaconazole coadministration
[e] Tacrolimus dose should be reduced 66% with voriconazole and posaconazole coadministration

unpredictable trough plasma voriconazole concentrations, ranging from ≤1 µg/ml in 25% to >5.5 µg/ml in 31%. Lack of response to therapy was significantly greater in patients with levels ≤1 µg/ml (46%, 6/13) than in those with levels >1 µg/ml (12%, 5/39) [13]. Smith et al. separately reported that of 28 patients who underwent TDM because of disease progression or drug toxicity, a random voriconazole concentration of >2.05 µg/ml was associated with a 100% favorable clinical response compared with a 44% (8/18) favorable response for patients with random plasma concentrations <2.05 µg/ml [12]. Of patients whose voriconazole dose was increased based on having a voriconazole level ≤1 µg/ml, 73% (8/11) survived. Finally, in an open-label treatment trial for IA, of the 5% of patients who had mean plasma levels consistently <0.25 µg/ml, none responded [14].

High levels of voriconazole have been associated with toxicity including visual symptoms [10, 16], hepatic dysfunction [14, 17], and encephalopathy [13, 18]. Based on data from ten clinical trials, 21% of patients receiving voriconazole experienced abnormal vision, color vision disturbance, or photophobia. Fortunately, these visual disturbances were reversible and rarely led to discontinuation of drug. More importantly, clinically significant transaminase elevations were seen in 12.4% (206/1655) of patients treated with voriconazole [10] and in an open-label voriconazole study, 6 of 22 patients with plasma concentrations >6 µg/ml experienced liver dysfunction or liver failure [14]. Finally, encephalopathy, which reversed upon drug discontinuation, was reported in 31% (5/16) of patients with a voriconazole trough level >5.5 µg/ml vs. none in patients with a level <5.5 µg/ml ($p=0.002$) [13].

Tests for voriconazole blood levels are becoming more widely available as high performance liquid chromatogrphy (HPLC), liquid chromatography-mass spectrometry (LC-MS), and bioassays have been developed [19, 20]. Of these, bioassays measure the antifungal effect of the patient's blood on a fungal strain and may give falsely high values, particularly if the patient is receiving other antifungal agents.

An international survey and proficiency study for measurement of antifungal azole plasma concentrations revealed that most laboratories used HPLC ($n=26/33$) or LC-MS ($n=6/33$) for drug level determination [20]. Overall, 82% ($n=57$) of voriconazole analyses were correctly reported within the predefined range and no statistically significant difference was found between methods. Voriconazole levels are available in many tertiary medical centers as well as from multiple reference laboratories which offer reasonable turnaround time [21, 22].

Voriconazole meets all important criteria for TDM: unpredictable blood levels due to variations in metabolism and significant drug interactions, evidence that low levels are associated with poor outcomes while high levels are associated with adverse effects, and an accurate and available test. With that said, studies rigorously establishing target drug levels or showing the efficacy of dose adjustment based upon drug level have not been conducted. Based upon the available data, we recommend voriconazole trough concentrations in patients with serious/life-threatening mycoses, in cases where there is concern about drug metabolism or interactions, or in cases of suspected treatment failure. Trough levels can be reliably checked 2–3 days after initiation of voriconazole, once steady-state levels are obtained (or at day 5 if no loading dose is given). Although the optimal concentration is not completely defined, we advocate a minimum target trough plasma level of 1 μg/ml. If levels are <1 μg/ml, we suggest increasing the dose by 50% and rechecking the level. In order to prevent toxicity, levels >5.5 μg/ml should be avoided.

Posaconazole

Posaconazole is only available orally and demonstrates moderate variability in absorption. Absorption is saturated at doses >800 mg and further increasing the dose has no affect on plasma concentrations. In healthy volunteers, a dosing interval of 200 mg 4 times per day demonstrated the greatest bioavailability [23, 24] and posaconazole C_{max} was increased with coadministration of an acidic beverage by 92% and with Boost® nutritional supplement by 60–137%. Posaconazole C_{max} was also increased by 96% when the drug was administered before and up to 337% when administered during or after a high-fat meal. Conversely, enhanced gastric motility and higher gastric pH decreased posaconazole maximum concentrations by 21 and 46%, respectively [25]. In a dose-finding study of 30 neutropenic, hematopoietic stem cell transplant (HSCT) recipients, interpatient pharmacokinetic variability ranged from 38 to 68% [26]. In a separate study conducted in HSCT recipients with graft versus host disease (GVHD), mean posaconazole concentrations (1.47 μg/ml) were 54% higher in patients with chronic GVHD ($n=82$) compared with those with acute GVHD ($n=158$, mean concentration 0.958 μg/ml) [27].

There are several important drug interactions with posaconazole (see Table 27.2). Posaconazole is primarily metabolized via UDP-glucuronidation and rifabutin, phenytoin, and efavirenz can decrease posaconazole C_{max} by 39–45% in healthy volunteers via induction of this pathway [28]. Although not metabolized by the hepatic cytochrome P450 system, posaconazole inhibits it. Specifically, it affects CYP3A4 and increases plasma concentrations of several important coadministered medications [28].

One published trial links efficacy with posaconazole plasma concentrations [29]. In an open-label salvage study of refractory invasive aspergillosis (IA), patients with mean posaconazole average plasma concentrations (C_{av}) in the lowest (0.134 μg/ml), second (0.411 μg/ml), third (0.852 μg/ml), and fourth (1.250 μg/ml) quartiles had 24% (4/17), 53% (9/17), 57% (9/17), and 75% (12/16) response to therapy, respectively. On the other hand, secondary analysis of a phase III posaconazole prophylaxis trial found no correlation between plasma levels and clinical outcome. This finding may have been due to a lack of statistical power rather than an absence of a true difference as the low number of breakthrough mould infections precluded formal statistical comparison. Interestingly, the C_{av} for the three patients with breakthrough infections were all below the mean C_{av} (0.586 μg/ml) of those free from breakthrough infection ($n=188$) [30]. In the new drug application process, the FDA also examined the drug-exposure relationship in both phase III prophylaxis studies and found a significant increase in breakthrough invasive fungal infections in patients with posaconazole C_{av} <0.7 μg/ml [31]. Based on this, a cautionary warning was placed in the posaconazole package insert that lower posaconazole concentrations may be associated with an increased risk of treatment failure [28].

Hepatic dysfunction is the most common serious adverse effect noted in the posaconazole prophylaxis trials [28], but no studies have correlated posaconazole levels with this or any other toxicity.

As with voriconazole, posaconazole drug levels are available through several reference laboratories [32]. However, in the international proficiency testing program for measurement of antifungal azole plasma concentrations previously mentioned, only 62% ($n=26$) of posaconazole analyses were within the targeted concentration range [20]. Thus, more work is needed to establish an accurate test method for clinical use.

Posaconazole therefore meets some, but not all, requirements for TDM. Plasma levels are unpredictable and efficacy has been linked to plasma concentration according to one published trial. On the other hand, toxicity has not been associated with plasma concentration and more work is needed to establish a reliable test method for determining blood concentrations. For these reasons, we do not suggest routine posaconazole TDM in prophylaxis and treatment. However, in cases of severe/life-threatening mycoses, concerns about drug bioavailability or interactions, and suspected clinical failure, we would recommend checking a steady-state level (3–5 h after a dose and ≥7 days after initiation of the drug). In such cases, concentrations <0.5–0.7 μg/ml should guide adjustment of the dosing schedule (e.g., switching the dosing interval from 2 to 4 times daily) or change to an alternative agent.

In Vitro Antifungal Susceptibility Testing for Yeasts and Moulds

Candida Species

Antifungal susceptibility testing first became important in the AIDS era when long-term fluconazole treatment for oral candidiasis bred clinical resistance [33]. Recognizing this, in 1982, the Clinical and Laboratory Standards Institute (CLSI, formerly NCCLS) formed the Subcommittee on Antifungal Susceptibility Testing (SAST). Based on a collaborative study documenting unacceptably low interlaboratory agreement in Minimal Inhibitory Concentration (MIC) results [34], the committee set out to standardize a reference method for testing yeasts and to establish reference MIC ranges for quality control organisms [35]. Over the ensuing years, less labor-intense, commercially available methods of testing including broth microdilution [36–38], agar dilution [39–42], and disk diffusion [34, 43] have been favorably compared with the CLSI reference method, thus allowing for susceptibility testing of yeasts in most clinical microbiology laboratories [44].

The CLSI SAST also worked to create interpretative categories for *Candida* susceptibility results to several antifungal agents. Developing interpretive breakpoints for any organism–drug combination requires integration of the MIC distribution of the organism, pharmacokinetic and pharmacodynamic properties of the drug, and the relationship between the in vitro activity and outcome from in vivo and clinical studies. Using data generated by standardized testing methods, interpretive breakpoints for fluconazole, itraconazole, flucy-tosine, voriconazole, and the echinocandins against *Candida* species have been established and/or proposed [15, 45, 46].

MIC interpretative criteria for fluconazole were first published by Rex et al. [47, 48] and recently confirmed by Pfaller et al. [49]. In 1997, tentative fluconazole MIC breakpoints in *Candida* infections of susceptible (S; ≤8 μg/ml), susceptible dependent upon dose (SDD; 16–32 μg/ml), and resistant (R; ≥64 μg/ml) were proposed [47]. Pooling the available clinical isolates, success rates for patients receiving fluconazole 100 mg/day were 98% (248/253), 78% (21/27), and 73% (16/22) for isolates with MICs ≤8, 16–32, and ≥64 μg/ml, respectively. For doses of fluconazole >100 mg/day, success rates for isolates with MICs ≤8, 16–32, and ≥64 μg/ml were 81% (122/150), 86% (24/28), and 46% (18/39), respectively. Because a dose of fluconazole >100 mg/day portended clinical success in the MIC 16–32 range as would be expected from pharmacokinetic analysis, the delineation of SDD was created.

Several caveats to the proposed breakpoints were noted. First, *Candida krusei* had higher MICs to and frequent clinical failure with fluconazole. Hence, *C. krusei* was deemed "intrinsically resistant" to fluconazole, obviating the need for MIC testing of this organism/drug combination [47, 50]. Second, the breakpoints were based mainly on cases of oropharyngeal candidiasis in HIV-infected patients (411/519 cases) and therefore needed confirmation in invasive disease. In 2006, the interpretive breakpoints for fluconazole and *Candida* were revisited using data accumulated in the interim from 12 clinical trials [49]. In the invasive candidiasis subset, successful treatment was seen in 77% (353/460), 71% (51/72), and 44% (31/71) for patients with isolates in the S, SDD, and R MIC ranges, respectively. The original breakpoints for fluconazole in *Candida* infection were thus confirmed.

Using an analytic plan similar to that employed for fluconazole, interpretive criteria for voriconazole have also been established. The MIC distribution for voriconazole was determined using a collection of 8,702 clinical isolates [15]. The MIC at which 90% of isolates were inhibited (MIC_{90}) was 0.25 μg/ml; 99% of isolates were inhibited at ≤1 μg/ml of voriconazole. Compiled data from 249 patients in phase III voriconazole trials revealed a significant correlation between MIC and investigator end-of-treatment assessment of outcome. For *Candida* species, the data supported the following MIC breakpoints for voriconazole: S ≤1 μg/ml; SDD 2 μg/ml; and R ≥4 μg/ml [15, 25].

Although the CLSI broth microdilution susceptibility testing method has been validated for posaconazole, the FDA has yet to approve a commercial test system for posaconazole and interpretive breakpoints for posaconazole to *Candida* have not yet been established. A study comparing MIC results for posaconazole to those for fluconazole and voriconazole against 10,807 isolates of *Candida* species was performed to examine the use of fluconazole or voriconazole as surrogate markers for posaconazole activity. Overall, the posaconazole MIC_{90} was 1 μg/ml; 96.9% of isolates had MIC ≤1 μg/ml. For comparative purposes only, investigators applied voriconazole breakpoints to the posaconazole MICs (S ≤1 μg/ml; SDD 2 μg/ml; R ≥4 μg/ml). Using this approach, over 99% of fluconazole-susceptible isolates were "susceptible" to posaconazole, while only 47% (127/272) of fluconazole-resistant isolates were "susceptible" to posaconazole. Similarly, 98% of voriconazole-susceptible isolates were "susceptible" to posaconazole, while only 4% (4/92) of voriconazole-resistant isolates were "susceptible" to posaconazole [51]. This analysis, together with population MIC distributions, suggested that fluconazole and voriconazole are fairly reliable surrogate markers to predict posaconazole activity and that posaconazole and voriconazole have similar susceptibility profiles against *Candida* species.

The currently available echinocandins, caspofungin, micafungin, and anidulafungin, are highly active against *Candida* species. The three drugs have similar spectrum and potency, and scatter plots comparing *Candida* population MICs for the three agents show a high degree of correlation. Of 5,346 *Candida* isolates tested, the overall MIC_{90} for caspofungin was 0.25 µg/ml and 99.9% of isolates were inhibited by ≤2 µg/ml of caspofungin [45]. Interestingly, the caspofungin MIC_{90} for *C. krusei* (0.25 µg/ml), *C. parapsilosis* (1 µg/ml), and *C. guilliermondii* (1 µg/ml) was considerably higher than that observed for the three most common species of *Candida* recovered from blood (*C. albicans*, *C. glabrata*, and *C. tropicalis*; each with caspofungin MIC_{90} 0.06 µg/ml). The mechanism for this bimodal "wild type" MIC distribution for the echinocandins appears to be polymorphisms within the FKS1 gene, which encodes essential components of the glucan synthesis enzyme complex. A naturally occurring proline-to-alanine amino acid change at position 660 (P660A) in FKS1p is thought to account for this reduced echinocandin susceptibility [45, 52]. Fortunately, in clinical trials this FKS1 gene polymorphism was not associated with decreased clinical response, leading to speculation that this specific mutation may also confer decreased fitness for the organism. The decreased fitness, coupled with the excellent pharmacokinetics of the drug, may enable effective treatment for infections due to *Candida* species with MICs as high as 2 µg/ml with this polymorphism.

Several alternative mutations in the FKS1 gene have been correlated with higher echinocandin MICs, typically >2 µg/ml and usually ≥8 µg/ml, and clinical failure [15, 45, 53–55]. These mutations conferred equally high MICs (>2 µg/ml) to caspofungin, anidulafungin, and micafungin. Among 14 strains with such mutant FKS1p enzymes studied, caspofungin appeared to be the best surrogate marker for echinocandin "class resistance" [56].

The CLSI standardized method of testing the echinocandins against *Candida* species provides reliable and reproducible MIC results with good separation of the "wild type" MIC distribution from isolates of *Candida* with mutations in the FKS1 gene which confer an MIC >2 µg/ml, and presumably, clinical resistance. Fortunately, the number of isolates with such mutations remains rare despite widespread use of the echinocandins. CLSI currently recommends a breakpoint for susceptibility of ≤2 µg/ml for the echinocandins. Because of the very small number of clinical isolates with an MIC >2 µg/ml, SDD and R categories have not been defined. Thus, until appropriate numbers of such isolates treated with echinocandins are available, any isolate with an MIC >2 µg/ml is currently considered "nonsusceptible" [45].

Interpretive breakpoints have not been established for *Candida* against amphotericin B (AMB) as the MIC population distribution is narrow (0.5–2 µg/ml) and studies have been unable to demonstrate a consistent clinical correlation within that range [35]. One demonstrative example is a series of clinical isolates from 107 patients treated with AMB for candidemia. Mean and median MICs for isolates from successfully treated patients were 0.33 and 0.5 µg/ml, respectively, which were almost identical to corresponding values for isolates from patients deemed clinical failures [57].

In summary, in vitro antifungal testing for *Candida* species correlates with clinical outcome and can offer important guidance in the care of patients. We recommend susceptibility testing for clinically relevant *Candida* species for which susceptibility is unpredictable (e.g., *C. glabrata* to fluconazole), isolates from patients with previous prolonged antifungal exposure, and isolates from patients demonstrating unexplained clinical resistance to a given agent.

Moulds

Standard methods for testing filamentous fungi have also been established [58]. However, caution is advised when correlating MIC data clinically as the relationship between in vitro and in vivo data has only been evaluated in animal models and case reports. The clinical relevance of testing moulds therefore remains uncertain and interpretive breakpoints of proven import have yet to be established.

Aspergillus Species

Per Table 27.3, the population MIC distributions of extended-spectrum azoles and AMB for *Aspergillus* spp. have been documented based on 2,088 clinical isolates from three different reports. The MIC_{90} of itraconazole, voriconazole, posaconazole, and AMB deoxycholate (dAMB) were 0.25–2, 0.5–1, 0.25–0.5, and 1–4 µg/ml, respectively [59–61].

Mechanisms to explain significant differences in MIC values among *Aspergillus* isolates for the extended-spectrum triazoles are beginning to be teased out. A review of all *Aspergillus fumigatus* isolates stored at a tertiary hospital in the Netherlands from 1994 to 2007 found that 2.6% (32/1219) of isolates had itraconazole MICs ≥4 µg/ml

Table 27.3 MIC_{90} for different antifungal agents to common fungal pathogens

Organism	MIC_{90} or MEC_{90}[a]					
	Fluconazole	Itraconazole	Voriconazole	Posaconazole	Caspofungin	AMB
Candida albicans	0.5	N/A	0.15–25	0.06	0.06	0.5–2
C. glabrata	32	N/A	1–4	2	0.12	1–2
C. tropicalis	2	N/A	0.25	0.12	0.06	1–2
C. parapsilosis	2	N/A	0.06	0.12	2	1–2
C. krusei	64[b]	N/A	0.5–1	1	2	2
Aspergillus fumigatus	N/A	0.5–2	0.5	0.5	0.06	1–2
A. flavus	N/A	0.25–1	0.5–1	0.5	0.06	2
A. terreus	N/A	0.25–0.5	0.5–1	0.25	0.06	2–4
Zygomycetes[c]	N/A	8–32	16–128	1–4	>16	0.5–2
Fusarium species[d]	N/A	>8	>0038	>8	>8	2–4; 32
Scedosporium apiospermum	N/A	1–32	0.25	1	NR	8
S. prolificans	N/A	16–64	8	32	NR	16–32

References [43, 45, 51, 57, 59–61, 64, 68, 73, 75, 139–143]
AMB amphotericin B; *NR* not reported; *N/A* not applicable

[a]Using CLSI methodology M27-A3 and M38-A2; note for echinocandins, MEC_{90} used for testing moulds and MIC_{90} used for testing *Candida*
[b]*C. krusei* is considered intrinsically resistant to fluconazole and thus need not be tested; however, it has generally been found to be susceptible to voriconazole and posaconazole
[c]The zygomycetes include many important pathogenic moulds and the MIC_{90} for Itraconazole, Posaconazole, and AMB varies considerably between species
[d]*Fusarium* isolates demonstrated differences in MIC_{90} among species. *F. oxysporum* and *F. monoliforme* demonstrated lower MIC_{90} than other *Fusarium* spp.

as well as elevated MICs to voriconazole, posaconazole, and ravuconazole [62]. Ninety-four percent (30/32) of these isolates had a *cyp51A* gene mutation, which included a leucine for histidine substitution at codon 98 in conjunction with two copies of a 34-bp sequence in tandem in the gene promoter (TR/L98H). In a separate report, Verweij et al. described the TR/L98H mutation in nine patients with IA [63]. Of those treated with voriconazole ($n=3$) or posaconazole ($n=1$) monotherapy, 50% (2/4) died while the five patients receiving alternate treatment survived suggesting that the TR/L98H mutation produced clinically significant cross-resistance among all extended-spectrum triazoles.

Further elucidation of the resistance mechanisms for *Aspergillus* to the triazoles comes from a report of 771 *Aspergillus* isolates, including multiple species from around the world. Itraconazole MICs ≥4 μg/ml were demonstrated in 2.2% ($n=17$) of isolates, but high MICs to itraconazole did not necessarily correspond to high voriconazole and posaconazole MICs [64]. This difference was subsequently explained in part by different mutations involving the *cyp51A* gene that conferred unique patterns of azole activity [65]. For example, G54 mutations led to high MICs for both itraconazole and posaconazole, while M220 resulted in high MICs for all four drugs [66]. Multiple different mechanisms of resistance, some of which are as yet unidentified, likely contribute to each organism's phenotypic profile. At this time, the CLSI broth microdilution method of testing appears to be reproducible enough to identify mould isolates with triazoles MICs ≥1 μg/ml [66].

Several studies have correlated high MICs to AMB with clinical failure, particularly for *A. terreus*. One study demonstrated that for *Aspergillus* spp. isolated from patients with invasive disease, AMB MICs <2 μg/ml were associated with survival (6/6), while MICs ≥2 μg/ml were associated with death (22/23). The latter group included all nine patients infected with *A. terreus* [67]. In a single-center review of proven IA cases, response to AMB was only 21% (5/24) for patients infected with *A. terreus*, which was significantly worse than the 48% (11/23) response for non-*terreus Aspergillus* infections [68]. In this study, of the 32 *A. terreus* isolates undergoing MIC determination, the MIC_{90} for AMB was 4 μg/ml compared with the voriconazole MIC_{90} of 1 μg/ml. Clinical confirmation of superior voriconazole activity for *A. terreus* came from a multicenter retrospective review of 83 cases of invasive *A. terreus* infection. Only 26.2% (11/42) receiving an AMB formulation as primary therapy survived vs. 64.7% (11/17) who received voriconazole as primary therapy ($p=0.01$) [69]. Unfortunately, MIC data for those cases were not available.

All echinocandins appear to be active in vitro against *Aspergillus*. In a large study of 372 *Aspergillus* species isolates, the caspofungin minimum effective concentration (MEC) at which 90% of isolates were inhibited was 0.06 μg/ml, while 98.4% of isolates were inhibited at ≤1 μg/ml [60]. There are only a few reports of *Aspergillus* in vitro resistance to the echinocandins. One study examined the echinocandin MECs of *Aspergillus* isolates from nine cases of caspofungin breakthrough infection in an allogeneic stem cell transplant population. Of the four isolates examined, *A. ustus* and

A. nidulans had higher MECs (8 and 4 μg/ml, respectively) compared with MECs of 1 and 0.25 μg/ml for the two *A. fumigatus* isolates. A search for specific mechanisms of resistance was not done [70]. A second study evaluated a single isolate from a patient who failed caspofungin. Interestingly, while the broth microdilution MEC for the isolate was 0.25 μg/ml, the Etest® and an animal model indicated reduced caspofungin activity. Furthermore, although no FKS gene mutation was present, its expression was increased in the presence of drug suggesting that it played some role [71]. In the laboratory, researchers induced an *A. fumigatus* FKS1p mutation in the "hot-spot" region (serine-678-proline) and found an MEC ≥8 for all mutants [72]. Evidence linking echinocandin clinical failures to *Aspergillus* MEC is slim.

Non-Aspergillus Moulds

The MIC_{90} of antifungal agents to several non-*Aspergillus* moulds is listed in Table 27.3. In general, AMB is the most active agent followed by posaconazole. For example, in vitro susceptibility testing of 217 zygomycetes revealed that, for *Rhizopus*, the MIC_{90} to dAMB was 0.5 μg/ml and 100% of the isolates had MICs ≤1 μg/ml ($n=86$), whereas for posaconazole, the MIC_{90} was 1 μg/ml and 80% of isolates had MICs ≤1 μg/ml ($n=66$) [73]. Although only eight isolates were tested, *Cunninghamella bertholletiae* had the highest MICs to dAMB compared with all other zygomycetes, which may account for the worse clinical outcomes reported with this infection [74]. By standardized testing methods, the echinocandins are inactive in vitro against zygomycetes and *Fusarium* species. In a compilation of two studies, the MEC of caspofungin to each zygomycosis tested ($n=113$) was ≥16 μg/ml [73, 75]. Also, in an exhaustive literature review, Espinel-Ingroff reported echinocandin MECs of ≥8 μg/ml to all 68 *Fusarium* spp. tested [76]. The data on echinocandin activity against other non-*Aspergillus* moulds are limited.

The most robust data correlating MIC with clinical outcomes for the non-*Aspergillus* moulds are from a report of in vitro susceptibility of 590 isolates collected from all phase III voriconazole trials [61]. The overall MIC_{90} for voriconazole was 1 μg/ml. The 34 isolates with a voriconazole MIC ≥4.0 μg/ml included 9/9 zygomycetes, 10/13 *Fusarium solani*, 9/11 *Scedosporium prolificans*, and one isolate each of *S. apiospermum*, *A. fumigatus*, *F. oxysporum*, *F. proliferatum*, *Microascus cineeus*, and *Scopulariopsis brevicaulis*. Of patients infected with these isolates with clinical data available, outcome was successful for only 38% (9/24) of patients infected with a mould with MIC ≥4.0 μg/ml compared with 52% (105/202) of those infected with a mould with MIC <4.0 μg/ml ($p=0.0899$). Correlation of in vitro data with clinical outcome for the echinocandins and AMB with non-*Aspergillus* moulds is scant.

Because of the laborious nature, lack of interpretive breakpoints, and unproven clinical correlation of mould in vitro susceptibility testing, most clinical laboratories do not routinely perform this testing, and similarly, we do not recommend routine in vitro susceptibility testing of filamentous fungi. More important in the selection of an appropriate antifungal agent is the correct identification of the mould, preferably to the species level, with choice of drug based on known population MIC distributions for the specific organism recovered. However, several notable exceptions for which susceptibility testing of filamentous moulds may help guide therapy include patients heavily pretreated with mould-active agents, patients failing to respond clinically, or patients with isolates for which MICs are not predictable. In such cases, a general rule of thumb for the triazoles and AMB is as follows: an MIC ≤1 μg/ml suggests that the drug may have in vivo activity against the organism and an MIC ≥4 μg/ml should prompt the choice of an alternative agent. Again, emphasis must be placed on the limitations of the data and that such information would be used only in conjunction with other parameters when deciding on treatment options.

Treatment of Zygomycosis

Historically, dAMB was the only active systemic antifungal agent for zygomycete infection. A literature review of 929 published cases of patients with zygomycete infection from 1940 to 2003 was performed, and in a multivariate model of risk factors for mortality, the odds ratio for dAMB vs. no antifungal therapy was 0.21 (95% CI 0.13–0.25, $p=<0.001$) and lipid AMB vs. no antifungal therapy was 0.10 (95% CI 0.04–0.24, $p=<0.0001$) [74]. Moreover, early antifungal therapy for this infection is critical. In a retrospective review of 70 consecutive hematology patients with invasive zygomycete infection, investigators found almost twofold higher mortality with delayed (≥6 days after diagnosis) AMB administration (49 vs. 83%) [77].

Unfortunately, the use of dAMB is accompanied by severe infusion reactions and renal toxicity. To minimize adverse effects, lipid formulations of AMB were developed. The currently available lipid AMB products include liposomal amphotericin B (LAMB), amphotericin B lipid complex (ABLC), and amphotericin B colloidal dispersion (ABCD). All three offer the broad antifungal activity of dAMB; however, ABCD is not frequently used secondary to increased infusion toxicity compared with dAMB [78]. No prospective head-to-head trial comparing the various AMB formulations in the treatment of invasive zygomycosis has been conducted.

While most experts now consider a lipid formulation of AMB to be first-line therapy for zygomycosis, there is no firm agreement regarding which of the lipid products (ABLC or LAMB) is preferable and whether the addition of other agents is beneficial. The following section examines these areas of controversy.

In Vitro Data

As previously discussed, AMB is the most active agent in vitro followed closely by posaconazole. Although not reflected in MIC, one study demonstrated an immunomodulatory activity of echinocandins against several moulds including *Rhizopus oryzae* [79]. In this study, administration of caspofungin increased mould cell wall β-glucan exposure and enhanced human neutrophil activity against the cell wall. Testing caspofungin in combination with posaconazole, Guembe et al. found a synergistic effect in all 12 zygomycete strains tested [80]. Perkhofer et al. tested 30 zygomycetes and found that combination of posaconazole and dAMB more often demonstrated a synergistic effect on zygomycete hyphae (40%) compared with zygomycete conidia (10%) [81].

Animal Data

The frequent central nervous system (CNS) involvement of zygomycete infection has engendered debate about which lipid formulation of AMB best penetrates the blood–brain barrier. Ibrahim et al. found that high-dose LAMB (15 mg/kg/day) was superior to LAMB 7.5 mg/kg/day and dAMB 1 mg/kg/day in a diabetic ketoacidosis (DKA) mouse model of disseminated zygomycosis [82]. In a recent head-to-head comparison of LAMB and ABLC in a disseminated *R. oryzae* mouse model, LAMB demonstrated significantly better survival in a DKA model and a nonsignificant trend towards improved survival in a neutropenic model [83]. CNS fungal burden in both models was significantly reduced with LAMB 15 mg/kg/day, ABLC 15 mg/kg/day, and LAMB 7.5 mg/kg/day, but not with ABLC 7.5 mg/kg/day as compared with placebo.

There are conflicting data regarding the activity of posaconazole in the mouse model. In both the DKA and neutropenic mouse models of disseminated *R. oryzae* infection, survival with posaconazole monotherapy was not significantly better than placebo and combination posaconazole plus LAMB added no benefit to LAMB alone [84]. However, in a neutropenic model of disseminated *R. oryzae* using two different strains, Rodriguez et al. showed that posaconazole monotherapy was better than placebo ($p<0.05$), but inferior to dAMB ($p<0.05$) [85]. In that model, the addition of posaconazole to dAMB enabled a lower dose of dAMB (0.3 mg/kg/day) to obtain a survival similar to the higher dose monotherapy of dAMB (0.8 mg/kg/day). CNS fungal burden for one of the two *Rhizopus* strains was decreased significantly with combination therapy. Finally, a third mouse model found a lack of posaconazole activity to *R. oryzae*, partial activity for *Absidia corymbifera*, and a clear dose–response effect for *R. microsporus* [86]. In summary, posaconazole had variable antizygomycete activity as a single agent, and for certain strains, posaconazole appeared synergistic when administered in combination with AMB.

Although not active in vitro, the echinocandins appear to have limited activity in murine models of disseminated zygomycete infection [87, 88]. Two reports of echinocandin–AMB synergy have been published, both of which demonstrated a significant improvement over AMB monotherapy in mouse survival [89, 90]. The first study used ABLC plus caspofungin, while the follow-up study demonstrated a class effect by testing LAMB in combination with micafungin and anidulafungin. Why low doses of caspofungin and micafungin (1 mg/kg/day) and high doses of anidulafungin (10 mg/kg/day) conferred this benefit while micafungin 3 mg/kg/day and anidulafungin 1 mg/kg/day did not remains unexplained.

Clinical Data

Treatment success in humans has been reported with all three lipid AMB products; however, prospective clinical trials directly comparing the agents are lacking [74, 91–95]. A large review of the Collaborative Exchange for Antifungal Research database demonstrated a 52% clinical response (33/64 cured or improved) in patients with zygomycete infection treated with ABLC [96]. A review of 59 cases of zygomycosis in hematology units in Italy demonstrated 64% (7/11) cure with LAMB vs. 32% (6/19) success with dAMB [95]. A retrospective review of cases in Los Angeles found higher success rates ($p=0.28$) with dAMB or LAMB (72%; 13/18) compared to ABLC (37%; 7/19) [97]. LAMB treatment success was 100% (4/4), but the small sample size and retrospective nature of the study considerably limit the strength of the finding. Although a dose–tolerance study found that LAMB could be given safely up to 15 mg/kg/day [98], studies of high-dose LAMB for the treatment of IA have shown increased toxicity compared to standard dosing [99].

The lack of an intravenous formulation and preclinical data suggesting less efficacy compared to lipid AMB has limited the use of posaconazole as first-line therapy for zygomycosis. With that said, the clinical experience with posaconazole has been much more encouraging. The bulk of support comes from a retrospective compassionate-use study of 91 cases of zygomycosis either refractory to prior antifungal therapy (48%), or intolerant of prior antifungal therapy (10%), or both (33%). In this difficult population, 60% of patients who received posaconazole had a favorable treatment outcome [100]. Importantly, investigators reported that the most deeply immunosuppressed patients received posaconazole plus lipid AMB in combination, and the favorable response rate in that subset was an encouraging 46% (6/13). Although not formally studied, the ability to give this agent orally as sequential therapy for patients who have responded to an initial course of lipid AMB has gained favor in many institutions.

Clinical data supporting the addition of an echinocandin to AMB are limited to a retrospective review of 34 patients with rhino-orbital-cerebral zygomycosis [97]. Most patients in the study had diabetes (83%) with only 10% having received a transplant. Treatment was successful for all six evaluable patients who received AMB–caspofungin combination therapy (one patient lost to follow-up) compared with 41% (14/34) in the AMB monotherapy group ($p=0.19$). Taken in conjunction with the promising preclinical data, this study does lend support for adding an echinocandin in zygomycete infection. However, we emphasize that this small study requires validation as it was retrospective, had a select group of patients, and used various AMB formulations.

Bottomline is that current evidence from mouse models and humans slightly favors the use of LAMB, although ABLC has proven antizygomycete activity and is an acceptable alternative. Currently, a phase II, noncomparative clinical trial is underway to investigate the efficacy of high-dose LAMB (10 mg/kg/day) which may help clarify whether a higher starting dose is preferable. Until more convincing data become available, we do not advocate the routine addition of an echinocandin to lipid AMB for invasive zygomycosis.

Adjunctive Therapy

Iron chelation with deferoxamine has long been known to be a risk factor for zygomycete infection by acting as a siderophore to enhance iron uptake by the organism and promote its growth [101]. Newer iron-chelating agents including deferasirox have the opposite effect and steal iron from the zygomycete. Deferasirox has shown impressive antimould activity in vitro and in mouse models, and this agent was successful in one dramatic case report [102–104]. However, a second case report of a disseminated zygomycosis refractory to LAMB, caspofungin, surgery, and deferasirox was less encouraging [105]. A randomized, double-blind, placebo-controlled phase II clinical trial is underway to more rigorously evaluate the utility of adding deferasirox to LAMB for the management of zygomycosis.

In addition to iron-chelating agents, several novel therapies have been used to treat zygomycosis, including hyperbaric oxygen, GM-CSF, IFNγ, and granulocyte transfusions.

The use of these other adjunct therapies is currently supported by biological plausibility, in vitro data, and uncontrolled small case series. These strategies have been discussed in several recent reviews [101, 104, 106–109] in detail and are addressed in this book (Sect. III, Chap. 29 on Immune Enhancement and Cytokine Therapy in Patients with Difficult-to-Treat Fungal Infections).

Combination Therapy for Invasive Aspergillosis (IA)

Much interest has been generated over the utility of combination therapy for the treatment of IA as outcomes with monotherapy remain poor despite recent advances. For example, in the landmark trial comparing voriconazole with dAMB as primary treatment of IA, successful outcome was achieved for only 52.8% (76/144) of patients treated with voriconazole and 31.6% (42/133) of patients treated with dAMB [110]. Also, treating with high doses of LAMB did not offer improved efficacy in a randomized trial comparing standard dose (3 mg/kg/day) with high-dose (10 mg/kg/day) LAMB for primary treatment of invasive fungal disease (96% IA). Favorable response at the end of study drug administration (median 14.5 days) was only 50 and 46% for the low- and high-dose groups, respectively [99]. Other drugs with clinical efficacy in IA have published response rates of 40–42% for posaconazole [29, 111], 42% for ABLC [93], and 45% for caspofungin [112] in the salvage setting. This begs the question: can we improve on this 50% clinical response by using combinations of antifungal drugs?

Steinbach et al. exhaustively reviewed the literature from 1966 to 2001, reporting 249 cases where combination or sequential therapy was used for IA [113]. The authors found that 23 different antifungal combinations were used, resulting in clinical improvement for 63% of patients. Notably, the largest combination therapy cohorts included only ten patients and the review predated the use of voriconazole, posaconazole, and the echinocandins in the treatment of IA. Here we will examine the contemporary clinical trials published, which focus on the subject and which are summarized in Table 27.4.

Preclinical Data

In vitro and animal model data are conflicting; antagonism was shown using azoles with AMB in vitro and in an animal model (Lewis RE AAC 2002; Meletiadis JID 2006), while echinocandin synergy with both azoles and AMB has been demonstrated [114–121]. Steinbach et al. found synergy,

Table 27.4 Clinical combination studies of IA, 1966–2008[a]

Author, year	Setting	Trial design	Study medications	EOT clinical response[b]	Day 90 survival[c]	Statistical significance?
Popp (1999)	Any cancer	Retrospective cohort	ITRA+dAMB	82% (9/11)	82% (9/11)	No (not powered to detect a difference)
			dAMB	50% (5/10)	50% (5/10)	
Kontoyiannis (2005)	Heme	Retrospective cohort	ITRA+lipid AMB	0% (0/11)	36% (4/11)	No ($p>0.05$)
			Lipid AMB	10% (10/101)	34 (34%)	
Chandrasekar (2005)	Any	Retrospective cohort	ITRA+ABLC	33% (30/90)	NR	NR
			ABLC	47% (132/278)	NR	
Marr (2004)	Heme/SCT	Retrospective cohort	CAS+VOR	NR	63% (10/16)	Yes (HR 0.42, $p=0.048$)
			VOR	NR	32% (10/31)	
Singh (2006)	SOT	Prospective, observational	CAS+VOR	NR	67.5% (27/40)	No (HR 0.58, $p=0.12$)
			LAMB	NR	51% (24/47)	
Maertens (2006)	Heme	Prospective open-label salvage	CAS+VOR	54% (15/28)	Overall 45%; groups not specified	NR
			CAS+AMB	50% (8/16)		
			CAS+ITRA	29% (2/7)		
Kontoyiannis (2003)	Heme/SCT	Retrospective cohort	CAS+LAMB	22% (5/23)	NR	N/A
Caillot (2007)	Heme	Prospective RCT	LAMB+CAS	66% (10/15)	100% (15/15)	Yes (EOT $p=0.028$) and No (Day 90 $p>0.05$)
			HD LAMB	27% (4/15)	80% (12/15)	
Raad (2008)	Heme/SCT	Retrospective cohort, open-label salvage	CAS+HD LAMB	11% (4/38)	26% (10/38)	Yes: POS vs. Both LAMB groups ($p<0.05$)[b]
			HD LAMB	8% (4/52)	35% (18/52)	
			POS	40% (21/53)	57% (30/53)	
Denning (2006)[d]	Any	Prospective, open-label (87% salvage)	MICA+OLAT	34% (65/191)	NR	NR
			MICA	44% (15/34)	NR	
Kontoyiannis (2009)[d]	SCT	Prospective, open-label (91% salvage)	MICA+OLAT	24% (22/90)	NR	NR
			MICA	38% (3/8)	NR	

References [111, 123–132]

NR not reported; *N/A* not applicable; *Heme* hematologic malignancies; *SOT* solid organ transplant; *SCT* stem cell transplant; *RCT* randomized control trial; *EOT* end-of-therapy; *HD LAMB* high-dose LAMB (10 mg/kg/day in Caillot 2007; ≥7.5 mg/kg/day in Raad 2008)

[a] Studies including 10 or more subjects

[b] In Popp 1999, clinical response and survival were determined at EOT. In Konyotyiannis 2005, survival was determined on day 30. In Maertens 2006, clinical response and survival were both assessed on day 84 (not EOT)

[c] In Raad 2008, LAMB 5 mg/kg/day was used alone or in combination for 80% of the primary antifungal therapy, potentially skewing the results for the HD LAMB group

[d] Kontoyiannis 2009 published the SCT subset of patients previously included in the cohort published by Denning 2006

additive effect, indifference, and antagonism in 36, 24, 28, and 11% of in vitro reports ($n=27$) and 14, 20, 51, and 14% of animal studies ($n=18$), respectively [113]. An important and relevant factor in interpreting and applying these results is that combination antifungal in vitro testing has not been standardized. In fact, a recent study sponsored by the CLSI SAST suggests checkerboard testing for combination antifungal activity is not reproducible across laboratories [122].

Clinical Data

In a retrospective review of patients who were treated for IA at Memorial Sloan-Kettering Cancer Center between 1995 and 1997, a favorable response was found in 82% (9/11) who received itraconazole (ITRA) plus dAMB vs. 50% (5/10) of those treated with dAMB alone [123]. Kontoyiannis et al. retrospectively compared treatment of IA in a hematologic cancer population with lipid AMB with and without ITRA and found similarly poor results with either strategy (0 vs. 10% favorable response, $p>0.05$) [124]. Finally, in a large retrospective analysis of ABLC use, the subset of patients receiving combination ITRA plus ABLC had a 33% (30/90) favorable response vs. the 47% favorable response seen in the ABLC monotherapy group [125]. In this study, there was a concern for selection bias: the investigators treating IA with combination therapy likely were doing so in response to the severity of the infection. Overall, there was neither clear antagonism nor synergy with combination ITRA plus AMB in these studies.

Marr et al. retrospectively reviewed 47 hematologic cancer patients with IA at Fred Hutchinson Cancer Research Center from 1997 to 2001 who received voriconazole (VOR) salvage therapy after failing either dAMB or LAMB primary therapy. Beginning in 2001, caspofungin (CAS) was administered in combination with voriconazole for salvage treatment routinely. The 63% (10/16) 3-month survival for the combination therapy group was statistically superior to 32% (10/31) in the voriconazole monotherapy group [126]. Combination VOR plus CAS vs. lipid AMB for primary therapy of IA was studied in solid organ transplant recipients in a prospective, multicenter observational study [127]. Ninety-day survival and percent successful outcome were comparable between the two groups. Lastly, in an open-labeled, noncomparative salvage study of IA in a hematologic patient population, CAS was administered with other antifungal agents. Although small numbers precluded formal statistical testing, day 84 treatment successes for CAS when combined with VOR, AMB, or ITRA were 54% (15/28), 50% (8/16), and 29% (2/7), respectively [128].

A retrospective analysis of 23 patients with hematologic malignancy and IA in 2001 evaluated the combination of CAS plus LAMB. Six patients received the combination as primary therapy, while 17 patients received salvage CAS plus LAMB after failing LAMB monotherapy. Unfortunately, overall clinical response at the end of therapy was a dismal 22% (5/23). Study limitations included evaluation of response to treatment at 20 days (median) at which time many patients were still neutropenic and absence of a monotherapy comparison group [129]. A second retrospective analysis of combination of CAS plus LAMB was performed by Raad et al. [111]. The three comparator groups included CAS plus high-dose (HD) LAMB (LAMB ≥7.5 mg/kg/day), HD LAMB alone, and posaconazole alone. End-of-therapy treatment success and 12-week survival were significantly worse in the HD LAMB plus CAS and HD LAMB monotherapy groups as compared to the patients who received posaconazole alone. Notably, 80% of patients had received primary therapy with LAMB 5 mg/kg/day either alone or in combination with other antifungal agents, which potentially skewed the data toward favoring posaconazole. The HD LAMB and HD LAMB plus CAS groups did not have significantly different outcomes.

The only randomized trial of combination anti-*Aspergillus* therapy published to date included 30 patients with hematologic malignancy and proven or probable IA. Patients were randomized to CAS plus LAMB 3 mg/kg/day vs. monotherapy with HD LAMB 10 mg/kg/day [130]. At end-of-therapy, the CAS plus LAMB group had a 66% (10/15) favorable response which was statistically superior to the 27% (4/15) clinical response in the monotherapy group. Nephrotoxicity was also more common in the HD LAMB group (23 vs. 7%); however, 12-week survival was not statistically different. Until further study, it is unknown whether the superiority of CAS plus LAMB was simply due to the lower dose of LAMB or the addition of caspofungin. At a minimum, the combination appeared to be well tolerated and the good outcomes were encouraging.

Micafungin (MICA) was evaluated in a study of treatment for pulmonary IA as either primary or salvage therapy and as either mono- or combination therapy from 1998 to 2002. One hundred ninety-one patients received micafungin in addition to the antifungal therapy they had already been failing, most commonly AMB or ITRA. Those receiving combination therapy in the salvage group had a 35% (60/174) favorable response [131]. The subset of stem cell transplant patients from this study was subsequently examined and found to have a 24% (22/90) vs. 38% (3/8) favorable response when comparing the MICA plus other licensed antifungal therapy vs. MICA monotherapy groups [132].

Studies demonstrating the safety of both inhaled ABLC [133, 134] and inhaled LAMB [135] in the setting of antifungal prophylaxis have been published. However, whether an inhaled AMB compound would penetrate tissue sufficiently to synergize with systemic antifungal therapy for documented invasive pulmonary aspergillosis has not yet been evaluated.

While it appears that combination antifungal therapy may confer some benefit in IA, this has not yet been rigorously tested in a randomized trial.

Summary

In conclusion a number of important factors are driving the use of echinocandins in combination with other antifungal agents, primarily voriconazole and lipid AMB, which include:

- The need for better clinical outcomes in IA
- The biologic plausibility of using a cell wall-active (AMB, azole) and a cell membrane-active (echinocandin) agent in tandem
- The favorable adverse effect and drug interaction profile of echinocandins
- In vitro and preclinical studies generally suggesting synergy without evidence of antagonism
- Noncomparative retrospective and prospective cohorts demonstrating benefit
- A single small prospective randomized trial showing benefit but having several limitations

Updated 2008 IDSA guidelines for IA state the following: "There are insufficient clinical data to support combination therapy as routine primary treatment of invasive pulmonary aspergillosis. Although initial laboratory studies, case reports, and retrospective case series indicate encouraging findings, the efficacy of primary combination antifungal therapy requires a prospective, randomized, clinical trial to justify this approach" [136]. We support this view as do two recent comprehensive reviews [121, 137]. A phase III prospective, randomized, double-blind trial comparing voriconazole monotherapy vs. combination voriconazole plus anidulafungin for primary therapy of proven or probable IA currently enrolling should help definitively conclude the efficacy of azole–echinocandin combination therapy for this disease. Until such data is available, combination therapy should be reserved for patients in whom voriconazole monotherapy has failed or is contraindicated and for high-risk patients with unusual or resistant isolates. In such cases, current data would suggest combination with an azole–echinocandin or LAMB–echinocandin to be reasonable options.

Acknowledgement This publication was made possible by Grant# 5 KL2 RR 024127 03 (Pfeiffer) from the National Center for Research Resources (NCRR), a component of the National Institutes of Health (NIH), and NIH Roadmap for Medical Research. Its contents are solely the responsibility of the authors and do not necessarily represent the official view of NCRR or NIH. Information on NCRR is available at http://www.ncrr.nih.gov/. Information on Re-engineering the Clinical Research Enterprise can be obtained from http://nihroadmap.nih.gov/clinicalresearch/overview-translational.asap. This publication was also supported in part by NIH-NIAID-1 K24 AI072522-01A1 (Alexander).

References

1. Smith J, Andes D. Therapeutic drug monitoring of antifungals: pharmacokinetic and pharmacodynamic considerations. Ther Drug Monit. 2008;30(2):167–72.
2. Theuretzbacher U, Ihle F, Derendorf H. Pharmacokinetic/pharmacodynamic profile of voriconazole. Clin Pharmacokinet. 2006;45(7):649–63.
3. Purkins L, Wood N, Ghahramani P, Greenhalgh K, Allen MJ, Kleinermans D. Pharmacokinetics and safety of voriconazole following intravenous- to oral-dose escalation regimens. Antimicrob Agents Chemother. 2002;46(8):2546–53.
4. Trifilio S, Pennick G, Pi J, et al. Monitoring plasma voriconazole levels may be necessary to avoid subtherapeutic levels in hematopoietic stem cell transplant recipients. Cancer. 2007;109(8):1532–5.
5. Trifilio S, Ortiz R, Pennick G, et al. Voriconazole therapeutic drug monitoring in allogeneic hematopoietic stem cell transplant recipients. Bone Marrow Transplant. 2005;35(5):509–13.
6. Hyland R, Jones BC, Smith DA. Identification of the cytochrome P450 enzymes involved in the N-oxidation of voriconazole. Drug Metab Dispos. 2003;31(5):540–7.
7. Weiss J, Ten HM, Burhenne J, et al. CYP2C19 genotype is a major factor contributing to the highly variable pharmacokinetics of voriconazole. J Clin Pharmacol. 2009;49:196–204.
8. Ikeda Y, Umemura K, Kondo K, Sekiguchi K, Miyoshi S, Nakashima M. Pharmacokinetics of voriconazole and cytochrome P450 2C19 genetic status. Clin Pharmacol Ther. 2004;75(6):587–8.
9. Goodwin ML, Drew RH. Antifungal serum concentration monitoring: an update. J Antimicrob Chemother. 2008;61(1):17–25.
10. VFend® [package insert]. New York: Pfizer Inc; 2008. 2009. Ref Type: Generic.
11. Sustiva® [package insert]. Princeton: Bristol-Myers Squibb Company; 2008. 2009. Ref Type: Generic.
12. Smith J, Safdar N, Knasinski V, et al. Voriconazole therapeutic drug monitoring. Antimicrob Agents Chemother. 2006;50(4):1570–2.
13. Pascual A, Calandra T, Bolay S, Buclin T, Bille J, Marchetti O. Voriconazole therapeutic drug monitoring in patients with invasive mycoses improves efficacy and safety outcomes. Clin Infect Dis. 2008;46(2):201–11.
14. Denning DW, Ribaud P, Milpied N, et al. Efficacy and safety of voriconazole in the treatment of acute invasive aspergillosis. Clin Infect Dis. 2002;34(5):563–71.
15. Pfaller MA, Diekema DJ, Rex JH, et al. Correlation of MIC with outcome for *Candida* species tested against voriconazole: analysis and proposal for interpretive breakpoints. J Clin Microbiol. 2006;44(3):819–26.
16. Boyd AE, Modi S, Howard SJ, Moore CB, Keevil BG, Denning DW. Adverse reactions to voriconazole. Clin Infect Dis. 2004;39(8):1241–4.
17. Lutsar I, Hodges MR, Tomaszewski K, Troke PF, Wood ND. Safety of voriconazole and dose individualization. Clin Infect Dis. 2003;36(8):1087–8.
18. Imhof A, Schaer DJ, Schanz U, Schwarz U. Neurological adverse events to voriconazole: evidence for therapeutic drug monitoring. Swiss Med Wkly. 2006;136(45–46):739–42.
19. Pascual A, Nieth V, Calandra T, et al. Variability of voriconazole plasma levels measured by new high-performance liquid chromatography and bioassay methods. Antimicrob Agents Chemother. 2007;51(1):137–43.
20. Bruggemann RJ, Touw DJ, Aarnoutse RE, Verweij PE, Burger DM. International interlaboratory proficiency testing program for measurement of antifungal azole plasma concentrations. Antimicrob Agents Chemother. 2009;53(1):303–5.

21. MiraVista Diagnostics. http://www.miravistalabs.com. Accessed 15 Feb 2009; The fungus testing laboratory. http://pathology.uthscsa.edu/strl/fungus/index.shtml. Accessed 15 Feb 2009. Ref Type: Generic.
22. The Fungus Testing Laboratory. 2009. http://pathology.uthscsa.edu/strl/fungus/index.shtml. Accessed 15 Feb 2009. Ref Type: Generic.
23. Courtney R, Pai S, Laughlin M, Lim J, Batra V. Pharmacokinetics, safety, and tolerability of oral posaconazole administered in single and multiple doses in healthy adults. Antimicrob Agents Chemother. 2003;47(9):2788–95.
24. Ezzet F, Wexler D, Courtney R, Krishna G, Lim J, Laughlin M. Oral bioavailability of posaconazole in fasted healthy subjects: comparison between three regimens and basis for clinical dosage recommendations. Clin Pharmacokinet. 2005;44(2):211–20.
25. Krishna G, Moton A, Ma L, Medlock MM, McLeod J. The pharmacokinetics and absorption of posaconazole oral suspension under various gastric conditions in healthy volunteers. Antimicrob Agents Chemother. 2009;53:958–66.
26. Gubbins PO, Krishna G, Sansone-Parsons A, et al. Pharmacokinetics and safety of oral posaconazole in neutropenic stem cell transplant recipients. Antimicrob Agents Chemother. 2006;50(6):1993–9.
27. Ullmann AJ, Lipton JH, Vesole DH, et al. Posaconazole or fluconazole for prophylaxis in severe graft-versus-host disease. N Engl J Med. 2007;356(4):335–47.
28. Noxafil® [package insert]. Schering Corporation: Kenilworth, NJ; 2008. 2009. Ref Type: Generic
29. Walsh TJ, Raad I, Patterson TF, et al. Treatment of invasive aspergillosis with posaconazole in patients who are refractory to or intolerant of conventional therapy: an externally controlled trial. Clin Infect Dis. 2007;44(1):2–12.
30. Krishna G, AbuTarif M, Xuan F, Martinho M, Angulo D, Cornely OA. Pharmacokinetics of oral posaconazole in neutropenic patients receiving chemotherapy for acute myelogenous leukemia or myelodysplastic syndrome. Pharmacotherapy. 2008;28(10):1223–32.
31. Center for Drug Evaluation and Research. Posaconazole (Noxafil®, Schering-Plough); Clinical Pharmacology and Biopharmaceutics Reviews. Application 22-003, 2005. 2009. http://www.fda.gov/cder/foi/nda/2006/022003s000_Noxafil_ClinPharmR.pdf. Accessed 17 Feb 2009. Ref Type: Generic.
32. MiraVista Diagnostics. Available at: http://www.miravistalabs.com. Accessed February 15, 2009; The Fungus Testing Laboratory. Available at http://pathology.uthscsa.edu/strl/fungus/index.shtml. Accessed February 15, 2009. Ref Type: Generic.
33. Johnson EM. Issues in antifungal susceptibility testing. J Antimicrob Chemother. 2008;61 Suppl 1:i13–8.
34. NCCLS document M44-A. NCCLS. Reference method for broth dilution antifungal susceptibility testing of yeasts; Approved Guideline. Wayne: National Committee for Clinical Laboratory Standards; 2004. 2009. Ref Type: Generic.
35. CLSI document M27-A3. CLSI. Method for antifungal disk diffusion susceptibility testing of yeasts; Approved Standard-Third Edition. Wayne: Clincal and Laboratory Standards Institute; 2008. 2009. Ref Type: Generic.
36. Sensititre YeastOne Test Panel®. Trek Diagnostic Systems, Inc.: Westlake, OH. 2009. Ref Type: Generic.
37. Davey KG, Holmes AD, Johnson EM, Szekely A, Warnock DW. Comparative evaluation of FUNGITEST and broth microdilution methods for antifungal drug susceptibility testing of Candida species and Cryptococcus neoformans. J Clin Microbiol. 1998; 36(4):926–30.
38. Espinel-Ingroff A, Pfaller M, Messer SA, Knapp CC, Holliday N, Killian SB. Multicenter comparison of the Sensititre YeastOne colorimetric antifungal panel with the NCCLS M27-A2 reference method for testing new antifungal agents against clinical isolates of Candida spp. J Clin Microbiol. 2004;42(2):718–21.
39. Etest®. AB Biodisk: Solna, Sweden. 2009. Ref Type: Generic
40. Diekema DJ, Messer SA, Hollis RJ, et al. Evaluation of Etest and disk diffusion methods compared with broth microdilution antifungal susceptibility testing of clinical isolates of Candida spp. against posaconazole. J Clin Microbiol. 2007;45(6):1974–7.
41. Pfaller MA, Messer SA, Mills K, Bolmstrom A, Jones RN. Evaluation of Etest method for determining caspofungin (MK-0991) susceptibilities of 726 clinical isolates of Candida species. J Clin Microbiol. 2001;39(12):4387–9.
42. Warnock DW, Johnson EM, Rogers TR. Multi-centre evaluation of the Etest method for antifungal drug susceptibility testing of Candida spp. and Cryptococcus neoformans. BSAC Working Party on Antifungal Chemotherapy. J Antimicrob Chemother. 1998;42(3):321–31.
43. Pfaller MA, Diekema DJ, Gibbs DL, et al. Results from the ARTEMIS DISK Global Antifungal Surveillance study, 1997 to 2005: an 8.5-year analysis of susceptibilities of Candida species and other yeast species to fluconazole and voriconazole determined by CLSI standardized disk diffusion testing. J Clin Microbiol. 2007;45(6):1735–45.
44. Alexander BD, Byrne TC, Smith KL, et al. Comparative evaluation of Etest and sensititre yeastone panels against the Clinical and Laboratory Standards Institute M27-A2 reference broth microdilution method for testing Candida susceptibility to seven antifungal agents. J Clin Microbiol. 2007;45(3):698–706.
45. Pfaller MA, Diekema DJ, Ostrosky-Zeichner L, et al. Correlation of MIC with outcome for Candida species tested against caspofungin, anidulafungin, and micafungin: analysis and proposal for interpretive MIC breakpoints. J Clin Microbiol. 2008; 46(8):2620–9.
46. Johnson E, Espinel-Ingroff A, Szekely A, Hockey H, Troke P. Activity of voriconazole, itraconazole, fluconazole and amphotericin B in vitro against 1,763 yeasts from 472 patients in the voriconazole phase III clinical studies. Int J Antimicrob Agents. 2008;32(6):511–4.
47. Rex JH, Pfaller MA, Galgiani JN, et al. Development of interpretive breakpoints for antifungal susceptibility testing: conceptual framework and analysis of in vitro-in vivo correlation data for fluconazole, itraconazole, and candida infections. Subcommittee on Antifungal Susceptibility Testing of the National Committee for Clinical Laboratory Standards. Clin Infect Dis. 1997; 24(2):235–47.
48. Rex JH, Pfaller MA. Has antifungal susceptibility testing come of age? Clin Infect Dis. 2002;35(8):982–9.
49. Pfaller MA, Diekema DJ, Sheehan DJ. Interpretive breakpoints for fluconazole and Candida revisited: a blueprint for the future of antifungal susceptibility testing. Clin Microbiol Rev. 2006;19(2):435–47.
50. Rex JH, Rinaldi MG, Pfaller MA. Resistance of Candida species to fluconazole. Antimicrob Agents Chemother. 1995;39(1):1–8.
51. Pfaller MA, Messer SA, Boyken L, Tendolkar S, Hollis RJ, Diekema DJ. Selection of a surrogate agent (fluconazole or voriconazole) for initial susceptibility testing of posaconazole against Candida spp.: results from a global antifungal surveillance program. J Clin Microbiol. 2008;46(2):551–9.
52. Garcia-Effron G, Katiyar SK, Park S, Edlind TD, Perlin DS. A naturally occurring proline-to-alanine amino acid change in Fks1p in Candida parapsilosis, Candida orthopsilosis, and Candida metapsilosis accounts for reduced echinocandin susceptibility. Antimicrob Agents Chemother. 2008;52(7):2305–12.
53. Perlin DS. Resistance to echinocandin-class antifungal drugs. Drug Resist Updat. 2007;10(3):121–30.
54. Balashov SV, Park S, Perlin DS. Assessing resistance to the echinocandin antifungal drug caspofungin in Candida albicans by profiling mutations in FKS1. Antimicrob Agents Chemother. 2006;50(6):2058–63.

55. Park S, Kelly R, Kahn JN, et al. Specific substitutions in the echinocandin target Fks1p account for reduced susceptibility of rare laboratory and clinical *Candida* sp. isolates. Antimicrob Agents Chemother. 2005;49(8):3264–73.
56. Garcia-Effron G, Park S, Perlin DS. Correlating echinocandin MIC and kinetic inhibition of fks1 mutant glucan synthases for *C. albicans*: implications for interpretive breakpoints. Antimicrob Agents Chemother. 2008;53:112–22.
57. Park BJ, Arthington-Skaggs BA, Hajjeh RA, et al. Evaluation of amphotericin B interpretive breakpoints for Candida bloodstream isolates by correlation with therapeutic outcome. Antimicrob Agents Chemother. 2006;50(4):1287–92.
58. CLSI document M38-A2. CLSI. Reference method for broth dilution antifungal susceptibility testing of filamentous fungi; Approved Standard-Second Edition. Wayne: Clincal and Laboratory Standards Institute; 2008. 2009. Ref Type: Generic.
59. Sabatelli F, Patel R, Mann PA, et al. In vitro activities of posaconazole, fluconazole, itraconazole, voriconazole, and amphotericin B against a large collection of clinically important molds and yeasts. Antimicrob Agents Chemother. 2006;50(6):2009–15.
60. Diekema DJ, Messer SA, Hollis RJ, Jones RN, Pfaller MA. Activities of caspofungin, itraconazole, posaconazole, ravuconazole, voriconazole, and amphotericin B against 448 recent clinical isolates of filamentous fungi. J Clin Microbiol. 2003;41(8):3623–6.
61. Espinel-Ingroff A, Johnson E, Hockey H, Troke P. Activities of voriconazole, itraconazole and amphotericin B in vitro against 590 moulds from 323 patients in the voriconazole Phase III clinical studies. J Antimicrob Chemother. 2008;61(3):616–20.
62. Snelders E, van der Lee HA, Kuijpers J, et al. Emergence of azole resistance in *Aspergillus fumigatus* and spread of a single resistance mechanism. PLoS Med. 2008;5(11):e219.
63. Verweij PE, Mellado E, Melchers WJ. Multiple-triazole-resistant aspergillosis. N Engl J Med. 2007;356(14):1481–3.
64. Pfaller MA, Messer SA, Boyken L, et al. In vitro survey of triazole cross-resistance among more than 700 clinical isolates of *Aspergillus* species. J Clin Microbiol. 2008;46(8):2568–72.
65. Garcia-Effron G, Dilger A, Alcazar-Fuoli L, Park S, Mellado E, Perlin DS. Rapid detection of triazole antifungal resistance in *Aspergillus fumigatus*. J Clin Microbiol. 2008;46(4):1200–6.
66. Rodriguez-Tudela JL, Alcazar-Fuoli L, Mellado E, Alastruey-Izquierdo A, Monzon A, Cuenca-Estrella M. Epidemiological cut-offs and cross-resistance to azole drugs in *Aspergillus fumigatus*. Antimicrob Agents Chemother. 2008;52(7):2468–72.
67. Lass-Florl C, Kofler G, Kropshofer G, et al. In-vitro testing of susceptibility to amphotericin B is a reliable predictor of clinical outcome in invasive aspergillosis. J Antimicrob Chemother. 1998;42(4):497–502.
68. Lass-Florl C, Griff K, Mayr A, et al. Epidemiology and outcome of infections due to *Aspergillus terreus*: 10-year single centre experience. Br J Haematol. 2005;131(2):201–7.
69. Steinbach WJ, Benjamin Jr DK, Kontoyiannis DP, et al. Infections due to *Aspergillus terreus*: a multicenter retrospective analysis of 83 cases. Clin Infect Dis. 2004;39(2):192–8.
70. Madureira A, Bergeron A, Lacroix C, et al. Breakthrough invasive aspergillosis in allogeneic haematopoietic stem cell transplant recipients treated with caspofungin. Int J Antimicrob Agents. 2007;30(6):551–4.
71. Arendrup MC, Perkhofer S, Howard SJ, et al. Establishing in vitro-in vivo correlations for *Aspergillus fumigatus*: the challenge of azoles versus echinocandins. Antimicrob Agents Chemother. 2008;52(10):3504–11.
72. Rocha EM, Garcia-Effron G, Park S, Perlin DS. A Ser678Pro substitution in Fks1p confers resistance to echinocandin drugs in *Aspergillus fumigatus*. Antimicrob Agents Chemother. 2007;51(11):4174–6.
73. Almyroudis NG, Sutton DA, Fothergill AW, Rinaldi MG, Kusne S. In vitro susceptibilities of 217 clinical isolates of zygomycetes to conventional and new antifungal agents. Antimicrob Agents Chemother. 2007;51(7):2587–90.
74. Roden MM, Zaoutis TE, Buchanan WL, et al. Epidemiology and outcome of zygomycosis: a review of 929 reported cases. Clin Infect Dis. 2005;41(5):634–53.
75. Torres-Narbona M, Guinea J, Martinez-Alarcon J, Pelaez T, Bouza E. In vitro activities of amphotericin B, caspofungin, itraconazole, posaconazole, and voriconazole against 45 clinical isolates of zygomycetes: comparison of CLSI M38-A, Sensititre YeastOne, and the Etest. Antimicrob Agents Chemother. 2007;51(3):1126–9.
76. Espinel-Ingroff A. In vitro antifungal activities of anidulafungin and micafungin, licensed agents and the investigational triazole posaconazole as determined by NCCLS methods for 12,052 fungal isolates: review of the literature. Rev Iberoam Micol. 2003;20(4):121–36.
77. Chamilos G, Lewis RE, Kontoyiannis DP. Delaying amphotericin B-based frontline therapy significantly increases mortality among patients with hematologic malignancy who have zygomycosis. Clin Infect Dis. 2008;47(4):503–9.
78. Bowden R, Chandrasekar P, White MH, et al. A double-blind, randomized, controlled trial of amphotericin B colloidal dispersion versus amphotericin B for treatment of invasive aspergillosis in immunocompromised patients. Clin Infect Dis. 2002;35(4):359–66.
79. Lamaris GA, Lewis RE, Chamilos G, et al. Caspofungin-mediated beta-glucan unmasking and enhancement of human polymorphonuclear neutrophil activity against Aspergillus and non-Aspergillus hyphae. J Infect Dis. 2008;198(2):186–92.
80. Guembe M, Guinea J, Pelaez T, Torres-Narbona M, Bouza E. Synergistic effect of posaconazole and caspofungin against clinical zygomycetes. Antimicrob Agents Chemother. 2007;51(9):3457–8.
81. Perkhofer S, Locher M, Cuenca-Estrella M, et al. Posaconazole enhances the activity of amphotericin B against hyphae of zygomycetes in vitro. Antimicrob Agents Chemother. 2008;52(7):2636–8.
82. Ibrahim AS, Avanessian V, Spellberg B, Edwards Jr JE. Liposomal amphotericin B, and not amphotericin B deoxycholate, improves survival of diabetic mice infected with *Rhizopus oryzae*. Antimicrob Agents Chemother. 2003;47(10):3343–4.
83. Ibrahim AS, Gebremariam T, Husseiny MI, et al. Comparison of lipid amphotericin B preparations in treating murine zygomycosis. Antimicrob Agents Chemother. 2008;52(4):1573–6.
84. Ibrahim AS, Gebremariam T, Schwartz JA, Edwards Jr JE, Spellberg B. Posaconazole mono- or combination therapy for the treatment of murine Zygomycosis. Antimicrob Agents Chemother. 2009;53:772–5.
85. Rodriguez MM, Serena C, Marine M, Pastor FJ, Guarro J. Posaconazole combined with amphotericin B, an effective therapy for a murine disseminated infection caused by *Rhizopus oryzae*. Antimicrob Agents Chemother. 2008;52(10):3786–8.
86. Dannaoui E, Meis JF, Loebenberg D, Verweij PE. Activity of posaconazole in treatment of experimental disseminated zygomycosis. Antimicrob Agents Chemother. 2003;47(11):3647–50.
87. Del PM, Schell WA, Perfect JR. In vitro antifungal activity of pneumocandin L-743, 872 against a variety of clinically important molds. Antimicrob Agents Chemother. 1997;41(8):1835–6.
88. Ibrahim AS, Bowman JC, Avanessian V, et al. Caspofungin inhibits *Rhizopus oryzae* 1,3-beta-D-glucan synthase, lowers burden in brain measured by quantitative PCR, and improves survival at a low but not a high dose during murine disseminated zygomycosis. Antimicrob Agents Chemother. 2005;49(2):721–7.
89. Ibrahim AS, Gebremariam T, Fu Y, Edwards Jr JE, Spellberg B. Combination echinocandin-polyene treatment of murine mucormycosis. Antimicrob Agents Chemother. 2008;52(4):1556–8.
90. Spellberg B, Fu Y, Edwards Jr JE, Ibrahim AS. Combination therapy with amphotericin B lipid complex and caspofungin acetate of

90. disseminated zygomycosis in diabetic ketoacidotic mice. Antimicrob Agents Chemother. 2005;49(2):830–2.
91. Herbrecht R, Letscher-Bru V, Bowden RA, et al. Treatment of 21 cases of invasive mucormycosis with amphotericin B colloidal dispersion. Eur J Clin Microbiol Infect Dis. 2001;20(7):460–6.
92. Strasser MD, Kennedy RJ, Adam RD. Rhinocerebral mucormycosis. Therapy with amphotericin B lipid complex. Arch Intern Med. 1996;156(3):337–9.
93. Walsh TJ, Hiemenz JW, Seibel NL, et al. Amphotericin B lipid complex for invasive fungal infections: analysis of safety and efficacy in 556 cases. Clin Infect Dis. 1998;26(6):1383–96.
94. Gleissner B, Schilling A, Anagnostopolous I, Siehl I, Thiel E. Improved outcome of zygomycosis in patients with hematological diseases? Leuk Lymphoma. 2004;45(7):1351–60.
95. Pagano L, Offidani M, Fianchi L, et al. Mucormycosis in hematologic patients. Haematologica. 2004;89(2):207–14.
96. Perfect JR. Treatment of non-Aspergillus moulds in immunocompromised patients, with amphotericin B lipid complex. Clin Infect Dis. 2005;40 Suppl 6:S401–8.
97. Reed C, Bryant R, Ibrahim AS, et al. Combination polyene-caspofungin treatment of rhino-orbital-cerebral mucormycosis. Clin Infect Dis. 2008;47(3):364–71.
98. Walsh TJ, Goodman JL, Pappas P, et al. Safety, tolerance, and pharmacokinetics of high-dose liposomal amphotericin B (AmBisome) in patients infected with Aspergillus species and other filamentous fungi: maximum tolerated dose study. Antimicrob Agents Chemother. 2001;45(12):3487–96.
99. Cornely OA, Maertens J, Bresnik M, et al. Liposomal amphotericin B as initial therapy for invasive mold infection: a randomized trial comparing a high-loading dose regimen with standard dosing (AmBiLoad trial). Clin Infect Dis. 2007;44(10):1289–97.
100. van Burik JA, Hare RS, Solomon HF, Corrado ML, Kontoyiannis DP. Posaconazole is effective as salvage therapy in zygomycosis: a retrospective summary of 91 cases. Clin Infect Dis. 2006;42(7):e61–5.
101. Chayakulkeeree M, Ghannoum MA, Perfect JR. Zygomycosis: the re-emerging fungal infection. Eur J Clin Microbiol Infect Dis. 2006;25(4):215–29.
102. Ibrahim AS, Gebermariam T, Fu Y, et al. The iron chelator deferasirox protects mice from mucormycosis through iron starvation. J Clin Invest. 2007;117(9):2649–57.
103. Reed C, Ibrahim A, Edwards Jr JE, Walot I, Spellberg B. Deferasirox, an iron-chelating agent, as salvage therapy for rhinocerebral mucormycosis. Antimicrob Agents Chemother. 2006;50(11):3968–9.
104. Spellberg B, Edwards Jr J, Ibrahim A. Novel perspectives on mucormycosis: pathophysiology, presentation, and management. Clin Microbiol Rev. 2005;18(3):556–69.
105. Soummer A, Mathonnet A, Scatton O, et al. Failure of deferasirox, an iron chelator agent, combined with antifungals in a case of severe zygomycosis. Antimicrob Agents Chemother. 2008;52(4):1585–6.
106. Walsh TJ, Kontoyiannis DP. Editorial commentary: what is the role of combination therapy in management of zygomycosis? Clin Infect Dis. 2008;47(3):372–4.
107. Rogers TR. Treatment of zygomycosis: current and new options. J Antimicrob Chemother. 2008;61 Suppl 1:i35–40.
108. Safdar A. Difficulties with fungal infections in acute myelogenous leukemia patients: immune enhancement strategies. Oncologist. 2007;12 Suppl 2:2–6.
109. Kauffman CA, Malani AN. Zygomycosis: an emerging fungal infection with new options for management. Curr Infect Dis Rep. 2007;9(6):435–40.
110. Herbrecht R, Denning DW, Patterson TF, et al. Voriconazole versus amphotericin B for primary therapy of invasive aspergillosis. N Engl J Med. 2002;347(6):408–15.
111. Raad II, Hanna HA, Boktour M, et al. Novel antifungal agents as salvage therapy for invasive aspergillosis in patients with hematologic malignancies: posaconazole compared with high-dose lipid formulations of amphotericin B alone or in combination with caspofungin. Leukemia. 2008;22(3):496–503.
112. Maertens J, Raad I, Petrikkos G, et al. Efficacy and safety of caspofungin for treatment of invasive aspergillosis in patients refractory to or intolerant of conventional antifungal therapy. Clin Infect Dis. 2004;39(11):1563–71.
113. Steinbach WJ, Stevens DA, Denning DW. Combination and sequential antifungal therapy for invasive aspergillosis: review of published in vitro and in vivo interactions and 6281 clinical cases from 1966 to 2001. Clin Infect Dis. 2003;37 Suppl 3:S188–224.
114. Kirkpatrick WR, Perea S, Coco BJ, Patterson TF. Efficacy of caspofungin alone and in combination with voriconazole in a Guinea pig model of invasive aspergillosis. Antimicrob Agents Chemother. 2002;46(8):2564–8.
115. Perea S, Gonzalez G, Fothergill AW, Kirkpatrick WR, Rinaldi MG, Patterson TF. In vitro interaction of caspofungin acetate with voriconazole against clinical isolates of Aspergillus spp. Antimicrob Agents Chemother. 2002;46(9):3039–41.
116. Lewis RE, Prince RA, Chi J, Kontoyiannis DP. Itraconazole preexposure attenuates the efficacy of subsequent amphotericin B therapy in a murine model of acute invasive pulmonary aspergillosis. Antimicrob Agents Chemother. 2002;46(10):3208–14.
117. Meletiadis J, Petraitis V, Petraitiene R, et al. Triazole-polyene antagonism in experimental invasive pulmonary aspergillosis: in vitro and in vivo correlation. J Infect Dis. 2006;194(7):1008–18.
118. MacCallum DM, Whyte JA, Odds FC. Efficacy of caspofungin and voriconazole combinations in experimental aspergillosis. Antimicrob Agents Chemother. 2005;49(9):3697–701.
119. Petraitis V, Petraitiene R, Sarafandi AA, et al. Combination therapy in treatment of experimental pulmonary aspergillosis: synergistic interaction between an antifungal triazole and an echinocandin. J Infect Dis. 2003;187(12):1834–43.
120. Arikan S, Lozano-Chiu M, Paetznick V, Rex JH. In vitro synergy of caspofungin and amphotericin B against Aspergillus and Fusarium spp. Antimicrob Agents Chemother. 2002;46(1):245–7.
121. Johnson MD, Perfect JR. Combination antifungal therapy: what can and should we expect? Bone Marrow Transplant. 2007;40(4):297–306.
122. Chaturvedi. 2009. Ref Type: Personal Communication.
123. Popp AI, White MH, Quadri T, Walshe L, Armstrong D. Amphotericin B with and without itraconazole for invasive aspergillosis: a three-year retrospective study. Int J Infect Dis. 1999;3(3):157–60.
124. Kontoyiannis DP, Boktour M, Hanna H, Torres HA, Hachem R, Raad II. Itraconazole added to a lipid formulation of amphotericin B does not improve outcome of primary treatment of invasive aspergillosis. Cancer. 2005;103(11):2334–7.
125. Chandrasekar PH, Ito JI. Amphotericin B lipid complex in the management of invasive aspergillosis in immunocompromised patients. Clin Infect Dis. 2005;40 Suppl 6:S392–400.
126. Marr KA, Boeckh M, Carter RA, Kim HW, Corey L. Combination antifungal therapy for invasive aspergillosis. Clin Infect Dis. 2004;39(6):797–802.
127. Singh N, Limaye AP, Forrest G, et al. Combination of voriconazole and caspofungin as primary therapy for invasive aspergillosis in solid organ transplant recipients: a prospective, multicenter, observational study. Transplantation. 2006;81(3):320–6.
128. Maertens J, Glasmacher A, Herbrecht R, et al. Multicenter, noncomparative study of caspofungin in combination with other antifungals as salvage therapy in adults with invasive aspergillosis. Cancer. 2006;107(12):2888–97.
129. Kontoyiannis DP, Hachem R, Lewis RE, et al. Efficacy and toxicity of caspofungin in combination with liposomal amphotericin B as

primary or salvage treatment of invasive aspergillosis in patients with hematologic malignancies. Cancer. 2003;98(2):292–9.
130. Caillot D, Thiebaut A, Herbrecht R, et al. Liposomal amphotericin B in combination with caspofungin for invasive aspergillosis in patients with hematologic malignancies: a randomized pilot study (Combistrat trial). Cancer. 2007;110(12):2740–6.
131. Denning DW, Marr KA, Lau WM, et al. Micafungin (FK463), alone or in combination with other systemic antifungal agents, for the treatment of acute invasive aspergillosis. J Infect. 2006;53(5):337–49.
132. Kontoyiannis DP, Ratanatharathorn V, Young JA, et al. Micafungin alone or in combination with other systemic antifungal therapies in hematopoietic stem cell transplant recipients with invasive aspergillosis. Transpl Infect Dis. 2009;11(1):89–93.
133. Alexander BD, Dodds Ashley ES, Addison RM, Alspaugh JA, Chao NJ, Perfect JR. Non-comparative evaluation of the safety of aerosolized amphotericin B lipid complex in patients undergoing allogeneic hematopoietic stem cell transplantation. Transpl Infect Dis. 2006;8(1):13–20.
134. Drew RH, Dodds AE, Benjamin Jr DK, Duane DR, Palmer SM, Perfect JR. Comparative safety of amphotericin B lipid complex and amphotericin B deoxycholate as aerosolized antifungal prophylaxis in lung-transplant recipients. Transplantation. 2004;77(2):232–7.
135. Rijnders BJ, Cornelissen JJ, Slobbe L, et al. Aerosolized liposomal amphotericin B for the prevention of invasive pulmonary aspergillosis during prolonged neutropenia: a randomized, placebo-controlled trial. Clin Infect Dis. 2008;46(9):1401–8.
136. Walsh TJ, Anaissie EJ, Denning DW, et al. Treatment of aspergillosis: clinical practice guidelines of the Infectious Diseases Society of America. Clin Infect Dis. 2008;46(3):327–60.
137. Maschmeyer G, Haas A, Cornely OA. Invasive aspergillosis: epidemiology, diagnosis and management in immunocompromised patients. Drugs. 2007;67(11):1567–601.
138. Clinical Pharmacology [database online]. Tampa, FL, Gold Standard, Inc. 2009. http://www.clinicalpharmacology.com. Accessed 30 Jan 2009. Ref Type: Generic.
139. Pfaller MA, Diekema DJ, Procop GW, Rinaldi MG. Multicenter comparison of the VITEK 2 antifungal susceptibility test with the CLSI broth microdilution reference method for testing amphotericin B, flucytosine, and voriconazole against *Candida* spp. J Clin Microbiol. 2007;45(11):3522–8.
140. Pfaller MA, Boyken L, Hollis RJ, Messer SA, Tendolkar S, Diekema DJ. In vitro susceptibilities of clinical isolates of *Candida* species, *Cryptococcus neoformans*, and *Aspergillus* species to itraconazole: global survey of 9,359 isolates tested by clinical and laboratory standards institute broth microdilution methods. J Clin Microbiol. 2005;43(8):3807–10.
141. Guinea J, Pelaez T, Alcala L, Bouza E. Comparison of Sensititre YeastOne with the NCCLS M38-A microdilution method to determine the activity of amphotericin B, voriconazole, and itraconazole against clinical isolates of *Aspergillus fumigatus*. Diagn Microbiol Infect Dis. 2006;56(1):53–5.
142. Dannaoui E, Meletiadis J, Mouton JW, Meis JF, Verweij PE. In vitro susceptibilities of zygomycetes to conventional and new antifungals. J Antimicrob Chemother. 2003;51(1):45–52.
143. Sun QN, Fothergill AW, McCarthy DI, Rinaldi MG, Graybill JR. In vitro activities of posaconazole, itraconazole, voriconazole, amphotericin B, and fluconazole against 37 clinical isolates of zygomycetes. Antimicrob Agents Chemother. 2002;46(5):1581–2.

Chapter 28
Fungal Drug Resistance and Pharmacologic Considerations of Dosing Newer Antifungal Therapies

Russell E. Lewis and David S. Perlin

Abstract Recent advances in hematopoietic cell transplantation and a broadening array of salvage chemotherapy options have extended the survival of patients with hematological cancers, but can result in prolonged periods of immunosuppression and susceptibility to invasive fungal infections. Among these high-risk patient populations, systemic antifungal therapy is administered episodically or sometimes continuously for months or even years, increasing concerns for the development of antifungal resistance. As newer triazoles (voriconazole and posaconazole) and echinocandins (anidulafungin, caspofungin, and micafungin) have supplanted amphotericin B formulations as the preferred antifungal therapies for primary and secondary prophylaxis, pharmacokinetic variability inherent to the triazoles as well as emerging patterns of intrinsic and acquired antifungal resistance are becoming increasingly important factors in the long-term management of invasive fungal infections. In this chapter, we review recent data concerning antifungal drug resistance for these newer azoles and echinocandins, as well as key considerations in drug dosing.

Keywords Echinocandins • Glucan synthase • Fks1 • Caspofungin • Anidulafungin • Micafungin • Triazoles • Fluconazole • Voriconazole • Posaconazole • Itraconazole • Erg11 • Pharmacodynamics • Therapeutic drug monitoring

Introduction

Invasive fungal infections continue to be a source of extensive morbidity and mortality in severely ill cancer patients due to limitations in diagnostics and treatment [1]. More antifungal agents are available to treat invasive fungal diseases than at any time in the past decades [2]. Yet, the management of these serious infections in cancer patients remains problematic because these agents represent restricted chemical classes and targets. The aggressive use of antifungal therapy, especially triazole antifungals, correlates with a shift in the epidemiology of fungal infections, as non-*albicans Candida* species, *Aspergillus* spp., and other moulds, which have emerged as leading causes of infection in the heavily immunosuppressed cancer patients [3–6]. Unfortunately, many of these emerging fungi are not only difficult to differentiate [diagnose] from more susceptible pathogens, but are also frequently less susceptible to other classes of antifungal agents.

The epidemiological landscape of invasive fungal infections in cancer patients has been further changed by new approaches towards chemotherapy of hematological malignancies and hematopoietic stem cell transplantation (HSCT). Expanding use of purine analogs (i.e., fludarabine, cladarabine) and antilymphocyte monoclonal antibodies (i.e., rituximab, alemtuzumab) as well as other targeted therapies have reduced early nonrelapse mortality associated with remission-induction or salvage chemotherapy, but can result in persistent lymphopenia lasting months after bone marrow recovery [7–9]. Likewise, infectious diseases mortality in the early phases of HSCT (day 0–40) has decreased with nonmyeloablative conditioning regimens, peripheral blood stem cell sources, and hematopoietic growth factors that are associated with more rapid engraftment and shorter periods of neutropenia [10, 11]. As a consequence, fungal infections (especially moulds) are now encountered much later after stem cell engraftment (i.e., days 100–300) when graft versus host disease and high-dose glucocorticoid therapy predominate as risk

R.E. Lewis (✉)
Department of Clinical Sciences and Administration,
College of Pharmacy, University of Houston,
Texas Medical Center Campus, 1441 Moursund Street,
#424, Houston, TX 77030, USA
and
Department of Infectious Disease, Infection Control,
and Employee Health, The University of Texas/M.D. Anderson
Cancer Center, Houston, TX, USA
e-mail: rlewis@uh.edu

factors for infection [12]. Metabolic factors in chronically immunosuppressed and transfusion-dependent patients, including hyperglycemia/malnutrition and iron-overload, further predispose this population to a widening array of fungal pathogens [13]. Cancer patients are more likely than ever to exhibit a complex mosaic of mixed immunosuppression and increased environmental exposures and are more likely to have received hundreds of days of antifungal therapy prior to developing a clinically evident invasive fungal infection [13, 14].

Overview of Antifungal Resistance Mechanisms

Successful therapy of invasive fungal infections is influenced by a variety of factors including host status, drug pharmacokinetic/pharmacodynamic properties, and pathogen drug susceptibility. Yet, it is the latter property of drug resistance that has the potential to broadly diminish the effectiveness of entire classes of therapeutics. Drug resistance is best defined as clinical failure following a standard therapeutic dose and course. Primary resistance is the most significant factor contributing to antifungal drug resistance and it results from the selection of inherently less susceptible species (Table 28.1). Secondary or acquired resistance is less prevalent and refers to the induction of a biochemical mechanism that confers reduced susceptibility on a previously susceptible strain. The emergence of drug resistance is multifactorial and is influenced by host immune status, duration of immunosuppression, underlying disease, and total drug exposure. Recent global antifungal surveillance studies demonstrate that resistance varies with geography, as well as clinical service and the severity of disease with hematology/oncology units often showing the highest levels [5]. Patient exposure to a prior antifungal agent is also a risk factor for the development of resistant mould infections [15]. In fact, the epidemiology of mould infections in the past decade reflects a shift toward drug-resistant non-*fumigatus* *Aspergillus* species, *Fusarium* species, and Zygomycetes [16–18]. Zygomycosis is now observed in nearly 7% of patients at autopsy [19]. Triazole resistance in susceptible species like *Aspergillus fumigatus* is more common than once thought with an annual prevalence of 1.7–6% observed in the Netherlands [20]. In addition, multitriazole resistance has been reported following primary therapy and/or prophylaxis [21–23].

Many aspects of secondary or acquired antifungal resistance are still poorly understood, particularly with respect to the in vivo regulation and expression of resistance mechanisms. Nevertheless, advances in molecular biology and genomic sequencing of pathogenic fungi have yielded progress in our understanding of mechanisms most frequently leading to antifungal resistance. These mechanisms can be broadly grouped into five general categories (Fig. 28.1):

- Decreased drug import or increased drug export (efflux) [1, 2]
- Overproduction or alteration of the drug target binding site [3, 6]
- Gain of function mutations in transcriptional regulators of antifungal resistance [4]
- Diminished intracellular drug activation or modification [5]
- Changes in biosynthetic pathways (especially sterol synthesis) that circumvent or attenuate the effects of antifungal inhibition or binding [7]

Importantly, multiple mechanisms are often expressed simultaneously and can result in cross-resistance (depending on the time, sequence, and length of antifungal exposure) between unrelated classes of antifungals [24]. For example, genome-wide profiling of *Candida albicans* during exposure to triazole antifungals have shown transient up-regulation of several resistance mechanisms simultaneously, including ergosterol biosynthesis *ERG3*, *ERG11*; efflux pumps-*CDR1*, *CDR2*; and a transcriptional regulator-*Tac1* that regulates the expression of efflux pumps [25]. Unlike resistance with antibacterials, the development of antifungal resistance is generally associated with longer courses of therapy and a more gradual accumulation of several resistance mechanisms that result in laboratory-detectable resistance [26].

Newer Triazole Antifungals and Fungal Susceptibility

The newer triazole antifungals, voriconazole and posaconazole, are synthetic derivatives of fluconazole and itraconazole with improved spectrum of activity against moulds (Table 28.1). Like other triazole antifungals, voriconazole and posaconazole inhibit ergosterol biosynthesis in susceptible fungi through inhibition of the fungal cytochrome p450 enzyme, 14α-demethylase (CYP51p) [27]. Inhibiting ergosterol biosynthesis results in the accumulation of toxic 14α-methylated sterols in the cell membrane, which disrupts phospholipid membrane fluidity and membrane-bound enzyme systems, arresting fungal cell growth [28]. Drug binding is mediated through interactions of nitrogen in the triazole rings with the CYP51p heme target site, while the remainder of the drug molecule binds to the apoprotein in a manner dependent on the individual structure of the azole. For posaconazole, extension of a lipophilic side-chain expands the potency and spectrum of the triazole against both yeast and moulds, including *Aspergillus* and some species associated with mucormycosis. For voriconazole, inclusion of an α-*O*-methyl group confers activity against *Aspergillus* and some *Fusarium* species (Table 28.1) [27].

Table 28.1 Systemic antifungals: spectrum of in vitro activity

	A. flavus	A. fumigatus	A. niger	A. lentulus	A. terreus	Fusarium	C. albicans	C. krusei	C. glabrata	C. parapsilosis	C. neoformans	Coccidioides spp.	Blastomyces spp.	Histoplasma spp.	S. apiospermum	Zygomycetes
Amphotericin B	+	+	+	−	+	+	+	+	+	+	+	+	+	+	+	±
Fluconazole	−	−	−	−	−	−	+	−	±	+	+	+	+	+	−	−
Itraconazole	+	+	−	−	−	−	+	±	±	+	+	+	+	+	−	±
Posaconazole	+	+	+	±	+	+	+	+	±	+	+	+	+	+	+	+
Voriconazole	+	+	+	±	+	±	+	±	±	+	+	+	+	+	+	−
Caspofungin	+	+	+	−	+	−	+	+	+	±	−	−	−	−	−	−
Micafungin	+	+	+	−	+	−	+	+	+	±	−	−	−	−	−	−
Anidulafungin	+	+	+	+	+	−	+	+	+	±	−	−	−	−	−	−

+ Susceptible; − nonsusceptible; ± mixed susceptibility

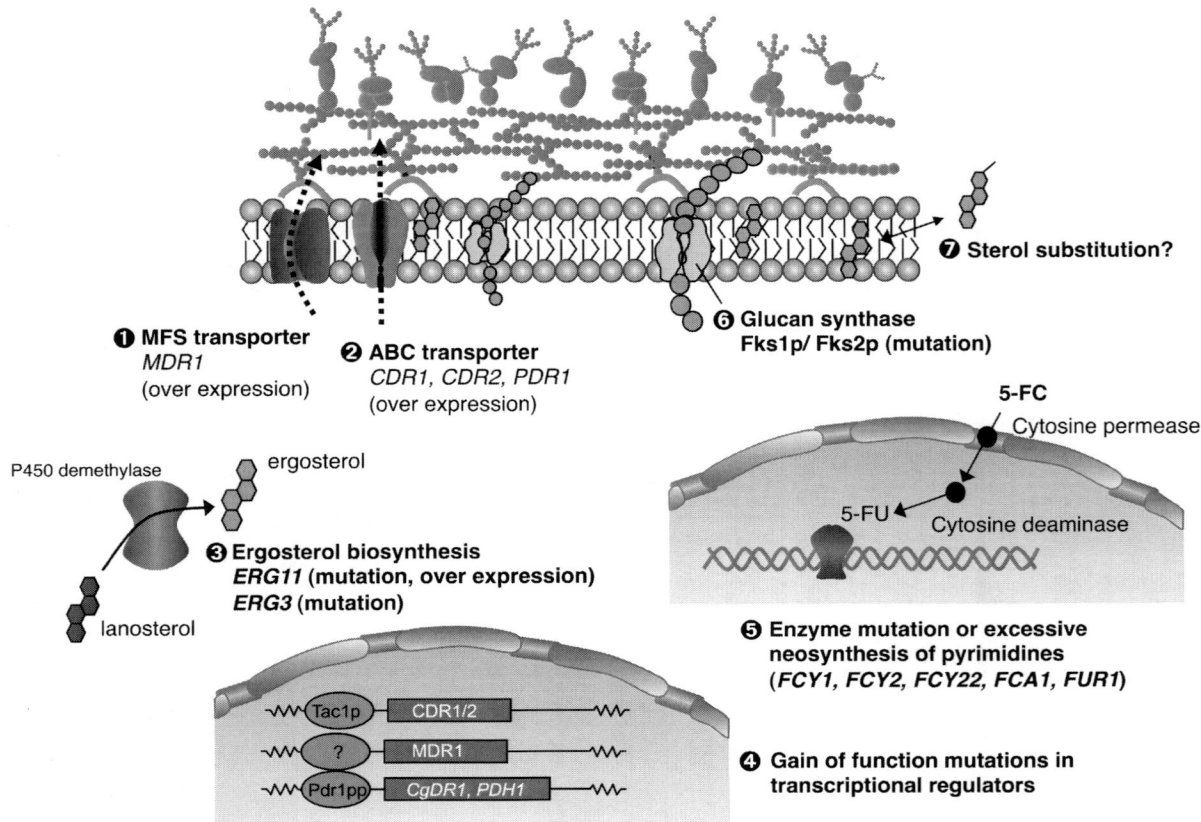

Fig. 28.1 Mechanisms of antifungal resistance

One drawback of exploiting fungal CYP-450 as a target for antifungal chemotherapy is the homology of these enzyme targets with mammalian CYP-450 involved in drug metabolism. Modifications to azole pharmacophore which enhance binding to the fungal CYP51p target (and improved spectrum) are frequently associated with increased binding to mammalian CYP-P450 enzymes, increasing the risk for drug interactions [29]. Both voriconazole and posaconazole inhibit human CYP3A4, the pathway responsible for the metabolism of 50% of clinically administered drugs [30]. Therefore, coadministration of voriconazole or posaconazole with drugs metabolized through CYP3A4 results in markedly decreased (i.e., 50–90%) metabolism/elimination of the second drug [29]. Similarly, administration of broad-spectrum triazoles with inducers of Phase I/II metabolism (rifamycins, phenytoin, carbamazepime, etc.) can result in low or undetectable levels of these antifungals [29]. While many of these interactions are not clinically significant, some interactions affecting the pharmacokinetics of drugs with a narrow therapeutic index for efficacy (e.g., chemotherapy agents, immunosuppressants used in transplantation) or the blood levels of antifungals needed to treat life-threatening fungal infections carry the potential for serious harm. Concurrent use of these drugs with voriconazole or posaconazole should either be avoided or proactively monitored with dosing guided by serum drug concentration monitoring [31, 32].

Pharmacokinetic Variability as a Contributor to Clinical Failure with Voriconazole

Voriconazole is available in both intravenous and oral formulation, which in healthy volunteers demonstrates excellent oral bioavailability (96%) [33, 34], but exhibits wide inter-subject pharmacokinetic variability due to the extensive saturable metabolism of this triazole. Several studies have demonstrated that most of this pharmacokinetic variability is due to differences in the ability of patients to metabolize voriconazole via CYP2C19 P450 enzyme [33–35]. Polymorphisms in the gene-encoding CYP2C19 are common and result in variable rates of voriconazole metabolism. Patients who are homozygous extensive metabolizers of

CYP2C19 have less than one-fourth the average voriconazole plasma concentrations of patients who are homozygous poor metabolizers and one-half the average plasma concentrations compared to patients who are heterozygous extensive metabolizers [36]. While these polymorphisms can occur in any individual, the homozygous poor metabolism genotype is found most frequently (14–19%) in patients of Asian descent [35, 37]. In contrast, the homozygous poor metabolism genotype is only found in 2–5% of caucasians, while 26–28% are heterozygous extensive metabolizers and 70–73% are homozygous extensive metabolizers [35, 37]. In the absence of individual genotyping, it may be difficult to predict a priori the dose of voriconazole that will result in therapeutic or potentially toxic drug concentrations in the bloodstream.

Beyond the genetic status, other factors that have been shown to influence voriconazole pharmacokinetics include age, liver disease, comedications that induce or inhibit CYP-P450 enzymes, and changes from intravenous (weight-based) therapy to a fixed oral dose of 200 mg twice daily. For example, the change from a standard intravenous maintenance dose of 4 mg/kg every 12 h to a fixed 200-mg tablet administered twice daily results in dose reduction of approximately 33% and significantly lower plasma drug concentrations [36].

Intra- and interpatient pharmacokinetic variability of voriconazole may be sufficiently large in patients with acute hematological malignancies or following HSCT to require drug dosing guided by plasma drug level monitoring [36]. In a series of articles from Northwestern Memorial Hospital (Chicago, IL), Trifilio et al. [38–40] found that 18–27% of adult allogeneic hematopoietic stem cell transplant recipients who receive standard oral voriconazole doses may have subtherapeutic drug exposures. Importantly, the subtherapeutic exposures could not be predicted based on daily or weight-based (mg/kg) dose of voriconazole alone (Fig. 28.2a) [38]. The investigators also noted a significant temporal effect of transplant on voriconazole plasma concentrations, with one

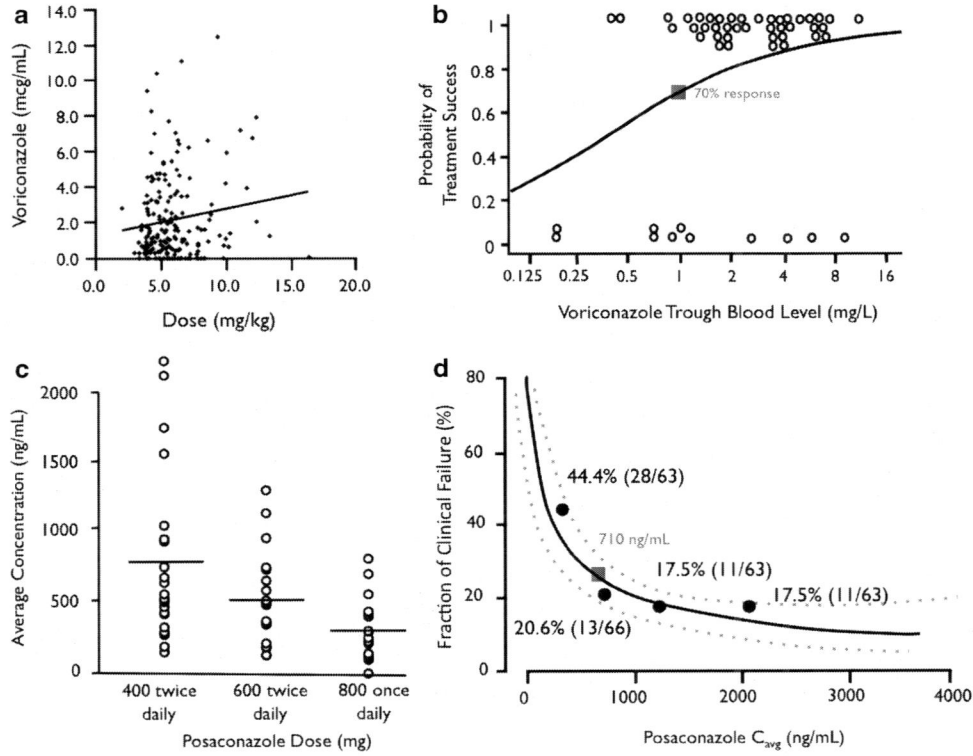

Fig. 28.2 Pharmacokinetic variability and relationship of plasma drug exposures to clinical failure for voriconazole and posaconazole. (**a**) Voriconazole trough concentrations exhibit a poor correlation with plasma trough concentrations [39]. (**b**) Logistic regression analysis of voriconazole trough concentrations from 52 patients receiving voriconazole for proven, probable, or possible invasive fungal infection demonstrating that log-transformed voriconazole trough level is a significant predictor of response to therapy: a twofold increase in blood level is associated with an OR for success of 1.8 (95% CI, 1.1–3.1; $P=0.03$). The logistic regression model indicates a 70% probability of response at a voriconazole trough concentration of 1 mg/L; [45] (**c**) Comparison of three posaconazole dosing schedule in febrile neutropenic patients revealing wide interpatient variability in drug exposure and dose-limited absorption; [54] (**d**) relationship between log-transformed posaconazole plasma exposures and risk of breakthrough invasive fungal infection during posaconazole prophylaxis; average drug concentrations <710 ng/mL were associated with an increased risk of breakthrough infection, $P<0.001$ [36]

Table 28.2 Provisional guidelines for therapeutic drug monitoring of mould-active triazoles

Drug	Indication	Time of first measurement	Target blood concentration (μg/mL)-trough concentrations	
			Efficacy	Safety
Itraconazole	Routine during first week of therapy, lack of clinical response, GI dysfunction, suspected drug interactions	4–7 days	Prophylaxis >0.5; treatment >1–2	NA
Voriconazole	Lack of clinical response; GI dysfunction; suspected drug interactions; pediatric patients; severe hepatopathy, unexplained neurological signs or symptoms; monotherapy for documented infection	4–7 days	Prophylaxis >0.5; for treatment >1–2	Trough of <6
Posaconazole	Lack of clinical response; suspected poor absorption or compliance, concurrent H_2 or proton pump inhibitor therapy, possible drug interactions	4–7 days	Prophylaxis >0.5; for treatment trough >0.5–1.5	NA

Adapted from Andes et al. [36]

third of patients who previously determined to have therapeutic concentrations becoming subtherapeutic with subsequent tests – hence acceptability of a concentration on one occasion cannot be extrapolated to future concentrations in the same patient [41]. Therefore, close therapeutic drug monitoring and dose adjustment may be important in patients who have received an allogeneic HSCT due to the frequent use of prolonged voriconazole and changing liver function with GvHD.

Pediatric patients who receive voriconazole are at high risk for subtherapeutic dosing, due to their linear nonsaturable metabolism of the drug [42]. Maintenance doses of 7–14 mg/kg every 12 h may be required to achieve effective blood concentrations in children compared to the 6 mg/kg every 12 h recommended for adults. Because variability and subtherapeutic values are frequently observed in this population, monitoring of voriconazole plasma concentrations may be necessary in all pediatric patients receiving voriconazole [43].

Treatment outcome has been statistically linked to voriconazole plasma concentrations in several single-center retrospective and prospective studies [40, 44, 45]. In a prospective evaluation of 52 patients with invasive fungal infections who had over 180 concentrations determinations over 2,000 treatment days, patients with trough concentrations <1 μg/mL had lower clinical responses compared to patients with trough concentrations >1 μg/mL (50% vs. 90%, respectively; Fig. 28.2) [45]. Interestingly, reversible neurologic symptoms (confusion, hallucination, myoclonia) were observed in four patients with voriconazole trough concentrations >5.5 μg/mL – all of the patients were receiving the 2C19 inhibitor omeprazole. The probability of neurological symptoms in patients with voriconazole trough concentrations of 8 μg/mL or greater was >90%. Therefore, signs of encephalopathy occurring during voriconazole therapy should follow drug discontinuation or, if available in a timely fashion, plasma drug concentration determinations to ensure the patient does not have excessively elevated voriconazole plasma concentrations.

Toxicodynamic evaluation of data from Phase II–III clinical trials for voriconazole have demonstrated similar relationships between voriconazole plasma concentrations, the probability of developing self-limiting photopsia, and liver function test (LFT) abnormalities [46]. The median voriconazole plasma concentration for patients who develop visual abnormalities was 3.52 μg/mL versus 2.52 μg/mL in the symptom-free patients. However, therapeutic drug monitoring to reduce the risk of visual changes is not justified, due to the self-limiting and fully reversible nature of this adverse effect [36]. Hepatotoxicity with voriconazole is a greater concern and often manifests in the setting of multiple aggregate insults (i.e., viral reactivation, graft vs. host disease, high-dose chemotherapy, other medications). Therefore, assessment of a plasma voriconazole level could help identify whether excessive voriconazole exposures are potentially contributing to an evolving hepatotoxicity [36]. A toxicodynamic evaluation of voriconazole exposures and LFT abnormalities revealed the risk of significant abnormalities (defined as ≥2× upper limit normal for aspartate transaminase (AST) or alanine transaminase (ALT) or ≥3 mg/dL for total bilirubin) by 7–17% for every 1 μg/mL increase in random plasma voriconazole concentrations [46]. However, the overall risk for hepatic toxicity was low (<10%), suggesting that routine therapeutic drug monitoring to *prevent* hepatotoxicity is probably not useful beyond select situations of severe hepatic toxicity [47]. Provisional guidelines for monitoring voriconazole are presented in Table 28.2.

Pharmacokinetic Variability as a Contributor to Clinical Failure with Posaconazole

Unlike voriconazole, pharmacokinetic variability with posaconazole is primarily due to the saturable oral absorption of the drug, which is maximized with administration with high-fat meals and in divided (three to four times daily) doses. Incomplete dissolution of the suspension in the gastrointestinal tract results in wide intra- and interpatient pharmacokinetic variability in both healthy volunteers and patient populations (Fig. 28.1c) [48–54]. Several factors have been shown to impact posaconazole absorption including high-fat meals, gastric pH (and the use of H_2 antagonists and proton pump inhibitors), mucositis, severe diarrhea, and the frequency of administration (due to saturable absorption) [36]. Administration of the oral posaconazole suspension with a high-fat meal (>50% of calories from fat) increases the mean AUC and maximum observed plasma concentrations (C_{max}) fourfold compared to fasted conditions [55]. Even a nonfat meal enhances posaconazole bioavailability, as mean AUC and C_{max} values increase 2.6- and 3-fold, respectively, compared with fasted conditions [55]. The importance of sufficient food intake for absorption of posaconazole can be problematic in cancer patients, particularly those who have nausea and vomiting, diarrhea and mucositis, or graft versus host disease involving the gut. Based on our clinical experience, one fourth to one third of patients with concomitant conditions or drugs that decrease posaconazole plasma concentrations have undetectable or near undetectable plasma concentrations at maximal doses (200 mg administered four times daily).

Although limited pharmacodynamic data are available, a single published trial that evaluated posaconazole as a salvage therapy reported the relationship of treatment response with randomly drawn plasma concentrations in a subset of 67 patients with refractory aspergillosis [56]. The patients in the lowest concentration quartile (≤0.13 µg/mL) had the poorest clinical response (20%). Patients with the highest response rates on salvage posaconazole therapy (70%) had average steady-state posaconazole concentrations of 1.25 µg/mL. Patients with plasma exposures in the middle two quartiles, 0.5–0.7 µg/mL, exhibited response rates of 53% [56].

A similar investigation of posaconazole plasma drug concentrations and risk of breakthrough fungal infection was explored in pivotal Phase III studies that examined the effectiveness of posaconazole prophylaxis in high-risk neutropenic patients or HSCT patients with graft versus host disease [57, 58]. Posaconazole concentrations were twofold lower in the cohort of patients who developed breakthrough invasive fungal infections ($n=5$) versus the cohort who did not develop infections ($n=241$; C_{avg} 0.611 vs. 0.922, respectively). Although these differences were not statistically significant due to the small numbers of patients who developed infection (2.4%), they do suggest that a threshold exposure level of posaconazole >0.6 µg/mL may be desirable to prevent the development of an invasive fungal infection [36]. Therefore, therapeutic drug monitoring of posaconazole should be considered in patients with documented fungal infection or patients with suspected malabsorption who are receiving posaconazole prophylaxis. Guidelines for potential therapeutic drug monitoring approaches are outlined in Table 28.2.

Echinocandin Drugs and Fungal Susceptibility

The echinocandin class drugs, caspofungin, micafungin, and anidulafungin, are cyclic lipopeptides that inhibit glucan synthase, which is responsible for the biosynthesis of β-1,3-D-glucan, the central building block of fungal cell walls. Caspofungin, the first of this class, received FDA approval in 2001 for treatment of patients unresponsive to or who could not tolerate standard therapies for invasive pulmonary aspergillosis (IPA); it was followed by an expanded indication for empirical therapy in febrile neutropenic patients. Micafungin was approved in 2005 for the treatment of esophageal candidiasis and prophylaxis of *Candida* infections in patients undergoing hematopoietic stem cell transplantation; the label was extended in 2008 to include patients with candidemia, acute disseminated candidiasis, *Candida* peritonitis, and abscesses. Anidulafungin was approved in 2006 for the treatment of candidemia, esophageal candidiasis, *Candida* peritonitis, and intra-abdominal abscesses. Overall, these drugs display consistent pharmacokinetic–pharmacodynamic properties and demonstrate excellent safety and tolerability with few drug-related adverse events [59–61].

The echinocandin drugs are fungicidal with yeasts, including azole-resistant *Candida* strains [62], but they are only mildly fungistatic with most moulds causing irregular cellular and colony morphologies [63]. Although only caspofungin received an indication for treatment of invasive aspergillosis, all three echinocandin drugs show efficacy against *A. fumigatus* in animal models [64–66]. As weak in vitro antifungal agents against *Aspergillus* spp., the effectiveness of echinocandin drugs in treating such mould infections may reflect drug-induced changes at the surface cell wall in exposure of epitopes, such as glucans, which promote strong local immunological responses through the dectin and toll-like receptors [67, 68], as has been reported for *C. albicans* [69, 70]. Overall, the echinocandins show a more limited spectrum of activity than polyene or triazole drugs (Table 28.1). They are not effective against *Cryptococcus* spp., *Trichosporon* spp., *Fusarium,* and most Zygomycetes [71, 72]. In addition, some *Aspergillus* spp. such as *A. lentulus* spp., a sibling species of *A. fumigatus,* are resistant to echinocandin drugs [73].

MIC and Epidemiology of Echinocandin Resistance

The echinocandin drugs are highly active against *Candida* spp. where in vitro susceptibility testing by either standard CLSI or EUCAST methodologies reveals MIC values for a majority of strains in the submicromolar range [72, 74–76]. For this reason, the emergence of clinical isolates of *Candida* spp. with reduced susceptibility in normally susceptible strains is a concern for successful therapy. Yet, a complex relationship exists between MIC and clinical success, and an elevated MIC does not always foretell therapeutic outcome [77–79]. Modeling of pharmacokinetic and pharmacodynamic parameters in a neutropenic candidemia model revealed that a strong relationship exists between exposure and effect related to MIC, and the apparent discordance between MIC and clinical outcome is most likely related to a narrow MIC distribution window [80].

To assess in vitro drug susceptibility trends, more than 5,300 clinical isolates of *Candida* spp. collected globally over a 6-year period were evaluated for susceptibility to anidulafungin, caspofungin, and micafungin (Table 28.3) [76]. Overall, infecting strains retained their susceptibility over this period. In fact, it was determined for a wide range of species that greater than 99% of isolates were inhibited at ≤2 mg/mL for all echinocandin drugs [76]. On this basis, the CLSI Antifungal Subcommittee established a MIC ≤2 mg/mL, as an interpretive breakpoint for susceptibility of *Candida* spp. for all licensed echinocandin drugs [79]. The emergence of high MIC isolates of *Candida* above the breakpoint for normally susceptible strains is a risk factor for therapeutic failure, but a resistance breakpoint per se could not be assigned because of the small number of isolates evaluated [79]. It is important to recognize that as echinocandin drugs are exclusively delivered by intravenous route, they are extensively bound (97–99%) to serum protein [81], which modulates their antifungal properties [82–84]. The CLSI protocol M27-A3 does not take into account the influence of serum protein binding on the relative efficacy of echinocandin drugs, since it is a parameter that is difficult to standardize.

Breakthrough Infections and Fks Mutations

Breakthrough infections involving high MIC strains are encountered uncommonly. When they occur, mechanism-specific resistance has been reported for clinical isolates of *C. albicans, C. glabrata, C. krusei, C. dubliniensis, C. tropicalis,* and *C. parapsilosis* [85–94]. Breakthrough mould infections have also been reported following therapy with anidulafungin [95] or caspofungin [96]. Resistant isolates show cross-resistance across the entire class of echinocandin drugs. These strains retain sensitivity to other antifungal agents, which is consistent with a separate mechanism of resistance [97]. It is now well recognized that high MIC isolates of *Candida* spp. from patients failing therapy often contain amino acid substitutions in Fks subunits (Fks1p and/or Fks2p), which comprise the 1,3-β-D-glucan synthase complex [98]. The high MIC phenotype resulting from mutations in Fks subunits is a direct consequence of decreased biochemical sensitivity of glucan synthase to drug. Depending on the mutation, the drug sensitivity of the enzyme can be reduced several log orders, which renders the infecting strain highly cross-resistant to all echinocandin drugs [99]. This decreased biochemical sensitivity is observed as a comparable rise in the ED99 values for reduction of fungal burdens in animal models [86]. Yet, the fold decrease in enzyme sensitivity, as reflected in kinetic parameters IC_{50} or K_i, does not strictly correlate with an equivalent fold rise in MIC. Nevertheless, there is an unambiguous linkage between increasing values for these kinetic constants and MIC [99]. This tightly coupled relationship between K_i and MIC has been used recently to independently validate the new CLSI breakpoint of echinocandin drugs for *C. albicans* [99]. For caspofungin, nearly all clinical isolates containing *fks1* mutations were captured at MIC values ≥2 mg/mL, which fully supported the CLSI breakpoint. However, a threshold MIC value of ≥2 mg/mL was less inclusive for anidulafungin and micafungin, which typically display lower cut-off values [99]. These subtle differences are eliminated when MIC values are determined in the presence of serum, which allows 100% capture of *fks1*-resistant isolates at a breakpoint value of ≥2 mg/mL.

Table 28.3 In vitro susceptibilities of 5,346 clinical isolates of *Candida* species to anidulafungin, caspofungin, and micafungin

Species	Number of isolates tested	Anidulafungin		Caspofungin		Micafungin	
		MIC_{90}	% ≤2	MIC_{90}	% ≤2	MIC_{90}	% ≤2
C. albicans	2,869	0.06	100	0.06	100	0.03	100
C. glabrata	747	0.12	99.9	0.06	99.9	0.015	100
C. tropicalis	625	0.06	100	0.06	99.8	0.06	100
C. krusei	136	0.06	100	0.25	100	0.12	100
C. parapsilosis	759	2	92.5	1	99.9	2	100
C. guillermondii	61	2	90.2	1	95.1	1	100
All *Candida* species	5,346	2	98.8	0.25	99.9	1	100

Adapted from Pfaller et al. [76]

Fks-Mediated Resistance

The Fks mechanism of resistance is widely distributed among fungi accounting for echinocandin resistance in common *Candida* spp. [98]. Mutations conferring resistance are clustered in two highly conserved hot-spot regions of Fks subunits (Fig. 28.3). Most fungi contain multiple genes encoding glucan synthase, but the genes *FKS1* and *FKS2* are the most highly expressed. In *C. albicans* and several other *Candida* spp., *FKS1* is the most highly expressed of the genes and accounts for all resistance mutations. Resistance is dominant and mutation of a single allele in *C. albicans* is sufficient to confer a resistant phenotype [86]. In *C. glabrata*, *FKS1* and *FKS2* are expressed in nearly equal proportions, and hot-spot mutations conferring resistance occur readily in both genes [87, 91].

The Fks mechanism also helps account for reduced susceptibility in *Candida* spp. such as *C. parapsilosis* group and its siblings species *C. orthopsilosis* and *C. metapsilosis*. Most infections due to *C. parapsilosis* respond to primary echinocandin therapy [100]. Although clinical failures have been reported [85], there is evidence linking caspofungin usage to increased incidence of *C. parapsilosis* candidemia [101]. There is also a concern that the elevated baseline drug susceptibility may provide an initial step toward clinical resistance, especially in regions of the world like Latin America where *C. parapsilosis* infections are more common [102, 103]. Recently, it was demonstrated that a polymorphism in *C. parapsilosis* and related species at the C-terminal region of FKS1 hot-spot 1 confer moderate reduced sensitivity of glucan synthase to drug, which most likely accounts for the observed reduced susceptibility [104].

The Fks resistance mechanism appears ubiquitous within the fungal kingdom. In *A. fumigatus*, mutation of *FKS1* confers strong resistance to all echinocandin drugs [105]. Such mutations in *A. fumigatus* have not been observed clinically. However, a clinical strain with reduced susceptibility isolated from a patient on caspofungin therapy did show hyperexpression of *FKS1*, suggesting that an increase in the expression of the target can confer reduced susceptibility in *Aspergillus* [106].

Elevated MICs and Non-Fks Mechanisms

Echinocandin drugs induce enormous selection pressure on most fungi, since glucan synthase is required for cell growth, cell wall remodeling, and development [107]. Partial or complete inhibition of glucan synthase induces a wide array of compensatory cellular processes including cell wall integrity pathway and the molecular chaperones, such as HSP90 [108]. Many of these processes are regulated by the ubiquitous G-protein Rho1 and MAP kinase signaling cascades, which help modulate the cell wall in response to environmental stresses. These compensatory biological responses help account elevated MIC values [98] and have been implicated in the paradoxical effect, in which certain strains of *Candida* [109–111] and *Aspergillus* [112] become insensitive to drug at high concentrations. In at least one strain, a replacement of glucan as the major cell wall carbohydrate with chitin helped account for the phenomenon [110]. As drug levels required are above the highest serum levels achieved during normal patient dosing, the significance of the paradoxical effect based on animal models and limited clinical data remains unclear [111–113].

Summary

There is now convincing evidence that pharmacokinetic variability with newer mould-active triazoles contributes to the risk of clinical failure, and echinocandin resistance in breakthrough strains arises from genetic changes in two defined regions of the Fks subunits of glucan synthase. Therefore, patients with suspect absorption, poor clinical response, or unexpected toxicity should have determination of voriconazole or posaconazole plasma concentrations to determine if unexpectedly high or low drug exposures are contributing factors to lack of efficacy or observed toxicity. For echinocandins, the new susceptibility breakpoint provides a valuable measure of potential clinical response and could prove a useful determinant of emerging echinocandin resistance in *Candida* species. Yet, a direct assessment of Fks1 mutations may provide a more precise indicator of clinical outcome.

Organism	FKS1 Hot Spot 1	FKS1 Hot Spot 2	FKS2 Hot Spot 1
C. albicans	FLTLSLRDP	DWIRRYTL	
C. kruseii	FLILSIRDP	DWIRRYTL	
C. glabrata	FLILSIRDP	DWIRRYTL	FLILSIRDP
C. guilliermondii	FMALSIRDP	DWIRRYTL	
C. lypolytica	FLILSIRDP	DWIRRCVL	
C. tropicalis	FLTLSIRDP	DWIRRYTL	
C. dubliniensis	FLTLSIRDP	DWIRRYTL	
C. parapsilosis	FLTLSIRDA	DWIRRYTL	
C. orthopsilosis	FLTLSIRDA	DWVRRYTL	
C. metapsilosis	FLTLSIRDA	DWIRRYTL	

Fig. 28.3 FKS mutations (*yellow*) and polymorphisms (*blue*) in hot-spot regions conferring reduced susceptibility among *Candida* spp. Mutations in *green* do not confer changes in drug sensitivity

References

1. Maertens J, Buve K, Anaissie E. Broad-spectrum antifungal prophylaxis in patients with cancer at high risk for invasive mold infections: counterpoint. J Natl Compr Canc Netw. 2008;6:183–9.
2. Krcmery V, Kalavsky E. Antifungal drug discovery, six new molecules patented after 10 years of feast: why do we need new patented drugs apart from new strategies? Recent Pat Antiinfect Drug Discov. 2007;2:182–7.
3. Bhatti Z, Shaukat A, Almyroudis NG, Segal BH. Review of epidemiology, diagnosis, and treatment of invasive mould infections in allogeneic hematopoietic stem cell transplant recipients. Mycopathologia. 2006;162:1–15.
4. Chamilos G, Luna M, Lewis RE, et al. Invasive fungal infections in patients with hematologic malignancies in a tertiary care cancer center: an autopsy study over a 15-year period (1989-2003). Haematologica. 2006;91:986–9.
5. Pfaller MA, Diekema DJ. Epidemiology of invasive candidiasis: a persistent public health problem. Clin Microbiol Rev. 2007;20:133–63.
6. Warnock DW. Trends in the epidemiology of invasive fungal infections. Nippon Ishinkin Gakkai Zasshi. 2007;48:1–12.
7. Maschmeyer G, Haas A. The epidemiology and treatment of infections in cancer patients. Int J Antimicrob Agents. 2008;31:193–7.
8. Thursky KA, Worth LJ, Seymour JF, Miles Prince H, Slavin MA. Spectrum of infection, risk and recommendations for prophylaxis and screening among patients with lymphoproliferative disorders treated with alemtuzumab*. Br J Haematol. 2006;132:3–12.
9. Elter T, Vehreschild JJ, Gribben J, Cornely OA, Engert A, Hallek M. Management of infections in patients with chronic lymphocytic leukemia treated with alemtuzumab. Ann Hematol. 2009;88:121–32.
10. Marr KA, Seidel K, White TC, Bowden RA. Candidemia in allogeneic blood and marrow transplant recipients: evolution of risk factors after the adoption of prophylactic fluconazole. J Infect Dis. 2000;181:309–16.
11. Upton A, Kirby KA, Carpenter P, Boeckh M, Marr KA. Invasive aspergillosis following hematopoietic cell transplantation: outcomes and prognostic factors associated with mortality. Clin Infect Dis. 2007;44:531–40.
12. Fukuda T, Boeckh M, Carter RA, et al. Risks and outcomes of invasive fungal infections in recipients of allogeneic hematopoietic stem cell transplants after nonmyeloablative conditioning. Blood. 2003;102:827–33.
13. Garcia-Vidal C, Upton A, Kirby KA, Marr KA. Epidemiology of invasive mold infections in allogeneic stem cell transplant recipients: biological risk factors for infection according to time after transplantation. Clin Infect Dis. 2008;47:1041–50.
14. Neofytos D, Horn D, Anaissie E, et al. Epidemiology and outcome of invasive fungal infection in adult hematopoietic stem cell transplant recipients: analysis of Multicenter Prospective Antifungal Therapy (PATH) Alliance registry. Clin Infect Dis. 2009;48:265–73.
15. Kontoyiannis DP, Lewis RE. Antifungal drug resistance of pathogenic fungi. Lancet. 2002;359:1135–44.
16. Kontoyiannis DP, Lionakis MS, Lewis RE, et al. Zygomycosis in a tertiary-care cancer center in the era of Aspergillus-active antifungal therapy: a case-control observational study of 27 recent cases. J Infect Dis. 2005;191:1350–60.
17. Kontoyiannis DP, Lewis RE. Invasive zygomycosis: update on pathogenesis, clinical manifestations, and management. Infect Dis Clin North Am. 2006;20:581–607, vi.
18. Malani AN, Kauffman CA. Changing epidemiology of rare mould infections: implications for therapy. Drugs. 2007;67:1803–12.
19. Brown J. Zygomycosis: an emerging fungal infection. Am J Health Syst Pharm. 2005;62:2593–6.
20. Snelders E, van der Lee HA, Kuijpers J, et al. Emergence of azole resistance in Aspergillus fumigatus and spread of a single resistance mechanism. PLoS Med. 2008;5:e219.
21. Howard SJ, Webster I, Moore CB, et al. Multi-azole resistance in Aspergillus fumigatus. Int J Antimicrob Agents. 2006;28:450–3.
22. Mellado E, Garcia-Effron G, Alcazar-Fuoli L, et al. A new Aspergillus fumigatus resistance mechanism conferring in vitro cross-resistance to azole antifungals involves a combination of cyp51A alterations. Antimicrob Agents Chemother. 2007;51:1897–904.
23. Verweij PE, Mellado E, Melchers WJ. Multiple-triazole-resistant aspergillosis. N Engl J Med. 2007;356:1481–3.
24. White TC, Marr KA, Bowden RA. Clinical, cellular, and molecular factors that contribute to antifungal drug resistance. Clin Microbiol Rev. 1998;11:382–402.
25. Liu TT, Lee RE, Barker KS, Wei L, Homayouni R, Rogers PD. Genome-wide expression profiling of the response to azole, polyene, echinocandin, and pyrimidine antifungal agents in Candida albicans. Antimicrob Agents Chemother. 2005;49:2226–36.
26. White TC. Mechanisms of resistance to antifungal agents. In: Murray PR, Baron EJ, Jorgensen JH, Pfaller MA, Yolken RH, editors. Manual of clinical microbiology. 8th ed. Washington, DC: ASM Press; 2003. p. 1869–79.
27. Sheehan DJ, Hitchcock CA, Sibley CM. Current and emerging azole antifungal agents. Clin Microbiol Rev. 1999;12:40–79.
28. Groll AH, Piscitelli SC, Walsh TJ. Clinical pharmacology of systemic antifungal agents: a comprehensive review of agents in clinical use, current investigational compounds, and putative targets for antifungal drug development. Adv Pharmacol. 1998;44:343–499.
29. Gubbins PO, McConnell SA, Amsden JR. Antifungal agents. In: Piscitelli SC, Rodvold KA, editors. Drug interactions in infectious diseases. 2nd ed. Totowa, NJ: Humana; 2005. p. 289–338.
30. Smith G, Stubbins MJ, Harries LW, Wolf CR. Molecular genetics of the human cytochrome P450 monooxygenase superfamily. Xenobiotica. 1998;28:1129–65.
31. Lewis RE, editor. Antifungal drug interactions. Washington, DC: ASM Press; 2009.
32. Lewis RE. Managing drug interactions in the patient with aspergillosis. Med Mycol. 2006;44(suppl):349–56.
33. Purkins L, Wood N, Ghahramani P, Greenhalgh K, Allen MJ, Kleinermans D. Pharmacokinetics and safety of voriconazole following intravenous- to oral-dose escalation regimens. Antimicrob Agents Chemother. 2002;46:2546–53.
34. Lazarus HM, Blumer JL, Yanovich S, Schlamm H, Romero A. Safety and pharmacokinetics of oral voriconazole in patients at risk of fungal infection: a dose escalation study. J Clin Pharmacol. 2002;42:395–402.
35. Hyland R, Jones BC, Smith DA. Identification of the cytochrome P450 enzymes involved in the N-oxidation of voriconazole. Drug Metab Dispos. 2003;31:540–7.
36. Andes D, Pascual A, Marchetti O. Antifungal therapeutic drug monitoring: established and emerging indications. Antimicrob Agents Chemother. 2009;53:24–34.
37. Ikeda Y, Umemura K, Kondo K, Sekiguchi K, Miyoshi S, Nakashima M. Pharmacokinetics of voriconazole and cytochrome P450 2C19 genetic status. Clin Pharmacol Ther. 2004;75:587–8.
38. Trifilio S, Ortiz R, Pennick G, et al. Voriconazole therapeutic drug monitoring in allogeneic hematopoietic stem cell transplant recipients. Bone Marrow Transplant. 2005;35:509–13.
39. Trifilio S, Pennick G, Pi J, et al. Monitoring plasma voriconazole levels may be necessary to avoid subtherapeutic levels in hematopoietic stem cell transplant recipients. Cancer. 2007;109:1532–5.

40. Trifilio S, Singhal S, Williams S, et al. Breakthrough fungal infections after allogeneic hematopoietic stem cell transplantation in patients on prophylactic voriconazole. Bone Marrow Transplant. 2007;40:451–6.
41. Trifilio SM, Yarnold PR, Scheetz MH, Pi J, Pennick G, Mehta J. Serial plasma voriconazole concentrations after allogeneic hematopoietic stem cell transplantation. Antimicrob Agents Chemother. 2009;53(5):1793–6.
42. Walsh TJ, Karlsson MO, Driscoll T, et al. Pharmacokinetics and safety of intravenous voriconazole in children after single- or multiple-dose administration. Antimicrob Agents Chemother. 2004;48:2166–72.
43. Pasqualotto AC, Shah M, Wynn R, Denning DW. Voriconazole plasma monitoring. Arch Dis Child. 2008;93:578–81.
44. Smith J, Safdar N, Knasinski V, et al. Voriconazole therapeutic drug monitoring. Antimicrob Agents Chemother. 2006;50:1570–2.
45. Pascual A, Calandra T, Bolay S, Buclin T, Bille J, Marchetti O. Voriconazole therapeutic drug monitoring in patients with invasive mycoses improves safety and efficacy outcomes. Clin Infect Dis. 2007;46:201–11.
46. Tan K, Brayshaw N, Tomaszewski K, Troke P, Wood N. Investigation of the potential relationships between plasma voriconazole concentrations and visual adverse events or liver function test abnormalities. J Clin Pharmacol. 2006;46:235–43.
47. Scherpbier HJ, Hilhorst MI, Kuijpers TW. Liver failure in a child receiving highly active antiretroviral therapy and voriconazole. Clin Infect Dis. 2003;37:828–30.
48. Courtney R, Pai S, Laughlin M, Lim J, Batra V. Pharmacokinetics, safety, and tolerability of oral posaconazole administered in single and multiple doses in healthy adults. Antimicrob Agents Chemother. 2003;47:2788–95.
49. Courtney R, Sansone A, Smith W, et al. Posaconazole pharmacokinetics, safety, and tolerability in subjects with varying degrees of chronic renal disease. J Clin Pharmacol. 2005;45:185–92.
50. Gubbins PO, Krishna G, Sansone-Parsons A, et al. Pharmacokinetics and safety of oral posaconazole in neutropenic stem cell transplant recipients. Antimicrob Agents Chemother. 2006;50:1993–9.
51. Krishna G, Martinho M, Chandrasekar P, Ullmann AJ, Patino H. Pharmacokinetics of oral posaconazole in allogeneic hematopoietic stem cell transplant recipients with graft-versus-host disease. Pharmacotherapy. 2007;27:1627–36.
52. Krishna G, Parsons A, Kantesaria B, Mant T. Evaluation of the pharmacokinetics of posaconazole and rifabutin following co-administration to healthy men. Curr Med Res Opin. 2007;23:545–52.
53. Lewis R, Hogan H, Howell A, Safdar A. Progressive fusariosis: unpredictable posaconazole bioavailability, and feasibility of recombinant interferon-gamma plus granulocyte macrophage-colony stimulating factor for refractory disseminated infection. Leuk Lymphoma. 2008;49:163–5.
54. Ullmann AJ, Cornely OA, Burchardt A, et al. Pharmacokinetics, safety, and efficacy of posaconazole in patients with persistent febrile neutropenia or refractory invasive fungal infection. Antimicrob Agents Chemother. 2006;50:658–66.
55. Courtney R, Radwanski E, Lim J, Laughlin M. Pharmacokinetics of posaconazole coadministered with antacid in fasting or nonfasting healthy men. Antimicrob Agents Chemother. 2004;48:804–8.
56. Walsh TJ, Raad I, Patterson TF, et al. Treatment of invasive aspergillosis with posaconazole in patients who are refractory to or intolerant of conventional therapy: an externally controlled trial. Clin Infect Dis. 2007;44:2–12.
57. Ullmann AJ, Lipton JH, Vesole DH, et al. Posaconazole or fluconazole for prophylaxis in severe graft-versus-host disease. N Engl J Med. 2007;356:335–47.
58. Cornely OA, Maertens J, Winston DJ, et al. Posaconazole vs. fluconazole or itraconazole prophylaxis in patients with neutropenia. N Engl J Med. 2007;356:348–59.
59. Betts R, Glasmacher A, Maertens J, et al. Efficacy of caspofungin against invasive Candida or invasive Aspergillus infections in neutropenic patients. Cancer. 2006;106:466–73.
60. Wagner C, Graninger W, Presterl E, Joukhadar C. The echinocandins: comparison of their pharmacokinetics, pharmacodynamics and clinical applications. Pharmacology. 2006;78:161–77.
61. Wiederhold NP, Lewis RE. The echinocandin antifungals: an overview of the pharmacology, spectrum and clinical efficacy. Expert Opin Investig Drugs. 2003;12:1313–33.
62. Pfaller MA, Boyken L, Hollis RJ, Messer SA, Tendolkar S, Diekema DJ. In vitro activities of anidulafungin against more than 2,500 clinical isolates of Candida spp., including 315 isolates resistant to fluconazole. J Clin Microbiol. 2005;43:5425–7.
63. Kurtz MB, Heath IB, Marrinan J, Dreikorn S, Onishi J, Douglas C. Morphological effects of lipopeptides against Aspergillus fumigatus correlate with activities against (1, 3)-beta-D-glucan synthase. Antimicrob Agents Chemother. 1994;38:1480–9.
64. Abruzzo GK, Gill CJ, Flattery AM, et al. Efficacy of the echinocandin caspofungin against disseminated aspergillosis and candidiasis in cyclophosphamide-induced immunosuppressed mice. Antimicrob Agents Chemother. 2000;44:2310–8.
65. Matsumoto S, Wakai Y, Nakai T, et al. Efficacy of FK463, a new lipopeptide antifungal agent, in mouse models of pulmonary aspergillosis. Antimicrob Agents Chemother. 2000;44:619–21.
66. Warn PA, Morrissey G, Morrissey J, Denning DW. Activity of micafungin (FK463) against an itraconazole-resistant strain of Aspergillus fumigatus and a strain of Aspergillus terreus demonstrating in vivo resistance to amphotericin B. J Antimicrob Chemother. 2003;51:913–9.
67. Hohl TM, Feldmesser M, Perlin DS, Pamer EG. Caspofungin modulates inflammatory responses to Aspergillus fumigatus through stage-specific effects on fungal beta-glucan exposure. J Infect Dis. 2008;198(2):176–85.
68. Lamaris GA, Lewis RE, Chamilos G, et al. Caspofungin-mediated beta-glucan unmasking and enhancement of human polymorphonuclear neutrophil activity against Aspergillus and non-Aspergillus hyphae. J Infect Dis. 2008;198:186–92.
69. Wheeler RT, Kombe D, Agarwala SD, Fink GR. Dynamic, morphotype-specific Candida albicans beta-glucan exposure during infection and drug treatment. PLoS Pathog. 2008;4:e1000227.
70. Wheeler RT, Fink GR. A drug-sensitive genetic network masks fungi from the immune system. PLoS Pathog. 2006;2:e35.
71. Uchida K, Nishiyama Y, Yokota N, Yamaguchi H. In vitro antifungal activity of a novel lipopeptide antifungal agent, FK463, against various fungal pathogens. J Antibiot (Tokyo). 2000;53:1175–81.
72. Espinel-Ingroff A. In vitro antifungal activities of anidulafungin and micafungin, licensed agents and the investigational triazole posaconazole as determined by NCCLS methods for 12,052 fungal isolates: review of the literature. Rev Iberoam Micol. 2003;20:121–36.
73. Balajee SA, Gribskov JL, Hanley E, Nickle D, Marr KA. Aspergillus lentulus sp. nov., a new sibling species of A. fumigatus. Eukaryot Cell. 2005;4:625–32.
74. Chryssanthou E, Cuenca-Estrella M. Comparison of the Antifungal Susceptibility Testing Subcommittee of the European Committee on Antibiotic Susceptibility Testing proposed standard and the E-test with the NCCLS broth microdilution method for voriconazole and caspofungin susceptibility testing of yeast species. J Clin Microbiol. 2002;40:3841–4.
75. Cuenca-Estrella M, Lee-Yang W, Ciblak MA, et al. Comparative evaluation of NCCLS M27-A and EUCAST broth microdilution procedures for antifungal susceptibility testing of Candida species. Antimicrob Agents Chemother. 2002;46:3644–7.
76. Pfaller MA, Boyken L, Hollis RJ, et al. In vitro susceptibility of invasive isolates of Candida spp. to anidulafungin, caspofungin, and micafungin: six years of global surveillance. J Clin Microbiol. 2008;46:150–6.

77. Kartsonis N, Killar J, Mixson L, et al. Caspofungin susceptibility testing of isolates from patients with esophageal candidiasis or invasive candidiasis: relationship of MIC to treatment outcome. Antimicrob Agents Chemother. 2005;49:3616–23.
78. Pfaller MA, Diekema DJ, Rinaldi MG, et al. Results from the ARTEMIS DISK Global Antifungal Surveillance Study: a 6.5-year analysis of susceptibilities of *Candida* and other yeast species to fluconazole and voriconazole by standardized disk diffusion testing. J Clin Microbiol. 2005;43:5848–59.
79. Pfaller MA, Diekema DJ, Ostrosky-Zeichner L, et al. Correlation of MIC with outcome for *Candida* species tested against caspofungin, anidulafungin, and micafungin: analysis and proposal for interpretive MIC breakpoints. J Clin Microbiol. 2008;46(8):2620–9.
80. Andes DR, Diekema DJ, Pfaller MA, Marchillo K, Bohrmueller J. In vivo pharmacodynamic target investigation for micafungin against *Candida albicans* and *C. glabrata* in a neutropenic murine candidiasis model. Antimicrob Agents Chemother. 2008;52:3497–503.
81. Wiederhold NP, Lewis II JS. The echinocandin micafungin: a review of the pharmacology, spectrum of activity, clinical efficacy and safety. Expert Opin Pharmacother. 2007;8:1155–66.
82. Odabasi Z, Paetznick V, Rex JH, Ostrosky-Zeichner L. Effects of serum on in vitro susceptibility testing of echinocandins. Antimicrob Agents Chemother. 2007;51:4214–6.
83. Paderu P, Garcia-Effron G, Balashov S, Delmas G, Park S, Perlin DS. Serum differentially alters the antifungal properties of echinocandin drugs. Antimicrob Agents Chemother. 2007;51:2253–6.
84. Wiederhold NP, Najvar LK, Bocanegra R, Molina D, Olivo M, Graybill JR. In vivo efficacy of anidulafungin and caspofungin against *Candida glabrata* and association with in vitro potency in the presence of sera. Antimicrob Agents Chemother. 2007;51:1616–20.
85. Moudgal V, Little T, Boikov D, Vazquez JA. Multiechinocandin- and multiazole-resistant *Candida parapsilosis* isolates serially obtained during therapy for prosthetic valve endocarditis. Antimicrob Agents Chemother. 2005;49:767–9.
86. Park S, Kelly R, Kahn JN, et al. Specific substitutions in the echinocandin target Fks1p account for reduced susceptibility of rare laboratory and clinical *Candida* sp. isolates. Antimicrob Agents Chemother. 2005;49:3264–73.
87. Katiyar S, Pfaller M, Edlind T. *Candida albicans* and *Candida glabrata* clinical isolates exhibiting reduced echinocandin susceptibility. Antimicrob Agents Chemother. 2006;50:2892–4.
88. Laverdiere M, Lalonde RG, Baril JG, Sheppard DC, Park S, Perlin DS. Progressive loss of echinocandin activity following prolonged use for treatment of *Candida albicans* oesophagitis. J Antimicrob Chemother. 2006;57:705–8.
89. Miller CD, Lomaestro BW, Park S, Perlin DS. Progressive esophagitis caused by *Candida albicans* with reduced susceptibility to caspofungin. Pharmacotherapy. 2006;26:877–80.
90. Kahn JN, Garcia-Effron G, Hsu MJ, Park S, Marr KA, Perlin DS. Acquired echinocandin resistance in a *Candida krusei* isolate due to modification of glucan synthase. Antimicrob Agents Chemother. 2007;51:1876–8.
91. Cleary JD, Garcia-Effron G, Chapman SW, Perlin DS. Reduced *Candida glabrata* susceptibility secondary to an FKS1 mutation developed during candidemia treatment. Antimicrob Agents Chemother. 2008;52:2263–5.
92. Desnos-Ollivier M, Bretagne S, Raoux D, Hoinard D, Dromer F, Dannaoui E. Mutations in the fks1 gene in *Candida albicans*, *C. tropicalis*, and *C. krusei* correlate with elevated caspofungin MICs uncovered in AM3 medium using the method of the European Committee on Antibiotic Susceptibility Testing. Antimicrob Agents Chemother. 2008;52:3092–8.
93. Thompson III GR, Wiederhold NP, Vallor AC, Villareal NC, Lewis II JS, Patterson TF. Development of caspofungin resistance following prolonged therapy for invasive candidiasis secondary to *Candida glabrata* infection. Antimicrob Agents Chemother. 2008;52:3783–5.
94. Wiederhold NP, Grabinski JL, Garcia-Effron G, Perlin DS, Lee SA. Pyrosequencing to detect mutations in FKS1 that confer reduced echinocandin susceptibility in *Candida albicans*. Antimicrob Agents Chemother. 2008;52:4145–8.
95. Wetzstein GA, Green MR, Greene JN. Mould breakthrough in immunosuppressed adults receiving anidulafungin: a report of 2 cases. J Infect. 2007;55:e131–3.
96. Arendrup MC, Garcia-Effron G, Buzina W, et al. Breakthrough *Aspergillus fumigatus* and *Candida albicans* double infection during caspofungin treatment: laboratory characteristics and implication for susceptibility testing. Antimicrob Agents Chemother. 2009;53(3):1185–93.
97. Niimi K, Maki K, Ikeda F, et al. Overexpression of *Candida albicans* CDR1, CDR2, or MDR1 does not produce significant changes in echinocandin susceptibility. Antimicrob Agents Chemother. 2006;50:1148–55.
98. Perlin DS. Resistance to echinocandin-class antifungal drugs. Drug Resist Updat. 2007;10:121–30.
99. Garcia-Effron G, Park S, Perlin DS. Correlating echinocandin MIC and kinetic inhibition of fks1 mutant glucan synthases for *Candida albicans*: implications for interpretive breakpoints. Antimicrob Agents Chemother. 2009;53:112–22.
100. Bennett JE. Echinocandins for candidemia in adults without neutropenia. N Engl J Med. 2006;355:1154–9.
101. Forrest GN, Weekes E, Johnson JK. Increasing incidence of *Candida parapsilosis* candidemia with caspofungin usage. J Infect. 2008;56:126–9.
102. Colombo AL, Nucci M, Park BJ, et al. Epidemiology of candidemia in Brazil: a nationwide sentinel surveillance of candidemia in eleven medical centers. J Clin Microbiol. 2006;44:2816–23.
103. Pfaller MA, Diekema DJ, Gibbs DL, et al. Geographic and temporal trends in isolation and antifungal susceptibility of *Candida parapsilosis*: a global assessment from the ARTEMIS DISK Antifungal Surveillance Program, 2001 to 2005. J Clin Microbiol. 2008;46:842–9.
104. Garcia-Effron G, Katiyar SK, Park S, Edlind TD, Perlin DS. A naturally occurring proline-to-alanine amino acid change in Fks1p in *Candida parapsilosis*, *Candida orthopsilosis*, and *Candida metapsilosis* accounts for reduced echinocandin susceptibility. Antimicrob Agents Chemother. 2008;52:2305–12.
105. Rocha EM, Garcia-Effron G, Park S, Perlin DS. A Ser678Pro substitution in Fks1p confers resistance to echinocandin drugs in *Aspergillus fumigatus*. Antimicrob Agents Chemother. 2007;51:4174–6.
106. Arendrup MC, Fuursted K, Gahrn-Hansen B, et al. Semi-national surveillance of fungaemia in Denmark 2004-2006: increasing incidence of fungaemia and numbers of isolates with reduced azole susceptibility. Clin Microbiol Infect. 2008;14:487–94.
107. Levin DE. Cell wall integrity signaling in *Saccharomyces cerevisiae*. Microbiol Mol Biol Rev. 2005;69:262–91.
108. Cowen LE, Lindquist S. Hsp90 potentiates the rapid evolution of new traits: drug resistance in diverse fungi. Science. 2005;309:2185–9.
109. Stevens DA, Espiritu M, Parmar R. Paradoxical effect of caspofungin: reduced activity against *Candida albicans* at high drug concentrations. Antimicrob Agents Chemother. 2004;48:3407–11.
110. Stevens DA, Ichinomiya M, Koshi Y, Horiuchi H. Escape of *Candida* from caspofungin inhibition at concentrations above the MIC (paradoxical effect) accomplished by increased cell wall chitin; evidence for beta-1, 6-glucan synthesis inhibition by caspofungin. Antimicrob Agents Chemother. 2006;50:3160–1.

111. Chamilos G, Lewis RE, Albert N, Kontoyiannis DP. Paradoxical effect of echinocandins across *Candida* species in vitro: evidence for echinocandin-specific and *Candida* species-related differences. Antimicrob Agents Chemother. 2007;51:2257–9.
112. Lewis RE, Albert ND, Kontoyiannis DP. Comparison of the dose-dependent activity and paradoxical effect of caspofungin and micafungin in a neutropenic murine model of invasive pulmonary aspergillosis. J Antimicrob Chemother. 2008;61: 1140–4.
113. Clemons KV, Espiritu M, Parmar R, Stevens DA. Assessment of the paradoxical effect of caspofungin in therapy of candidiasis. Antimicrob Agents Chemother. 2006;50:1293–7.

Chapter 29
Immunotherapy for Difficult-to-Treat Invasive Fungal Diseases

Brahm H. Segal, Amar Safdar, and David A. Stevens

Abstract Opportunistic fungal diseases occur most commonly in highly immunocompromised patients, such as those with prolonged neutropenia or transplant recipients treated with intensive immunosuppression. Significant advances have been made in antifungal agents, which have led to improved therapeutic outcomes as well as a greater emphasis on antifungal prophylaxis targeted to the highly immunocompromised. In addition, we are gaining more knowledge about how our immune system recognizes fungi and protects us from fungal disease, while limiting potentially injurious inflammation and allergy. This knowledge has led to novel experimental approaches for immunotherapy. Progress in paving the way from promising preclinical approaches and limited clinical experience to properly conducted clinical trials has been poor – a reflection of invasive fungal diseases being relatively uncommon and the heterogeneity of the patient populations at risk, and insufficient funding for multicenter clinical immunotherapeutic trials. We describe our approaches to immunotherapy for severe and refractory invasive fungal diseases, realizing that important gaps in knowledge exist regarding benefit and toxicity. Future perspectives on immunotherapy are discussed.

Keywords Aspergillosis • Candidiasis • Fungal infection • Immunotherapy • Interferon-γ • Cytokines

Patients at Risk for Invasive Fungal Diseases

Yeasts and Dimorphic Fungi

Risk factors for invasive fungal diseases vary based on the specific fungal pathogen. *Candida* species are endogenous flora that colonize the skin, gastrointestinal, and vaginal mucosa. Candidemia generally requires disruption of barriers of the skin (e.g., from a central venous or dialysis catheter) or bowel mucosa (e.g., from mucotoxic chemotherapy or radiation) [1, 2]. Diseases caused by dimorphic fungi (e.g., histoplasmosis and coccidioidomycosis) occur in immunocompetent persons, but are more likely to be severe or disseminated in patients with compromised cellular immunity (e.g., HIV infection, transplant recipients) [3]. Host genes among different ethnic groups also appear to affect susceptibility to coccidioidomycosis [4]. *Cryptococcus neoformans* and *Pneumocystis jiroveci* (formerly *Pneumocystis carinii*) principally cause disease in patients with severe impairment in cellular immunity (Table 29.1).

Aspergillosis and Other Moulds

Risk factors for invasive aspergillosis and other moulds are complex. Patients at risk for invasive aspergillosis include those with prolonged neutropenia (e.g., following induction therapy for acute leukemia), hematopoietic stem cell transplant (HSCT) recipients, solid organ transplant recipients, advanced AIDS, and chronic granulomatous disease (CGD) [5].

In neutropenic patients, the degree and duration of neutropenia predict the risk of invasive mould diseases [6, 7]. Among allogeneic HSCT recipients, the early period of risk of invasive mould diseases corresponds to neutropenia following the conditioning regimen and later periods correspond to the intensity of immunosuppressive therapy required to control graft-versus-host disease (GVHD) [8]. In severe GVHD, global immune impairment occurs that affects both innate phagocyte function and cellular and humoral immunity. Several studies have reported the predominance of invasive aspergillosis cases occurring in the post-engraftment rather than in the neutropenic period in allogeneic HSCT recipients [9–16], with immunosuppressive therapy for GVHD and T-cell depletion [17] being principal risk factors.

B.H. Segal (✉)
Department of Medicine and Immunology, Roswell Park Cancer Institute, Department of Medicine, School of Medicine and Biomedical Sciences, University of Buffalo, Elm & Carlton Streets, Buffalo, NY, USA
e-mail: brahm.segal@roswellpark.org

Table 29.1 Host defense deficits predisposing to invasive fungal diseases

Underlying diseases	Host defense impairment	Principal fungal pathogens
Acute myelogenous leukemia (AML), myelodysplastic syndrome, aplastic anemia	Neutropenia	*Candida* sp., *Aspergillus* sp., rarer moulds (e.g., zygomycetes, *Fusarium* spp., dark-walled moulds)
Acute lymphoblastic leukemia	Neutropenia; impaired cellular immunity due to corticosteroids	Similar spectrum as AML, plus *Pneumocystis jiroveci*
HTLV-1-associated hematological malignancies	Neutropenia; T-cell impairment	Similar spectrum as AML, plus *P. jiroveci*, *Cryptococcus neoformans*
Hematopoietic stem cell transplantation (HSCT) during neutropenia	Neutropenia	Similar spectrum as AML
HSCT during graft-versus-host disease	Global impairment in innate and antigen-driven immunity; risk of opportunistic infections related to intensity of immunosuppressive therapy for GVHD	*Candida* sp., *Aspergillus* sp., rarer moulds (e.g., zygomycetes, *Fusarium* sp., dark-walled moulds), *P. jiroveci*, dimorphic fungi, *C. neoformans*
Solid organ transplantation	Similar to allogeneic HSCT; risk of opportunistic infections related to intensity of immunosuppressive therapy to prevent allograft rejection	Similar spectrum as HSCT with GVHD
AIDS	T-cell impairment	Mucosal candidiasis, *P. jiroveci*, *C. neoformans*, dimorphic fungi; invasive aspergillosis is an uncommon complication of advanced AIDS (CD4 count <100 per μl; concurrent risk factors, e.g., neutropenia)
Collagen vascular diseases	Risk of opportunistic infections related to intensity of immunosuppression, e.g., dose and duration of corticosteroids, use of alkylating agents, TNF-α inhibition	Mucosal candidiasis, *P. jiroveci*, *C. neoformans*, dimorphic fungi; invasive aspergillosis is an uncommon complication
Chronic granulomatous disease	NADPH oxidase deficiency	Aspergillosis, rarer moulds

Purine analogues and alemtuzumab used to treat hematological malignancies (e.g., chronic lymphocytic leukemia) cause prolonged T-cell suppression that can persist from months to more than a year. Prophylaxis to prevent *P. jiroveci* infection is standard among alemtuzumab recipients. Indeed, multiple host defense pathways may be disabled by immunodeficiencies associated with the primary malignancy and cytotoxic and immunosuppressive agents.

Among solid organ transplant recipients, the intensity of immunosuppression to control graft rejection is the major predictor of opportunistic fungal and viral diseases. The incidence of invasive aspergillosis is higher after lung transplantation compared to other allografts [18]. *Aspergillus* species colonizing the airways in end-stage lung disease may be a source of fungal infection following single-lung transplantation [19].

The phagocyte NADPH oxidase is essential in host defense against aspergillosis and rarer moulds, as illustrated by chronic granulomatous disease (CGD), an inherited disorder of the NADPH oxidase complex in which phagocytes are defective in generating the superoxide anion and downstream reactive oxidant intermediates, hydrogen peroxide, hydroxyl anion, and hypohalous acid. CGD patients suffer from recurrent life-threatening bacterial and fungal infections, with invasive aspergillosis being a major cause of mortality [20, 21].

Principles and Challenges for Immunotherapy

The first decision point when considering immunotherapy for an invasive fungal disease is whether iatrogenic immunosuppression (e.g., corticosteroids) could be reduced or eliminated. This may not be feasible. For example, a certain level of immunosuppression is required for allograft survival following solid organ transplantation.

Immunotherapy must be tailored to the specific immunodeficiency that exists in a given patient population. This concept is straightforward for neutropenia in which the aim is to augment neutrophil number, e.g., by colony stimulating factors (CSF) or granulocyte transfusions. In GVHD, the immune impairment is more complex; the immunotherapeutic strategy may at best ameliorate some features of the immunocompromised state, but would not reconstitute for a sustained period all of the disabled host defense pathways. In addition, a potential exists that attempts to augment anti-fungal immunity may exacerbate GVHD (or prime allograft rejection in solid organ transplant recipients).

Finally, there is no adjunctive immunotherapy for invasive fungal diseases that has established efficacy. In the absence of modern, randomized, clinical trials, decisions about using

Table 29.2 Evidence supporting immune augmentation strategies to prevent and treat invasive fungal diseases

Host defense impairment	Immune augmentation (rating[a])
Neutropenia (absolute neutrophil count <500 per μl)	• Prophylactic G-CSF or GM-CSF in patients with at least 20% risk of developing neutropenic fever (2A) [28] • G-CSF or GM-CSF as adjunctive treatment for patients with fever and neutropenia (not routinely recommended) [28] • G-CSF or GM-CSF as adjunctive therapy for an invasive fungal disease (guidelines vary between 2A and 2B) [28, 98, 99] • Prophylactic granulocyte transfusions (not recommended) • Granulocyte transfusions as adjunctive therapy for an invasive fungal disease refractory to standard antifungal therapy (2B) [98, 99] • Prophylactic rIFN-γ (not recommended) • rIFN-γ as adjunctive therapy for an invasive fungal disease refractory to standard antifungal therapy (2B) [98]
Allogeneic HSCT recipients without neutropenia	• Reduce intensity of immunosuppressive therapy if feasible (uniform agreement) • Prophylactic G-CSF, GM-CSF, or rIFN-γ (not recommended) • G-CSF, GM-CSF, rIFN-γ, or combination as adjunctive therapy for an invasive fungal disease refractory to standard antifungal therapy (2B) [98]
Solid organ transplant recipients	• Reduce intensity of immunosuppressive therapy if feasible (uniform agreement)
AIDS	• Highly active antiretroviral therapy is the most effective mode to reconstitute immunity; be aware of immune reconstitution inflammatory syndrome [100] • rIFN-γ as adjunctive therapy for AIDS-associated cryptococcal meningitis (2B) [59]
Chronic granulomatous disease	• Prophylactic rIFN-γ (1A) [58] • Adjunctive rIFN-γ for invasive fungal disease (2B) • Granulocyte transfusions as adjunctive therapy for an invasive fungal disease refractory to standard antifungal therapy (2B) [101] • Adjunctive colony-stimulating factors (not routinely recommended)

[a]Level 1, uniform consensus based on high level of evidence (e.g., randomized trial); 2A, lower level of evidence than randomized trial, but recommended in authoritative guidelines; 2B, recommendation based on clinical experience, with lack of expert consensus

adjunctive immunotherapy reasonably entail consideration of a number of factors, including the following: (1) immunotherapy may be used as a salvage approach when standard antifungal agents fail; (2) the use of immunotherapy may be supported by in vitro studies and animal models; (3) limited support may exist from retrospective studies or early phase clinical trial data. Table 29.2 summarizes the level of evidence supporting immune-based therapies in specific patient populations.

Augmentation of Neutrophil Number

Colony Stimulating Factors

Normal myelopoiesis requires stem cell factor, interleukin 3 (IL-3), and granulocyte-macrophage colony-stimulating factor (GM-CSF), which give rise to the colony forming unit-granulocyte/macrophage (CFU-GM). Granulocyte-colony-stimulating factor (G-CSF) acts at a later stage in concert with other growth factors to specifically drive granulopoiesis. The rationale for administration of recombinant CSFs is to accelerate myeloid recovery in patients with marrow failure either from an underlying hematological disorder or, more commonly, from cytotoxic chemotherapy.

CSFs can be administered as prophylaxis (prior to the onset of infection or neutropenia), or as adjunctive therapy to treat a suspected or documented infection. There is a substantial randomized database on use of prophylactic CSFs in patients receiving cytotoxic antineoplastic chemotherapy [22]. Primary (prophylactic) administration of colony stimulating factors CSFs has reduced the incidence of febrile neutropenia by approximately 50% in randomized trials in adults in whom the incidence of neutropenic fever was greater than 40% in the control group [23]. In patients with acute myelogenous leukemia, CSFs produce a modest decrease in the duration of neutropenia associated with induction chemotherapy, which in some studies has translated into a reduction in the duration of fever, use of antibiotics, and hospitalization [24, 25]. In one randomized study in patients receiving chemotherapy for acute myelogenous leukemia, prophylaxis with granulocyte-macrophage colony-stimulating factor (GM-CSF) led to a lower frequency of fatal fungal infections compared to placebo (1.9 versus 19%, respectively) and reduced overall early mortality [26, 27]. This degree of reduction in invasive fungal diseases has not been observed in other randomized studies of prophylactic CSFs; in addition, the value of CSFs in preventing fungal diseases in patients receiving mould-active prophylaxis has not been established.

The American Society of Clinical Oncology (ASCO) [28] and National Comprehensive Cancer Network [29] have established authoritative guidelines related to which patients should receive prophylactic CSFs. The principal rationale for prophylactic CSFs is to reduce the incidence of neutropenic fever. ASCO guidelines advise a prophylactic CSF when the risk of neutropenic fever is approximately 20% and no other equally effective regimen that does not require CSFs is available [28].

The rationale for CSFs for established infections (referred to as adjunctive therapy, as opposed to prophylaxis) stems from both the quantitative and qualitative effects of these agents on phagocytic cells. In neutropenic patients with life-threatening infections, survival is strongly influenced by the rapidity of neutrophil recovery [30]. Although the benefit of a CSF for established infections in neutropenic patients is unproven, ASCO guidelines reasonably advise that a CSF be considered in serious infections, such as invasive fungal diseases [28].

Some studies in vitro [31] and in animal models [32, 33] show that G-CSF or GM-CSF add to antifungal activity when combined with antifungal agents. A Phase II randomized study of G-CSF plus fluconazole for invasive candidiasis and candidemia in non-neutropenic patients showed the safety of G-CSF, but was not powered for efficacy [34].

There are insufficient data to guide whether G-CSF or GM-CSF is preferred as adjunctive therapy for an invasive fungal disease. G-CSFs act only on neutrophils, whereas GM-CSF also accelerates the proliferation of the monocyte–macrophage system, and is a potent activator of monocytes and macrophages [35]. We do not know if the broader effect of GM-CSF on innate effector cells translates to clinical benefit in patients with invasive fungal diseases.

In allogeneic HSCT recipients, G-CSF, but not GM-CSF, may result in Th2 skewing of lymphocytes and promote the development of T regulatory cells, which could dampen a desired pro-inflammatory effect [36, 37]. G-CSF given after T-cell depleted haplotype-mismatched transplantation was associated with faster neutrophil recovery, but prolonged cellular immune dysfunction [38]. Prospective, randomized trials are required to assess the short-term benefits versus long-term immune consequences of CSFs in allogeneic HSCT.

Another gap in knowledge is whether CSFs are safe and effective as either prophylaxis or adjunctive therapy in non-leukopenic patients with severe impairment in phagocyte function. GM-CSF has been demonstrated to reverse the steroid-induced depression of macrophage activity against *Aspergillus* conidia [39]. However, in case reports of patients with neutropenia, CSF therapy has been linked to pulmonary hemorrhage in patients with pulmonary aspergillosis [40]. Triggering of inflammatory reactions by CSFs could produce undesirable deterioration of organ functions. Intensive immunosuppressive corticosteroid-based regimens for GVHD cause global impairment of phagocyte effector functions and disable reconstitution of antigen-specific immunity, though circulating neutrophil counts are generally normal. There are no clinical data to support prophylactic CSFs in non-neutropenic patients, and they should not be used as prophylaxis in this setting in the absence of supporting clinical trial data. In severely immunocompromised non-neutropenic patients (e.g., allogeneic HSCT recipient) with a refractory invasive fungal disease, it is reasonable to consider adjunctive GM-CSF to augment qualitative macrophage and neutrophil functions. We emphasize that the data on safety of CSFs in non-neutropenic patients is retrospective [41] and, outside of a clinical trial, should generally be reserved for when standard therapy fails.

Granulocyte Transfusions

The rationale for granulocyte transfusions is to provide transient elevations in circulating neutrophil counts for the neutropenic patient with a life-threatening infection until myeloid recovery occurs. Important concerns about the toxicity of granulocyte transfusions exist, including acute pulmonary reactions, HLA alloimmunization (which could render patients refractory to platelet transfusions and potentially impair myeloid engraftment following HSCT), and transfusion-associated infections, such as cytomegalovirus (CMV).

With more effective antibiotics, the interest in granulocyte transfusions waned in the 1980s. In the 1990s, the impetus to reexamine the role of granulocyte transfusions stemmed from improvements in donor mobilization methods. G-CSF and dexamethasone mobilization leads to as much as a tenfold increase in the yield of granulocytes that translates to improved levels of circulating neutrophils in neutropenic recipients [42]. The increase in circulating neutrophils tends to be sustained for 24–30 h following transfusion, as a consequence of prolonged circulating half-life of G-CSF mobilized granulocytes [43]. The qualitative functions of G-CSF- and steroid-mobilized neutrophils are intact based on in vitro bactericidal activity, respiratory burst, migration to experimental skin chambers, and localization to sites of inflammation.

Price et al. [44] conducted a phase I/II study of granulocyte transfusions derived from unrelated, non-HLA-matched, community donors, following G-CSF and dexamethasone mobilization. Chills, fever, and oxygen desaturation of ≥3% occurred in association with 7% of transfusions, but did not limit therapy. Eight of 11 patients with bacterial infections or candidemia survived, but all eight patients with invasive mould infection died. This study showed the safety and feasibility of using community donors for granulocytapheresis donations. The Transfusion Medicine and Hemostasis network of the National Heart Lung and Blood Institute is currently in the planning stages of a randomized study of adjunctive granulocyte transfusions in neutropenic patients with severe bacterial and fungal infections.

Currently, there is no justification outside of a clinical trial to use granulocyte transfusions either as prophylaxis or in cases of documented infections that are likely to respond to conventional therapy. We reserve granulocyte transfusions for patients with prolonged neutropenia and life-threatening infections refractory to conventional therapy. Filamentous fungi are likely to constitute the majority of such refractory infections. Infusions of amphotericin B should be separated by several hours from granulocyte transfusions to avoid pulmonary toxicity [45]. In some highly alloimmunized patients, transfused granulocytes are rapidly consumed and are likely to have more toxicity than benefit [46]. Monitoring of post-transfusion granulocyte counts is advised. CMV-seronegative granulocyte donors should be used in allogeneic HSCT recipients where both the allograft donor and recipient are CMV-seronegative [47].

Recombinant Interferon-γ

Interferons are immune modulators that regulate the expression of numerous genes that mediate inflammation. Interferon-α is a cornerstone of therapy for chronic hepatitis C infection [48]. Several laboratories have shown that interferon (IFN)-γ augments the antifungal activity of effector cells (macrophages and neutrophils) ex-vivo against a variety of fungal pathogens, including *Candida albicans*, *Histoplasma capsulatum*, *Coccidioides* species, *C. neoformans*, and *Aspergillus* species [49–51]. Data in mouse models using cytokine depletion, gene knockout mice, and administration of exogenous cytokines have been instrumental in establishing the conceptual basis for immunotherapy in invasive mycoses and in paving the way to early clinical trials [52]. We will focus our discussion on rIFN-γ because the database is the most developed.

IFN-γ is produced by lymphocytes (CD4+, CD8+, and NK cells) as well as macrophages and perhaps neutrophils [53]. It is induced by a number of signals, including IL-12 and IL-18 [54, 55] and in turn induces hundreds of genes, including its own inducers [56, 57]. Exposure to various pathogens can stimulate at least two patterns of cytokine production by CD4+ T cells. Th1 cells are defined by production of IFN-γ, lymphotoxin and IL-2, and Th2 cells by production of IL-4, IL-5, IL-9, IL-10, and IL-13. The antimicrobial activity induced by IFN-γ encompasses intracellular and extracellular parasites, bacteria, fungi, and viruses. In patients with hematologic malignancies, use of rIFN-γ as adjunctive therapy for invasive fungal diseases has attracted substantial interest.

Recombinant IFN-γ is licensed as a prophylactic agent in patients with CGD based on a randomized trial in which IFN-γ reduced the number and severity of infections in CGD by about 70%, regardless of antibiotic prophylaxis or genetic subtype of CGD [58]. Despite the widespread use of prophylactic rIFN-γ in CGD, invasive fungal diseases have remained a persistent problem with an incidence of 0.1 fungal infections per patient year predating routine mould-active prophylaxis [20].

The value of rIFN-γ as adjunctive therapy for established fungal infection is unknown. Pappas et al. [59] conducted a phase II placebo-controlled study of adjunctive rIFN-γ in patients with AIDS-associated cryptococcal meningitis. rIFN-γ was well tolerated and the IFN-treated group showed a trend toward improved combined clinical and mycologic success.

Studies in vitro, in animal models [60], and limited patient data provide a rationale for adjunctive IFN-γ for invasive aspergillosis [61]. rIFN-γ augmented human neutrophil oxidative response and killing of *Aspergillus fumigatus* hyphae in vitro and acted additively with G-CSF [62]. It prevented corticosteroid-mediated suppression of neutrophil killing of hyphae [63]. rIFN-γ also enhanced killing of *A. fumigatus* hyphae by human monocytes [64]. Administration of rIFN-γ to CGD patients augmented ex vivo neutrophil-mediated damage of *A. fumigatus* hyphae [65].

Dignani et al. [66] reported successful outcomes using rIFN-g paired with CSFs in four patients with leukemia and refractory fungal disease. One concern about rIFN-γ in allogeneic HSCT recipients is the potential for worsening GVHD. Safdar et al. [67] retrospectively evaluated rIFN-γ use in 25 allogeneic HSCT recipients with proven or suspected invasive fungal disease. rIFN-γ was well-tolerated and did not result in marrow suppression or worsening of GVHD. In another retrospective analysis, combination granulocyte transfusions and rIFN-γ appeared to be safe in neutropenic patients with hematological malignancies and severe infections [68]. This database is exploratory and does not permit conclusions about efficacy of rIFN-γ as the sole immune adjuvant or paired with CSFs and/or granulocyte transfusions.

We reserve rIFN-γ for patients with life-threatening invasive mould infections refractory to standard antifungal therapy. Such decisions are necessarily based on retrospective analyses and anecdotal data. Pairing rIFN-γ with G-CSF or GM-CSF is another reasonable option in the setting of refractory fungal disease, though we emphasize that the clinical experience is anecdotal and that the efficacy of this approach is not established.

Antifungal Agents as Immunomodulators

Another area of research interest relates to the immunomodulatory effect of antifungals. Fungal cell wall constituents on opportunistic fungi are ligands for Toll-like receptors (TLR) and other innate pathogen recognition receptors [50, 69, 70]. Recognition of pathogen-associated molecular patterns by

TLRs, either alone or in cooperation with other TLR or non-TLR receptors (e.g. Dectin-1), induces signals responsible for the activation of the innate immune response. Several studies have demonstrated a crucial involvement of TLRs in the recognition of fungal pathogens such as *C. albicans*, *A. fumigatus*, and *C. neoformans* [50, 70–74]. In vivo, antifunga;s decrease the antigen load, which alone can help restore Th1 responses.

One example of the immunologic effect of antifungals is the infusional toxicity of amphotericin B that likely results from release of proinflammatory cytokines from monocytes [75, 76]. Other antifungal agents may have more indirect effects on host cell responses. Amphotericin B deoxycholate and liposomal amphotericin B have distinct effects on TLR signaling and antifungal activity of murine neutrophils [77]. Empty liposomes attenuated the immunopathology in experimental aspergillosis [78]. Echinocandins cause structural changes in the fungal cell wall, including blebbing and cell wall rupture [79, 80]. The beta-glucan constituent of the fungal cell wall is recognized by specific host cell pathogen recognition receptors and elicits immunologic responses [69, 81–85]. Echinocandins can unmask the beta-glucan constituents of fungal cell walls of Candida and filamentous fungi, leading to modulation of the immune response in macrophages and neutrophils [86–88]. In addition, compensatory cell wall synthesis pathways are likely to be induced by beta-glucan depletion [89], which may further alter antigenic cell wall epitopes. Other possibilities for antifungal-cytokine interactions includes the probability that cytokines can enhance uptake of antifungals by effector cells, and that effector cell antifungal mechanisms (e.g., oxidative metabolites) act synergistically with antifungal effects on fungi. Antifungals also appear to increase pro-inflammatory cytokines at a transcriptional level, inhibit anti-inflammatory cytokines, act synergistically with cytokines to induce protective pro-inflammatory responses, and prime effector cells for a second signal from cytokines. In vivo, antifungals decrease the antigen load, which alone can help restore Th1 responses.

We do not know the clinical significance of the immunomodulatory properties of antifungal agents. To gain at least correlative data, it would be useful if immunologic studies were included as secondary endpoints in future clinical trials.

Summary

There is currently insufficient proof that any immune-based therapy is effective for invasive fungal diseases. Knowledge of the immunopathogenesis of fungal infections has paved the way to promising strategies for immunotherapy at the preclinical level. These include strategies that increase phagocyte number, activate innate host defense pathways in phagocytes and dendritic cells, and stimulate antigen-specific immunity, such as vaccines [90–94]. Newer approaches, with supporting preclinical data, include infusion of donor T cells sensitized against *Aspergillus*, the use of monoclonal antibodies directed against protein and/or carbohydrate epitopes of pathogenic fungi, or against cytokines which depress the Th1 response, synthetic immunomodulators which act as TLR agonists [95], the therapeutic use of collectins, such as mannose-binding lectin [96], or gene therapy to deliver cytokines to the infected host [96a]. Studies of adjunctive immunotherapy for established infection should target specific well-defined patient groups to maximize the likelihood of detecting a treatment effect. Kullberg et al. [97] reasonably suggest that Phase I and II studies of immunotherapies focus on laboratory surrogates likely to predict efficacy (e.g. augmenting neutrophil number or type I cytokine responses) that would pave the way to larger studies that evaluate clinically relevant endpoints (e.g., survival, successful control of infection).

References

1. Blumberg HM, Jarvis WR, Soucie JM, et al. Risk factors for candidal bloodstream infections in surgical intensive care unit patients: the NEMIS prospective multicenter study. The National Epidemiology of Mycosis Survey. Clin Infect Dis. 2001;33:177–86.
2. Bow EJ, Loewen R, Cheang MS, Shore TB, Rubinger M, Schacter B. Cytotoxic therapy-induced D-xylose malabsorption and invasive infection during remission-induction therapy for acute myeloid leukemia in adults. J Clin Oncol. 1997;15:2254–61.
3. Galgiani JN, Ampel NM, Blair JE, et al. IDSA guidelines: coccidioidomycosis. Clin Infect Dis. 2005;41:1217–23.
4. Louie L, Ng S, Hajjeh R, et al. Influence of host genetics on the severity of coccidioidomycosis. Emerg Infect Dis. 1999;5:672–80.
5. Segal BH. Aspergillosis. N Engl J Med. 2009;360:1870–84.
6. Gerson SL, Talbot GH, Hurwitz S, Strom BL, Lusk EJ, Cassileth PA. Prolonged granulocytopenia: the major risk factor for invasive pulmonary aspergillosis in patients with acute leukemia. Ann Intern Med. 1984;100:345–51.
7. Weinberger M, Elattar I, Marshall D, et al. Patterns of infection in patients with aplastic anemia and the emergence of Aspergillus as a major cause of death. Medicine (Baltimore). 1992;71:24–43.
8. Marty FM, Rubin RH. The prevention of infection post-transplant: the role of prophylaxis, preemptive and empiric therapy. Transpl Int. 2006;19:2–11.
9. Wald A, Leisenring W, van Burik JA, Bowden RA. Epidemiology of Aspergillus infections in a large cohort of patients undergoing bone marrow transplantation. J Infect Dis. 1997;175:1459–66.
10. Baddley JW, Stroud TP, Salzman D, Pappas PG. Invasive mold infections in allogeneic bone marrow transplant recipients. Clin Infect Dis. 2001;32:1319–24.
11. Grow WB, Moreb JS, Roque D, et al. Late onset of invasive aspergillus infection in bone marrow transplant patients at a university hospital. Bone Marrow Transplant. 2002;29:15–9.
12. Jantunen E, Ruutu P, Niskanen L, et al. Incidence and risk factors for invasive fungal infections in allogeneic BMT recipients. Bone Marrow Transplant. 1997;19:801–8.

13. McWhinney PH, Kibbler CC, Hamon MD, et al. Progress in the diagnosis and management of aspergillosis in bone marrow transplantation: 13 years' experience. Clin Infect Dis. 1993;17:397–404.
14. Yuen KY, Woo PC, Ip MS, et al. Stage-specific manifestation of mold infections in bone marrow transplant recipients: risk factors and clinical significance of positive concentrated smears. Clin Infect Dis. 1997;25:37–42.
15. Marr KA, Carter RA, Boeckh M, Martin P, Corey L. Invasive aspergillosis in allogeneic stem cell transplant recipients: changes in epidemiology and risk factors. Blood. 2002;100:4358–66.
16. Shaukat A, Bakri F, Young P, et al. Invasive filamentous fungal infections in allogeneic hematopoietic stem cell transplant recipients after recovery from neutropenia: clinical, radiologic, and pathologic characteristics. Mycopathologia. 2005;159:181–8.
17. van Burik JA, Carter SL, Freifeld AG, et al. Higher risk of cytomegalovirus and aspergillus infections in recipients of T cell-depleted unrelated bone marrow: analysis of infectious complications in patients treated with T cell depletion versus immunosuppressive therapy to prevent graft-versus-host disease. Biol Blood Marrow Transplant. 2007;13:1487–98.
18. Morgan J, Wannemuehler KA, Marr KA, et al. Incidence of invasive aspergillosis following hematopoietic stem cell and solid organ transplantation: interim results of a prospective multicenter surveillance program. Med Mycol. 2005;43 Suppl 1:S49–58.
19. Hadjiliadis D, Sporn TA, Perfect JR, Tapson VF, Davis RD, Palmer SM. Outcome of lung transplantation in patients with mycetomas. Chest. 2002;121:128–34.
20. Winkelstein JA, Marino MC, Johnston RBJr, et al. Chronic granulomatous disease: report on a national registry of 368 patients. Medicine (Baltimore). 2000;79:155–69.
21. Segal BH, Leto TL, Gallin JI, Malech HL, Holland SM. Genetic, biochemical, and clinical features of chronic granulomatous disease. Medicine (Baltimore). 2000;79:170–200.
22. Rowe JM. Concurrent use of growth factors and chemotherapy in acute leukemia. Curr Opin Hematol. 2000;7:197–202.
23. Ozer H, Armitage JO, Bennett CL, et al. 2000 update of recommendations for the use of hematopoietic colony-stimulating factors: evidence-based, clinical practice guidelines. American Society of Clinical Oncology Growth Factors Expert Panel. J Clin Oncol. 2000;18:3558–85.
24. Godwin JE, Kopecky KJ, Head DR, et al. A double-blind placebo-controlled trial of granulocyte colony-stimulating factor in elderly patients with previously untreated acute myeloid leukemia: a Southwest Oncology Group study (9031). Blood. 1998;91:3607–15.
25. Heil G, Hoelzer D, Sanz MA, et al. A randomized, double-blind, placebo-controlled, phase III study of filgrastim in remission induction and consolidation therapy for adults with de novo acute myeloid leukemia. The International Acute Myeloid Leukemia Study Group. Blood. 1997;90:4710–8.
26. Giles FJ. Monocyte-macrophages, granulocyte-macrophage colony-stimulating factor, and prolonged survival among patients with acute myeloid leukemia and stem cell transplants. Clin Infect Dis. 1998;26:1282–9.
27. Rowe JM, Andersen JW, Mazza JJ, et al. A randomized placebo-controlled phase III study of granulocyte- macrophage colony-stimulating factor in adult patients (> 55 to 70 years of age) with acute myelogenous leukemia: a study of the Eastern Cooperative Oncology Group (E1490). Blood. 1995;86:457–62.
28. Smith TJ, Khatcheressian J, Lyman GH, et al. 2006 update of recommendations for the use of white blood cell growth factors: an evidence-based clinical practice guideline. J Clin Oncol. 2006;24:3187–205.
29. Lyman GH, Kleiner JM. Summary and comparison of myeloid growth factor guidelines in patients receiving cancer chemotherapy. J Natl Compr Canc Netw. 2007;5:217–28.
30. Bodey GP, Buckley M, Sathe YS, Freireich EJ. Quantitative relationships between circulating leukocytes and infection in patients with acute leukemia. Ann Intern Med. 1966;64:328–40.
31. Vora S, Purimetla N, Brummer E, Stevens DA. Activity of voriconazole, a new triazole, combined with neutrophils or monocytes against Candida albicans: effect of granulocyte colony-stimulating factor and granulocyte-macrophage colony-stimulating factor [published erratum appears in Antimicrob Agents Chemother 1998 Aug;42(8):2152]. Antimicrob Agents Chemother. 1998;42:907–10.
32. Sionov E, Mendlovic S, Segal E. Experimental systemic murine aspergillosis: treatment with polyene and caspofungin combination and G-CSF. J Antimicrob Chemother. 2005;56:594–7.
33. Sionov E, Segal E. Polyene and cytokine treatment of experimental aspergillosis. FEMS Immunol Med Microbiol. 2003;39:221–7.
34. Kullberg BJ, Vandewoude K, Herbrecht R, Jacobs F, Aoun M, Kujath P. A double-blind, randomized, placebo-controlled phase II study of filgrastim (recombinant granulocyte colony-stimulating factor) in combination with fluconazole for treatment of invasive candidiasis and candidemia in nonneutropenic patients. In: 38th Interscience Conference on Antimicrobial Agents and Chemotherapy. San Diego, CA; 1998. p. J-100.
35. Nemunaitis J. Use of macrophage colony-stimulating factor in the treatment of fungal infections. Clin Infect Dis. 1998;26:1279–81.
36. Sloand EM, Kim S, Maciejewski JP, et al. Pharmacologic doses of granulocyte colony-stimulating factor affect cytokine production by lymphocytes in vitro and in vivo. Blood. 2000;95:2269–74.
37. Rutella S, Pierelli L, Bonanno G, et al. Role for granulocyte colony-stimulating factor in the generation of human T regulatory type 1 cells. Blood. 2002;100:2562–71.
38. Volpi I, Perruccio K, Tosti A, et al. Postgrafting administration of granulocyte colony-stimulating factor impairs functional immune recovery in recipients of human leukocyte antigen haplotype-mismatched hematopoietic transplants. Blood. 2001;97:2514–21.
39. Choi JH, Brummer E, Kang YJ, Jones PP, Stevens DA. Inhibitor kappaB and nuclear factor kappaB in granulocyte-macrophage colony-stimulating factor antagonism of dexamethasone suppression of the macrophage response to Aspergillus fumigatus conidia. J Infect Dis. 2006;193:1023–8.
40. Groll A, Renz S, Gerein V, et al. Fatal haemoptysis associated with invasive pulmonary aspergillosis treated with high-dose amphotericin B and granulocyte-macrophage colony-stimulating factor (GM-CSF). Mycoses. 1992;35:67–75.
41. Safdar A, Rodriguez G, Rolston KV, et al. High-dose caspofungin combination antifungal therapy in patients with hematologic malignancies and hematopoietic stem cell transplantation. Bone Marrow Transplant. 2007;39:157–64.
42. Bensinger WI, Price TH, Dale DC, et al. The effects of daily recombinant human granulocyte colony-stimulating factor administration on normal granulocyte donors undergoing leukapheresis [see comments]. Blood. 1993;81:1883–8.
43. Dale DC, Liles WC, Llewellyn C, Rodger E, Price TH. Neutrophil transfusions: kinetics and functions of neutrophils mobilized with granulocyte-colony stimulating factor and dexamethasone [see comments]. Transfusion. 1998;38:713–21.
44. Price TH, Bowden RA, Boeckh M, et al. Phase I/II trial of neutrophil transfusions from donors stimulated with G-CSF and dexamethasone for treatment of patients with infections in hematopoeitic stem cell transplantation. Blood. 2000;95:3302–9.
45. Wright DG, Robichaud KJ, Pizzo PA, Deisseroth AB. Lethal pulmonary reactions associated with the combined use of amphotericin B and leukocyte transfusions. N Engl J Med. 1981;304:1185–9.
46. Stroncek DF, Leonard K, Eiber G, Malech HL, Gallin JI, Leitman SF. Alloimmunization after granulocyte transfusions. Transfusion. 1996;36:1009–15.

47. Nichols WG, Price T, Boeckh M. Cytomegalovirus infections in cancer patients receiving granulocyte transfusions. Blood. 2002;99: 3483–4.
48. Schalm SW, Weiland O, Hansen BE, et al. Interferon-ribavirin for chronic hepatitis C with and without cirrhosis: analysis of individual patient data of six controlled trials. Eurohep Study Group for Viral Hepatitis. Gastroenterology. 1999;117:408–13.
49. Stevens DA. Combination immunotherapy and antifungal chemotherapy. Clin Infect Dis. 1998;26:1266–9.
50. Segal BH, Kwon-Chung J, Walsh TJ, et al. Immunotherapy for fungal infections. Clin Infect Dis. 2006;42:507–15.
51. Segal BH, Holland SM. Interferon-gamma in infectious diseases. In: Kawakami K, Stevens DA, editors. Immunomodulators as promising therapeutic agents against infectious diseases. Kerala, India: Research Signpost; 2004. p. 23–54.
52. Stevens DA, Brummer E, Clemons KV. Interferon-gamma as an antifungal. J Infect Dis. 2006;194 Suppl 1:S33–7.
53. Wang J, Wakeham J, Harkness R, Xing Z. Macrophages are a significant source of type 1 cytokines during mycobacterial infection. J Clin Invest. 1999;103:1023–9.
54. Mountford AP, Coulson PS, Cheever AW, Sher A, Wilson RA, Wynn TA. Interleukin-12 can directly induce T-helper 1 responses in interferon-gamma (IFN-gamma) receptor-deficient mice, but requires IFN-gamma signalling to downregulate T-helper 2 responses. Immunology. 1999;97:588–94.
55. Tomura M, Maruo S, Mu J, et al. Differential capacities of CD4+, CD8+, and CD4-CD8- T cell subsets to express IL-18 receptor and produce IFN-gamma in response to IL-18. J Immunol. 1998;160:3759–65.
56. Boehm U, Klamp T, Groot M, Howard JC. Cellular responses to interferon-gamma. Annu Rev Immunol. 1997;15:749–95.
57. Pien GC, Satoskar AR, Takeda K, Akira S, Biron CA. Cutting edge: selective IL-18 requirements for induction of compartmental IFN-gamma responses during viral infection. J Immunol. 2000;165:4787–91.
58. The International Chronic Granulomatous Disease Cooperative Study Group. A controlled trial of interferon gamma to prevent infection in chronic granulomatous disease. N Engl J Med. 1991;324:509–16.
59. Pappas PG, Bustamante B, Ticona E, et al. Recombinant interferon-gamma 1b as adjunctive therapy for AIDS-related acute cryptococcal meningitis. J Infect Dis. 2004;189:2185–91.
60. Nagai H, Guo J, Choi H, Kurup V. Interferon-gamma and tumor necrosis factor-alpha protect mice from invasive aspergillosis. J Infect Dis. 1995;172:1554–60.
61. Stevens DA. Th1/Th2 in aspergillosis. Med Mycol. 2006;44:S229–35.
62. Roilides E, Uhlig K, Venzon D, Pizzo PA, Walsh TJ. Enhancement of oxidative response and damage caused by human neutrophils to *Aspergillus fumigatus* hyphae by granulocyte colony-stimulating factor and gamma interferon. Infect Immun. 1993;61: 1185–93.
63. Roilides E, Uhlig K, Venzon D, Pizzo PA, Walsh TJ. Prevention of corticosteroid-induced suppression of human polymorphonuclear leukocyte-induced damage of *Aspergillus fumigatus* hyphae by granulocyte colony-stimulating factor and gamma interferon. Infect Immun. 1993;61:4870–7.
64. Roilides E, Holmes A, Blake C, Venzon D, Pizzo PA, Walsh TJ. Antifungal activity of elutriated human monocytes against *Aspergillus fumigatus* hyphae: enhancement by granulocyte-macrophage colony-stimulating factor and interferon-gamma. J Infect Dis. 1994;170:894–9.
65. Rex JH, Bennett JE, Gallin JI, Malech HL, DeCarlo ES, Melnick DA. In vivo interferon-gamma therapy augments the in vitro ability of chronic granulomatous disease neutrophils to damage Aspergillus hyphae. J Infect Dis. 1991;163:849–52.
66. Dignani MC, Rex JH, Chan KW, et al. Immunomodulation with interferon-gamma and colony stimulating factors for refractory fungal infections in patients with leukemia. Cancer. 2005;104: 199–204.
67. Safdar A, Rodriguez G, Ohmagari N, et al. The safety of interferon-gamma-1b for invasive fungal infections after hematopoietic stem cell transplantation. Cancer. 2005;103:731–9.
68. Safdar A, Rodriguez GH, Lichtiger B, et al. Recombinant interferon gamma1b immune enhancement in 20 patients with hematologic malignancies and systemic opportunistic infections treated with donor granulocyte transfusions. Cancer. 2006;106:2664–71.
69. Brown GD. Dectin-1: a signalling non-TLR pattern-recognition receptor. Nat Rev Immunol. 2006;6:33–43.
70. Romani L. Immunity to fungal infections. Nat Rev Immunol. 2004;4:1–23.
71. Netea MG, Van der Graaf C, Van der Meer JW, Kullberg BJ. Recognition of fungal pathogens by Toll-like receptors. Eur J Clin Microbiol Infect Dis. 2004;23:672–6.
72. Bellocchio S, Moretti S, Perruccio K, et al. TLRs govern neutrophil activity in aspergillosis. J Immunol. 2004;173:7406–15.
73. Bellocchio S, Montagnoli C, Bozza S, et al. The contribution of the Toll-like/IL-1 receptor superfamily to innate and adaptive immunity to fungal pathogens in vivo. J Immunol. 2004;172:3059–69.
74. Romani L, Montagnoli C, Bozza S, et al. The exploitation of distinct recognition receptors in dendritic cells determines the full range of host immune relationships with *Candida albicans*. Int Immunol. 2004;16:149–61.
75. Arning M, Kliche KO, Heer-Sonderhoff AH, Wehmeier A. Infusion-related toxicity of three different amphotericin B formulations and its relation to cytokine plasma levels. Mycoses. 1995;38:459–65.
76. Rogers PD, Kramer RE, Chapman SW, Cleary JD. Amphotericin B-induced interleukin-1beta expression in human monocytic cells is calcium and calmodulin dependent. J Infect Dis. 1999;180: 1259–66.
77. Bellocchio S, Gaziano R, Bozza S, et al. Liposomal amphotericin B activates antifungal resistance with reduced toxicity by diverting Toll-like receptor signalling from TLR-2 to TLR-4. J Antimicrob Chemother. 2005;55:214–22.
78. Lewis RE, Chamilos G, Prince RA, Kontoyiannis DP. Pretreatment with empty liposomes attenuates the immunopathology of invasive pulmonary aspergillosis in corticosteroid-immunosuppressed mice. Antimicrob Agents Chemother. 2007;51:1078–81.
79. Petraitis V, Petraitiene R, Groll AH, et al. Antifungal efficacy, safety, and single-dose pharmacokinetics of LY303366, a novel echinocandin B, in experimental pulmonary aspergillosis in persistently neutropenic rabbits. Antimicrob Agents Chemother. 1998;42:2898–905.
80. Dennis CG, Greco WR, Brun Y, et al. Effect of amphotericin B and micafungin combination on survival, histopathology, and fungal burden in experimental aspergillosis in the p47phox-/- mouse model of chronic granulomatous disease. Antimicrob Agents Chemother. 2006;50:422–7.
81. Gantner BN, Simmons RM, Canavera SJ, Akira S, Underhill DM. Collaborative induction of inflammatory responses by dectin-1 and Toll-like receptor 2. J Exp Med. 2003;197:1107–17.
82. Gersuk GM, Underhill DM, Zhu L, Marr KA. Dectin-1 and TLRs permit macrophages to distinguish between different *Aspergillus fumigatus* cellular states. J Immunol. 2006;176:3717–24.
83. Netea MG, Gow NA, Munro CA, et al. Immune sensing of *Candida albicans* requires cooperative recognition of mannans and glucans by lectin and Toll-like receptors. J Clin Invest. 2006;116(6): 1642–50.
84. Hohl TM, Van Epps HL, Rivera A, et al. *Aspergillus fumigatus* triggers inflammatory responses by stage-specific beta-glucan display. PLoS Pathog. 2005;1:e30.

85. Graham LM, Tsoni SV, Willment JA, et al. Soluble Dectin-1 as a tool to detect beta-glucans. J Immunol Methods. 2006;314:164–9.
86. Hohl TM, Feldmesser M, Perlin DS, Pamer EG. Caspofungin modulates inflammatory responses to *Aspergillus fumigatus* through stage-specific effects on fungal beta-glucan exposure. J Infect Dis. 2008;198:176–85.
87. Lamaris GA, Lewis RE, Chamilos G, et al. Caspofungin-mediated beta-glucan unmasking and enhancement of human polymorphonuclear neutrophil activity against Aspergillus and non-Aspergillus hyphae. J Infect Dis. 2008;198:186–92.
88. Wheeler RT, Fink GR. A drug-sensitive genetic network masks fungi from the immune system. PLoS Pathog. 2006;2:e35.
89. Popolo L, Gilardelli D, Bonfante P, Vai M. Increase in chitin as an essential response to defects in assembly of cell wall polymers in the ggp1delta mutant of *Saccharomyces cerevisiae*. J Bacteriol. 1997;179:463–9.
90. Spellberg BJ, Ibrahim AS, Avenissian V, et al. The anti-*Candida albicans* vaccine composed of the recombinant N terminus of Als1p reduces fungal burden and improves survival in both immunocompetent and immunocompromised mice. Infect Immun. 2005;73:6191–3.
91. Torosantucci A, Bromuro C, Chiani P, et al. A novel glycoconjugate vaccine against fungal pathogens. J Exp Med. 2005;202:597–606.
92. Bozza S, Montagnoli C, Gaziano R, et al. Dendritic cell-based vaccination against opportunistic fungi. Vaccine. 2004;22:857–64.
93. Stevens DA. Vaccinate against aspergillosis! A call to arms of the immune system. Clin Infect Dis. 2004;38:1131–6.
94. Cox RA, Magee DM. Coccidioidomycosis: host response and vaccine development. Clin Microbiol Rev. 2004;17:804–39. table of contents.
95. Brummer E, Antonysamy MA, Bythadka L, Gullikson GW, Stevens DA. Effect of 3M-003, an imidazoquinoline analog of imiquimod, on phagocyte candidacidal activity directly and via peripheral blood mononuclear cell cytokines. FEMS Immunol Med Microbiol. 2010;59(1):81–9.
96. Brummer E, Stevens DA. Collectins and fungal pathogens: roles of surfactant proteins and mannose binding lectin in host resistance. Med Mycol. 2010;48(1):16–28.
96a. Clemons KV, Kamberi P, Chiller TM, et al. Effects of interferon-gamma gene therapy in the murine central nervous system and concentrations in cerebrospinal fluid after intrathecal or intracerebral administration. Biotechnology 2005;4:11–18.
97. Kullberg BJ, Oude Lashof AM, Netea MG. Design of efficacy trials of cytokines in combination with antifungal drugs. Clin Infect Dis. 2004;39 Suppl 4:S218–23.
98. Walsh TJ, Anaissie EJ, Denning DW, et al. Treatment of aspergillosis: clinical practice guidelines of the Infectious Diseases Society of America. Clin Infect Dis. 2008;46:327–60.
99. Segal BH, Freifeld AG, Baden LR, et al. Prevention and treatment of cancer-related infections. J Natl Compr Canc Netw. 2008;6:122–74.
100. Singh N, Perfect JR. Immune reconstitution syndrome associated with opportunistic mycoses. Lancet Infect Dis. 2007;7:395–401.
101. Buescher ES, Gallin JI. Leukocyte transfusions in chronic granulomatous disease: persistence of transfused leukocytes in sputum. N Engl J Med. 1982;307:800–3.

Chapter 30
Cytomegalovirus in Patients with Cancer

Morgan Hakki, Per Ljungman, and Michael Boeckh

Abstract Human cytomegalovirus (CMV) is a common opportunistic infection after hematopoietic cell transplant (HCT) and is less frequently encountered among patients undergoing cytotoxic chemotherapy for various malignancies. Both primary infection and reactivation can result in substantial morbidity and mortality in the immunocompromised host. Therefore, the prompt recognition and treatment of CMV infection is critical. This chapter will outline the diagnosis, prevention, and treatment of CMV, focusing on the HCT recipient since it is this population that is at greatest risk for, and bears the largest burden of, CMV infection and disease.

Keywords Cytomegalovirus • Cancer • Stem cell transplant

Virus Structure and Replication

CMV, along with human herpesvirus (HHV)-6 and HHV-7, is a member of the beta (β) subfamily of the herpesviridae. The virion consists of a double-stranded DNA genome encased in an icosahedral capsid. Surrounding the capsid are the tegument (or matrix) and an outermost lipid membrane.

The genome contains approximately 230,000 base pairs of DNA that encode approximately 200 proteins [1, 2]. CMV genes are named based on their position within each segment of the genome. For example, UL97 is the 97th open reading frame (ORF) in the unique long segment. Some genes also have names based on historical usage or homologies to genes of other herpesviruses; UL55, for example, is also known as glycoprotein B.

CMV grows in a limited number of cell lines in the laboratory, such as diploid human fibroblasts, endothelial cells, and macrophages. During human infection, however, CMV has been found in a wide range of cells, including endothelial cells, epithelial cells, blood cells including neutrophils, and smooth muscle cells [3]. The presence of CMV in these cells may contribute to dissemination and transmission.

The ability to persist in a latent state in which evidence of viral replication is undetectable but replication-competent virus is present is a hallmark of herpesviruses. In the case of CMV, little is known about the site or mechanisms of latency. Since CMV can be transmitted from seropositive blood donors, a blood component is likely to be one site of latency. Several studies indicate that cells of the granulocyte-monocyte lineage harbor latent CMV [4–6]. Transplantation of solid organs clearly can transmit CMV, so it is possible that cells other than those mentioned above can harbor and transmit latent CMV.

CMV and Host Immunity

Adaptive Immunity

The importance of a competent immune system in controlling CMV replication is manifested by the clear association of immunosuppression with CMV infection and disease. The role of humoral immunity in controlling CMV replication is not clear. While antibodies to multiple different CMV proteins, primarily glycoproteins B (gB), and H (gH), develop during infection, they do not appear to prevent primary infection in adults, but rather may function to limit disease severity [7–11].

CMV provokes a robust CD8+ cytotoxic T lymphocyte (CTL) response and the percentage of circulating CD8+ T cells in healthy individuals that are CMV-specific may be as high 40% [12–17]. The most dominant proteins targeted by CD8+ T-cell responses are the products of UL123 (IE-1), UL122 (IE-2), and UL83 (pp65) [14, 17–23]. The importance of intact T-cell mediated cellular immunity in controlling CMV replication is demonstrated by studies correlating the lack of CMV-specific CD8+ CTL responses with CMV

M. Hakki (✉)
Division of Infectious Diseases,
Oregon Health & Science University, Portland, OR, USA
e-mail: hakki@ohsu.edu

infection, and the reconstitution of CMV-specific CD8+ CTL responses with protection from CMV [24–28]. The presence of multifunctional CMV-specific CD8+ T cells have been associated with less recurrent CMV reactivation in seropositive hematopoietic cell transplant (HCT) recipients.

After HCT, detectable CMV-specific CD4+ T-cell responses are associated with protection from CMV disease [24, 29–31]. The lack of CMV-specific CD4+ T-cell is associated with late CMV disease and death in patients who have undergone HCT [32]. CMV-specific CD4+ cells likely function at least in part by helping to maintain robust CMV-specific CD8+ cell responses [28, 33].

Innate Immunity

Less is known about the role of innate immunity in controlling CMV replication, but evidence exists indicating that this arm of the immune response is indeed required to control CMV replication. CMV triggers cellular inflammatory cytokine production upon binding to the target cell, mediated in part by the interaction of gB and gH with toll-like receptor (TLR) 2 [34–36]. Polymorphisms in TLR2 have been associated with CMV infection after liver transplantation [37]. In mouse studies, TLR3 and TLR9 proved to be important components in limiting murine cytomegalovirus (MCMV) replication [38, 39].

Natural killer (NK) cells represent another arm of the innate immune response and have been shown to limit MCMV replication in mice [25, 40–44]. In humans, a deficiency in NK cells is associated with severe CMV infection (among other herpesviruses) [45]. The genotype of the donor activating killer immunoglobulin-like receptor (aKIR), which regulates NK cell function, is associated with the development of CMV infection after allogeneic HCT [46–48]. These findings require validation in independent cohorts.

Finally, polymorphisms in chemokine receptor 5 (CCR5), IL-10, and monocyte chemoattractant protein 1 (MCP-1) have been associated with CMV reactivation and disease after allogeneic HCT [49]. Validation of these associations in independent cohorts is lacking at this time.

Immune Evasion

Numerous CMV-encoded genes function in immune evasion by inhibiting apoptosis [50], MHC-I restricted antigen presentation [51], and interferon-mediated pathways [52–55]. CMV also encodes several homologues of cellular proteins, including MHC class-I molecules, chemokine receptors, IL-10, TNF receptors, and CXC-1 homologues, that function to help CMV evade the host immune response [56–60].

Diagnostic Methods

Several assays are available to assist in the diagnosis of CMV. The strengths and limitations of these assays are summarized in Table 30.1. The serologic determination of IgG and IgM has an important role in determining a patient's risk for CMV infection after transplantation (see below, Section E)

Table 30.1 Methods utilized in the diagnosis of CMV infection and disease

Assay	Turnaround time	Advantages	Disadvantages
Histology	24–48 h	Specific	Low sensitivity
		Useful in determining invasive disease	Utility limited to tissue biopsy specimens
Serology	<24 h	Provides prognostic information regarding risk of CMV during HCT	Not useful in diagnosis of acute infection or disease
Culture	Up to 6 weeks	Specific	Low sensitivity
		Allows for phenotypic antiviral susceptibility testing	Long assay time
Shell vial	24–48 h	Specific	Low sensitivity compared to molecular assays
		More rapid than culture	
		Test of choice on BAL fluid	
pp65 antigenemia	<24 h	Rapid	Unable to perform in setting of profound neutropenia
		More sensitive than culture	Not as sensitive as PCR
		Provides approximate quantitation of viral load	Only validated on whole blood
Quantitative DNA PCR (qPCR)	<24 h	Most sensitive assay	Requires technical expertise
		Highly specific	Not validated on BAL fluid, tissue biopsy specimens Interlaboratory variability
		Provides direct quantitation of viral load	
pp67 mRNA NASBA	<24 h	More sensitive than culture	Less sensitive than DNA qPCR
		Specific for replicating virus	Qualitative
			Requires technical expertise

or during immunosuppressive therapy, but is not useful in the diagnosis of CMV infection or disease. Growth of CMV in tissue culture takes several weeks, limiting its clinical usefulness as a diagnostic tool. Culture-proven viremia is highly predictive of CMV disease, but is of limited utility for screening since this finding frequently coincides with the onset of symptomatic disease [61–63].

The shell vial technique, in which monoclonal antibodies are used to detect CMV immediate-early proteins in cultured cells, can be performed within 18–24 h after inoculation. This assay is not sensitive enough to use for routine blood monitoring [62], but is highly useful on bronchoalveolar lavage (BAL) fluid in the diagnosis of CMV pneumonia and in tissue samples to diagnose CMV gastrointestinal disease [64].

The presence of characteristic CMV "owl's eye" nuclear inclusions in tissue specimens is useful in the diagnosis of invasive CMV disease (Fig. 30.1a). This method has relatively low sensitivity, but can be enhanced by use of immunohistochemical techniques to identify CMV antigens (Fig. 30.1b) even when classic inclusions may not be evident.

Advances in molecular diagnostic techniques that do not rely on the growth in CMV in tissue culture have dramatically improved our ability to diagnose CMV.

The detection of the CMV pp65 tegument phosphoprotein in peripheral blood leukocytes offers a rapid, sensitive, and specific method of diagnosing CMV viremia. In this assay, peripheral leukocytes are spread on a glass slide and stained with a fluorescent antibody directed against pp65. The number of positive cells is reported per number of total leukocytes on the slide, thereby providing a rough quantitative assessment of the circulating viral load. In the transplant setting, a positive CMV pp65 assay has been shown to predict the development of invasive disease [65, 66]. Since this assay relies on the detection of pp65 in circulating leukocytes, it may not be reliable in patients with profound leukopenia. The predictive value of this assay has not been validated when performed on other body fluids such as BAL fluid.

Quantitative polymerase chain reaction (qPCR) relies on the amplification and quantitative measurement of CMV DNA. qPCR testing has become the standard method for detecting CMV in blood (either whole blood or plasma) and spinal fluid at many, if not most, institutions, for several reasons. PCR is the most sensitive method for detecting CMV [67], thereby prompting treatment initiation in cases of CMV disease that have been missed with the pp65 antigenemia assay [68]. At the same time, qPCR maintains high specificity. In addition, it is very rapid, with results usually available within 24 h. qPCR also provides a direct quantitative measurement of CMV viral load and viral load kinetics, which are accurate predictors of CMV disease after transplantation [32, 69–72]. This facet of qPCR may enable the development of institution-specific viral load thresholds for beginning treatment, thereby avoiding unnecessary treatment of patients who are at low risk of progression to disease.

Although PCR has been used on BAL fluid [73], viral load cut-offs have not been defined, and while the sensitivity and negative predictive values are very high, the specificity and positive predictive values are not known.

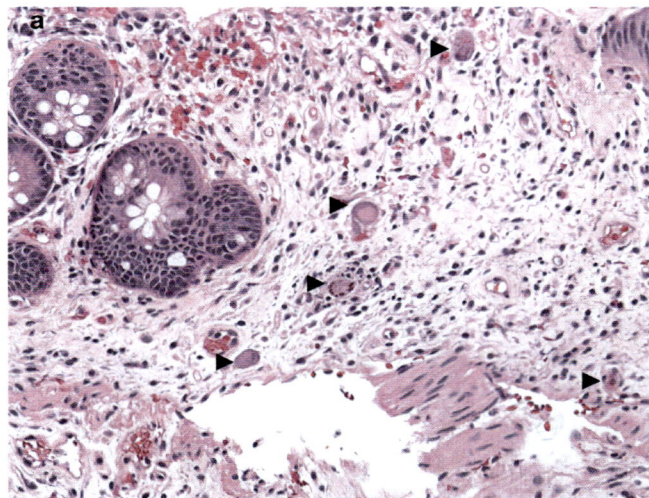 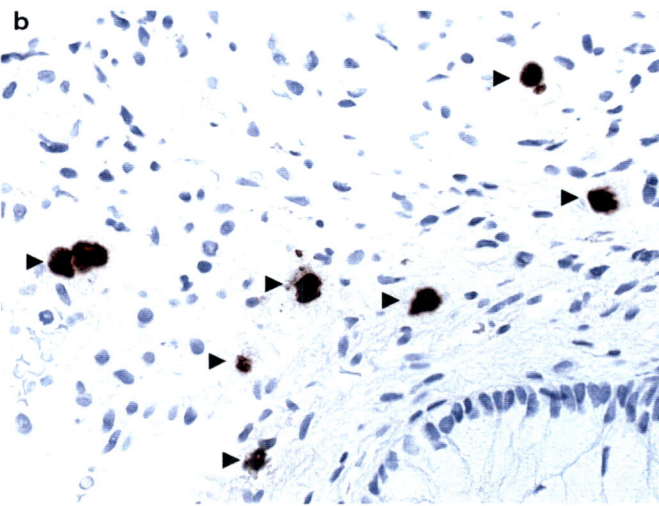

Fig. 30.1 (a) Hematoxylin and eosin (H&E) stain (20× magnification) of a transverse colon biopsy specimen from a patient day +46 after HCT demonstrating nuclear and cytoplasmic inclusions in CMV-infected cells (*arrowheads*). (b) Anti-CMV immunostaining (Dako, 40× magnification) of the same specimen, demonstrating CMV-infected cells (*arrowheads*). Photomicrographs courtesy of Dr. Howard Shulman (Fred Hutchinson Cancer Research Center)

The detection of CMV mRNA by nucleic acid sequence-based amplification (NASBA) on blood samples has proven to be as useful as DNA PCR or p65 antigenemia for guiding pre-emptive therapy after HCT [74, 75]. However, this method has not been as widely adopted as the pp65 antigenemia- or PCR-based assays.

Clinical Manifestations

Care must be taken to distinguish CMV "infection" from CMV "disease." CMV infection simply indicates the detection of CMV in plasma, whole blood, urine, or throat samples in asymptomatic CMV-seronegative patient (primary infection) or CMV-seropositive patients (reactivation of latent virus or superinfection with another strain of CMV) [76, 77].

International definitions of CMV disease have been published and generally denote the presence of symptoms and signs compatible with CMV end-organ involvement along with the detection of CMV using a validated method in the appropriate clinical specimen [78]. Almost any organ can be involved in CMV disease and therefore CMV infection has protean manifestations. Fever is perhaps the most common manifestation, but may be absent in patients receiving high-dose immunosuppression.

Pneumonia is the most important clinical manifestation of CMV disease due to its high associated mortality. Patients who have undergone autologous or allogeneic HCT have mortality rates of 60–90% [79–81]. This unacceptably high mortality rate has not changed much in the past 20 years, indicating that the management of these patients has not yet been optimized.

CMV pneumonia often manifests with fever, nonproductive cough, hypoxia, and interstitial infiltrates on radiography (Fig. 30.2a, b). Rarely, nodules may be observed on radiography (Fig. 30.2c). The onset of symptoms can occur over 1–2 weeks, often times with rapid progression to respiratory failure and the requirement for mechanical ventilation.

The diagnosis of CMV pneumonia is established by detection of CMV by shell vial, culture, or histology in BAL or lung biopsy specimens. While pulmonary shedding of CMV is common, the detection of CMV in BAL fluid from asymptomatic patients who underwent routine BAL screening at day 35 after HCT was predictive of subsequent CMV pneumonia in approximately two-thirds of cases [82]. Therefore, the presence of CMV in a BAL specimen in the absence of clinical evidence of CMV disease must be interpreted with caution.

We do not recommend PCR testing on BAL fluid since there is little data correlating CMV DNA detection by PCR in BAL fluid with CMV pneumonia. However, due to the high negative predictive value afforded by its high sensitivity, a negative PCR result can be used to rule out the diagnosis of CMV pneumonia [73].

CMV can affect any part of the gastrointestinal tract from the esophagus to the colon. Esophagitis typically results in odynophagia, while abdominal pain and hematochezia occur with colitis. Ulcers extending deep into the submucosal layers are seen on endoscopy, and visual differentiation of these lesions from other processes that may affect the gastrointestinal tract in these populations, such as graft-versus-host disease, is often difficult. The diagnosis of gastrointestinal disease relies on detection of CMV in biopsy specimens by culture and/or histology (Fig. 30.1a, b). Given the relative lack of sensitivity of each method, both methods should be used on biopsy specimens to diagnose CMV disease. Notably, gastrointestinal disease can occur in the absence of CMV detection in the blood [83, 84].

Retinitis is relatively uncommon after HCT [85–88]. Decreased visual acuity or blurred vision are typical presenting symptoms, and approximately 60% of patients will have involvement of both eyes [86]. Most cases present later than

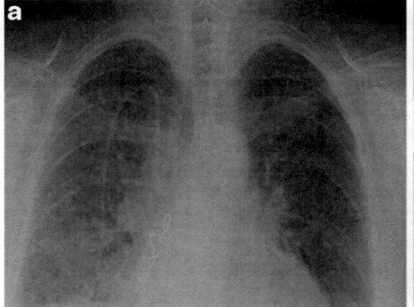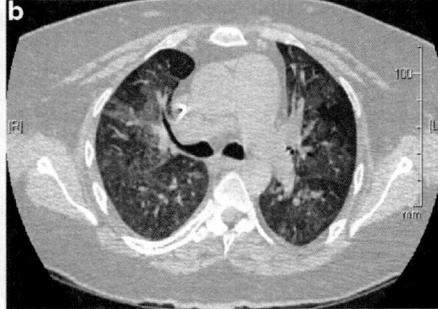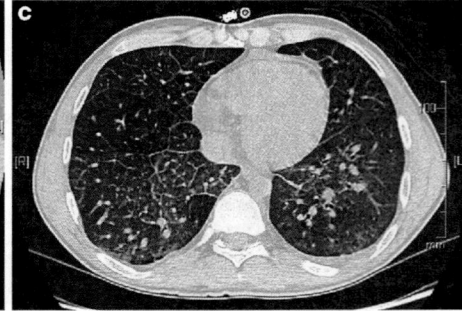

Fig. 30.2 (a) Chest radiograph demonstrating bilateral infiltrates in a patient post-HCT with CMV pneumonia. (b) Chest computed tomography of the same patient in (a). (c) Chest computed tomography demonstrating lower lobe nodules in a different patient, also post-HCT, with CMV pneumonia

day 100 after transplantation and are associated with prior CMV reactivation, delayed lymphocyte engraftment, and graft-versus-host disease (GVHD) [86].

Other manifestations, including hepatitis, encephalitis, and infection of the bone marrow resulting in myelosuppression, are all rare with current preventative strategies.

Risk Factors

Allogeneic HCT Recipients

In the setting of allogeneic HCT, the most important risk factor is the serological status of the donor and recipient. CMV-seronegative patients who receive stem cells from a CMV-seronegative donor (D−/R−) have a very low risk of primary infection. Primary infection can still occur if CMV is transmitted in transfused blood products or is acquired via sexual contact or through contact with another individual with primary CMV infection (e.g., via saliva).

Approximately 30% of seronegative recipients who receive stem cells from a seropositive donor (D+/R−) will develop primary CMV infection due to transmission of latent CMV via the allograft. While the risk of CMV disease is low due to pre-emptive treatment of CMV infection, mortality due to bacterial and fungal infections in these patients is higher than in similarly matched D−/R− transplants (18.3 versus 9.7%, respectively) [89]. The reason for this is not entirely clear, one hypothesis being that CMV infection after HCT has additional immunomodulating effects ("indirect effects") that increase a patient's susceptibility to infection with other, unrelated organisms.

Without prophylaxis, approximately 80% of CMV-seropositive patients will experience CMV infection after allogeneic HCT. Again, current preventative strategies have resulted in a substantial decrease in the incidence of CMV disease, which had historically occurred in 20–35% of these patients [90]. While a CMV-seropositive recipient is at higher risk for non-relapse mortality (NRM) than a seronegative recipient [91, 92], the impact of donor serostatus when the recipient in seropositive remains controversial. Some studies have reported a beneficial effect of having seropositive donor with regards to a reduction in relapse- or NRM, whereas other studies have found no such benefit [93–104]. A large CIBMTR study is presently underway to reconcile these controversial findings. However, although the effects on NRM and overall survival are controversial, the D−/R+ serological combination has been reported as a risk factor for delayed CMV-specific immune reconstitution [105–108], CMV reactivation [106, 109], late CMV recurrence [110], and CMV disease [72, 106, 111].

Other risk factors for CMV infection after allogeneic include the use of mismatched or unrelated donors, recipient HSV serostatus, malignant (versus nonmalignant) underlying disease, T-cell depletion, as well as posttransplant factors such as the use of steroids at doses greater than 1 mg/kg body weight/day and acute and chronic GVHD [69, 72, 111–117]. Whether the source of stem cells (peripheral blood versus bone marrow) has a significant impact on the development of CMV infection and disease is not clear, as several studies have yielded conflicting results [111, 115, 116, 118, 119]. Interestingly, the use of sirolimus for GVHD prophylaxis appears to protect against CMV infection, possibly due to the inhibition of cellular signaling pathways that are co-opted by CMV during infection for synthesis of viral proteins [111, 120].

Late CMV Infection After Allogeneic HCT

Whereas, CMV was typically seen by 100 days after allogeneic HCT [121], in the current era of pre-emptive ganciclovir therapy, it has become a significant problem after day 100 following allogeneic HCT [32, 110, 122]. In the absence of specific preventative measures, 15–30% of allogeneic HCT patients will experience late CMV infection and 6–18% will consequently develop disease [32, 69, 110, 123–125]. Late CMV infection is strongly associated with NRM [110].

Several factors predict the development of late CMV infection, including early (before day 100) CMV infection or disease, lack of CMV-specific immune reconstitution, acute or chronic GVHD, and lymphopenia [24, 30, 32, 110, 112]. Measures such as prolonged courses of therapy and continued weekly surveillance are warranted in these patients in order to reduce the risk of late CMV disease [32, 125, 126].

Nonmyeloablative HCT

The use of matched, related nonmyeloablative conditioning regimens generally results in a less CMV infection and disease early after HCT compared to standard myeloablative regimens [113, 126]. However, by 1 year after HCT, the risk of CMV infection and disease is similar among nonmyeloablative and myeloablative groups [116, 126, 127]. Conditioning regimens that include T-cell depletion show no reduction in CMV after nonmyeloablative transplantation compared to myeloablative regimens [128], and matched, unrelated nonmyeloablative transplantation carries the same risk of CMV infection and disease as does myeloablative transplantation [126].

Autologous HCT and Umbilical Cord Blood Transplantation

After autologous transplantation, approximately 40% of seropositive patients will have detectable CMV infection [79, 129]. While CMV disease is rare after autologous transplantation [118, 130–132], the outcome of CMV pneumonia is similar to that after allogeneic HCT [79, 133, 134]. Risk factors for CMV disease after autologous transplantation include CD34+ selection, high-dose corticosteroids, and the use of total-body irradiation or fludarabine as part of the conditioning regimen [118]. Therefore, while CMV is not typically considered a significant pathogen after autologous HCT, certain patients who are at high risk for CMV in this setting merit routine surveillance and pre-emptive therapy.

Umbilical cord blood transplantation (CBT) is a technique that is now utilized when a suitable donor for bone marrow or peripheral blood stem cell transplantation is not available [135]. Since most infants are born without CMV infection, the transplanted allograft is almost always CMV-negative. Among CMV-seropositive recipients who do not receive antiviral prophylaxis, the rate of CMV infection after CBT is 40–80%, with one study reporting 100% [136–140]. When patients receive prophylaxis with high-dose valacyclovir after CBT, it does not appear that CBT entails a significantly greater risk of CMV infection and disease than does peripheral blood stem cell or bone marrow transplantation [115, 141].

Prevention of CMV Infection and Disease

Pretransplant Risk Reduction

CMV serological status of the recipient and donor should be assessed as early as possible prior to HCT, as this is the most important predictor of subsequent CMV infection. For the seronegative recipient, the main goal is to prevent primary CMV infection. Therefore, recipients who are CMV-seronegative before allogeneic HCT should ideally receive a graft from a CMV-negative donor. Weighing the factor of donor CMV serostatus compared to other relevant donor factors, such as HLA-match, is difficult. No data exists indicating whether study HLA-matching is more important compared to CMV serostatus in affecting a good outcome for the patient. Given the choice, an antigen-matched donor for HLA-A, B, or DR would most likely be preferred to a CMV-negative donor. For lesser degrees of mismatch, (allele-mismatches or mismatches on HLA-C, DQ, or DP), the CMV serostatus of donor should be considered as a factor even if the match was poorer. Compared to other donor factors such as age or blood group, a CMV-seronegative donor would have preference.

The transfusion of blood products represents a significant source for CMV transmission in D−/R− patients [142]. To reduce this risk, blood products from CMV-seronegative donors or leukocyte-reduced, filtered blood products should be used in this setting [143–145]. It is not clear which strategy is the most effective [146, 147], and no controlled study has investigated whether there is an extra benefit from the use of both methods.

Posttransplant Risk Reduction

Immunoprophylaxis

Intravenous immune globulin (IVIG) is not reliably effective as prophylaxis against primary CMV infection [148, 149]. Similarly, negative results were observed using a CMV-specific monoclonal antibody [150]. Likewise, the effect of immunoglobulin on reducing CMV infection in seropositive patients is modest, and no survival benefit among those receiving immunoglobulin has been reported in any study or meta-analysis [151–156]. Therefore, the prophylactic use of immune globulin is not recommended [157].

Antiviral Prophylaxis and Pre-Emptive Therapy

The prophylactic or pre-emptive use of antiviral agents after HCT has markedly reduced the incidence of early CMV disease and has improved survival among certain high-risk populations [62, 68, 112]. Prophylaxis denotes the routine administration of antivirals to all at-risk patients regardless of the presence of active CMV infection. Pre-emptive therapy, on the other hand, withholds antiviral therapy until CMV infection is detected, but prior to the development of CMV disease.

Both approaches have their benefits and drawbacks. Since prophylaxis involves the treatment of all at-risk patients, close monitoring is not required when ganciclovir or foscarnet are used, making this the easier strategy conceptually and useful in situations where rapid, sensitive CMV diagnostic methods are not available. Additionally, prophylaxis may prevent the indirect effects associated with CMV infection. However, since not all at-risk patients will experience CMV infection, prophylaxis strategies result in some patients receiving the drug unnecessarily, thereby exposing the patient to potential drug-related toxicities without discernable benefit. This is not an issue with pre-emptive treatment, since by definition all patients who receive treatment will have active CMV infection.

The success of the pre-emptive treatment strategy is largely dependent on the early detection of viremia. This, in turn, depends on access to rapid, sensitive CMV surveillance methods, and on strict adherence to a surveillance testing schedule. By allowing a limited amount of viral replication, pre-emptive therapy may stimulate immune responses and thereby promote CMV-specific immune reconstitution [24]. Since both strategies are equally effective in preventing CMV disease [68], most transplant centers have moved towards pre-emptive strategies as pp65 antigenemia and DNA PCR-based diagnostics techniques have become readily available [158–160]. The quantitative nature of modern PCR assays now allows to define threshold of viral load for different risk situation, thereby taking full advantage of the high sensitivity of the assay and, at the same time, limiting the use of antiviral drug treatment [161].

More recently, there has been great interest in utilizing methods to determine CMV-specific immune reconstitution after HCT as an additional means to stratify risk of CMV infection and disease ("immune monitoring") and further tailor surveillance and pre-emptive therapy strategies. The types of assays used, their strengths and limitations, and their predictive value in terms of CMV infection and disease after transplantation have been extensively reviewed elsewhere [12, 162]. The utility of measuring T-cell responses as a guide for withholding therapy was evaluated in a small pilot study involving HCT recipients more than 100 days after transplant [105]. While promising, the use of immune monitoring in this fashion requires validation in larger, randomized trials before it can be recommended.

Antiviral Agents

Several antiviral drugs with activity against CMV are available once the decision is made to employ either prophylaxis or pre-emptive treatment (Table 30.2). High-dose acyclovir reduces the risk for CMV infection and possibly disease [163, 164]. Valacyclovir is the valin-ester prodrug of acyclovir and is better absorbed, thereby attaining higher serum concentrations than acyclovir. High-dose valacyclovir is more effective than acyclovir in reducing CMV infection and the need for pre-emptive therapy with ganciclovir after HCT, although the impact of this on survival after HCT is not clear [165]. Routine monitoring for CMV infection is still required if valacyclovir or acyclovir prophylaxis is used. Ganciclovir is a nucleoside analog of guanosine that acts as a competitive inhibitor of deoxyguanosine triphosphate incorporation into viral DNA. A CMV gene, UL97, encodes a phoptotransferase that converts ganciclovir to ganciclovir monophosphate. Cellular enzymes then convert ganciclovir monophosphate to the active triphosphate form. Ganciclovir is currently the first-line agent for CMV prophylaxis and pre-emptive treatment barring contraindications. Intravenous ganciclovir has been demonstrated to reduce the risk of CMV infection and disease compared to placebo, but did not improve overall survival [68, 166–168]. Neutropenia occurs in up to 30% of HCT recipients during ganciclovir therapy [169], thereby placing the patient at risk of invasive bacterial and fungal infections [68, 166, 169]. Neutropenia often responds to dose reduction and support with granulocyte-colony stimulating factor, but occasionally discontinuation

Table 30.2 Antiviral agents used for prophylaxis, pre-emptive therapy, and treatment of CMV disease after HSCT

Agent	Toxicities	Dose based on reason for use		
		Prophylaxis	Pre-emptive therapy	Treatment of disease
Acyclovir	Local injection reactions (IV), nephrotoxicity, headache, neuropsychiatric, nausea	IV: 500 mg/m^2 t.i.d. PO: 800 mg 4×/day or 600 mg/m^2 4×/day if <40 kg	Not recommended	Not recommended
Valacyclovir	Gastrointestinal up set, neutropenia, neuropsychiatric, nephrotoxicity, TTP/HUS	2 g 3–4×/day (>40 kg)	Not recommended	Not recommended
Ganciclovir	Neutropenia, anemia, thrombocytopenia, nephrotoxicity	Induction: 5 mg/kg b.i.d. Maintenance: 5 mg/kg/day	Induction: 5 mg/kg b.i.d. Maintenance: 5 mg/kg/day	Induction: 5 mg/kg b.i.d. Maintenance: 5 mg/kg/day
Valganciclovir	Neutropenia, headache, nausea, diarrhea, nephrotoxicity	Not established	Induction: 900 mg b.i.d. (>40 kg) Maintenance: 900 mg q.d. (>40 kg)	Not established
Cidofovir	Nephrotoxicity, neutropenia, ocular hypotony, uveitis, acidosis	Not established	Induction: 5 mg/kg/week × 2 doses Maintenance: 5 mg/kg every other week	Induction: 5 mg/kg every other week Maintenance: 5 mg/kg/every other week
Foscarnet	Nephrotoxicity, metabolic abonormalities, urethral irritation, anemia	Induction: 60 mg/kg b.i.d. Maintenance: 90–120	Induction: 60 mg/kg b.i.d. Maintenance: 90 mg/kg/day	Induction: 60 mg/kg t.i.d. Maintenance: 90 mg/kg/day

of ganciclovir is required, in which case foscarnet is typically the second-line agent of choice. Measurement of ganciclovir concentrations can be helpful to guide therapy and reduce the risk for toxicity especially in the situation of preexisting renal impairment.

Valganciclovir is the orally available prodrug of ganciclovir and achieves serum concentrations at least equivalent to intravenous ganciclovir [170–172]. The results of several uncontrolled studies suggest that valganciclovir is comparable to intravenous ganciclovir in terms of efficacy and safety when used as pre-emptive therapy after allogeneic HCT [170, 173–175]. As of the writing of this chapter, no data comparing valganciclovir to intravenous ganciclovir in the setting of a randomized, controlled trial have been published. Preliminary data from a randomized trial has been presented indicating little or no difference in efficacy or toxicity compared to intravenous ganciclovir [176]. Until more data is available, caution should be exercised when choosing valganciclovir as pre-emptive therapy.

Foscarnet is a pyrophosphate analog that binds directly to and competitively inhibits the CMV DNA polymerase. Foscarnet is generally considered to be as effective as ganciclovir for pre-emptive therapy after allogeneic transplantation [177]. However, three uncontrolled studies have documented cases of breakthrough CMV disease during foscarnet therapy [178–180]. These findings, combined with commonly encountered toxicities of foscarnet, have led to the use of foscarnet as a second-line agent when ganciclovir is contraindicated or not tolerated.

Cidofovir is a cytosine nucleotide analog that does not require phosphorylation by viral enzymes for antiviral activity. Cellular enzymes convert cidofovir to cidofovir triphosphate, which then inhibits the CMV DNA polymerase. The long half-life of cidofovir allows a once-per-week dosing schedule. However, the major toxicity with cidofovir – acute renal tubular necrosis – limits its utility after HCT and it should therefore be considered third-line therapy after ganciclovir and foscarnet [181].

Monitoring for CMV Infection and Initiation of Pre-Emptive Therapy

The current approach to prophylaxis and pre-emptive therapy has been recently summarized [157]. With the exception of those receiving ganciclovir prophylaxis, all patients who have undergone allogeneic HCT, regardless of pretransplant donor and recipient serostatus [182], should be monitored on a weekly basis for CMV infection using pp65 antigenemia, DNA PCR, or mRNA NASBA. If a pre-emptive strategy is used, the initial detection of CMV in peripheral blood after allogeneic HCT should prompt the initiation of antiviral therapy and a thorough evaluation of the patient in order to assess for signs and symptoms concerning for CMV disease [183].

Various durations of pre-emptive antiviral treatment have been explored. Initial studies administered ganciclovir until day 100 after engraftment, which ultimately entailed approximately 6–8 weeks of therapy in the average recipient. Studies from the mid 1990s using short courses (2–3 week) of ganciclovir based on negative PCR assays at the end of therapy were generally effective; however, resumption of pre-emptive therapy was necessary in approximately 30% of patients [62, 177, 184]. Most centers now continue antiviral treatment until the designated viral marker is negative and the patient has received at least 2 weeks of antiviral therapy [161]. If less sensitive markers than DNA PCR, such as the pp65 antigenemia assay, are used, then pre-emptive therapy should be continued until two negative assays are obtained [177]. If a patient is still viremic by PCR or pp65 antigenemia assay after 2 weeks of therapy, treatment should be extended at maintenance dosing until clearance is achieved. It has been shown that a low rate of viral load decrease is a risk factor for later-occurring CMV disease [72].

Monitoring is generally performed until day 100 after engraftment or longer in patients at risk for late CMV disease. The ideal duration and frequency of CMV monitoring in the later transplantation periods have not been determined [125, 126].

Routine monitoring of autograft recipients is not recommended, with the exception being high-risk patients as described above [159, 160, 183].

Special Populations

Patients with CMV infection occurring prior to planned allogeneic HCT have a very high risk of death after transplantation [185]. After transplantation, a patient with documented pretransplant CMV infection should either be monitored for CMV very closely (i.e., twice weekly), or be given prophylaxis with ganciclovir or foscarnet.

The optimal approach to CMV after CBT is not clear. One study described successful pre-emptive treatment with ganciclovir [140], while others combined high-dose valacyclovir prophylaxis with continued monitoring and pre-emptive therapy [115]. Due to initial experience in Seattle suggesting a high rate of infection and disease early posttransplant, the latter approach, coupled with ganciclovir prophylaxis for the week prior to transplant and continued CMV surveillance posttransplant, has been adopted.

Antiviral Resistance

Drug resistance is relatively uncommon after HCT but can occur with all drugs used for the treatment and prophylaxis of CMV and can be fatal [186]. Risk factors for drug resistance include prolonged (months) antiviral therapy, intermittent low-level viral replication in the presence of drug due to profound immunosuppression or suboptimal drug levels, and lack of prior immunity to CMV [187]. Drug resistance should be suspected in patients that are on an appropriate dosage of an antiviral drug and who have increasing quantitative viral loads for more than 2 weeks. After start of antiviral therapy in treatment-naïve patients, an increase in the viral load will occur in approximately one-third of patients and is likely due to the underlying immunosuppression, not true drug resistance [66]. If a patient has received ganciclovir before transplantation or if viral load increases occur in the late setting where most patients are not antiviral drug naïve anymore, drug resistance should be suspected.

An approach to the patient with suspected drug-resistant CMV is presented in Fig. 30.3. Since ganciclovir is used as a first-line agent in most cases of CMV infection, resistance to this antiviral is the most commonly encountered problem. Resistance is due most often to mutations in the UL97 gene, and less often to mutations in the UL54-encoded DNA polymerase. UL97 mutations that confer resistance have been described and genotypic assays are available for diagnostic analysis in reference laboratories [188]. Phenotypic testing can be performed, but this type of assay is time-consuming and is therefore not as helpful as rapid genotypic testing in guiding patient management. However, since different UL97 mutations confer varying degrees of ganciclovir resistance, some cases of genotypically-defined ganciclovir-resistant CMV may still respond to ganciclovir therapy, especially at higher doses [189]; therefore care must be taken in interpreting genotype results.

If ganciclovir resistance is documented or suspected, foscarnet is generally the second-line agent of choice. Unlike ganciclovir, foscarnet activity is not dependent on phosphorylation by the UL97 gene product; thus, CMV that has acquired ganciclovir resistance due to UL97 mutations will still be susceptible to foscarnet [190]. Studies evaluating the utility of combination therapy of foscarnet and ganciclovir for ganciclovir-resistant CMV disease have been inconclusive and therefore this strategy is not routinely recommended [191]. Resistance to foscarnet can occur and is due to

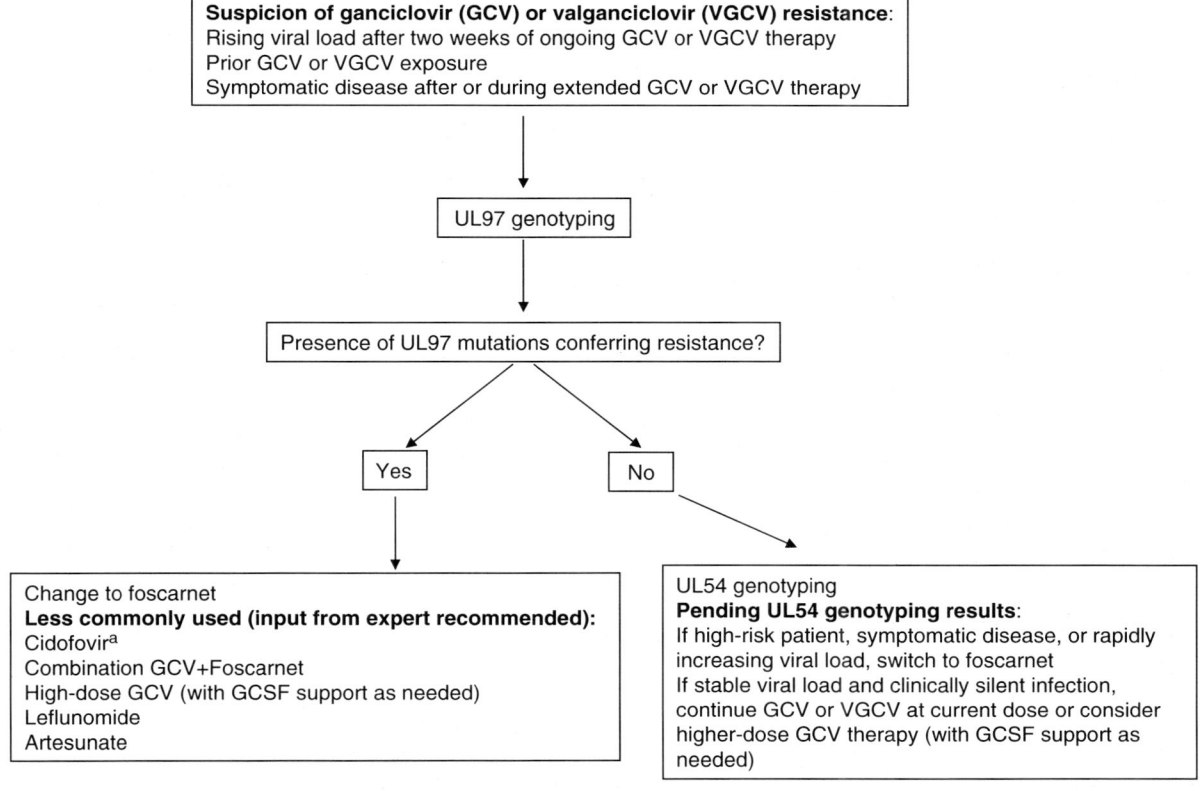

Fig. 30.3 Approach to the patient with suspected ganciclovir- or valganciclovir-resistant CMV

mutations in UL54. Interestingly, cross-resistance between foscarnet and ganciclovir does not occur, as mutations in UL54 conferring resistance to foscarnet occur in regions distinct from those conferring ganciclovir resistance [192].

Since cidofovir is not phosphorylated by the CMV UL97 gene product, it is active against ganciclovir-resistant UL97 mutants. However, certain UL54 mutations can confer causes cross-resistance between ganciclovir and cidofovir [190, 192]. Therefore, additional genotype testing of UL54 is indicated to evaluate for potential cross-resistance conferring mutations. There is limited experience with cidofovir for treatment of ganciclovir-resistant CMV, and its toxicity profile precludes its routine use as second-line treatment for ganciclovir-resistant CMV.

Drugs presently under evaluation, such as maribavir (especially at high doses), CMX001, an oral cidofovir derivative, and AIC 246, a inhibitor for late DNA synthesis, may also provide therapeutic options in the future [193–195]. Other licensed drugs with possible anti-CMV activity include the arthritis drug leflunomide and the antimalaria compound artesunate [196–198]. None of these are approved by European or American regulatory authorities for the treatment of CMV. Another potentially useful approach is to use the immunosuppressive drug sirolimus as adjunct therapy since it may impair CMV replication by regulating cellular signaling pathways, and has in fact been shown to reduce the risk of CMV reactivation after HCT and renal transplantation [111, 120].

Vaccination

Given the costs and toxicities associated with antiviral therapy, a vaccine to prevent CMV infection would be of substantial benefit. Indeed, the Institute of Medicine has given the development of a CMV vaccine highest priority [199]. Thus far, most vaccine candidates have yielded mixed results [200]. Recently, a phase I trial of a bivalent vaccine containing plasmids encoding gB and pp65 showed promising results in CMV-seronegative vaccine recipients, but not CMV-seropositive recipients, which is a limitation common to many CMV vaccine candidates [201]. Since it is the seropositive transplant patient who is at greatest risk for CMV infection, more work is required to provide protective immunity in these patients after HCT.

Management of CMV Disease

As mentioned earlier, the diagnosis of CMV disease requires documenting the presence of CMV in the appropriate diagnostic specimen, coupled with symptoms and signs consistent with CMV. For gastrointestinal disease, standard therapy generally entails induction treatment with an intravenous antiviral, most often ganciclovir, for 3–4 weeks followed by several weeks of maintenance. Shorter courses of induction therapy (2 weeks) are not as effective [202]. There is no role for concomitant intravenous immunoglobulin (IVIG) in the treatment of gastrointestinal disease [203]. Recurrence of GI disease may occur in approximately 30% of patients in the setting of continued immunosuppression and such patients may benefit from secondary prophylaxis with maintenance antivirals until immunosuppression has been reduced. Foscarnet can be used as an alternative if neutropenia is present. Valganciclovir as maintenance treatment for gastrointestinal disease has not been well studied but may be reasonable if symptoms are improved, systemic viremia is suppressed, and there are no factors that would impair the absorption of an orally-administered medication, such as severe gastrointestinal GVHD.

Several studies established the current standard of care for CMV pneumonia, which is treatment with ganciclovir (or foscarnet as an alternative agent) in combination with IVIG [204–207]. These studies showed improved survival rates compared to historical outcome results. There does not appear to be a specific advantage of CMV-specific immune globulin (CMV-Ig) compared to pooled immunoglobulin [205]. However, in specific clinical situations, such as volume overload, CMV-Ig may be preferred. Several studies have raised doubt regarding the beneficial effect of concomitant IVIG [208, 209]. However, while the use of IVIG remains a controversial topic, it is still considered as standard of care at many centers until more data regarding its utility is available.

CMV retinitis is typically treated with systemic ganciclovir, foscarnet, or cidofovir, with or without intraocular ganciclovir injections or implants [86, 210–212]. Fomivirsen is an antisense RNA molecule that targets mRNA encoded by CMV and is approved as second-line therapy for CMV retinitis in patients with AIDS [213].

Other manifestations of CMV disease, such as hepatitis and encephalitis, are uncommon and are typically managed with intravenous ganciclovir. The duration of therapy for these manifestations has not been well-established and should be tailored to the individual patient.

Adoptive Immunotherapy

HCMV-specific T cells can be generated via several different mechanisms in attempts to passively restore cellular immunity after transplantation [12]. Several groups have reported a beneficial impact of adoptive immunotherapy on HCMV viral loads in patients who had undergone HCT [214]. Despite these seemingly promising results, scientific questions remain unanswered (such as the optimal cell type and dose for infusion) and technical hurdles persist (widespread availability of clinical grade reagents) that preclude adoptive immunotherapy from becoming a routine clinical procedure at the current time.

CMV in the Non-HCT Setting

While not typically thought of as a commonly-occurring opportunistic infection among non-HCT cancer patients, the incidence of CMV disease increased between the years 1964 and 1990, likely due to the development of fludarabine and high-dose cyclophosphamide based regimens for the treatment of leukemia and lymphoma [215–219]. The highest rates, 8.8 and 11.4%, were seen in patients with chronic lymphoblastic leukemia and lymphoblastic lymphoma, respectively. More recently, the incidence of CMV disease, specifically pneumonia, appears to have declined, perhaps due to improved preventative strategies [220].

The increasing use of immunomodulating monoclonal antibodies poses a new and perhaps the greatest risk for CMV infection outside of the HCT setting [221]. Alemtuzumab is an anti-CD52 monoclonal antibody that results in CD4+ and CD8+ lymphopenia that can last for up to 9 months after administration. CMV infection typically occurs during the period of maximal immunosuppression, which is 3–6 weeks after alemtuzumab therapy [222, 223]. When alemtuzumab is used for the treatment of CLL, NHL, and T cell prolymphocytic leukemic, the rate of CMV reactivation typically ranges from 10 to 66%, depending on the underlying disease and whether alemtuzumab is given as first-line or salvage therapy [224–228], although one study reported 100% [229]. Approximately, 4–29% of CMV infections in this population will be symptomatic, manifesting primarily with fevers [222, 225, 229]. The precise incidence of visceral CMV disease in this population is not known.

The optimal approach to the patient being treated with alemtuzumab is not clear. Several studies have documented the efficacy of prophylactic valganciclovir or ganciclovir in preventing CMV infection during alemtuzumab therapy [230–232]. Other studies used pre-emptive therapy with oral ganciclovir or valganciclovir once CMV was detected, in addition to withholding further alemtuzumab treatment, to successfully prevent CMV disease [225, 233]. Which strategy is superior in this population is not known. If routine prophylaxis is not used, patients receiving alemtuzumab should be monitored for CMV infection for a period of approximately 2 months after receipt of the last dose [183, 222, 234]. Detection of CMV by either PCR or pp65 antigenemia during alemtuzumab therapy should prompt a thorough evaluation for evidence of end-organ disease. Symptomatic infection or the presence of visceral disease always requires treatment, but the optimal management of asymptomatic infection is not clear, as many patients with asymptomatic CMV infection may not develop CMV disease despite the absence of anti-CMV therapy. Options in the latter situation include the administration of antivirals versus continued close viral monitoring combined with clinical observation [159]. Controversy also exists regarding the question of whether to withhold further alemtuzumab therapy in the setting of CMV infection. Some do not feel that asymptomatic CMV infection requires discontinuation of alemtuzumab [183, 222, 229, 235, 236], but several studies have withheld alemtuzumab treatment during CMV viremia [225, 231] and therefore this practice has been advocated by some groups [237]. Thus, the optimal approach to the patient receiving alemtuzumab is not clear at the present time and will certainly require further study.

Routine screening of asymptomatic patients with hematological malignancies undergoing treatment with conventional chemotherapy, hyperCVAD, fludarabine, or rituximab is not recommended due to the relatively low rate of CMV disease [238].

Summary

While much progress has been made in the prevention of CMV disease after HCT over the past decade, several issues remain. Increasing the specificity of pre-emptive therapy by combining detection of viremia with monitoring of CMV-specific T-cell immunity merits evaluation in a randomized trial. CMV pneumonia still carries a poor prognosis that outcome has not significantly changed in the past 20 years. Therefore, other strategies, such as combination antiviral therapy, should be studied in this setting in order to improve outcome. Additionally, the benefit provided by IVIG in the treatment of CMV pneumonia needs to be determined. New treatment and vaccination options for CMV are urgently needed because the currently available drugs have major limitations, such as toxicity and resistance. Novel drugs such as lipid cidofovir [239], a novel nonnucleoside inhibitor [194], as well as leflunomide and artesunate, deserve a systematic evaluation. Vaccination may also play an increasing role in the future prevention of CMV infection and disease.

Acknowledgments Per Ljungman had support from Karolinska Institutet research funds and the Swedish Children's Cancer Fund. Michael Boeckh had support from the National Institute of Health (NIH CA 18029, HL93294).

References

1. Mocarski ES, Shenk T, Pass RF. Cytomegaloviruses. In: Knipe DM, Howley PM, editors. Fields virology. 5th ed. Philadelphia: Lippincott Williams & Wilkins; 2007. p. 2701–72.
2. Murphy E, Yu D, Grimwood J, et al. Coding potential of laboratory and clinical strains of human cytomegalovirus. Proc Natl Acad Sci USA. 2003;100(25):14976–81.
3. Sinzger C, Digel M, Jahn G. Cytomegalovirus cell tropism. Curr Top Microbiol Immunol. 2008;325:63–83.
4. Bolovan-Fritts CA, Mocarski ES, Wiedeman JA. Peripheral blood CD14(+) cells from healthy subjects carry a circular conformation of latent cytomegalovirus genome. Blood. 1999;93(1):394–8.
5. Kondo K, Kaneshima H, Mocarski ES. Human cytomegalovirus latent infection of granulocyte-macrophage progenitors. Proc Natl Acad Sci USA. 1994;91(25):11879–83.
6. Taylor-Wiedeman J, Sissons JG, Borysiewicz LK, Sinclair JH. Monocytes are a major site of persistence of human cytomegalovirus in peripheral blood mononuclear cells. J Gen Virol. 1991;72(Pt 9):2059–64.
7. Britt WJ, Vugler L, Butfiloski EJ, Stephens EB. Cell surface expression of human cytomegalovirus (HCMV) gp55-116 (gB): use of HCMV-recombinant vaccinia virus-infected cells in analysis of the human neutralizing antibody response. J Virol. 1990;64(3):1079–85.
8. Marshall GS, Rabalais GP, Stout GG, Waldeyer SL. Antibodies to recombinant-derived glycoprotein B after natural human cytomegalovirus infection correlate with neutralizing activity. J Infect Dis. 1992;165(2):381–4.
9. Rasmussen L, Matkin C, Spaete R, Pachl C, Merigan TC. Antibody response to human cytomegalovirus glycoproteins gB and gH after natural infection in humans. J Infect Dis. 1991;164(5):835–42.
10. Boppana SB, Britt WJ. Antiviral antibody responses and intrauterine transmission after primary maternal cytomegalovirus infection. J Infect Dis. 1995;171(5):1115–21.
11. Jonjic S, Pavic I, Lucin P, Rukavina D, Koszinowski UH. Efficacious control of cytomegalovirus infection after long-term depletion of CD8+ T lymphocytes. J Virol. 1990;64(11):5457–64.
12. Crough T, Khanna R. Immunobiology of human cytomegalovirus: from bench to bedside. Clin Microbiol Rev. 2009;22(1):76–98, Table of Contents.
13. Gillespie GM, Wills MR, Appay V, et al. Functional heterogeneity and high frequencies of cytomegalovirus-specific CD8(+) T lymphocytes in healthy seropositive donors. J Virol. 2000;74(17):8140–50.
14. Khan N, Cobbold M, Keenan R, Moss PA. Comparative analysis of CD8+ T cell responses against human cytomegalovirus proteins pp 65 and immediate early 1 shows similarities in precursor frequency, oligoclonality, and phenotype. J Infect Dis. 2002;185(8):1025–34.
15. Khan N, Hislop A, Gudgeon N, et al. Herpesvirus-specific CD8 T cell immunity in old age: cytomegalovirus impairs the response to a coresident EBV infection. J Immunol. 2004;173(12):7481–9.
16. Ouyang Q, Wagner WM, Wikby A, et al. Large numbers of dysfunctional CD8+ T lymphocytes bearing receptors for a single dominant CMV epitope in the very old. J Clin Immunol. 2003;23(4):247–57.
17. Sylwester AW, Mitchell BL, Edgar JB, et al. Broadly targeted human cytomegalovirus-specific CD4+ and CD8+ T cells dominate the memory compartments of exposed subjects. J Exp Med. 2005;202(5):673–85.
18. Elkington R, Walker S, Crough T, et al. Ex vivo profiling of CD8+-T-cell responses to human cytomegalovirus reveals broad and multispecific reactivities in healthy virus carriers. J Virol. 2003;77(9):5226–40.
19. Kern F, Bunde T, Faulhaber N, et al. Cytomegalovirus (CMV) phosphoprotein 65 makes a large contribution to shaping the T cell repertoire in CMV-exposed individuals. J Infect Dis. 2002;185(12):1709–16.
20. Kern F, Surel IP, Faulhaber N, et al. Target structures of the CD8(+)-T-cell response to human cytomegalovirus: the 72-kilodalton major immediate-early protein revisited. J Virol. 1999;73(10):8179–84.
21. Khan N, Best D, Bruton R, Nayak L, Rickinson AB, Moss PA. T cell recognition patterns of immunodominant cytomegalovirus antigens in primary and persistent infection. J Immunol. 2007;178(7):4455–65.
22. Khan N, Bruton R, Taylor GS, et al. Identification of cytomegalovirus-specific cytotoxic T lymphocytes in vitro is greatly enhanced by the use of recombinant virus lacking the US2 to US11 region or modified vaccinia virus Ankara expressing individual viral genes. J Virol. 2005;79(5):2869–79.
23. Kondo E, Akatsuka Y, Kuzushima K, et al. Identification of novel CTL epitopes of CMV-pp 65 presented by a variety of HLA alleles. Blood. 2004;103(2):630–8.
24. Li CR, Greenberg PD, Gilbert MJ, Goodrich JM, Riddell SR. Recovery of HLA-restricted cytomegalovirus (CMV)-specific T-cell responses after allogeneic bone marrow transplant: correlation with CMV disease and effect of ganciclovir prophylaxis. Blood. 1994;83(7):1971–9.
25. Polic B, Hengel H, Krmpotic A, et al. Hierarchical and redundant lymphocyte subset control precludes cytomegalovirus replication during latent infection. J Exp Med. 1998;188(6):1047–54.
26. Quinnan Jr GV, Kirmani N, Rook AH, et al. Cytotoxic t cells in cytomegalovirus infection: HLA-restricted T-lymphocyte and non-T-lymphocyte cytotoxic responses correlate with recovery from cytomegalovirus infection in bone-marrow-transplant recipients. N Engl J Med. 1982;307(1):7–13.
27. Reusser P, Cathomas G, Attenhofer R, Tamm M, Thiel G. Cytomegalovirus (CMV)-specific T cell immunity after renal transplantation mediates protection from CMV disease by limiting the systemic virus load. J Infect Dis. 1999;180(2):247–53.
28. Reusser P, Riddell SR, Meyers JD, Greenberg PD. Cytotoxic T-lymphocyte response to cytomegalovirus after human allogeneic bone marrow transplantation: pattern of recovery and correlation with cytomegalovirus infection and disease. Blood. 1991;78(5):1373–80.
29. Hebart H, Daginik S, Stevanovic S, et al. Sensitive detection of human cytomegalovirus peptide-specific cytotoxic T-lymphocyte responses by interferon-gamma-enzyme-linked immunospot assay and flow cytometry in healthy individuals and in patients after allogeneic stem cell transplantation. Blood. 2002;99(10):3830–7.
30. Krause H, Hebart H, Jahn G, Muller CA, Einsele H. Screening for CMV-specific T cell proliferation to identify patients at risk of developing late onset CMV disease. Bone Marrow Transplant. 1997;19(11):1111–6.
31. Ljungman P, Aschan J, Azinge JN, et al. Cytomegalovirus viraemia and specific T-helper cell responses as predictors of disease after allogeneic marrow transplantation. Br J Haematol. 1993;83(1):118–24.
32. Boeckh M, Leisenring W, Riddell SR, et al. Late cytomegalovirus disease and mortality in recipients of allogeneic hematopoietic stem cell transplants: importance of viral load and T-cell immunity. Blood. 2003;101(2):407–14.
33. Einsele H, Roosnek E, Rufer N, et al. Infusion of cytomegalovirus (CMV)-specific T cells for the treatment of CMV infection not responding to antiviral chemotherapy. Blood. 2002;99(11):3916–22.
34. Boehme KW, Guerrero M, Compton T. Human cytomegalovirus envelope glycoproteins B and H are necessary for TLR2 activation in permissive cells. J Immunol. 2006;177(10):7094–102.

35. Compton T, Kurt-Jones EA, Boehme KW, et al. Human cytomegalovirus activates inflammatory cytokine responses via CD14 and Toll-like receptor 2. J Virol. 2003;77(8):4588–96.
36. Juckem LK, Boehme KW, Feire AL, Compton T. Differential initiation of innate immune responses induced by human cytomegalovirus entry into fibroblast cells. J Immunol. 2008;180(7):4965–77.
37. Kijpittayarit S, Eid AJ, Brown RA, Paya CV, Razonable RR. Relationship between Toll-like receptor 2 polymorphism and cytomegalovirus disease after liver transplantation. Clin Infect Dis. 2007;44(10):1315–20.
38. Delale T, Paquin A, Asselin-Paturel C, et al. MyD88-dependent and -independent murine cytomegalovirus sensing for IFN-alpha release and initiation of immune responses in vivo. J Immunol. 2005;175(10):6723–32.
39. Tabeta K, Georgel P, Janssen E, et al. Toll-like receptors 9 and 3 as essential components of innate immune defense against mouse cytomegalovirus infection. Proc Natl Acad Sci USA. 2004; 101(10):3516–21.
40. Brown MG, Dokun AO, Heusel JW, et al. Vital involvement of a natural killer cell activation receptor in resistance to viral infection. Science. 2001;292(5518):934–7.
41. Bukowski JF, Warner JF, Dennert G, Welsh RM. Adoptive transfer studies demonstrating the antiviral effect of natural killer cells in vivo. J Exp Med. 1985;161(1):40–52.
42. Bukowski JF, Woda BA, Habu S, Okumura K, Welsh RM. Natural killer cell depletion enhances virus synthesis and virus-induced hepatitis in vivo. J Immunol. 1983;131(3):1531–8.
43. Scalzo AA, Fitzgerald NA, Simmons A, La Vista AB, Shellam GR. Cmv-1, a genetic locus that controls murine cytomegalovirus replication in the spleen. J Exp Med. 1990;171(5):1469–83.
44. Scalzo AA, Fitzgerald NA, Wallace CR, et al. The effect of the Cmv-1 resistance gene, which is linked to the natural killer cell gene complex, is mediated by natural killer cells. J Immunol. 1992;149(2):581–9.
45. Biron CA, Byron KS, Sullivan JL. Severe herpesvirus infections in an adolescent without natural killer cells. N Engl J Med. 1989;320(26):1731–5.
46. Chen C, Busson M, Rocha V, et al. Activating KIR genes are associated with CMV reactivation and survival after non-T-cell depleted HLA-identical sibling bone marrow transplantation for malignant disorders. Bone Marrow Transplant. 2006;38(6):437–44.
47. Cook M, Briggs D, Craddock C, et al. Donor KIR genotype has a major influence on the rate of cytomegalovirus reactivation following T-cell replete stem cell transplantation. Blood. 2006;107(3):1230–2.
48. Zaia JA, Sun JY, Gallez-Hawkins GM, et al. The effect of single and combined activating killer immunoglobulin-like receptor genotypes on cytomegalovirus infection and immunity after hematopoietic cell transplantation. Biol Blood Marrow Transplant. 2009;15(3):315–25.
49. Loeffler J, Steffens M, Arlt EM, et al. Polymorphisms in the genes encoding chemokine receptor 5, interleukin-10, and monocyte chemoattractant protein 1 contribute to cytomegalovirus reactivation and disease after allogeneic stem cell transplantation. J Clin Microbiol. 2006;44(5):1847–50.
50. Goldmacher VS, Bartle LM, Skaletskaya A, et al. A cytomegalovirus-encoded mitochondria-localized inhibitor of apoptosis structurally unrelated to Bcl-2. Proc Natl Acad Sci USA. 1999;96(22):12536–41.
51. Basta S, Bennink JR. A survival game of hide and seek: cytomegaloviruses and MHC class I antigen presentation pathways. Viral Immunol. 2003;16(3):231–42.
52. Abate DA, Watanabe S, Mocarski ES. Major human cytomegalovirus structural protein pp 65 (ppUL83) prevents interferon response factor 3 activation in the interferon response. J Virol. 2004;78(20):10995–1006.
53. Child SJ, Hakki M, De Niro KL, Geballe AP. Evasion of cellular antiviral responses by human cytomegalovirus TRS1 and IRS1. J Virol. 2004;78(1):197–205.
54. Taylor RT, Bresnahan WA. Human cytomegalovirus immediate-early 2 gene expression blocks virus-induced beta interferon production. J Virol. 2005;79(6):3873–7.
55. Taylor RT, Bresnahan WA. Human cytomegalovirus immediate-early 2 protein IE86 blocks virus-induced chemokine expression. J Virol. 2006;80(2):920–8.
56. Benedict CA, Butrovich KD, Lurain NS, et al. Cutting edge: a novel viral TNF receptor superfamily member in virulent strains of human cytomegalovirus. J Immunol. 1999;162(12): 6967–70.
57. Chapman TL, Heikeman AP, Bjorkman PJ. The inhibitory receptor LIR-1 uses a common binding interaction to recognize class I MHC molecules and the viral homolog UL18. Immunity. 1999;11(5):603–13.
58. Gao JL, Murphy PM. Human cytomegalovirus open reading frame US28 encodes a functional beta chemokine receptor. J Biol Chem. 1994;269(46):28539–42.
59. Kotenko SV, Saccani S, Izotova LS, Mirochnitchenko OV, Pestka S. Human cytomegalovirus harbors its own unique IL-10 homolog (cmvIL-10). Proc Natl Acad Sci USA. 2000;97(4):1695–700.
60. Penfold ME, Dairaghi DJ, Duke GM, et al. Cytomegalovirus encodes a potent alpha chemokine. Proc Natl Acad Sci USA. 1999;96(17):9839–44.
61. Boeckh M, Boivin G. Quantitation of cytomegalovirus: methodologic aspects and clinical applications. Clin Microbiol Rev. 1998;11(3):533–54.
62. Einsele H, Ehninger G, Hebart H, et al. Polymerase chain reaction monitoring reduces the incidence of cytomegalovirus disease and the duration and side effects of antiviral therapy after bone marrow transplantation. Blood. 1995;86(7):2815–20.
63. Meyers JD, Ljungman P, Fisher LD. Cytomegalovirus excretion as a predictor of cytomegalovirus disease after marrow transplantation: importance of cytomegalovirus viremia. J Infect Dis. 1990;162(2):373–80.
64. Crawford SW, Bowden RA, Hackman RC, Gleaves CA, Meyers JD, Clark JG. Rapid detection of cytomegalovirus pulmonary infection by bronchoalveolar lavage and centrifugation culture. Ann Intern Med. 1988;108(2):180–5.
65. Boeckh M, Bowden RA, Goodrich JM, Pettinger M, Meyers JD. Cytomegalovirus antigen detection in peripheral blood leukocytes after allogeneic marrow transplantation. Blood. 1992;80(5): 1358–64.
66. Nichols WG, Corey L, Gooley T, et al. Rising pp 65 antigenemia during preemptive anticytomegalovirus therapy after allogeneic hematopoietic stem cell transplantation: risk factors, correlation with DNA load, and outcomes. Blood. 2001;97(4):867–74.
67. Boeckh M, Huang M, Ferrenberg J, et al. Optimization of quantitative detection of cytomegalovirus DNA in plasma by real-time PCR. J Clin Microbiol. 2004;42(3):1142–8.
68. Boeckh M, Gooley TA, Myerson D, Cunningham T, Schoch G, Bowden RA. Cytomegalovirus pp 65 antigenemia-guided early treatment with ganciclovir versus ganciclovir at engraftment after allogeneic marrow transplantation: a randomized double-blind study. Blood. 1996;88(10):4063–71.
69. Einsele H, Hebart H, Kauffmann-Schneider C, et al. Risk factors for treatment failures in patients receiving PCR-based preemptive therapy for CMV infection. Bone Marrow Transplant. 2000; 25(7):757–63.
70. Emery VC, Griffiths PD. Prediction of cytomegalovirus load and resistance patterns after antiviral chemotherapy. Proc Natl Acad Sci USA. 2000;97(14):8039–44.
71. Gor D, Sabin C, Prentice HG, et al. Longitudinal fluctuations in cytomegalovirus load in bone marrow transplant patients: relationship

between peak virus load, donor/recipient serostatus, acute GVHD and CMV disease. Bone Marrow Transplant. 1998;21(6): 597–605.
72. Ljungman P, Perez-Bercoff L, Jonsson J, et al. Risk factors for the development of cytomegalovirus disease after allogeneic stem cell transplantation. Haematologica. 2006;91(1):78–83.
73. Cathomas G, Morris P, Pekle K, Cunningham I, Emanuel D. Rapid diagnosis of cytomegalovirus pneumonia in marrow transplant recipients by bronchoalveolar lavage using the polymerase chain reaction, virus culture, and the direct immunostaining of alveolar cells. Blood. 1993;81(7):1909–14.
74. Gerna G, Lilleri D, Baldanti F, et al. Human cytomegalovirus immediate-early mRNAemia versus pp 65 antigenemia for guiding pre-emptive therapy in children and young adults undergoing hematopoietic stem cell transplantation: a prospective, randomized, open-label trial. Blood. 2003;101(12):5053–60.
75. Hebart H, Ljungman P, Klingebiel T, et al. Prospective comparison of PCR-based versus late mRNA-based preemptive antiviral therapy for HCMV infection in patients after allogeneic stem cell transplantation. Blood. 2003;102(11):195a.
76. Collier AC, Chandler SH, Handsfield HH, Corey L, McDougall JK. Identification of multiple strains of cytomegalovirus in homosexual men. J Infect Dis. 1989;159(1):123–6.
77. Manuel O, Pang XL, Humar A, Kumar D, Doucette K, Preiksaitis JK. An assessment of donor-to-recipient transmission patterns of human cytomegalovirus by analysis of viral genomic variants. J Infect Dis. 2009;199(11):1621–8.
78. Ljungman P, Griffiths P, Paya C. Definitions of cytomegalovirus infection and disease in transplant recipients. Clin Infect Dis. 2002;34(8):1094–7.
79. Boeckh M, Stevens-Ayers T, Bowden RA. Cytomegalovirus pp 65 antigenemia after autologous marrow and peripheral blood stem cell transplantation. J Infect Dis. 1996;174(5):907–12.
80. Konoplev S, Champlin RE, Giralt S, et al. Cytomegalovirus pneumonia in adult autologous blood and marrow transplant recipients. Bone Marrow Transplant. 2001;27(8):877–81.
81. Ljungman P. Cytomegalovirus pneumonia: presentation, diagnosis, and treatment. Semin Respir Infect. 1995;10(4):209–15.
82. Schmidt GM, Horak DA, Niland JC, Duncan SR, Forman SJ, Zaia JA. A randomized, controlled trial of prophylactic ganciclovir for cytomegalovirus pulmonary infection in recipients of allogeneic bone marrow transplants; The City of Hope-Stanford-Syntex CMV Study Group. N Engl J Med. 1991;324(15):1005–11.
83. Jang EY, Park SY, Lee EJ, et al. Diagnostic performance of the cytomegalovirus (CMV) antigenemia assay in patients with CMV gastrointestinal disease. Clin Infect Dis. 2009;48(12):e121–4.
84. Mori T, Okamoto S, Matsuoka S, et al. Risk-adapted pre-emptive therapy for cytomegalovirus disease in patients undergoing allogeneic bone marrow transplantation. Bone Marrow Transplant. 2000;25(7):765–9.
85. Coskuncan NM, Jabs DA, Dunn JP, et al. The eye in bone marrow transplantation. VI. Retinal complications. Arch Ophthalmol. 1994;112(3):372–9.
86. Crippa F, Corey L, Chuang EL, Sale G, Boeckh M. Virological, clinical, and ophthalmologic features of cytomegalovirus retinitis after hematopoietic stem cell transplantation. Clin Infect Dis. 2001;32(2):214–9.
87. Eid AJ, Bakri SJ, Kijpittayarit S, Razonable RR. Clinical features and outcomes of cytomegalovirus retinitis after transplantation. Transpl Infect Dis. 2008;10(1):13–8.
88. Larsson K, Lonnqvist B, Ringden O, Hedquist B, Ljungman P. CMV retinitis after allogeneic bone marrow transplantation: a report of five cases. Transpl Infect Dis. 2002;4(2):75–9.
89. Nichols WG, Corey L, Gooley T, Davis C, Boeckh M. High risk of death due to bacterial and fungal infection among cytomegalovirus (CMV)-seronegative recipients of stem cell transplants from seropositive donors: evidence for indirect effects of primary CMV infection. J Infect Dis. 2002;185(3):273–82.
90. Boeckh M. Current antiviral strategies for controlling cytomegalovirus in hematopoietic stem cell transplant recipients: prevention and therapy. Transpl Infect Dis. 1999;1(3):165–78.
91. Broers AE, van Der Holt R, van Esser JW, et al. Increased transplant-related morbidity and mortality in CMV- seropositive patients despite highly effective prevention of CMV disease after allogeneic T-cell-depleted stem cell transplantation. Blood. 2000;95(7):2240–5.
92. Craddock C, Szydlo RM, Dazzi F, et al. Cytomegalovirus seropositivity adversely influences outcome after T-depleted unrelated donor transplant in patients with chronic myeloid leukaemia: the case for tailored graft-versus-host disease prophylaxis. Br J Haematol. 2001;112(1):228–36.
93. Behrendt CE, Rosenthal J, Bolotin E, Nakamura R, Zaia J, Forman SJ. Donor and recipient CMV serostatus and outcome of pediatric allogeneic HSCT for acute leukemia in the era of CMV-preemptive therapy. Biol Blood Marrow Transplant. 2009;15(1):54–60.
94. Boeckh M, Nichols WG. The impact of cytomegalovirus serostatus of donor and recipient before hematopoietic stem cell transplantation in the era of antiviral prophylaxis and preemptive therapy. Blood. 2004;103(6):2003–8.
95. Bordon V, Bravo S, Van Renterghem L, et al. Surveillance of cytomegalovirus (CMV) DNAemia in pediatric allogeneic stem cell transplantation: incidence and outcome of CMV infection and disease. Transpl Infect Dis. 2008;10(1):19–23.
96. Cwynarski K, Roberts IA, Iacobelli S, et al. Stem cell transplantation for chronic myeloid leukemia in children. Blood. 2003;102(4):1224–31.
97. Erard V, Guthrie KA, Riddell S, Boeckh M. Impact of HLA A2 and cytomegalovirus serostatus on outcomes in patients with leukemia following matched-sibling myeloablative allogeneic hematopoietic cell transplantation. Haematologica. 2006;91(10):1377–83.
98. Grob JP, Grundy JE, Prentice HG, et al. Immune donors can protect marrow-transplant recipients from severe cytomegalovirus infections. Lancet. 1987;1(8536):774–6.
99. Jacobsen N, Badsberg JH, Lonnqvist B, et al. Graft-versus-leukaemia activity associated with CMV-seropositive donor, posttransplant CMV infection, young donor age and chronic graft-versus-host disease in bone marrow allograft recipients. The Nordic Bone Marrow Transplantation Group. Bone Marrow Transplant. 1990;5(6):413–8.
100. Kollman C, Howe CW, Anasetti C, et al. Donor characteristics as risk factors in recipients after transplantation of bone marrow from unrelated donors: the effect of donor age. Blood. 2001;98(7): 2043–51.
101. Ljungman P, Einsele H, Frassoni F, Niederwieser D, Cordonnier C. Donor CMV serological status influences the outcome of CMVseropositive recipients after unrelated donor stem cell transplantation; an EBMT Megafile analysis. Blood. 2003;102: 4255–60.
102. Nachbaur D, Clausen J, Kircher B. Donor cytomegalovirus seropositivity and the risk of leukemic relapse after reduced-intensity transplants. Eur J Haematol. 2006;76(5):414–9.
103. Ringden O, Schaffer M, Le Blanc K, et al. Which donor should be chosen for hematopoietic stem cell transplantation among unrelated HLA-A, -B, and -DRB1 genomically identical volunteers? Biol Blood Marrow Transplant. 2004;10(2):128–34.
104. Jernberg AG, Remberger M, Ringden O, Winiarski J. Risk factors in pediatric stem cell transplantation for leukemia. Pediatr Transplant. 2004;8(5):464–74.
105. Avetisyan G, Aschan J, Hagglund H, Ringden O, Ljungman P. Evaluation of intervention strategy based on CMV-specific immune responses after allogeneic SCT. Bone Marrow Transplant. 2007;40(9):865–9.

106. Ganepola S, Gentilini C, Hilbers U, et al. Patients at high risk for CMV infection and disease show delayed CD8+ T-cell immune recovery after allogeneic stem cell transplantation. Bone Marrow Transplant. 2007;39(5):293–9.
107. Lilleri D, Fornara C, Chiesa A, Caldera D, Alessandrino EP, Gerna G. Human cytomegalovirus-specific CD4+ and CD8+ T-cell reconstitution in adult allogeneic hematopoietic stem cell transplant recipients and immune control of viral infection. Haematologica. 2008;93(2):248–56.
108. Moins-Teisserenc H, Busson M, Scieux C, et al. Patterns of cytomegalovirus reactivation are associated with distinct evolutive profiles of immune reconstitution after allogeneic hematopoeitic stem cell transplantation. J Infect Dis. 2008;198(6):818–26.
109. Lin TS, Zahrieh D, Weller E, Alyea EP, Antin JH, Soiffer RJ. Risk factors for cytomegalovirus reactivation after CD6+ T-cell-depleted allogeneic bone marrow transplantation. Transplantation. 2002;74(1):49–54.
110. Ozdemir E, Saliba R, Champlin R, et al. Risk factors associated with late cytomegalovirus reactivation after allogeneic stem cell transplantation for hematological malignancies. Bone Marrow Transplant. 2007;40(2):125–36.
111. Marty FM, Bryar J, Browne SK, et al. Sirolimus-based graft-versus-host disease prophylaxis protects against cytomegalovirus reactivation after allogeneic hematopoietic stem cell transplantation: a cohort analysis. Blood. 2007;110(2):490–500.
112. Ljungman P, Aschan J, Lewensohn-Fuchs I, et al. Results of different strategies for reducing cytomegalovirus-associated mortality in allogeneic stem cell transplant recipients. Transplantation. 1998;66(10):1330–4.
113. Martino R, Rovira M, Carreras E, et al. Severe infections after allogeneic peripheral blood stem cell transplantation: a matched-pair comparison of unmanipulated and CD34+ cell-selected transplantation. Haematologica. 2001;86(10):1075–86.
114. Miller W, Flynn P, McCullough J, et al. Cytomegalovirus infection after bone marrow transplantation: an association with acute graft-v-host disease. Blood. 1986;67(4):1162–7.
115. Walker CM, van Burik JA, De For TE, Weisdorf DJ. Cytomegalovirus infection after allogeneic transplantation: comparison of cord blood with peripheral blood and marrow graft sources. Biol Blood Marrow Transplant. 2007;13(9):1106–15.
116. Nakamae H, Kirby KA, Sandmaier BM, et al. Effect of conditioning regimen intensity on CMV infection in allogeneic hematopoietic cell transplantation. Biol Blood Marrow Transplant. 2009;15(6):694–703.
117. Islam MS, Anoop P, Rice P, et al. Early cytomegalovirus infections following allogeneic stem cell transplantation: a comparison between non-malignant and malignant haematological disorders. Hematology. 2010;15(1):4–10.
118. Holmberg LA, Boeckh M, Hooper H, et al. Increased incidence of cytomegalovirus disease after autologous CD34-selected peripheral blood stem cell transplantation. Blood. 1999;94(12):4029–35.
119. Trenschel R, Ross S, Husing J, et al. Reduced risk of persisting cytomegalovirus pp 65 antigenemia and cytomegalovirus interstitial pneumonia following allogeneic PBSCT. Bone Marrow Transplant. 2000;25(6):665–72.
120. Kudchodkar SB, Yu Y, Maguire TG, Alwine JC. Human cytomegalovirus infection alters the substrate specificities and rapamycin sensitivities of raptor- and rictor-containing complexes. Proc Natl Acad Sci USA. 2006;103(38):14182–7.
121. Einsele H, Steidle M, Vallbracht A, Saal JG, Ehninger G, Muller CA. Early occurrence of human cytomegalovirus infection after bone marrow transplantation as demonstrated by the polymerase chain reaction technique. Blood. 1991;77(5):1104–10.
122. Nguyen Q, Champlin R, Giralt S, et al. Late cytomegalovirus pneumonia in adult allogeneic blood and marrow transplant recipients. Clin Infect Dis. 1999;28(3):618–23.
123. Machado CM, Menezes RX, Macedo MC, et al. Extended antigenemia surveillance and late cytomegalovirus infection after allogeneic BMT. Bone Marrow Transplant. 2001;28(11):1053–9.
124. Osarogiagbon RU, Defor TE, Weisdorf MA, Erice A, Weisdorf DJ. CMV antigenemia following bone marrow transplantation: risk factors and outcomes. Biol Blood Marrow Transplant. 2000;6(3):280–8.
125. Peggs KS, Preiser W, Kottaridis PD, et al. Extended routine polymerase chain reaction surveillance and pre-emptive antiviral therapy for cytomegalovirus after allogeneic transplantation. Br J Haematol. 2000;111(3):782–90.
126. Junghanss C, Boeckh M, Carter RA, et al. Incidence and outcome of cytomegalovirus infections following nonmyeloablative compared with myeloablative allogeneic stem cell transplantation, a matched control study. Blood. 2002;99(6):1978–85.
127. Safdar A, Rodriguez GH, Mihu CN, et al. Infections in non-myeloablative hematopoietic stem cell transplantation patients with lymphoid malignancies: spectrum of infections, predictors of outcome and proposed guidelines for fungal infection prevention. Bone Marrow Transplant. 2010;45(2):339–47.
128. Chakrabarti S, Mackinnon S, Chopra R, et al. High incidence of cytomegalovirus infection after nonmyeloablative stem cell transplantation: potential role of Campath-1H in delaying immune reconstitution. Blood. 2002;99(12):4357–63.
129. Hebart H, Schroder A, Loffler J, et al. Cytomegalovirus monitoring by polymerase chain reaction of whole blood samples from patients undergoing autologous bone marrow or peripheral blood progenitor cell transplantation. J Infect Dis. 1997;175(6):1490–3.
130. Bilgrami S, Aslanzadeh J, Feingold JM, et al. Cytomegalovirus viremia, viruria and disease after autologous peripheral blood stem cell transplantation: no need for surveillance. Bone Marrow Transplant. 1999;24(1):69–73.
131. Boeckh M, Gooley TA, Reusser P, Buckner CD, Bowden RA. Failure of high-dose acyclovir to prevent cytomegalovirus disease after autologous marrow transplantation. J Infect Dis. 1995;172(4):939–43.
132. Singhal S, Powles R, Treleaven J, et al. Cytomegaloviremia after autografting for leukemia: clinical significance and lack of effect on engraftment. Leukemia. 1997;11(6):835–8.
133. Enright H, Haake R, Weisdorf D, et al. Cytomegalovirus pneumonia after bone marrow transplantation. Risk factors and response to therapy. Transplantation. 1993;55(6):1339–46.
134. Reusser P, Fisher LD, Buckner CD, Thomas ED, Meyers JD. Cytomegalovirus infection after autologous bone marrow transplantation: occurrence of cytomegalovirus disease and effect on engraftment. Blood. 1990;75(9):1888–94.
135. Schoemans H, Theunissen K, Maertens J, Boogaerts M, Verfaillie C, Wagner J. Adult umbilical cord blood transplantation: a comprehensive review. Bone Marrow Transplant. 2006;38(2):83–93.
136. Albano MS, Taylor P, Pass RF, et al. Umbilical cord blood transplantation and cytomegalovirus: posttransplantation infection and donor screening. Blood. 2006;108(13):4275–82.
137. Matsumura T, Narimatsu H, Kami M, et al. Cytomegalovirus infections following umbilical cord blood transplantation using reduced intensity conditioning regimens for adult patients. Biol Blood Marrow Transplant. 2007;13(5):577–83.
138. Saavedra S, Sanz GF, Jarque I, et al. Early infections in adult patients undergoing unrelated donor cord blood transplantation. Bone Marrow Transplant. 2002;30(12):937–43.
139. Takami A, Mochizuki K, Asakura H, Yamazaki H, Okumura H, Nakao S. High incidence of cytomegalovirus reactivation in adult recipients of an unrelated cord blood transplant. Haematologica. 2005;90(9):1290–2.
140. Tomonari A, Takahashi S, Ooi J, et al. Preemptive therapy with ganciclovir 5 mg/kg once daily for cytomegalovirus infection after unrelated cord blood transplantation. Bone Marrow Transplant. 2008;41(4):371–6.

141. Beck JC, Wagner JE, DeFor TE, et al. Impact of cytomegalovirus (CMV) reactivation after umbilical cord blood transplantation. Biol Blood Marrow Transplant. 2010;16(2):215–22.
142. Bowden RA, Sayers M, Flournoy N, et al. Cytomegalovirus immune globulin and seronegative blood products to prevent primary cytomegalovirus infection after marrow transplantation. N Engl J Med. 1986;314(16):1006–10.
143. Bowden R, Cays M, Schoch G, et al. Comparison of filtered blood (FB) to seronegative blood products (SB) for prevention of cytomegalovirus (CMV) infection after marrow transplant. Blood. 1995;86:3598–603.
144. Ljungman P, Larsson K, Kumlien G, et al. Leukocyte depleted, unscreened blood products give a low risk for CMV infection and disease in CMV seronegative allogeneic stem cell transplant recipients with seronegative stem cell donors. Scand J Infect Dis. 2002;34(5):347–50.
145. Nichols WG, Price TH, Gooley T, Corey L, Boeckh M. Transfusion-transmitted cytomegalovirus infection after receipt of leukoreduced blood products. Blood. 2003;101(10):4195–200.
146. Blajchman MA, Goldman M, Freedman JJ, Sher GD. Proceedings of a consensus conference: prevention of post-transfusion CMV in the era of universal leukoreduction. Transfus Med Rev. 2001;15(1):1–20.
147. Ratko TA, Cummings JP, Oberman HA, et al. Evidence-based recommendations for the use of WBC-reduced cellular blood components. Transfusion. 2001;41(10):1310–9.
148. Bowden RA, Fisher LD, Rogers K, Cays M, Meyers JD. Cytomegalovirus (CMV)-specific intravenous immunoglobulin for the prevention of primary CMV infection and disease after marrow transplant [see comments]. J Infect Dis. 1991;164(3):483–7.
149. Ruutu T, Ljungman P, Brinch L, et al. No prevention of cytomegalovirus infection by anti-cytomegalovirus hyperimmune globulin in seronegative bone marrow transplant recipients. The Nordic BMT Group. Bone Marrow Transplant. 1997;19(3):233–6.
150. Boeckh M, Bowden R, Storer B, et al. Randomized, placebo-controlled, double-blind study of a cytomegalovirus-specific monoclonal antibody (MSL-109) for prevention of cytomegalovirus infection after allogeneic hematopoietic stem cell transplantation. Biol Blood Marrow Transplant. 2001;7(6):343–51.
151. Bass E, Powe N, Goodman S, et al. Efficacy of immune globulin in preventing complications of bone marrow transplantation: a meta-analysis. Bone Marrow Transplant. 1993;12:179–83.
152. Messori A, Rampazzo R, Scroccaro G, Martini N. Efficacy of hyperimmune anti-cytomegalovirus immunoglobulins for the prevention of cytomegalovirus infection in recipients of allogeneic bone marrow transplantation: a meta analysis. Bone Marrow Transplant. 1994;13:163–8.
153. Raanani P, Gafter-Gvili A, Paul M, Ben-Bassat I, Leibovici L, Shpilberg O. Immunoglobulin prophylaxis in haematopoietic stem cell transplantation: systematic review and meta-analysis. J Clin Oncol. 2009;27(5):770–81.
154. Sullivan KM, Kopecky KJ, Jocom J, et al. Immunomodulatory and antimicrobial efficacy of intravenous immunoglobulin in bone marrow transplantation. N Engl J Med. 1990;323(11):705–12.
155. Winston DJ, Ho WG, Lin CH, et al. Intravenous immune globulin for prevention of cytomegalovirus infection and interstitial pneumonia after bone marrow transplantation. Ann Intern Med. 1987;106(1):12–8.
156. Zikos P, Van Lint MT, Lamparelli T, et al. A randomized trial of high dose polyvalent intravenous immunoglobulin (HDIgG) vs. cytomegalovirus (CMV) hyperimmune IgG in allogeneic hemopoietic stem cell transplants (HSCT). Haematologica. 1998;83(2):132–7.
157. Tomblyn M, Chiller T, Einsele H, et al. Guidelines for preventing infectious complications among hematopoietic cell transplantation recipients: a global perspective. Biol Blood Marrow Transplant. 2009;15(10):1143–238.
158. Avery RK, Adal KA, Longworth DL, Bolwell BJ. A survey of allogeneic bone marrow transplant programs in the United States regarding cytomegalovirus prophylaxis and pre-emptive therapy. Bone Marrow Transplant. 2000;26(7):763–7.
159. Ljungman P. CMV infections after hematopoietic stem cell transplantation. Bone Marrow Transplant. 2008;42 Suppl 1:S70–2.
160. Ljungman P, Reusser P, de la Camara R, et al. Management of CMV infections: recommendations from the infectious diseases working party of the EBMT. Bone Marrow Transplant. 2004;33(11):1075–81.
161. Boeckh M, Ljungman P. How we treat cytomegalovirus in hematopoietic cell transplant recipients. Blood. 2009;113(23):5711–9.
162. Lacey SF, Diamond DJ, Zaia JA. Assessment of cellular immunity to human cytomegalovirus in recipients of allogeneic stem cell transplants. Biol Blood Marrow Transplant. 2004;10(7):433–47.
163. Meyers JD, Reed EC, Shepp DH, et al. Acyclovir for prevention of cytomegalovirus infection and disease after allogeneic marrow transplantation. N Engl J Med. 1988;318(2):70–5.
164. Prentice HG, Gluckman E, Powles RL, et al. Impact of long-term acyclovir on cytomegalovirus infection and survival after allogeneic bone marrow transplantation. European Acyclovir for CMV Prophylaxis Study Group. Lancet. 1994;343(8900):749–53.
165. Ljungman P, De La Camara R, Milpied N, et al. A randomised study of valaciclovir as prophylaxis against CMV reactivation in allogeneic bone marrow transplant recipients. Blood. 2002;73:930–6.
166. Goodrich JM, Bowden RA, Fisher L, Keller C, Schoch G, Meyers JD. Ganciclovir prophylaxis to prevent cytomegalovirus disease after allogeneic marrow transplant. Ann Intern Med. 1993;118(3):173–8.
167. Winston DJ, Ho WG, Bartoni K, et al. Ganciclovir prophylaxis of cytomegalovirus infection and disease in allogeneic bone marrow transplant recipients. Results of a placebo-controlled, double-blind trial. Ann Intern Med. 1993;118(3):179–84.
168. Winston DJ, Yeager AM, Chandrasekar PH, Snydman DR, Petersen FB, Territo MC. Randomized comparison of oral valacyclovir and intravenous ganciclovir for prevention of cytomegalovirus disease after allogeneic bone marrow transplant. Clin Infect Dis. 2003;36(6):749–58.
169. Salzberger B, Bowden RA, Hackman RC, Davis C, Boeckh M. Neutropenia in allogeneic marrow transplant recipients receiving ganciclovir for prevention of cytomegalovirus disease: risk factors and outcome. Blood. 1997;90(6):2502–8.
170. Busca A, de Fabritiis P, Ghisetti V, et al. Oral valganciclovir as preemptive therapy for cytomegalovirus infection post allogeneic stem cell transplantation. Transpl Infect Dis. 2007;9(2):102–7.
171. Einsele H, Reusser P, Bornhauser M, et al. Oral valganciclovir leads to higher exposure to ganciclovir than intravenous ganciclovir in patients following allogeneic stem cell transplantation. Blood. 2006;107(7):3002–8.
172. Winston DJ, Baden LR, Gabriel DA, et al. Pharmacokinetics of ganciclovir after oral valganciclovir versus intravenous ganciclovir in allogeneic stem cell transplant patients with graft-versus-host disease of the gastrointestinal tract. Biol Blood Marrow Transplant. 2006;12(6):635–40.
173. Allice T, Busca A, Locatelli F, Falda M, Pittaluga F, Ghisetti V. Valganciclovir as pre-emptive therapy for cytomegalovirus infection post-allogenic stem cell transplantation: implications for the emergence of drug-resistant cytomegalovirus. J Antimicrob Chemother. 2009;63(3):600–8.
174. Ayala E, Greene J, Sandin R, et al. Valganciclovir is safe and effective as pre-emptive therapy for CMV infection in allogeneic hematopoietic stem cell transplantation. Bone Marrow Transplant. 2006;37(9):851–6.

175. Takenaka K, Eto T, Nagafuji K, et al. Oral valganciclovir as preemptive therapy is effective for cytomegalovirus infection in allogeneic hematopoietic stem cell transplant recipients. Int J Hematol. 2009;89(2):231–7.
176. Volin L, Barkholt L, Nihtinen A, et al. An open-label randomised study of oral valganciclovir versus intravenous ganciclovir for pre-emptive therapy of cytomegalovirus infection after allogeneic stem cell transplantation. In: 34th Annual Meeting of the European Group for Blood and Marrow Transplantation, Florence, Italy; 2008.
177. Reusser P, Einsele H, Lee J, et al. Randomized multicenter trial of foscarnet versus ganciclovir for preemptive therapy of cytomegalovirus infection after allogeneic stem cell transplantation. Blood. 2002;99(4):1159–64.
178. Bacigalupo A, Tedone E, Van Lint MT, et al. CMV prophylaxis with foscarnet in allogeneic bone marrow transplant recipients at high risk of developing CMV infections. Bone Marrow Transplant. 1994;13(6):783–8.
179. Bregante S, Bertilson S, Tedone E, et al. Foscarnet prophylaxis of cytomegalovirus infections in patients undergoing allogeneic bone marrow transplantation (BMT): a dose-finding study. Bone Marrow Transplant. 2000;26(1):23–9.
180. Reusser P, Gambertoglio JG, Lilleby K, Meyers JD. Phase I-II trial of foscarnet for prevention of cytomegalovirus infection in autologous and allogeneic marrow transplant recipients [see comments]. J Infect Dis. 1992;166(3):473–9.
181. Ljungman P, Deliliers GL, Platzbecker U. Cidofovir for cytomegalovirus infection and disease in allogeneic stem cell transplant recipients. The Infectious Diseases Working Party of the European Group for Blood and Marrow Transplantation. Blood. 2001;97(2):388–92.
182. Nichols WG, Price T, Boeckh M. Donor serostatus and CMV infection and disease among recipients of prophylactic granulocyte transfusions. Blood 2003;101(12):5091–2; author reply 2.
183. Ljungman P, de la Camara R, Cordonnier C, et al. Management of CMV, HHV-6, HHV-7 and Kaposi-sarcoma herpesvirus (HHV-8) infections in patients with hematological malignancies and after SCT. Bone Marrow Transplant. 2008;42(4):227–40.
184. Ljungman P, Lore K, Aschan J, et al. Use of a semi-quantitative PCR for cytomegalovirus DNA as a basis for pre-emptive antiviral therapy in allogeneic bone marrow transplant patients. Bone Marrow Transplant. 1996;17(4):583–7.
185. Fries BC, Riddell SR, Kim HW, et al. Cytomegalovirus disease before hematopoietic cell transplantation as a risk for complications after transplantation. Biol Blood Marrow Transplant. 2005;11(2):136–48.
186. Arslan F, Tabak F, Avsar E, et al. Ganciclovir-resistant cytomegalovirus encephalitis in a hematopoietic stem cell transplant recipient. J Neurovirol. 2010;16(2):174–8.
187. Chou SW. Cytomegalovirus drug resistance and clinical implications. Transpl Infect Dis. 2001;3 Suppl 2:20–4.
188. Chou S. Cytomegalovirus UL97 mutations in the era of ganciclovir and maribavir. Rev Med Virol. 2008;18(4):233–46.
189. Iwasenko JM, Scott GM, Rawlinson WD, Keogh A, Mitchell D, Chou S. Successful valganciclovir treatment of post-transplant cytomegalovirus infection in the presence of UL97 mutation N597D. J Med Virol. 2009;81(3):507–10.
190. Prichard MN, Britt WJ, Daily SL, Hartline CB, Kern ER. Human cytomegalovirus UL97 kinase is required for the normal intranuclear distribution of pp 65 and virion morphogenesis. J Virol. 2005;79(24):15494–502.
191. Drew WL. Is combination antiviral therapy for CMV superior to monotherapy? J Clin Virol. 2006;35(4):485–8.
192. Chou S, Lurain NS, Thompson KD, Miner RC, Drew WL. Viral DNA polymerase mutations associated with drug resistance in human cytomegalovirus. J Infect Dis. 2003;188(1):32–9.
193. Andrei G, De Clercq E, Snoeck R. Novel inhibitors of human CMV. Curr Opin Investig Drugs. 2008;9(2):132–45.
194. Lischka P, Hewlett G, Wunberg T, et al. In vitro and in vivo activities of the novel anticytomegalovirus compound AIC246. Antimicrob Agents Chemother. 2010;54(3):1290–7.
195. Winston DJ, Young JA, Pullarkat V, et al. Maribavir prophylaxis for prevention of cytomegalovirus infection in allogeneic stem cell transplant recipients: a multicenter, randomized, double-blind, placebo-controlled, dose-ranging study. Blood. 2008;111(11):5403–10.
196. Avery RK, Bolwell BJ, Yen-Lieberman B, et al. Use of leflunomide in an allogeneic bone marrow transplant recipient with refractory cytomegalovirus infection. Bone Marrow Transplant. 2004;34(12):1071–5.
197. Battiwalla M, Paplham P, Almyroudis NG, et al. Leflunomide failure to control recurrent cytomegalovirus infection in the setting of renal failure after allogeneic stem cell transplantation. Transpl Infect Dis. 2007;9(1):28–32.
198. Efferth T, Romero M, Wolf D, Stamminger T, Marin J, Marschall M. The antiviral activities of artemisinin and artesunate. Clin Infect Dis. 2008;47:804–11.
199. Arvin AM, Fast P, Myers M, Plotkin S, Rabinovich R. Vaccine development to prevent cytomegalovirus disease: report from the National Vaccine Advisory Committe. Clin Infect Dis. 2004;39(2):233–9.
200. Adler SP. Human CMV vaccine trials: what if CMV caused a rash? J Clin Virol. 2008;41(3):231–6.
201. Wloch MK, Smith LR, Boutsaboualoy S, et al. Safety and immunogenicity of a bivalent cytomegalovirus DNA vaccine in healthy adult subjects. J Infect Dis. 2008;197(12):1634–41.
202. Reed EC, Wolford JL, Kopecky KJ, et al. Ganciclovir for the treatment of cytomegalovirus gastroenteritis in bone marrow transplant patients. A randomized, placebo-controlled trial. Ann Intern Med. 1990;112(7):505–10.
203. Ljungman P, Cordonnier C, Einsele H, et al. Use of intravenous immune globulin in addition to antiviral therapy in the treatment of CMV gastrointestinal disease in allogeneic bone marrow transplant patients: a report from the European Group for Blood and Marrow Transplantation (EBMT). Infectious Diseases Working Party of the EBMT. Bone Marrow Transplant. 1998;21(5):473–6.
204. Emanuel D, Cunningham I, Jules-Elysee K, et al. Cytomegalovirus pneumonia after bone marrow transplantation successfully treated with the combination of ganciclovir and high-dose intravenous immune globulin. Ann Intern Med. 1988;109(10):777–82.
205. Ljungman P, Engelhard D, Link H, et al. Treatment of interstitial pneumonitis due to cytomegalovirus with ganciclovir and intravenous immune globulin: experience of European Bone Marrow Transplant Group. Clin Infect Dis. 1992;14(4):831–5.
206. Reed EC, Bowden RA, Dandliker PS, Lilleby KE, Meyers JD. Treatment of cytomegalovirus pneumonia with ganciclovir and intravenous cytomegalovirus immunoglobulin in patients with bone marrow transplants. Ann Intern Med. 1988;109(10):783–8.
207. Schmidt GM, Kovacs A, Zaia JA, et al. Ganciclovir/immunoglobulin combination therapy for the treatment of human cytomegalovirus-associated interstitial pneumonia in bone marrow allograft recipients. Transplantation. 1988;46(6):905–7.
208. Erard V, Gutherie KA, Smith J, Chien J, Corey L, Boeckh M. Cytomegalovirus pneumonia (CMV-IP) after hematopoeitic cell transplantation (HCT): outcomes and factors associated with mortality (abstract V-1379). In: 47th Interscience Conference on Antimicrobial Agents and Chemotherapy, Chicago, IL; 2007.
209. Machado CM, Dulley FL, Boas LS, et al. CMV pneumonia in allogeneic BMT recipients undergoing early treatment of pre-emptive ganciclovir therapy. Bone Marrow Transplant. 2000;26(4):413–7.
210. Chang M, Dunn JP. Ganciclovir implant in the treatment of cytomegalovirus retinitis. Expert Rev Med Devices. 2005;2(4):421–7.

211. Okamoto T, Okada M, Mori A, et al. Successful treatment of severe cytomegalovirus retinitis with foscarnet and intraocular infection of ganciclovir in a myelosuppressed unrelated bone marrow transplant patient. Bone Marrow Transplant. 1997;20(9):801–3.
212. Ganly PS, Arthur C, Goldman JM, Schulenburg WE. Foscarnet as treatment for cytomegalovirus retinitis following bone marrow transplantation. Postgrad Med J. 1988;64(751):389–91.
213. Biron KK. Antiviral drugs for cytomegalovirus diseases. Antiviral Res. 2006;71(2–3):154–63.
214. Einsele H, Kapp M, Grigoleit GU. CMV-specific T cell therapy. Blood Cells Mol Dis. 2008;40(1):71–5.
215. Eizuru Y, Tamura K, Minamishima Y, et al. Cytomegalovirus infections in adult T-cell leukemia patients. J Med Virol. 1987;23(2):123–33.
216. Mera JR, Whimbey E, Elting L, et al. Cytomegalovirus pneumonia in adult nontransplantation patients with cancer: review of 20 cases occurring from 1964 through 1990. Clin Infect Dis. 1996;22(6):1046–50.
217. Nguyen Q, Estey E, Raad I, et al. Cytomegalovirus pneumonia in adults with leukemia: an emerging problem. Clin Infect Dis. 2001;32(4):539–45.
218. Suzumiya J, Marutsuka K, Nabeshima K, et al. Autopsy findings in 47 cases of adult T-cell leukemia/lymphoma in Miyazaki prefecture, Japan. Leuk Lymphoma. 1993;11(3–4):281–6.
219. Yoshioka R, Yamaguchi K, Yoshinaga T, Takatsuki K. Pulmonary complications in patients with adult T-cell leukemia. Cancer. 1985;55(10):2491–4.
220. Torres HA, Aguilera E, Safdar A, et al. Fatal cytomegalovirus pneumonia in patients with haematological malignancies: an autopsy-based case-control study. Clin Microbiol Infect. 2008;14(12):1160–6.
221. Koo S, Baden LR. Infectious complications associated with immunomodulating monoclonal antibodies used in the treatment of hematologic malignancy. J Natl Compr Canc Netw. 2008;6(2):202–13.
222. O'Brien SM, Keating MJ, Mocarski ES. Updated guidelines on the management of cytomegalovirus reactivation in patients with chronic lymphocytic leukemia treated with alemtuzumab. Clin Lymphoma Myeloma. 2006;7(2):125–30.
223. Orlandi EM, Baldanti F, Citro A, Pochintesta L, Gatti M, Lazzarino M. Monitoring for cytomegalovirus and Epstein-Barr virus infection in chronic lymphocytic leukemia patients receiving i.v. fludarabine-cyclophosphamide combination and alemtuzumab as consolidation therapy. Haematologica. 2008;93(11):1758–60.
224. Keating MJ, Flinn I, Jain V, et al. Therapeutic role of alemtuzumab (Campath-1H) in patients who have failed fludarabine: results of a large international study. Blood. 2002;99(10):3554–61.
225. Laurenti L, Piccioni P, Cattani P, et al. Cytomegalovirus reactivation during alemtuzumab therapy for chronic lymphocytic leukemia: incidence and treatment with oral ganciclovir. Haematologica. 2004;89(10):1248–52.
226. Lundin J, Kimby E, Bjorkholm M, et al. Phase II trial of subcutaneous anti-CD52 monoclonal antibody alemtuzumab (Campath-1H) as first-line treatment for patients with B-cell chronic lymphocytic leukemia (B-CLL). Blood. 2002;100(3):768–73.
227. Lundin J, Osterborg A, Brittinger G, et al. CAMPATH-1H monoclonal antibody in therapy for previously treated low-grade non-Hodgkin's lymphomas: a phase II multicenter study. European Study Group of CAMPATH-1H Treatment in Low-Grade Non-Hodgkin's Lymphoma. J Clin Oncol. 1998;16(10):3257–63.
228. Nguyen DD, Cao TM, Dugan K, Starcher SA, Fechter RL, Coutre SE. Cytomegalovirus viremia during Campath-1H therapy for relapsed and refractory chronic lymphocytic leukemia and prolymphocytic leukemia. Clin Lymphoma. 2002;3(2):105–10.
229. Cheung WW, Tse E, Leung AY, Yuen KY, Kwong YL. Regular virologic surveillance showed very frequent cytomegalovirus reactivation in patients treated with alemtuzumab. Am J Hematol. 2007;82(2):108–11.
230. Hwang YY, Cheung WW, Leung AY, Tse E, Au WY, Kwong YL. Valganciclovir thrice weekly for prophylaxis against cytomegalovirus reactivation during alemtuzumab therapy. Leukemia. 2009;23:800–1.
231. Visani G, Mele A, Guiducci B, et al. An observational study of once weekly intravenous ganciclovir as CMV prophylaxis in heavily pre-treated chronic lymphocytic leukemia patients receiving subcutaneous alemtuzumab. Leuk Lymphoma. 2006;47(12):2542–6.
232. O'Brien S, Ravandi F, Riehl T, et al. Valganciclovir prevents cytomegalovirus reactivation in patients receiving alemtuzumab-based therapy. Blood. 2008;111(4):1816–9.
233. Gonzalez H, Vernant JP, Caumes E. Successful oral valganciclovir treatment of cytomegalovirus infection during Campath-1H therapy. Leukemia. 2005;19(3):478.
234. Thursky KA, Worth LJ, Seymour JF, Miles Prince H, Slavin MA. Spectrum of infection, risk and recommendations for prophylaxis and screening among patients with lymphoproliferative disorders treated with alemtuzumab*. Br J Haematol. 2006;132(1):3–12.
235. Osterborg A, Foa R, Bezares RF, et al. Management guidelines for the use of alemtuzumab in chronic lymphocytic leukemia. Leukemia. 2009;23:1980–8.
236. Worth LJ, Thursky KA. Cytomegalovirus reactivation in patients with chronic lymphocytic leukemia treated with alemtuzumab: prophylaxis vs. pre-emptive strategies for prevention. Leuk Lymphoma. 2006;47(12):2435–6.
237. Brugiatelli M, Bandini G, Barosi G, et al. Management of chronic lymphocytic leukemia: practice guidelines from the Italian Society of Hematology, the Italian Society of Experimental Hematology and the Italian Group for Bone Marrow Transplantation. Haematologica. 2006;91(12):1662–73.
238. Ng AP, Worth L, Chen L, et al. Cytomegalovirus DNAemia and disease: incidence, natural history and management in settings other than allogeneic stem cell transplantation. Haematologica. 2005;90(12):1672–9.
239. Williams-Aziz SL, Hartline CB, Harden EA, et al. Comparative activities of lipid esters of cidofovir and cyclic cidofovir against replication of herpesviruses in vitro. Antimicrob Agents Chemother. 2005;49(9):3724–33.

Chapter 31
Epstein-Barr Virus, Varicella Zoster Virus, and Human Herpes Viruses-6 and -8

Mini Kamboj and David M. Weinstock

Abstract Epstein-Barr virus (EBV), varicella zoster virus (VZV), and human herpes viruses-6 (HHV-6) and -8 (HHV-8) present unique management challenges to clinicians who care for patients with cancer. Although latent infection by these organisms is either common (HHV-8, VZV) or essentially ubiquitous (EBV, HHV-6), clinical manifestations vary widely in frequency and severity. Syndromes caused by EBV, VZV, HHV-6, and HHV-8 span from highly contagious infections (e.g., varicella) to monoclonal malignant populations (e.g., endemic Burkitt's lymphoma). Within this broad spectrum are polyclonal cellular proliferations (e.g., Multicentric Castleman's disease) that obscure the traditional boundary between infection and cancer. Despite the availability of acyclovir and related compounds, these Herpes viruses continue to cause significant morbidity and mortality in patients with cancer. Newer therapies that modulate the host immune response, either by vaccination or the infusion of targeted lymphocytes, have generated significant interest and are already available in some centers.

Keywords Herpes • Cancer • Infection • Epstein-Barr virus • Varicella zoster virus • Human herpes virus-6 • Human herpes virus-8

Introduction

Eight herpes viruses are known to cause clinical syndromes in humans: herpes simplex viruses 1 and 2, varicella zoster virus (VZV), Epstein-Barr virus (EBV), cytomegalovirus (see Chap. 30), and human herpes viruses-6 (HHV-6), -7 (HHV-7), and -8 (HHV-8). These organisms have double-stranded DNA genomes within an icosadeltahedral capsid and a glycoprotein envelope derived from the membrane of infected cells.

Upon entry into a human host, Herpes viruses can establish lifelong infection that roughly divides into three phases. First (primary infection), viral replication within host cells leads to cell lysis, viral dissemination, and further cellular infection. Primary infection can be subclinical or produce a syndrome with characteristics that vary based on the immune competence, genetic background, and age of the host. Primary infection is resolved by the host's innate immune system and results in the production of neutralizing antibodies.

In the second phase (latency), the organism achieves a quiescent equilibrium with the host adaptive immune response, primarily by reducing the number of genes expressed from the viral genome. Other factors that contribute to viral persistence within latently infected cells include viral microRNA, chemokine homologs, cytokines, and modulators of immune recognition.

In the third phase (reactivation), the organism reestablishes lytic viral replication by expressing genes necessary for the production and release of infectious virus. The balance between lytic and latent infection is highly complex and poorly understood. In fact, subclinical lytic infection can be either continuous or episodic for many Herpes viruses and results in asymptomatic viral shedding in saliva and other fluids. Characteristic clinical syndromes (e.g., herpes zoster) manifest when the extent of lytic viral infection exceeds an ill-defined threshold. The loss of immune competence, specifically the cytotoxic T-cell response, generally favors symptomatic lytic reactivation and more severe clinical complications. Acyclovir (and related antivirals) are only effective against lytic infection (primary or reactivation), as viral kinases that phosphorylate acyclovir to its active form are not expressed during latency.

The γ-herpes viruses HHV-8 and EBV are notable for their ability to induce both nonmalignant and malignant proliferations of latently infected cells. These proliferations are a teleologic conundrum, as they create a selective disadvantage for hosts infected by the organism without favoring viral transmission. The γ-herpes viruses utilize a vast array of mechanisms to promote cellular survival and replication. Yet, only a miniscule fraction of latently infected cells

---

D.M. Weinstock (✉)
Department of Medical Oncology, Dana-Farber Cancer Institute,
450 Brookline Avenue, DA510B, Boston, MA, 02215, USA
e-mail: davidm_weinstock@dfci.harvard.edu

progress to become pathologic proliferations. The rarity of these proliferations argues that tumors derived from latently infected cells represent an unintended by-product of the latent program that requires additional factors, including the stochastic acquisition of complementary mutations and the failure of immune surveillance.

In this chapter, we will review aspects of infection caused by VZV, HHV-6, EBV, and HHV-8, which are pertinent to clinicians who care for patients with cancer. We will focus on the diagnosis, management, and prevention of traditional infections. The panoply of cellular proliferations, both malignant and nonmalignant, that are associated with γ-herpes viruses has been reviewed elsewhere [1–4]. HSV-1 and HSV-2 will also not be further discussed, although primary and reactivation syndromes caused by these organisms occur frequently in immunocompetent and immunocompromised patients with cancer. Finally, HHV-7 does not appear to be a common cause of morbidity in patients with cancer [5].

Varicella Zoster Virus

Epidemiology and risk factors. VZV infections occur worldwide. The organism produces two distinct clinical syndromes, primary varicella (chicken pox) and herpes zoster (shingles). Primary varicella is mostly a disease of childhood in temperate areas and of adolescent to early adulthood years in tropical areas [6]. Primary varicella is highly contagious and, unlike other Herpes viruses, is transmissible via the respiratory route.

During primary varicella, the virus establishes latency in the afferent neurons of dorsal root and cranial ganglia. Reactivation can manifest as herpes zoster (i.e., shingles), although only 15% of persons infected with VZV ever develop herpes zoster [7, 8]. VZV reactivation induces a profound anti-VZV T-cell response. Thus, second episodes of herpes zoster are rare in the general population, but occur more frequently in persons with impaired cell-mediated immunity [9].

Immunodeficiency, either from cancer or its treatment, is a risk factor for VZV disease and dissemination. In a population study of adult patients within 5 years after cancer diagnosis [10], the cumulative incidence of VZV disease was 625/100,000 person-years, a rate 5 times higher than the general population [11]. However, the incidence of VZV disease among patients with cancer varies widely based on several factors that primarily affect immune competence, including patient age, underlying tumor type, and cancer treatment.

Cell-mediated, rather than innate or humoral, immunity is the primary protector against VZV reactivation. Patients with underlying solid tumors treated with standard doses of cytotoxic agents (e.g., platinum compounds, vinca alkaloids, taxanes, and anthracyclines) generally have rates of VZV disease which are similar to age-matched controls, and complications other than postherpetic neuralgia are rare [12–14]. Dose-intensive regimens that include these agents increase the risk for VZV disease [15–18], although marginally. Even among patients with acute myelogenous leukemia, who typically retain some extent of adaptive immunity, less than 2% develop VZV disease [14, 19–22].

In contrast, patients with underlying lymphoproliferative disorders [20, 23–25] are at high-risk for VZV disease and severe complications. In the absence of routine acyclovir prophylaxis, 10–25% of adult and pediatric patients with acute lymphocytic leukemia (ALL) or Hodgkin's lymphoma develop VZV disease [14, 19–21, 25], with an annual incidence of approximately 6% and the highest attack rates among patients who receive combined chemotherapy and radiation. Among the latter, disseminated infection develops in approximately one quarter of cases and up to 15% experience a second episode of herpes zoster.

Newer chemotherapies that profoundly suppress cell-mediated immunity can *markedly* increase the risk for VZV disease. These include the purine analogs fludarabine, pentostatin and cladribine [26–28], alemtuzumab [29], temozolomide [30, 31], and bortezomib [32, 33]. Routine chemoprophylaxis against VZV should be strongly considered in patients treated with these compounds.

The widespread use of varicella vaccine (Varivax) to prevent infection by wild-type VZV has already reduced the overall incidence of VZV disease among children in the US [34]. As the age of vaccinated patients increases, it is likely that the epidemiology of VZV disease among patients with cancer will undergo dramatic shifts. Presumably, the lower rates of latent infection by wild-type VZV will result in fewer and less severe episodes of herpes zoster among vaccinated patients. However, the possibility also exists that immunity among vaccinated patients may be reduced compared to patients who experienced wild-type varicella, placing them at higher risk for "reinfection" by wild-type strains during or after cancer therapy. Epidemiologic studies to discern the effects of childhood VZV vaccination on the risk for VZV disease among patients with cancer will be essential for developing future prophylaxis and treatment strategies.

Hematopoietic stem cell transplant (HSCT) recipients. VZV disease among HSCT recipients typically occurs more than 30 days after transplant, when myelopoiesis and innate immunity are restored, but adaptive immunity is highly deficient. The median time to the onset of VZV disease after HSCT is approximately 5 months (Table 31.1), but varies widely between centers based on differences in the duration of prophylaxis after HSCT with acyclovir or related agents. Symptomatic VZV disease develops in 16.6–46% of HSCT recipients within 2 years after transplant [35–42].

Table 31.1 Summary of reports describing varicella zoster virus (VZV)-related illness in hematopoietic stem cell transplant (HSCT) recipients

References	Years	Population	Graft type	N	Rate	Timing of VZV-related illness after HSCT	Comments
Safdar et al. [40]	1996–2005	Adult and pediatric	UCB	97	11%	100% after day +100	All seven cases had chronic GVHD
Koc et al. [37]	1992–1997	Adult	Allogeneic	100	41%	12% by day +100 88% by +24 months	Disseminated infection in 17% of cases
Leung et al. [38]	1991–1998	Pediatric	Autologous and allogeneic	109	30%	73% by +12 months	11% visceral and 48% cutaneous dissemination
Schuchter et al. [41]	1983–1987	Adult and pediatric	Autologous	153	28%	60% by +6 months 91% by +12 months	5% visceral, 15% cutaneous dissemination Acyclovir used in 79% of cases
Wacker et al. [42]	1979–1987	Pediatric	Autologous	236	23%	87% by +6 months	13% cutaneous dissemination Antiviral used in 85%
Han et al. [36]	1974–1989	Adult and pediatric	Autologous and allogeneic	1,186	18.3%	15% by +6 months 86% by +18 months	6% visceral, 26% cutaneous dissemination
Atkinson et al. [35]	1970–1976	Adult and pediatric	Allogeneic and syngeneic	89	46%	Median onset +5 months	
Locksley et al. [39]	1969–1982	Adult and pediatric	Autologous and allogeneic	1,394	16.6%	80% by +9 months	13% visceral, 23% cutaneous dissemination Acyclovir used in 9.6% of cases

GVHD graft-versus-host disease; *UCB* umbilical cord blood; *disseminated* cutaneous dissemination

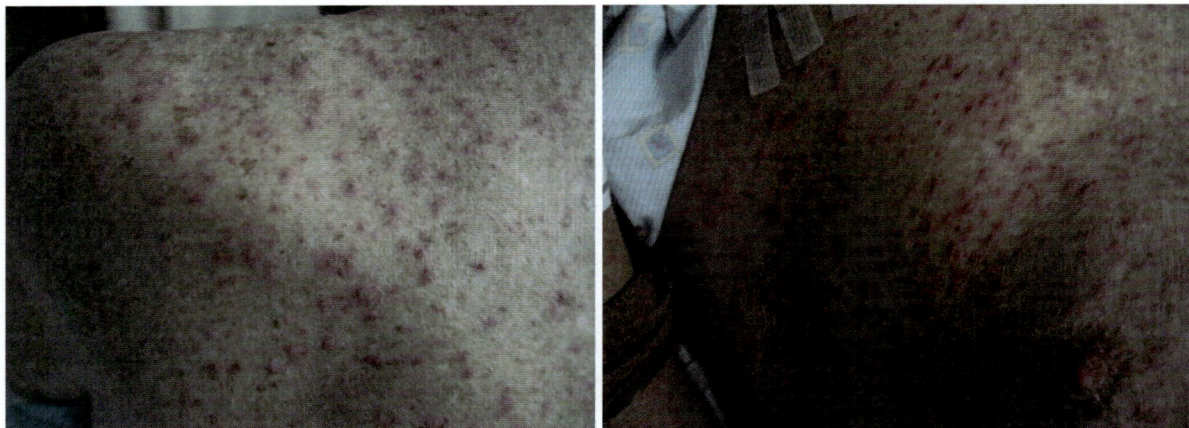

Fig. 31.1 Herpes zoster with cutaneous dissemination (courtesy of Dr. Ying Taur, Memorial Sloan-Kettering Cancer Center, New York, NY)

However, a large fraction of the remaining patients experience subclinical VZV reactivations that can be inferred by the acquisition of VZV IgG within the years after HSCT [43].

Like other herpes viruses, recipient-derived virus causes the vast majority of VZV disease after allogeneic HSCT. Thus, prior infection of the recipient by VZV is the strongest predictor of VZV reactivation after transplant. Some studies have reported that graft-versus-host disease (GVHD) and its treatment increase the risk for VZV reactivation and disseminated disease [37, 39]. Among autologous HSCT recipients, type of underlying malignancy appears to be an important factor, with the highest incidence of VZV infection among patients with underlying lymphoma [41].

Clinical manifestations. The clinical manifestations from VZV disease among persons with and without cancer largely overlap, although immunocompromised patients have a higher risk for cutaneous and visceral dissemination. Visceral VZV dissemination typically manifests as pneumonitis, hepatitis, and/or encephalitis [44–50]. Additional neurologic complications include vasculitis, meningitis, leukoencephalopathy, ganglionitis, postherpetic neuralgia, polyradiculopathy, myelitis, ventriculitis, and necrotizing angitis [47, 48, 51, 52]. Pulmonary and neurologic symptoms typically develop a week after the onset of rash [44].

A rare, but important, syndrome results from visceral involvement in the absence of cutaneous lesions [53, 54]. A delay in antiviral treatment is commonly fatal in these cases, so VZV should be considered in highly immunocompromised patients who present with idiopathic severe abdominal pain, unexplained transaminitis, or the syndrome of inappropriate antidiuretic hormone (SIADH) [55–58].

A few unique aspects of VZV infection have been reported in patients with cancer. For example, herpes zoster may have a predilection for previously irradiated areas or sites of tumor involvement [10, 14, 24]. Disseminated herpes zoster can also mimic primary varicella in immunocompromised patients [39, 44]. This is known as "atypical generalized zoster" and is characterized by skin lesions that appear in a nondermatomal distribution and have the same umbilicated "dew-drop" appearance classically seen with primary varicella (Fig. 31.1). Finally, VZV reinfection has been described in patients with cancer, although the distinction between a second episode of primary varicella and atypical generalized zoster can be exceedingly difficult [59]. Cases of reinfection described in the literature have generally been mild and seldom encountered in clinical practice [59, 60].

Laboratory diagnosis. Tissue culture remains the gold standard for the diagnosis of VZV infection. Direct immunofluorescence assays that use a monoclonal antibody against glycoprotein E are widely available. These assays have largely supplanted the Tzanck smear, as their turnaround time is a few hours and they can reliably distinguish between VZV, HSV, and pox viruses [61]. PCR is commercially available and is useful for identifying VZV DNA in cerebrospinal fluid [62–64], bronchoalveolar lavage [65], and tissue. PCR in conjunction with restriction fragment length polymorphism (RFLP) analysis is the most common approach for strain identification, either in the setting of a suspected outbreak or to distinguish between wild-type and vaccine strains [66, 67].

Serological testing remains the standard for identifying immunity and is routinely performed in HSCT candidates and other patients at high-risk, especially when considering chemoprophylaxis. A number of serological tests are available, including latex agglutination [68] and enzyme-linked immunosorbent (ELISA) assays. Fluorescent-antibody staining of membrane antigen (FAMA) [69, 70] is the most sensitive assay for VZV IgG, but remains only an investigational tool [70].

Treatment. Acyclovir was licensed in the United States in 1982 based on studies demonstrating its superior activity when compared to vidarabine (Ara-A) for the treatment of VZV disease. Despite its widespread use in the general population, acyclovir-resistant VZV remains exceedingly uncommon.

Among immunocompromised patients with herpes zoster, acyclovir is associated with fewer treatment failures compared to vidarabine. Acyclovir also shortens both the duration of culture positivity and the interval to clinical resolution [71–74]. In a placebo-controlled, double-blinded study of immunocompromised patients with herpes zoster, acyclovir 1,500 mg/m^2/day reduced cutaneous dissemination and visceral spread. Acyclovir curtailed disease even when started more than 3 days after the onset of rash [74].

High-dose oral acyclovir (800 mg five times daily) has comparable efficacy to intravenous acyclovir in selected patients with cancer and localized herpes zoster [75]. The newer antivirals, valacyclovir and famciclovir, have largely replaced high-dose acyclovir for this indication because of their superior bioavailability. Famciclovir, an oral prodrug of penciclovir, administered at 500 mg three times daily has comparable efficacy to high-dose oral acyclovir for the treatment of localized zoster in HSCT recipients and patients with cancer who are >12 years old [76].

Valacyclovir is a prodrug of acyclovir with 3–5-fold higher bioavailability. In a recent study, patients with solid tumors actively receiving chemotherapy and/or radiation and patients with lymphoma were randomized to receive treatment for VZV disease with valacyclovir dosed at either 1 or 2 g thrice daily. No differences were noted between the doses in median time to crusting of lesions or zoster-associated neurasthenia [77].

Studies of oral antivirals in patients with cancer are limited to the treatment of localized zoster in selected patients. As such, there are no definitive criteria for which cancer patients can be safely treated with oral therapy. In the authors' experience, cancer patients with primary varicella or disseminated herpes zoster should receive an initial course of intravenous therapy. Among patients with herpes zoster involving only a single dermatome, those with solid tumors who are not actively receiving cytotoxic chemotherapy, those with hematologic malignancies who are in complete remission and have not received therapy for more than 6 months, and HSCT recipients who are not receiving immunosuppressive therapy can be safely treated with oral therapy. Many patients who do not satisfy these criteria can be treated with a brief course of intravenous therapy until no further lesions have developed and older lesions have begun to crust, and then switched to oral therapy to complete a 7–14 day course. More immunocompromised patients (e.g., active lymphoid malignancy, HSCT recipient) may benefit from continuing therapy until all lesions are crusted.

Antiviral therapy with acyclovir in immunocompromised patients with primary varicella decreases the risk of progression to pneumonitis [78, 79]. Among immunocompetent persons, this effect appears to depend on the institution of therapy in the first 72 h after the onset of rash. Whether the delay of therapy beyond 72 h negates any benefit in immunocompromised hosts is not known. However, it is likely that, similar to the treatment of herpes zoster in these patients, "better late than never" applies. The recommended dose for treating primary varicella is 10 mg/kg every 8 h. In children, the starting dose should be 500 mg/m^2 every 8 h. Continuous infusion with acyclovir 2 mg/kg/h has been tried in severe infections, although the data to support its use are sparse [80]. The total duration of intravenous or oral therapy depends upon the degree of underlying immunosuppression and response, following the same tenets as outlined for herpes zoster.

Humoral immunity to VZV is important for protecting against primary infection, but its role in limiting the extent of either primary or reactivation disease appears to be negligible. Thus, the use of adoptive VZV immune globulin (VZIG or VariZIG) to treat infection or prevent the dissemination of localized disease is not recommended [81, 82]. VZV immunoglobulin preparations remain in limited supply and should be reserved for scenarios where their application offers a demonstrated benefit.

Prevention and infection control. Nosocomial transmission of VZV has occurred frequently between patients with cancer. Aggressive infection control efforts to prevent and mitigate this transmission are essential [83–85]. Guidelines published in 2000 from the Infectious Disease Society of America, American Society for Blood and Marrow Transplantation, and Centers for Disease Control include several recommendations for infection control efforts pertinent to VZV [86], including the use of barrier precautions in patients with known or suspected VZV infection and postexposure prophylaxis for patients possibly exposed to VZV.

Patients with VZV are potentially infectious beginning 4 days prior to the onset of rash. Because primary and disseminated VZV can be transmitted by the airborne route, patients with VZV disease should be isolated with airborne (negative pressure room, N95 or higher level respirators or masks) and contact (gowns and gloves) precautions, in addition to standard precautions. After an exposure, VZV antibody testing should be performed as quickly as possible. Susceptible (i.e., VZV nonimmune) but asymptomatic patients should be isolated with appropriate precautions beginning 10 days after exposure and continuing until 21 days after the last exposure. VZV immune globulin (Ig) administered within 96 h after exposure has moderate efficacy in the prevention and mitigation of primary infection [87, 88]. VZV Ig can lengthen the period from exposure to the onset of symptoms. Thus, isolation should be lengthened to 28 days after exposure for patients who receive VZV Ig.

Because reinfection is very uncommon, seropositive patients do not require VZV Ig prophylaxis unless there is a substantial concern that antibodies were passively acquired, such as through the administration of intravenous immune globulin (IVIG) [59, 88]. VZV Ig is recommended for all HSCT recipients whose serostatus in unknown or who are seronegative after an exposure [86]. VZV Ig should be considered in all nonimmune patients with cancer, especially adults and those with impaired cell-mediated immunity, as primary varicella causes significant morbidity and mortality [89]. Nonspecific IVIG is a reasonable substitute if VZV Ig is unavailable [81, 90].

Antivirals. Acyclovir and the newer antivirals are an attractive alternative to VZV Ig for postexposure prophylaxis, as they are readily available and inexpensive. The data to support their use is primarily limited to studies of healthy children [91–93]. Nonetheless, chemoprophylaxis with these agents is likely to be beneficial in immunocompromised patients. In addition to VZV Ig (if available), the authors offer valacyclovir 1 g tid prophylaxis to nonimmune, immunocompromised adults (including allogeneic HSCT recipients) exposed to VZV until 22 days after exposure (or 28 days if VZV Ig is also administered) [59, 94].

Vaccination to prevent VZV disease. Both VZV vaccines that are currently licensed by the FDA contain live VZV derived from the attenuated Oka strain. Thus, immunocompromised patients who receive these vaccines could develop VZV infections caused by the vaccine virus.

Varicella vaccine. Between the two vaccines, Varivax contains a lower titer of virus and is approved for the prevention of primary varicella. Varivax is immunogenic in selected children with lymphoreticular malignancies, acute leukemias, and autologous HSCT recipients [95–99]. The incidence of zoster among patients with acute leukemia who had received varicella vaccine has been lower than or similar to patients with a history of wild-type varicella [100–102]. One study of 13 children with ALL receiving maintenance chemotherapy tested two doses of Varivax 3 months apart. The seroconversion rate increased from 19 to 94% with a second dose of vaccine. One of the 13 children developed a possible case of vaccine strain varicella [103]. In a second study, five of 52 children with ALL developed varicella-like illness after receiving Varivax [104]. Postmarketing surveillance identified six additional cases of disseminated Oka strain infection in immunocompromised patients [105].

A 4-year-old girl with ALL developed fatal disseminated varicella from Oka strain virus, despite vaccination 5 months after achieving a complete remission. She presented with fulminant hepatic failure 5 weeks after receiving the vaccine [106]. Although varicella vaccination may be considered in selected patients with underlying cancer, more studies are needed before the safety and timing of varicella vaccine in high-risk patients are defined. Nonfatal, secondary transmission of vaccine strain virus has also been reported in immunocompromised patients [107, 108].

Zoster vaccine. In 2006, a higher dose of Oka strain vaccine (Zostavax) was licensed in the US for the prevention of herpes zoster in adults more than 60 years old. The titer of virus in Zostavax is at least 14 times greater than the titer in Varivax, which is believed to correlate with a higher likelihood of causing symptomatic VZV disease. As such, Zostavax is contraindicated in HSCT recipients and persons with hematologic malignancies other than leukemia in remission. The vaccine may be administered to selected patients with other cancers, although at least 1 month prior to the initiation of therapy or no sooner than 3 months after the completion of treatment [109]. The authors are generally reluctant to administer Zostavax to any patient with cancer within 1 year after receiving chemotherapy or radiation. Although the prevention of herpes zoster remains a priority from a public health perspective, the potential risk of Zostavax in this population remains too poorly defined.

Other preventive strategies. Vaccination of close contacts and healthcare workers, aggressive outbreak investigation, and postexposure prophylaxis and furloughing for nonimmune healthcare workers are mainstays for reducing nosocomial VZV transmission [86]. Although the risk for transmission of vaccine strain virus is low, healthcare workers who develop a rash after VZV vaccination (Varivax or Zostavax) should avoid all contact with immunocompromised patients until the rash has cleared [110]. If inadvertent exposure to a vaccine recipient with a rash occurs, postexposure prophylaxis may be considered for highly immunocompromised, nonimmune patients who are not receiving acyclovir or other antiviral medications with activity against VZV. The vaccine strain virus is sensitive to acyclovir and related compounds.

Antiviral prophylaxis. Widespread use of chemoprophylaxis with acyclovir and related compounds has substantially reduced the rate of visceral dissemination and mortality related to VZV among high-risk patients [39, 42, 73, 111, 112]. Yet, even considering the considerable morbidity of herpes zoster in immunocompromised patients, antiviral prophylaxis against VZV reactivation is generally not recommended [113]. Studies of long-term antiviral prophylaxis are primarily limited to HSCT recipients and have confirmed that acyclovir reduces the incidence of herpes zoster during the treatment period [114–121]. Unfortunately, a significant fraction of patients will develop herpes zoster within a year after discontinuing antiviral prophylaxis, such that the overall rate of herpes zoster is not significantly reduced by a limited period of prophylaxis. Presumably, chemoprophylaxis suppresses VZV reactivation, which prevents VZV-specific immune reconstitution. In contrast with HSCT recipients, other patients with cancer at high-risk for developing VZV due to immunosuppressive chemotherapy are likely to reestablish immunity upon the cessation of immune suppression. Therefore, the same "rebound" in VZV incidence may not be observed in these patients.

Although the overall fraction of HSCT recipients who experience VZV reactivation was not reduced in the prophylaxis studies, the VZV disease that developed after discontinuing prophylaxis (typically 6–12 months after HSCT) was generally localized and mild [117, 119]. Allogeneic HSCT recipients who required immunosuppression after stopping antiviral prophylaxis had a greater likelihood of developing VZV disease. That increased risk was reduced by continuing antiviral prophylaxis [114, 115, 119–121].

In general, the authors favor long-term prophylaxis to prevent VZV reactivation among very high-risk patients, including HSCT recipients and those receiving alemtuzumab, purine analogs, or high-dose corticosteroids. For example, we use acyclovir (1,200–1,600 mg daily in divided doses) or valacyclovir (500 mg twice daily) prophylaxis in all VZV-seropositive allogeneic HSCT recipients who are receiving immunosuppressive drugs, including those receiving systemic therapy for GVHD. Patients who received T-cell depleted or CD34-selected allografts are typically offered prophylaxis against VZV for at least 12 months after HSCT. The duration of prophylaxis may also be guided by the measurement of T-cell immune responses [122].

Human Herpes Virus-6 (HHV-6)

HHV-6 is an essentially ubiquitous β-Herpes virus that causes exanthema subitum (roseola) in children. Symptomatic reactivation is believed to be exceedingly rare in immunocompetent hosts, but can develop during periods of severe immunodeficiency. HHV-6 reactivation can cause hepatitis, pneumonitis, encephalitis, and a viremic syndrome characterized by fever, rash, and myelosuppression.

HHV-6 encephalitis classically manifests as anterograde amnesia and seizures that result from limbic involvement [123], possibly reflecting a viral tropism for hippocampal astrocytes [124]. Pleocytosis and elevated protein are present in the cerebrospinal fluid of one half to two thirds of patients with HHV-6 encephalitis. In these patients, characteristic abnormalities on MRI include nonenhancing, low attenuation lesions involving the gray matter and occasionally the white matter. These findings can be quite subtle and not visible by CT scanning [125, 126].

Recently, several studies have reported high rates of HHV-6 reactivation among allogeneic HSCT recipients [5, 123, 127–131]. Serial PCR monitoring of serum identified HHV-6 DNA in 50–70% of unselected allogeneic HSCT recipients within 30 days after transplant. In most cases, these reactivations were asymptomatic and associated with only a single positive sample, although higher DNA titers were predicted for GVHD, CMV reactivation and nonrelapse mortality. The highest incidence (80–100%) of reactivation was observed among recipients of umbilical cord blood grafts, as these grafts presumably lack any pathogen-specific immunity.

HHV-6 is susceptible to ganciclovir, foscarnet, and cidofovir in vitro, but has reduced susceptibility to acyclovir. Because the diagnosis of HHV-6 is often presumptive and a positive serum PCR does not prove causality, the decision whether to institute one of these drugs can be extremely difficult. Ganciclovir is myelosuppressive and both foscarnet and cidofovir are highly nephrotoxic, especially in combination with calcineurin inhibitors. Nonetheless, some centers routinely perform preemptive serum PCR screening for HHV-6 among umbilical cord blood transplant recipients and institute foscarnet in those with a positive PCR and symptoms consistent with HHV-6 disease, including persistent fever, delayed engraftment, or neurologic symptoms. No randomized data are available to evaluate the benefit of this approach.

Epstein-Barr Virus (EBV)

EBV infects more than 95% of humans in the first two decades of life. Transmission of EBV is most frequently horizontal through the passage of infected saliva. Vertical, sexual, blood, and transplant-mediated transmission also occur. Among children, primary infection is typically asymptomatic. Infection in adolescence or later in life is frequently accompanied by infectious mononucleosis, a syndrome of lymphocytosis, lymphadenopathy, and splenomegaly caused by the vigorous primary CD8 T-cell response against EBV-infected B cells.

B cells are believed to be essential for EBV persistence as patients with X-linked agammaglobulinemia (who lack B cells) do not develop persistent EBV infection. EBV gains entry into B cells via the CD21 receptor on the B-cell surface. The mechanism for EBV entry into epithelial, mesenchymal, and T cells, which lack CD21, remains unclear.

EBV is associated with a wide array of lymphoid and nonlymphoid proliferations in both immunocompetent and immunocompromised hosts (Table 31.2). The clonality of these proliferations can be determined by assaying the number of tandem repeats present in the episomal EBV genome. Proliferations whose cells contain a common number of tandem repeats are monoclonal, while proliferations that include variable numbers of repeats are polyclonal.

In immunocompetent hosts, the diagnosis of EBV infection can be made by assaying for heterophile antibodies. PCR of serum, plasma, or whole blood can be useful for diagnosing EBV reactivation or latent proliferations, although PCR assays vary widely and the benefit of preemptive PCR screening in high-risk patients remains largely unproven [132, 133].

EBV proliferations in highly immunocompromised hosts. EBV causes a range of pathologic disorders in immunocompromised patients, from fever to posttransplant lymphoproliferative disorder (PTLD) to monoclonal non-Hodgkin's

Table 31.2 Abridged compilation of malignant and nonmalignant proliferations associated with the γ-herpes viruses, Epstein-Barr virus (EBV) and human herpes virus-8 (HHV-8) [1, 2]

Epstein-Barr virus	Human herpes virus-8
Nonmalignant disease	
Infectious mononucleosis	Bone marrow failure syndrome
Chronic active infection	
Oral hairy leukoplakia	Multicentric Castleman's disease
Malignant lymphoid disease	
Immunodeficiency-associated B cell lymphomas	Plasmablastic lymphoma
	Germinotropic lymphoma
Posttransplantation lymphoproliferative disorder	Endemic lymphoma
	Primary effusion lymphoma
Lymphomatoid granulomatosis	Secondary effusion lymphoma
Primary effusion lymphoma	
Burkitt lymphoma	
Classical Hodgkin lymphoma	
Extranodal NK/T cell lymphoma, nasal type	
Virus-associated hemophagocytic syndrome	
Malignant nonlymphoid disease	
Lymphoepithelioma-like carcinoma	Kaposi's sarcoma
Nasopharyngeal carcinoma	
Breast carcinoma	
Hepatocellular carcinoma	
Leiomyosarcoma	
Follicular dendritic cell sarcoma	

lymphoma. A wide variety of immunodeficiency-associated B cell lymphomas occur in immunocompromised patients. Among primary effusion lymphomas, EBV is found in some cases, while HHV-8 is present in all cases. These arise from either lytic reactivation or the outgrowth of latently infected B cells.

Among HSCT recipients, the highest incidence for EBV-related proliferations occurs in the first 6 months after transplant, and the vast majority of cases develop during the first year. In allogeneic HSCT recipients, the virus is typically derived from the recipient while the B cells are donor-derived. Risk factors for EBV-related pathology in these patients are primarily related to T-cell immunodeficiency, including transplantation from an unrelated or HLA-mismatched donor, in vitro T-cell depletion of the allograft, the use of anti-T-cell antibodies, and chronic GVHD.

Treatment. Primary EBV can be highly fatal in patients with severe T cell defects. In these cases, acyclovir or related compounds may be beneficial, although published evidence is lacking. Available treatments for EBV-related B cell proliferations are either cytotoxic (i.e., chemotherapy and radiation) or immune-mediated. Among the latter, the anti-CD20 monoclonal antibody rituximab induces long-term remission in approximately half of HSCT recipients with EBV reactivation [133], but is less effective for solid organ transplant recipients. For the latter, withdrawing immunosuppression can induce complete responses.

In patients who lack EBV-specific immunity, either due to immunoablation or primary immunodeficiency, adoptive cellular therapy can provide EBV-specific immunity and engender responses against EBV-associated proliferations [134]. In the allogeneic HSCT setting, immunity against EBV can be transferred by donor lymphocyte infusion [135]. However, nonselected donor lymphocytes also place the recipient at high-risk for developing GVHD. An alternative is to generate allogeneic EBV-specific T cells in vitro, a method now widely used at a few centers and associated with essentially no risk for causing GVHD. The group at Baylor University has pioneered the development of multivalent T cell products with activity against EBV, cytomegalovirus, and adenovirus [136]. A possibility currently being tested is that partially or fully HLA-matched, third-party (i.e., not from the donor or recipient) EBV-specific T cells will retain activity against EBV proliferations in the recipient. If so, T cells specific to EBV or other infectious agents could be taken "off-the-shelf" and given to a wide range of affected patients.

Human Herpes Virus 8 (HHV-8)

Although Moritz Kaposi first described his eponymous sarcoma in 1872, it was not until the early 1990s that epidemiologic studies suggested Kaposi's sarcoma (KS) is a sexually transmitted disease, and not until 1994 that the organism was identified by subtraction cloning [137]. Like EBV, HHV-8 is a γ-herpes virus that maintains latency in B cells and is associated with a variety of malignant and nonmalignant proliferations (Table 31.2). Also like EBV, transmission of HHV-8 is primarily through infected saliva, but can occur via other routes.

Unlike EBV, HHV-8 infects only 1–5% of persons in developed countries and up to 50% of persons in other regions, most notably Africa. Serum serology is the standard assay for demonstrating prior exposure (and latent infection), while immunohistochemistry on tissue sections is useful to confirm the presence of HHV-8 in Castleman's disease, KS, or non-Hodgkin lymphoma. HHV-8 infection can be diagnosed by serum PCR, although this method may be overly sensitive. Previous PCR studies have erroneously implicated HHV-8 in a variety of diseases where it is unlikely to be involved [2].

Primary HHV-8 infection is probably asymptomatic in most cases, although a mononucleosis-like illness has been reported. Among immunodeficient hosts, HHV-8 can widely disseminate and infect endothelial cells and a variety of bloodborne mononuclear cells. Dissemination can cause a syndrome of severe myelosuppression in transplant recipients [138, 139].

HHV-8 is susceptible to ganciclovir, foscarnet, and cidofovir in vitro, although like EBV, there is sparse evidence demonstrating its efficacy in patients. Immune reconstitution is effective in reversing KS in patients with AIDS and, when this is a viable option, is likely to be the most effective therapy against many HHV-8 associated processes in patients with cancer.

References

1. Kutok JL, Wang F. Spectrum of Epstein-Barr virus-associated diseases. Annu Rev Pathol. 2006;1:375–404.
2. Laurent C, Meggetto F, Brousset P. Human herpesvirus 8 infections in patients with immunodeficiencies. Hum Pathol. 2008;39:983–93.
3. Hengge UR, Ruzicka T, Tyring SK, et al. Update on Kaposi's sarcoma and other HHV8 associated diseases. Part 2: pathogenesis, Castleman's disease, and pleural effusion lymphoma. Lancet Infect Dis. 2002;2:344–52.
4. Hengge UR, Ruzicka T, Tyring SK, et al. Update on Kaposi's sarcoma and other HHV8 associated diseases. Part 1: epidemiology, environmental predispositions, clinical manifestations, and therapy. Lancet Infect Dis. 2002;2:281–92.
5. Zerr DM, Corey L, Kim HW, Huang ML, Nguy L, Boeckh M. Clinical outcomes of human herpesvirus 6 reactivation after hematopoietic stem cell transplantation. Clin Infect Dis. 2005;40:932–40.
6. Seward J, Galil K, Wharton M. Epidemiology of varicella. In: Arvin AM, Gershon AA, editors. Varicella zoster virus: virology and clinical management. Cambridge: Cambridge University Press; 2000. p. 187–205.
7. Hambleton S, Gershon AA. Preventing varicella-zoster disease. Clin Microbiol Rev. 2005;18:70–80.
8. Donahue JG, Choo PW, Manson JE, Platt R. The incidence of herpes zoster. Arch Intern Med. 1995;155:1605–9.
9. Dworkin RH, Johnson RW, Breuer J, et al. Recommendations for the management of herpes zoster. Clin Infect Dis. 2007;44 Suppl 1:S1–26.
10. Rusthoven JJ, Ahlgren P, Elhakim T, et al. Varicella-zoster infection in adult cancer patients. A population study. Arch Intern Med. 1988;148:1561–6.
11. Ragozzino MW, Melton III LJ, Kurland LT, Chu CP, Perry HO. Population-based study of herpes zoster and its sequelae. Medicine (Baltimore). 1982;61:310–6.
12. Markman M, Abeloff MD. No predisposition to herpes zoster with chemotherapy of breast cancer. N Engl J Med. 1981;304:789.
13. Morison WL. Letter: herpes simplex and herpes zoster in neoplasia. Lancet. 1974;1:1293.
14. Schimpff S, Serpick A, Stoler B, et al. Varicella-zoster infection in patients with cancer. Ann Intern Med. 1972;76:241–54.
15. Feld R, Evans WK, DeBoer G. Herpes zoster in patients with small-cell carcinoma of the lung receiving combined modality treatment. Ann Intern Med. 1980;93:282–3.
16. Huberman M, Fossieck Jr BE, Bunn Jr PA, Cohen MH, Ihde DC, Minna JD. Herpes zoster and small cell bronchogenic carcinoma. Am J Med. 1980;68:214–8.
17. Feld R, Evans WK, DeBoer G. Herpes zoster in patients with carcinoma of the lung. Am J Med. 1982;73:795–801.
18. Dunst J, Steil B, Furch S, Fach A, Bormann G, Marsch W. Herpes zoster in breast cancer patients after radiotherapy. Strahlenther Onkol. 2000;176:513–6.
19. Feldman S, Hughes WT, Kim HY. Herpes zoster in children with cancer. Am J Dis Child. 1973;126:178–84.
20. Mazur MH, Dolin R. Herpes zoster at the NIH: a 20 year experience. Am J Med. 1978;65:738–44.
21. Novelli VM, Brunell PA, Geiser CF, Narkewicz S, Frierson L. Herpes zoster in children with acute lymphocytic leukemia. Am J Dis Child. 1988;142:71–2.
22. Rusthoven JJ, Ahlgren P, Elhakim T, Pinfold P, Stewart L, Feld R. Risk factors for varicella zoster disseminated infection among adult cancer patients with localized zoster. Cancer. 1988;62:1641–6.
23. Pancoast HK, Pendergrass EP. The occurence of herpes zoster in Hodgkin's disease. Am J Med Sci. 1924;168:326–34.
24. Sokal JE, Firat D. Varicella-zoster infection in Hodgkin's disease: clinical and epidemiological aspects. Am J Med. 1965;39:452–63.
25. Guinee VF, Guido JJ, Pfalzgraf KA, et al. The incidence of herpes zoster in patients with Hodgkin's disease. An analysis of prognostic factors. Cancer. 1985;56:642–8.
26. Anaissie EJ, Kontoyiannis DP, O'Brien S, et al. Infections in patients with chronic lymphocytic leukemia treated with fludarabine. Ann Intern Med. 1998;129:559–66.
27. Cheson BD. Infectious and immunosuppressive complications of purine analog therapy. J Clin Oncol. 1995;13:2431–48.
28. Buss DH, Scharyj M, White DR. Visceral herpesvirus infections in leukemic patients receiving cytarabine. JAMA. 1980;243:1903–5.
29. Laros-van Gorkam BA, Huisman CA, Wijermans PW, Schipperus MR. Experience with alemtuzumab in treatment of chronic lymphocytic leukaemia in the Netherlands. Neth J Med. 2007;65:333–8.
30. Schwarzberg AB, Stover EH, Sengupta T, et al. Selective lymphopenia and opportunistic infections in neuroendocrine tumor patients receiving temozolomide. Cancer Invest. 2007;25:249–55.
31. Su YB, Sohn S, Krown SE, et al. Selective CD4+ lymphopenia in melanoma patients treated with temozolomide: a toxicity with therapeutic implications. J Clin Oncol. 2004;22:610–6.
32. Kim SJ, Kim K, Kim BS, et al. Bortezomib and the increased incidence of herpes zoster in patients with multiple myeloma. Clin Lymphoma Myeloma. 2008;8:237–40.
33. Chanan-Khan A, Sonneveld P, Schuster MW, et al. Analysis of herpes zoster events among bortezomib-treated patients in the phase III APEX study. J Clin Oncol. 2008;26:4784–90.
34. Marin M, Meissner HC, Seward JF. Varicella prevention in the United States: a review of successes and challenges. Pediatrics. 2008;122:e744–51.
35. Atkinson K, Meyers JD, Storb R, Prentice RL, Thomas ED. Varicella zoster virus infection after marrow transplantation for aplastic anemia or leukemia. Transplantation. 1980;29:47–50.
36. Han CS, Miller W, Haake R, Weisdorf D. Varicella zoster infection after bone marrow transplantation: incidence, risk factors and complications. Bone Marrow Transplant. 1994;13:277–83.
37. Koc Y, Miller KB, Schenkein DP, et al. Varicella zoster virus infections following allogeneic bone marrow transplantation: frequency, risk factors, and clinical outcome. Biol Blood Marrow Transplant. 2000;6:44–9.
38. Leung TF, Chik KW, Li CK, et al. Incidence, risk factors and outcome of varicella-zoster virus infection in children after haematopoietic stem cell transplantation. Bone Marrow Transplant. 2000;25:167–72.
39. Locksley RM, Flournoy N, Sullivan KM, Meyers JD. Infection with varicella-zoster virus after marrow transplantation. J Infect Dis. 1985;152:1172–81.
40. Safdar A, Rodriguez GH, De Lima MJ, et al. Infections in 100 cord blood transplantations: spectrum of early and late posttransplant infections in adult and pediatric patients 1996–2005. Medicine (Baltimore). 2007;86:324–33.
41. Schuchter LM, Wingard JR, Piantadosi S, Burns WH, Santos GW, Saral R. Herpes zoster infection after autologous bone marrow transplantation. Blood. 1989;74:1424–7.

42. Wacker P, Hartmann O, Benhamou E, Salloum E, Lemerle J. Varicella-zoster virus infections after autologous bone marrow transplantation in children. Bone Marrow Transplant. 1989;4:191–4.
43. Ljungman P, Lonnqvist B, Gahrton G, Ringden O, Sundqvist VA, Wahren B. Clinical and subclinical reactivations of varicella-zoster virus in immunocompromised patients. J Infect Dis. 1986;153:840–7.
44. Gnann Jr JW. Varicella-zoster virus: atypical presentations and unusual complications. J Infect Dis. 2002;186 Suppl 1:S91–8.
45. David DS, Tegtmeier BR, O'Donnell MR, Paz IB, McCarty TM. Visceral varicella-zoster after bone marrow transplantation: report of a case series and review of the literature. Am J Gastroenterol. 1998;93:810–3.
46. Chien JW, Johnson JL. Viral pneumonias. Infection in the immunocompromised host. Postgrad Med. 2000;107:67–70, 64–73, 77–80.
47. Tauro S, Toh V, Osman H, Mahendra P. Varicella zoster meningoencephalitis following treatment for dermatomal zoster in an alloBMT patient. Bone Marrow Transplant. 2000;26:795–6.
48. Hughes BA, Kimmel DW, Aksamit AJ. Herpes zoster-associated meningoencephalitis in patients with systemic cancer. Mayo Clin Proc. 1993;68:652–5.
49. Weaver S, Rosenblum MK, DeAngelis LM. Herpes varicella zoster encephalitis in immunocompromised patients. Neurology. 1999;52:193–5.
50. Mantadakis E, Anagnostatou N, Danilatou V, et al. Fulminant hepatitis due to varicella zoster virus in a girl with acute lymphoblastic leukemia in remission: report of a case and review. J Pediatr Hematol Oncol. 2005;27:551–3.
51. Kennedy PGE. Neurological complications of varicella zoster virus. In: Kennedy PGE, Johnson RT, editors. Infections of the nervous system. London: Butterworths; 1987. p. 177–208.
52. Ojeda VJ, Peters DM, Spagnolo DV. Giant cell granulomatous angiitis of the central nervous system in a patient with leukemia and cutaneous herpes zoster. Am J Clin Pathol. 1984;81:529–32.
53. Rogers SY, Irving W, Harris A, Russell NH. Visceral varicella zoster infection after bone marrow transplantation without skin involvement and the use of PCR for diagnosis. Bone Marrow Transplant. 1995;15:805–7.
54. Stemmer SM, Kinsman K, Tellschow S, Jones RB. Fatal noncutaneous visceral infection with varicella-zoster virus in a patient with lymphoma after autologous bone marrow transplantation. Clin Infect Dis. 1993;16:497–9.
55. Ohara F, Kobayashi Y, Akabane D, et al. Abdominal pain and syndrome of inappropriate antidiuretic hormone secretion as a manifestation of visceral varicella zoster virus infection in a patient with non-Hodgkin's lymphoma. Am J Hematol. 2007;82:416.
56. Schiller GJ, Nimer SD, Gajewski JL, Golde DW. Abdominal presentation of varicella-zoster infection in recipients of allogeneic bone marrow transplantation. Bone Marrow Transplant. 1991;7:489–91.
57. Leena M, Ville V, Veli-Jukka A. Visceral varicella zoster virus infection after stem cell transplantation: a possible cause of severe abdominal pain. Scand J Gastroenterol. 2006;41:242–4.
58. Berman JN, Wang M, Berry W, Neuberg DS, Guinan EC. Herpes zoster infection in the post-hematopoietic stem cell transplant pediatric population may be preceded by transaminitis: an institutional experience. Bone Marrow Transplant. 2006;37:73–80.
59. Weinstock DM, Boeckh M, Boulad F, et al. Postexposure prophylaxis against varicella-zoster virus infection among recipients of hematopoietic stem cell transplant: unresolved issues. Infect Control Hosp Epidemiol. 2004;25:603–8.
60. Gershon AA, Steinberg SP, Gelb L. Clinical reinfection with varicella-zoster virus. J Infect Dis. 1984;149:137–42.
61. Gershon A, LaRussa P, Steinberg S. Varicella zoster virus. In: Murray PR, Baron EJ, Jorgenson JH, Pfaller MA, Yolken RH, editors. Manual of clinical microbiology. 8th ed. Washington: ASM Press; 2003. p. 1319–30.
62. Ihekwaba UK, Kudesia G, McKendrick MW. Clinical features of viral meningitis in adults: significant differences in cerebrospinal fluid findings among herpes simplex virus, varicella zoster virus, and enterovirus infections. Clinical Infect Dis. 2008;47:783–9.
63. Calvario A, Bozzi A, Scarasciulli M, et al. Herpes Consensus PCR test: a useful diagnostic approach to the screening of viral diseases of the central nervous system. J Clin Virol. 2002;25 Suppl 1:S71–8.
64. DeBiasi RL, Kleinschmidt-DeMasters BK, Weinberg A, Tyler KL. Use of PCR for the diagnosis of herpesvirus infections of the central nervous system. J Clin Virol. 2002;25 Suppl 1:S5–11.
65. Cowl CT, Prakash UB, Shawn Mitchell P, Migden MR. Varicella-zoster virus detection by polymerase chain reaction using bronchoalveolar lavage specimens. Am J Respir Crit Care Med. 2000;162:753–4.
66. LaRussa P, Steinberg S, Arvin A, et al. Polymerase chain reaction and restriction fragment length polymorphism analysis of varicella-zoster virus isolates from the United States and other parts of the world. J Infect Dis. 1998;178 Suppl 1:S64–6.
67. Levy O, Orange JS, Hibberd P, et al. Disseminated varicella infection due to the vaccine strain of varicella-zoster virus, in a patient with a novel deficiency in natural killer T cells. J Infect Dis. 2003;188:948–53.
68. Gershon AA, Larussa P, Steinberg S. Detection of antibodies to varicella-zoster virus using a latex agglutination assay. Clin Diagn Virol. 1994;2:271–7.
69. Gershon AA, Krugman S. Seroepidemiologic survey of varicella: value of specific fluorescent antibody test. Pediatrics. 1975;56:1005–8.
70. Saiman L, LaRussa P, Steinberg SP, et al. Persistence of immunity to varicella-zoster virus after vaccination of healthcare workers. Infect Control Hosp Epidemiol. 2001;22:279–83.
71. Selby PJ, Powles RL, Janeson B, et al. Parenteral acyclovir therapy for herpesvirus infections in man. Lancet. 1979;2:1267–70.
72. Shepp DH, Dandliker PS, Meyers JD. Current therapy of varicella zoster virus infection in immunocompromised patients. A comparison of acyclovir and vidarabine. Am J Med. 1988;85:96–8.
73. Shepp DH, Dandliker PS, Meyers JD. Treatment of varicella-zoster virus infection in severely immunocompromised patients. A randomized comparison of acyclovir and vidarabine. N Engl J Med. 1986;314:208–12.
74. Balfour Jr HH, Bean B, Laskin OL, et al. Acyclovir halts progression of herpes zoster in immunocompromised patients. N Engl J Med. 1983;308:1448–53.
75. Ljungman P, Lonnqvist B, Ringden O, Skinhoj P, Gahrton G. A randomized trial of oral versus intravenous acyclovir for treatment of herpes zoster in bone marrow transplant recipients. Nordic Bone Marrow Transplant Group. Bone Marrow Transplant. 1989;4:613–5.
76. Tyring S, Belanger R, Bezwoda W, Ljungman P, Boon R, Saltzman RL. A randomized, double-blind trial of famciclovir versus acyclovir for the treatment of localized dermatomal herpes zoster in immunocompromised patients. Cancer Invest. 2001;19:13–22.
77. Arora A, Mendoza N, Brantley J, Yates B, Dix L, Tyring S. Double-blind study comparing 2 dosages of valacyclovir hydrochloride for the treatment of uncomplicated herpes zoster in immunocompromised patients 18 years of age and older. J Infect Dis. 2008;197:1289–95.
78. Feldman S, Lott L. Varicella in children with cancer: impact of antiviral therapy and prophylaxis. Pediatrics. 1987;80:465–72.
79. Prober CG, Kirk LE, Keeney RE. Acyclovir therapy of chickenpox in immunosuppressed children – a collaborative study. J Pediatr. 1982;101:622–5.
80. Kakinuma H, Itoh E. A continuous infusion of acyclovir for severe hemorrhagic varicella. N Engl J Med. 1997;336:732–3.
81. Stevens DA, Merigan TC. Zoster immune globulin prophylaxis of disseminated zoster in compromised hosts. A randomized trial. Arch Intern Med. 1980;140:52–4.

82. Groth KE, McCullough J, Marker SC, et al. Evaluation of zoster immune plasma. Treatment of cutaneous disseminated zoster in immunocompromised patients. JAMA. 1978;239:1877–9.
83. Meyers JD, MacQuarrie MB, Merigan TC, Jennison MH. Nosocomial varicella. Part I: outbreak in oncology patients at a children's hospital. West J Med. 1979;130(3):196–9.
84. Morens DM, Bregman DJ, West CM, et al. An outbreak of varicella-zoster virus infection among cancer patients. Ann Intern Med. 1980;93:414–9.
85. Kavaliotis J, Loukou I, Trachana M, Gombakis N, Tsagaropoulou-Stigga H, Koliouskas D. Outbreak of varicella in a pediatric oncology unit. Med Pediatr Oncol. 1998;31(3):166–9.
86. Dykewicz CA, National Center for Infectious Diseases, Centers for Disease Control and Prevention, Infectious Diseases Society of America, American Society for Blood and Marrow Transplantation. Guidelines for preventing opportunistic infections among hematopoietic stem cell transplant recipients. MMWR Recomm Rep. 2000;49:1–125, CE121–7.
87. Geiser CF, Bishop Y, Myers M, Jaffe N, Yankee R. Prophylaxis of varicella in children with neoplastic disease: comparative results with zoster immune plasma and gamma globulin. Cancer. 1975;35:1027–30.
88. Zaia JA, Levin MJ, Preblud SR, et al. Evaluation of varicella-zoster immune globulin: protection of immunosuppressed children after household exposure to varicella. J Infect Dis. 1983;147:737–43.
89. Centers for Disease Control. Prevention of varicella: recommendations of the Advisory Committee on Immunization Practices (ACIP). MMWR Recomm Rep. 2007;56:1–40.
90. Paryani SG, Arvin AM, Koropchak CM, et al. Varicella zoster antibody titers after the administration of intravenous immune serum globulin or varicella zoster immune globulin. Am J Med. 1984;76:124–7.
91. Asano Y, Yoshikawa T, Suga S, et al. Postexposure prophylaxis of varicella in family contact by oral acyclovir. Pediatrics. 1993;92:219–22.
92. Suga S, Yoshikawa T, Ozaki T, Asano Y. Effect of oral acyclovir against primary and secondary viraemia in incubation period of varicella. Arch Dis Child. 1993;69:639–42; discussion 633–42.
93. Lin TY, Huang YC, Ning HC, Hsueh C. Oral acyclovir prophylaxis of varicella after intimate contact. Pediatr Infect Dis J. 1997;16:1162–5.
94. Weinstock DM, Boeckh M, Sepkowitz KA. Postexposure prophylaxis against varicella zoster virus infection among hematopoietic stem cell transplant recipients. Biol Blood Marrow Transplant. 2006;12:1096–7.
95. Gershon AA, Steinberg S, Galasso G, et al. Live attenuated varicella vaccine in children with leukemia in remission. Biken J. 1984;27:77–81.
96. Brunell PA, Shehab Z, Geiser C, Waugh JE. Administration of live varicella vaccine to children wtih leukaemia. Lancet. 1982;2:1069–73.
97. Gershon AA, Steinberg SP, Gelb L. Live attenuated varicella vaccine use in immunocompromised children and adults. Pediatrics. 1986;78:757–62.
98. LaRussa P, Steinberg S, Gershon AA. Varicella vaccine for immunocompromised children: results of collaborative studies in the United States and Canada. J Infect Dis. 1996;174 Suppl 3:S320–3.
99. Ljungman P, Wang FZ, Nilsson C, Solheim V, Linde A. Vaccination of autologous stem cell transplant recipients with live varicella vaccine: a pilot study. Support Care Cancer. 2003;11:739–41.
100. Brunell PA, Taylor-Wiedeman J, Geiser CF, Frierson L, Lydick E. Risk of herpes zoster in children with leukemia: varicella vaccine compared with history of chickenpox. Pediatrics. 1986;77:53–6.
101. Hardy I, Gershon AA, Steinberg SP, LaRussa P. The incidence of zoster after immunization with live attenuated varicella vaccine. A study in children with leukemia. Varicella Vaccine Collaborative Study Group. N Engl J Med. 1991;325:1545–50.
102. Lawrence R, Gershon AA, Holzman R, Steinberg SP. The risk of zoster after varicella vaccination in children with leukemia. N Engl J Med. 1988;318:543–8.
103. Leung TF, Li CK, Hung EC, et al. Immunogenicity of a two-dose regime of varicella vaccine in children with cancers. Eur J Haematol. 2004;72:353–7.
104. Brunell PA, Geiser CF, Novelli V, Lipton S, Narkewicz S. Varicella-like illness caused by live varicella vaccine in children with acute lymphocytic leukemia. Pediatrics. 1987;79:922–7.
105. Galea SA, Sweet A, Beninger P, et al. The safety profile of varicella vaccine: a 10-year review. J Infect Dis. 2008;197 Suppl 2:S165–9.
106. Schrauder A, Henke-Gendo C, Seidemann K, et al. Varicella vaccination in a child with acute lymphoblastic leukaemia. Lancet. 2007;369:1232.
107. Hughes P, LaRussa P, Pearce JM, Lepow M, Steinberg S, Gershon A. Transmission of varicella-zoster virus from a vaccinee with leukemia, demonstrated by polymerase chain reaction. J Pediatr. 1994;124:932–5.
108. Tsolia M, Gershon AA, Steinberg SP, Gelb L. Live attenuated varicella vaccine: evidence that the virus is attenuated and the importance of skin lesions in transmission of varicella-zoster virus. National Institute of Allergy and Infectious Diseases Varicella Vaccine Collaborative Study Group. J Pediatr. 1990;116:184–9.
109. Harpaz R, Ortega-Sanchez IR, Seward JF. Prevention of herpes zoster: recommendations of the Advisory Committee on Immunization Practices (ACIP). MMWR Recomm Rep. 2008;57:1–30; quiz CE32–4.
110. Kamboj M, Sepkowitz KA. Risk of transmission associated with live attenuated vaccines given to healthy persons caring for or residing with an immunocompromised patient. Infect Control Hosp Epidemiol. 2007;28:702–7.
111. Whitley RJ, Gnann Jr JW, Hinthorn D, et al. Disseminated herpes zoster in the immunocompromised host: a comparative trial of acyclovir and vidarabine. The NIAID Collaborative Antiviral Study Group. J Infect Dis. 1992;165:450–5.
112. Meyers JD, Wade JC, Shepp DH, Newton B. Acyclovir treatment of varicella-zoster virus infection in the compromised host. Transplantation. 1984;37:571–4.
113. Sullivan KM, Dykewicz CA, Longworth DL, et al. Preventing opportunistic infections after hematopoietic stem cell transplantation: the Centers for Disease Control and Prevention, Infectious Diseases Society of America, and American Society for Blood and Marrow Transplantation Practice Guidelines and beyond. Hematology Am Soc Hematol Educ Program. 2001;1:392–421.
114. Kanda Y, Mineishi S, Saito T, et al. Long-term low-dose acyclovir against varicella-zoster virus reactivation after allogeneic hematopoietic stem cell transplantation. Bone Marrow Transplant. 2001;28:689–92.
115. Ljungman P, Wilczek H, Gahrton G, et al. Long-term acyclovir prophylaxis in bone marrow transplant recipients and lymphocyte proliferation responses to herpes virus antigens in vitro. Bone Marrow Transplant. 1986;1:185–92.
116. Selby PJ, Powles RL, Easton D, et al. The prophylactic role of intravenous and long-term oral acyclovir after allogeneic bone marrow transplantation. Br J Cancer. 1989;59:434–8.
117. Sempere A, Sanz GF, Senent L, et al. Long-term acyclovir prophylaxis for prevention of varicella zoster virus infection after autologous blood stem cell transplantation in patients with acute leukemia. Bone Marrow Transplant. 1992;10:495–8.
118. Steer CB, Szer J, Sasadeusz J, Matthews JP, Beresford JA, Grigg A. Varicella-zoster infection after allogeneic bone marrow transplantation: incidence, risk factors and prevention with low-dose aciclovir and ganciclovir. Bone Marrow Transplant. 2000;25:657–64.
119. Thomson KJ, Hart DP, Banerjee L, Ward KN, Peggs KS, Mackinnon S. The effect of low-dose aciclovir on reactivation of

119. varicella zoster virus after allogeneic haemopoietic stem cell transplantation. Bone Marrow Transplant. 2005;35:1065–9.
120. Boeckh M, Kim HW, Flowers ME, Meyers JD, Bowden RA. Long-term acyclovir for prevention of varicella zoster virus disease after allogeneic hematopoietic cell transplantation – a randomized double-blind placebo-controlled study. Blood. 2006;107:1800–5.
121. Erard V, Guthrie KA, Varley C, et al. One-year acyclovir prophylaxis for preventing varicella-zoster virus disease after hematopoietic cell transplantation: no evidence of rebound varicella-zoster virus disease after drug discontinuation. Blood. 2007;110:3071–7.
122. Boeckh M. Prevention of VZV infection in immunosuppressed patients using antiviral agents. Herpes. 2006;13:60–5.
123. Seeley WW, Marty FM, Holmes TM, et al. Post-transplant acute limbic encephalitis: clinical features and relationship to HHV6. Neurology. 2007;69:156–65.
124. Fotheringham J, Donati D, Akhyani N, et al. Association of human herpesvirus-6B with mesial temporal lobe epilepsy. PLoS Med. 2007;4:e180.
125. Singh N, Paterson DL. Encephalitis caused by human herpesvirus-6 in transplant recipients: relevance of a novel neurotropic virus. Transplantation. 2000;69:2474–9.
126. Ljungman P, de la Camara R, Cordonnier C, et al. Management of CMV, HHV-6, HHV-7 and Kaposi-sarcoma herpesvirus (HHV-8) infections in patients with hematological malignancies and after SCT. Bone Marrow Transplant. 2008;42:227–40.
127. Wang LR, Dong LJ, Zhang MJ, Lu DP. Correlations of human herpesvirus 6B and CMV infection with acute GVHD in recipients of allogeneic haematopoietic stem cell transplantation. Bone Marrow Transplant. 2008;42:673–7.
128. Wang LR, Dong LJ, Zhang MJ, Lu DP. The impact of human herpesvirus 6B reactivation on early complications following allogeneic hematopoietic stem cell transplantation. Biol Blood Marrow Transplant. 2006;12:1031–7.
129. Yamane A, Mori T, Suzuki S, et al. Risk factors for developing human herpesvirus 6 (HHV-6) reactivation after allogeneic hematopoietic stem cell transplantation and its association with central nervous system disorders. Biol Blood Marrow Transplant. 2007;13:100–6.
130. de Pagter PJ, Schuurman R, Visscher H, et al. Human herpes virus 6 plasma DNA positivity after hematopoietic stem cell transplantation in children: an important risk factor for clinical outcome. Biol Blood Marrow Transplant. 2008;14:831–9.
131. Wang FZ, Linde A, Hagglund H, Testa M, Locasciulli A, Ljungman P. Human herpesvirus 6 DNA in cerebrospinal fluid specimens from allogeneic bone marrow transplant patients: does it have clinical significance? Clin Infect Dis. 1999;28:562–8.
132. van Esser JW, Niesters HG, van der Holt B, et al. Prevention of Epstein-Barr virus-lymphoproliferative disease by molecular monitoring and preemptive rituximab in high-risk patients after allogeneic stem cell transplantation. Blood. 2002;99:4364–9.
133. Weinstock DM, Ambrossi GG, Brennan C, Kiehn TE, Jakubowski A. Preemptive diagnosis and treatment of Epstein-Barr virus-associated post transplant lymphoproliferative disorder after hematopoietic stem cell transplant: an approach in development. Bone Marrow Transplant. 2006;37:539–46.
134. O'Reilly RJ, Small TN, Papadopoulos E, Lucas K, Lacerda J, Koulova L. Biology and adoptive cell therapy of Epstein-Barr virus-associated lymphoproliferative disorders in recipients of marrow allografts. Immunol Rev. 1997;157:195–216.
135. Papadopoulos EB, Ladanyi M, Emanuel D, et al. Infusions of donor leukocytes to treat Epstein-Barr virus-associated lymphoproliferative disorders after allogeneic bone marrow transplantation. N Engl J Med. 1994;330:1185–91.
136. Leen AM, Heslop HE. Cytotoxic T lymphocytes as immunetherapy in haematological practice. Br J Haematol. 2008;143:169–79.
137. Chang Y, Cesarman E, Pessin MS, et al. Identification of herpesvirus-like DNA sequences in AIDS-associated Kaposi's sarcoma. Science. 1994;266:1865–9.
138. Luppi M, Barozzi P, Schulz TF, et al. Bone marrow failure associated with human herpesvirus 8 infection after transplantation. N Engl J Med. 2000;343:1378–85.
139. Cuzzola M, Irrera G, Iacopino O, et al. Bone marrow failure associated with herpesvirus 8 infection in a patient undergoing autologous peripheral blood stem cell transplantation. Clin Infect Dis. 2003;37:e102–6.

Chapter 32
Respiratory Viruses

Roy F. Chemaly, Dhanesh B. Rathod, and Robert Couch

Abstract The respiratory viruses as a group are the most common cause of an acute infectious illness in developed societies. The immunocompromised state of many cancer patients constitutes the basis for the frequent failure of the host to promote a normal and rapid recovery from an acute respiratory viral infection and results in a more severe and prolonged infection that causes significant morbidity and mortality in these patients. Those respiratory viruses that are most prevalent and most prone to produce lower respiratory illnesses and pneumonia in healthy hosts, RSV, influenza viruses, and parainfluenza viruses, are those most likely to cause severe illness and pneumonia leading to hospitalization in immunocompromised persons. However, viruses less prone to produce a lower respiratory illness but that are highly prevalent, such as rhinoviruses, may frequently be associated with severe illness. The limited availability of antivirals and vaccines for the acute respiratory viruses means that these infections will continue to be important for many years and dictate a need for utilizing infection control procedures as much as possible, particularly in hospitals and institutions, so as to minimize spread. Efforts to develop specific vaccines are important as their use could prevent as well as reduce exposure of cancer patients to these viruses. Development of specific antivirals is important for use in immunocompromised patients as normal recovery mechanisms may be seriously impaired.

Keywords Influenza • Cancer • Transplant • RSV • Adenovirus • Metapneumovirus

Introduction

Community respiratory virus infections were once primarily considered to be infections of children and generally nonserious. However, over the past two decades, it has become clear that these viruses can cause serious infections that require medical attention, particularly in infant, elderly, and immunocompromised patients. Historically, the most common causes of respiratory infections in cancer patients were thought to be opportunistic bacteria and fungi, but newer diagnostic methods have revealed that respiratory viruses can cause serious morbidity and mortality in such patients, including leukemia patients and hematopoietic stem cell transplant (HSCT) recipients.

Many viruses are known to cause respiratory tract infections, but the most common in hospitalized cancer patients are influenza viruses, respiratory syncytial virus (RSV), and parainfluenza viruses (PIV) [1, 2]. However, all respiratory viruses can cause respiratory infections in cancer patients including rhinoviruses, enteroviruses, coronaviruses, human metapneumoviruses (hMPVs), adenoviruses, as well as cytomegaloviruses, herpes simplex, and varicella zoster viruses. In this chapter, we discuss the common clinical presentations, diagnostic methods, treatments, and prevention measures for respiratory virus infections in general and in cancer patients in particular (Table 32.1).

Data from September 2008 to February 2010 (18-month period) at our institution (Fig. 32.1) demonstrate the cyclical pattern of the three major respiratory viruses: RSV, influenza, and PIV. During the 2009–2010 season, influenza infections in our cancer patients were reported starting July 2009 with a peak in October 2009 due to the pandemic A (H1N1) influenza virus. More recently, a total of 181 cases of influenza, parainfluenza, and RSV were identified at our institution between 1 September 2009 and 28 February 2010 (Fig. 32.2). Of these cases, most were in HSCT recipients (45%).

Respiratory Syncytial Virus

Most RSV infections occur in infants and young children throughout the world [2, 3]. In the United States, these infections usually occur from late fall to the end of spring, with a peak from January to February; few cases are reported during

R.F. Chemaly (✉)
Department of Infectious Diseases, Infection Control, and Employee Health, The University of Texas M.D. Anderson Cancer Center, 1515 Holcombe Boulevard, Unit 1460, Houston, TX 77030, USA
e-mail: rfchemaly@mdanderson.org

Table 32.1 Syndromes and their commonly associated viruses

Syndrome	Commonly associated viruses	Less commonly associated viruses
Common cold	Rhinoviruses, coronaviruses	Influenza and parainfluenza viruses, enteroviruses, adenoviruses
Influenza-like illness	Influenza viruses	Parainfluenza viruses, adenoviruses
Croup/laryngitis	Parainfluenza viruses	Influenza viruses, respiratory syncytial virus, adenoviruses
Bronchitis/bronchiolitis	Respiratory syncytial virus	Influenza and parainfluenza viruses, adenovirus
Pneumonia	Influenza viruses, respiratory syncytial virus, adenoviruses	Parainfluenza viruses, measles, cytomegalovirus, varicella zoster virus, herpes simplex virus

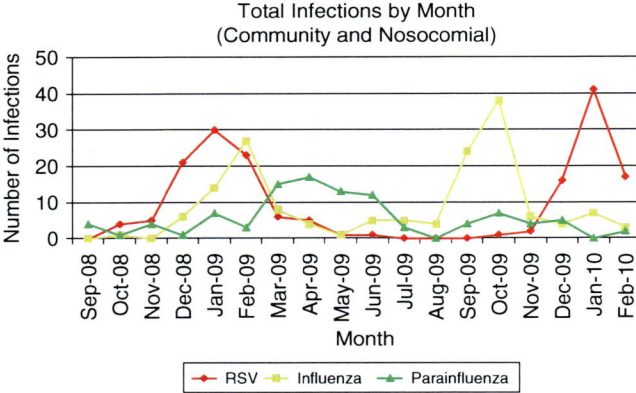

Fig. 32.1 Community and nosocomial infections per month for RSV, influenza, and parainfluenza virus at M.D. Anderson Cancer Center between September 2008 and February 2010

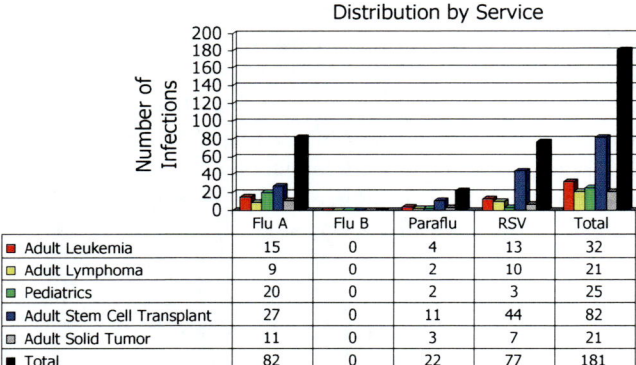

Fig. 32.2 Distribution of the infections caused by RSV, influenza, and parainfluenza virus by different services at M.D. Anderson Cancer Center that occurred between September 2009 and February 2010

Clinical Presentations

RSV infections can present with a wide array of upper or lower respiratory symptoms. The incubation period is 4–6 days in adults. In infants and young children, the primary infection starts in the upper respiratory tract, with rhinorrhea, low-grade fever, and cough; it may progress to lower respiratory infection (LRI) (bronchiolitis or pneumonia), at which stage most patients seek medical attention [3, 6]. It is also likely to involve the sinuses and the middle ear. RSV is known to cause apnea in infants, although the mechanism of this action remains unknown. Older children and adults typically present with upper respiratory tract symptoms, but may also have constitutional symptoms such as fever and malaise [3, 7]. RSV upper respiratory infections (URIs) can also progress to the lower respiratory tract, particularly in institutionalized adults and those with severe combined immunodeficiency, leukemia, HSCT, and in lung transplant recipients [2, 8, 9]. These patients may present with wheezing and shortness of breath, with or without underlying comorbidities or known hyperactive airways. Almost 35% of elderly patients with RSV infections report wheezing [8–11].

Infections in Immunocompromised Patients

Patients with weakened immune systems because of malignancy, chemotherapy, steroid use, HSCT, or solid organ transplantation are at high risk for developing severe illnesses. They also tend to have a longer duration of infection, with a varied presentation [12, 13]. Leukemia patients and solid organ and stem cell transplant recipients are particularly at risk, with the latter being at high risk for pneumonia and death prior to engraftment [11].

Leukemia Patients and HSCT Recipients

RSV infections begin as URI, but progress to LRI in 30–60% of HSCT recipients, leading to respiratory failure with significant morbidity and mortality; some early studies described a mortality rate of 70–100% [14, 15]. In HSCT recipients, the risk factors for progression to LRI

the summer [2–4]. RSV is a member of the *Paramyxoviridae* family and the genus *Pneumovirus*. It is an enveloped single-stranded RNA virus approximately 150–300 nm in diameter that is contained in a helical nucleocapsid surrounded by a lipid envelope. This envelope bears two glycoproteins: the G protein, which attaches to the cell surface, and the F (fusion) protein, which enables the internal components to enter the cell after fusion of host and viral membranes and to initiate replication. Both glycoproteins are integral to pathogenesis [2, 3, 5]. There are two groups of RSV viruses, groups A and B [2–5].

include lymphopenia, older age, stage of malignancy, graft-versus-host disease, and no ribavirin treatment [16–19]. Torres et al. [20] found that a high APACHE II score and not giving aerosolized ribavirin treatment were independent predictors of progression to pneumonia in leukemia patients; those with URI who were treated with aerosolized ribavirin were less likely than untreated patients to develop pneumonia (68 vs. 96%, $p<0.01$) and die with RSV infection (6 vs. 36%, $p=0.1$). The overall mortality rate in the study was 10% [20].

Solid Organ Transplant Recipients

Solid organ transplantation patients with RSV infection may present with dyspnea, cough, fever, and wheezing which progress to pneumonia in more than 70% of patients [21]. In lung transplant recipients, a higher frequency of RSV pneumonia has been reported, but the mortality rate is low; the mortality rate is also low in kidney transplant recipients [21]. In pediatric liver transplant patients, Pohl et al. reported a mortality rate of 17% for RSV pneumonia with early infection onset and preexisting lung disease as predictors of severe disease [22].

Other Immunocompromised Patients

In children, genetic polymorphisms in cytokine and chemokine-related genes (interleukin [IL]-4, IL-8, IL-10, IL-13, and CCR5) and genes related to potential virus-cell surface interactions or cell signaling (TLR-4, CX3CR1, SP-A, and SP-D) have been associated with severe RSV infections [23].

Data on HIV patients with RSV infections are scarce; however, a cohort study by Miller et al. [24] performed in the winter of 1994–1995 found no evidence of influenza, RSV, parainfluenza, adenovirus, or enterovirus infections in the bronchoscopic alveolar lavage fluids of 44 HIV-1-positive patients.

Diagnosis

RSV can be diagnosed on the basis of the clinical presentation in infants with LRI during an outbreak period [3]. RSV infections in adults cannot be clinically differentiated from other viral infections that cause upper respiratory symptoms. For a specific diagnosis, RSV must be detected in respiratory secretions. Nasal aspirates or washes are most likely to give a positive RSV test in young children. If a nasal aspirate or wash cannot be obtained, a nasopharyngeal swab or throat swab may be used. Because immunocompromised or intubated patients are more likely to develop an LRI due to RSV, tracheal aspiration or bronchoalveolar lavage should be performed [8, 25]. The gold standard for diagnosing RSV remains the identification of virus causing typical syncytia in cultures of HEp-2 cells [25]. Viral cultures may take 2 days (shell vial cultures) and up to 2 weeks (routine cultures) to become positive, making isolation less relevant in most clinical settings. Other available methods include antigen detection by enzyme-linked immunosorbent assay (ELISA), immunoflourescence assay, and polymerase chain reaction (PCR) tests. Fan et al. [26] reported a sensitivity of 65–95% for RSV detection using rapid antigen testing with ELISA. PCR tests have been shown to be more sensitive than direct antigen detection [27, 28].

Treatment

For most immunocompromised patients, RSV treatment is focused on reducing symptom severity and preventing progression to LRIs. Nonsteroidal anti-inflammatory drugs and antihistamines have been used in patients with a URI. Ribavirin, a nucleoside analog, has in vitro activity against RSV and has been approved by the United States Food and Drug Administration for the treatment of RSV infections in children. Two schedules of aerosolized ribavirin have been used in immunocompromised patients: continuous and intermittent. On the continuous schedule, a daily dose of 6 g (concentration, 20 mg/mL) is delivered over 18 h via a small particle aerosol generator unit, administered via a face mask in a tent. On the intermittent schedule, a concentration of 60 mg/mL is delivered over 3 h every 8 h.

Aerosolized ribavirin may be beneficial in certain adults and children with LRIs. Its early use has been shown in some retrospective studies to reduce morbidity and mortality in HSCT recipients [3, 29] and patients with hematologic malignancies, particularly when the infection is treated early on [30]. However, its effectiveness in solid organ transplantation patients remains unknown [31]. An RSV-specific monoclonal antibody (Palivizumab) did not demonstrate a therapeutic benefit in a major study conducted in children [32]. Although the combination of ribavirin and intravenous immunoglobulin (IVIG) or palivizumab has not been evaluated in a randomized trial, it is sometimes used in severely ill patients with RSV pneumonia, especially HSCT recipients, given that they have high mortality rates from this infection [3, 11, 14]. In patients at risk for progression to LRI, aerosolized ribavirin should be considered at an early stage. A recent trial demonstrated that both the intermittent and continuous schedules of aerosolized ribavirin were effective at preventing progression to LRIs in 91% and 80% of patients with RSV URIs and hematologic malignancies (including HSCT recipients), respectively [33].

Prevention/Vaccination

RSV infection may be acquired nosocomially, thus specific infection control measures should be implemented when dealing with patients with known or suspected infections. Briefly, patients should be isolated in private rooms when possible, and appropriate personnel protective equipments should be used (i.e., disposable gloves, masks, and gowns) [34]. No licensed vaccine is available for RSV; however, two agents, RSV-IVIG and palivizumab, have been used to prevent RSV infection. RSV-IVIG has been studied in children younger than 24 months with severe lung disease and those who were born prematurely [35], but it was removed from the market in 2003. A randomized double-blind placebo-controlled study in children found that palivizumab recipients had a 45% relative reduction in RSV hospitalizations ($p = 0.003$). Twenty-one children (3.3%) died in the palivizumab group vs. 27 (4.2%) in the placebo group with no deaths attributable to palivizumab [36]. Palivizumab is easier to administer than regular IVIG, which must be given over 4–6 h, and does not interfere with other vaccinations. However, RSV-IVIG and IVIG may provide additional protection against other respiratory viruses as well [35, 37, 38].

Influenza Viruses

Influenza viruses infect both the upper and lower respiratory tracts. Outbreaks are common every winter, although the severity of the disease varies considerably. Influenza viruses belong to the *Orthomyxoviridae* family, with influenza types A, B, and C constituting one genus. These RNA viruses are enveloped and measure about 80–120 nm in diameter. The designation of the viruses into types is based on the stable antigenic characteristics of the nucleoprotein and the matrix protein antigens. Influenza A and B viruses have surface glycoproteins known as hemagglutinins (HA) and neuraminidase (NA). Three hemagglutinin subtypes (H1, H2, and H3) and two neuraminidase subtypes (N1 and N2) have been described for the influenza A viruses that infect humans. Major antigenic changes in the glycoprotein (basis for new subtypes) are called antigenic shift and can cause pandemics; minor antigenic changes occur frequently, are called antigenic drift, and cause the annual epidemics. Influenza B has only exhibited minor antigenic drift [3, 39]. The 2009 pandemic influenza A (H1N1) contains segments present in North American swine for years, but is a new reassortant virus that acquired M and NA gene segments from a Eurasian adamantane-resistant swine influenza virus [40].

Clinical Presentation

Influenza typically has a short incubation period and an abrupt onset of symptoms, such as headache, fever, chills, myalgia, and malaise, along with respiratory symptoms of runny nose, cough, and sore throat. It can also present as a febrile URI or with constitutional manifestations only or with few-to-no respiratory symptoms.

Influenza can progress to pneumonia in otherwise healthy persons, but particularly in patients with comorbidities such as lung diseases, heart disease, diabetes mellitus, renal diseases, and hemoglobinopathies, in immunocompromised individuals, residents of nursing homes or chronic care facilities, and in individuals over 65 years of age [41].

Primary pneumonia occurs when the influenza virus directly involves the lung and should be suspected when clinical symptoms progress to high fever, dyspnea, and hypoxemia [42]. Influenza virus infections also affect the epithelium of the tracheobronchial tree, leading to impaired defense and a secondary bacterial pneumonia.

Infections in Immunocompromised Patients

Influenza infections can increase morbidity and mortality rates in cancer patients [2].

Leukemia Patients and HSCT Recipients

In a study of leukemia patients with influenza infections, 39% of patients developed pneumonia [43], with cough and dyspnea being the most common manifestations. Half of the patients had lymphopenia [43]. The incidence of influenza infection in HSCT recipients is reported as 0.4% [44], with a mortality rate up to 38% [43], mainly due to respiratory failure. In one study [44], 17% of patients who developed influenza after HSCT presented with pneumonia; of those who presented with URIs, 14% experienced progression to LRI. Risk factors associated with progression to LRI were lymphopenia and days from transplantation (i.e., pneumonia developed more commonly among those infected earlier after transplantation); whereas use of systemic steroids and autologous stem cell transplantation appeared to be protective. X-ray findings include a diffuse interstitial pattern or focal pulmonary infiltrates [45].

Solid Organ Transplant Patients

Among patients with solid organ transplantation, lung transplant recipients are at the highest risk for influenza virus infection [46]. The initial presentation in these patients may not always be in the respiratory tract, as illness can present with nonspecific gastrointestinal symptoms; however, patients who required hospitalization always presented with pneumonia [47]. Progression to bronchiolitis obliterans, which is a characteristic of chronic lung rejection after infection, was also reported. In patients postrenal transplantation, influenza pneumonia is often acute, with high fever, cough, dyspnea, cyanosis, leukopenia, and thrombocytopenia [48].

Diagnosis

Influenza infection can only be diagnosed clinically in persons exhibiting the classic syndrome during an epidemic. However, because other viruses can produce the same syndrome and influenza infection can produce other respiratory syndromes, a confirmatory test detecting the virus or viral antigens in nasal washes, throat swabs, respiratory tract secretions, or bronchoalveolar lavage specimens is needed in sporadic cases and in immunocompromised patients. Viral culture remains the gold standard for diagnosis, but can take up to 72 h to yield results [49]. Sputum and nasal washes or nose swabs are superior to throat swabs for diagnosis [50]. Rapid antigen testing using immunoflourescence assays, enzyme immunoassays, and PCR-based testing are used frequently in clinical settings [51]. The results of these tests can be obtained in hours and can have good sensitivity (72–95%) and specificity (76–84%) if obtained early from those with more severe illnesses [52]. PCR-based assays are more sensitive than rapid antigen testing for diagnosing influenza A and B, but are not often used because of availability and cost [51]. Samples should be obtained within 24–48 h of the appearance of symptoms for the most accurate results.

Treatment

Two classes of drugs are available to treat influenza infections [53]: the neuraminidase inhibitors, zanamivir and oseltamivir, which are active against influenza A and B viruses; and the M2 inhibitors, amantadine and rimantadine, which are only active against influenza A viruses [54]. Amantadines are not effective against influenza B and resistance has been reported for 2009 novel H1N1 virus; resistance to oseltamivir has increased for the seasonal H1N1 virus (Table 32.2) [55, 56].

Table 32.2 Recent antiviral resistance pattern for different influenza strains[a,b]

	Oseltamivir	Zanamivir	M2 inhibitors[c]
2009 H1N1	Susceptible	Susceptible	Resistant
Seasonal H1N1	Mostly resistant	Susceptible	Mostly susceptible
Seasonal H3N2	Susceptible	Susceptible	Susceptible
Influenza B	Susceptible	Susceptible	Resistant
Avian H5N1	Susceptible	Susceptible	Variable

[a]Centers for Disease Control and Prevention. http://www.cdc.gov/h1n1flu/recommendations.htm
[b]WHO Guidelines for the Pharmacologic Management of Pandemic (H1N1) 2009 influenza and other influenza viruses. http://www.who.int/csr/resources/publications/swineflu/h1n1_use_antivirals_20090820/en/index.html
[c]Amantadine and rimantadine

Therapy should be initiated as early as possible, preferably within 48 h after symptom onset [57]. Zanamivir and oseltamivir have been used extensively to treat both influenza A and B; both were shown to reduce the mean duration of symptoms by 1 day when used within 48 h of symptom onset [58]. Both neuraminidase inhibitors have been shown to significantly decrease the incidence of complications associated with influenza such as development of pneumonia when compared to placebo [59]. The most common side effects of oseltamivir are nausea and vomiting, although other toxicities have been reported. Central nervous system side effects such as anxiety, insomnia, impaired thinking, confusion, lightheadedness, and hallucinations have been reported with amantadine use. Newer NI inhibitors including parenteral preparations are under development [60].

Prevention/Vaccination

The mainstay of influenza prophylaxis in the general population is the administration of influenza vaccine. Annual vaccination has been recommended for many years for people at high risk for complications, including those older than 65 years, residents of nursing homes or other facilities, adults and children with chronic pulmonary or cardiovascular conditions, adults and children hospitalized during the previous year, women in the second and the third trimesters of pregnancy, immunocompromised patients, healthcare workers, and family member of those at high risk prior to the onset of influenza season [41]. The American Committee on Immunization Practices has recently recommended vaccination for all persons for whom there is no contraindication [61].

Currently, there are two types of vaccines available, an intramuscular (inactivated virus vaccine) and an intranasal (attenuated virus vaccine). The intranasal form is to be used only in healthy individuals between the ages of 2 and 49 years;

it should not be used to vaccinate immunocompromised patients [62]. Individuals with a significant allergy to eggs or those with acute febrile illness should not be given vaccine [63]. The Advisory Committee on Immunization Practices recommends that immunocompromised individuals be vaccinated prior to influenza season and receive daily chemoprophylaxis with an antiviral medication during community outbreaks [41].

Influenza chemoprophylaxis may be used in patients at high risk for complications if the vaccine is contraindicated or not likely to be completely protective. Antiviral drugs should be administered to patients within the first 6 months of HSCT, those with documented graft-versus-host disease, unvaccinated healthcare workers who care for immunocompromised individuals, and residents of long-term care institutions during outbreak periods [64]. The American Society for Blood and Marrow Transplantation (ASBMT) 2009 guidelines [65] for prevention of infection in HSCT recipients recommend annual inactivated influenza vaccine before the beginning of the season and before stem cell transplant. The vaccine may be given 4–6 months after HSCT. They also recommended prophylaxis and preemptive treatment during community and nosocomial outbreaks of influenza A for HSCT recipients regardless of the vaccination status in those who are within 24 months of the transplant or in those with more than 24 months posttransplant, but have GVHD and/or are on immunosuppression. The drug to be used for chemoprophylaxis depends on the susceptibility pattern of the outbreak virus.

Parainfluenza Viruses

PIV are enveloped, single-stranded RNA viruses that belong to the *Paramyxoviridae* family. The envelope contains two glycoproteins, one with both HA and neuraminidase activity and the other with fusion activity. There are five types that share certain antigens with other members of the *Paramyxoviridae* family [3, 66]. Of the five, PIV-3 is the most prevalent, with most adults demonstrating the presence of antibodies [67]. PIV-3 infections may be epidemic in the spring and summer, but may also occur through the year; PIV-3 is associated with pneumonia and bronchiolitis in infants. PIV-1 and 2 are associated with croup in children which occurs as outbreaks every 2 years in the fall; PIV-4A and 4B cause only mild illnesses [67, 68].

Clinical Presentation

PIV infections have a wide spectrum of presentations, from a simple URI to a life-threatening complication such as pneumonia. The incubation period is usually 2–6 days. Young children may present with coryza, sore throat, hoarseness, and cough with chest X-rays revealing interstitial infiltrates. In adults, most infections are mild, but in immunocompromised individuals, the infection can progress to a lower respiratory tract illness including pneumonia and cause prolonged illness and even death [3, 67, 69].

Infections in Immunocompromised Patients

Immunocompromised individuals are at risk for a PIV infection that can progress to pneumonia. A study at our institution found a higher rate of progression among leukemia patients than among HSCT recipients [70].

Leukemia Patients and HSCT Recipients

PIV usually presents as an URI. In a large study in HSCT recipients over several years, PIV infections were documented in 7.1% of cases, with 78% being community-acquired [71]. Patients who have undergone HSCT are at particular risk for developing severe PIV-associated pneumonia [71–74]; Wendt et al. [72] reported a mortality rate up to 30%. Coinfections (*Aspergillus fumigatus* being the most common) and mechanical ventilation were found to be significant risk factors for PIV pneumonia-associated mortality in one study [71]. Other factors associated with progression include neutropenia within 1 month prior to infection, an APACHE II score higher than 15, and pulmonary coinfection; this study also found a mortality rate around 20%, with no difference between those treated and those not treated with aerosolized ribavirin [70].

Solid Organ Transplant Patients

Patients who have undergone solid organ transplantation do not appear to be at increased risk for developing severe PIV illness, but only a few studies have been reported [75, 76]. One of these studies in lung transplant patients found PIV infections in 11% of patients, all of whom developed pneumonia, but the majority (74%) were treated with aerosolized ribavirin and all but one recovered [75].

Diagnosis

Except for croup in young children, the clinical pattern of PIV infection is similar to that of other respiratory viruses and cannot be distinguished on the basis of symptoms alone. During a community outbreak, a presumptive diagnosis can be made; however, confirmation in laboratory tests may be appropriate in immunocompromised individuals. The virus can be detected in respiratory tract secretions, nasal washes, nasal swabs, throat swabs, and bronchoalveolar lavage specimens. Viral culture remains the gold standard for diagnosis, but can take days to yield a result [3, 77]. Rapid antigen detection by immunofluorescence or ELISA is most commonly used and can have a sensitivity of as high as 75–95% [78]. Recent PCR-based assays have sensitivities up to 100%, with high specificity [26, 79].

Treatment

Management of PIV infection is mostly supportive as no PIV-directed antiviral therapy has been licensed by the U.S. Food and Drug Administration. Ribavirin has been shown to be active against the virus in vitro and in animal models and has been used occasionally to treat immunocompromised patients with severe PIV infections [80]. One case series reported a decrease in PIV viral loads and clinical improvement after aerosolized ribavirin treatment in children with severe immunodeficiency [81]. Nichols et al. [71] reported that aerosolized ribavirin did not reduce viral shedding or mortality rates in HSCT recipients after the infection had progressed to the lower respiratory tract. Our data also showed no apparent benefit of aerosolized ribavirin on the mortality rate in HSCT recipients and leukemia patients [70]. On the other hand, a combination of methylprednisolone and intravenous or oral ribavirin has, apparently, been used successfully to treat PIV pneumonia in a HSCT and a heart transplant recipient, respectively [82, 83].

Prevention/Vaccination

Currently, no licensed vaccine is available for the prevention of PIV infection. Hence, infection control measures play an important role in containing the spread of the infection. Patients with suspected or confirmed infections should be isolated, and personnel protective equipment should be used.

Adenovirus

Human adenoviruses are DNA viruses belonging to the *Mastadenovirus* genus of the Adenoviridae family which measure about 70–80 nm in diameter [3, 84]. There are at least 51 known human serotypes divided into subgenera A to F based on the DNA genome and pattern of hemagglutination [84]. Adenovirus infections are reported most frequently in infants and children and can occur throughout the year; however, they may cause serious infections in immunocompromised patients. After a primary infection in childhood, adenoviruses establish latency in adenoidal tissues along with lifelong persistence of specific antibodies [84, 85].

Clinical Presentation

Adenovirus infections are transmitted by either inhalation of aerosolized virus, inoculation of the virus into conjunctival sac, or through the fecal-oral route [3, 84]. Subgroup A, type 31 and various types from subgroups B and C have been associated with pneumonia and hepatitis [86]. Serotypes 4, 7, 14, and 21 are associated with outbreaks of acute respiratory disease in military recruits, mostly in winter and spring [3]. Types 1, 2, 5, and 6 are most common in children and present as an acute upper respiratory tract illness which can progress to lower respiratory disease; types 3 and 7 are less common, but can cause severe disease. In adults, infections due to adenovirus are characterized by sore throat and gradual onset of fever. Cough, coryza, and regional lymphadenopathy are commonly seen. The most common clinical symptoms besides respiratory symptoms are fever and diarrhea [3].

Infections in Immunocompromised Patients

Leukemia Patients and HSCT Recipients

Adenovirus infections are common after HSCT and can occur as a localized illness or as part of a disseminated disease. It has been associated with delayed engraftment and graft failure. Infections due to adenovirus in HSCT recipients have a reported incidence of 0.5–3% [87, 88] and are more commonly reported in allogeneic HSCT recipients than in autologous transplant recipients (6 vs. 0.92%) [87]; however, the mortality rate can be as high as 75% in both groups [87, 89]. Some reports also suggest that the incidence of adenovirus infection in patients after HSCT may be rising due to transplantation practices [90, 91]. Disseminated infection may occur without respiratory tract symptoms and disease can develop in almost any organ causing gastrointestinal disease, hepatitis, nephritis, pneumonia, conjunctivitis, thrombotic thrombocytopenic purpura, pancreatitis, or hemorrhagic cystitis. Viremia may be present, but is not detected in all cases of disseminated disease [92].

Adenovirus is known to be fatal even in the absence of any respiratory tract involvement; however, if pneumonia is present, the mortality has been reported to be higher (80 vs. 50%) [87]. Coinfections with *Aspergillus* spp. and bacteria such as Nocardia, *Legionella* spp., and *Mycobacterium tuberculous* are frequently seen in this patient population [90, 93]. Risk factors for adenovirus infections include GVHD, unrelated donor, total body irradiation, T-cell depletion, younger age (<7 years old), chronic disease, and recent transplantation [90, 91, 94, 95]; the degree of T-cell depletion and posttransplant suppression of T-cell function are the most important ones [92]. Adenovirus types 5 and 21 are associated with severe infections in HSCT recipients [95].

Solid Organ Transplant Patients

There are a few reports of adenovirus infections in solid organ transplant patients in whom the virus involved the donor organ and led to pneumonia, hepatitis, hemorrhagic cystitis, nephritis, enterocolitis, or disseminated disease. In patients with previous liver transplantation, adenovirus pneumonia had a reported prevalence of 1.5% with a mortality rate of 66% [96]. Serotype 5 is known to be associated with hepatitis [96, 97], whereas serotypes 1 and 2 are more commonly associated with pneumonia. In lung transplant recipients, one study found adenovirus infection to be an early complication following surgery with a prevalence rate of 1.3% [98]. Progressive adenovirus infections are known to be associated with graft loss, progression to bronchiolitis obliterans, or death [99].

Diagnosis

Adenovirus infection should be suspected in cases of acute respiratory disease in military recruits or during outbreaks. In most cases, infection caused by the virus cannot be differentiated from those caused by other respiratory viruses from the clinical presentation alone [3]. A definitive diagnosis can be established by viral culture or the detection of specific viral antigens.

Viral culture remains the gold standard for identification of adenovirus. Nasopharyngeal aspirate or swab, throat swab, sputum samples, or bronchoalveolar lavage can be used, depending on the site of the infection. A cytopathic effect is seen in human cell lines such as HeLa (cervix), A549 (lung), HEK (human embryonic kidney), and HEp-2 (larynx) by strains of adenovirus except for types 40 and 41. Adenovirus 40 and 41 grow well in HEK 293 cells. Adenovirus-specific Enzyme Immunoassay (ELISA) or immunofluorescence assay can be used to detect the presence of virus in clinical samples. These rapid tests suffer from a sensitivity of only about 50%; PCR-based assays can detect adenovirus DNA from a variety of clinical specimens and has better sensitivity [100, 101]. Viral load quantification is a useful tool to measure prognosis and monitor clinical response [102, 103]. Viral loads higher than 1×10^6 copies/mL have been associated with an increased likelihood of death [104, 105].

Treatment

There have been no randomized clinical trials for the treatment of adenovirus infection in immunocompromised patients. Most patients are managed using symptom-based treatment and supportive therapy. Cidofovir is currently being used in immunocompromised patients since it has been shown to decrease plasma viral loads in HSCT recipients [106]. Although cidofovir is active against all strains of adenovirus in vitro, only retrospective data are available on the efficacy of cidofovir in HSCT [106–109] and solid organ transplant recipients [110]. Nephrotoxicity is commonly encountered with this drug and it should be used with caution. There are two accepted regimens: 5 mg/kg every 1–2 weeks, or 1 mg/kg 3 times per week, with the latter being associated with less nephrotoxicity [110]. Orally active ether lipid-ester prodrugs of cidofovir (S)-HPMPA are under development with some promising results in in vitro experiments and phase I trials [111]. When tested against five adenovirus serotypes, they were shown to be more active than the unmodified parent compounds [111].

Intravenous ribavirin has been used in a few reported cases, but results were conflicting [112–114]. Finally, another treatment option using adenovirus-specific donor T-cells infusion has been shown to be feasible and effective in protecting children from complications due to adenovirus infection and causing a significant decrease in viral loads [115].

Prevention/Vaccination

Currently, there are no vaccines available for adenovirus infection other than the oral partially attenuated vaccines contained in enteric-coated capsules with use restricted to the military [116]. Only routine infection control practices are recommended for civilian populations where special precautions must be taken for contact and droplet exposure. In HSCT recipients at high risk from adenovirus infection, weekly PCR surveillance of viremia and preemptive treatment with cidofovir can be used [92, 117].

Rhinovirus

Rhinoviruses are members of the *Picornaviridae* family. They are nonenveloped, single-stranded RNA viruses that measure about 15–30 nm. The capsid of the virus is icosahedral and contains 60 copies of four polypeptides each. A canyon on the viral surface contains the attachment site for the host-cell receptor, with most rhinoviruses using this site to attach to the intercellular adhesion molecule-1 receptor expressed on the surface of host cells [3, 118]. More than 100 serotypes of the virus have been isolated, making a vaccine unlikely in the near future [3, 119, 120].

Rhinoviruses are proven to cause 15–40% of common colds in adults [3]. Each year, adults experience 2 or 3 colds, whereas children may experience 8–12 [3, 120]. Children are the major reservoir for rhinoviruses with infection rates decreasing with age. Although infections occur throughout the year, peaks may occur in the fall and spring. This infection is primarily due to the deposition of the virus on the nasal mucosa. This can occur via self-inoculation or contact with infected secretions such as small- and large-particle aerosols (respiratory droplets) [3, 118, 120].

Clinical Presentation

Individuals with rhinovirus infections may be asymptomatic. When symptoms occur, they are typically those of the common cold: most commonly rhinorrhea and sneezing, which are associated with nasal congestion. Infections due to rhinovirus have an incubation period of 1–4 days. Adults characteristically experience sneezing, nasal obstruction and discharge along with cough, and a sore or scratchy throat. Sinuses are commonly involved so that the illness is rhinosinusitis. Symptoms may last for 4–9 days and usually resolve with no complications. Fever is not usually associated with adult illness [3, 121]. Children, on the other hand, may experience fever, cough, and nasal discharge and obstruction. In addition, the duration of symptoms may be longer. Although bronchitis, bronchiolitis, and bronchopneumonia have been reported in children, rhinovirus is not usually a major cause of lower respiratory illness [3, 122]. However, they are an important cause of exacerbations of asthma and chronic obstructive pulmonary disease in children and adults and of LRI in the elderly [3, 119].

Infections in Immunocompromised Patients

Leukemia Patients and HSCT Recipients

A retrospective study in adults with rhinovirus infections who had undergone HSCT found that 32% of patients developed and eventually died of pneumonia [123]. One patient was found to have a coinfection with *Aspergillus* spp. on autopsy; most of the other patients had interstitial pneumonitis and/or acute respiratory distress syndrome [123]. A study performed at another institution reported that 55% of HSCT recipients with rhinovirus infections developed pneumonia and 33% died [124].

Other Immunocompromised Patients

In a study of community-acquired pneumonia in immunocompromised patients (after HSCT or solid organ transplantation, with HIV infection, or receiving steroids or chemotherapy), rhinovirus was responsible for about 12% of cases, with a mortality rate of 18% [125]. These findings suggest that rhinovirus may cause more severe complications in immunocompromised patients than previously thought.

Diagnosis

Many viruses cause common cold symptoms, and a definitive diagnosis cannot be made only on the basis of the presenting symptoms but rhinoviruses are most commonly associated with colds. A definitive diagnosis can be made by isolating the virus from nasal washes or other nasal secretion specimens in tissue culture. Newer diagnostic methods such as real-time reverse-transcription PCR (RT-PCR) have been used; however, these tests are not frequently performed given the self-limited nature of most infections.

Treatment

No specific antiviral treatment is available for rhinovirus infections. Most cases are managed with supportive care using antihistamines, decongestants, and nonsteroidal anti-inflammatory drugs.

Prevention

Given the number of rhinovirus serotypes known to cause infection, an effective vaccine is unlikely to be developed in the near future. Infection control measures such as hand washing and isolating patients who are known or suspected to have rhinovirus infections can help contain the spread of the virus.

Human Metapneumovirus

hMPV belongs to the subfamily *Pneumovirinae* of the *Paramyxoviridae* family. The virus was discovered in 2001 and is genetically similar to RSV. hMPV is an enveloped RNA virus that is known to cause URIs and LRIs in all age groups [126]. Although hMPV infections are more common in children, a recent study revealed an infection rate of 4.5% in adults with acute upper respiratory illness; 11% of patients required hospitalization [127].

Clinical Presentation

hMPV usually causes a mild infection of short duration (about 3–5 days) and is self-limiting. The incubation period is 4–6 days [128]. The most common presenting symptoms in adults are cough, nasal congestion, rhinorrhea, dyspnea, hoarseness, and wheezing [127]. Children often present with cough, rhinitis, fever, and wheezing [129, 130].

Infections in Immunocompromised Patients

A recent study of patients with hematologic malignancies revealed a 9% incidence of hMPV infection. Nine of the 22 patients who had undergone HSCT had pneumonia; three of these patients died [131]. Another study in HSCT recipients detected the presence of hMPV in 3% (in 5 out of 163) of bronchoalveolar lavage specimens. These 5 patients presented with fever, cough, nasal congestion, and sore throat within the first 40 days after transplantation. The infection progressed to respiratory failure, pulmonary hemorrhage, and culture-negative septic shock. The mortality rate was 80% (4 of 5 patients) [132].

Diagnosis

hMPV's growth in culture is slow and unreliable, which makes this method of diagnosis impractical. The presenting symptoms are similar to those of other infections that cause an acute respiratory illness, making clinical diagnosis impossible. PCR-based methods have been used to diagnose the infection in some centers.

Treatment

No specific antiviral therapy exists for hMPV infections. In vitro studies have demonstrated that ribavirin has activity against the virus [133]; however, no clinical studies have been reported. Immune serum globulins may neutralize the virus as demonstrated in one in vitro study [133]. Anecdotally, a lung transplant recipient with respiratory failure secondary to hMPV pneumonia was treated successfully with aerosolized ribavirin [134].

Prevention

The use of general preventive measures for patients with known or suspected hMPV infections can help reduce the rate of transmission. No vaccine is currently available for this virus.

Coronavirus

Coronaviruses are single-stranded RNA viruses that measure about 80–160 nm in diameter. They are enveloped with club-shaped projections, giving them a crown-like appearance – hence the name [3, 135]. Coronaviruses can cause diarrhea in infants and may play a role in demyelinating diseases of the central nervous system [3, 136]. Coronaviruses are difficult to grow in vitro; some strains can only be grown in human tracheal organ cultures. The major antigenic types that cause diseases in humans are 229E, OC43, HK, and NL63 viruses which cause common colds and may also cause lower respiratory tract illnesses in young children, and SARS-CoV, which causes a severe acute respiratory syndrome [3, 137, 138].

Coronaviruses are found in all tropical, subtropical, and temperate climates. Most infections occur in the late fall, winter, and early spring [3, 139]. Cyclical outbreaks of these infections may occur every 2–4 years. Respiratory infections due to HCoV-229E and HCoV-OC43 strains probably spread in a manner similar to rhinovirus, i.e., via direct contact with infected secretions or aerosol droplets [3].

Clinical Presentation

The clinical manifestations of coronavirus infections are similar to those of rhinovirus infections. The most common symptoms are rhinorrhea, throat congestion, and fever. The middle ear may also be affected, leading to effusions and acute otitis media, especially in children [3, 135]. The incubation period is 1–3 days and the duration of the illness is shorter than that of rhinovirus infections, a mean of 6–7 days. The subtype SARS-CoV has a slightly longer incubation period of 4–5 days.

Infections in Immunocompromised Patients

In immunocompromised adults, coronaviruses can cause lower respiratory tract infections [3, 140]. A recent case series found that the infection rate among immunocompromised patients was significantly higher when compared to immunocompetent patients (8.8 vs. 4.5%) [141]. No large studies have been conducted in cancer patients or other immunocompromised individuals, but a few cases have been reported. Folz and Elkordy [140] reported a patient who had undergone autologous HSCT and was diagnosed with a coronavirus LRI. The patient developed a fever, sore throat, cough, and severe hypoxia and was treated successfully using supportive measures. Kumar et al. [142] described a patient who developed a fatal severe acute respiratory syndrome (SARS) after liver transplantation.

Diagnosis

Epidemiologically, these infections should be suspected during the late fall or winter or during an outbreak. However, no practical method is available to confirm the infection except PCR-based tests. These are used to diagnose coronavirus infections at some institutions [3, 143].

Treatment

Similar to rhinovirus, no specific antiviral therapy is available for coronavirus. Most patients respond well to supportive treatment with nonsteroidal anti-inflammatory drugs, decongestants and antihistamines.

Prevention

General preventive measures must be used around patients with coronavirus infections; hand washing, disposing of infected material carefully, and proper disinfection can help prevent the spread of the virus. No vaccine against the virus has been developed.

Enterovirus

Enteroviruses are single-stranded RNA viruses that can multiply in the gastrointestinal tract. They belong to the *Picornaviridae* family, but are relatively stable at a low pH. The virus is surrounded by an icosahedral capsid comprising four viral proteins. It has no lipid envelope and is not susceptible to alcohol, ether, or detergents. Poliovirus is the prototype of this group, but nonpolio enteroviruses have a wide spectrum of manifestations including acute respiratory illnesses [3, 144].

Enterovirus infections are more common in developing countries and socioeconomically depressed areas and are associated with poor hygiene and sanitation. They can occur throughout the year, but the peak occurs in the summer and fall [3, 145]. They can be transmitted by direct contact with feces during activities such as cleaning and diaper handling.

Clinical Presentation

The clinical picture of enterovirus infections is similar to that of rhinovirus infections; no specific symptoms are associated with the virus.

Infections in Immunocompromised Patients

Immunocompromised patients have been reported to develop central nervous system infections, chronic disseminated infections, and a dermatomyositis-like syndrome with enterovirus infection. In a study of respiratory tract infections in hematologic malignancy patients, 3% of patients had enterovirus infections; most (66%) were HSCT recipients with 33% of these developing pneumonia [131]. A study from Spain reported on four HSCT recipients who developed enterovirus infections, with a mortality rate of 75% (3 of 4) [146]. These findings demonstrate that immunocompromised patients may be at risk for lower respiratory tract infections and death from an enterovirus infection [3, 131, 146].

Diagnosis

Most enteroviruses can be isolated in cell cultures from nasopharyngeal or throat swabs. PCR-based testing is used to amplify the viral RNA from throat swabs, cerebrospinal fluid, and tissues. For diagnosis, isolation of the virus from the throat is more clinically significant than from stool because this virus has a shorter duration of shedding from the throat.

Treatment

Most enterovirus infections are self-limiting and do not require specific treatment. Intensive care may be required for central nervous system, cardiac, and hepatic infections. IVIGs have been used in some patients with severe infections, but no specific antiviral therapies are available [3, 147].

Prevention

General infection control measures must be undertaken around patients with enterovirus infections. Special attention must be paid to hand hygiene. Material in contact with or soiled by feces should be handled carefully and discarded with proper precautions.

Summary Comments

The respiratory viruses as a group are the most common cause of an acute infectious illness in developed societies. The variety of viruses that can cause infection and illness in all age groups and their presence in high frequencies throughout the year describe the risk of exposure of all persons at all times including immunocompromised persons residing in the community. The immunocompromised state of many cancer patients constitutes the basis for the frequent failure of the host to promote a normal and rapid recovery from an acute respiratory viral infection and results in a more severe and prolonged infection that causes significant morbidity and mortality in these patients. Those respiratory viruses that are most prevalent and most prone to produce lower respiratory illnesses and pneumonia in healthy hosts, RSV, influenza viruses and PIV, are those most likely to cause severe illness and pneumonia leading to hospitalization in immunocompromised persons. However, viruses less prone to produce a lower respiratory illness but that are highly prevalent, such as rhinoviruses, may frequently be associated with severe illness. Although not generally considered respiratory viruses, the Herpes viruses are known to produce respiratory infection and disease, sometimes severe, in immunocompromised patients (Table 32.1). A historically important virus, measles virus, is now rarely encountered because of widespread vaccination.

The limited availability of antivirals and vaccines for the acute respiratory viruses means that these infections will continue to be important for many years and dictate a need for utilizing infection control procedures as much as possible, particularly in hospitals and institutions, so as to minimize spread. Efforts to develop specific vaccines are important as their use could prevent as well as reduce exposure of cancer patients to these viruses. Development of specific antivirals is important for use in immunocompromised patients as normal recovery mechanisms may be seriously impaired.

References

1. Whimbey E, Englund JA, Couch RB. Community respiratory virus infections in immunocompromised patients with cancer. Am J Med. 1997;102(3A):10–8.
2. Hicks KL, Chemaly RF, Kontoyiannis DP. Common community respiratory viruses in patients with cancer: more than just "common colds". Cancer. 2003;97(10):2576–87.
3. Kasper DL, Braunwald E, Hauser S, Longo D, Jameson JL, Fauci AS. Harrison's principles of internal medicine. 16th ed. New York: McGraw-Hill; 2001. p. 1120–43.
4. Peret TC, Hall CB, Schnabel KC, Golub JA, Anderson LJ. Circulation patterns of genetically distinct group A and B strains of human respiratory syncytial virus in a community. J Gen Virol. 1998;79(9):2221–9.
5. Hall CB. Respiratory syncytial virus and parainfluenza virus. N Engl J Med. 2001;344(25):1917–28.
6. Glezen WP, Taber LH, Frank AL, Kasel JA. Risk of primary infection and reinfection with respiratory syncytial virus. Am J Dis Child. 1986;140:543.
7. Hall CB, Long CE, Schnabel KC. Respiratory syncytial virus infections in previously healthy working adults. Clin Infect Dis. 2001;33:792.
8. Walsh EE, Falsey AR, Hennessey PA. Respiratory syncytial and other virus infections in persons with chronic cardiopulmonary disease. Am J Respir Crit Care Med. 1999;160:791.
9. Wald TG, Miller BA, Shult P, et al. Can respiratory syncytial virus and influenza A be distinguished clinically in institutionalized older persons? J Am Geriatr Soc. 1995;43:170.
10. O'Shea MK, Ryan MA, Hawksworth AW, et al. Symptomatic respiratory syncytial virus infection in previously healthy young adults living in a crowded military environment. Clin Infect Dis. 2005;41:311.
11. Wendt CH, Hertz MI. Respiratory syncytial virus and parainfluenza virus infections in the immunocompromised host. Semin Respir Infect. 1995;10(4):224–31.
12. Couch RB, Englund JA, Whimbey E. Respiratory virus infections in immunocompetent and immunocompromised persons. Am J Med. 1997;102:2–9.
13. Falsey AR, Walsh EE. Respiratory syncytial virus infection in adults. Clin Microbiol Rev. 2000;13:371–84.
14. Hertz M, Englund J, Snover D, et al. Respiratory syncytial virus-induced acute lung injury in adult patients with bone marrow transplants. Medicine. 1989;68:269.
15. Whimbey E, Champlin R, Englund J, et al. Combination therapy with aerosolized ribavirin and intravenous immunoglobulin for respiratory syncytial virus disease in adult bone marrow transplant recipients. Bone Marrow Transplant. 1995;16:393.
16. Englund JA. Diagnosis and epidemiology of community-acquired respiratory virus infections in the immunocompromised host. Biol Blood Marrow Transplant. 2001;7:2S–4.
17. Ljungman P, Ward KN, Crooks BN, et al. Respiratory virus infections after stem cell transplantation: a prospective study from the Infectious Diseases Working Party of the European Group for Blood and Marrow Transplantation. Bone Marrow Transplant. 2001;28(5):479–84.
18. Whimbey E, Bodey GP. Viral pneumonia in the immunocompromised adult with neoplastic disease: the role of common community respiratory viruses. Semin Respir Infect. 1992;7:122–31.
19. Whimbey E, Champlin RE, Couch RB, et al. Community respiratory virus infections among hospitalized adult bone marrow transplant recipients. Clin Infect Dis. 1996;22(5):778–82.
20. Torres HA, Aguilera EA, Mattiuzzi GN, et al. Characteristics and outcome of respiratory syncytial virus infection in patients with leukemia. Haematologica. 2007;92(9):1216–23.
21. Kim YJ, Boeckh M, Englund JA. Community respiratory virus infections in immunocompromised patients: hematopoietic stem cell and solid organ transplant recipients and individuals with human immunodeficiency virus infection. Semin Respir Crit Care Med. 2007;28:222–42.
22. Pohl C, Green M, Wald ER, Ledesma-Medina J. Respiratory syncytial virus infections in pediatric liver transplant recipients. J Infect Dis. 1992;165(1):166–9.
23. Collins PL, Graham BD. Viral and host factors in human respiratory syncytial virus pathogenesis. J Virol. 2008;82(5):2040–55.
24. Miller RF, Loveday C, Holton J, Sharvell Y, Patel G, Brink NS. Community-based respiratory viral infections in HIV-positive patients with lower respiratory tract disease: a prospective bronchoscopic study. Genitourin Med. 1996;72(1):9–11.
25. Englund JA, Piedra PA, Jewell A, et al. Rapid diagnosis of respiratory syncytial virus infections in immunocompromised adults. J Clin Microbiol. 1996;34:1649.
26. Fan J, Henrickson KJ, Savatski LL. Rapid simultaneous diagnosis of infections with respiratory syncytial viruses A and B, influenza viruses A and B, and human parainfluenza virus types 1, 2, and 3 by multiplex quantitative reverse transcription-polymerase chain reaction-enzyme hybridization assay (Hexaplex). Clin Infect Dis. 1998;26(6):1397–402.
27. Casiano-Colon AE, Hulbert BB, Mayer TK, et al. Lack of sensitivity of rapid antigen tests for the diagnosis of respiratory syncytial virus infection in adults. J Clin Virol. 2003;28:169.
28. Moore C, Valappil M, Corden S, Westmoreland D. Enhanced clinical utility of the NucliSens EasyQ RSV A+B Assay for rapid

detection of respiratory syncytial virus in clinical samples. Eur J Clin Microbiol Infect Dis. 2006;25:167.
29. McColl MD, Corser RB, Bremner J, Chopra R. Respiratory syncytial virus infection in adult BMT recipients: effective therapy with short duration nebulised ribavirin. Bone Marrow Transplant. 1998;21:423.
30. Chemaly RF, Ghosh S, Bodey GP, et al. Respiratory viral infections in adults with hematologic malignancies and human stem cell transplantation recipients: a retrospective study at a major cancer center. Medicine (Baltimore). 2006;85(5):278–87.
31. Krinzman S, Basgoz N, Kradin R, et al. Respiratory syncytial virus-associated infections in adult recipients of solid organ transplants. J Heart Lung Transplant. 1998;17:202.
32. Saez-Llorens X, Moreno MT, Ramilo O, et al. Safety and pharmacokinetics of palivizumab therapy in children hospitalized with respiratory syncytial virus infection. Pediatr Infect Dis J. 2004;23:707.
33. Rathod DB, Torres HA, Munsell MF, et al. Continuous versus intermittent dose schedule of aerosolized ribavirin for treatment of RSV upper respiratory tract infection (URI) in patients with hematological malignancies: an adaptive randomized trial. In: Oral presentation at the 49th annual ICAAC meeting, San Francisco, Sept 2009.
34. Tablan OC, Anderson LJ, Besser R, et al. Guidelines for preventing health-care-associated pneumonia, 2003: recommendations of CDC and the Healthcare Infection Control Practices Advisory Committee. MMWR Recomm Rep. 2004;53(RR-3):1–36.
35. PREVENT Study Group. Reduction of respiratory syncytial virus hospitalization among premature infants and infants with bronchopulmonary dysplasia using respiratory syncytial virus immune globulin prophylaxis. Pediatrics. 1997;99:93–9.
36. Feltes TF, Cabalka AK, Meissner HC, et al. Palivizumab prophylaxis reduces hospitalization due to respiratory syncytial virus in young children with hemodynamically significant congenital heart disease. J Pediatr. 2003;143(4):532–40.
37. Robinson RF, Nahata MC. Respiratory syncytial virus (RSV) immune globulin and palivizumab for prevention of RSV infection. Am J Health Syst Pharm. 2000;57:259–67.
38. Groothuis JR, Simoes EA, Levin MJ, et al. Prophylactic administration of respiratory syncytial virus immune globulin to high-risk infants and young children. N Engl J Med. 1993;329:1524–30.
39. Gubareva LV, Kaiser L, Hayden FG. Influenza virus neuraminidase inhibitors. Lancet. 2000;355:827.
40. Deyde VM, Sheu TG, Trujillo AA, et al. Detection of molecular markers of drug resistance in 2009 pandemic influenza A (H1N1) viruses by pyrosequencing. Antimicrob Agents Chemother. 2010;54(3):1102–10.
41. Prevention and Control of Seasonal Influenza with Vaccines. Recommendations of the advisory committee on immunization practices (ACIP). 2009. Retrieved from Feb 24, 2010. http://www.cdc.gov/mmwr/preview/mmwrhtml/rr5808a1.htm?s_cid=rr5808a1_e.
42. Martin CM, Kunin CM, Gottlieb LS, et al. Asian influenza A in Boston, 1957–1958. Arch Intern Med. 1959;103:516.
43. Chemaly RF, Torres HA, Aguilera EA, et al. Neuraminidase inhibitors improve outcome of patients with leukemia and influenza: an observational study. Clin Infect Dis. 2007;44(7):964–7.
44. Nichols WG, Guthrie KA, Corey L, Boeckh M. Influenza infections after hematopoietic stem cell transplantation: risk factors, mortality, and the effect of antiviral therapy. Clin Infect Dis. 2004;39(9):1300–6.
45. Scott JD, Englund JA, Myerson D, Geballe AP. Influenza A pneumonia presenting as progressive focal infiltrates in a stem cell transplant recipient. J Clin Virol. 2004;31(2):96–9.
46. Vilchez RA, McCurry K, Dauber J, Lacono A, Griffith B, Fung J, et al. Influenza virus infection in adult solid organ transplant recipients. Am J Transplant. 2002;2(3):287–91.
47. Garantziotis S, Howell DN, McAdams HP, Davis RD, Henshaw NG, Palmer SM. Influenza pneumonia in lung transplant recipients: clinical features and association with bronchiolitis obliterans syndrome. Chest. 2001;119(4):1277–80.
48. Karalakulasingam R, Schacht RA, Lansing AM, Raff MJ. Influenza virus pneumonia after renal transplant. Postgrad Med. 1977;62(2):164–7.
49. Treanor JJ. Influenza virus. In: Mandell GL, Bennett JE, Dolin R, editors. Principles and practice of infectious diseases. 6th ed. Philadelphia: Churchill Livingstone; 2005. p. 2060.
50. Covalciuc KA, Webb KH, Carlson CA. Comparison of four clinical specimen types for detection of influenza A and B viruses by optical immunoassay (FLU OIA test) and cell culture methods. J Clin Microbiol. 1999;37:3971.
51. Ellis JS, Zambon MC. Molecular diagnosis of influenza. Rev Med Virol. 2002;12(6):375–89.
52. Rodriguez WJ, Schwartz RH, Thorne MM. Evaluation of diagnostic tests for influenza in a pediatric practice. Pediatr Infect Dis J. 2002;21(3):193–6.
53. Fiore AE, Shay DK, Broder K, et al. Prevention and control of influenza. Recommendations of the Advisory Committee on Immunization Practices (ACIP). MMWR Recomm Rep. 2008;57:1.
54. Ong AK, Hayden FG, John F. Enders lecture 2006: antivirals for influenza. J Infect Dis. 2007;196:181.
55. Sheu TG, Deyde VM, Okomo-Adhiambo M, et al. Surveillance for neuraminidase inhibitor resistance among human influenza A and B viruses circulating worldwide from 2004 to 2008. Antimicrob Agents Chemother. 2008;52(9):3284–92.
56. Okomo-Adhiambo M, Nguyen HT, Sleeman K, et al. Host cell selection of influenza neuraminidase variants: implications for drug resistance monitoring in A(H1N1) viruses. Antiviral Res. 2010;85(2):381–8.
57. Updated Interim Recommendations. Special considerations for clinicians regarding 2009 H1N1 influenza in severely immunosuppressed patients. Retrieved from Feb 24, 2010. http://www.flu.gov/individualfamily/healthconditions/immunosuppression.html.
58. Cooper NJ, Sutton AJ, Abrams KR, Wailoo A, Turner D, Nicholson KG. Effectiveness of neuraminidase inhibitors in treatment and prevention of influenza A and B: systematic review and meta-analyses of randomised controlled trials. BMJ. 2003;326(7401):1235–40.
59. Nicholson KG, Aoki FY, Osterhaus ME, et al. Efficacy and safety of oseltamivir in treatment of acute influenza: a randomized controlled trial. Lancet. 2000;355:1845–50.
60. Beigel J, Bray M. Current and future antiviral therapy of severe seasonal and avian influenza. Antiviral Res. 2008;78(1):91–102.
61. ACIP provisional recommendations for the use of influenza vaccines. Feb 24, 2010. http://www.cdc.gov/vaccines/recs/provisional/downloads/flu-vac-mar-2010-508.pdf.
62. Kamboj M, Sepkowitz KA. Risk of transmission associated with live attenuated vaccines given to healthy persons caring for or residing with an immunocompromised patient. Infect Control Hosp Epidemiol. 2007;28(6):702–7.
63. Influenza vaccine 2005–2006. Med Lett Drugs Ther. 2005;47:85.
64. Van Voris LP, Newell PM. Antivirals for the chemoprophylaxis and treatment of influenza. Semin Respir Infect. 1992;7:61–70.
65. Tomblyn M, Chiller T, Einsele H, Gress R, Sepkowitz K, Storek J, et al. Guidelines for preventing infectious complications among hematopoietic cell transplant recipients: a global perspective. Bone Marrow Transplant. 2009;44(8):453–558.
66. Henrickson KJ, Savatski LL. Genetic variation and evolution of human parainfluenza virus type 1 hemagglutinin neuraminidase: analysis of 12 clinical isolates. J Infect Dis. 1992;166:995.
67. Walker TA, Khurana S, Tilden SJ. Viral respiratory infections. Pediatr Clin North Am. 1994;41:1365.
68. Henrickson K, Ray R, Belshe R. Parainfluenza viruses. In: Mandell GL, Bennett JE, Dolin R, editors. Principles and practice of infectious diseases. 4th ed. New York: Churchill Livingstone; 1995. p. 1489.

69. Fiore AE, Iverson C, Messmer T, Erdman D, Lett SM, Talkington DF, et al. Outbreak of pneumonia in a long-term care facility: antecedent human parainfluenza virus 1 infection may predispose to bacterial pneumonia. J Am Geriatr Soc. 1998;46(9):1112–7.
70. Hanmod SH, Rathod DB, Doshi A, et al. The outcome of parainfluenza virus (PIV) infection in patients with leukemia and recipients of hematopoietic stem cell transplantation (HSCT). In: Abstract presented at the 46th annual IDSA/48th annual ICAAC meeting, Washington, Oct 2008.
71. Nichols WG, Corey L, Gooley T, et al. Parainfluenza virus infections after hematopoietic stem cell transplantation: risk factors, response to antiviral therapy, and effect on transplant outcome. Blood. 2001;98:573.
72. Wendt CH, Weisdorf DJ, Jordan MC, et al. Parainfluenza virus respiratory infection after bone marrow transplantation. N Engl J Med. 1992;326:921.
73. Taylor CE, Osman HK, Turner AJ, et al. Parainfluenza virus and respiratory syncytial virus infection in infants undergoing bone marrow transplantation for severe combined immunodeficiency. Commun Dis Public Health. 1998;1:202.
74. Zambon M, Bull T, Sadler CJ, et al. Molecular epidemiology of two consecutive outbreaks of parainfluenza 3 in a bone marrow transplant unit. J Clin Microbiol. 1998;36:2289.
75. Wendt CH, Fox JM, Hertz MI. Paramyxovirus infection in lung transplant recipients. J Heart Lung Transplant. 1995;14(3):479–85.
76. Vilchez R, McCurry K, Dauber J, Iacono A, Keenan R, Griffith B, et al. Influenza and parainfluenza respiratory viral infection requiring admission in adult lung transplant recipients. Transplantation. 2002;73(7):1075–8.
77. Frank AL, Couch RB, Griffis CA, Baxter BD. Comparison of different tissue cultures for isolation and quantitation of influenza and parainfluenza viruses. J Clin Microbiol. 1979;10:32.
78. Ray CG, Minnich LL. Efficiency of immunofluorescence for rapid detection of common respiratory viruses. J Clin Microbiol. 1987;25:355.
79. Osiowy C. Direct detection of respiratory syncytial virus, parainfluenza virus, and adenovirus in clinical respiratory specimens by a multiplex reverse transcription-PCR assay. J Clin Microbiol. 1998;36:3149.
80. Gilbert BE, Knight V. Biochemistry and clinical applications of ribavirin. Antimicrob Agents Chemother. 1986;30:201–5.
81. McIntosh K, Kurachek SC, Goodspeed B. Treatment of respiratory viral infection in an immunodeficient infant with ribavirin aerosol. Am J Dis Child. 1984;138:305–8.
82. Wright JJ, O'driscoll G. Treatment of parainfluenza virus 3 pneumonia in a cardiac transplant recipient with intravenous ribavirin and methylprednisolone. J Heart Lung Transplant. 2005;24(3):343–6.
83. Shima T, Yoshimoto G, Nonami A, Yoshida S, Kamezaki K, Iwasaki H, et al. Successful treatment of parainfluenza virus 3 pneumonia with oral ribavirin and methylprednisolone in a bone marrow transplant recipient. Int J Hematol. 2008;88(3):336–40.
84. Boeckh M. The challenge of respiratory virus infections in hematopoietic cell transplant recipients. Br J Haematol. 2008;143(4):455–67.
85. Horwitz MS. Adenovirus. In: Knipe DM, Howley PM, editors. Field virology. Philadelphia: Lippincott Williams & Wilkins; 2001. p. 2301–26.
86. South MA, Dolen J, Beach DK, Mirkovic RR. Fatal adenovirus hepatic necrosis in severe combined immune deficiency. Pediatr Infect Dis. 1982;1(6):416–9.
87. La Rosa AM, Champlin RE, Mirza N, et al. Adenovirus infections in adult recipients of blood and marrow transplants. Clin Infect Dis. 2001;32(6):871–6.
88. Raboni SM, Nogueira MB, Tsuchiya LR, et al. Respiratory tract viral infections in bone marrow transplant patients. Transplantation. 2003;76(1):142–6.
89. Ljungman P. Respiratory virus infections in bone marrow transplant recipients: the European perspective. Am J Med. 1997;102(3A): 44–7.
90. Flomenberg P, Babbitt J, Drobyski WR, et al. Increasing incidence of adenovirus disease in bone marrow transplant recipients. J Infect Dis. 1994;169(4):775–81.
91. Bruno B, Gooley T, Hackman RC, Davis C, Corey L, Boeckh M. Adenovirus infection in hematopoietic stem cell transplantation: effect of ganciclovir and impact on survival. Biol Blood Marrow Transplant. 2003;9(5):341–52.
92. Lion T, Baumgartinger R, Watzinger F, Matthes-Martin S, Suda M, Preuner S, et al. Molecular monitoring of adenovirus in peripheral blood after allogeneic bone marrow transplantation permits early diagnosis of disseminated disease. Blood. 2003;102(3):1114–20.
93. Shields AF, Hackman RC, Fife KH, Corey L, Meyers JD. Adenovirus infections in patients undergoing bone-marrow transplantation. N Engl J Med. 1985;312(9):529–33.
94. Baldwin A, Kingman H, Darville M, Foot AB, Grier D, Cornish JM, et al. Outcome and clinical course of 100 patients with adenovirus infection following bone marrow transplantation. Bone Marrow Transplant. 2000;26(12):1333–8.
95. Gray GC, McCarthy T, Lebeck MG, et al. Genotype prevalence and risk factors for severe clinical adenovirus infection, United States 2004–2006. Clin Infect Dis. 2007;45(9):1120–31.
96. McGrath D, Falagas ME, Freeman R, et al. Adenovirus infection in adult orthotopic liver transplant recipients: incidence and clinical significance. J Infect Dis. 1998;177(2):459–62.
97. Michaels MG, Green M, Wald ER, Starzl TE. Adenovirus infection in pediatric liver transplant recipients. J Infect Dis. 1992;165(1):170–4.
98. Ohori NP, Michaels MG, Jaffe R, Williams P, Yousem SA. Adenovirus pneumonia in lung transplant recipients. Hum Pathol. 1995;26(10):1073–9.
99. Bridges ND, Spray TL, Collins MH, Bowles NE, Towbin JA. Adenovirus infection in the lung results in graft failure after lung transplantation. J Thorac Cardiovasc Surg. 1998;116(4):617–23.
100. Raboni SM, Siqueira MM, Portes SR, Pasquini R. Comparison of PCR, enzyme immunoassay and conventional culture for adenovirus detection in bone marrow transplant patients with hemorrhagic cystitis. J Clin Virol. 2003;27(3):270–5.
101. Raty R, Kleemola M, Melen K, Stenvik M, Julkunen I. Efficacy of PCR and other diagnostic methods for the detection of respiratory adenoviral infections. J Med Virol. 1999;59(1):66–72.
102. Lankester AC, Heemskerk B, Claas EC, et al. Effect of ribavirin on the plasma viral DNA load in patients with disseminating adenovirus infection. Clin Infect Dis. 2004;38(11):1521–5.
103. Leruez-Ville M, Minard V, Lacaille F, et al. Real-time blood plasma polymerase chain reaction for management of disseminated adenovirus infection. Clin Infect Dis. 2004;38(1):45–52.
104. Claas EC, Schilham MW, de Brouwer CS, et al. Internally controlled real-time PCR monitoring of adenovirus DNA load in serum or plasma of transplant recipients. J Clin Microbiol. 2005;43(4):1738–44.
105. Schilham MW, Claas EC, van Zaane W, et al. High levels of adenovirus DNA in serum correlate with fatal outcome of adenovirus infection in children after allogeneic stem-cell transplantation. Clin Infect Dis. 2002;35(5):526–32.
106. Neofytos D, Ojha A, Mookerjee B, et al. Treatment of adenovirus disease in stem cell transplant recipients with cidofovir. Biol Blood Marrow Transplant. 2007;13(1):74–81.
107. Hoffman JA, Shah AJ, Ross LA, Kapoor N. Adenoviral infections and a prospective trial of cidofovir in pediatric hematopoietic stem cell transplantation. Biol Blood Marrow Transplant. 2001;7(7):388–94.
108. Legrand F, Berrebi D, Houhou N, et al. Early diagnosis of adenovirus infection and treatment with cidofovir after bone marrow transplantation in children. Bone Marrow Transplant. 2001;27(6):621–6.

109. Ljungman P, Ribaud P, Eyrich M, et al. Cidofovir for adenovirus infections after allogeneic hematopoietic stem cell transplantation: a survey by the Infectious Diseases Working Party of the European Group for Blood and Marrow Transplantation. Bone Marrow Transplant. 2003;31(6):481–6.
110. Doan ML, Mallory GB, Kaplan SL, et al. Treatment of adenovirus pneumonia with cidofovir in pediatric lung transplant recipients. J Heart Lung Transplant. 2007;26(9):883–9.
111. Hartline CB, Gustin KM, Wan WB, et al. Ether lipid-ester prodrugs of acyclic nucleoside phosphonates: activity against adenovirus replication in vitro. J Infect Dis. 2005;191(3):396–9.
112. Liles WC, Cushing H, Holt S, Bryan C, Hackman RC. Severe adenoviral nephritis following bone marrow transplantation: successful treatment with intravenous ribavirin. Bone Marrow Transplant. 1993;12(4):409–12.
113. Chakrabarti S, Collingham KE, Fegan CD, Milligan DW. Fulminant adenovirus hepatitis following unrelated bone marrow transplantation: failure of intravenous ribavirin therapy. Bone Marrow Transplant. 1999;23(11):1209–11.
114. Bordigoni P, Carret AS, Venard V, Witz F, Le Faou A. Treatment of adenovirus infections in patients undergoing allogeneic hematopoietic stem cell transplantation. Clin Infect Dis. 2001;32(9):1290–7.
115. Feuchtinger T, Matthes-Martin S, Richard C, Lion T, Fuhrer M, Hamprecht K, et al. Safe adoptive transfer of virus-specific T-cell immunity for the treatment of systemic adenovirus infection after allogeneic stem cell transplantation. Br J Haematol. 2006;134(1):64–76.
116. Gaydos CA, Gaydos JC. Adenovirus vaccines in the US military. Milit Med. 1995;160:300–4.
117. Yusuf U, Hale GA, Carr J, Gu Z, Benaim E, Woodard P, et al. Cidofovir for the treatment of adenoviral infection in pediatric hematopoietic stem cell transplant patients. Transplantation. 2006;81(10):1398–404.
118. Hendley JO. Clinical virology of rhinoviruses. Adv Virus Res. 1999;54:453.
119. Heymann P, Platts-Mills T, Johnston SL. Role of viral infections, atopy and antiviral immunity in the etiology of wheezing exacerbations among children and young adults. Pediatr Infect Dis J. 2005;24:S217.
120. Winther B, Gwaltney Jr JM, Mygind N, Hendley JO. Viral-induced rhinitis. Am J Rhinol. 1998;12:17.
121. Gwaltney Jr JM, Hendley JO, Simon G, Jordan Jr WS. Rhinovirus infections in an industrial population. II. Characteristics of illness and antibody response. JAMA. 1967;202:494.
122. Pappas DE, Hendley JO, Hayden FG, Winther B. Symptom profile of common colds in school-aged children. Pediatr Infect Dis J. 2008;27:8.
123. Ghosh S, Champlin R, Couch R, et al. Rhinovirus infections in myelosuppressed adult blood and marrow transplant recipients. Clin Infect Dis. 1999;29(3):528–32.
124. Hassan IA, Chopra R, Swindell R, Mutton KJ. Respiratory viral infections after bone marrow/peripheral stem-cell transplantation: the Christie hospital experience. Bone Marrow Transplant. 2003;32(1):73–7.
125. Camps Serra M, Cervera C, Pumarola T, et al. Virological diagnosis in community-acquired pneumonia in immunocompromised patients. Eur Respir J. 2008;31(3):618–24.
126. Van den Hoogen BG, de Jong JC, Groen J, et al. A newly discovered human pneumovirus isolated from young children with respiratory tract disease. Nat Med. 2001;7:719.
127. Falsey A, Erdman D, Anderson LJ, Walsh EE. Human metapneumovirus infections in young and elderly adults. J Infect Dis. 2003;187:785.
128. Alto WA. Human metapneumovirus: a newly described respiratory tract pathogen. J Am Board Fam Pract. 2004;17(6):466–9.
129. Williams JV, Harris PA, Tollefson SJ, et al. Human metapneumovirus and lower respiratory tract disease in otherwise healthy infants and children. N Engl J Med. 2004;350:443.
130. Esper F, Martinello RA, Boucher D, et al. A 1-year experience with human metapneumovirus in children aged <5 years. J Infect Dis. 2004;189:1388.
131. Williams JV, Martino R, Rabella N, et al. A prospective study comparing human metapneumovirus with other respiratory viruses in adults with hematologic malignancies and respiratory tract infections. J Infect Dis. 2005;192:1061.
132. Englund JA, Boeckh M, Kuypers J, et al. Brief communication: fatal human metapneumovirus infection in stem-cell transplant recipients. Ann Intern Med. 2006;144(5):344–9.
133. Wyde PR, Chetty SN, Jewell AM, Boivin G, Piedra PA. Comparison of the inhibition of human metapneumovirus and respiratory syncytial virus by ribavirin and immune serum globulin in vitro. Antiviral Res. 2003;60(1):51–9.
134. Raza K, Ismailjee SB, Crespo M, et al. Successful outcome of human metapneumovirus (hMPV) pneumonia in a lung transplant recipient treated with intravenous ribavirin. J Heart Lung Transplant. 2007;26(8):862–4.
135. Pitkaranta A, Jero J, Arruda E, et al. Polymerase chain reaction-based detection of rhinovirus, respiratory syncytial virus, and coronavirus in otitis media with effusion. J Pediatr. 1998;133:390.
136. Arbour N, Talbot PJ. Persistent infection of neural cell lines by human coronaviruses. Adv Exp Med Biol. 1998;440:575.
137. Kolb AF, Hegyi A, Siddell SG. Identification of residues critical for the human coronavirus 229E receptor function of human aminopeptidase N. J Gen Virol. 1997;78(pt 11):2795.
138. Vlasak R, Luytjes W, Spaan W, Palese P. Human and bovine coronaviruses recognize sialic acid-containing receptors similar to those of influenza C viruses. Proc Natl Acad Sci USA. 1988;85:4526.
139. Lina B, Valette M, Foray S, et al. Surveillance of community-acquired viral infections due to respiratory viruses in Rhone-Alpes (France) during winter 1994 to 1995. J Clin Microbiol. 1996;34:3007.
140. Folz RJ, Elkordy MA. Coronavirus pneumonia following autologous bone marrow transplantation for breast cancer. Chest. 1999;115:901.
141. Gerna G, Campanini G, Rovida F, Percivalle E. Genetic variability of human coronavirus OC43-, 229E-, and NL63-like strains and their association with lower respiratory tract infections of hospitalized infants and immunocompromised patients. J Med Virol. 2006;78:938–49.
142. Kumar D, Tellier R, Draker R, Levy G, Humar A. Severe acute respiratory syndrome (SARS) in a liver transplant recipient and guidelines for donor SARS screening. Am J Transplant. 2003;3(8):977–81.
143. West JA, Dakhama A, Khan MA, et al. Community study using a polymerase chain reaction panel to determine the prevalence of common respiratory viruses in asthmatic and nonasthmatic children. J Asthma. 1999;36:605.
144. Oberste MS, Maher K, Kilpatrick DR, et al. Typing of human enteroviruses by partial sequencing of VP1. J Clin Microbiol. 1999;37:1288.
145. Moore M. Enteroviral disease in the United States. J Infect Dis. 1982;146:103.
146. González Y, Martino R, Badell I, et al. Pulmonary enterovirus infections in stem cell transplant recipients. Bone Marrow Transplant. 1999;23(5):511–3.
147. Mease PJ, Ochs HD, Wedgwood RJ. Successful treatment of echovirus meningoencephalitis and myositis-fasciitis with intravenous immune globulin therapy in a patient with X-linked agammaglobulinemia. N Engl J Med. 1981;304:1278.

Chapter 33
BK, JC, and Parvovirus Infections in Patients with Hematologic Malignancies

Véronique Erard and Michael Boeckh

Abstract The polyomaviruses, BK and JC virus, as well as parvoviruses are emerging infections in patients with hematologic malignancies and hematopoietic cell transplant recipients. BK virus has a predilection to the urinary tract and may cause hemorrhagic cystitis and nephritis. BK viremia appears to be an important marker and predictor for BK disease in immunocompromised patients. No well-established treatment options exist, but cidofovir has been used in addition to supportive care measures. JC virus is the cause of progressive multifocal leukoencephalopathy in immunosuppressed patients. The optimal treatment is not defined. There is increasing evidence that parvoviruses may also cause serious disease in immunocompromised patients, including anemia, pericarditis, myocarditis, hepatitis, pneumonitis, and neurologic disease. The frequency of these complications of parvoviruses is presently poorly defined. Treatment consists of intravenous immunoglobulin; no specific antiviral treatment exists. This chapter will review the epidemiology, disease manifestations, and diagnostic and management options for polyomaviruses and parvoviruses in patients with hematologic malignancies.

Keywords Polyomavirus • BKV • JC virus • Viremia • Progressive multifocal leukoencephalopathy • Immunosuppressed patients • Cancer • Stem cell transplantation • Hemorrhagic cystitis • Nephritis

BK Virus

Polyomavirus BK was first reported to be a human pathogen in 1971, when a renal transplant recipient, with initials BK, presented with ureteric stenosis [1]. Reports of the role of BK virus infection in clinical disease increased with the advent of more potent immunosuppressive medication. In the last decade, BK virus became an emerging pathogen in the setting of kidney transplantation by its propensity to cause severe nephritis in the allograft resulting in graft loss in up to 80% [2, 3]. In the bone marrow and stem cell transplant population, the association of BK virus infection and hemorrhagic cystitis (HC) was reported first in the mid-1980s [4, 5]. In this review, we will focus on BK-associated HC, the main manifestation of BK virus in patients with hematological malignancies and following hematopoietic stem cell transplantation (HCT), as well as on nephritis, which can also occasionally occur in these settings.

Virologic Aspects

BK virus is a small (diameter 40 nm) nonenveloped virus with a double-stranded DNA genome. It belongs to the Papovaviridae family together with JC virus and the simian virus (SV) 40. The viral icosahedric capsid is composed of three structural proteins, VP1, VP2, and VP3. The viral DNA is a supercoiled (like plasmid DNA), circular, double-stranded DNA of 5,300 base pairs and shares approximately 75% of homology with the JC virus and 69% with the SV40 [6]. The genome is organized in three regions (early, late, and regulatory region), each of which has specific functions. The early region encodes the large tumor antigen (TAg) and small tumor antigen (tAg); the late region encodes the viral capsid proteins VP1, VP2, and VP3 and the nonstructural agnoprotein; and the noncoding control region contains promoter elements for both the early and late regions and the origin of DNA replication [6]. Currently, there are four known seroypes of BKV in the human population. Sequences variation within the VL1 gene accounts for the antigenic differences of the BKV genotypes [6].

The details of the many steps leading to productive BKV infection remain incompletely defined. At the cellular level, the entry of BK virus into the cells remains partially known and is described in recent reports [7–13]. After attachment

V. Erard (✉)
Médecin Adjointe, Infectiologie, HFR-Fribourg, Switzerland
e-mail: ErardV@h-fr.ch
and
M. Boeckh (✉)
Vaccine and Infectious Disease Division, University of Washington,
Fred Hutchinson Cancer Research Center,
1100 Fairview Avenue N Seattle, WA 98109, USA
e-mail: mboeckh@fhcrc.org

to the surface of the cell membrane, the virions induce the formation of vesicles called caveolae [10, 14] and are transported eventually to the nucleus. BK virus employs specific trafficking pathways, relying on various cellular components, to establish a productive infection [8]. However, the details of the many steps leading to productive BKV infection remain incompletely defined.

Transmission and Pathogenesis

The mode of transmission of BK virus is not yet well defined; however, the reports in the literature suggest the respiratory route as the main mechanism of transmission. BK virus seroprevalence is reported to reach up to 90% in adolescents and adults around the world [15]. Potential alternative modes of transmission include transplacental transmission [16–18], fecal–oral [19, 20], or organ transplantation [21, 22].

Primary infection with BK virus during childhood is generally asymptomatic or associated with fever and mild upper respiratory symptoms [23], and occasionally followed self-limited hemorrhagic cystitis [24]. Primary infection is followed by viral dissemination to the sites of persistent infection. The sites of latency are principally the cells of the kidney and urinary tract [25–27].

Intermittent replication may occur as evidenced by periodic excretion of BK virus in the urine in immunocompetent individuals and pregnant women [18, 28–30]. The control of persistent infection by the host innate, humoral, and cellular immunity is incompletely understood. Initial studies suggest a role of cell-mediated immunity [2].

BK Virus-Associated Disease

Polyomavirus replication is lytic, and hence, cytopathic. Depending on the state of the immune system, host cellular lysis may elicit nonspecific inflammatory response or specific cellular and humoral immune response. Thus, polyomavirus infections have been associated with diverse pattern according to the cytopathic, inflammatory, and immunologic features. The pathogenesis of tissue damage in BK virus-infected tissues is to date only partially understood and principally described in kidney transplant recipients. The preferential manifestation of BK virus nephropathy in the allograft kidney of renal transplants as compared to other allografts or to autologous kidneys of other organ transplants suggests that organ tissue and immunologic factors interplay [25, 31–33].

In cancer patients, BK virus has been mainly associated with hemorrhagic cystitis following HCT [34]. In recent years, cases of BK nephritis have been reported sporadically in HCT recipients and patients with leukemia [35–40].

Hemorrhagic Cystitis

Definition. HC is characterized by hemorrhagic inflammation of the bladder mucosa leading to painful micturation, urinary frequency, and urgency with hematuria. HC can be ranging from a mild and brief (Grade I) to a severe and life-threatening (Grade IV) complication [41, 42]. In the HCT setting, HC occurs early (before engraftment) or late (after engraftment) after transplantation. Early manifestation has been linked to the toxicity of the conditioning regimen containing high dose of cyclophosphamide, especially when administered in association with busulfan or irradiation [43–46]. The administration of 2-mercaptoethane sodium sulfonate (MESNA), polyuric diurese, bladder irrigation, and alkalization are the various protective measures in the prevention of hemorrhagic cystitis after allogeneic HCT [41, 47–50] (Table 33.1).

In the HCT settings, late onset of HC is attributed mainly to viral infection such as BK virus, adenovirus, and rarely, cytomegalovirus (CMV). Other factors that have been associated with late HC include myeloablative conditioning regimen, HLA mismatch, and graft versus host disease [43, 63–66].

BK virus-associated HC. The association of BK virus infection with HC was first reported two decades ago in the HCT population. These early studies reported a qualitative association between BK viruria and late HC [4, 41, 67]. BK viruria was often present in patients with HC and preceded the onset of disease. However, a significant percentage of patients presented with persistent BK viruria without hemorrhagic cystitis. Subsequent studies demonstrated a quantitative association between HC and BK viruria [68–70]. BK viremia has been shown to be a sensitive and specific indicator of BK virus nephritis in kidney transplant recipients [71]. An association of BK viremia with HC has also been observed [34, 46, 55, 71]. The association seems to be particularly strong with high viral load in plasma [46]. However, this observation was not found in all studies [72, 73]. A recent seroepidemiologic study has identified that patients who developed a higher peak of viruria and hence an increased risk of HC were more likely to have higher anti-BK virus antibody titers before HCT [70].

Given that BK viruria occurs frequently in HCT recipients who remained free of hemorrhagic cystitis, it is thought that other factors are likely to contribute to the development of BK virus-associated HC [72, 73]. Several theories of the pathogenesis of BK virus-associated HC have been proposed [2, 69]. First, chemotherapeutic agents and/or irradiation damage the uroepithelium providing a supportive environment

Table 33.1 Studies and Case reports of BK virus-associated disease in patients with hematologic malignancies

First authors, year	Study design	Study population	Disease	Incidence[a]
Leung, 2002 [44]	Prospective cohort s	HCT adults, $n=50$	Hemorrhagic cystitis (HC)	12%
Erard, 2004 [51]	Retrospective cohort	HCT adults/children, $n=132$	HC	14%
Gorczynska, 2005 [52]	Retrospective cohort	HCT children, $n=102$	HC	25%
Fioriti, 2005 [53]	Prospective cohort	HCT, $n=20$	HC	25%
Giraud, 2008 [54]	Prospective cohort	HCT adults/children, $n=175$	HC	12%
Cesaro, 2008 [55]	Prospective cohort	HCT children, $n=15$	HC	30%
Park, 2009 [56]	Retrospective cohort	HCT adults, $n=12$ (alemtuzumab); $N=18$ (ATG)	HC	42% (ALTZ) 6% (ATG)
Gaziev, 2010 [57]	Prospective cohort	HCT children, $n=117$	HC (with/without BK infection)	26% 58% (ATG) 17% (no ATG)
De Padua Silva, 2010 [58]	Prospective cohort	HCT adults, $n=209$	HC	12%
Strake, 2003 [59]	Case report	HCT adult, $n=1$	Nephritis	–
Lekakis, 2009 [37]	Case report	HCT adult, $n=1$	HC and nephritis	–
Verghese, 2009 [60]	Case report	HCT children, $n=2$	HC and nephritis	–
Galan, 2005 [61]	Case report	LLC adult, $n=1$[b]	Fatal pneumonia	–
Sandler, 1997 [62]	Case report	HCT child, $n=1$	Fatal pneumonia	–

HCT hematopoietic cell transplant, ALTX alemtuzumab, ATG antithymocyte globulin
[a] Incidence figures may refer to the overall rate of HC or that related to BK virus; see references for details
[b] Patient had received chemotherapy for chronic lymphatic leukemia

for BK virus replication, which proceeds in the absence of functional immunity. The restoration of immunity occurring at engraftment further increases the mucosal damage induced by the cytopathic effects of viral replication [2]. No animal model has yet verified the hypothesis of an immune reconstitution disease. Furthermore, the role of immune reconstitution in pathogenesis remains controversial, as late HC has been reported in patients with very low lymphocytes counts, occurs with antithymocyte globulin- and alemtuzumab-based conditioning regimens [56, 57], and does not appear to be modified by steroids administration [46, 56] (Table 33.1). A direct lytic effect of the virus on the urothelium is possible, as BK virus has been detected in tissue samples from patients with HC [74]. Thus, to date the exact pathogenic link between BK virus and hemorrhagic cystitis remains enigmatic, mainly because a gold standard for the diagnosis of BK virus-associated cystitis does not exist.

Diagnosis of BK virus-associated HC. The diagnosis of BK virus-associated HC is indirect in most situations by testing urine and blood. Definite diagnosis requires a bladder biopsy. Most cases of BK-associated HC occur after engraftment. Cytology of the urine can detect polyomavirus-infected cells, the decoy cells. These cells are characterized by an enlarged nucleus containing basophilic intranuclear inclusion easily seen by phase-contrast microscopy [75]. The limitations of cytology to diagnose BK virus disease include that adenovirus or JC virus infection will produce similar cytology [76–78]. Viral cultures are not useful for detection of BK virus replication because the growth of the virus in tissue culture may take several weeks [79]. Currently, the method of choice for detecting BK virus in urine is the detection of DNA by quantitative PCR. The primer selection is important for optimal sensitivity of the PCR assay [80]. However, BK viruria has a low BK virus disease specificity. Other characteristics of BK virus replication may be utilized to diagnose BK virus-associated HC. Indeed, high peak urine viral loads (10^9 to 10^{10} copies/ml), BK viruria increasing by more than $3 \log_{10}$ from baseline, or the presence of BK viremia, particularly greater than 10^4 copies/ml of plasma, have all been linked to an increased risk of hemorrhagic cystitis [55]. Therefore, as suggested in a recent review [81], patients who develop late-onset HC should be tested for BK virus in the urine followed by blood if the urine is positive and other causes should be ruled out, i.e., adenovirus, and to a lesser degree, CMV [82, 83].

Treatment. The management of hemorrhagic cystitis depends on the severity of the disease. In the majority of the cases, the treatment is supportive including analgesia, hyperhydratation, and forced diuresis, as well as continuous bladder irrigation in order to prevent clot formation. Furthermore, measures to control and alleviate bleeding, including platelet and red blood cell transfusions, may be required. In the case of urinary tract obstruction following severe bleeding, cystoscopy for clots removal and possible cauthrization should be considered. In the extreme situation of intractable bleeding, a cystectomy may be the only alternative [45, 84].

Despite the emergence of BK virus-associated nephropathy in the kidney transplant population over the last decade, antiviral drugs with specific activity against BK virus have not been approved for treatment. However, several drugs, including cidofovir, leflunomide, fluoroquinolones, and intravenous immunoglobulins (IVIg), have been tested in small clinical series involving kidney and HCT recipients [37, 52, 57, 85–91] (Table 33.2).

Cidofovir is a nucleotide analog of cytosine active against a large number of DNA viruses. Cidofovir has emerged as the most selective antipolyomavirus agent; however, its mechanism of antiviral action is uncertain [96]. The drug is licensed for the treatment of CMV retinitis in patients with acquired immunodeficiency syndrome (AIDS). Nephrotoxicity and hematotoxicity can occur after multiple dosing (especially with higher doses) and limit routine use following HCT.

Leflunomide is an immunosuppressive agent, acting by the inhibition of several enzyme involved in the pyrimidine synthesis and lymphocytes signaling pathways [88]. It is licensed for the treatment of rheumatoid arthritis [97]. It has in vitro anti-CMV and anti-BK virus action [37, 86, 98, 99]. The mechanism of antiviral action is unknown.

Fluoroquinolones have been shown to inhibit the helicase, an essential enzyme for replication of SV40 in vitro [100].

Intravenous immunoglobulin (*IVIg*) has immunomodulatory properties and contains polyomavirus-reactive antibodies [101]. However, the role of antibody-mediated immunity in polyomavirus control remains unclear, as majority of patients with active BK virus infection have high level of specific antibodies.

Clinical results. A recent review of treatment for BK virus-associated nephropathy in kidney transplant recipients [102] reported 184 patients treated with cidofovir (0.25–1 mg/kg per dose, every 2–3 weeks). The clearance of viremia was 49% and the graft loss 23%. Other studies show no results of low-dose cidofovir [95]. Patients treated with leflunomide ($n=189$) had the same rate of viremia clearance, but a lower percentage of graft loss (12%). The authors stress that a high dose of leflunomide (~40 mg per day) is required to achieve a therapeutic effect. None of the patients treated with fluoroquinolones ($n=14$) achieved viremia clearance. Patients treated with IVIG ($n=29$) at a dose of 2 g/kg divided over 2–5 days had a 52% rate of viremia clearance and only 7% had allograft loss, but the majority of patients received concomitant treatment with leflunomide ($n=16$) or cidofovir ($n=1$). The results are difficult to interpret because of the lack of adequate controls.

In HCT settings, systemic administration of cidofovir has achieved some success to treat BK virus-associated HC; however, none of the studies were randomized or included a control group with multivariate modeling to evaluate the role of supportive care alone [57, 85, 91, 103]. Savona et al. reported clinical response in 84% of patients treated with weekly low dose of cidofovir; however, a decreased viral load in urine was observed in only 47% [91]. In a retrospective study, Cesaro et al. reported a complete clinical response in 67% of patients and among them a viral clearance in 81% and 20% of patients from blood and urine, respectively.

Cidofovir was given for a median number of doses of 4 (1–15) at a dose ranging from 0.5 to 5 mg/kg, with renal toxic effect observed in only a few patients [85]. A recent study by Gaziev et al. showed an increase of HC in children receiving ATG as part of their conditioning regimen and a response to cidofovir [57]; patients receiving supportive care alone also recovered; however, the treated and untreated patients differed in terms of disease severity making interpretation of the results difficult.

Intravesical administration of cidofovir leading to clinical improvement and reduction of viruria has been reported in few cases and has been suggested as an alternative to systemic therapy in patients with kidney dysfunction [93, 104, 105], 0.5–5 mg/kg, 1–15 doses) [85].

In HCT recipients, leflunomide has been used to treat refractory CMV infection with variable success [106, 107]. A recent report by Lekakis et al. describes the case of a HCT recipient with BK virus-associated cystitis and nephritis, treated by leflunomide in combination with *IVIg* [37]. Treatment was effective in reducing hemorrhagic cystitis symptoms and stabilizing kidney function [37]. Nevertheless, the requirement of high doses of leflunomide to achieve a therapeutic effect, the unpredictable relationship between drug dose and blood level, and the myelosuppressive and hepatotoxic properties of the drug limit its use in HCT population.

Leung et al. observed that ciprofloxacin decreases BK virus shedding in urine [92]; however, the clinical significance of fluoroquinolones in BK virus-associated HC was not convincing. Furthermore, based on the limited antiviral activity of fluoroquinolones observed in vitro, authors have suggested that fluoroquinolones may be more effective as prophylactic agents against BK virus-associated hemorrhagic cystitis rather than therapeutic agents [81, 108]. A single nonrandomized clinical study investigated the effect of prophylactic ciprofloxacin (500 mg orally/200 mg IV twice a day) on BK viruria and incidence of severity of postengraftment HC in adult HCT recipients [108]. In this trial, ciprofloxacin decreased the peak of BK viruria, but did not reduce the HC incidence. However, Rhandawa et al. demonstrated that ciprofloxacin had a modest antiviral activity and expressed a low selectivity index (defined as the ratio of the 50% in the host cell replication value to the 50% virus inhibitory concentration value) [109]. This observation let the author conclude that the drug may have a prophylactic effect, but its low selectivity index makes its efficacy very uncertain in a established disease characterized by high viral load. *IVIg* has been used in BK disease after kidney transplantation with variable success (Table 33.2); however, to date, there are no published data on the efficacy of *IVIg* for BK virus-associated disease in HCT setting.

Overall, to date no conclusive evidence from randomized trials or multivariate analyses of larger clinical cohorts exists

Table 33.2 Potential preventive and medical therapeutic interventions in BK virus-associated diseases

Interventions	References	Study design	Population	Disease	Controls	Key outcome	Comment
Prevention							
Ciprofloxacin	Leung, 2005 [92]	Prospective	Allogeneic HCT recipients	HC	Nonrandomized control: cephalosporines	Reduction in BK peak viral load in urine	Small sample size; nonrandomized; no effect on HC
MESNA versus hyperhydratation	Bedi, 1995 [41]	Prospective	Allogeneic HCT recipients	HC	Randomized	Both methods equally effective	Important trial
Continuous bladder irrigation	Hadjibabaie, 2008 [48]	Prospective	Allogeneic HCT recipients	HC	Nonrandomized control: no irrigation	Continuous irrigation was additive to MESNA, hydration, and alkalization	Relatively small sample size, nonrandomized
Therapeutic							
Cidofovir (high dose)	Gorczynska, 2005 [52]	Prospective	Allogeneic pediatric HCT recipients	HC	None	Clinical response in 15/19 children; eradication of viremia in all responders; one progression on cidofovir	Small series; no controls; no significant toxicities
Cidofovir (low-high dose)	Cesaro, 2009 [85]	Retrospective	Allogeneic HCT recipients	HC	None	Complete response in 67%; renal toxicity in 6/57; neutropenia 1/57	Larger series ($N=57$) but no controls
Cidofovir (high dose)	Gaziev, 2010 [57]	Prospective	Allogeneic HCT recipients (pediatric)	HC	Nonrandomized Untreated controls	Complete clinical response in treated and untreated patients	Small sample size; treated and untreated patients differed in severity of disease
Cidofovir (low dose)	Savona, 2007 [91]	Retrospective	Allogeneic HCT recipients	HC	None	Clinical response in 16/19; 14/19 no increase in serum creatinine	Small sample size, no controls
Cidofovir intravesical	Rao, 2009 [93]	Case series retrospective	Allogeneic HCT recipients	HC	None	Resolution of symptoms; no renal toxicity but mild pain	Small sample size, no controls
Cidofovir intravesical	Cesaro, 2009 [85]	Case series retrospective	Allogeneic HCT recipients	HC	None	Complete response in 3/6 patients; partial response in 1/6; bladder spasm in 1/6	Small sample size; no controls; poorly tolerated in one patient
Leflunomide	Canivet, 2009 [30]	Pilot	Kidney transplant recipients	Nephritis	None	Clearance or reduction in viral load in 9/12 patients; one organ loss	Small sample size; no controls
Immunoglobulin	Sener, 2006 [94]	Case series	Kidney transplant recipients	Nephritis	None	Response in 7/8 patients	Small sample size; no controls
Immunoglobulin	Wadei, 2006 [95]	Case series	Kidney transplant recipients	Nephritis	Analysis of various treatments, including low-dose cidofovir	No clear effect on functional decline and viral clearance	Small sample size; no controls

MESNA 2-mercaptoethane sodium sulfonate, *HC* hemorrhagic cystitis, *HCT* hematopoietic cell transplant

demonstrating that treatment with cidofovir (at any dose) or any other therapeutic is superior to supportive care.

Others Manifestation of BK Virus Disease After HCT

BK virus nephritis. Over the past few years, BK virus-associated nephritis has been sporadically reported in the native kidneys of HCT recipients, not always accompanied by hemorrhagic cystitis [37–40, 42]. This complication was always severe, leading to permanent renal failure in all cases despite treatment. Therefore, any unexplained significant deteriorating kidney function should be evaluated for BK virus involvement. A rational diagnostic algorithm may include initial testing in urine and blood followed by a renal biopsy with immunostaining for BK virus. The optimal treatment of BK virus nephritis in HCT population is currently unknown. If feasible, a reduction of immunosuppression should be attempted. Correction of hypogammaglobulinemia, low-dose cidofovir (0.25–1 mg/kg up to twice a week) without probenecid, and/or use of leflunomide with careful monitoring for possible adverse events are available for treatment; however, none of these therapies have been systematically evaluated.

Other organ manifestations. Clinical manifestations of BK virus infection in hemato-oncologic patients (with or without AIDS) outside the genitourinary tract have been reported in selected cases, including disseminated disease, meningitis, encephalitis, and pneumonitis [39, 61, 62, 110, 111]. A systematic evaluation of the significance of BK virus in disease manifestations outside the urinary tract has not been performed.

JC Virus

JC virus is a nonenveloped DNA virus and also classified as polyomavirus. JC virus is the cause of progressive multifocal leukoencephalopathy in immunosuppressed patients. Several cases have been reported after HCT and in patients with hematologic malignancies [112–116]. Overall, the frequency of this complication seems to be very rare. PCR detection of JC virus in the cerebrospinal fluid is used for diagnosis [117]; however, its sensitivity is not 100%. Therefore, brain biopsies may be required; plasma PCR may also be useful [116]. The optimal treatment is not defined. Cidofovir has activity in vitro; however, little is known about its in vivo efficacy in HCT recipients [118]. A study in HIV-infected individuals failed to show a therapeutic effect of cidofovir. Other treatment options include IL-2, cytarabine, chlorpromazine, or the antipsychotic drugs ziprasidone, risperidone, and olanzapine [116, 119]; however, only individual patients have been treated with these drugs, thus making an assessment of efficacy difficult [120]. CMX-001, an oral derivative of cidofovir, is highly active against JC virus in vitro [121]. The compound is presently undergoing clinical testing in immunosuppressed patients for BK virus and CMV disease.

Parvovirus B19

Parvoviruses are small, naked, single-stranded DNA viruses. Parvovirus B19 is the best-studied virus; however, other parvoviruses exist and may cause human disease. Human parvovirus can be isolated from asymptomatic blood donors and be detected by PCR, but transmission via blood products (especially when viral load is low) is uncommon [122]. Seroepidemiolocal studies showed evidence of past infection in approximately 60% of young adults. The virus is most likely spread by respiratory transmission or by blood. Parvovirus B19 can infect erythroid progenitor cells. Parvovirus B19 commonly is associated with aplastic crisis in patients with hemolytic anemia. It is also the cause of erythema infectiosum, a self-limited disease of childhood characterized by fever, fatigue, myalgias, a lace-like rash, and a "slapped-cheek" appearance. Parvovirus B19 has also been associated with some cases of rheumatoid arthritis.

Besides hematologic complications (anemia, thrombocytopenia, engraftment failure), clinical manifestations that have been associated with parvovirus immunocompromised patients include transient prolonged viremia pancytogenia, chronic anemia, pericarditis, myocarditis, hepatitis, pneumonitis, and neurologic disease [123–127]. Neurologic diseases, including encephalitis, meningitis, stroke, and peripheral neuropathy, have been reported to occur in both immunocompetent and immunosuppressed individuals [128]. The basis for these reports is the detection of parvovirus in patients with disease; however, more work is needed to conclusively establish parvovirus as a pathogen in these disease manifestations.

PCR is useful as a diagnostic tool [124]. These associations have been seen in case reports or small series. A more systematic evaluation of parvovirus as a cause of these clinical syndromes is needed for most of these manifestations.

IVIg is effective in treating parvovirus B19 symptomatic infection [129]. Prophylactic *IVIg* seems to have a protective effect against parvovirus B19, although this has not been established in a randomized study [130]. *IVIg* has also been used for treatment (e.g. 400 mg/kg for 5 days) and reduction of immunosuppression, if feasible, has been advocated [127], however, no systematic evaluation of these strategies is available. At this time, there is no antiviral drug treatment available for parvovirus infection.

Summary

BK virus has emerged as an important pathogen in the solid organ and hematopoietic cell transplant population. With the rising development of immunosuppressive drugs and the increasing population of immunocompromised patients, the incidence and diversity of BK virus manifestations are expected to increase. Although therapies for BK virus have been described, the quality of the evidence supporting their use is poor and randomized studies are urgently needed to determine the efficacy of the currently available antiviral drugs. Furthermore, the development of more effective and specific antiviral agents is needed. A candidate antiviral agent, HDP-cidofovir (CMX001), an oral derivative of cidofovir with significantly enhanced activity against BK virus, is presently undergoing clinical testing. Also, studies are needed to better understand the interaction of the virus with the host to answer unresolved questions in BK virus pathogenesis.

It should also be emphasized that besides hemorrhagic cystitis, nephritis appears to be of increasing importance in HCT recipients. The optimal management of this disease remains unknown; however, low dose of cidofovir, reduction of immunosuppression, correction of hypogammaglobulinemia, and perhaps leflunomide might be reasonable options. Regarding late-onset hemorrhagic cystitis, because of the transient nature of the condition in most cases and the toxicity of available antiviral drugs, optimal supportive treatment seems to be a nonnocere approach, especially for mild-to-moderate disease. Any further interventions for more severe disease would have to be considered on an individual basis for a given clinical scenario, balancing benefits and risks.

No proven treatment options exist for JC virus and the outcome of JC virus disease is often devastating. Agents under development (CMX001) are promising based on their in vitro susceptibility, but no clinical data exist at this point.

Parvoviruses have long been associated with hematologic complications. However, recent reports also occasionally implicate this virus in cardiac, lung, hepatic, and neurologic disease. More systematic evaluation to establish the role of parvovirus as a true pathogen is needed.

Acknowledgments Michael Boeckh was supported in part by National Institute of Health grants CA18029 and HL93294.

References

1. Gardner SD, Field AM, Coleman DV, Hulme B. New human papovavirus (B.K.) isolated from urine after renal transplantation. Lancet. 1971;1(7712):1253–7.
2. Hirsch HH, Steiger J, Polyomavirus BK. Lancet Infect Dis. 2003;3:611–23.
3. Randhawa PS, Demetris AJ. Nephropathy due to polyomavirus type BK. N Engl J Med. 2000;342(18):1361–3.
4. Apperley JF, Rice SJ, Bishop JA, et al. Late-onset hemorrhagic cystitis associated with urinary excretion of polyomaviruses after bone marrow transplantation. Transplantation. 1987;43(1):108–12.
5. Arthur RR, Shah KV, Charache P, Saral R. BK and JC virus infections in recipients of bone marrow transplants. J Infect Dis. 1988;158(3):563–9.
6. Cubitt CL. Molecular genetics of the BK virus. Adv Exp Med Biol. 2006;577:85–95.
7. Drachenberg CB, Papadimitriou JC, Wali R, Cubitt CL, Ramos E. BK polyoma virus allograft nephropathy: ultrastructural features from viral cell entry to lysis. Am J Transplant. 2003;3(11):1383–92.
8. Jiang M, Abend JR, Tsai B, Imperiale MJ. Early events during BK virus entry and disassembly. J Virol. 2009;83(3):1350–8.
9. Moriyama T, Sorokin A. BK virus (BKV): infection, propagation, quantitation, purification, labeling, and analysis of cell entry. Curr Protoc Cell Biol. 2009;Chapter 26:Unit 26.2.
10. Marsh M, Helenius A. Virus entry: open sesame. Cell. 2006;124(4):729–40.
11. Eash S, Querbes W, Atwood WJ. Infection of vero cells by BK virus is dependent on caveolae. J Virol. 2004;78(21):11583–90.
12. Ashok A, Atwood WJ. Virus receptors and tropism. Adv Exp Med Biol. 2006;577:60–72.
13. Low JA, Magnuson B, Tsai B, Imperiale MJ. Identification of gangliosides GD1b and GT1b as receptors for BK virus. J Virol. 2006;80(3):1361–6.
14. Moriyama T, Marquez JP, Wakatsuki T, Sorokin A. Caveolar endocytosis is critical for BK virus infection of human renal proximal tubular epithelial cells. J Virol. 2007;81(16):8552–62.
15. Knowles WA. Discovery and epidemiology of the human polyomaviruses BK virus (BKV) and JC virus (JCV). Adv Exp Med Biol. 2006;577:19–45.
16. Pietropaolo V, Di Taranto C, Degener AM, et al. Transplacental transmission of human polyomavirus BK. J Med Virol. 1998;56(4):372–6.
17. Shah K, Daniel R, Madden D, Stagno S. Serological investigation of BK papovavirus infection in pregnant women and their offspring. Infect Immun. 1980;30(1):29–35.
18. Coleman DV, Wolfendale MR, Daniel RA, et al. A prospective study of human polyomavirus infection in pregnancy. J Infect Dis. 1980;142(1):1–8.
19. Vanchiere JA, Nicome RK, Greer JM, Demmler GJ, Butel JS. Frequent detection of polyomaviruses in stool samples from hospitalized children. J Infect Dis. 2005;192(4):658–64.
20. Bofill-Mas S, Formiga-Cruz M, Clemente-Casares P, Calafell F, Girones R. Potential transmission of human polyomaviruses through the gastrointestinal tract after exposure to virions or viral DNA. J Virol. 2001;75(21):10290–9.
21. Bohl DL, Storch GA, Ryschkewitsch C, et al. Donor origin of BK virus in renal transplantation and role of HLA C7 in susceptibility to sustained BK viremia. Am J Transplant. 2005;5(9):2213–21.
22. Hirsch HH. Polyomavirus BK nephropathy: a (re-)emerging complication in renal transplantation. Am J Transplant. 2002;2:25–30.
23. Goudsmit J, Wertheim-van Dillen P, van Strien A, van der Noordaa J. The role of BK virus in acute respiratory tract disease and the presence of BKV DNA in tonsils. J Med Virol. 1982;10(2):91–9.
24. Feder Jr HM, Solomon B, Gavin LD. Polyoma virus hemorrhagic cystitis in an otherwise normal child. Pediatr Infect Dis J. 2008;27(10):948–9.
25. Nickeleit V, Singh HK, Mihatsch MJ. Polyomavirus nephropathy: morphology, pathophysiology, and clinical management. Curr Opin Nephrol Hypertens. 2003;12(6):599–605.
26. Monini P, Rotola A, Di Luca D, et al. DNA rearrangements impairing BK virus productive infection in urinary tract tumors. Virology. 1995;214(1):273–9.

27. Doerries K. Human polyomavirus JC and BK persistent infection. Adv Exp Med Biol. 2006;577:102–16.
28. Arthur RR, Dagostin S, Shah KV. Detection of BK virus and JC virus in urine and brain tissue by the polymerase chain reaction. J Clin Microbiol. 1989;27(6):1174–9.
29. Chang D, Wang M, Ou WC, Lee MS, Ho HN, Tsai RT. Genotypes of human polyomaviruses in urine samples of pregnant women in Taiwan. J Med Virol. 1996;48(1):95–101.
30. Egli A, Infanti L, Dumoulin A, et al. Prevalence of polyomavirus BK and JC infection and replication in 400 healthy blood donors. J Infect Dis. 2009;199(6):837–46.
31. Hirsch HH, Brennan DC, Drachenberg CB, et al. Polyomavirus-associated nephropathy in renal transplantation: interdisciplinary analyses and recommendations. Transplantation. 2005;79(10):1277–86.
32. Hirsch HH, Drachenberg CB, Steiger J, Ramos E. Polyomavirus-associated nephropathy in renal transplantation: critical issues of screening and management. Adv Exp Med Biol. 2006;577:160–73.
33. Nickeleit V, Mihatsch MJ. Polyomavirus allograft nephropathy and concurrent acute rejection: a diagnostic and therapeutic challenge. Am J Transplant. 2004;4(5):838–9.
34. O'Donnell PH, Swanson K, Josephson MA. BK virus infection is associated with hematuria and renal impairment in recipients of allogeneic hematopoetic stem cell transplants. Biol Blood Marrow Transplant. 2009;15(9):1038–48. e1.
35. Inaba H, Jones DP, Gaber LW, et al. BK virus-induced tubulointerstitial nephritis in a child with acute lymphoblastic leukemia. J Pediatr. 2007;151(2):215–7.
36. van der Bij A, Betjes M, Weening J, et al. BK virus nephropathy in an immunodeficient patient with chronic lymphocytic leukemia. J Clin Virol. 2009;45(4):341–4.
37. Lekakis LJ, Macrinici V, Baraboutis IG, Mitchell B, Howard DS. BK virus nephropathy after allogeneic stem cell transplantation: a case report and literature review. Am J Hematol. 2009;84(4):243–6.
38. Limaye AP, Smith KD, Cook L, et al. Polyomavirus nephropathy in native kidneys of non-renal transplant recipients. Am J Transplant. 2005;5(3):614–20.
39. Shapiro S, Robin M, Esperou H, et al. Polyomavirus nephropathy in the native kidneys of an unrelated cord blood transplant recipient followed by a disseminated polyomavirus infection. Transplantation. 2006;82(2):292–3.
40. Bruno B, Zager R, Boeckh M, Gooley T, Myerson DH, Huang M, et al. Adenovirus nephritis in hematopoietic stem cell transplantation. Transplantation. 2004;77:1049–57.
41. Bedi A, Miller CB, Hanson JL, et al. Association of BK virus with failure of prophylaxis against hemorrhagic cystitis following bone marrow transplantation. J Clin Oncol. 1995;13(5):1103–9.
42. Iwamoto S, Azuma E, Hori H, et al. BK virus-associated fatal renal failure following late-onset hemorrhagic cystitis in an unrelated bone marrow transplantation. Pediatr Hematol Oncol. 2002;19(4):255–61.
43. Seber A, Shu XO, Defor T, Sencer S, Ramsay N. Risk factors for severe hemorrhagic cystitis following BMT. Bone Marrow Transplant. 1999;23(1):35–40.
44. Leung AY, Mak R, Lie AK, et al. Clinicopathological features and risk factors of clinically overt haemorrhagic cystitis complicating bone marrow transplantation. Bone Marrow Transplant. 2002;29(6):509–13.
45. Hu RQ, Mehter H, Nadasdy T, et al. Severe hemorrhagic cystitis associated with prolonged oral cyclophosphamide therapy: case report and literature review. Rheumatol Int. 2008;28(11):1161–4.
46. Erard V, Kim HW, Corey L, et al. BK DNA viral load in plasma: evidence for an association with hemorrhagic cystitis in allogeneic hematopoietic cell transplant recipients. Blood. 2005;106(3):1130–2.
47. Schuchter LM, Hensley ML, Meropol NJ, Winer EP. 2002 update of recommendations for the use of chemotherapy and radiotherapy protectants: clinical practice guidelines of the American Society of Clinical Oncology. J Clin Oncol. 2002;20(12):2895–903.
48. Hadjibabaie M, Alimoghaddam K, Shamshiri AR, et al. Continuous bladder irrigation prevents hemorrhagic cystitis after allogeneic hematopoietic cell transplantation. Urol Oncol. 2008;26(1):43–6.
49. Shepherd JD, Pringle LE, Barnett MJ, Klingemann HG, Reece DE, Phillips GL. Mesna versus hyperhydration for the prevention of cyclophosphamide-induced hemorrhagic cystitis in bone marrow transplantation. J Clin Oncol. 1991;9(11):2016–20.
50. Garcia Ligero J, Mora Peris B, Garcia Garcia F. Hemorrhagic cystitis caused by BK and JC polyomavirus in patients treated with bone marrow transplantation: clinical features and urologic management. Actas Urol Esp. 2002;26(2):104–10.
51. Erard V, Storer B, Corey L, et al. BK virus infection in hematopoietic stem cell transplant recipients: frequency, risk factors, and association with postengraftment hemorrhagic cystitis. Clin Infect Dis. 2004;39(12):1861–5.
52. Gorczynska E, Turkiewicz D, Rybka K, et al. Incidence, clinical outcome, and management of virus-induced hemorrhagic cystitis in children and adolescents after allogeneic hematopoietic cell transplantation. Biol Blood Marrow Transplant. 2005;11(10):797–804.
53. Fioriti D, Degener AM, Mischitelli M, et al. BKV infection and hemorrhagic cystitis after allogeneic bone marrow transplant. Int J Immunopathol Pharmacol. 2005;18(2):309–16.
54. Giraud G, Priftakis P, Bogdanovic G, et al. BK-viruria and haemorrhagic cystitis are more frequent in allogeneic haematopoietic stem cell transplant patients receiving full conditioning and unrelated-HLA-mismatched grafts. Bone Marrow Transplant 2008.
55. Cesaro S, Facchin C, Tridello G, et al. A prospective study of BK-virus-associated haemorrhagic cystitis in paediatric patients undergoing allogeneic haematopoietic stem cell transplantation. Bone Marrow Transplant. 2008;41(4):363–70.
56. Park SH, Choi SM, Lee DG, et al. Infectious complications associated with alemtuzumab use for allogeneic hematopoietic stem cell transplantation: comparison with anti-thymocyte globulin. Transpl Infect Dis. 2009;11:413–23.
57. Gaziev J, Paba P, Miano R, et al. Late-onset hemorrhagic cystitis in children after hematopoietic stem cell transplantation for thalassemia and sickle cell anemia: a prospective evaluation of polyoma (BK) virus infection and treatment with cidofovir. Biol Blood Marrow Transplant. 2010;16(5):662–71.
58. De Padua Silva L, Patah PA, Saliba RM, et al. Hemorrhagic cystitis after allogeneic hematopoietic stem cell transplants is the complex result of BK virus infection, preparative regimen intensity and donor type. Haematologica 2010.
59. Stracke S, Helmchen U, von Muller L, Bunjes D, Keller F. Polyoma virus-associated interstitial nephritis in a patient with acute myeloic leukaemia and peripheral blood stem cell transplantation. Nephrol Dial Transplant. 2003;18(11):2431–3.
60. Verghese PS, Finn LS, Englund JA, Sanders JE, Hingorani SR. BK nephropathy in pediatric hematopoietic stem cell transplant recipients. Pediatr Transplant. 2009;13(7):913–8.
61. Galan A, Rauch CA, Otis CN. Fatal BK polyoma viral pneumonia associated with immunosuppression. Hum Pathol. 2005;36(9):1031–4.
62. Sandler ES, Aquino VM, Goss-Shohet E, Hinrichs S, Krisher K. BK papova virus pneumonia following hematopoietic stem cell transplantation. Bone Marrow Transplant. 1997;20(2):163–5.
63. Asano Y, Kanda Y, Ogawa N, et al. Male predominance among Japanese adult patients with late-onset hemorrhagic cystitis after hematopoietic stem cell transplantation. Bone Marrow Transplant. 2003;32(12):1175–9.
64. Bielorai B, Shulman LM, Rechavi G, Toren A. CMV reactivation induced BK virus-associated late onset hemorrhagic cystitis after

peripheral blood stem cell transplantation. Bone Marrow Transplant. 2001;28(6):613–4.
65. Basquiera AL, Calafat P, Parodi JM, De Diller AB, Zlocowski JC, Caeiro JP. Cytomegalovirus-induced haemorrhagic cystitis in a patient with neurogenic bladder. Scand J Infect Dis. 2003;35(11–12):902–4.
66. Priftakis P, Bogdanovic G, Kokhaei P, Mellstedt H, Dalianis T. BK virus quantification in urine samples of bone marrow transplanted patients is helpful for diagnosis of hemorrhagic cystitis, although wide individual variations exist. J Clin Virol. 2002.
67. Arthur RR, Shah KV, Baust SJ, Santos GW, Saral R. Association of BK viruria with hemorrhagic cystitis in recipients of bone marrow transplants. N Engl J Med. 1986;315(4):230–4.
68. Bogdanovic G, Priftakis P, Giraud G, et al. Association between a high BK virus load in urine samples of patients with graft-versus-host disease and development of hemorrhagic cystitis after hematopoietic stem cell transplantation. J Clin Microbiol. 2004;42(11):5394–6.
69. Leung AY, Chan M, Tang SC, Liang R, Kwong YL. Real-time quantitative analysis of polyoma BK viremia and viruria in renal allograft recipients. J Virol Methods. 2002;103(1):51–6.
70. Wong AS, Chan KH, Cheng VC, Yuen KY, Kwong YL, Leung AY. Relationship of pretransplantation polyoma BK virus serologic findings and BK viral reactivation after hematopoietic stem cell transplantation. Clin Infect Dis. 2007;44(6):830–7.
71. Hirsch HH, Knowles W, Dickenmann M, et al. Prospective study of polyomavirus type BK replication and nephropathy in renal-transplant recipients. N Engl J Med. 2002;347(7):488–96.
72. Leung AY, Suen CK, Lie AK, Liang RH, Yuen KY, Kwong YL. Quantification of polyoma BK viruria in hemorrhagic cystitis complicating bone marrow transplantation. Blood. 2001;98(6):1971–8.
73. Xie Y, Han Y, Wu DP. The role of BK polyomavirus in the development of hemorrhagic cystitis after hematopoietic stem cell transplantation. Zhonghua Nei Ke Za Zhi. 2008;47(9):746–9.
74. Parkin RK, Boeckh MJ, Erard V, Huang ML, Myerson D. Specific delineation of BK polyomavirus in kidney tissue with a digoxigenin-labeled DNA probe. Mol Cell Probes. 2005;19(2):87–92.
75. Fogazzi GB, Cantu M, Saglimbeni L. 'Decoy cells' in the urine due to polyomavirus BK infection: easily seen by phase-contrast microscopy. Nephrol Dial Transplant. 2001;16(7):1496–8.
76. Boldorini R, Veggiani C, Barco D, Monga G. Kidney and urinary tract polyomavirus infection and distribution: molecular biology investigation of 10 consecutive autopsies. Arch Pathol Lab Med. 2005;129(1):69–73.
77. Hiraoka A, Ishikawa J, Kitayama H, et al. Hemorrhagic cystitis after bone marrow transplantation: importance of a thin sectioning technique on urinary sediments for diagnosis. Bone Marrow Transplant. 1991;7(2):107–11.
78. Randhawa P, Vats A, Shapiro R. Monitoring for polyomavirus BK and JC in urine: comparison of quantitative polymerase chain reaction with urine cytology. Transplantation. 2005;79(8):984–6.
79. Semple K, Lovchik J, Drachenberg C. Identification of polyoma BK virus in kidney transplant recipients by shell vial cell culture assay and urine cytology. Am J Clin Pathol. 2006;126(3):444–7.
80. Hoffman NG, Cook L, Atienza EE, Limaye AP, Jerome KR. Marked variability of BK virus load measurement using quantitative real-time PCR among commonly used assays. J Clin Microbiol. 2008;46(8):2671–80.
81. Dropulic LK, Jones RJ. Polyomavirus BK infection in blood and marrow transplant recipients. Bone Marrow Transplant. 2008;41(1):11–8.
82. Ambinder RF, Burns W, Forman M, et al. Hemorrhagic cystitis associated with adenovirus infection in bone marrow transplantation. Arch Intern Med. 1986;146(7):1400–1.
83. Spach DH, Bauwens JE, Myerson D, Mustafa MM, Bowden RA. Cytomegalovirus-induced hemorrhagic cystitis following bone marrow transplantation. Clin Infect Dis. 1993;16(1):142–4.
84. Fergany AF, Moussa AS, Gill IS. Laparoscopic cystoprostatectomy for radiation-induced hemorrhagic cystitis. J Endourol. 2009;23(2):275–8.
85. Cesaro S, Hirsch HH, Faraci M, et al. Cidofovir for BK virus-associated hemorrhagic cystitis: a retrospective study. Clin Infect Dis. 2009;49(2):233–40.
86. Williams JW, Javaid B, Kadambi PV, et al. Leflunomide for polyomavirus type BK nephropathy. N Engl J Med. 2005;352(11):1157–8.
87. Farasati NA, Shapiro R, Vats A, Randhawa P. Effect of leflunomide and cidofovir on replication of BK virus in an in vitro culture system. Transplantation. 2005;79(1):116–8.
88. Josephson MA, Gillen D, Javaid B, et al. Treatment of renal allograft polyoma BK virus infection with leflunomide. Transplantation. 2006;81(5):704–10.
89. Josephson MA, Williams JW, Chandraker A, Randhawa PS. Polyomavirus-associated nephropathy: update on antiviral strategies. Transpl Infect Dis. 2006;8(2):95–101.
90. Lamoth F, Pascual M, Erard V, Venetz JP, Nseir G, Meylan P. Low-dose cidofovir for the treatment of polyomavirus-associated nephropathy: two case reports and review of the literature. Antivir Ther. 2008;13(8):1001–9.
91. Savona MR, Newton D, Frame D, Levine JE, Mineishi S, Kaul DR. Low-dose cidofovir treatment of BK virus-associated hemorrhagic cystitis in recipients of hematopoietic stem cell transplant. Bone Marrow Transplant. 2007;39(12):783–7.
92. Leung AY, Chan MT, Yuen KY, et al. Ciprofloxacin decreased polyoma BK virus load in patients who underwent allogeneic hematopoietic stem cell transplantation. Clin Infect Dis. 2005;40(4):528–37.
93. Rao KV, Buie LW, Shea T, et al. Intravesicular cidofovir for the management of BK virus-associated cystitis. Biol Blood Marrow Transplant. 2009;15(3):391–2.
94. Sener A, House AA, Jevnikar AM, et al. Intravenous immunoglobulin as a treatment for BK virus associated nephropathy: one-year follow-up of renal allograft recipients. Transplantation. 2006;81(1):117–20.
95. Wadei HM, Rule AD, Lewin M, et al. Kidney transplant function and histological clearance of virus following diagnosis of polyomavirus-associated nephropathy (PVAN). Am J Transplant. 2006;6(5 Pt 1):1025–32.
96. Bernhoff E, Gutteberg TJ, Sandvik K, Hirsch HH, Rinaldo CH. Cidofovir inhibits polyomavirus BK replication in human renal tubular cells downstream of viral early gene expression. Am J Transplant. 2008;8(7):1413–22.
97. Rho YH, Oeser A, Chung CP, Milne GL, Stein CM. Drugs used in the treatment of rheumatoid arthritis: relationship between current use and cardiovascular risk factors. Arch Drug Inf. 2009;2(2):34–40.
98. Canivet C, Rostaing L, Galvani S, et al. Polyoma BK virus-associated nephropathy in kidney-transplant patients: effects of leflunomide on T-cell functions and disease outcome. Int Immunopharmacol. 2009;9(9):1131–6.
99. Faguer S, Hirsch HH, Kamar N, et al. Leflunomide treatment for polyomavirus BK-associated nephropathy after kidney transplantation. Transpl Int. 2007;20(11):962–9.
100. Ali SH, Chandraker A, DeCaprio JA. Inhibition of simian virus 40 large T antigen helicase activity by fluoroquinolones. Antivir Ther. 2007;12(1):1–6.
101. Puliyanda D AN, Dhavan A, et al. Heart and bone marrow transplant recipients are at low risk for BK viremia and nephropathy. Am J Transplant. 2003;3:510.
102. Hilton R, Tong CY. Antiviral therapy for polyomavirus-associated nephropathy after renal transplantation. J Antimicrob Chemother. 2008;62(5):855–9.

103. Held TK, Biel SS, Nitsche A, et al. Treatment of BK virus-associated hemorrhagic cystitis and simultaneous CMV reactivation with cidofovir. Bone Marrow Transplant. 2000;26(3):347–50.
104. Bridges B, Donegan S, Badros A. Cidofovir bladder instillation for the treatment of BK hemorrhagic cystitis after allogeneic stem cell transplantation. Am J Hematol. 2006;81(7):535–7.
105. Walden O, Hartel C, Doehn C, Jocham D. Intravesical cidofovir – instillation therapy for polyomavirus-associated hemorrhagic cystitis after bone marrow transplantation. Urologe A. 2007;46(5):535–7.
106. Avery RK, Bolwell BJ, Yen-Lieberman B, et al. Use of leflunomide in an allogeneic bone marrow transplant recipient with refractory cytomegalovirus infection. Bone Marrow Transplant. 2004;34(12):1071–5.
107. Ehlert K, Groll AH, Kuehn J, Vormoor J. Treatment of refractory CMV-infection following hematopoietic stem cell transplantation with the combination of foscarnet and leflunomide. Klin Pädiatr. 2006;218(3):180–4.
108. Leung AYHY, K.Y, Kwong YL. Anti-BK virus activity of ciprofloxacin and related antibiotics. 2005.
109. Randhawa PS. Anti-BK virus activity of ciprofloxacin and related antibiotics. Clin Infect Dis. 2005;41(9):1366–7.
110. Stoner GL, Alappan R, Jobes DV, Ryschkewitsch CF, Landry ML. BK virus regulatory region rearrangements in brain and cerebrospinal fluid from a leukemia patient with tubulointerstitial nephritis and meningoencephalitis. Am J Kidney Dis. 2002;39(5):1102–12.
111. Lesprit P, Chaline-Lehmann D, Authier FJ, Ponnelle T, Gray F, Levy Y. BK virus encephalitis in a patient with AIDS and lymphoma. AIDS. 2001;15(9):1196–9.
112. Coppo P, Laporte JP, Aoudjhane M, et al. Progressive multifocal leucoencephalopathy with peripheral demyelinating neuropathy after autologous bone marrow transplantation for acute myeloblastic leukemia (FAB5). Bone Marrow Transplant. 1999;23(4):401–3.
113. Re D, Bamborschke S, Feiden W, et al. Progressive multifocal leukoencephalopathy after autologous bone marrow transplantation and alpha-interferon immunotherapy. Bone Marrow Transplant. 1999;23(3):295–8.
114. Holzapfel C, Kellinghaus C, Luttmann R, et al. Progressive multifocal leukoencephalopathy (PML) in chronic lymphatic leukemia (CLL). Review of the literature and case report. Nervenarzt. 2002;73(6):543–7.
115. Seong D, Bruner JM, Lee KH, et al. Progressive multifocal leukoencephalopathy after autologous bone marrow transplantation in a patient with chronic myelogenous leukemia. Clin Infect Dis. 1996;23(2):402–3.
116. Kharfan-Dabaja MA, Ayala E, Greene J, Rojiani A, Murtagh FR, Anasetti C. Two cases of progressive multifocal leukoencephalopathy after allogeneic hematopoietic cell transplantation and a review of the literature. Bone Marrow Transplant. 2007;39(2):101–7.
117. Taoufik Y, Gasnault J, Karaterki A, et al. Prognostic value of JC virus load in cerebrospinal fluid of patients with progressive multifocal leukoencephalopathy. J Infect Dis. 1998;178(6):1816–20.
118. Houston S, Roberts N, Mashinter L. Failure of cidofovir therapy in progressive multifocal leukoencephalopathy unrelated to human immunodeficiency virus. Clin Infect Dis. 2001;32:150–2.
119. Focosi D, Fazzi R, Montanaro D, Emdin M, Petrini M. Progressive multifocal leukoencephalopathy in a haploidentical stem cell transplant recipient: a clinical, neuroradiological and virological response after treatment with risperidone. Antivir Res. 2007;74(2):156–8.
120. Przepiorka D, Jaeckle KA, Birdwell RR, et al. Successful treatment of progressive multifocal leukoencephalopathy with low-dose interleukin-2. Bone Marrow Transplant. 1997;20(11):983–7.
121. Dal Pozzo F, Andrei G, Lebeau I. In vitro evaluation of the anti-orf virus activity of alkoxyalkyl esters of CDV, cCDV and (S)-HPMPA. Antivir Res. 2007;75(1):52–7.
122. Kleinman SH, Glynn SA, Lee TH, et al. A linked donor-recipient study to evaluate parvovirus B19 transmission by blood component transfusion. Blood. 2009;114(17):3677–83.
123. Azzi A, Fanci R, Ciappi S, Zakrzewska K, Bosi A. Human parvovirus B19 infection in bone marrow transplantation patients. Am J Hematol. 1993;44(3):207–9.
124. Schleuning M, Jager G, Holler E, et al. Human parvovirus B19-associated disease in bone marrow transplantation. Infection. 1999;27(2):114–7.
125. Florea AV, Ionescu DN, Melhem MF. Parvovirus B19 infection in the immunocompromised host. Arch Pathol Lab Med. 2007;131(5):799–804.
126. Eid AJ, Brown RA, Patel R, Razonable RR. Parvovirus B19 infection after transplantation: a review of 98 cases. Clin Infect Dis. 2006;43(1):40–8.
127. Eid AJ, Posfay-barbe KM, AST Infectious Diseases Community of Practice. Parvovirus B19 in solid organ transplant recipients. Am J Transplant. 2009;9 Suppl 4:S147–50.
128. Douvoyiannis M, Litman N, Goldman DL. Neurologic manifestations associated with parvovirus B19 infection. Clin Infect Dis. 2009;48(12):1713–23.
129. Kurtzman G, Frickhofen N, Kimball J, Jenkins DW, Nienhuis AW, Young NS. Pure red-cell aplasia of 10 years' duration due to persistent parvovirus B19 infection and its cure with immunoglobulin therapy [see comments]. N Engl J Med. 1989;321(8):519–23.
130. Frickhofen N, Arnold R, Hertenstein B, Wiesneth M, Young NS. Parvovirus B19 infection and bone marrow transplantation. Ann Hematol. 1992;64(Suppl):A121–4.

Chapter 34
Antiviral Resistance and Implications for Prophylaxis

Robin K. Avery

Abstract Development of prophylactic, preemptive, and therapeutic strategies has reduced the morbidity and mortality of viral infections after HSCT. However, the future success of such strategies is threatened by the increasing emergence of antiviral-resistant virus strains. In some cases, resistance is common enough to warrant changes in recommendations for prophylaxis (e.g., influenza in the 2008–2009 season). In other cases (HSV, VZV, CMV, HBV), resistance has not yet altered the primary class of agent(s) utilized for prophylaxis or preemptive therapy at the majority of centers, but clinicians should have a heightened awareness of the possibility of antiviral resistance and a low threshold to alter therapy in the setting of high viral loads, unusual clinical presentations, or refractoriness to standard therapy. A detailed overview of the scope of this problem and strategies for managing patients with these difficult-to-treat infections is presented in this chapter.

Keywords Viral drug resistance • Influenza virus • CMV • Herpes simplex virus • Varicella-zoster virus • Hepatitis B virus

Background

Viruses, like bacteria and fungi, are becoming more resistant to standard antimicrobial agents over time. One of the cornerstones of successful infection prevention programs in HSCT recipients has been the use of antiviral agents, principally derivatives of acyclovir and ganciclovir for prevention or suppression of herpesvirus infections, including cytomegalovirus (CMV), herpes simplex virus (HSV), and varicella-zoster virus (VZV) [1] (Table 34.1). Genotypic antiviral resistance appears to be increasing for all three of these

R.K. Avery (✉)
Department of Infectious Disease, Cleveland Clinic Foundation, Lerner College of Medicine of Case Western Reserve University, 9500 Euclid Avenue, Mail Code G21, Cleveland, OH 44195, USA
e-mail: averyr@ccf.org

viruses, but alternative agents such as foscarnet and cidofovir have potential adverse effects such as nephrotoxicity. Agents on the horizon include the investigational benzimidazole agent maribavir (for CMV and EBV); the rheumatoid arthritis drug leflunomide (for CMV, BK polyomavirus, and HSV); and the antimalarial drug artesunate (for CMV). One of the most rapidly changing viruses with respect to resistance is influenza A, which developed widespread oseltamivir resistance (in the seasonal H1N1 group) between the 2007–2008 and the 2008–2009 seasons, but then pandemic H1N1 influenza was almost entirely oseltamivir-sensitive. In addition, hepatitis B virus strains resistant to lamivudine are increasingly appearing, a development particularly affecting HSCT programs in areas endemic for HBV.

For the most part, with the exception of influenza A (H1N1) viruses [2], these trends toward more resistance have not as yet led to abandonment of one or more standard agents or other major changes in recommendations [1]. However, the transplant community should be aware that antiviral prophylaxis for the viruses mentioned above, as well as possibly others, may become less efficacious over time, and future guidelines may be altered accordingly. Increasing reliance on early detection, newer agents, and other strategies may result. Interventions to restore pathogen-specific immunity without precipitating graft-versus-host disease will be welcome developments.

Herpes Simplex Virus

Herpes simplex virus (HSV) is an important pathogen after HSCT, causing mucosal ulcerations of the oropharynx, esophagus, genital, and perianal areas, as well as at times, visceral infection such as hepatitis, pneumonitis, and meningoencephalitis. Prophylaxis against HSV is frequently administered to HSCT recipients in the form of acyclovir or ganciclovir derivatives (which have activity against acyclovir-sensitive HSV). The investigational drug maribavir lacks intrinsic activity against HSV and VZV, and in future,

Table 34.1 Viruses with genotypic resistance of importance in HSCT

Virus	Resistance mutation types[a]	Primary agent(s) that resistance affects	Therapy for antiviral-resistant viral infections
HSV	Thymidine kinase, DNA polymerase	Thymidine kinase: acyclovir, ganciclovir DNA polymerase: acyclovir, ganciclovir, foscarnet	Foscarnet, cidofovir ?Leflunomide
VZV	Thymidine kinase, DNA polymerase	Thymidine kinase: acyclovir, ganciclovir DNA polymerase: acyclovir, ganciclovir, foscarnet	Foscarnet, cidofovir
CMV	UL97 kinase UL54 DNA polymerase UL27	UL97: acyclovir, ganciclovir; maribavir (different loci) UL54: acyclovir, ganciclovir, foscarnet, cidofovir UL27: maribavir	Foscarnet, cidofovir ?Maribavir, ?Leflunomide, ?Artesunate
Influenza A	Adamantane resistance Neuraminidase	Adamantane resistance: amantadine, rimantadine Neuraminidase: oseltamivir (possibly zanamivir in future)	Zanamivir or rimantadine for H1N1 viruses; oseltamivir for H3N2 or influenza B; zanamivir or rimantadine/oseltamivir for unknown type
HBV	Precore, core promoter, YMDD	YMDD: lamivudine	Adefovir, entecavir, adefovir/lamivudine

[a]Resistance is not invariably conferred by mutations in these regions

patients who are receiving CMV prophylaxis with maribavir may need a coadministered agent with anti-HSV and VZV activity.

The activity of acyclovir depends upon phosphorylation by a viral thymidine kinase to acyclovir triphosphate, which in turn inhibits viral replication. In the early 1980s, acyclovir resistance due to a thymidine kinase-deficient strain was reported, producing reduced phosphorylation of acyclovir [3–5]; shortly thereafter, resistance at the level of viral DNA polymerase was described, conferring reduced affinity for acyclovir triphosphate [6]. The thymidine kinase pathway is the more common one and can occur by a variety of mechanisms including insertion and deletion of nucleotides and point mutations [7]. Resistance to acyclovir has been described primarily in HSCT recipients [5, 8–16] and in persons with AIDS [17–19]. Although initially it was thought that such viruses might be attenuated, soon descriptions emerged of clinically significant disease, such as severe mucocutaneous lesions of the anogenital region [17], progressively severe esophagitis [20], bilateral keratitis [21], and meningoencephalitis [22]. Surprisingly, an acyclovir-sensitive infection can follow an acyclovir-resistant one [9]. Often, development of acyclovir-resistant HSV has followed suppressive courses of acyclovir prophylaxis or therapy [3, 16]. Ljungman and colleagues described three HSCT recipients with severe pneumonia due to acyclovir-resistant HSV, after receiving prophylaxis and repeated courses of therapy with acyclovir for previously acyclovir-sensitive HSV [23]. Although most reports describe the emergence of resistance after transplant, there is one report of a pediatric HSCT recipient who had pretransplant acyclovir-resistant HSV that reactivated posttransplant and acquired resistance to foscarnet as well [24]. In another case report, a pediatric HSCT recipient developed HSV 11 days after transplantation and was found to have acyclovir-resistant HSV 8 days later [25]. HSCT clinicians should be alert to the possibility of acyclovir resistance even early after transplant.

Large single- and multicenter surveillance studies have shown concerning trends. In one study of 207 HSV isolates from a tertiary care center, resistance was detected in 7/148 isolates from immunocompromised patients (4.7%), but in none of the isolates from immunocompetent patients [26]. However, there are now reports of acyclovir resistance in the immunocompetent population [27, 28]. As early as 1996, 25% of European oncology centers reported acyclovir-resistant HSV [29]. In 2004, a network of 15 virology laboratories evaluated HSV isolates from 3,357 patients [30]. This study found acyclovir-resistant strains in 0.32% of immunocompetent and 3.5% of immunocompromised patients from whom HSV was isolated, with the highest incidence being in the HSCT population (10.9% of strains from this group) [30]. A study from the Netherlands assessed 542 isolates and also found a low incidence of resistance in immunocompetent patients (0.27%), but 7% resistance in strains from immunocompromised patients, and again, the highest incidence of acyclovir resistance in HSCT recipients (14.3% of isolates from this group) [31]. Multidrug resistance may be increasing; in one study of 196 HSCT recipients, 14 developed acyclovir-resistant HSV of whom seven also had foscarnet resistance (3 initially, and 4 developing on therapy) [10]. Although virologic cidofovir resistance was not seen in this study, clinical responses to cidofovir were noted in only three of seven patients [10].

Risk factors identified for development of resistant HSV include severe GVHD [32], T-cell depletion [12], and unrelated donor HSCT [10]. Regarding the length of acyclovir prophylaxis, Erard and colleagues performed a large retrospective study in three consecutive cohorts of HSCT recipients (total $n=2,049$); cohort 1 received acyclovir for 30 days, cohort 2 for 1 year, and cohort 3 for >1 year after HSCT [8].

The 2-year probability of HSV disease was 31.6%, 3.9%, and 0% in the three cohorts, respectively. Acyclovir resistance developed in ten patients in cohort 1 (1.3%), two patients in cohort 2 (0.2%), and no patients in cohort 3. The authors concluded that longer-term acyclovir suppression appears to prevent drug resistance in HSV [8]. Thus, although it might be thought that increasing exposure to acyclovir would predispose to development of resistance, it appears that effective suppression during the period of time of maximum immunosuppression can overcome this.

Diagnosis of acyclovir-resistant HSV with the rapidity required for clinical decision-making has been problematic, since phenotypic assays traditionally have been time-consuming, often requiring 7–10 days [33]. A colorimetric phenotypic assay has been developed that is easier to perform and is suitable for large-scale screening [34]. Most recently, development of genotypic assays has been facilitated by an increasing understanding of the types of mutations leading to resistance [15, 31, 33, 35]. Many are thymidine kinase rather than DNA polymerase mutations and can be characterized by sequencing of the thymidine kinase gene directly from clinical specimens [35].

Therapy of acyclovir-resistant HSV has usually been with foscarnet [10, 17, 18] or cidofovir [10, 36, 37], and considerable experience with these drugs has been derived from the treatment of patients with AIDS and CMV retinitis [18, 38, 39] as well as HSV [17, 36]. Vidarabine was used in some early reports [40], but a controlled trial of foscarnet versus vidarabine revealed that foscarnet was more efficacious and less toxic [41]. Vidarabine and trifluridine are available in topical ophthalmic preparations for herpes simplex keratitis [42], a clinical entity displaying increasing acyclovir resistance even in immunocompetent patients (6.4% in one study) [43].

As described above, foscarnet resistance can emerge during therapy [10]. A case report of cidofovir therapy treating both BKV-associated hemorrhagic cystitis and acyclovir-resistant HSV in an HSCT recipient has been described, illustrating the versatility of cidofovir's broad spectrum of antiviral activity [44].

Systemic toxicity of foscarnet makes long-term therapy with this drug challenging [38]. Adverse effects include nephrotoxicity, electrolyte disturbances (potassium, phosphate, magnesium), and genitourinary ulcerations. In addition, it is available only in intravenous form. Multiple daily doses as well as intravenous hydration make this a cumbersome agent to use for home intravenous therapy. Topical foscarnet has been reported to be useful in the treatment of mucocutaneous HSV lesions unresponsive to acyclovir [19], but this formulation of foscarnet is not currently licensed in the US or Europe.

Cidofovir is also potentially nephrotoxic, particularly in the higher dosing range used for CMV (3–5 mg/kg/dose), although less so in the dose range used for BK polyomavirus therapy (0.3–1.0 mg/kg/dose). It has a broad spectrum of antiviral activity and has been used for adenovirus therapy as well as herpesviruses and BK virus. Possible adverse effects also include cytopenias including neutropenia and ophthalmologic side effects including uveitis and a complete loss of ocular pressure. Currently, only the intravenous formulation is licensed in the US and Europe.

The rheumatoid arthritis drug leflunomide has been reported to have novel anti-HSV activity as well as activity against CMV and BK virus [45, 46], although controlled clinical trials are lacking. Leflunomide should be used with caution in HSCT recipients with abnormal liver function [45].

Recent intriguing in vitro studies have reported that hydroxyurea, a ribonucleotide reductase inhibitor, can increase the susceptibility of antiviral-resistant HSV strains to acyclovir and cidofovir [47, 48], but not foscarnet [48]. The possibility of inhibition of viral ribonucleotide reductases encoded by HSV was described as far back as 1985 [49]. A ribonucleotide reductase-null HSV mutant has been described with enhanced sensitivity to antivirals [50]. Further data on the clinical utility of hydroxyurea as a potentiator of antiviral activity in drug-resistant viral infections would be of interest. Adverse effects would have to be closely monitored because of the issue of bystander cytotoxicity [51]; in fact, HSV thymidine kinase plus ganciclovir is under evaluation as an antitumor strategy [52] and as a therapy for graft-versus-host disease (in which HSV thymidine kinase is introduced into donor lymphocytes via retroviral transfer before allogeneic transplantation, and then these cells can be removed by ganciclovir after transplantation) [53].

Varicella-Zoster Virus

As with HSV, resistance to acyclovir in VZV was described in the early 1980s. An in vitro study demonstrated that VZV could acquire resistance to acyclovir through serial passaging in culture media containing acyclovir; as with HSV, most of these mutants showed loss of virus-specific thymidine kinase activity, but less commonly viral DNA polymerase mutations were seen [54].

VZV lesions resistant to acyclovir have been described in a non-HIV positive leukemic infant [55]. In this patient, the lesions were atypical, becoming hyperkeratotic and verrucous after initially presenting as vesicular and necrotic [55]. The infant responded to foscarnet therapy. This underscores the importance of clinical suspicion of resistant VZV infection even when lesions are not typical and when the patient is on prophylaxis. Further reports have included persistent disseminated hyperkeratotic papules in four patients with AIDS who were receiving long-term acyclovir therapy [56]. VZV with altered or absent thymidine kinase was isolated from each of these [56]. A report of foscarnet therapy in five

AIDS patients with acyclovir-resistant VZV lesions noted complete healing in four, although foscarnet resistance developed in serial specimens from one patient [57]. Another study of 18 patients with acyclovir-resistant VZV reported responses to foscarnet in 10/13 patients, but later relapses in 5/10 of the foscarnet-treated patients [58]. On the other hand, not all apparently clinically refractory VZV infections are due to resistant strains. Of 11 AIDS patients with persistent VZV after 10 days of acyclovir therapy, only three were acyclovir-resistant on further testing [59].

Of concern was the development of acyclovir-resistant VZV meningoradiculoneuritis in an AIDS patient with recurrent multidermatomal zoster who received several courses of acyclovir; during the last episode, the VZV strain from cutaneous lesions was still sensitive to acyclovir, but the VZV from the CSF was subsequently found to be acyclovir-resistant [60]. There are two reports of pediatric oncology patients developing acyclovir-resistant VZV of the Oka strain after varicella vaccination [61]. Clinicians should maintain high suspicion for varicella-zoster infection with any persistent vesicular or atypical verrucous eruption and should consider testing for antiviral resistance when VZV lesions do not respond to acyclovir. Visceral VZV infection is more difficult to diagnose, particularly when rash is absent, but testing of CSF and other body fluids by PCR as in the case above can be useful. The possibility of resistance developing after several courses of therapy should always be considered, even when the initial VZV strain was sensitive to standard antivirals.

Cytomegalovirus

A tremendous amount of basic, clinical, and translational research has gone into defining the cellular and molecular basis, risk factors, outcome, and therapies for ganciclovir-resistant CMV (GCV-R CMV) infection. Ganciclovir has been the mainstay of CMV therapy, but its use can be limited by hematologic toxicity including neutropenia and thrombocytopenia. GCV-R CMV was described in the early 1990s in the setting of AIDS patients on long-term ganciclovir therapy for CMV retinitis [62]. Then, Limaye and colleagues reported GCV-R CMV in high-risk solid organ transplant recipients who were receiving oral ganciclovir prophylaxis [63]. The risk for GCV-R CMV appears to be a function of the viral load as well as exposure to incompletely suppressive levels of antivirals [64]. Although it has been claimed that preemptive therapy (as opposed to prophylaxis) would lessen the risk of resistance by decreasing exposure to antivirals [65], GCV resistance has been described in lung transplant patients receiving preemptive therapy as well [66]. Valganciclovir, an oral derivative of ganciclovir, was found to be associated with decreased risk for GCV resistance when compared with oral ganciclovir in a randomized trial of 3 months of prophylaxis in high-risk solid organ recipients [67, 68]. However, GCV resistance after valganciclovir therapy has also been described (see below) [69].

Ganciclovir resistance occurs in relation to two different types of mutations: in the UL97 region (kinase) and the UL54 region (DNA polymerase) [70]. Mutations in the UL97 region, the most common sources of GCV resistance, affect the phosphorylation of ganciclovir to ganciclovir triphosphate; these affect only ganciclovir, acyclovir, and their derivatives and occur usually at codons 460, 520, or 591–596 [71]. By contrast, UL54 mutations affect the viral DNA polymerase and may confer resistance to foscarnet, cidofovir, or ganciclovir and its derivatives [72]. Multidrug resistance has been described [45, 73–76]. However, not all mutations in these regions are associated with antiviral resistance. The investigational drug maribavir, a benzimidazole agent which inhibits the UL97 kinase, is active at a different point of the virus's life cycle and is potentially active against CMV resistant to other agents [77]. However, maribavir resistance due to mutations in the UL27 and UL97 regions of CMV has already been described (with the UL97 mutations in a different region from those conferring ganciclovir resistance) [78, 79].

In hematopoietic stem cell transplantation, antiviral-resistant CMV poses an increasingly difficult problem. As early as 1996, a European survey found that 28% of HSCT centers reported GCV-R CMV [29]. It is important, however, to recognize that sustained, recurrent, or even increasing viral loads do not necessarily mean resistance in this context [80]. One report of three pediatric patients receiving T-cell depleted HSCT who developed GCV-R CMV (one also had resistance to foscarnet) emphasized that such infections do not necessarily have devastating outcomes [81]. On the other hand, these infections can be clinically severe, as in the description of two pediatric HSCT recipients who developed antiviral-resistant CMV, one with resistance to GCV and one to foscarnet, with a mutation conferring multidrug resistance [75]. In a case report by Hamprecht et al., an HSCT recipient developed CMV retinitis and fatal CMV encephalitis; several in vivo viral variants were noted, and the effect of oral ganciclovir therapy with a rapidly rising viral load in blood (10^6) serves as a cautionary reminder of the potential for mutation in the setting of exposure to antivirals that are not completely suppressive [82].

Although valganciclovir is associated with decreased risk for resistance as compared with oral ganciclovir prophylaxis in solid organ transplant recipients [68], Marfori and colleagues reported on two allogeneic HSCT recipients who developed rising CMV antigenemia after 4–5 months of preemptive therapy with valganciclovir, including one with fatal CMV pneumonia [69]. One recipient was found to have a newly described UL97 mutation; the other had a known UL97 mutation and a newly described UL54 mutation which conferred resistance to ganciclovir and cidofovir [69].

The availability of rapid genotyping assays [83] is an advance over previous phenotypic testing, which required growth of the virus in tissue culture prior to phenotype determinations (and could take weeks). A genotypic assay for resistance is helpful in the setting of tissue-invasive or high viral load CMV infection that is not clinically responding to ganciclovir. On the other hand, clinicians should also be alert for GCV-R CMV in the patient with multiple recurrences of CMV viremia with lower viral loads. Sending a rapid genotyping assay can allow for prompt changes in therapy, avoiding progression of CMV disease and the toxicity of continuing ganciclovir derivatives.

As discussed in the HSV section above, the principal alternatives to ganciclovir derivatives for therapy of active CMV are foscarnet and cidofovir, with the toxicities listed above, including nephrotoxicity (both) and electrolyte disturbances (foscarnet). The combination of foscarnet and cidofovir has also been used successfully for treatment of GCV-R CMV retinitis and encephalitis in an HSCT patient [84]. Maribavir, an investigational benzimidazole agent which is active against CMV and EBV (but not HSV and VZV), has recently been studied in a randomized trial of CMV prophylaxis [85]. In this study, 111 CMV seropositive HSCT recipients were randomized to receive maribavir at one of three dosing levels, or placebo. CMV infection as measured by plasma CMV DNA was decreased in the maribavir groups (7–19%) as compared with placebo (46%) [85]. CMV disease occurred in three patients receiving placebo, but none receiving maribavir [85]. Maribavir will likely be useful in the future due to its lack of hematologic toxicity, as compared with ganciclovir derivatives, with which neutropenia is common. It should be emphasized, however, that the study described above did not compare maribavir prophylaxis with ganciclovir derivatives, but rather with placebo. Further comparative studies will be of interest, as well as information on use of maribavir as therapy for active CMV, in addition to prophylaxis.

Other drugs with anti-CMV activity include the rheumatoid arthritis drug leflunomide, which has activity against CMV, HSV, and BK virus [45, 86–88]. One case report of an HSCT recipient with CMV refractory to ganciclovir, foscarnet, and leflunomide showed a marked reduction in viral load due to leflunomide, but subsequent worsening of liver function in the setting of preexisting GVHD of the liver [45]. Another report concerned a pediatric HSCT recipient who had CMV refractory to cidofovir, but who responded to a combination of foscarnet and leflunomide [89]. Although leflunomide may prove to be helpful in a subset of patients with complex CMV syndromes, its toxicities in HSCT recipients should be closely monitored (especially hepatic and hematologic), keeping in mind that leflunomide has a long half-life and may be detectable for weeks to months after discontinuation.

The most recent addition to the anti-CMV armamentarium is the antimalarial drug artesunate. Shapira et al. reported on an HSCT recipient with ganciclovir- and foscarnet-resistant CMV due to a DNA polymerase mutation, who responded to artesunate therapy with a 1.7–2.1 log decrease in viral load by day 7 [90]. This promising therapy warrants further study, but artesunate is not routinely available in the US at this time.

Strategies for preventing GCV resistance have also included use of antivirals other than ganciclovir derivatives for preemptive therapy. Such strategies have also been used during the neutropenic phase of HSCT when ganciclovir administration is problematic. Preemptive therapy with cidofovir has been studied in a pilot study, in which two of four HSCT patients treated with cidofovir developed CMV disease and one developed uveitis as a side effect of cidofovir [91]. On the other hand, in another study of cidofovir as second-line therapy in pediatric HSCT recipients who had already been treated with another agent, responses were seen in five of eight patients receiving cidofovir, with an acceptable toxicity profile [92]. Foscarnet has also been studied as a preemptive therapy agent, with less than expected toxicity in a 14-day course in a group of 15 HSCT patients monitored by CMV PCR [93]. In this group, electrolyte disturbances were common, but decreasing renal function requiring dose adjustment occurred in only two patients [93]. Neither foscarnet nor cidofovir has yet replaced ganciclovir derivatives as first-line preemptive therapy, and therapy for active disease, at most centers. However, if the incidence of GCV-R CMV increases, these strategies may become more widespread.

Influenza Viruses

Influenza viruses are classified into two main varieties, influenza A and influenza B, and are further categorized into subtypes according to their hemagglutinin type (H) and neuraminidase type (N). The influenza vaccine each year contains antigens corresponding to two influenza A types and one influenza B type. The composition of the vaccine is different each year because of changes in circulating strains from one year to the next.

Antiviral therapy for influenza in the past has consisted of the adamantanes (amantadine and rimantadine), which are effective only against influenza A, and the newer neuraminidase inhibitors oseltamivir and zanamivir, which are effective against both influenza A and B. For many years, the adamantanes were the only antiviral therapy available for influenza and were most frequently used for therapy of severely symptomatic disease, but sometimes also for chemoprophylaxis of an entire unit (e.g., a bone marrow transplant unit) in the setting of an outbreak. Resistance to the adamantanes has limited their use in recent years; from January 2006 onward, only the neuraminidase inhibitors were recommended for therapy and chemoprophylaxis. Prolonged excretion of an amantadine-resistant virus for one month after cessation of antiviral therapy in an immunocompromised patient underscores the potential for antiviral-resistant viruses to spread within oncology and HSCT units [94].

Oseltamivir and zanamivir were welcomed when they were first introduced, both because of their therapeutic potential for influenza B and because of widespread resistance to amantadine and rimantadine. In particular, oseltamivir has been widely used, because zanamivir is available only in an inhaled formulation. In addition, oseltamivir was widely hailed as a possible therapy for avian influenza. During the 2008–2009 respiratory virus season, however, oseltamivir resistance became widespread among H1N1 influenza A viruses (standard, not pandemic flu). However, pandemic 2009 H1N1 influenza was oseltamivir-sensitive with rare exceptions; and in the 2010–2011 influenza season, circulating H1N1 influenza is almost all pandemic H1N1 and therefore oseltamivir-sensitive. The CDC has issued a set of recommendations regarding therapy and chemoprophylaxis 95. The two circulating strains of influenza A so far fall into the H1N1 subtype resistant to adamantanes but susceptible to oseltamivir or the H3N2 subtype (resistant to adamantanes but susceptible to oseltamivir); influenza B also remains susceptible to oseltamivir. If oseltamivir resistance is suspected due to clinical refractoriness or viral persistence on testing, however, zanamivir should be used. This would potentially apply to severely ill immunocompromised patients. It may be difficult to administer zanamivir in an intubated or critically ill patient, and it is not indicated for children under 7 years of age, persons with chronic airways disease, or others who cannot use the zanamivir inhalation device.

The underlying mechanisms responsible for rapid development of resistance to antiviral drugs have been elucidated [95, 96]. Although the majority of currently circulating H3N2 viruses are susceptible to oseltamivir, a novel mutation in the neuraminidase gene of an H3N2 virus has been described that confers resistance to oseltamivir [97]. Resistance to oseltamivir occurring while on therapy has been described, particularly in seasonal H1N1 viruses [96]. Newer antiviral drug development is urgently needed; there are neuraminidase inhibitors which are not yet clinically available, which have activity against influenza resistant to oseltamivir [98].

Diagnosis of influenza itself is not difficult as rapid PCR testing on nasopharyngeal swabs is now widely available. Testing to distinguish H1N1 from H3N2 viruses is being developed, so as to target therapy to the strain detected and to avoid use of agents to which the particular strain is not susceptible.

It is clear that therapy and chemoprophylaxis of influenza is not a static issue and the rapidity with which strains develop resistance will likely make each year's recommendations different. Clinicians are encouraged to consult the CDC's website, www.cdc.gov, for additional recommendations. Chemoprophylaxis is still encouraged in institutional outbreaks or when a person at high risk for influenza complications has recent household or close contact with a person with laboratory-confirmed influenza, but the specific nature of prophylaxis administered should be in accordance with the most recent guidelines. Use of vaccination remains extremely important. Meticulous attention to infection control guidelines, including the 2007 Guideline for Isolation Precautions [99], remains crucial in protecting the oncology ward or HSCT unit from hospital-associated spread of influenza and other infections.

Hepatitis B Virus

Hepatitis B virus infection in the HSCT recipient poses a risk for posttransplant reactivation which is sometimes fulminant. Patients who are hepatitis B surface antigen (HBsAg)-positive chronic carriers are at risk for reactivation with development of severe liver disease and cirrhosis [100], but even patients who are HBsAg-negative with serologic antibody evidence of past HBV can undergo "reverse seroconversion," in which previous antibodies to HBV are lost, in conjunction with the emergence of HBsAg positivity and sometimes clinical hepatitis [101]. In addition, in parts of the world where HBV is highly endemic, the donor pool may also have a high incidence of HBV carriage [102].

Prophylactic and therapeutic strategies have been developed which mostly center on the antiviral drug lamivudine, which is effective in many circumstances [103, 104]. For example, one study assessed patients who underwent HSCT from HBsAg+ donors with and without prophylaxis using lamivudine therapy for both donor and recipient and recipient vaccination posttransplant [102]. With this strategy, HBV-related hepatitis developed in only 6.9% of recipients, compared with 48% of those transplanted without prophylaxis, and death from HBV-related liver disease was 0% versus 24% [102]. This study also identified HBV DNA positivity in the donor as a risk factor for posttransplant HBV [102]. Occasionally, hepatitis B immune globulin (HBIg) has been combined with lamivudine for prevention of posttransplant HBV reactivation [105], but HBIg is costly. Duration of lamivudine therapy remains an issue, and severe hepatitis following lamivudine withdrawal has been described [104, 106].

Despite the success of lamivudine as described above, emergence of lamivudine-resistant mutants, particularly at the YMDD locus, is an increasing problem [107]. Other mutations have also been described. In 1994 and 1997, HBV infection due to precore mutants was described in HSCT recipients [108, 109], in one instance refractory to alpha-interferon [108], and in the other, causing fatal fibrosing cholestatic hepatitis after HSCT [109]. Lamivudine-resistant HBV due to a YMDD mutation was described in an HSCT recipient receiving lamivudine prophylaxis after transplant from an HBsAg-positive donor [110]. Fatal fulminant hepatitis refractory to lamivudine was described in a patient with reverse seroconversion who was found to have a mutation in the core promoter region [111]. A study comparing HSCT recipients with HBV with nontransplanted HBV carriers found an increased incidence of core promoter and precore mutations in the HSCT recipients as well as an increase in decompensated liver disease [112]. In one study of lamivudine prophylaxis before and after HSCT, in which patients received lamivudine for a median duration of 73 weeks, 10 of 16 patients (63%) developed lamivudine resistance mutations, although there were no cases of severe hepatitis or death due to HBV [113].

As yet there is a paucity of data regarding newer anti-HBV agents (e.g., adefovir, tenofovir, entecavir) in the setting of HSCT. However, there is a growing experience with these agents in the setting of liver transplantation, either for salvage therapy of patients with lamivudine-resistant HBV or for prophylaxis to prevent posttransplant reinfection [114–117]. In addition to monotherapy, combinations of anti-HBV drugs with or without HBIg are also options in the liver transplant setting [115]. It appears that adding adefovir to lamivudine for lamivudine-resistant HBV, rather than switching to adefovir as monotherapy, can delay the appearance of resistance to adefovir [118]. Lessons learned from liver transplantation will likely be applied to HSCT in the future. For now, if an HSCT candidate is known to be HBsAg+ with a lamivudine-resistant strain of HBV, posttransplant prophylaxis with another agent or combination of agents should be considered and close monitoring of HBV DNA, HBsAg, and liver function tests is indicated.

Vaccination of the donor against HBV (in case of a related donor) has been cited as an intervention for prevention of reactivation of HBV after transplant [119, 120], but should not be relied upon as the sole intervention [101]; development of HBV reactivation with a novel surface mutation despite donor vaccination has been described [107]. The role of donor viral load reduction pretransplant for HBsAg+ donors is being explored as part of combination prophylaxis [121]. Posttransplant HBV vaccination of the recipient with a 3-dose series after cessation of immunosuppression has also been reported to help prevent HBV reverse seroconversion after HSCT [122]. In an era of increasing resistance, more randomized trials of different prophylaxis strategies from HBV-endemic areas are anticipated.

Summary

Development of prophylactic, preemptive, and therapeutic strategies has reduced the morbidity and mortality of viral infections after HSCT. However, the future success of such strategies is threatened by the increasing emergence of antiviral-resistant virus strains. In some cases, resistance is common enough to warrant changes in recommendations for prophylaxis (e.g., influenza). In other cases (HSV, VZV, CMV, HBV), resistance has not yet altered the primary class of agent(s) utilized for prophylaxis or preemptive therapy at the majority of centers, but clinicians should have a heightened awareness of the possibility of antiviral resistance and a low threshold to alter therapy in the setting of high viral loads, unusual clinical presentations, or refractoriness to standard therapy. Patients at higher than average risk for reactivation of viruses posttransplant may benefit from close monitoring by a sensitive molecular detection method. More rapid technologies for performing genotyping for detection of resistance mutations are helping clinicians to make treatment decisions in a more timely fashion.

References

1. Guidelines for preventing opportunistic infections among hematopoietic stem cell transplant recipients. MMWR Recomm Rep. 2000;49(RR-10):1–125, CE121–7.
2. CDC issues interim recommendations for the use of influenza antiviral medications in the setting of oseltamivir resistance among circulating influenza A (H1N1) viruses, 2008–09 influenza season. CDC Health Advisory, distributed via Health Alert Network. 12/19/08; http://www2a.cdc.gov/HAN/ArchiveSys/ViewMsgV.asp?AlertNum=00279 (2009). Accessed 22 Jan 2009.
3. Schnipper LE, Crumpacker CS, Marlowe SI, Kowalsky P, Hershey BJ, Levin MJ. Drug-resistant herpes simplex virus in vitro and after acyclovir treatment in an immunocompromised patient. Am J Med. 1982;73(1A):387–92.
4. Field HJ, Larder BA, Darby G. Isolation and characterization of acyclovir-resistant strains of herpes simplex virus. Am J Med. 1982;73(1A):369–71.
5. Burns WH, Saral R, Santos GW. Isolation and characterisation of resistant Herpes simplex virus after acyclovir therapy. Lancet. 1982;1(8269):421–3.
6. Darby G, Churcher MJ, Larder BA. Cooperative effects between two acyclovir resistance loci in herpes simplex virus. J Virol. 1984;50(3):838–46.
7. Gaudreau A, Hill E, Balfour Jr HH, Erice A, Boivin G. Phenotypic and genotypic characterization of acyclovir-resistant herpes simplex viruses from immunocompromised patients. J Infect Dis. 1998;178(2):297–303.

8. Erard V, Wald A, Corey L, Leisenring WM, Boeckh M. Use of long-term suppressive acyclovir after hematopoietic stem-cell transplantation: impact on herpes simplex virus (HSV) disease and drug-resistant HSV disease. J Infect Dis. 2007;196(2):266–70.
9. Arnulf B, Chebbi F, Lefrere F, Ait-Arkoub Z, Varet B, Fillet AM. Multiple herpes simplex virus infections with various resistance patterns in a matched unrelated donor transplant recipient. Bone Marrow Transplant. 2001;28(8):799–801.
10. Chen Y, Scieux C, Garrait V, et al. Resistant herpes simplex virus type 1 infection: an emerging concern after allogeneic stem cell transplantation. Clin Infect Dis. 2000;31(4):927–35.
11. Collins P, Larder BA, Oliver NM, Kemp S, Smith IW, Darby G. Characterization of a DNA polymerase mutant of herpes simplex virus from a severely immunocompromised patient receiving acyclovir. J Gen Virol. 1989;70(Pt 2):375–82.
12. Langston AA, Redei I, Caliendo AM, et al. Development of drug-resistant herpes simplex virus infection after haploidentical hematopoietic progenitor cell transplantation. Blood. 2002;99(3):1085–8.
13. Morfin F, Bilger K, Boucher A, et al. HSV excretion after bone marrow transplantation: a 4-year survey. J Clin Virol. 2004;30(4):341–5.
14. Morfin F, Souillet G, Bilger K, Ooka T, Aymard M, Thouvenot D. Genetic characterization of thymidine kinase from acyclovir-resistant and -susceptible herpes simplex virus type 1 isolated from bone marrow transplant recipients. J Infect Dis. 2000;182(1):290–3.
15. Stranska R, van Loon AM, Polman M, et al. Genotypic and phenotypic characterization of acyclovir-resistant herpes simplex viruses isolated from haematopoietic stem cell transplant recipients. Antivir Ther. 2004;9(4):565–75.
16. Wade JC, McLaren C, Meyers JD. Frequency and significance of acyclovir-resistant herpes simplex virus isolated from marrow transplant patients receiving multiple courses of treatment with acyclovir. J Infect Dis. 1983;148(6):1077–82.
17. Erlich KS, Jacobson MA, Koehler JE, et al. Foscarnet therapy for severe acyclovir-resistant herpes simplex virus type-2 infections in patients with the acquired immunodeficiency syndrome (AIDS). An uncontrolled trial. Ann Intern Med. 1989;110(9):710–3.
18. Hardy WD. Foscarnet treatment of acyclovir-resistant herpes simplex virus infection in patients with acquired immunodeficiency syndrome: preliminary results of a controlled, randomized, regimen-comparative trial. Am J Med. 1992;92(2A):30S–5.
19. Javaly K, Wohlfeiler M, Kalayjian R, et al. Treatment of mucocutaneous herpes simplex virus infections unresponsive to acyclovir with topical foscarnet cream in AIDS patients: a phase I/II study. J Acquir Immune Defic Syndr. 1999;21(4):301–6.
20. Sacks SL, Wanklin RJ, Reece DE, Hicks KA, Tyler KL, Coen DM. Progressive esophagitis from acyclovir-resistant herpes simplex. Clinical roles for DNA polymerase mutants and viral heterogeneity? Ann Intern Med. 1989;111(11):893–9.
21. Bodaghi B, Mougin C, Michelson S, et al. Acyclovir-resistant bilateral keratitis associated with mutations in the HSV-1 thymidine kinase gene. Exp Eye Res. 2000;71(4):353–9.
22. Gateley A, Gander RM, Johnson PC, Kit S, Otsuka H, Kohl S. Herpes simplex virus type 2 meningoencephalitis resistant to acyclovir in a patient with AIDS. J Infect Dis. 1990;161(4):711–5.
23. Ljungman P, Ellis MN, Hackman RC, Shepp DH, Meyers JD. Acyclovir-resistant herpes simplex virus causing pneumonia after marrow transplantation. J Infect Dis. 1990;162(1):244–8.
24. Saijo M, Yasuda Y, Yabe H, et al. Bone marrow transplantation in a child with Wiskott-Aldrich syndrome latently infected with acyclovir-resistant (ACV(r)) herpes simplex virus type 1: emergence of foscarnet-resistant virus originating from the ACV(r) virus. J Med Virol. 2002;68(1):99–104.
25. Morfin F, Thouvenot D, Aymard M, Souillet G. Reactivation of acyclovir-resistant thymidine kinase-deficient herpes simplex virus harbouring single base insertion within a 7 Gs homopolymer repeat of the thymidine kinase gene. J Med Virol. 2000;62(2):247–50.
26. Englund JA, Zimmerman ME, Swierkosz EM, Goodman JL, Scholl DR, Balfour Jr HH. Herpes simplex virus resistant to acyclovir. Ann Intern Med. 1990;112(6):416–22.
27. Kriesel JD, Spruance SL, Prichard M, Parker JN, Kern ER. Recurrent antiviral-resistant genital herpes in an immunocompetent patient. J Infect Dis. 2005;192(1):156–61.
28. Swetter SM, Hill EL, Kern ER, et al. Chronic vulvar ulceration in an immunocompetent woman due to acyclovir-resistant, thymidine kinase-deficient herpes simplex virus. J Infect Dis. 1998;177(3):543–50.
29. Reusser P, Cordonnier C, Einsele H, et al. European survey of herpesvirus resistance to antiviral drugs in bone marrow transplant recipients. Infectious Diseases Working Party of the European Group for Blood and Marrow Transplantation (EBMT). Bone Marrow Transplant. 1996;17(5):813–7.
30. Danve-Szatanek C, Aymard M, Thouvenot D, et al. Surveillance network for herpes simplex virus resistance to antiviral drugs: 3-year follow-up. J Clin Microbiol. 2004;42(1):242–9.
31. Stranska R, Schuurman R, Nienhuis E, et al. Survey of acyclovir-resistant herpes simplex virus in the Netherlands: prevalence and characterization. J Clin Virol. 2005;32(1):7–18.
32. Chakrabarti S, Pillay D, Ratcliffe D, Cane PA, Collingham KE, Milligan DW. Resistance to antiviral drugs in herpes simplex virus infections among allogeneic stem cell transplant recipients: risk factors and prognostic significance. J Infect Dis. 2000;181(6):2055–8.
33. Frobert E, Thouvenot D, Lina B, Morfin F. Genotyping diagnosis of acyclovir resistant herpes simplex virus. Pathol Biol. 2007;55(10):504–11.
34. Danve C, Morfin F, Thouvenot D, Aymard M. A screening dye-uptake assay to evaluate in vitro susceptibility of herpes simplex virus isolates to acyclovir. J Virol Methods. 2002;105(2):207–17.
35. Frobert E, Cortay JC, Ooka T, et al. Genotypic detection of acyclovir-resistant HSV-1: characterization of 67 ACV-sensitive and 14 ACV-resistant viruses. Antiviral Res. 2008;79(1):28–36.
36. Lalezari JP, Drew WL, Glutzer E, et al. Treatment with intravenous (S)-1-[3-hydroxy-2-(phosphonylmethoxy)propyl]-cytosine of acyclovir-resistant mucocutaneous infection with herpes simplex virus in a patient with AIDS. J Infect Dis. 1994;170(3):570–2.
37. Bryant P, Sasadeusz J, Carapetis J, Waters K, Curtis N. Successful treatment of foscarnet-resistant herpes simplex stomatitis with intravenous cidofovir in a child. Pediatr Infect Dis J. 2001;20(11):1083–6.
38. Balfour Jr HH, Drew WL, Hardy WD, Heinemann MH, Polsky B. Therapeutic algorithm for treatment of cytomegalovirus retinitis in persons with AIDS. A roundtable summary. J Acquir Immune Defic Syndr. 1992;5 Suppl 1:S37–44.
39. Lalezari JP, Stagg RJ, Kuppermann BD, et al. Intravenous cidofovir for peripheral cytomegalovirus retinitis in patients with AIDS. A randomized, controlled trial. Ann Intern Med. 1997;126(4):257–63.
40. Washio M, Hamada T, Goda H, et al. Acyclovir-resistant herpes zoster encephalitis successfully treated with vidarabine: a case report. Fukuoka Igaku Zasshi. 1993;84(10):436–9.
41. Safrin S, Crumpacker C, Chatis P, et al. A controlled trial comparing foscarnet with vidarabine for acyclovir-resistant mucocutaneous herpes simplex in the acquired immunodeficiency syndrome. The AIDS Clinical Trials Group. N Engl J Med. 1991;325(8):551–5.
42. Wilhelmus KR. Therapeutic interventions for herpes simplex virus epithelial keratitis. *Cochrane Database Syst Rev.* 2008(1):CD002898.
43. Duan R, de Vries RD, Osterhaus AD, Remeijer L, Verjans GM. Acyclovir-resistant corneal HSV-1 isolates from patients with herpetic keratitis. J Infect Dis. 2008;198(5):659–63.
44. Andrei G, Fiten P, Goubau P, et al. Dual infection with polyomavirus BK and acyclovir-resistant herpes simplex virus successfully treated with cidofovir in a bone marrow transplant recipient. Transpl Infect Dis. 2007;9(2):126–31.

45. Avery RK, Bolwell BJ, Yen-Lieberman B, et al. Use of leflunomide in an allogeneic bone marrow transplant recipient with refractory cytomegalovirus infection. Bone Marrow Transplant. 2004;34(12):1071–5.
46. Knight DA, Hejmanowski AQ, Dierksheide JE, Williams JW, Chong AS, Waldman WJ. Inhibition of herpes simplex virus type 1 by the experimental immunosuppressive agent leflunomide. Transplantation. 2001;71(1):170–4.
47. Neyts J, De Clercq E. Hydroxyurea potentiates the antiherpesvirus activities of purine and pyrimidine nucleoside and nucleoside phosphonate analogs. Antimicrob Agents Chemother. 1999;43(12):2885–92.
48. Sergerie Y, Boivin G. Hydroxyurea enhances the activity of acyclovir and cidofovir against herpes simplex virus type 1 resistant strains harboring mutations in the thymidine kinase and/or the DNA polymerase genes. Antiviral Res. 2008;77(1):77–80.
49. Spector T. Inhibition of ribonucleotide reductases encoded by herpes simplex viruses. Pharmacol Ther. 1985;31(3):295–302.
50. Yamada Y, Yamamoto N, Daikoku T, Nishiyama Y. Susceptibility of a herpes simplex virus ribonucleotide reductase null mutant to deoxyribonucleosides and antiviral nucleoside analogs. Microbiol Immunol. 1991;35(8):681–6.
51. Gentry BG, Boucher PD, Shewach DS. Hydroxyurea induces bystander cytotoxicity in cocultures of herpes simplex virus thymidine kinase-expressing and nonexpressing HeLa cells incubated with ganciclovir. Cancer Res. 2006;66(7):3845–51.
52. Wahlfors T, Karppinen A, Janne J, Alhonen L, Wahlfors J. Polyamine depletion and cell cycle manipulation in combination with HSV thymidine kinase/ganciclovir cancer gene therapy. Int J Oncol. 2006;28(6):1515–22.
53. Garin MI, Garrett E, Tiberghien P, et al. Molecular mechanism for ganciclovir resistance in human T lymphocytes transduced with retroviral vectors carrying the herpes simplex virus thymidine kinase gene. Blood. 2001;97(1):122–9.
54. Biron KK, Fyfe JA, Noblin JE, Elion GB. Selection and preliminary characterization of acyclovir-resistant mutants of varicella zoster virus. Am J Med. 1982;73(1A):383–6.
55. Crassard N, Souillet AL, Morfin F, Thouvenot D, Claudy A, Bertrand Y. Acyclovir-resistant varicella infection with atypical lesions in a non-HIV leukemic infant. Acta Paediatr. 2000;89(12):1497–9.
56. Jacobson MA, Berger TG, Fikrig S, et al. Acyclovir-resistant varicella zoster virus infection after chronic oral acyclovir therapy in patients with the acquired immunodeficiency syndrome (AIDS). Ann Intern Med. 1990;112(3):187–91.
57. Safrin S, Berger TG, Gilson I, et al. Foscarnet therapy in five patients with AIDS and acyclovir-resistant varicella-zoster virus infection. Ann Intern Med. 1991;115(1):19–21.
58. Breton G, Fillet AM, Katlama C, Bricaire F, Caumes E. Acyclovir-resistant herpes zoster in human immunodeficiency virus-infected patients: results of foscarnet therapy. Clin Infect Dis. 1998;27(6):1525–7.
59. Saint-Leger E, Caumes E, Breton G, et al. Clinical and virologic characterization of acyclovir-resistant varicella-zoster viruses isolated from 11 patients with acquired immunodeficiency syndrome. Clin Infect Dis. 2001;33(12):2061–7.
60. Snoeck R, Gerard M, Sadzot-Delvaux C, et al. Meningoradiculoneuritis due to acyclovir-resistant varicella-zoster virus in a patient with AIDS. J Infect Dis. 1993;168(5):1330–1.
61. Levin MJ, Dahl KM, Weinberg A, Giller R, Patel A, Krause PR. Development of resistance to acyclovir during chronic infection with the Oka vaccine strain of varicella-zoster virus, in an immunosuppressed child. J Infect Dis. 2003;188(7):954–9.
62. Drew WL, Miner RC, Busch DF, et al. Prevalence of resistance in patients receiving ganciclovir for serious cytomegalovirus infection. J Infect Dis. 1991;163(4):716–9.
63. Limaye AP, Corey L, Koelle DM, Davis CL, Boeckh M. Emergence of ganciclovir-resistant cytomegalovirus disease among recipients of solid-organ transplants. Lancet. 2000;356(9230):645–9.
64. Drew WL. Ganciclovir resistance: a matter of time and titre. Lancet. 2000;356(9230):609–10.
65. Singh N. Late-onset cytomegalovirus disease as a significant complication in solid organ transplant recipients receiving antiviral prophylaxis: a call to heed the mounting evidence. Clin Infect Dis. 2005;40(5):704–8.
66. Limaye AP, Raghu G, Koelle DM, Ferrenberg J, Huang ML, Boeckh M. High incidence of ganciclovir-resistant cytomegalovirus infection among lung transplant recipients receiving preemptive therapy. J Infect Dis. 2002;185(1):20–7.
67. Paya C, Humar A, Dominguez E, et al. Efficacy and safety of valganciclovir vs. oral ganciclovir for prevention of cytomegalovirus disease in solid organ transplant recipients. Am J Transplant. 2004;4(4):611–20.
68. Boivin G, Goyette N, Gilbert C, et al. Absence of cytomegalovirus-resistance mutations after valganciclovir prophylaxis, in a prospective multicenter study of solid-organ transplant recipients. J Infect Dis. 2004;189(9):1615–8.
69. Marfori JE, Exner MM, Marousek GI, Chou S, Drew WL. Development of new cytomegalovirus UL97 and DNA polymerase mutations conferring drug resistance after valganciclovir therapy in allogeneic stem cell recipients. J Clin Virol. 2007;38(2):120–5.
70. Drew WL, Paya CV, Emery V. Cytomegalovirus (CMV) resistance to antivirals. Am J Transplant. 2001;1(4):307–12.
71. Chou S, Guentzel S, Michels KR, Miner RC, Drew WL. Frequency of UL97 phosphotransferase mutations related to ganciclovir resistance in clinical cytomegalovirus isolates. J Infect Dis. 1995;172(1):239–42.
72. Chou S, Lurain NS, Thompson KD, Miner RC, Drew WL. Viral DNA polymerase mutations associated with drug resistance in human cytomegalovirus. J Infect Dis. 2003;188(1):32–9.
73. Scott GM, Weinberg A, Rawlinson WD, Chou S. Multidrug resistance conferred by novel DNA polymerase mutations in human cytomegalovirus isolates. Antimicrob Agents Chemother. 2007;51(1):89–94.
74. Baldanti F, Lilleri D, Campanini G, et al. Human cytomegalovirus double resistance in a donor-positive/recipient-negative lung transplant patient with an impaired CD4-mediated specific immune response. J Antimicrob Chemother. 2004;53(3):536–9.
75. Springer KL, Chou S, Li S, et al. How evolution of mutations conferring drug resistance affects viral dynamics and clinical outcomes of cytomegalovirus-infected hematopoietic cell transplant recipients. J Clin Microbiol. 2005;43(1):208–13.
76. Blackman SC, Lurain NS, Witte DP, Filipovich AH, Groen P, Schleiss MR. Emergence and compartmentalization of fatal multidrug-resistant cytomegalovirus infection in a patient with autosomal-recessive severe combined immune deficiency. J Pediatr Hematol Oncol. 2004;26(9):601–5.
77. Drew WL, Miner RC, Marousek GI, Chou S. Maribavir sensitivity of cytomegalovirus isolates resistant to ganciclovir, cidofovir or foscarnet. J Clin Virol. 2006;37(2):124–7.
78. Chou S. Cytomegalovirus UL97 mutations in the era of ganciclovir and maribavir. Rev Med Virol. 2008;18(4):233–46.
79. Chou S, Marousek GI, Senters AE, Davis MG, Biron KK. Mutations in the human cytomegalovirus UL27 gene that confer resistance to maribavir. J Virol. 2004;78(13):7124–30.
80. Gilbert C, Roy J, Belanger R, et al. Lack of emergence of cytomegalovirus UL97 mutations conferring ganciclovir (GCV) resistance following preemptive GCV therapy in allogeneic stem cell transplant recipients. Antimicrob Agents Chemother. 2001;45(12):3669–71.
81. Eckle T, Prix L, Jahn G, et al. Drug-resistant human cytomegalovirus infection in children after allogeneic stem cell transplantation may have different clinical outcomes. Blood. 2000;96(9):3286–9.

82. Hamprecht K, Eckle T, Prix L, Faul C, Einsele H, Jahn G. Ganciclovir-resistant cytomegalovirus disease after allogeneic stem cell transplantation: pitfalls of phenotypic diagnosis by in vitro selection of an UL97 mutant strain. J Infect Dis. 2003;187(1):139–43.
83. Lurain NS, Weinberg A, Crumpacker CS, Chou S. Sequencing of cytomegalovirus UL97 gene for genotypic antiviral resistance testing. Antimicrob Agents Chemother. 2001;45(10):2775–80.
84. Hubacek P, Keslova P, Formankova R, et al. Cytomegalovirus encephalitis/retinitis in allogeneic haematopoietic stem cell transplant recipient treated successfully with combination of cidofovir and foscarnet. *Pediatr Transplant.* 2008.
85. Winston DJ, Young JA, Pullarkat V, et al. Maribavir prophylaxis for prevention of cytomegalovirus infection in allogeneic stem cell transplant recipients: a multicenter, randomized, double-blind, placebo-controlled, dose-ranging study. Blood. 2008;111(11):5403–10.
86. Chong AS, Zeng H, Knight DA, et al. Concurrent antiviral and immunosuppressive activities of leflunomide in vivo. Am J Transplant. 2006;6(1):69–75.
87. Levi ME, Mandava N, Chan LK, Weinberg A, Olson JL. Treatment of multidrug-resistant cytomegalovirus retinitis with systemically administered leflunomide. Transpl Infect Dis. 2006;8(1):38–43.
88. John GT, Manivannan J, Chandy S, et al. A prospective evaluation of leflunomide therapy for cytomegalovirus disease in renal transplant recipients. Transplant Proc. 2005;37(10):4303–5.
89. Ehlert K, Groll AH, Kuehn J, Vormoor J. Treatment of refractory CMV-infection following hematopoietic stem cell transplantation with the combination of foscarnet and leflunomide. Klin Padiatr. 2006;218(3):180–4.
90. Shapira MY, Resnick IB, Chou S, et al. Artesunate as a potent antiviral agent in a patient with late drug-resistant cytomegalovirus infection after hematopoietic stem cell transplantation. Clin Infect Dis. 2008;46(9):1455–7.
91. Chakrabarti S, Collingham KE, Osman H, Fegan CD, Milligan DW. Cidofovir as primary pre-emptive therapy for post-transplant cytomegalovirus infections. Bone Marrow Transplant. 2001;28(9):879–81.
92. Cesaro S, Zhou X, Manzardo C, et al. Cidofovir for cytomegalovirus reactivation in pediatric patients after hematopoietic stem cell transplantation. J Clin Virol. 2005;34(2):129–32.
93. Ljungman P, Oberg G, Aschan J, et al. Foscarnet for pre-emptive therapy of CMV infection detected by a leukocyte-based nested PCR in allogeneic bone marrow transplant patients. Bone Marrow Transplant. 1996;18(3):565–8.
94. Boivin G, Goyette N, Bernatchez H. Prolonged excretion of amantadine-resistant influenza a virus quasi species after cessation of antiviral therapy in an immunocompromised patient. Clin Infect Dis. 2002;34(5):E23–5.
95. Centers for Disease Control and Prevention. Antiviral agents for the treatment and chemoprophylaxis of influenza. Recommendations of the Advisory Committee on Immunization Practices (ACIP). MMWR Recomm Rep. 2011;60(1):1–26.
96. Stephenson I, Democratis J, Lackenby A, et al. Neuraminidase inhibitor resistance after oseltamivir treatment of acute influenza A and B in children. Clin Infect Dis. 2009;48:389–96.
97. Abed Y, Baz M, Boivin G. A novel neuraminidase deletion mutation conferring resistance to oseltamivir in clinical influenza A/H3N2 virus. J Infect Dis. 2009;199(2):180–3.
98. Abed Y, Nehme B, Baz M, Boivin G. Activity of the neuraminidase inhibitor A-315675 against oseltamivir-resistant influenza neuraminidases of N1 and N2 subtypes. Antiviral Res. 2008;77(2):163–6.
99. Siegel JD, Rhinehart E, Jackson M, Chiarello L. 2007 Guideline for isolation precautions: preventing transmission of infectious agents in health care settings. Am J Infect Control. 2007;35(10 Suppl 2):S65–164.
100. Hui CK, Lie A, Au WY, et al. A long-term follow-up study on hepatitis B surface antigen-positive patients undergoing allogeneic hematopoietic stem cell transplantation. Blood. 2005;106(2):464–9.
101. Kaloyannidis P, Batsis I, Yannaki E, et al. Allografted recipients immunized against hepatitis B virus are at high risk of gradual surface antibody (HbsAb) disappearance post transplant, regardless of adoptive immunity transfer. Biol Blood Marrow Transplant. 2007;13(9):1049–56.
102. Hui CK, Lie A, Au WY, et al. Effectiveness of prophylactic Anti-HBV therapy in allogeneic hematopoietic stem cell transplantation with HBsAg positive donors. Am J Transplant. 2005;5(6):1437–45.
103. Nakagawa M, Simizu Y, Suemura M, Sato B. Successful long-term control with lamivudine against reactivated hepatitis B infection following intensive chemotherapy and autologous peripheral blood stem cell transplantation in non-Hodgkin's lymphoma: experience of 2 cases. Am J Hematol. 2002;70(1):60–3.
104. Moses SE, Lim ZY, Sudhanva M, et al. Lamivudine prophylaxis and treatment of hepatitis B Virus-exposed recipients receiving reduced intensity conditioning hematopoietic stem cell transplants with alemtuzumab. J Med Virol. 2006;78(12):1560–3.
105. Tavil B, Kuskonmaz B, Kasem M, Demir H, Cetin M, Uckan D. Hepatitis B immunoglobulin in combination with lamivudine for prevention of hepatitis B virus reactivation in children undergoing bone marrow transplantation. Pediatr Transplant. 2006;10(8):966–9.
106. Lin PC, Poh SB, Lee MY, Hsiao LT, Chen PM, Chiou TJ. Fatal fulminant hepatitis B after withdrawal of prophylactic lamivudine in hematopoietic stem cell transplantation patients. Int J Hematol. 2005;81(4):349–51.
107. Knoll A, Boehm S, Hahn J, Holler E, Jilg W. Long-term surveillance of haematopoietic stem cell recipients with resolved hepatitis B: high risk of viral reactivation even in a recipient with a vaccinated donor. J Viral Hepat. 2007;14(7):478–83.
108. Miura Y, Takamatsu H, Okumura H, Yoshida T, Nakao S, Matsuda T. Allogeneic bone marrow transplantation for a patient complicated by chronic hepatitis due to precore mutant hepatitis B virus: failure of management with interferon-alpha therapy. Am J Hematol. 1997;54(4):344–5.
109. McIvor C, Morton J, Bryant A, Cooksley WG, Durrant S, Walker N. Fatal reactivation of precore mutant hepatitis B virus associated with fibrosing cholestatic hepatitis after bone marrow transplantation. Ann Intern Med. 1994;121(4):274–5.
110. Lee YC, Young KC, Su WC, Tsao CJ, Chen TY. Emergence of YMDD mutant hepatitis B virus after allogeneic stem cell transplantation from a HBsAG-positive donor during lamivudine prophylaxis. Haematologica. 2004;89(4):ECR09.
111. Kitano K, Kobayashi H, Hanamura M, et al. Fulminant hepatitis after allogenic bone marrow transplantation caused by reactivation of hepatitis B virus with gene mutations in the core promotor region. Eur J Haematol. 2006;77(3):255–8.
112. Chen PM, Yao NS, Wu CM, et al. Detection of reactivation and genetic mutations of the hepatitis B virus in patients with chronic hepatitis B infections receiving hematopoietic stem cell transplantation. Transplantation. 2002;74(2):182–8.
113. Hsiao LT, Chiou TJ, Liu JH, et al. Extended lamivudine therapy against hepatitis B virus infection in hematopoietic stem cell transplant recipients. Biol Blood Marrow Transplant. 2006;12(1):84–94.
114. Neff GW, Nery J, Lau DT, et al. Tenofovir therapy for lamivudine resistance following liver transplantation. Ann Pharmacother. 2004;38(12):1999–2004.
115. Angus PW, Patterson SJ, Strasser SI, McCaughan GW, Gane E. A randomized study of adefovir dipivoxil in place of HBIG in combination with lamivudine as post-liver transplantation hepatitis B prophylaxis. Hepatology. 2008;48(5):1460–6.
116. Schiff ER, Lai CL, Hadziyannis S, et al. Adefovir dipivoxil therapy for lamivudine-resistant hepatitis B in pre- and post-liver transplantation patients. Hepatology. 2003;38(6):1419–27.
117. Limquiaco JL, Wong J, Wong VW, et al. Lamivudine monoprophylaxis and adefovir salvage for liver transplantation in chronic hepatitis B: a seven-year follow-up study. J Med Virol. 2009;81(2):224–9.

118. van der Poorten D, Prakoso E, Khoo TL, et al. Combination adefovir-lamivudine prevents emergence of adefovir resistance in lamivudine-resistant hepatitis B. J Gastroenterol Hepatol. 2007;22(9):1500–5.
119. Lindemann M, Barsegian V, Runde V, et al. Transfer of humoral and cellular hepatitis B immunity by allogeneic hematopoietic cell transplantation. Transplantation. 2003;75(6):833–8.
120. Dhedin N, Douvin C, Kuentz M, et al. Reverse seroconversion of hepatitis B after allogeneic bone marrow transplantation: a retrospective study of 37 patients with pretransplant anti-HBs and anti-HBc. Transplantation. 1998;66(5):616–9.
121. Sobhonslidsuk A, Ungkanont A. A prophylactic approach for bone marrow transplantation from a hepatitis B surface antigen-positive donor. World J Gastroenterol. 2007;13(7):1138–40.
122. Onozawa M, Hashino S, Darmanin S, et al. HB vaccination in the prevention of viral reactivation in allogeneic hematopoietic stem cell transplantation recipients with previous HBV infection. Biol Blood Marrow Transplant. 2008;14(11):1226–30.

Chapter 35
Management of Gram-Positive Bacterial Disease: *Staphylococcus aureus*, Streptococcal, Pneumococcal and Enterococcal Infections

Samuel Shelburne and Daniel M. Musher

Abstract Gram-positive bacteria are a diverse group of organisms that are a major source of morbidity and mortality in patients with cancer. The increasing use of long-term indwelling central catheters and cytotoxic chemotherapies has contributed to the emergence of Gram-positive bacteria as the leading cause of bacteremia in cancer patients. These organisms are also among the foremost causes of pneumonia, skin and soft-tissue infections, osteomyelitis, and central nervous system infections in cancer patients. Gram-positive organisms have a remarkable ability to develop resistance to many of the currently available antimicrobials, but the predilection to become antimicrobial resistant varies substantially for particular organisms and for individual antimicrobial agents. Therefore physicians treating cancer patients need to be familiar with the common clinical manifestations, complications, and treatment options for a wide variety of diseases caused by Gram-positive bacteria.

Keywords Staphylococcus aureus • Streptococcal, pneumococcal, and enterococcal Infections • Cancer • Antibiotic resistance

Historical Perspective

Historically, Gram-negative rods were the predominant bacterial pathogens causing invasive disease in patients with cancer [1, 2]. However, a major rise in the incidence of Gram-positive infections occurred in the mid- to late-1980s such that Gram-positive organisms now cause the majority of invasive bacterial disease in patients with cancer (Fig. 35.1) [3–13]. Reasons for the increase in Gram-positive infections include, but are not limited to, antimicrobial prophylaxis strategies, increased use of long-term in-dwelling catheters, and advances in chemotherapeutic regimens [5, 14, 15]. Regardless of the causal factors for the escalation of Gram-positive infections, physicians caring for patients with cancer need to be familiar with the epidemiology and clinical manifestations of, and the treatment options for, infections due to Gram-positive bacteria. In this chapter, we will examine the major Gram-positive bacterial genera that cause invasive disease in cancer patients (Table 35.1).

Staphylococci

Staphylococci are the predominant Gram-positive pathogens causing serious infections in patients with cancer (Fig. 35.2) [16–19]. Staphylococci can be divided into two main classes depending on their ability to coagulate rabbit plasma, with *Staphylococcus aureus* being coagulase positive and the remainder of species grouped together as coagulase-negative staphylococci (CNS). *S. aureus* has the ability to cause a broad array of serious diseases, whereas CNS are plainly less virulent pathogens [20, 21].

Staphylococcus aureus

Epidemiology

S. aureus is a common commensal that can be isolated at any given time from 20 to 40% of humans [22, 23]. *S. aureus* is a leading cause of both community-onset and nosocomial infections and is commonly divided into methicillin-sensitive (MSSA) and methicillin-resistant (MRSA) depending on sensitivity to β-lactam antimicrobials [24]. Prior to 2000, a reasonable rule of thumb was that MSSA caused disease in the community whereas MRSA caused nosocomial infections [25]. The rise of community-associated MRSA (CA-MRSA), however, in many parts of the world means that MRSA now causes the majority of *S. aureus* disease in

S. Shelburne (✉)
Department of Infectious Diseases, The University of Texas, M.D. Anderson Cancer Center, 1515 Holcombe Blvd., Unit 1460, Houston, TX 77030, USA
e-mail: sshelburne@mdanderson.org

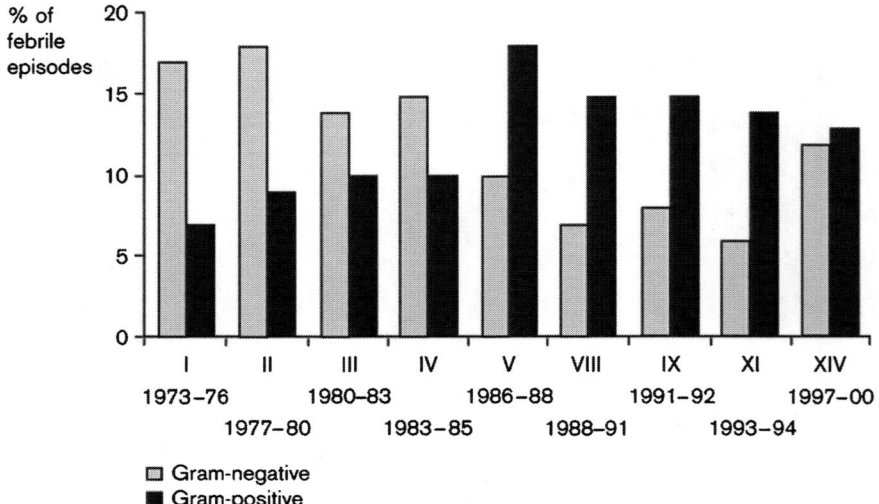

Fig. 35.1 Data demonstrating percent of infection in patients with neutropenia caused by Gram-negative (*gray bars*) and Gram-positive (*black bars*) bacteria. Note the increase in Gram-positive infection beginning in mid-1980s. Data graphs are single organism bacteremias in International Antimicrobial Therapy Group of the European Organization for Research and Treatment of Cancer trials of febrile neutropenia. Reprinted with permission from ref. [3]

Table 35.1 Summary of major Gram-positive pathogens causing invasive infections in patients with cancer

Bacteria	Risk factors	Typical infections	Treatment options	Comments
Staphylococcus aureus	Breaks in skin, mechanical ventilation, and indwelling venous catheters	Skin and soft-tissue infection, pneumonia, osteomyelitis, and catheter-related bacteremia	β-lactams vancomycin	Surgical intervention often necessary
Coagulase-negative staphylococci	Indwelling venous catheters and prosthetic devices	Catheter-related bacteremia and prosthetic device infection	Vancomycin	Generally cause healthcare related infections
Viridans group streptococci	Neutropenia and mucositis	Septicemia and pneumonia	β-lactams vancomycin	Cause of septic shock in neutropenic patients
β-hemolytic streptococci	Breaks in skin and chronic disease	Skin and soft-tissue infection, septic shock, and osteomyelitis	Penicillin	Surgical intervention needed for necrotizing soft tissue infections
Streptococcus pneumoniae	Chronic medical diseases, impaired immunoglobulin production	Pneumonia and meningitis	β-lactams, vancomycin, and fluoroquinolones	Consider vaccination
Enterococci	Broad-spectrum antimicrobials, surgery, and prolonged hospital stay	Catheter-related bacteremia and catheter-related urinary tract infections	β-lactams, vancomycin; Q/D,[a] and daptomycin for VRE[b]	Low virulence pathogens

[a] *Q/D* quinupristin/dalfopristin
[b] *VRE* vancomycin resistant enterococci

both the community and healthcare settings, including patients with cancer [26–28].

Most invasive *S. aureus* disease in patients with cancer occurs when mechanical defense barriers are breached, for example due to breaks in the skin resulting from catheter placement or bypassing of airway defenses by the insertion of an endotracheal tube [29]. Compared to the general population, patients with cancer have a nearly 13-fold increase of invasive disease due to *S. aureus* with major additional risk factors including graft-versus-host disease, receipt of corticosteroids, surgery, mechanical ventilation, neutropenia, diabetes mellitus, and hemodialysis [29–31].

Clinical Manifestations/Diagnosis

Although many *S. aureus* infections are confined to the skin and soft-tissue, a considerable number of patients, especially

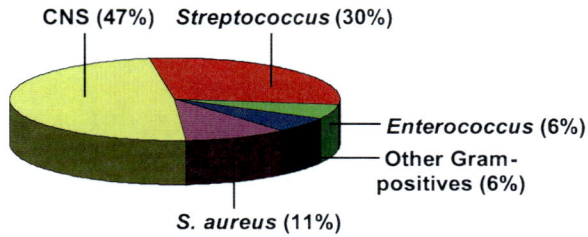

Fig. 35.2 Epidemiology of Gram-positive organisms causing bloodstream infections in patients with neutropenia. Data are from compiled from refs. [4, 6–8]. *CNS* coagulase-negative staphylococci

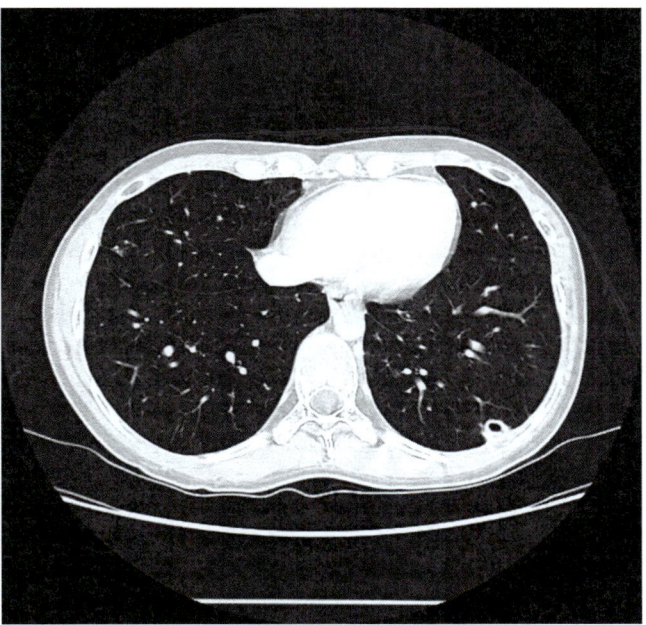

Fig. 35.3 Chest computerized tomography demonstrating cavitary pneumonia due to *S. aureus* that resulted from hematogenous seeding due to an infected Hickman catheter in a 30-year-old man with osteosarcoma

those who are immune-compromised, develop more invasive disease [4, 24]. *S. aureus* is a leading cause of catheter-related bacteremia, prosthetic joint infections, and postsurgical infections [21]. Among patients with cancer, suppurative complications such as infective endocarditis, bacteremic pneumonia, and osteomyelitis often result from *S. aureus* bacteremia [32, 33]. Necrotizing pneumonia due to *S. aureus* in patients with malignancy usually occurs in mechanically-ventilated patients, but can affect healthy patients in the community especially following an antecedent influenza infection or in patients with long-term in-dwelling catheters (Fig. 35.3) [34, 35]. The rise of CA-MRSA has been especially concerning given that CA-MRSA isolates can cause devastating invasive infection such as necrotizing fasciitis and necrotizing pneumonia even in otherwise healthy hosts and more so in patients with cancer [36]. *S. aureus* is commonly isolated from cancer patients with pyomyositis, septic arthritis, and septic bursitis either as a result of contiguous infection or hematogenous seeding [32].

The diagnosis of *S. aureus* infection is relatively straightforward as the organism is hardy, grows well in the microbiology laboratory, and is easily identified. The isolation of *S. aureus* from a sterile site should almost always be taken as evidence of invasive disease with the exception that, on occasion, *S. aureus* may contaminate blood cultures [37]. In light of the propensity of *S. aureus* to colonize, the isolation of *S. aureus* from nonsterile samples such as an endotracheal aspirate does not, in and of itself, indicate an infectious process [38]. Serologic or antigen assays have not proven to be clinically helpful in the diagnosis of an *S. aureus* infection.

Treatment

Therapy of *S. aureus* disease consists of a combination approach involving antimicrobials and surgical drainage when indicated [39]. The importance of drainage of pus and/or surgical removal of dead tissue cannot be overemphasized as many patients will respond to surgery alone, whereas few patients will be cured with antimicrobials alone when pus is undrained or nonviable tissue is present [40, 41]. Similarly if foreign-material, such as an indwelling venous catheter or an infected prosthetic joint, remains in place, then therapeutic success rates are markedly reduced [42, 43].

Antibiotic treatment of *S. aureus* infection is complicated by extensive antimicrobial resistance. When the organism is sensitive, β-lactam antibiotics are the drugs of choice for *S. aureus* infections with typically used agents including nafcillin, oxacillin, and cefazolin [44–46]. Optimal treatment for invasive MRSA infections is an area of intense debate with the most experience having been accumulated with vancomycin [47]. Treatment of bacteremic MRSA infection with vancomycin is associated with a substantial failure rate – perhaps 15–20%, although overt vancomycin resistance is not responsible [48]. These failures have motivated a search for alternative anti-MRSA agents [49, 50] and, during the past decade, new drugs active against MRSA have been developed including quinupristin-dalfopristin, linezolid, tigecycline, and daptomycin [49–52]. Each of these agents has significant limitations and none has been proven superior to vancomycin in a clinical trial setting.

The duration of therapy for *S. aureus* infection is highly individualized, but a minimum of 2 weeks is typical given for uncomplicated catheter-related bacteremia [53]. Patients with complicated disease such as infective endocarditis, necrotizing pneumonia, septic arthritis, and osteomyelitis are generally treated with between 4 and 8 weeks of antimicrobials [54, 55]. The therapy is usually all intravenous for more serious infections whereas some portion of treatment may be oral for nonlife threatening infections such as lower extremity osteomyelitis [56]. Regardless of treatment duration, complications, such as a new suppurative focus, may arise during therapy or for a significant period of time thereafter meaning that patients with serious *S. aureus* infections need to be closely monitored [57].

Coagulase Negative Staphylococci

Epidemiology

CNS are part of the normal flora of the human mucosa and skin with up to 90% of persons being colonized with CNS at any given time [58]. In contrast to patients without cancer, patients with cancer are especially vulnerable to CNS infection as a result of their damaged immune response, extensive contact with the healthcare system, and high frequency of use of medical devices [17, 18]. When species studies are performed, *Staphylococcus epidermidis* is generally the leading cause of invasive CNS in patients with cancer [59].

The major CNS diseases in cancer patients are bloodstream infections in patients with indwelling catheters and postsurgical infections (Fig. 35.2) [60, 61]. The pathogenesis of device-related CNS infection is thought to stem from their capacity to form biofilms on indwelling catheters [62]. CNS are also the leading cause of cerebrospinal fluid (CSF) shunt infections which are a significant issue for cancer patients with primary or metastatic central nervous system tumors [63].

Clinical Manifestations/Diagnosis

Catheter-related bacteremia due to CNS generally presents as fever without an apparent site of infection [64]. Infected catheters may have little to no evidence of purulence or surrounding erythema, and patients with CNS bacteremia may appear relatively asymptomatic [65]. Complications of CNS catheter-related bacteremia include infective endocarditis and hematogenous osteomyelitis among others, but complications of CNS-related bacteremia are rare compared to more virulent organisms such as *S. aureus* or Gramnegative rods [66]. CNS are the leading cause of prosthetic valve endocarditis, and endocarditis must be considered in all patients with a prosthetic valve and CNS bacteremia [67]. Prosthetic valve endocarditis due to CNS often presents with valve dysfunction or intracardiac abscess [68].

The clinical presentation of CNS infection of prosthetic devices other than venous catheters depends on the device involved and the level of the inflammatory response. For example, CNS infection of CSF shunt may present with overt meningitis, but often the presentation is more subtle with only low-grade temperature, alteration in mental function, or shunt-malfunction [63]. Pleocytosis of the CSF may be mild or the cell count may even be normal. Similarly, CNS infection of prosthetic joints may present with symptoms ranging from mild pain or joint dysfunction to a prominent, localized inflammatory response [42].

The diagnosis of CNS infection relies on isolation of the organism from appropriately obtained specimens. Because CNS are present on the skin of patients and healthcare workers, false-positive cultures from blood and other sterile sites are exceedingly common and lead to substantial difficulty in physician interpretation [69]. Good data on the reliability of blood cultures come from studies of CNS catheter-related bacteremia [43]. If a catheter is the source of infection, then quantitative cultures generally show fourfold higher numbers of colony forming units for blood drawn through the catheter compared to peripheral blood [64]. Similarly, cultures of blood drawn through an affected catheter tends to turn positive in automated blood culture systems at least 2 h earlier compared to those obtained from peripheral blood [64, 70]. The diagnosis of CNS infection from sources other than blood needs to be considered on a patient-specific basis with full knowledge that CNS is both the most common culture contaminant and a leading cause of prosthetic device infection.

Treatment

Because of the propensity of CNS to adhere to foreign material, optimal treatment of CNS infection includes removal of the infected device when possible [71]. The vast majority of CNS causing healthcare-associated infections are resistant to β-lactams [72]. Vancomycin is the drug for which most experience is available for CNS infection [73]. Because rifampin is active against CNS in the biofilm state, rifampin may be added for serious CNS infections such as prosthetic valve endocarditis although there is no clear proof of its efficacy [68, 74]. CNS are usually susceptible to recently developed antimicrobials such as quinupristin/dalfopristin, linezolid, and daptomycin [60]. With the exceptions of prosthetic valve endocarditis and prosthetic joint infection, most CNS infections respond readily to antimicrobials especially when the infected device is removed [10, 75]. Guidelines suggest that 7 days is adequate treatment for uncomplicated CNS catheter-related bacteremia after catheter removal and relapse rates are generally lower than those observed for *S. aureus* [43].

Streptococci

The streptococci are a heterogeneous group of pathogens with a confusing and oft-changing nomenclature [76]. For the purposes of this chapter, we will follow the approach of the clinical microbiology laboratory, stratifying streptococci into viridans group streptococci (VGS), β-hemolytic streptococci, and *Streptococcus pneumoniae*. Streptococci not classified into these groups rarely cause invasive disease in patients with cancer and thus will not be discussed further herein.

Viridans Group Streptococci

Epidemiology

VGS are a diverse group of bacteria that commonly colonize the human oropharynx, upper respiratory tract, gastrointestinal tract, and female genital tract [77]. Viridans, derived from Latin, *viridis*, means green and refers to the tendency of these organisms to break down hemoglobin in blood or chocolate agar plates (α-hemolysis) causing a greenish color to appear. Most clinical microbiology laboratories do not routinely speciate α-hemolytic streptococci beyond determining whether *S. pneumoniae* is present, with non-*S. pneumoniae* α-hemolytic streptococci being broadly labeled as VGS. The major VGS responsible for invasive disease in cancer patients belong to the *mitis* group and include *S. mitis*, *S. oralis*, *S. sanguis*, and *S. parasanguis* [78–80].

VGS are considered to have low intrinsic virulence and rarely cause disease other than endocarditis in immunocompetent individuals [81]. Similar to CNS, VGS are far more likely to cause disease in patients with cancer, and these organisms are consistently identified as among the leading if not the most common cause of bloodstream infection in neutropenic individuals (Fig. 35.2) [82–84]. VGS bacteremia occurs almost exclusively in patients receiving aggressive cytoreduction therapy for such conditions as acute leukemia or following bone marrow transplantation [85, 86]. It is believed that the development of mucositis allows for translocation of colonizing VGS from the oropharynx or gastrointestinal tract into the bloodstream [87]. VGS bacteremia has been correlated with the use of prophylactic antimicrobials that have limited anti-VGS activity such as trimethoprim-sulfamethoxazole and fluoroquinolones [88].

Clinical Presentation/Diagnosis

Most patients with invasive VGS disease present with fever in the setting of mucositis and profound neutropenia [89]. Approximately 25% of patients present with a fulminant septic shock syndrome characterized by hypotension, rash, and adult respiratory distress syndrome (Fig. 35.4); *S. mitis* is the VGS species most commonly isolated from these patients [78, 89, 90]. Whether the dramatic clinical presenta-

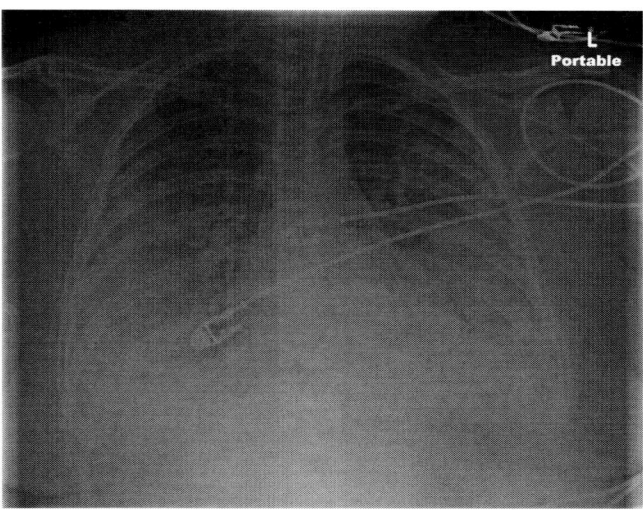

Fig. 35.4 Anterior-posterior chest X-ray demonstrating features consistent with adult respiratory distress syndrome (ARDS) that occurred following viridans group streptococcal bacteremia in a 23-year-old woman being treated for acute lymphoblastic leukemia

tion in such patients is due to host susceptibility, *S. mitis* toxin elaboration or a combination of both is not currently understood. VGS bacteremia only rarely leads to endocarditis in patients with neutropenia, perhaps because of concomitant thrombocytopenia [65, 81].

The diagnosis of VGS disease relies on culturing the organism from a sterile site, usually the bloodstream. Isolating VGS from the skin or mucosal sites has no diagnostic significance given that these organisms are common colonizers. VGS may contaminate blood cultures [91]. But should be considered true pathogens in the appropriate clinical setting, i.e. in patients with neutropenia, mucositis, and fever. Serologic or antigen tests have no utility in diagnosing invasive VGS disease.

Treatment

Therapy of VGS disease is hampered by increasing resistance to β-lactam antimicrobials [92, 93]. When isolated from patients with neutropenia, VGS susceptibility to penicillin may be as low as 40% [86]. β-lactams remain the drugs of choice for invasive VGS disease if the organisms are susceptible. VGS isolates are uniformly susceptible to vancomycin, and vancomycin is commonly prescribed when invasive VGS is suspected [94]. Isolates from VGS infections that develop in patients receiving fluoroquinolone prophylaxis are often fluoroquinolone resistant [88, 95]. VGS bacteremia is generally treated for 10–14 days with longer course reserved for complicated cases, such as endocarditis. Whether agents such as intravenous immunoglobulin would help patients with fulminant VGS sepsis is not known [96].

β-Hemolytic Streptococci

The β-hemolytic streptococci are so-called because of their ability to fully lyse red blood cells during growth on blood agar plates. Most cancer-related β-hemolytic streptococcal infections are caused by group A β-hemolytic streptococci (*S. pyogenes*), group B β-hemolytic streptococci (*S. agalactiae*), and groups C and G β-hemolytic streptococci (*S. dysgalactiae* subspecies *equisimilis*) [97–99]. For purpose of clarity, herein we will call these organisms GAS, GBS, GCS, and GGS for group A, B, C, and G *Streptococcus* respectively.

Epidemiology

β-hemolytic streptococci are ubiquitous colonizers of the human skin and mucous membranes and a major cause of invasive disease in patients with and without cancer [100]. The main sites of GAS colonization in humans are the oropharynx and skin [101, 102]. GBS commonly colonizes the perineal area, whereas GCS and GGS can be isolated from the throat and skin [103, 104]. The vast majority of infections due to these organisms have a community onset [64]. Having a malignancy markedly increases the risk of invasive disease due to β-hemolytic streptococci compared to the general population [105, 106]. The risk of cellulitis due to β-hemolytic streptococci is even further increased in patients with cancer who have had disruption of lymphatic drainage by, for example, a lymph node dissection [107]. Limited systematic studies have suggested that GBS is the most common of the invasive β-hemolytic streptococci isolated from persons with cancer followed by GAS, GCS, and GGS [108, 109]. The development of invasive GAS disease, however, carries an especially poor prognosis with mortality rates of >50% [110].

Clinical Manifestations/Diagnosis

Most β-hemolytic streptococcal infections in adult cancer patients are skin and soft-tissue related. Disease may range from relatively uncomplicated cellulitis to necrotizing fasciitis and toxic shock syndrome especially when the etiologic agent is GAS. Cellulitis due to β-hemolytic streptococci tends to develop rapidly, spread quickly, and be accompanied by systemic manifestations such as chills and fever [111]. Erysipelas is a form of cellulitis caused by β-hemolytic streptococci in which disease is restricted to the dermis. Lesions are raised above the level of the surrounding tissue, and there is a clear demarcation of involved from uninvolved tissue [112]. This infection tends to occur – and, importantly – to recur in areas of damaged lymphatic drainage, which explains the propensity for recurrent infection in the ipsilateral arm after breast resection and lymph node dissection. Among children, GAS along with GCS and GGS are the leading bacterial causes of pharyngitis which is usually uncomplicated, although invasive disease, such as peritonsillar abscess and cervical lymphadentis, may occur [102].

Although less common than uncomplicated cellulitis or pharyngitis, infection of deeper tissues by β-hemolytic streptococci causes substantial morbidity and mortality in cancer patients [110]. Large skin lesions (>5 cm), pain out of proportion to abnormal findings on physical examination, systemic toxicity, skin discoloration, and the development of bullae all raise concern for deep tissue involvement and mandate consideration of invasive β-hemolytic infection [113]. Toxin elaboration by β-hemolytic streptococci, especially GAS, leads to profound tissue destruction and rapidly expanding disease. Streptococcal toxic shock syndrome has also been described among cancer patients with mortality rates exceeding 50% [109]. Hematogenous osteomyelitis is a common presentation of invasive GBS disease, especially among patients with diabetes mellitus [114].

Culture is the mainstay of diagnosis for β-hemolytic streptococcal infection. Rapid antigen tests when positive are reliable in diagnosing GAS pharyngitis when the ordered in patients with a high pretest probability of having the disease [115]. Recovery of β-hemolytic streptococci from a sterile site should be taken as indication of a true infection, whereas the isolation of β-hemolytic streptococci from mucous membranes and skin are often without clinical significance. An exception to this rule is toxic shock syndrome, which can occur in the absence of invasive disease; thus a diagnosis of GAS-related toxic shock syndrome can be supported by isolation of the organism from a mucosal site [116]. Serologic tests are not useful in the acute setting in diagnosing disease due to β-hemolytic streptococci. Acute and convalescent serum for antibodies to streptolysin O or DNase can be sent to determine whether an infection with GAS has occurred although these tests are rarely used in a clinical setting [117].

Treatment

β-hemolytic streptococci remain susceptible to penicillin and other β-lactam antibiotics, and these agents remain the drugs of choice for the treatment of infections due to β-hemolytic streptococci [118]. For patients who cannot receive β-lactams vancomycin is recommended although consideration should also be given to carbapenems if the penicillin allergy is not life threatening [119]. Macrolide and lincosamide resistance rates are highly variable, and these agents should not be used for serious infections without knowing strain susceptibility [120]. Many isolates are resistant to tetracyclines and trimethoprim-sulfamethoxazole [121, 122]. Experience with newer Gram-positive agents such as daptomycin, linezolid, quinupristin-dalfopristin, and tigecycline is limited although in vitro data are promising [123, 124]. In cases of serious soft tissue infection, especially toxic shock syndrome, clindamycin is added to reduce toxin production by slowly dying GAS [125]. Uncomplicated bacteremia due to β-hemolytic streptococci can be treated with a 10-day course of antibiotics whereas complicated disease mandates longer therapy. Surgical debridement of devitalized tissue is mandatory when these agents cause necrotizing soft-tissue infections [113].

Streptococcus pneumoniae

Epidemiology

Although genetically quite closely related to VGS, *S. pneumoniae* is generally considered distinct because of its prominent role as a major pathogen of both immunocompetent and immunocompromised humans. Pneumococci colonize the nasopharynx of 20–40% of children and 10–20% of healthy adults at any given time [126]. As indicated by its name, *S. pneumoniae* is among the leading causes of community-acquired pneumonia [127]. *S. pneumoniae* is the also the most common etiology of bacterial meningitis [128]. Risk factors for *S. pneumoniae* infection include extremes of age, comorbid illnesses such as chronic obstructive pulmonary disease and chronic kidney disease, and deficiencies in humoral immunity such as in patients with B cell neoplasms like chronic lymphocytic leukemia, non-Hodgkin's B cell lymphoma or multiple myeloma and following splenectomy or in patients with human immunodeficiency virus infection [129]. Malignancy itself is a risk factor for invasive disease due to *S. pneumoniae* with persons with leukemia or lymphoma, those having undergone a hematopoietic stem cell transplant, and those receiving corticosteroids being at highest risk [130–132]. *S. pneumoniae* causes high rates of invasive disease in children less than 5 years of age so young children with cancer have a particularly increased chance of being infected [133].

Clinical Presentations/Diagnosis

S. pneumoniae is a major cause of infection in all parts of the respiratory tract and contiguous structures including the middle ear, sinuses, bronchi, and lungs [134]. Community-acquired pneumonia is the most common serious pneumococcal infection among patients with malignancy and generally presents with cough, fatigue, fever, chills, and shortness of breath [135]. Patients with pneumococcal meningitis may or may not have concomitant pneumonia and tend to present with fever, headache, stiff neck, and altered sensorium or obtundation.

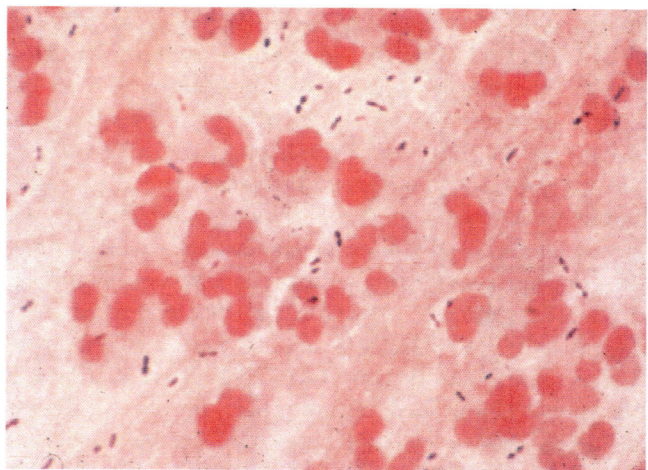

Fig. 35.5 Gram stain of sputum sample from patient with pneumococcal pneumonia. Note diploid organisms surrounded by polymorphonuclear cell infiltrate

Unlike staphylococci or even other streptococci, *S. pneumoniae* can be difficult to identify by sputum culture, and the value of diagnostic cultures is significantly reduced with prior antibiotic administration [136]. When a valid sputum sample can be obtained (this is possible in about two-thirds of pneumonia patients) and the patient has not received prior antibiotics, there is an 85% likelihood of identifying pneumococci in a Gram-stained specimen (Fig. 35.5) and a 90% likelihood of identifying the organism by culture. A subset of patients will have bacteremia along with pneumonia, but blood cultures are positive in only approximately 20% of pneumococcal pneumonia [134]. Serologic studies are not helpful acutely in making a diagnosis of invasive disease due to *S. pneumoniae*. A recently described test (BINAX-NOW) that detects C-polysaccharide in the urine is positive in 75–85% of adult patients with bacteremia pneumococcal pneumonia and a lower proportion of non-bacteremia cases; This test in adults is almost never falsely positive [137]. Patients with pneumococcal meningitis have a leukocytosis with polymorphonuclear predominance, low glucose, and high protein in the CSF. CSF Gram-stain and culture establish the diagnosis in nearly all patients who have not received antibiotics [134].

Treatment

The definition of penicillin susceptibility of *S. pneumoniae* has recently been redefined to include consideration of the site of infection and the route by which antibiotics are being delivered [138]. *S. pneumoniae* causing an infection that does not involve the central nervous system and will be treated with intravenous penicillin is considered susceptible if it is inhibited by ≤2 μg/mL penicillin; in the United States at the present time, about 95% of all pneumococci are susceptible by this definition [138]. In a case of meningitis, inhibition by <0.06 µg/mL penicillin defines susceptibility; an MIC of ≥0.12 µg/mL is defined as resistance with about 75% of pneumococcal isolates causing meningitis in the USA being susceptible by these criteria [138]. Pneumococcal isolates are universally susceptible to vancomycin and usually susceptible to quinolones for which there is extensive experience in treating most *S. pneumoniae* infections, except for meningitis [139]. *S. pneumoniae* resistance to macrolides, clindamycin, trimethoprim-sulfamethoxazole and tetracyclines ranges from 20 to 40% in the USA, and these drugs should not be used in treating cancer patients who have invasive pneumococcal disease [140] unless susceptibility has been proven by in vitro testing. There are increasing data indicating that linezolid is effective for *S. pneumoniae* infections whereas daptomycin is not used to treat pneumonia because it is inactivated by pulmonary surfactant [141]. Although mortality for invasive pneumococcal disease remains around 15% for the first 7 days after admission, most infections respond to relatively short course of antimicrobials with longer courses reserved for meningitis, empyema, and complicated bacteremia [134].

Of all the pathogens discussed in this chapter, *S. pneumoniae* is the only one for which a vaccine is available. A vaccine consisting of capsular polysaccharides from 23 serologic types of pneumococcus is licensed for use in adults [142]. Vaccination is indicated in all adults ≥65 years of age and at any age for patients with malignancy who have an increased risk of pneumococcal disease such as those with lymphoma, multiple myeloma, transplant recipients, and those receiving chronic glucocorticoids [143]. Unfortunately, it is these very adults who are least likely to respond to such vaccination [144]. In the past decade a protein-conjugated vaccine that includes capsular polysaccharides from seven pneumococcal types has been licensed for use in children. Widespread use of this vaccine in infants and toddlers has reduced the incidence of pneumococcal disease in the entire population; however, replacement by other pneumococcal types has eroded vaccine efficacy in the population at large [129].

Enterococcus

Epidemiology

Similar to CNS and viridans group streptococci, enterococci cause a disproportionate amount of disease in patients with cancer compared to the general population [145]. The two main species causing disease in humans are *Enterococcus faecalis* and *Enterococcus faecium* [146]. As their name implies, enterococci are common colonizers of the gastrointestinal tract. The vast majority of enterococcal infections are nosocomial in origin [146]. The major risk factors for serious enterococcal disease include general debilitation, a prolonged hospital stay, recent surgery, neutropenia, presence of indwelling catheters, and receipt of broad-spectrum antimicrobials [147, 148]. Patients with malignancy appear to have especially high risk for infection with vancomycin resistant enterococci (VRE) perhaps because of broad use of vancomycin and agents with anti-anaerobic activity in this patient population [147].

Clinical Presentation/Diagnosis

Enterococci may cause catheter-related urinary tract infection, bacteremia (either catheter-related or from a gastrointestinal source), intra-abdominal infections, wound infections, and meningitis in patients with in-dwelling CSF catheters [149]. Enterococci are considered to be low virulence pathogens, and enterococcal infections often have a minimal inflammatory component [150]. Fever may or may not be present even in cases of bacteremia [151]. Culture is the mainstay of diagnosis with serologic or antigen tests being of no value. The isolation of enterococci from nonsterile specimens such as urine, sputum, or draining wounds usually represents colonization or subclinical infection rather than infection that requires treatment. Prescribing antibiotics in this situation generally fails to eradicate the organism while promoting the development of antimicrobial resistance and exposing the patient to potentially serious side effects [152]. Even when isolated from sterile sites, such as the abdominal cavity, enterococci are usually present along with one or more other organisms [153], and treatment of more virulent pathogens has been shown to cure such infections even in the absence of targeted enterococcal therapy [151]. This concept is illustrated by the highly effective nature of cephalosporins in treating intra-abdominal infections despite having no anti-enterococcal activity [154].

Treatment

Treatment of enterococcal infection is complicated by some unusual antimicrobial resistance. Most *E. faecalis* isolates remain relatively susceptible to penicillins, specifically penicillin, ampicillin, amoxicillin, and piperacillin (not nafcillin) and carbapenems (for example, imipenem), but are intrinsically resistant to cephalosporins [155]. In contrast, penicillin resistance among *E. faecium* isolates exceeds 50% [155]. Enterococci are generally resistant to macrolides, trimethoprim-sulfamethoxazole, and fluoroquinolones [156]. Vancomycin has been the drug of choice for treating enterococci resistant to β-lactam agents, but rates of VRE have increased dramatically over the past 20 years [152]. Enterococci are tolerant to β-lactam antibiotics, meaning that they are inhibited but not killed by them; this becomes clinically meaningful in treating endocarditis and, perhaps, infections in neutropenic patients, as well [152]. A bactericidal effect may be achieved against some isolates by the addition of an aminoglycoside. Because, in this instance, the killing is attributable to the aminoglycosides, no synergy occurs against strains that are highly resistant to aminoglycosides, and such resistance has been increasing [157]. The emergence of VRE has left physicians with relatively few treatment options. Linezolid and quinupristin/dalfopristin are the only drugs approved by the United States Food and Drug Administration for treatment of infections due to VRE, although both drugs have significant limitations such as a lack of efficacy of quinupristin/dalfopristin against *E. faecalis* [158]. In vitro data with daptomycin and tigecycline are encouraging although emergence of resistance and reports of clinical failures are concerning [159]. The lack of clear clinical data regarding VRE treatment has recently led the Infectious Diseases Society of America to declare that determining optimal VRE treatment strategies is an area of paramount importance [160].

The Effect of the Emergence of Gram-Positive Infections on Empiric Antimicrobial Therapy for Patients with Malignancy

For many years empiric antimicrobial treatment of cancer patients with possible bacterial infections focused on Gram-negative pathogens, because bacteremic infection with these organisms was associated with a high risk of death [75]. The increased rates of isolation of Gram-positive pathogens has led many physicians to add an anti-Gram-positive antimicrobial, such as vancomycin or linezolid, when treating cancer patients with suspected infection [161], even though the same risk for death has not been documented for Gram-positive compared with Gram-negative bacteremia [66, 162]. In fact, clinical trials demonstrate no clinical benefit for the addition of targeted anti-Gram positive antimicrobials in empiric treatment regimens [94, 163, 164]. Widespread use of vancomycin and other targeted anti-Gram-positive agents is a major factor contributing to the emergence of such multidrug resistant organisms as VRE [165]. Nonetheless, the practice of adding vancomycin or other targeted Gram-positive antimicrobials empirically in neutropenic patients with fever and, by extension, in many other cancer patients who are not neutropenic, remains pervasive [166]. Taken together, these factors have led to specific recommendations against adding empiric anti-Gram-positive treatment in patients with cancer and suspected infection [94]. Institutional attempts to limit additional empiric anti-Gram-positive antimicrobial treatment to patients with specific risk factors have had limited success to date, but provide some hope for minimizing the overuse of antimicrobial agents [4]. Historically, a broad array of Gram-positive pathogens have shown the remarkable ability to overcome any widely prescribed antimicrobial, and thus antimicrobial conservation may play a pivotal role in the long-term control of these prevalent organisms [167].

References

1. Klastersky J. Science and pragmatism in the treatment and prevention of neutropenic infection. J Antimicrob Chemother. 1998;41(Suppl D):13–24.
2. Frei III E et al. The nature and control of infections in patients with acute leukemia. Cancer Res. 1965;25(9):1511–5.
3. Viscoli C, Castagnola E. Treatment of febrile neutropenia: what is new? Curr Opin Infect Dis. 2002;15(4):377–82.
4. Cordonnier C et al. Epidemiology and risk factors for gram-positive coccal infections in neutropenia: toward a more targeted antibiotic strategy. Clin Infect Dis. 2003;36(2):149–58.
5. Zinner SH. Changing epidemiology of infections in patients with neutropenia and cancer: emphasis on gram-positive and resistant bacteria. Clin Infect Dis. 1999;29(3):490–4.
6. Winston DJ et al. Randomized, double-blind, multicenter trial comparing clinafloxacin with imipenem as empirical monotherapy for febrile granulocytopenic patients. Clin Infect Dis. 2001;32(3):381–90.
7. Feld R et al. Meropenem versus ceftazidime in the treatment of cancer patients with febrile neutropenia: a randomized, double-blind trial. J Clin Oncol. 2000;18(21):3690–8.
8. Del Favero A et al. A multicenter, double-blind, placebo-controlled trial comparing piperacillin-tazobactam with and without amikacin as empiric therapy for febrile neutropenia. Clin Infect Dis. 2001;33(8):1295–301.
9. Rubio M et al. Predominance of gram-positive microorganisms as a cause of septicemia in patients with hematological malignancies. Infect Control Hosp Epidemiol. 1994;15(2):101–4.
10. Ortega M et al. Bacterial and fungal bloodstream isolates from 796 hematopoietic stem cell transplant recipients between 1991 and 2000. Ann Hematol. 2005;84(1):40–6.
11. Koll BS, Brown AE. The changing epidemiology of infections at cancer hospitals. Clin Infect Dis. 1993;17 Suppl 2:S322–8.
12. Safdar A et al. Changing trends in etiology of bacteremia in patients with cancer. Eur J Clin Microbiol Infect Dis. 2006; 25(8):522–6.
13. Ramphal R. Changes in the etiology of bacteremia in febrile neutropenic patients and the susceptibilities of the currently isolated pathogens. Clin Infect Dis. 2004;39 Suppl 1:S25–31.
14. Oppenheim BA. The changing pattern of infection in neutropenic patients. J Antimicrob Chemother. 1998;41(Suppl D):7–11.
15. Viscoli C, Varnier O, Machetti M. Infections in patients with febrile neutropenia: epidemiology, microbiology, and risk stratification. Clin Infect Dis. 2005;40 Suppl 4:S240–5.
16. Rolston KV et al. The spectrum of Gram-positive bloodstream infections in patients with hematologic malignancies, and the in vitro activity of various quinolones against Gram-positive bacteria isolated from cancer patients. Int J Infect Dis. 2006; 10(3):223–30.
17. Kanamaru A, Tatsumi Y. Microbiological data for patients with febrile neutropenia. Clin Infect Dis. 2004;39 Suppl 1:S7–10.

18. Wisplinghoff H et al. Current trends in the epidemiology of nosocomial bloodstream infections in patients with hematological malignancies and solid neoplasms in hospitals in the United States. Clin Infect Dis. 2003;36(9):1103–10.
19. Puig N et al. A study of incidence and characteristics of infections in 476 patients from a single center undergoing autologous blood stem cell transplantation. Int J Hematol. 2007;86(2):186–92.
20. Archer GL, Climo MW. Staphylococcus epidermidis and other coagulase-negative staphylococci. In: Mandell GL, Bennett JE, Dolin R, editors. Principles and practice of infectious diseases. Philadelphia: Elsevier; 2005. p. 2352–9.
21. Moreillon P, Que YA, Glauser MP. Staphylococcus aureus (including staphylococcal toxic shock). In: Mandell GL, Bennett JE, Dolin R, editors. Principles and practice of infectious diseases. Philadelphia: Elsevier; 2005. p. 2321–51.
22. Dossi CM, Zepeda FG, Ledermann DW. Nasal carriage of Staphylococcus aureus in a cohort of children with cancer. Rev Chilena Infectol. 2007;24(3):194–8.
23. Kuehnert MJ et al. Prevalence of Staphylococcus aureus nasal colonization in the United States, 2001–2002. J Infect Dis. 2006;193(2):172–9.
24. Klevens RM et al. Invasive methicillin-resistant Staphylococcus aureus infections in the United States. JAMA. 2007;298(15):1763–71.
25. Boucher HW, Corey GR. Epidemiology of methicillin-resistant Staphylococcus aureus. Clin Infect Dis. 2008;46 Suppl 5:S344–9.
26. Navarro MB, Huttner B, Harbarth S. Methicillin-resistant Staphylococcus aureus control in the 21st century: beyond the acute care hospital. Curr Opin Infect Dis. 2008;21(4):372–9.
27. Ghanem G et al. The role of molecular methods in the prevention of nosocomial methicillin-resistant Staphylococcus aureus clusters in cancer patients. Am J Infect Control. 2008;36(9):656–60.
28. Rolston KV. Challenges in the treatment of infections caused by gram-positive and gram-negative bacteria in patients with cancer and neutropenia. Clin Infect Dis. 2005;40 Suppl 4:S246–52.
29. Laupland KB, Ross T, Gregson DB. Staphylococcus aureus bloodstream infections: risk factors, outcomes, and the influence of methicillin resistance in Calgary, Canada, 2000–2006. J Infect Dis. 2008;198(3):336–43.
30. Mihu CN et al. Risk factors for late Staphylococcus aureus bacteremia after allogeneic hematopoietic stem cell transplantation: a single-institution, nested case-controlled study. Biol Blood Marrow Transplant. 2008;14(12):1429–33.
31. Wang FD et al. Risk factors and mortality in patients with nosocomial Staphylococcus aureus bacteremia. Am J Infect Control. 2008;36(2):118–22.
32. Ghanem GA et al. Catheter-related Staphylococcus aureus bacteremia in cancer patients: high rate of complications with therapeutic implications. Medicine (Baltimore). 2007;86(1):54–60.
33. Raad I et al. Serious complications of vascular catheter-related Staphylococcus aureus bacteremia in cancer patients. Eur J Clin Microbiol Infect Dis. 1992;11(8):675–82.
34. Rolston KV. The spectrum of pulmonary infections in cancer patients. Curr Opin Oncol. 2001;13(4):218–23.
35. Rubinstein E, Kollef MH, Nathwani D. Pneumonia caused by methicillin-resistant Staphylococcus aureus. Clin Infect Dis. 2008;46 Suppl 5:S378–85.
36. Miller LG et al. Necrotizing fasciitis caused by community-associated methicillin-resistant Staphylococcus aureus in Los Angeles. N Engl J Med. 2005;352(14):1445–53.
37. Denniston S, Riordan FA. Staphylococcus aureus bacteraemia in children and neonates: a 10 year retrospective review. J Infect. 2006;53(6):387–93.
38. Ewig S et al. Bacterial colonization patterns in mechanically ventilated patients with traumatic and medical head injury. Incidence, risk factors, and association with ventilator-associated pneumonia. Am J Respir Crit Care Med. 1999;159(1):188–98.
39. Moellering Jr RC. Current treatment options for community-acquired methicillin-resistant Staphylococcus aureus infection. Clin Infect Dis. 2008;46(7):1032–7.
40. Lee MC et al. Management and outcome of children with skin and soft tissue abscesses caused by community-acquired methicillin-resistant Staphylococcus aureus. Pediatr Infect Dis J. 2004;23(2):123–7.
41. Lowy FD. Staphylococcus aureus infections. N Engl J Med. 1998;339(8):520–32.
42. Zimmerli W, Trampuz A, Ochsner PE. Prosthetic-joint infections. N Engl J Med. 2004;351(16):1645–54.
43. Mermel LA et al. Guidelines for the management of intravascular catheter-related infections. Clin Infect Dis. 2001;32(9):1249–72.
44. Chang FY et al. Staphylococcus aureus bacteremia: recurrence and the impact of antibiotic treatment in a prospective multicenter study. Medicine (Baltimore). 2003;82(5):333–9.
45. Stryjewski ME et al. Use of vancomycin or first-generation cephalosporins for the treatment of hemodialysis-dependent patients with methicillin-susceptible Staphylococcus aureus bacteremia. Clin Infect Dis. 2007;44(2):190–6.
46. Ruotsalainen E et al. Methicillin-sensitive Staphylococcus aureus bacteraemia and endocarditis among injection drug users and non-addicts: host factors, microbiological and serological characteristics. J Infect. 2008;56(4):249–56.
47. Daum RS. Clinical practice. Skin and soft-tissue infections caused by methicillin-resistant Staphylococcus aureus. N Engl J Med. 2007;357(4):380–90.
48. Chang FY et al. A prospective multicenter study of Staphylococcus aureus bacteremia: incidence of endocarditis, risk factors for mortality, and clinical impact of methicillin resistance. Medicine (Baltimore). 2003;82(5):322–32.
49. Fowler Jr VG et al. Daptomycin versus standard therapy for bacteremia and endocarditis caused by Staphylococcus aureus. N Engl J Med. 2006;355(7):653–65.
50. Weigelt J et al. Linezolid versus vancomycin in treatment of complicated skin and soft tissue infections. Antimicrob Agents Chemother. 2005;49(6):2260–6.
51. Fagon J et al. Treatment of gram-positive nosocomial pneumonia. Prospective randomized comparison of quinupristin/dalfopristin versus vancomycin. Nosocomial Pneumonia Group. Am J Respir Crit Care Med. 2000;161(3 Pt 1):753–62.
52. Postier RG et al. Results of a multicenter, randomized, open-label efficacy and safety study of two doses of tigecycline for complicated skin and skin-structure infections in hospitalized patients. Clin Ther. 2004;26(5):704–14.
53. Kim AI, Adal KA, Schmitt SK. Staphylococcus aureus bacteremia: using echocardiography to guide length of therapy. Cleve Clin J Med. 2003;70(6):517, 520–1, 525–6 passim.
54. Livorsi DJ et al. Outcomes of treatment for hematogenous Staphylococcus aureus vertebral osteomyelitis in the MRSA ERA. J Infect. 2008;57(2):128–31.
55. Murray RJ. Staphylococcus aureus infective endocarditis: diagnosis and management guidelines. Intern Med J. 2005;35 Suppl 2:S25–44.
56. Daver NG et al. Oral step-down therapy is comparable to intravenous therapy for Staphylococcus aureus osteomyelitis. J Infect. 2007;54(6):539–44.
57. Kaplan SL. Community-acquired methicillin-resistant Staphylococcus aureus infections in children. Semin Pediatr Infect Dis. 2006;17(3):113–9.
58. Costa SF et al. Colonization and molecular epidemiology of coagulase-negative Staphylococcal bacteremia in cancer patients: a pilot study. Am J Infect Control. 2006;34(1):36–40.
59. Persson L et al. Phenotypic and genotypic characterization of coagulase-negative staphylococci isolated in blood cultures from patients with haematological malignancies. Eur J Clin Microbiol Infect Dis. 2006;25(5):299–309.

60. Kirby JT, Fritsche TR, Jones RN. Influence of patient age on the frequency of occurrence and antimicrobial resistance patterns of isolates from hematology/oncology patients: report from the Chemotherapy Alliance for Neutropenics and the Control of Emerging Resistance Program (North America). Diagn Microbiol Infect Dis. 2006;56(1):75–82.
61. Ashour HM, el-Sharif A. Microbial spectrum and antibiotic susceptibility profile of gram-positive aerobic bacteria isolated from cancer patients. J Clin Oncol. 2007;25(36):5763–9.
62. von Eiff C, Peters G, Heilmann C. Pathogenesis of infections due to coagulase-negative staphylococci. Lancet Infect Dis. 2002;2(11):677–85.
63. Conen A et al. Characteristics and treatment outcome of cerebrospinal fluid shunt-associated infections in adults: a retrospective analysis over an 11-year period. Clin Infect Dis. 2008;47(1):73–82.
64. Raad I, Hanna H, Maki D. Intravascular catheter-related infections: advances in diagnosis, prevention, and management. Lancet Infect Dis. 2007;7(10):645–57.
65. Yusuf SW et al. Culture-positive and culture-negative endocarditis in patients with cancer: a retrospective observational study, 1994–2004. Medicine (Baltimore). 2006;85(2):86–94.
66. Klastersky J et al. Bacteraemia in febrile neutropenic cancer patients. Int J Antimicrob Agents. 2007;30 Suppl 1:S51–9.
67. Wang A et al. Contemporary clinical profile and outcome of prosthetic valve endocarditis. JAMA. 2007;297(12):1354–61.
68. Chu V et al. Coagulase-negative staphylococcal prosthetic valve endocarditis: a contemporary update based on the International Collaboration on Endocarditis – Prospective Cohort Study. Heart. 2009;95:570–6.
69. Beekmann SE, Diekema DJ, Doern GV. Determining the clinical significance of coagulase-negative staphylococci isolated from blood cultures. Infect Control Hosp Epidemiol. 2005;26(6):559–66.
70. Bouza E et al. A randomized and prospective study of 3 procedures for the diagnosis of catheter-related bloodstream infection without catheter withdrawal. Clin Infect Dis. 2007;44(6):820–6.
71. Raad I et al. Impact of central venous catheter removal on the recurrence of catheter-related coagulase-negative staphylococcal bacteremia. Infect Control Hosp Epidemiol. 1992;13(4):215–21.
72. Mutnick AH, Kirby JT, Jones RN. CANCER resistance surveillance program: initial results from hematology-oncology centers in North America. Chemotherapy Alliance for Neutropenics and the Control of Emerging Resistance. Ann Pharmacother. 2003;37(1):47–56.
73. Kloos WE, Bannerman TL. Update on clinical significance of coagulase-negative staphylococci. Clin Microbiol Rev. 1994;7(1): 117–40.
74. Karchmer AW, Archer GL, Dismukes WE. Rifampin treatment of prosthetic valve endocarditis due to *Staphylococcus epidermidis*. Rev Infect Dis. 1983;5 Suppl 3:S543–8.
75. Elting LS et al. Outcomes of bacteremia in patients with cancer and neutropenia: observations from two decades of epidemiological and clinical trials. Clin Infect Dis. 1997;25(2):247–59.
76. Facklam R. What happened to the streptococci: overview of taxonomic and nomenclature changes. Clin Microbiol Rev. 2002;15(4):613–30.
77. Johnson CC, Tunkel AR. Viridans group streptococci, groups C and G streptococci, and Gemella morbilliform. In: Mandell GL, Bennett JE, Dolin R, editors. Principles and practice of infectious diseases. Philadelphia: Elsevier; 2005. p. 2434–50.
78. Han XY, Kamana M, Rolston KV. Viridans streptococci isolated by culture from blood of cancer patients: clinical and microbiologic analysis of 50 cases. J Clin Microbiol. 2006;44(1):160–5.
79. Husain E et al. Viridans streptococci bacteremia in children with malignancy: relevance of species identification and penicillin susceptibility. Pediatr Infect Dis J. 2005;24(6):563–6.
80. Lyytikainen O et al. Nosocomial bloodstream infections due to viridans streptococci in haematological and non-haematological patients: species distribution and antimicrobial resistance. J Antimicrob Chemother. 2004;53(4):631–4.
81. Fowler Jr VG et al. *Staphylococcus aureus* endocarditis: a consequence of medical progress. JAMA. 2005;293(24):3012–21.
82. Castagnola E et al. A prospective study on the epidemiology of febrile episodes during chemotherapy-induced neutropenia in children with cancer or after hemopoietic stem cell transplantation. Clin Infect Dis. 2007;45(10):1296–304.
83. Shenep JL. Viridans-group streptococcal infections in immunocompromised hosts. Int J Antimicrob Agents. 2000;14(2): 129–35.
84. Ahmed R et al. Viridans streptococcus bacteremia in children on chemotherapy for cancer: an underestimated problem. Pediatr Hematol Oncol. 2003;20(6):439–44.
85. Paganini H et al. Viridans streptococci bacteraemia in children with fever and neutropenia: a case-control study of predisposing factors. Eur J Cancer. 2003;39(9):1284–9.
86. Tunkel AR, Sepkowitz KA. Infections caused by viridans streptococci in patients with neutropenia. Clin Infect Dis. 2002;34(11): 1524–9.
87. Richard P et al. Viridans streptococcal bacteraemia in patients with neutropenia. Lancet. 1995;345(8965):1607–9.
88. Prabhu RM et al. Emergence of quinolone resistance among viridans group streptococci isolated from the oropharynx of neutropenic peripheral blood stem cell transplant patients receiving quinolone antimicrobial prophylaxis. Eur J Clin Microbiol Infect Dis. 2005;24(12):832–8.
89. Marron A et al. Serious complications of bacteremia caused by viridans streptococci in neutropenic patients with cancer. Clin Infect Dis. 2000;31(5):1126–30.
90. Elting LS, Bodey GP, Keefe BH. Septicemia and shock syndrome due to viridans streptococci: a case-control study of predisposing factors. Clin Infect Dis. 1992;14(6):1201–7.
91. Richter SS et al. Minimizing the workup of blood culture contaminants: implementation and evaluation of a laboratory-based algorithm. J Clin Microbiol. 2002;40(7):2437–44.
92. Huang WT et al. Clinical features and complications of viridans streptococci bloodstream infection in pediatric hemato-oncology patients. J Microbiol Immunol Infect. 2007;40(4):349–54.
93. Collin BA et al. Evolution, incidence, and susceptibility of bacterial bloodstream isolates from 519 bone marrow transplant patients. Clin Infect Dis. 2001;33(7):947–53.
94. Hughes WT et al. 2002 guidelines for the use of antimicrobial agents in neutropenic patients with cancer. Clin Infect Dis. 2002;34(6):730–51.
95. Razonable RR et al. Bacteremia due to viridans group streptococci with diminished susceptibility to levofloxacin among neutropenic patients receiving levofloxacin prophylaxis. Clin Infect Dis. 2002;34(11):1469–74.
96. Ohuoba EF et al. Failure of viridans group streptococci causing bacteremia in pediatric oncology patients to express superantigens. J Pediatr Hematol Oncol. 2006;28(9):627–9.
97. Sylvetsky N et al. Bacteremia due to beta-hemolytic Streptococcus group G: increasing incidence and clinical characteristics of patients. Am J Med. 2002;112(8):622–6.
98. Nielsen HU, Kolmos HJ, Frimodt-Moller N. Beta-hemolytic streptococcal bacteremia: a review of 241 cases. Scand J Infect Dis. 2002;34(7):483–6.
99. Colford Jr JM, Mohle-Boetani J, Vosti KL. Group B streptococcal bacteremia in adults. Five years' experience and a review of the literature. Medicine (Baltimore). 1995;74(4):176–90.
100. Bisno AL, Ruoff KL. *Streptococcus pyogenes*. In: Mandell GL, Bennett JE, Dolin R, editors. Principles and practice of infectious diseases. Philadelphia: Elsevier; 2005. p. 2362–79.
101. Peter G, Smith AL. Group A streptococcal infections of the skin and pharynx (second of two parts). N Engl J Med. 1977;297(7): 365–70.

102. Peter G, Smith AL. Group A streptococcal infections of the skin and pharynx (first of two parts). N Engl J Med. 1977;297(6):311–7.
103. Edwards MS et al. Group B streptococcal colonization and serotype-specific immunity in healthy elderly persons. Clin Infect Dis. 2005;40(3):352–7.
104. McDonald MI et al. Low rates of streptococcal pharyngitis and high rates of pyoderma in Australian aboriginal communities where acute rheumatic fever is hyperendemic. Clin Infect Dis. 2006;43(6):683–9.
105. Lamagni TL et al. Epidemiology of severe Streptococcus pyogenes disease in Europe. J Clin Microbiol. 2008;46(7):2359–67.
106. Phares CR et al. Epidemiology of invasive group B streptococcal disease in the United States, 1999–2005. JAMA. 2008;299(17): 2056–65.
107. Simon MS, Cody RL. Cellulitis after axillary lymph node dissection for carcinoma of the breast. Am J Med. 1992;93(5):543–8.
108. Awada A et al. Streptococcal and enterococcal bacteremia in patients with cancer. Clin Infect Dis. 1992;15(1):33–48.
109. Ekelund K et al. Invasive group A, B, C and G streptococcal infections in Denmark 1999–2002: epidemiological and clinical aspects. Clin Microbiol Infect. 2005;11(7):569–76.
110. Sharkawy A et al. Severe group A streptococcal soft-tissue infections in Ontario: 1992–1996. Clin Infect Dis. 2002;34(4):454–60.
111. Gabillot-Carre M, Roujeau JC. Acute bacterial skin infections and cellulitis. Curr Opin Infect Dis. 2007;20(2):118–23.
112. Bonnetblanc JM, Bedane C. Erysipelas: recognition and management. Am J Clin Dermatol. 2003;4(3):157–63.
113. Wong CH, Wang YS. The diagnosis of necrotizing fasciitis. Curr Opin Infect Dis. 2005;18(2):101–6.
114. Solis-Garcia del Pozo J et al. Vertebral osteomyelitis caused by Streptococcus agalactiae. J Infect. 2000;41(1):84–90.
115. Bisno AL et al. Practice guidelines for the diagnosis and management of group A streptococcal pharyngitis. Infectious Diseases Society of America. Clin Infect Dis. 2002;35(2):113–25.
116. The Working Group on Severe Streptococcal Infections. Defining the group A streptococcal toxic shock syndrome. Rationale and consensus definition. JAMA. 1993;269(3):390–1.
117. Shet A, Kaplan EL. Clinical use and interpretation of group A streptococcal antibody tests: a practical approach for the pediatrician or primary care physician. Pediatr Infect Dis J. 2002;21(5):420–6. quiz 427–30.
118. Kaplan EL. Recent evaluation of antimicrobial resistance in beta-hemolytic streptococci. Clin Infect Dis. 1997;24 Suppl 1:S89–92.
119. Sodhi M et al. Is it safe to use carbapenems in patients with a history of allergy to penicillin? J Antimicrob Chemother. 2004;54(6):1155–7.
120. Martin JM et al. Erythromycin-resistant group A streptococci in schoolchildren in Pittsburgh. N Engl J Med. 2002;346(16):1200–6.
121. Ayer V et al. Tetracycline resistance in group A streptococci: emergence on a global scale and influence on multiple-drug resistance. Antimicrob Agents Chemother. 2007;51(5):1865–8.
122. Traub WH, Leonhard B. Comparative susceptibility of clinical group A, B, C, F, and G beta-hemolytic streptococcal isolates to 24 antimicrobial drugs. Chemotherapy. 1997;43(1):10–20.
123. King A, Phillips I. The in vitro activity of daptomycin against 514 Gram-positive aerobic clinical isolates. J Antimicrob Chemother. 2001;48(2):219–23.
124. Jones RN et al. United States resistance surveillance results for linezolid (LEADER Program for 2007). Diagn Microbiol Infect Dis. 2008;62(4):416–26.
125. Russell NE, Pachorek RE. Clindamycin in the treatment of streptococcal and staphylococcal toxic shock syndromes. Ann Pharmacother. 2000;34(7–8):936–9.
126. Garcia-Rodriguez JA, Fresnadillo Martinez MJ. Dynamics of nasopharyngeal colonization by potential respiratory pathogens. J Antimicrob Chemother. 2002;50(Suppl S2):59–73.
127. Mandell LA et al. Infectious Diseases Society of America/American Thoracic Society consensus guidelines on the management of community-acquired pneumonia in adults. Clin Infect Dis. 2007;44 Suppl 2:S27–72.
128. Scarborough M et al. Corticosteroids for bacterial meningitis in adults in sub-Saharan Africa. N Engl J Med. 2007;357(24): 2441–50.
129. Lexau CA et al. Changing epidemiology of invasive pneumococcal disease among older adults in the era of pediatric pneumococcal conjugate vaccine. JAMA. 2005;294(16):2043–51.
130. Kyaw MH et al. The influence of chronic illnesses on the incidence of invasive pneumococcal disease in adults. J Infect Dis. 2005;192(3):377–86.
131. Kulkarni S et al. Chronic graft versus host disease is associated with long-term risk for pneumococcal infections in recipients of bone marrow transplants. Blood. 2000;95(12):3683–6.
132. Engelhard D et al. Early and late invasive pneumococcal infection following stem cell transplantation: a European Bone Marrow Transplantation survey. Br J Haematol. 2002;117(2):444–50.
133. Meisel R et al. Increased risk for invasive pneumococcal diseases in children with acute lymphoblastic leukaemia. Br J Haematol. 2007;137(5):457–60.
134. Musher DM. Streptococcus pneumoniae. In: Mandell GL, Bennett JE, Dolin R, editors. Principles and practice of infectious diseases. Philadelphia: Elsevier; 2005. p. 2392–410.
135. Youssef S et al. Streptococcus pneumoniae infections in 47 hematopoietic stem cell transplantation recipients: clinical characteristics of infections and vaccine-breakthrough infections, 1989–2005. Medicine (Baltimore). 2007;86(2):69–77.
136. Le Monnier A et al. Microbiological diagnosis of empyema in children: comparative evaluations by culture, polymerase chain reaction, and pneumococcal antigen detection in pleural fluids. Clin Infect Dis. 2006;42(8):1135–40.
137. Klugman KP, Madhi SA, Albrich WC. Novel approaches to the identification of Streptococcus pneumoniae as the cause of community-acquired pneumonia. Clin Infect Dis. 2008;47 Suppl 3:S202–6.
138. Centers for Disease Control and Prevention. Effects of new penicillin susceptibility breakpoints for Streptococcus pneumoniae – United States, 2006–2007. MMWR Morb Mortal Wkly Rep. 2008;57(50):1353–5.
139. Jones RN et al. Gatifloxacin used for therapy of outpatient community-acquired pneumonia caused by Streptococcus pneumoniae. Diagn Microbiol Infect Dis. 2002;44(1):93–100.
140. Sahm DF et al. Tracking resistance among bacterial respiratory tract pathogens: summary of findings of the TRUST Surveillance Initiative, 2001–2005. Postgrad Med. 2008;120(3 Suppl 1):8–15.
141. San Pedro GS et al. Linezolid versus ceftriaxone/cefpodoxime in patients hospitalized for the treatment of Streptococcus pneumoniae pneumonia. Scand J Infect Dis. 2002;34(10):720–8.
142. Targonski PV, Poland GA. Pneumococcal vaccination in adults: recommendations, trends, and prospects. Cleve Clin J Med. 2007;74(6):401–6, 408–10, 413–4.
143. Centers for Disease Control and Prevention. Prevention of pneumococcal disease: recommendations of the Advisory Committee on Immunization Practices (ACIP). MMWR Recomm Rep. 1997;46(RR-8):1–24.
144. Safdar A et al. Multiple-dose granulocyte-macrophage-colony-stimulating factor plus 23-valent polysaccharide pneumococcal vaccine in patients with chronic lymphocytic leukemia: a prospective, randomized trial of safety and immunogenicity. Cancer. 2008;113(2):383–7.
145. Sader HS, Fritsche TR, Jones RN. Frequency of occurrence and daptomycin susceptibility rates of Gram-positive organisms causing bloodstream infections in cancer patients. J Chemother. 2008;20(5):570–6.

146. Moellering Jr RC. Enterococcus species, *Streptococcus bovis, and* Leuconostoc species. In: Mandell GL, Bennett JE, Dolin R, editors. Principles and practice of infectious diseases. Philadelphia: Elsevier; 2005. p. 2411–2.
147. Ghanem G et al. Outcomes for and risk factors associated with vancomycin-resistant *Enterococcus faecalis* and vancomycin-resistant *Enterococcus faecium* bacteremia in cancer patients. Infect Control Hosp Epidemiol. 2007;28(9):1054–9.
148. Vergis EN et al. Determinants of vancomycin resistance and mortality rates in enterococcal bacteremia. A prospective multicenter study. Ann Intern Med. 2001;135(7):484–92.
149. Cetinkaya Y, Falk P, Mayhall CG. Vancomycin-resistant enterococci. Clin Microbiol Rev. 2000;13(4):686–707.
150. Mundy LM, Sahm DF, Gilmore M. Relationships between enterococcal virulence and antimicrobial resistance. Clin Microbiol Rev. 2000;13(4):513–22.
151. Maki DG, Agger WA. Enterococcal bacteremia: clinical features, the risk of endocarditis, and management. Medicine (Baltimore). 1988;67(4):248–69.
152. Murray BE. Vancomycin-resistant enterococcal infections. N Engl J Med. 2000;342(10):710–21.
153. Rolston KV, Bodey GP, Safdar A. Polymicrobial infection in patients with cancer: an underappreciated and underreported entity. Clin Infect Dis. 2007;45(2):228–33.
154. Fry DE. Third generation cephalosporin antibiotics in surgical practice. Am J Surg. 1986;151(2):306–13.
155. Weinstein MP. Comparative evaluation of penicillin, ampicillin, and imipenem MICs and susceptibility breakpoints for vancomycin-susceptible and vancomycin-resistant *Enterococcus faecalis* and *Enterococcus faecium*. J Clin Microbiol. 2001;39(7):2729–31.
156. Deshpande LM et al. Antimicrobial resistance and molecular epidemiology of vancomycin-resistant enterococci from North America and Europe: a report from the SENTRY antimicrobial surveillance program. Diagn Microbiol Infect Dis. 2007;58(2):163–70.
157. Chow JW. Aminoglycoside resistance in enterococci. Clin Infect Dis. 2000;31(2):586–9.
158. Raad I et al. Prospective, randomized study comparing quinupristin-dalfopristin with linezolid in the treatment of vancomycin-resistant *Enterococcus faecium* infections. J Antimicrob Chemother. 2004;53(4):646–9.
159. Grim SA et al. Daptomycin for the treatment of vancomycin-resistant enterococcal infections. J Antimicrob Chemother. 2009;63:414–6.
160. Boucher HW et al. Bad bugs, no drugs: no ESKAPE! An update from the Infectious Diseases Society of America. Clin Infect Dis. 2009;48(1):1–12.
161. Jaksic B et al. Efficacy and safety of linezolid compared with vancomycin in a randomized, double-blind study of febrile neutropenic patients with cancer. Clin Infect Dis. 2006;42(5):597–607.
162. Feld R. Bloodstream infections in cancer patients with febrile neutropenia. Int J Antimicrob Agents. 2008;32 Suppl 1:S30–3.
163. Cometta A et al. Vancomycin versus placebo for treating persistent fever in patients with neutropenic cancer receiving piperacillin-tazobactam monotherapy. Clin Infect Dis. 2003;37(3):382–9.
164. Paul M et al. Additional anti-Gram-positive antibiotic treatment for febrile neutropenic cancer patients. Cochrane Database Syst Rev. 2005;3:CD003914.
165. Camins BC et al. A population-based investigation of invasive vancomycin-resistant Enterococcus infection in metropolitan Atlanta, Georgia, and predictors of mortality. Infect Control Hosp Epidemiol. 2007;28(8):983–91.
166. Kirst HA, Thompson DG, Nicas TI. Historical yearly usage of vancomycin. Antimicrob Agents Chemother. 1998;42(5):1303–4.
167. Irfan S et al. Emergence of carbapenem resistant Gram negative and vancomycin resistant Gram positive organisms in bacteremic isolates of febrile neutropenic patients: a descriptive study. BMC Infect Dis. 2008;8:80.

Chapter 36
Infections Caused by Aerobic and Anaerobic Gram-Negative Bacilli

Kenneth V.I. Rolston, David E. Greenberg, and Amar Safdar

Abstract Many cancer treatment centers have documented a decline in the proportion of bacterial infections caused by aerobic Gram-negative bacilli in the past 2 decades. Nevertheless, these organisms still cause a wide spectrum of infection (from benign colonization to disseminated disease) and are associated with substantial morbidity and mortality in patients with cancer, particularly during episodes of neutropenia. The most significant problem developed in the recent years has been the emergence of resistance among most Gram-negative pathogens, with some organisms acquiring multiple resistance mechanisms, which render them multi-drug-resistant. Exacerbating this problem is the fact that the pipeline for new drug development is relatively dry. This has led to the increased use of combination regimens and the revival of older agents such as colistin. Greater emphasis needs to be placed on antimicrobial stewardship and on strict adherence to infection control policies, in order to reduce the frequency of and limit the spread of these organisms. Bacteroides and other anaerobic Gram-negative bacteria may lead to life-threatening infections, presence of refractory hypotension, high-grade fever, acute intravascular hemolysis and disseminated coagulation, and early onset of tissue necrosis are the hallmark of this devastating disease. A high level of suspicion and prompt systemic therapy coupled with surgical excision of devitalized tissue when possible may improve outcomes.

Keywords Cancer • Pseudomonas • Stenotrophomonas • Drug-resistance • Antimicrobial therapy • *E. coli*

negative component [2]. Since polymicrobial infections now account for 25–30% of documented bacterial infections (a proportion that has been increasing over the last 2 decades), Gram-negative bacilli are isolated from ~50% of bacterial infections in this patient population. This occurs despite the use of antimicrobial prophylaxis directed primarily against Gram-negative bacilli in high-risk neutropenic patients. The majority of Gram-negative pathogens are residents of the human intestinal tract, although some are acquired from environmental or other sources. In general, Gram-negative, and polymicrobial infections are associated with greater morbidity and mortality than Gram-positive infections. Consequently, the prompt administration of empiric, broad-spectrum, parenteral, antimicrobial therapy is the standard of care for most febrile neutropenic patients [3]. Unfortunately, neutropenic episodes occur often, and the frequent use of antimicrobial agents for prophylaxis and therapy has led to the emergence of resistant organisms [4–6]. Some organisms acquire multiple resistance mechanisms that render them multi-drug-resistant (MDR) – defined as resistance to at least three different classes of antimicrobial agents that are expected to be active against a particular pathogen. MDR Gram-negative pathogens pose a significant problem, especially since the pipeline for new drug development is relatively dry, as outlined by several recent publications from the Infectious Diseases Society of America [7, 8]. This chapter will deal with Gram-negative infections overall, and with specific Gram-negative organisms of particular importance.

Introduction

Aerobic Gram-negative bacilli account for 15–20% of documented bacterial infections in neutropenic patients [1]. Furthermore, ~80% of polymicrobial infections have a Gram-

K.V.I. Rolston (✉)
Department of Infectious Diseases, Infection Control, and Employee Health, The University of Texas M.D. Anderson Cancer Center, 1515 Holcombe Blvd., Unit 1460, Houston, TX 77030, USA
e-mail: krolston@mdanderson.org

Current Spectrum of Gram-Negative Organisms

Most cancer treatment centers have documented a decline in the proportion of bacterial infections caused by aerobic Gram-negative bacilli over the past 2–3 decades, with a corresponding increase in Gram-positive infections [1, 9, 10]. Of late, some centers are reporting a shift back toward a predominance of Gram-negative infections [11, 12]. Unfortunately, most epidemiologic studies focus primarily

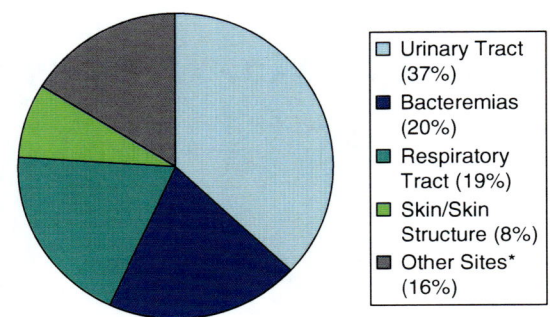

Fig. 36.1 Most common sites for Gram-negative infection in cancer patients

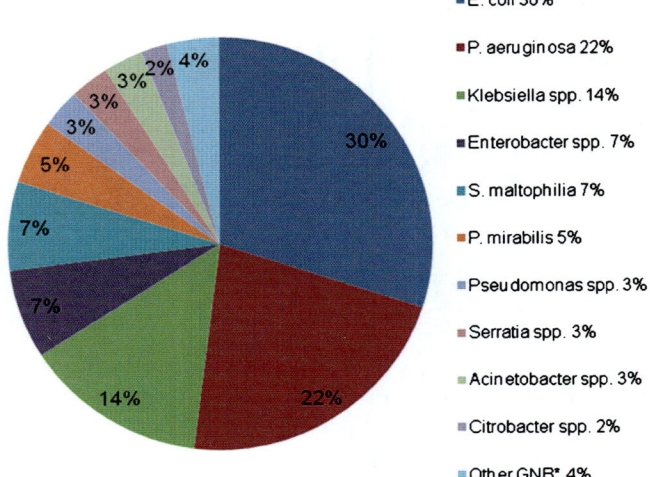

Fig. 36.2 Proportion of various Gram-negative bacilli causing infection in cancer patients

on single-organism (monomicrobial) bacteremias, and fail to provide data on polymicrobial infections and on sites of infection other than the bloodstream (e.g., urinary tract, respiratory tract, skin/skin structure, intestinal/hepato-biliary tract). Since bacteremias account for only 15–25% of infections in such patients, these data paint an incomplete picture. Whereas Gram-positive organisms predominate as the cause of bacteremias (up to 80% in some reports), Gram-negative organisms predominate at most other sites of infection [10, 13]. Additionally, ~80% of polymicrobial infections have a Gram-negative component, and 30–35% are caused by multiple Gram-negative species [2, 14]. Consequently, when all sites of infection, and polymicrobial infections are taken into account, a substantially different epidemiologic picture, with a greater proportion of infections being caused by Gram-negative organisms, emerges. The most common sites of infection are depicted in Fig. 36.1. These include urinary tract infections (37%), bacteremias (20%), respiratory tract infections (19%), and skin/skin structure infections (8%). Other, less common but important sites include the hepato-biliary tract, pleural fluid, peritoneal fluid, and cerebrospinal fluid. It is also commonly accepted that many cancer patients with clinically documented infections (e.g., pneumonia, neutropenic enterocolitis) and with episodes of unexplained fever have undocumented Gram-negative infections, especially if they are receiving prophylactic antibiotics.

Studies from various parts of the globe consistently show that *Escherichia coli*, Klebsiella species, and *Psuedomonas aeurginosa* are the three most common Gram-negative organisms isolated from cancer patients [1, 9, 10, 13, 15–17]. Other Enterobacteriaceae, Acinetobacter species, *Stenotrophomonas maltophilia*, and non-aeruginosa Pseudomonas species are less common but important pathogens that often develop multiple mechanisms of resistance to commonly used antibiotics. Local and interinstitutional differences do occur. It is therefore important to conduct periodic epidemiologic/surveillance studies in order to determine the most current spectrum of infections and susceptibility/resistance patterns. In our most recent survey, isolates from 903 consecutive, monomicrobial Gram-negative infections were collected for susceptibility testing. The most frequently isolated Gram-negative species were *E. coli* (268 – 30%), *P. aeruginosa* (200 – 20%), Klebsiella spp. (122 – 14%), Enterobacter spp. (62 – 7%), and *S. maltophilia* (61 – 7%) (Fig. 36.2). This spectrum is virtually identical to previous surveys we have conducted with the exception of a substantial increase in the proportion of infections caused by *S. maltophilia* from 3% in 1993 to 7% in the latest survey [18, 19]. *S. maltophilia* is isolated even more frequently from patients treated in our intensive care unit – being the third most common Gram-negative pathogen in that setting (unpublished data from the MDACC antimicrobial stewardship program). The remainder of this chapter will focus on individual Gram-negative pathogens.

The Enterobacteriaceae

Bacteria from the family Enterobacteriaceae are among the most common human pathogens, affecting all populations (immunosuppressed and immunocompetent). They cause syndromes ranging in severity from simple cystitis to widely disseminated infection. The Enterobacteriaceae are part of the normal intestinal flora. They are, however, opportunistic pathogens with infection usually being spread by fecal-oral contact routes. In cancer patients receiving chemotherapy, translocation of bacteria from the intestinal lumen to the bloodstream is common across damaged mucosal surfaces. This has led to the practice of administering antimicrobial prophylaxis to high-risk patients.

E. coli is the most frequent Gram-negative pathogen isolated from cancer patients. Infections frequently caused by *E. coli* include urinary tract infection, bacteremias, neutropenic

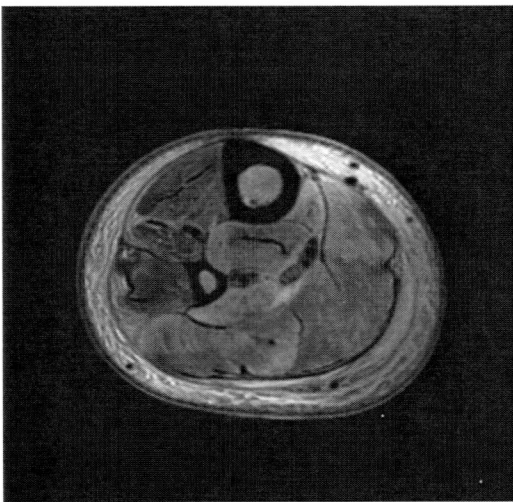

Fig. 36.3 Magnetic resonance image showing massive edema of leg muscles associated with *E. coli* pyomyositis

Table 36.1 Spectrum of infections caused by Gram-negative bacilli

Bacteremia – primary and catheter related
Pneumonia
Urinary tract infections – primary and catheter related
Enterocolitis/typhlitis/perirectal infection
Meningitis/brain abscess
Wound infection
Cholangitis/biliary tract infection
Abdominal/pelvic/hepatic abscess
Otitis externa/mastoiditis
Keratitis/endophthalmitis
Empyema
Prostatic infection
Osteomyelitis/device-related infection
Septic arthritis
Skin/ecthyma gangrenosum

enterocolitis, perirectal infections, and infections of the hepatobiliary tract. Investigators at The University of M.D. Anderson Cancer Center have recently described several cases of pyomositis caused by *E. coli* [20, 21]. All patients who developed pyomositis were receiving chemotherapy for hematologic malignancies and had profound neutropenia. The areas most often involved were the muscles of the calves and thighs. Septic shock (50%) was common. Magnetic resonance imaging showed diffuse abnormality of the musculature including edema, consistent with pyomositis (Fig. 36.3). Frank abscesses were present in 50% of these patients, and *E. coli* was the only pathogen isolated from these abscesses. All these isolates were resistant to fluoroquinolones and 55% produced extended spectrum beta-lactamases. The mortality was 33%, higher than in patients with other *E. coli* infections.

Klebsiella species have consistently been the second most frequent Gram-negative organisms isolated from cancer patients. The two most frequent pathogens are *Klebsiella pneumoniae* and Klebsiella oxytoca. The spectrum of infections caused by these organisms is similar to that caused by *E. coli* and other Gram-negatives (Table 36.1). Other, less frequent Enterobacteriaceae causing infections in cancer patients include Enterobacter species, Citrobacter species, and Serratia species. Collectively, they cause ~60% of monomicrobial Gram-negative infections in this patient population. *Serratia marcescens* has been the source of many healthcare-associated outbreaks, generally as the result of contamination of products such as medical devices, disinfectants, hand soaps, and medication vials. The last such incident was a 9-state outbreak of 162 cases of *S. marcescens* bacteremia associated with prefilled heparin and/or saline syringes made by a specific manufacturer [22]. Cultures of unopened prefilled heparin and saline syringes from this source grew *S. marcescens* during the subsequent investigation of the outbreak. Of the 83 *S. marcescens* blood culture isolates from patients in this outbreak, 84% were genetically related to the strain isolated from the prefilled syringe. A US Food and Drug Administration inspection revealed that the manufacturer was not in compliance with quality systems regulations. A voluntary, national recall of the prefilled syringes led to termination of the outbreak. This incident shows the importance of clinical vigilance and cooperation among multiple agencies entrusted with investigating such outbreaks.

Historically, bacteria from the family Enterobacteriaceae have been susceptible to a wide range of antimicrobial agents. During the past 2 decades however, multidrug resistance has become widespread. Resistance is mediated primarily via acquired genes that code for extended-spectrum-beta-lactamases (ESBLs) [23]. The ESBLs confer resistance to penicillins, cephalosporins, and aztreonam. However, these isolates typically remain susceptible to the carbapenems (imipenem, meropenem, ertapenem), and these agents are considered the drugs of choice for treating infections due to ESBL-producing bacteria. Data from our institution, the only comprehensive cancer center to participate in the Meropenem Yearly Susceptibility Testing Information Collection (MYSTIC) study, have shown that the proportion of ESBL producing *E. coli* rose from 4.5% in 1999 to 19.4% in 2008 [6]. This increase was disproportionate when compared to other participating institutions.

E. coli isolates have generally also been susceptible to most agents used for prophylaxis in cancer patients [18, 24–26]. With the widespread and increasing use of fluoroquinolones for antimicrobial prophylaxis in neutropenic patients, the emergence of *E. coli* strains that are resistant to the fluoroquinolones and other frontline agents has become commonplace [4–6, 20]. This is not only true for patients with hematological malignancies but also for those with solid tumors as well [27, 28]. Most individual studies of fluoroquinolone prophylaxis failed to demonstrate reduced mortality as a result of this strategy [29, 30]. However, one recent meta-analysis of several studies suggests that the use of fluoroquinolones prophylaxis reduces mortality in neutropenic patients [31, 32]. The potential benefits of prophylaxis need to be weighed against the substantial risk of the development of resistance, not only among *E. coli* but also many other important Gram-negative species such as *P. aeurginosa*. Most guidelines caution against the routine use of quinolone prophylaxis for all neutropenic patients, and recommend this strategy only for high-risk patients with prolonged neutropenia [3, 33]. Fortunately, many quinolone-resistant isolates remain susceptible to the aminoglycosides, broad-spectrum beta-lactam agents, and tigecycline.

The most alarming recent development has been the emergence of carbapenem-resistant Enterobacteriaceae [34, 35]. In 1996, a carbapenem-resistant *K. pneumoniae* was recovered from a patient in North Carolina. This isolate produced a class A beta-lactamase which hydrolyzes penicillins, cephalosporins, aztreonam, and carbapenems and is named *Klebsiella pneumoniae* carbapenemase (KPC). Since then, many other KPC producing Enterobacteriaceae have been isolated from various sources. Some of these organisms produce metallo-β-lactamase VIM enzymes as well, which also confer carbapenem resistance [36–38]. The gene coding for these enzymes is carried by plasmids that often carry other resistance factors, resulting in extensively-drug-resistance (XDR) organisms, severely limiting our capability to treat them effectively.

Nonfermentative Gram-Negative Bacilli

Despite an overall decline in the frequency of Gram-negative infections in cancer patients, there has been an increase in the proportion of such infections caused by nonfermentative Gram-negative bacilli (NFGNB) [39]. Collectively, NFGNB cause ~36% of documented Gram negative infections in this patient population (Table 36.2). *P. aeruginosa* is the most frequently isolated and most important pathogenic NFGNB. Non-aeruginosa pseudomonas species are less common and are associated with lower morbidity and mortality. The frequency of infections caused by *S. maltophilia* has risen dramatically over the past 2 decades and may be related to the widespread use of the carbapenems as monotherapy in febrile neutropenic patients [40]. Acinetobacter species are still relatively uncommon but are often MDR, and difficult to treat. These pathogens will be discussed in greater detail below.

Pseudomonas aeruginosa

P. aeruginosa emerged as a common cause of bacterial infection in neutropenic cancer patients during the 1960s, and before the availability of agents such as carbenicillin, was associated with mortality rates in excess of 90%. Since then, the availability of potent antipseudomonal agents along with significant improvements in critical and supportive care has reduced the mortality to approximately 25–30%. Substantial regional and institutional differences in the frequency of infections caused by *P. aeruginosa* have been documented [19]. Consequently, knowledge of local epidemiology and susceptibility/resistance patterns is important.

A recent large review of *P. aeruginosa* infection in cancer patients identified several risk factors [41]. Most patients (54%) had an underlying hematologic malignancy – usually a variant of acute leukemia. *P. aeruginosa* bacteremia was 27 times more common in patients with acute leukemia than in patients with solid tumors. During the 2 weeks prior to documentation of *P. aeruginosa* bacteremia, 89% of patients received some form of antineoplastic therapy (mostly chemotherapy), and 43% underwent an invasive procedure or placement of a medical device (urinary or intravascular catheters, or Ommaya reservoir). Additionally, during the 7 days preceding the onset of *P. aeruginosa* bacteremia, 36% of patients had received antibiotics for presumed or proven infections. The practice of administering intensive chemotherapy in the outpatient setting has had an impact on Pseudomonas infections. In the study cited above, 50% of patients with *P. aeruginosa* were not hospitalized. However, 9% had been discharged from the hospital during the preceding 3 days and, 25% had been discharged during the preceding week.

P. aeruginosa has the potential for developing resistance to antimicrobial agents by multiple resistance mechanisms. A recent study demonstrated that the risk factors associated with multidrug-resistant *P. aeruginosa* infection were the use of a carbapenem for ≥7 days, a history of *P. aeruginosa* infection during the preceding year, and a history of chronic obstructive pulmonary disease [42].

As mentioned, these infections are more common in patients with hematologic malignancies, and are often polymicrobial. While pseudomonal infections are documented less frequently in patients with solid tumors, a much wider spectrum is seen [43]. This is because most of these infections are associated with catheters or other foreign medical

Table 36.2 Increasing the frequency of infections caused by NFGNB[a] in cancer patients

References,[b]	Year	Total Gram-negative isolates – *n*	NFGNB,[a] *n* (%)
Bodey et al. [24]	1985	941	245 (26)
Bodey et al. [24]	1986	851	220 (26)
Rolston et al. [25]	1993	679	159 (23)
Jacobson et al. [26]	1996	758	225 (30)
Rolston et al. [18]	2002	903	329 (36)

[a]*NFGNB* nonfermentative Gram-negative bacilli
[b]Data from epidemiologic/surveillance studies conducted at The University of Texas M.D. Anderson Cancer Center

devices, surgical procedures, and the presence of obstructive lesions or devitalized tissues caused by the presence of large and rapidly growing tumors. Specific infections depend on the location of the tumor or foreign device. *P. aeruginosa* is often isolated from surgical wounds. Patients who have obstructive pulmonary lesions due to primary or metastatic tumors develop postobstructive necrotizing pneumonias, lung abscess, broncho-pleural fistula, or empyema. *P. aeruginosa* is a common pathogen in these settings, especially in patients requiring prolonged hospitalization, broad-spectrum antibiotics, or mechanical ventilation. Patients with hepato-biliary, gastro-intestinal, and gynecological malignancies develop localized infections such as abdominal, pelvic, or hepatic abscesses, and ascending cholangitis. These infections are predominantly polymicrobial with *P. aeruginosa* being among the most common isolates [2]. Genito-urinary infections including prostatitis are common in patients with prostate cancer and other tumors causing local obstruction. Finally, with the increased use of vascular access devices, urinary and other catheters, stents, and a variety of other foreign medical devices, an increasing number of pseudomonal infections are being documented.

Stenotrophomonas maltophilia

S. maltophilia colonization/infection rates in patients with cancer have substantially increased over the past 2 decades. Surveillance studies conducted at the University of Texas M.D. Anderson Cancer Center in Houston have documented an increase in the proportion of *S. maltophilia* from 2% of all Gram-negative bacilli isolated in 1986 to 7% in 2002 [18]. During this time, *S. maltophilia* increased from being the ninth most common Gram-negative isolate, to the fifth most common. Patients with prolonged neutropenia, exposure to broad spectrum antibiotics, particularly the carbapenems, and those requiring mechanical ventilation have a higher risk of infection [44–46]. However, these infections are being documented more often even in patients without these risk factors [47]. Some of these infections appear to be community acquired as they are being documented in patients not previously exposed to the healthcare system.

The most common clinical manifestation of *S. maltophilia* infection include bacteremia, which is often catheter-related, respiratory tract infection, skin and skin structure infection, and complicated urinary tract infection usually in the presence of obstruction of foreign medical devices. Furthermore, at our institution a significant increase (13%) in moderate to high-grade bacteremia (>100 cfu/mL) caused by *S. maltophilia* has occurred, and may reflect the increasing severity of these infections (Table 36.3).

Recovery of the *S. maltophilia* does not always indicate the presence of infection. Skin and intestinal colonization

Table 36.3 Frequency of moderate-to-high-grade bacteremia[a] in cancer patients at MDACC[b]

	Moderate to high-grade bacteremia	
	No. (%) of isolates	
Organisms	1998	2004
Gram-negative isolates	111 (39)[c]	78 (42)[d]
S. maltophilia	4 (4)	13 (17)
P. aeruginosa	14 (13)	8 (10)
Acinetobacter spp.	7 (6)	8 (10)

[a] Moderate: 101–500 CFU/mL; high-grade: >500 CFU/mL
[b] *MDACC* M.D. Anderson Cancer Center
[c] From a total of 284 Gram-negative bacilli
[d] From a total of 186 Gram-negative bacilli

occur most often. Intestinal colonization may occur after fluoroquinolone prophylaxis. In a recent surveillance study, *S. maltophilia* colonization was demonstrated in 10% of hospitalized neutropenic patients [48]. *S. maltophilia* respiratory tract colonization occurs frequently in patients with (a) prolonged stay in an intensive care unit, (b) presence of a tracheostomy, and (c) prolonged exposure to broad-spectrum antibiotics, and often precedes infection.

Trimethoprim/sulfamethoxazole (TMP/SMX) has had the most potent and reliable in vitro activity against *S. maltophilia*, but resistance rates appear to be increasing [49]. Several beta-lactams have been reported to have variable activity (ranging from 35 to 70%) against *S. maltophilia* including ceftazidime, cefepime, ticarcillin/clavulanate, and piperacillin/tazobactam [50]. The aminoglycosides have poor activity against these organisms. The quinolones have variable activity, with the newer agents such as moxifloxacin being more active than older ones such as ciprofloxacin [51]. Minocycline and the novel glycecycline agent tigecycline are also active against most *S. maltophilia* isolates [52].

Acinetobacter baumannii

Acinetobacter baumannii is being increasingly recognized worldwide as a significant cause of morbidity and mortality. *A. baumannii* usually causes infections in those who are immunosuppressed, with cancer patients being one of the groups who are most at risk [53]. Centers from around the world have reported high rates of *Acinetobacter* isolation. In one Brazilian cancer hospital, *A. baumannii* represented 9.3% of bloodstream infections among solid organ cancer patients during a 2-year study period [28]. This rate slightly surpassed that of *P. aeruginosa*. At the National Cancer Institute in Cairo, Egypt, *Acinetobacter* species comprised 6.9% of over 770 isolates from patients with either hematologic malignancies or solid tumors [54]. *Acinetobacter* is also seen in the pediatric population. In one study of 92 bloodstream isolates of *Acinetobacter* spp. over a 5-year period, ~50% of cases were in children with malignancies (both solid and hematologic) or transplants (solid organ and bone marrow). In a multivariate analysis, having a solid organ malignancy was associated with a greater risk of developing *Acinetobacter* infection [55].

The clinical manifestations of *Acinetobacter* infections are similar to those seen with other Gram-negative bacilli. Frequently seen infections include bacteremia, pneumonia, wound, and urine infections [56]. Although having cancer is an important risk factor for *Acinetobacter* infections, it is not clear if patients with cancer have higher attributable mortality due to *Acinetobacter* infections than those without cancer.

The increasing levels of antibiotic resistance that have been seen with other Gram-negative bacilli are also being seen in *Acinetobacter* isolates. In one large European study of antimicrobial susceptibility of bacterial isolates between 2004 and 2007, ~16% of all the *A. baumannii* isolates were considered multidrug resistant [57]. Due to the development of multidrug-resistant Gram-negative organisms, including *Acinetobacter* pp., older drugs such as colistin, which had been used infrequently due to toxicities, are now making a comeback. However, resistance to colistin has developed as well. In a recent study looking at colistin resistance among *A. baumannii* strains from across the world, 23% were found to be colistin heteroresistant [58]. In another recent study, the in vitro activity of tigecycline, minocycline, and colistin-tigecycline combination against clinical *A. baumannii* isolates including colistin-resistant isolates was evaluated [59]. Tigecycline showed better activity than minocycline even against pan-drug resistant strains.

Approximately, 4% of all Gram-negative infections are caused by other, less common, but important NFGNB including Achromobacter and Alcaligenes species, Chryseobacterium species, Burkholderia species, and non-aeruginosa Pseudomonas species [18]. Achromobacter and Alcaligenes species are ubiquitous organisms, and most infections can be traced to a common source such as contaminated dialysis fluid, deionized water, chlorhexidine solution, mechanical ventilators, and incubators [60]. Patients with cancer, those undergoing hematopoietic or solid organ transplantation, HIV/AIDS and other immunocompromised patients are at increased risk, and these infections can present as life-threatening events in such individuals. Primary uncomplicated bacteremia represents the most common clinical manifestation although infected indwelling catheters, pneumonia, and meningitis have also been reported. These organisms are uniformly resistant to the fluoroquinolones, and the impact of widespread fluoroquinolone prophylaxis on the frequency of these infections needs to be investigated. Most isolates are susceptible to TMP/SMX and the carbapenems [61]. Some combinations have been shown to be synergistic in vitro and may be preferred for therapy in neutropenic patients with sepsis and multiorgan dysfunction [62].

Chryseobacterium species (*C. indologenes* and *C. meningosepticum*) are rare pathogens but can cause life-threatening infections such as bacteremia and meningitis, especially in immunocompromised individuals [63–65]. *C. meningosepticun* is a waterborne saprophytic organism, ubiquitous in the natural and hospital environment. *C. indologenes* is also widely distributed in nature (plants, water, and soil). Antimicrobial susceptibility is variable with most isolates being resistant to the aminoglycosides, and many beta-lactams [66, 67]. The organisms may be susceptible to minocycline, TMP/SMX, rifampin, piperacillin/tazobactam, cefoperazone/sulbactam, and vancomycin. Combination therapy may be prudent in most cases. Burkholderia cepacia complex (BCC) is opportunistic pathogens that occasionally cause outbreaks in patients with cancer, which are generally traced to contaminated intravenous solutions, disinfectants such as chlorhexidine and povidone-iodine solution, ultrasound gel, mouthwashes, and aerosols [68–70]. They are often susceptible to TMP/SMX, the carbapenems, the quinolones, and extended spectrum cephalosporin and penicillins.

Pseudomonas fluorescens and Pseudomonas putida are members of the fluorescent pseudomonad group. Unlike *P. aeruginosa*, these organisms have low levels of virulence. They do colonize the skin in some individuals and can cause pseudobacteremia or procedure-related infections. The association between *P. fluorescens* and contaminated blood products has been well described [71–73]. They are also present in commercial bottled water, which can be a source of infection in neutropenic patients [74]. Catheter-related bacteremia and pneumonia are the most common clinical manifestations [75–77]. The carbapenems have the most reliable activity against these organisms. The activity of other beta-lactams and the quinolones is variable. The overall mortality associated with these organisms is low. Many patients respond to removal of the offending catheter alone, and most respond to appropriate antimicrobial therapy.

Treatment and Outcome

The treatment of Gram-negative infections in neutropenic patients, especially those caused by *P. aeruginosa*, has been the subject of considerable debate. There are two schools of thought. One school advocates the administration of combination therapy (preferably a synergistic combination) in all patients with documented Gram-negative infections, while the other considers treatment with a single, bactericidal, broad-spectrum agent with antipseudomonal activity to be adequate [78, 79]. It is likely that different approaches may be applicable for initial empiric therapy and for the treatment of documented Gram-negative infections [3, 80].

Empiric Therapy

Antipseudomonal coverage is an essential component of empiric therapy in neutropenic cancer patients [3]. This can be achieved using either combination antibiotic regimens or broad spectrum agents alone, as monotherapy. Traditionally, combination regimens have included an aminoglycoside and an antipseudomonal beta-lactam. Agents commonly used as monotherapy include the cephalosporins, ceftazidime, and cefepime; the carbapenems, imipenem, and meropenem; and piperacillin/tazobactam [3]. Several randomized trials in this setting have found monotherapy to be as effective as combination therapy, while some studies have hinted at the superiority of combination regimens [81–86]. A recent meta-analysis concluded that several broad-spectrum agents (ceftazidime, piperacillin/tazobactam, imipenem, and meropenem) were suitable as monotherapy in this setting [87]. Unfortunately, the number of documented pseudomonal infections in these trials was too small to draw firm conclusions regarding the treatment of this specific organism. Some authors have cautioned against the use of cefepime as monotherapy apparently due to an increase in all cause mortality associated with this agent compared to other beta-lactams, as published in a recent systemic review and meta-analysis [88]. Other authors have questioned the methods used to arrive at this conclusion [89, 90]. The FDA has conducted its own analysis which did not confirm this association, and deemed cefepime to be a suitable agent for monotherapy [91]. Monotherapy using an aminoglycoside is suboptimal in neutropenic patients whether used empirically or for the treatment of documented Gram-negative infections shown to be aminoglycoside susceptible in vitro [92].

Therapy of Documented Infections

As mentioned previously, the main debate regarding the treatment of documented Gram-negative infections is whether or not one needs to always use combination regimens, particularly for infections caused by *P. aeruginosa*. Two large studies collectively evaluating 665 episodes of *P. aeruginosa* bacteremia have been published from the M.D. Anderson Cancer Center [41, 93]. Both demonstrated that there was no significant difference in response rates between patients receiving monotherapy with an antipseudomonal beta-lactam and those receiving combination therapy. The overall response rate in the more recent study was 80%, a significant improvement over the 62% response rate in the earlier study. This probably reflects the availability of more potent antipseudomonal agents and advances in supportive care in recent years. Factors associated with an unfavorable outcome included (a) delay in the administration of appropriate therapy, (b) persistent and severe neutropenia, (c) severe sepsis including septic shock, and (d) the presence of tissue-based infections (pneumonia, enterocolitis/typhlitis, perirectal infections). The response rate was 97% in patients whose neutrophil count increased above 0.10×10^4/L during treatment compared to 62% if the neutrophil count persisted below this level. Patients with persistent neutropenia might benefit from the administration of hematopoietic growth factors (G-CSF, GM-CSF) or white blood cell transfusions although clear guidelines for the use of these modalities have not been established.

In a large study (covering 2 decades of experience) of the outcomes of bacteremia in neutropenic cancer patients, Elting et al. characterized bacteremia as simple and complex [94]. Simple bacteremias included those without any tissue site or those associated with minor infections such as cystitis, cellulitis, or bronchitis. Complex bacteremias were those that had sites of infection in major organs (lung, liver, spleen, colon, bones, joints, meninges) and extensive soft-tissue infections (>5 cc in size or with necrosis). The cure rate for simple bacteremia was 95% compared to 50% for complex bacteremias. Although the overall mortality was not significantly increased when patients with bacteremia due to Gram-negative organisms initially received monotherapy, this strategy increased the duration of therapy by 25%. These researchers also demonstrated that certain regimens considered therapeutically equivalent based on conventional response rates associated with them may differ drastically when time to clinical response is taken into consideration [95].

Clearly, there is no uniform strategy to treat Gram-negative infections in patients with or without neutropenia. One of the biggest problems in prospectively evaluating different therapeutic approaches has been the small number of documented Gram-negative infections even in large trials. Organizations such as the IDSA and NCCN have published guidelines for antimicrobial usage in neutropenic patients [3, 33]. Both sets of guidelines consider empiric monotherapy to be as effective as combination therapy. Opinion regarding the treatment of documented *P. aeruginosa* infection remains divided [96]. Although monotherapy might be effective for simple pseudomonal infections, most clinicians are more comfortable using combination regimens for complex pseudomonal infections [3, 33, 96]. In addition to increased efficacy as a result of synergy, other potential advantages of combination therapy might be a reduction in the emergence of resistance, and a quicker time to defervescence [3, 94, 95].

Antimicrobial Stewardship

Increasing rates of antimicrobial resistance among Gram-negative pathogens have been documented at most cancer centers [1, 3, 9, 10]. One method of combating this problem has been the development of novel agents that have activity against these resistant pathogens. Currently, however, the

Table 36.4 Antimicrobial stewardship strategies

- Create Multidisciplinary Antimicrobial Stewardship Team (MAST)
- Determine real time institutional epidemiology and susceptibility resistance patterns
- Know institutional formulary make up and prescribing habits
- Limit chemoprophylaxis to high-risk patients
- Encourage targeted therapy (not always feasible in neutropenic patients)
- Conduct prospective audits of antimicrobial usage
- Provide feedback (positive and/or negative) to prescribers
- Consider formulary restriction and/or preauthorization of certain agents
- Create institutional guidelines and pathways
- Consider antimicrobial heterogeneity
- Streamline (de-escalate) initial broad-spectrum regimen (when possible)
- Dose optimization and appropriate duration of therapy
- Education activities
- Strict adherence to infection control policies

Adapted from refs. [97–99]

pipeline for novel agents with potent activity against resistant Gram-negatives is relatively dry [7, 8]. Consequently, the judicious use of currently available antimicrobial agents (antimicrobial stewardship) to prevent the emergence of resistant organisms and strict adherence to infection control practices to reduce the spread of resistant organisms have become important strategies in the overall management of high-risk patients. The Infectious Diseases Society of America and the Society for Healthcare Epidemiology of America have published joint guidelines for developing institutional antimicrobial stewardship programs [96]. Collecting baseline data at the onset of a stewardship program is necessary as institutional differences do exist. These data include local epidemiologic and susceptibility/resistance patterns, and knowledge of hospital formulary and institutional prescribing habits. Armed with these data, several strategies can be implemented, Table 36.4. These include limiting the use of antibacterial prophylaxis, dose optimization, targeted therapy when possible, de-escalation or streamlining of the initial broad spectrum regimen, antibiotic heterogeneity, and educational/prospective feedback sessions. These strategies already have been implemented with considerable success at several cancer centers [97, 98].

Anaerobic Bacterial Infections

The majority of anaerobic Gram-Negative bacilli belong to *Bacteroides fragilis* group. Infections mostly originate from orointestinal tract. Adults with systemic Bacteroides infections often have hematologic malignancy, such as refractory leukemia, myelodysplastic syndrome, aplastic anemia, or have recently undergone surgery for bowel or gynecologic cancer [100, 101]. Presence of intestinal obstruction, poorly controlled diabetes mellitus, and intestinal epithelial damage due to cytotoxic drug or radiation therapy also increases risk for systemic GN anaerobic bacterial infection. Patients receiving high-dose systemic corticosteroids and those with high-grade graft-versus-host disease following allogeneic stem cell transplantation are also among the high-risk group [102]. Direct inoculation of a surgical wound is another well-recognized source of anaerobic wound and deep tissue infections [100]. Central venous catheter is an uncommon source of anaerobic bacteremia. Patients with neutropenic enterocolitis with a hematologic malignancy may also have a higher risk for anaerobic bacteremia [102].

Bacteroides and other anaerobic Gram-negative bacteria may lead to life-threatening infections, presence of refractory hypotension, high-grade fever, acute intravascular hemolysis and disseminated coagulation, and early onset of tissue necrosis are the hallmark of this devastating disease [100]. A dusk pallor tissue that is cold to touch heralds severe underlying tissue damage; crepitus on palpation may not be evident in patients with deep tissue involvement are most frequently seen in patients with clostridial myonecrosis. Muscle necrosis accompanies loss of arterial supply and sensation to the distal tissue in patients with proximal limb infection. In these patients, infection may have originated from the lower intestinal tract and spread via retroperitoneal facial planes. A high level of suspicion and prompt systemic therapy coupled with urgent surgical excision of devitalized tissue when possible improves outcomes. In select cases, adjuvant treatment with intravenous hyperimmunoglobulin and ribosomal active antimicrobials for arresting exotoxin production may also be attempted. In severely neutropenic patients with refractory neutropenia, recombinant myeloid growth factors and G-CSF primed donor-derived granulocyte transfusions need further evaluation and are presently used as salvage therapy. However, it is critical to emphasize that this disease progresses with lightening speed; therefore, any ameliorative measures and antimicrobial therapy require to be administered in most urgent manner.

Summary

Aerobic Gram-negative bacilli continue to be important pathogens in cancer patients with and without neutropenia, and are still associated with substantial morbidity and mortality despite significant advances in supportive care. Although the overall frequency of infections caused by these organisms has declined, the spectrum of organisms causing infection has expanded. The most important development impacting the treatment of Gram-negative bacterial infections has been the emergence of antimicrobial resistance. Some organisms such as Acinetobacter species, Klebsiella species, *P. aeruginosa*, and *S. maltophilia* have developed multiple mechanisms of resistance leaving very limited treatment options when they are isolated. This problem will continue to challenge clinicians for the foreseeable future, despite the implementation of antimicrobial stewardship and infection control programs. Bacteroides and other anaerobic Gram-negative bacteria may lead to life-threatening infections, presence of refractory hypotension, high-grade fever, acute intravascular hemolysis and disseminated coagulation, and early onset of tissue necrosis are the hallmark of this devastating disease. A high level of suspicion and prompt systemic therapy coupled with surgical excision of devitalized tissue when possible may improve outcomes.

References

1. Wisplinghoff H, Seifert H, Wenzel RP, Edmond MB. Current trends in the epidemiology of nosocomial bloodstream infections in patients with hematological malignancies and solid neoplasms in hospitals in the United States. Clin Infect Dis. 2003;36:1103–10.
2. Rolston KV, Bodey GP, Safdar A. Polymicrobial infection in patients with cancer: an underappreciated and underreported entity. Clin Infect Dis. 2007;45:228–33.
3. Hughes WT, Armstrong D, Bodey GP, et al. 2002 guidelines for the use of antimicrobial agents in neutropenic patients with cancer. Clin Infect Dis. 2002;34:730–51.
4. Rangaraj G, Granwehr BP, Jiang Y, Hachem R, Raad I. Perils of quinolone exposure in cancer patients: breakthrough bacteremia with multidrug-resistant organisms. Cancer. 2010;116:967–73.
5. Cattaneo C, Quaresmini G, Casari S, et al. Recent changes in bacterial epidemiology and the emergence of fluoroquinolone-resistant *Escherichia coli* among patients with haematological malignancies: results of a prospective study on 823 patients at a single institution. J Antimicrob Chemother. 2008;61:721–8.
6. Rolston K, Mihu CN, Tarrand J. Current microbiology of surgical site infections associated with breast cancer surgery. WOUNDS: A Compendium of Clinical Research and Practice. 2010;22:132–5.
7. Talbot GH, Bradley J, Edwards Jr JE, Gilbert D, Scheld M, Bartlett JG. Bad bugs need drugs: an update on the development pipeline from the Antimicrobial Availability Task Force of the Infectious Diseases Society of America. Clin Infect Dis. 2006; 42:657–68.
8. Boucher HW, Talbot GH, Bradley JS, et al. Bad bugs, no drugs: no ESKAPE! An update from the Infectious Diseases Society of America. Clin Infect Dis. 2009;48:1–12.
9. Zinner SH. Changing epidemiology of infections in patients with neutropenia and cancer: emphasis on gram-positive and resistant bacteria. Clin Infect Dis. 1999;29:490–4.
10. Yadegarynia D, Tarrand J, Raad I, Rolston K. Current spectrum of bacterial infections in patients with cancer. Clin Infect Dis. 2003;37:1144–5.
11. Ramphal R. Changes in the etiology of bacteremia in febrile neutropenic patients and the susceptibilities of the currently isolated pathogens. Clin Infect Dis. 2004;39 Suppl 1:S25–31.
12. Paul M, Gafter-Gvili A, Leibovici L, et al. The epidemiology of bacteremia with febrile neutropenia: experience from a single center, 1988–2004. Isr Med Assoc J. 2007;9:424–9.
13. Klastersky J, Ameye L, Maertens J, et al. Bacteraemia in febrile neutropenic cancer patients. Int J Antimicrob Agents. 2007;30 Suppl 1:S51–9.
14. Elting LS, Bodey GP, Fainstein V. Polymicrobial septicemia in the cancer patient. Medicine (Baltimore). 1986;65:218–25.
15. Greenberg D, Moser A, Yagupsky P, et al. Microbiological spectrum and susceptibility patterns of pathogens causing bacteraemia in paediatric febrile neutropenic oncology patients: comparison between two consecutive time periods with use of different antibiotic treatment protocols. Int J Antimicrob Agents. 2005;25:469–73.
16. Chen CY, Tsay W, Tang JL, et al. Epidemiology of bloodstream infections in patients with haematological malignancies with and without neutropenia. Epidemiol Infect. 2010;138:1044–51.
17. Gupta A, Singh M, Singh H, et al. Infections in acute myeloid leukemia: an analysis of 382 febrile episodes. Med Oncol. 2010;27:1037–45.
18. Rolston KVI, Kontoyiannis DP, Raad I, LeBlanc BJ, Streeter HL, Ho DH. Susceptibility surveillance among gram-negative bacilli at a comprehensive cancer center [A-004]. In: Program and abstracts of the 103rd general meeting of American Society of Microbiology. Washington: American Society of Microbiology; 2003.
19. Rolston KV, Tarrand JJ. *Pseudomonas aeruginosa* – still a frequent pathogen in patients with cancer: 11-year experience at a comprehensive cancer center. Clin Infect Dis. 1999;29:463–4.
20. Vigil KJ, Adachi JA, Aboufaycal H, et al. Multidrug-resistant *Escherichia coli* bacteremia in cancer patients. Am J Infect Control. 2009;37:741–5.
21. Vigil KJ, Johnson JR, Johnston BD, et al. *Escherichia coli* Pyomyositis: an emerging infectious disease among patients with hematologic malignancies. Clin Infect Dis. 2010;50:374–80.
22. Blossom D, Noble-Wang J, Su J, et al. Multistate outbreak of *Serratia marcescens* bloodstream infections caused by contamination of prefilled heparin and isotonic sodium chloride solution syringes. Arch Intern Med. 2009;169:1705–11.
23. Pitout JD, Laupland KB. Extended-spectrum beta-lactamase-producing Enterobacteriaceae: an emerging public-health concern. Lancet Infect Dis. 2008;8:159–66.
24. Bodey GP, Ho DH, Elting L. Survey of antibiotic susceptibility among gram-negative bacilli at a cancer hospital. Am J Med. 1988;85:49–51.
25. Rolston KV, Elting L, Waguespack S, Ho DH, LeBlanc B, Bodey GP. Survey of antibiotic susceptibility among gram-negative bacilli at a cancer center. Chemotherapy. 1996;42:348–53.
26. Jacobson K, Rolston K, Elting L, LeBlanc B, Whimbey E, Ho DH. Susceptibility surveillance among gram-negative bacilli at a cancer center. Chemotherapy. 1999;45:325–34.
27. Valdez JM, Scheinberg P, Young NS, Walsh TJ. Infections in patients with aplastic anemia. Semin Hematol. 2009;46:269–76.
28. Velasco E, Byington R, Martins CA, Schirmer M, Dias LM, Goncalves VM. Comparative study of clinical characteristics of neutropenic and non-neutropenic adult cancer patients with bloodstream infections. Eur J Clin Microbiol Infect Dis. 2006;25:1–7.
29. Bucaneve G, Micozzi A, Menichetti F, et al. Levofloxacin to prevent bacterial infection in patients with cancer and neutropenia. N Engl J Med. 2005;353:977–87.
30. Cullen M, Steven N, Billingham L, et al. Antibacterial prophylaxis after chemotherapy for solid tumors and lymphomas. N Engl J Med. 2005;353:988–98.
31. Gafter-Gvili A, Fraser A, Paul M, Leibovici L. Meta-analysis: antibiotic prophylaxis reduces mortality in neutropenic patients. Ann Intern Med. 2005;142:979–95.
32. Leibovici L, Paul M, Cullen M, et al. Antibiotic prophylaxis in neutropenic patients: new evidence, practical decisions. Cancer. 2006;107:1743–51.

33. Segal BH, Freifeld AG, Baden LR, et al. Prevention and treatment of cancer-related infections. J Natl Compr Canc Netw. 2008;6:122–74.
34. Quale J. Global spread of Carbapenemase-producing *Klebsiella pneumoniae*. Microbe. 2008;3:516–20.
35. Paterson DL, Ko WC, Von Gottberg A, et al. Antibiotic therapy for *Klebsiella pneumoniae* bacteremia: implications of production of extended-spectrum beta-lactamases. Clin Infect Dis. 2004;39:31–7.
36. Yigit H, Queenan AM, Anderson GJ, et al. Novel carbapenem-hydrolyzing beta-lactamase, KPC-1, from a carbapenem-resistant strain of *Klebsiella pneumoniae*. Antimicrob Agents Chemother. 2001;45:1151–61.
37. Queenan AM, Bush K. Carbapenemases: the versatile beta-lactamases. Clin Microbiol Rev. 2007;20:440–58.
38. Lee K, Chong Y, Shin HB, Kim YA, Yong D, Yum JH. Modified hodge and EDTA-disk synergy tests to screen metallo-beta-lactamase-producing strains of Pseudomonas and Acinetobacter species. Clin Microbiol Infect. 2001;7:88–91.
39. Rolston KV, Kontoyiannis DP, Yadegarynia D, Raad II. Nonfermentative gram-negative bacilli in cancer patients: increasing frequency of infection and antimicrobial susceptibility of clinical isolates to fluoroquinolones. Diagn Microbiol Infect Dis. 2005;51:215–8.
40. Sanyal SC, Mokaddas EM. The increase in carbapenem use and emergence of *Stenotrophomonas maltophilia* as an important nosocomial pathogen. J Chemother. 1999;11:28–33.
41. Chatzinikolaou I, Abi-Said D, Bodey GP, Rolston KV, Tarrand JJ, Samonis G. Recent experience with *Pseudomonas aeruginosa* bacteremia in patients with cancer: retrospective analysis of 245 episodes. Arch Intern Med. 2000;160:501–9.
42. Ohmagari N, Hanna H, Graviss L, et al. Risk factors for infections with multidrug-resistant *Pseudomonas aeruginosa* in patients with cancer. Cancer. 2005;104:205–12.
43. Rolston KVI. Infections in patients with solid tumors. In: Rolston KVI, Rubenstein EB, editors. Textbook of febrile neutropenia. London: Martin Dunitz; 2001. p. 91–109.
44. Safdar A, Rolston KV. *Stenotrophomonas maltophilia*: changing spectrum of a serious bacterial pathogen in patients with cancer. Clin Infect Dis. 2007;45:1602–9.
45. Sefcick A, Tait RC, Wood B. *Stenotrophomonas maltophilia*: an increasing problem in patients with acute leukaemia. Leuk Lymphoma. 1999;35:207–11.
46. Micozzi A, Venditti M, Monaco M, et al. Bacteremia due to *Stenotrophomonas maltophilia* in patients with hematologic malignancies. Clin Infect Dis. 2000;31:705–11.
47. Aisenberg G, Rolston KV, Dickey BF, Kontoyiannis DP, Raad II, Safdar A. *Stenotrophomonas maltophilia* pneumonia in cancer patients without traditional risk factors for infection, 1997–2004. Eur J Clin Microbiol Infect Dis. 2007;26:13–20.
48. Apisarnthanarak A, Fraser VJ, Dunne WM, et al. *Stenotrophomonas maltophilia* intestinal colonization in hospitalized oncology patients with diarrhea. Clin Infect Dis. 2003;37:1131–5.
49. Vartivarian S, Anaissie E, Bodey G, Sprigg H, Rolston K. A changing pattern of susceptibility of Xanthomonas maltophilia to antimicrobial agents: implications for therapy. Antimicrob Agents Chemother. 1994;38:624–7.
50. Krueger TS, Clark EA, Nix DE. In vitro susceptibility of *Stenotrophomonas maltophilia* to various antimicrobial combinations. Diagn Microbiol Infect Dis. 2001;41:71–8.
51. Lecso-Bornet M, Pierre J, Sarkis-Karam D, Lubera S, Bergogne-Berezin E. Susceptibility of *Xanthomonas maltophilia* to six quinolones and study of outer membrane proteins in resistant mutants selected in vitro. Antimicrob Agents Chemother. 1992;36:669–71.
52. Noskin GA. Tigecycline: a new glycylcycline for treatment of serious infections. Clin Infect Dis. 2005;41 Suppl 5:S303–14.
53. Karageorgopoulos DE, Falagas ME. Current control and treatment of multidrug-resistant *Acinetobacter baumannii* infections. Lancet Infect Dis. 2008;8:751–62.
54. Ashour HM, El-Sharif A. Species distribution and antimicrobial susceptibility of gram-negative aerobic bacteria in hospitalized cancer patients. J Transl Med. 2009;7:14.
55. Segal SC, Zaoutis TE, Kagen J, Shah SS. Epidemiology of and risk factors for Acinetobacter species bloodstream infection in children. Pediatr Infect Dis J. 2007;26:920–6.
56. Gales AC, Jones RN, Forward KR, Linares J, Sader HS, Verhoef J. Emerging importance of multidrug-resistant Acinetobacter species and *Stenotrophomonas maltophilia* as pathogens in seriously ill patients: geographic patterns, epidemiological features, and trends in the SENTRY Antimicrobial Surveillance Program (1997–1999). Clin Infect Dis. 2001;32 Suppl 2:S104–13.
57. Norskov-Lauritsen N, Marchandin H, Dowzicky MJ. Antimicrobial susceptibility of tigecycline and comparators against bacterial isolates collected as part of the TEST study in Europe (2004–2007). Int J Antimicrob Agents. 2009;34:121–30.
58. Yau W, Owen RJ, Poudyal A, et al. Colistin hetero-resistance in multidrug-resistant *Acinetobacter baumannii* clinical isolates from the Western Pacific region in the SENTRY antimicrobial surveillance programme. J Infect. 2009;58:138–44.
59. Arroyo LA, Mateos I, Gonzalez V, Aznar J. In vitro activities of tigecycline, minocycline, and colistin-tigecycline combination against multi- and pandrug-resistant clinical isolates of *Acinetobacter baumannii* group. Antimicrob Agents Chemother. 2009;53:1295–6.
60. Aisenberg G, Rolston KV, Safdar A. Bacteremia caused by Achromobacter and Alcaligenes species in 46 patients with cancer (1989–2003). Cancer. 2004;101:2134–40.
61. Rolston KV, Messer M. The in-vitro susceptibility of Alcaligenes denitrificans subsp. xylosoxidans to 40 antimicrobial agents. J Antimicrob Chemother. 1990;26:857–60.
62. Saiman L, Chen Y, Gabriel PS, Knirsch C. Synergistic activities of macrolide antibiotics against *Pseudomonas aeruginosa*, *Burkholderia cepacia*, *Stenotrophomonas maltophilia*, and *Alcaligenes xylosoxidans* isolated from patients with cystic fibrosis. Antimicrob Agents Chemother. 2002;46:1105–7.
63. Bloch KC, Nadarajah R, Jacobs R. *Chryseobacterium meningosepticum*: an emerging pathogen among immunocompromised adults. Report of 6 cases and literature review. Medicine (Baltimore). 1997;76:30–41.
64. Lin JT, Wang WS, Yen CC, et al. *Chryseobacterium indologenes* bacteremia in a bone marrow transplant recipient with chronic graft-versus-host disease. Scand J Infect Dis. 2003;35:882–3.
65. Adachi A, Mori T, Shimizu T, et al. *Chryseobacterium meningosepticum* septicemia in a recipient of allogeneic cord blood transplantation. Scand J Infect Dis. 2004;36:539–40.
66. Hsueh PR, Hsiue TR, Wu JJ, et al. *Flavobacterium indologenes* bacteremia: clinical and microbiological characteristics. Clin Infect Dis. 1996;23:550–5.
67. Chang JC, Hsueh PR, Wu JJ, Ho SW, Hsieh WC, Luh KT. Antimicrobial susceptibility of flavobacteria as determined by agar dilution and disk diffusion methods. Antimicrob Agents Chemother. 1997;41:1301–6.
68. Heo ST, Kim SJ, Jeong YG, Bae IG, Jin JS, Lee JC. Hospital outbreak of Burkholderia stabilis bacteraemia related to contaminated chlorhexidine in haematological malignancy patients with indwelling catheters. J Hosp Infect. 2008;70:241–5.
69. Pegues DA, Carson LA, Anderson RL, et al. Outbreak of Pseudomonas cepacia bacteremia in oncology patients. In: 1992 epidemic intelligence service (EIS) Conference. Atlanta: Centers for Disease Control; 1992.
70. Yamagishi Y, Fujita J, Takigawa K, Negayama K, Nakazawa T, Takahara J. Clinical features of Pseudomonas cepacia pneumonia in an epidemic among immunocompromised patients. Chest. 1993;103:1706–9.
71. Puckett A, Davison G, Entwistle CC, Barbara JA. Post transfusion septicaemia 1980–1989: importance of donor arm cleansing. J Clin Pathol. 1992;45:155–7.

72. Scott J, Boulton FE, Govan JR, Miles RS, McClelland DB, Prowse CV. A fatal transfusion reaction associated with blood contaminated with *Pseudomonas fluorescens*. Vox Sang. 1988;54:201–4.
73. Simor AE, Ricci J, Lau A, Bannatyne RM, Ford-Jones L. Pseudobacteremia due to *Pseudomonas fluorescens*. Pediatr Infect Dis. 1985;4:508–12.
74. Wilkinson FH, Kerr KG. Bottled water as a source of multi-resistant Stenotrophomonas and Pseudomonas species for neutropenic patients. Eur J Cancer Care (Engl). 1998;7:12–4.
75. Hsueh PR, Teng LJ, Pan HJ, et al. Outbreak of *Pseudomonas fluorescens* bacteremia among oncology patients. J Clin Microbiol. 1998;36:2914–7.
76. Anaissie E, Fainstein V, Miller P, et al. Pseudomonas putida. Newly recognized pathogen in patients with cancer. Am J Med. 1987;82:1191–4.
77. Martino R, Martinez C, Pericas R, et al. Bacteremia due to glucose non-fermenting gram-negative bacilli in patients with hematological neoplasias and solid tumors. Eur J Clin Microbiol Infect Dis. 1996;15:610–5.
78. Bodey GP. Synergy. Should it determine antibiotic selection in neutropenic patients? Arch Intern Med. 1985;145:1964–6.
79. Sculier JP, Klastersky J. Significance of serum bactericidal activity in gram-negative bacillary bacteremia in patients with and without granulocytopenia. Am J Med. 1984;76:429–35.
80. Finberg RW, Moellering RC, Tally FP, et al. The importance of bactericidal drugs: future directions in infectious disease. Clin Infect Dis. 2004;39:1314–20.
81. Cometta A, Calandra T, Gaya H, et al. Monotherapy with meropenem versus combination therapy with ceftazidime plus amikacin as empiric therapy for fever in granulocytopenic patients with cancer. The International Antimicrobial Therapy Cooperative Group of the European Organization for Research and Treatment of Cancer and the Gruppo Italiano Malattie Ematologiche Maligne dell'Adulto Infection Program. Antimicrob Agents Chemother. 1996;40:1108–15.
82. Raad II, Abi-Said D, Rolston KV, Karl CL, Bodey GP. How should imipenem-cilastatin be used in the treatment of fever and infection in neutropenic cancer patients? Cancer. 1998;82:2449–58.
83. Del Favero A, Menichetti F, Martino P, et al. A multicenter, double-blind, placebo-controlled trial comparing piperacillin-tazobactam with and without amikacin as empiric therapy for febrile neutropenia. Clin Infect Dis. 2001;33:1295–301.
84. Rolston KV, Berkey P, Bodey GP, et al. A comparison of imipenem to ceftazidime with or without amikacin as empiric therapy in febrile neutropenic patients. Arch Intern Med. 1992;152:283–91.
85. Feld R, DePauw B, Berman S, Keating A, Ho W. Meropenem versus ceftazidime in the treatment of cancer patients with febrile neutropenia: a randomized, double-blind trial. J Clin Oncol. 2000;18:3690–8.
86. Raad II, Escalante C, Hachem RY, et al. Treatment of febrile neutropenic patients with cancer who require hospitalization: a prospective randomized study comparing imipenem and cefepime. Cancer. 2003;98:1039–47.
87. Paul M, Soares-Weiser K, Leibovici L. Beta lactam monotherapy versus beta lactam-aminoglycoside combination therapy for fever with neutropenia: systematic review and meta-analysis. BMJ. 2003;326:1111.
88. Yahav D, Paul M, Fraser A, Sarid N, Leibovici L. Efficacy and safety of cefepime: a systematic review and meta-analysis. Lancet Infect Dis. 2007;7:338–48.
89. Nguyen TD, Williams B, Ocampo N. Cefepime and all-cause mortality reply. Clin Infect Dis. 2009;49:641–2.
90. Rolston KV, Bodey GP. Comment on: empirical antibiotic monotherapy for febrile neutropenia: systematic review and meta-analysis of randomized controlled trials. J Antimicrob Chemother. 2006;58:478. author reply 9–80.
91. Information for Healthcare Professionals: Cefepime (marketed by Maxipime). FDA alert. http://wwwfdagov/Drugs/DrugSafety/PostmarketDrugSafetyInformationforPatients. Accessed 17 June 2009.
92. Bodey GP, Middleman E, Umsawadi T, Rodriguez V. Infections in cancer patients. Results with gentamicin sulfate therapy. Cancer. 1972;29:1697–701.
93. Bodey GP, Jadeja L, Elting L. Pseudomonas bacteremia. Retrospective analysis of 410 episodes. Arch Intern Med. 1985;145:1621–9.
94. Elting LS, Rubenstein EB, Rolston KV, Bodey GP. Outcomes of bacteremia in patients with cancer and neutropenia: observations from two decades of epidemiological and clinical trials. Clin Infect Dis. 1997;25:247–59.
95. Elting LS, Rubenstein EB, Rolston K, et al. Time to clinical response: an outcome of antibiotic therapy of febrile neutropenia with implications for quality and cost of care. J Clin Oncol. 2000;18:3699–706.
96. Safdar N, Handelsman J, Maki DG. Does combination antimicrobial therapy reduce mortality in Gram-negative bacteraemia? A meta-analysis. Lancet Infect Dis. 2004;4:519–27.
97. Dellit TH, Owens RC, McGowan Jr JE, et al. Infectious Diseases Society of America and the Society for Healthcare Epidemiology of America guidelines for developing an institutional program to enhance antimicrobial stewardship. Clin Infect Dis. 2007;44:159–77.
98. Paskovaty A, Pflomm JM, Myke N, Seo SK. A multidisciplinary approach to antimicrobial stewardship: evolution into the 21st century. Int J Antimicrob Agents. 2005;25:1–10.
99. Adachi JA, Perego C, Vigil KJ, Mulanovich V, Chemaly R, Rolston KVI. Antibiotic stewardship initiative in the intensive care unit (ICU): evidence from a quality improvement project supporting the development of a multidisciplinary antimicrobial stewardship team (MAST) (Abst. #08-059). In: Multinational association for supportive care in cancer (MASCC/ISOO) 2008 international symposium. Houston, 26–28 June 2008.
100. Kagnoff MF, Armstrong D, Blevins A. Bacteroides bacteremia. Experience in a hospital for neoplastic diseases. Cancer. 1972;29:245–51.
101. Singer C, Kaplan MH, Armstrong D. Bacteremia and fungemia complicating neoplastic disease. A study of 364 cases. Am J Med. 1977;62:731–42.
102. Spánik S, Trupl J, Kunová A, Pichna P, Helpianska L, Ilavská I, et al. Bloodstream infections due to anaerobic bacteria in cancer patients: epidemiology, etiology, risk factors, clinical presentation and outcome of anaerobic bacteremia. Neoplasma. 1996;43:235–8.

Chapter 37
Listeriosis and Nocardiosis

Heather E. Clauss and Bennett Lorber

Abstract The bacterium *Listeria monocytogenes* infrequently causes illness in the general population. In some groups, however, including pregnant women, newborns, elderly persons, and those with impaired cell-mediated immunity, including many cancer patients, it is an important cause of invasive disease, particularly bacteremia, meningitis, encephalitis, and brain abscess. *Nocardia* species are aerobic, Gram-positive, branching, filamentous, bacterial rods, which are most often found in the environment in soil, water, and vegetable matter. The key host defense against developing nocardiosis is cell-mediated immunity; the humoral immune response offers little protection. These organisms are considered opportunistic pathogens, causing infection in patients with impaired cell-mediated immune response, including patients with lymphoreticular neoplasia, organ transplantation, HIV/AIDS, diabetes mellitus, and alcoholism. In particular, there is a well-documented association between nocardiosis and chronic granulomatous disease (CGD). In this chapter, we present a detailed review of epidemiology, clinical presentation, and management of these opportunistic infections in immunosuppressed patients with cancer.

Keywords Listeriosis • Nocardiosis • Brain abscess • Meningitis • Bacteremia • Antibiotic therapy • Refractory disease

Listeriosis

Introduction

The bacterium *Listeria monocytogenes* infrequently causes illness in the general population. In some groups, however, including pregnant women, newborns, elderly persons, and those with impaired cell-mediated immunity, including many cancer patients, it is an important cause of invasive disease, particularly bacteremia, meningitis, encephalitis, and brain abscess [1–3]. Additionally, listeriae may cause other clinical syndromes, including in utero infection typically resulting in miscarriage or stillbirth, as well as focal infections of the eye, skin, heart valves, joints, liver, and spleen, and a self-limited febrile gastroenteritis [4].

L. monocytogenes is a small, Gram-positive rod that is facultatively anaerobic, nonsporulating, and grows readily on blood agar where it produces incomplete beta-hemolysis [5]. The bacterium exhibits characteristic tumbling motility at room temperature and, unlike most bacteria, grows well at refrigerator temperatures (4–10°C). In clinical specimens, the organisms may be gram-variable and may look like diphtheroids, cocci, or diplococci leading to misdiagnosis. The isolation of a "diphtheroid" from blood or CSF should always alert one to the possibility that the organism is really *L. monocytogenes*.

Pathogenesis

Human-to-human transmission of *L. monocytogenes* has not been reported aside from vertical transmission between mother and child and sporadic cross contamination in neonatal nurseries [6]. Most commonly, listeriae are transmitted via the ingestion of contaminated food. In mammals $\geq 10^9$ organisms are required for infection [7]. Alkalinization of the stomach with antacids, H_2 blockers, proton pump inhibitors, or the achlorhydria associated with advanced age may promote infection [8]. The incubation period for invasive disease (bacteremia, meningitis) is not well established, but evidence from cases related to specific ingestions points to a range from 11 to 70 days (mean 31 days) [9].

Once inside an enterocyte or macrophage, *L. monocytogenes* uses its major virulence factor, listeriolysin O, to escape from the phagosome [10]. Through other novel mechanisms, it then can move from cell to cell without entering the extracellular space, thus avoiding contact with

B. Lorber (✉)
Department of Medicine, Section of Infectious Diseases, Temple University School of Medicine, Philadelphia, PA 19140, USA
e-mail: bennett.lorber@temple.edu

complement, antibodies, and neutrophils [11]. There is no increased frequency of listeriosis in those with deficiencies in neutrophil numbers or function, splenectomy, complement deficiency, or immunoglobulin disorders, the latter not surprising given that *L. monocytogenes* can be passed from cell to cell without being exposed to antibody.

Listeriae have a particular predilection for the central nervous system (CNS). Experimental data indicate that *L. monocytogenes* can use several different mechanisms to invade the CNS: (a) transportation of bacteria to the CNS within circulating leukocytes in a phagocyte-facilitated (Trojan horse) mechanism as described above, (b) via direct invasion of endothelial cells of the blood–brain barrier by blood-borne bacteria, or (c) via a neural route whereby bacteria are inoculated into oral tissues when abrasive food is chewed, followed by tissue macrophage phagocytosis of the bacteria making possible the invasion of cranial nerves [12]. In the latter case, bacteria move in a retrograde direction through the nerve axons, eventually reaching the CNS where they continue to spread intercellularly to the parenchyma.

Another important virulence factor for *L. monocytogenes* is the ability to scavenge iron. In vitro, iron enhances organism growth [13]. In animal models of listeria infection, iron overload is associated with enhanced susceptibility to infection and iron supplementation with enhanced lethality, whereas prolonged survival results from iron depletion [14]. Iron overload states are risk factors for listerial infection, and clinical correlates include outbreaks of listerial infection in patients receiving hemodialysis who have transfusion-induced iron overload and patients with hemochromatosis [9].

Epidemiology

L. monocytogenes is readily isolated from soil and decaying vegetation and has been found to be present in the feces of many mammals [15]. The organism has been isolated from the stool of ~5% of healthy adults [16]. Many foods are contaminated with *L. monocytogenes*; recovery rates of 15–70% have been found from raw vegetables, unpasteurized milk, fish, poultry, and meats [17]. Ingestion of listeriae must be a common occurrence. Numerous foodborne outbreaks have occurred with vehicles including unpasteurized soft cheeses, hot dogs, and deli-style ready-to-eat sliced poultry products. In October 2002, *L. monocytogenes* was found in sliced deli-style turkey meat, the ingestion of which produced illness in 54 patients in 9 states, resulting in the largest recall of meat ever in the United States (more than 30 million pounds of food products) [18].

The highest infection rates of invasive listeriosis are seen in adults >60 years of age and in infants <1 month old [19]. The rate of infection declines sharply between the ages of 1 and 11 months. Pregnant women account for approximately 27% of all cases of listerial bacteremia and 60% of cases in the 10–40-year age group. It is noteworthy, that although pregnancy is a clear risk factor for bacteremia, for unknown reasons, listerial meningitis is exceedingly rare during pregnancy unless a second risk factor, such as corticosteroid therapy, is present. Sixty-nine percent of nonperinatal infections occur in patients with impairments in cell-mediated immunity. Seemingly, normal persons may develop invasive disease, particularly those older than age 60.

The major risk factor for listeriosis is impaired cell-mediated immunity whether due to a specific disease or due to immunosuppressive therapy. Specific risk factors for developing listeriosis include corticosteroid treatment, organ transplantation, hematologic malignancy, AIDS, pregnancy, liver failure, solid malignancy, diabetes, and age >60 [20]. Reports continue to be published on *L. monocytogenes* meningitis presenting as an opportunistic infection in AIDS [21] and as a complication of solid organ transplantation [22]. One new risk factor for listerial infection is the use of antitumor necrosis factor alpha (TNF-α) agents. Case reports describe listerial meningitis complicating infliximab treatment for Crohn's disease [23] as well as etanercept treatment for Still's disease [24]. An interesting basic science correlate of these clinical events is the observation that, in a murine model, TNF was found to play a crucial role in the intracerebral control of *L. monocytogenes* infection [25].

Major Clinical Syndromes

The species name derives from the fact that an extract of the *L. monocytogenes* cell membrane has potent monocytosis-producing activity in rabbits [26], but monocytosis is a very rare feature of human infection.

Infection in Pregnancy and the Neonatal Period

Pregnant women are prone to develop listerial bacteremia with an estimated 17-fold increase in risk [27]. Listeriae proliferate in the placenta in areas that appear to be unreachable by usual defense mechanisms [28], and cell-to-cell spread facilitates maternal–fetal transmission [29]. For unexplained reasons, CNS infection, a commonly recognized form of listeriosis in other groups, is extremely rare during pregnancy in the absence of other risk factors [27, 30]. Bacteremia is manifested clinically as an acute febrile illness, often accompanied by myalgias, arthralgias, headache, and backache. Twenty-two percent of human perinatal infections result in stillbirth or neonatal death; spontaneous abortion is common. Untreated bacteremia is generally self-limited, although if there is a complicating amnionitis, fever in the mother may persist until the fetus is spontaneously or therapeutically aborted. Among women who have listeriosis during pregnancy, two thirds of surviving infants develop clinical neonatal listeriosis. Early diagnosis and antimicrobial treatment of the infected woman can result in the birth of a healthy infant [9, 27].

Similar to disease due to Group B streptococcus, neonatal infections manifest as early-onset sepsis with disseminated infection, typically in premature infants, or late-onset meningitis, typically in term infants who were healthy at birth.

Bacteremia

Bacteremia without an evident focus is the most common manifestation of listeriosis after the neonatal period [20]. Clinical manifestations are similar to those seen in bacteremia with other causes and typically include fever and myalgias; a prodromal illness with diarrhea and nausea may occur [9].

Central Nervous System Infection

The organisms that cause bacterial meningitis most frequently *(Streptococcus pneumoniae, Neisseria meningitidis, Haemophilus influenzae)* rarely cause parenchymal brain infections such as cerebritis and brain abscess. By contrast, *L. monocytogenes* has tropism for the brain itself, particularly the brain stem, as well as for the meninges [2, 3, 31]. Many patients with meningitis have altered consciousness, seizures, or movement disorders, or all of these, and truly have a meningoencephalitis.

Meningitis

In an active meningitis surveillance study [32], *L. monocytogenes* accounted for 20% of cases in neonates and 20% in those older than 60 years. Worldwide, *L. monocytogenes* is one of the three major causes of neonatal meningitis; is second only to pneumococcus as a cause of bacterial meningitis in adults older than 50 years; and is the most common cause of bacterial meningitis in patients with lymphomas [33], organ transplant recipients, or those receiving corticosteroid immunosuppression for any reason [9].

Clinically, meningitis caused by *L. monocytogenes* is usually similar to that due to more common causes [34, 35]; features particular to listerial meningitis are summarized in Table 37.1. Despite the name "monocytogenes," the CSF pleocytosis is more often neutrophilic than monocytic.

The first prospective study of meningitis due to *L. monocytogenes* recently was reported from the Netherlands [36]. In this nationwide cohort study of 30 adults, notable clinical

Table 37.1 Features particular to listerial meningitis as compared to more common bacterial etiologie.s (adapted from refs. [9, 34, 36])

Feature	Frequency (%)
Presentation can be subacute >24 h[a]	~60
Absense of stiff neck is more common	25
Movement disorders (ataxia, tremors, myoclonus) are more common	15–20
Seizures are more common	10–25
Fluctuating mental status is more common	~75
Focal neurologic findings are more common	35–40
Positive blood culture is more common	50–75
Cerebrospinal fluid (CSF)	
Positive Gram stain is less common	30–40
Normal CSF glucose is more common	>60
Mononuclear cell predominance is more common	~30

[a]May be several days or more and mimic tuberculous meningitis in ~10–30%

features of listerial meningitis included headache in 88%, nausea in 83%, and fever in 90%; but only 75% of patients had a stiff neck at the time of presentation. A focal neurologic deficit was present in 37% (many patients with meningitis have simultaneous infection of the brain parenchyma and truly have a meningoencephalitis). Only 43% had the classic meningitis triad of fever, neck stiffness, and change in mental status. At the time of presentation, 19 out of 30 patients had symptoms persisting for greater than 24 h, and 8 had symptoms for ≥4 days. Remarkable CSF findings included a median white blood cell count of 620 (range 24–16,003) and protein of 2.52 g/L. Spinal fluid Gram stain revealed a Gram-positive rod in only 28% of patients while blood cultures were positive for *L. monocytogenes* in 46% of patients. These data illustrate how difficult it can be to make a definitive diagnosis of listerial meningitis at initial presentation.

Mortality from listerial meningitis has variously been reported at 15% in a CDC active surveillance study [32], 27% in the Massachusetts General Hospital review [34], and 17% in the prospective study from the Netherlands [36]. In the last report, all deaths occurred within 3 days of being admitted to the hospital. Mortality is low (0–13%) for adults without serious underlying disease or immunosuppressive treatment [31].

Brain Stem Encephalitis (Rhombencephalitis)

An unusual form of listerial encephalitis involves the brain stem [37]. In contrast to other listerial CNS infections, this illness usually occurs in healthy adults. The typical clinical picture is one of a biphasic illness with a prodrome of fever, headache, nausea, and vomiting lasting about 4 days followed by the abrupt onset of asymmetric cranial nerve deficits, cerebellar signs, and hemiparesis or hemisensory deficits, or both. About 40% of patients develop respiratory failure. Nuchal rigidity is present in about one half, and CSF findings are only mildly abnormal with a positive CSF culture in about one third. Almost two-thirds of patients are bacteremic. Magnetic resonance imaging is superior to computed tomography for demonstrating brain stem encephalitis [38]. Mortality is high, and serious sequelae are common in survivors.

Brain Abscess

Macroscopic brain abscesses account for about 10% of CNS listerial infections. Bacteremia is almost always present, and concomitant meningitis with isolation of *L. monocytogenes* from the CSF is found in 25–40%; both these features are rare in other forms of bacterial brain abscess [39]. Most cases occur in known risk groups for listerial infection [40]. Subcortical abscesses located in the thalamus, pons, and medulla are common; these sites are exceedingly rare when abscesses are caused by other bacteria. Mortality is high, and survivors usually have serious sequelae.

Listeriosis in Cancer Patients

Louria, in 1967 [41], was the first to point out the strong association between opportunistic listerial infection and malignancies, particularly Hodgkins disease being treated with corticosteroids. He described 18 cases of invasive listerial infection, 16 of which had underlying hematologic malignancies. Twelve of the 18 cases were receiving corticosteroids at the time of diagnosis.

L. monocytogenes infection occurred in 94 patients during 1955–1997 at Memorial Sloan-Kettering Cancer Center; the incidence was 0.5 (1955–1966), 0.96 (1970–1979), and 0.14 (1985–1997) cases per 1,000 new admissions [33]. Eighty-five of ninety-four (90%) patients had listerial bacteremia, and 34/94 (36%) had evidence of intracranial infection. Listeriosis in these patients with cancer occurred most often in individuals receiving antineoplastic therapy for advanced or relapsed malignancy (77%), and systemic corticosteroids (68%). In another study, combined treatment with fludarabine and prednisone in patients with chronic lymphocytic leukemia decreased their CD4+ T-lymphocyte counts and increased their incidence of listeriosis; fludarabine alone was not associated with listeriosis [42].

In a comprehensive review [34] of 33 years experience at Massachusetts General Hospital with CNS listeriosis outside of the neonatal period and pregnancy, including a case series of 41 patients and 776 episodes from the literature, the most common predisposing factor for developing listerial meningitis was malignancy (both solid tumor and hematologic), occurring in 24% of patients.

At another institution, from 1990 to 2001, 34 cancer patients with listeriosis were reviewed and 20 (59%) had an underlying hematologic malignancy [43]. In 11 patients, listeriosis complicated bone marrow transplantation (BMT). Twenty-six patients received prior corticosteroids. Here again, bacteremia was the most common presentation of listeriosis (74%), followed by meningoencephalitis (21%). The rate of response to antimicrobial therapy was 79%, and no relapses were identified. Listeriosis contributed to death in 9 (75%) of the 12 patients who died. In the Memorial Sloan-Kettering study [33], 37 (39%) of the 94 patients died of listeriosis; in more than one third of deaths occurred within the first 48 h after *L. monocytogenes* cultures were obtained.

Another interesting relationship exists between listeriosis and cancer. Listerial endocarditis, not bacteremia per se, in an otherwise healthy person, may be an indicator of underlying gastrointestinal tract pathology, including colon cancer [44].

Diagnosis

The key to making a diagnosis of listerial infection and initiating early, appropriate treatment is knowing when it should be considered. CNS listeriosis should be a major consideration as part of the differential diagnosis in the following clinical settings:

1. Meningitis or parenchymal brain infection in:

    - Patients with hematologic malignancy, AIDS, organ transplantation, corticosteroid immunosuppression, or those receiving anti-TNF agents
    - Patients with a subacute presentation of meningitis
    - Neonates and adults >50 years of age
    - Those in whom CSF shows Gram-positive rods or is reported to have "diphtheroids" on Gram stain or culture

2. Simultaneous infection of the meninges and brain parenchyma.
3. Subcortical brain abscess.
4. Spinal symptoms in the setting of acute bacterial meningitis of uncertain etiology.
5. Fever during pregnancy, particularly in the third trimester.
6. Blood, CSF, or other normally sterile specimen reported to have "diphtheroids" on Gram stain or culture.
7. Foodborne outbreak of febrile gastroenteritis when routine cultures fail to identify a pathogen.

Diagnosis requires isolation of *L. monocytogenes* from a normally sterile site such as blood or CSF and identification through standard microbiologic techniques. Antibodies to listeriolysin O have proved useful during investigation of outbreaks of febrile gastroenteritis [45] but have not proved useful in invasive disease [46]. *L. monocytogenes* DNA in

CSF and tissue can be detected specifically by polymerase chain reaction (PCR) assays, though these have not proved to be useful clinically to diagnose invasive disease [47]. MRI is superior to CT for demonstrating parenchymal brain involvement, especially in the brainstem [37, 38].

Treatment

Many antimicrobials show in vitro activity against listerial isolates, but only a few agents have been proved clinically efficacious. Ampicillin has been the most widely used agent in the treatment of *L. monocytogenes* infections and generally is considered the preferred agent [2, 35]. Synergy has been demonstrated both in vitro and in animal models when an aminoglycoside is added to ampicillin or penicillin, and many authorities recommend the addition of an aminoglycoside to ampicillin for at least in the first week of treatment of CNS infection [9].

In the absence of a positive CSF Gram stain, initial therapy for bacterial meningitis in adults older than age 50 should include an antilisterial agent (either ampicillin or trimethoprim-sulfamethoxazole [TMP-SMX]). Due to the high affinity of *L. monocytogenes* for the CNS, meningitis doses of the chosen antibiotic should be used for all bacteremic patients, even in the absence of CNS findings, until the CSF is examined. An exception is bacteremia in pregnancy without another risk factor, since, in this group, CNS infection is almost never present. Relapses are reported in those with meningitis treated for less than 2 weeks; therefore, treatment for 3 weeks is recommended for all cases of listerial meningitis. Bacteremic patients with normal CSF may be treated for 2 weeks. Patients with brain abscess, cerebritis, or rhombencephalitis should be treated for at least 6 weeks and followed with repeated brain imaging studies. In cases of listerial brain abscess, surgical intervention may not be necessary; numerous case reports describe successful treatment with antimicrobial therapy alone.

In those with penicillin hypersensitivity, TMP-SMX is the treatment of choice and appears to be bactericidal and as effective as the combination of ampicillin and gentamicin. Cephalosporins have limited activity against listeriae. Many reports document treatment failures with cephalosporins, and patients have developed listerial meningitis while receiving cephalosporins for other reasons. Chloramphenicol has also been shown to have unacceptable failure and relapse rates and should not be used. Erythromycin and tetracycline have been reported to be effective, but are unreliable therapeutic options and should be avoided. Vancomycin has been successfully used in penicillin-allergic patients, but listerial meningitis has developed in patients being treated with vancomycin. Both imipenem and meropenem have also been used successfully to treat cases of listeriosis, but caution is advised because both drugs lower the seizure threshold, imipenem was less effective than ampicillin in a mouse model [48], and meropenem clinical failure has been documented [49].

In an animal model of listerial meningitis, the addition of rifampin to ampicillin was no better than ampicillin alone. While some newer quinolones and linezolid show good in vitro activity, clinical experience is mixed [50–52], and, to date, too limited to support recommending these antimicrobials.

Although adjunctive corticosteroids have become the standard of care in the initial management of bacterial meningitis, their value in listerial infection remains unknown. Listeriae use iron as a virulence factor; therefore, in patients with iron deficiency, it seems prudent to withhold iron replacement until treatment of infection is completed.

Prevention

Cancer patients with hematological malignancies and/or those on corticosteroids should be advised to avoid certain foods. People at high risk for listeriosis may choose to avoid soft cheeses. It is best to avoid foods from deli counters, such as prepared salads, meats, and cheeses. Those at risk who choose to eat these high-risk foods should be instructed to thoroughly cook them, avoid cross-contamination, and only refrigerate cooked perishable foods for short periods of time [53].

Except from infected mother to fetus, human-to-human transmission of listeriosis does not occur; therefore, patients do not need to be isolated.

Listerial infections are effectively prevented by TMP-SMX given as *Pneumocystis* prophylaxis to those on long-term corticosteroids [54].

Nocardiosis

Introduction

Nocardia species are aerobic, Gram-positive, branching, filamentous, bacterial rods, which are beaded appearing and stain variably with the modified acid-fast Kinyoun stain. They fragment into pleomorphic, rod-shaped, or coccoid pieces. Their relatively slow growth can result in the cultures being discarded before the colonies can be seen. Nocardia are found most often in the environment in soil, water, and vegetable matter.

The key host defense against developing nocardiosis is cell-mediated immunity; the humoral immune response offers little protection. These organisms are considered opportunistic pathogens, causing infection in patients with impaired cell-mediated immune response, including patients with lymphoreticular neoplasia, organ transplantation, HIV/AIDS, diabetes mellitus, and alcoholism. In particular, there is a well-documented association between nocardiosis and chronic granulomatous disease (CGD) [55]. *Nocardia asteroides, N. farcinica, N. nova,* and *N. brasiliensis* are the most important causes of human infection.

Clinical Syndromes

Clinical syndromes caused by *Nocardia* species include nodular lymphangitis, systemic disease, pulmonary masses, nodules, infiltrates and cavities, and brain abscesses. Primary infection occurs via inhalation or direct inoculation of skin and soft tissues. Then, bloodstream dissemination can cause metastatic infection throughout the body, most commonly to the CNS. Sites of metastasis can include virtually any other anatomic site.

The most important site of primary infection is the lung. Common clinical symptoms include a subacute course (over days to weeks) of fever, cough, purulent sputum production, malaise, and dyspnea on exertion. Oxygenation is usually preserved at rest until disease has advanced. Chest radiograph findings can include focal or multifocal disease, nodules, or consolidations that can progress to cavities [56]. In one study from Spain, predisposing conditions for 31 pulmonary nocardiosis patients were transplantation (29%), HIV infection (19%), and treatment with steroids (64.5%) [57]. In this study, the median time to diagnosis was 42 days, and the mortality rate for pulmonary nocardiosis was 41 and 64% for disseminated nocardiosis.

In all cases of pulmonary nocardiosis, an MRI of the brain should be performed to evaluate for CNS infection. Like *L. monocytogenes, Nocardia* species have a particular tropism for the brain and spinal cord. CNS involvement is seen in 44% of cases of disseminated nocardiosis [58]. These lesions can be seen throughout the brain, and there may be meningitis with or without involvement of other portions of the brain. Clinical presentation is usually subacute to chronic, as with the pulmonary infection. One should consider brain biopsy for diagnosis in an immunosuppressed patient with a CNS lesion.

Nocardiosis in Cancer Patients

At M.D. Anderson Cancer Center between 1988 and 2001, 42 cancer patients were diagnosed with nocardiosis [59]. Twenty-seven patients (64%) had hematologic malignancies, and in 13 patients, nocardiosis complicated BMT. Patients had received steroids in 25 (58%) episodes of nocardiosis and had received chemotherapy within 30 days before the onset of nocardiosis in 10 (23%) episodes. Pulmonary nocardiosis was diagnosed in 30 of 43 cases (70%), while only one (2%) patient developed CNS nocardial infection. The mortality rate in this study was 60%.

In bone marrow transplant patients at one institution, the rate of nocardiosis was 1/554 (0.2%) among autologous BMT recipients and 5/302 (1.7%) in allogeneic BMT recipients from 1980 to 1994 [60]. Interestingly, three of the patients developed nocardiosis despite taking TMP-SMX for *Pneumocystis* prophylaxis. In a retrospective study of 27 patients with nocardiosis, 40% had taken TMP-SMX regularly prior to developing nocardiosis [61]. In another study of *Nocardia* infection in organ transplant recipients, 69% (24/35) of the case patients developed their infection while on TMP-SMX [62]. Clearly TMP-SMX is not protective against nocardial infections in patients the same way it is protective against listerial infections in the HIV positive population.

Diagnosis

The mainstay of diagnosing nocardiosis is to inform the laboratory that this diagnosis is being considered. The organism must be isolated from a clinical specimen, noting that *Nocardia* species are not common lab contaminants or oral flora. However, some patients with chronic lung disease can have transient nocardial carriage, which must be interpreted with caution. Often this diagnosis requires an invasive procedure such as a lung biopsy, skin biopsy, or brain biopsy. All biopsies should be evaluated by Gram stain, modified acid fast staining, culture, and pathology. Blood cultures for *Nocardia* species require prolonged incubation. The organism usually grows in 3–5 days.

Treatment

The mainstay of treatment of nocardiosis is TMP-SMX. High doses are used for patients with high disease burden or CNS disease. Second line therapy includes the combination of imipenem/cilastin and amikacin. Common recommendations for treatment include 3–6 weeks of intravenous therapy, followed by several months of oral therapy (1–3 months for nonimmunosuppressed and 6 months for immunosuppressed). In patients with CNS infection, a minimum of 12–15 months would be appropriate [63]. A recent report describes six cases of nocardiosis successfully treated with linezolid [64].

References

1. Bucholz U, Mascola L. Transmission, pathogenesis, and epidemiology of *Listeria monocytogenes*. Infect Dis Clin Pract. 2001;10:34–41.
2. Lorber B. Listeriosis. In: Goldfine H, Shen H, editors. Listeria monocytogenes: pathogenesis and host response. New York: Springer; 2007. p. 13–31.
3. Painter J, Slutsker L. Listeriosis in humans. In: Ryser ET, Marth EH, editors. Listeria, listeriosis and food safety. 3rd ed. Boca Raton: CRC Press; 2007. p. 85–109.
4. Ooi ST, Lorber B. Gastroenteritis due to *Listeria monocytogenes*. Clin Infect Dis. 2005;40:1327–32.
5. Bille J. *Listeria* and *erysipelothrix*. In: Murray PR, Baron EJ, Jorgensen JH, et al., editors. Manual of clinical microbiology. 9th ed. Washington, DC: American Society for Microbiology Press; 2007. p. 474–84.
6. Colodner R, Sakran W, Miron D, Teitler N, Khavalevsky E, Kopelowitz J. *Listeria monocytogenes* cross-contamination in a nursery. Am J Infect Control. 2003;31:322–4.
7. Farber JM, Daley E, Coates F, Beausoleil N, Fournier J. Feeding trials of *Listeria monocytogenes* with a nonhuman primate model. J Clin Microbiol. 1991;29:2606–8.
8. Schlech III WF, Chase DP, Badley A. A model of food-borne *Listeria monocytogenes* infection in the Sprague-Dawley rat using gastric inoculation: development and effect of gastric acidity on infective dose. Int J Food Microbiol. 1993;18:15–24.
9. Lorber B. Listeriosis. Clin Infect Dis. 1997;24:1–11.
10. Schnupf P, Portnoy DA. Listeriolysin O: a phagosome-specific lysin. Microbes Infect. 2007;9:1176–87.
11. Hamon M, Bierne H, Cossart P. *Listeria monocytogenes*: a multifaceted model. Nat Rev. 2006;4:423–34.
12. Drevets DA, Leenen PJ, Greenfield RA. Invasion of the central nervous system by intracellular bacteria. Clin Microbiol Rev. 2004;17:323–47.
13. Dramsi S, Lévi S, Triller A, Cossart P. Entry of *Listeria monocytogenes* into neurons occurs by cell-to-cell spread: an in vitro study. Infect Immun. 1998;66:4461–8.
14. Ampel NM, Bejarano GC, Saavedra Jr M. Deferoxamine increases the susceptibility of beta-thalassemic, iron-overloaded mice to infection with *Listeria monocytogenes*. Life Sci. 1992;50:1327–32.
15. Schuchat A, Swaminathan B, Broome CV. Epidemiology of human listeriosis. Clin Microbiol Rev. 1991;4:169–83.
16. Schlech III WF, Lavigne PM, Bortolussi RA, Allen AC, Haldane EV, Wort AJ, et al. Epidemic listeriosis – evidence for transmission by food. N Engl J Med. 1983;308:203–6.
17. Farber JM, Peterkin PI. *Listeria monocytogenes*, a food-borne pathogen. Microbiol Rev. 1991;55:476–511.
18. Gottlieb SL, Newbern EC, Griffin PM, Graves LM, Hoekstra RM, Baker NL, et al. Multistate outbreak of listeriosis linked to turkey deli meat and subsequent changes in US regulatory policy. Clin Infect Dis. 2006;42:29–36.
19. Tappero JW, Schuchat A, Deaver KA, Mascola L, Wenger JD. Reduction in the incidence of human listeriosis in the United States. Effectiveness of prevention efforts? The Listeriosis Study Group. JAMA. 1995;273:1118–22.
20. Swaminathan B, Gerner-Smidt P. The epidemiology of human listeriosis. Microbes Infect. 2007;9:1236–43.
21. Patil AB, Nadiger S, Chandrasekhar MR, Halesh LH, Kumar M. *Listeria monocytogenes* meningitis: an uncommon opportunistic infection in HIV/AIDS. Ind J Pathol Microbiol. 2007;50:671–3.
22. Mizuno S, Zendejas IR, Reed AI, Kim RD, Howard RJ, Hemming AW, et al. *Listeria monocytogenes* following orthotopic liver transplantation: central nervous system involvement and review of the literature. World J Gastroenterol. 2007;13:4391–3.
23. Williams G, Khan AA, Schweiger F. Listeria meningitis complicating infliximab treatment for Crohn's disease. Can J Infect Dis Microbiol. 2005;16:289–92.
24. La Montagna G, Valentini G. *Listeria monocytogenes* meningitis in a patient receiving etanercept for Still's disease. Clin Exp Rheumatol. 2005;23:121.
25. Virna S, Deckert M, Lütjen S, Soltek S, Foulds KE, Shen H, et al. TNF is important for pathogen control and limits brain damage in murine cerebral listeriosis. J Immunol. 2006;177:3972–82.
26. Stanley NF. Studies of *Listeria monocytogenes*. I. Isolation of a monocytosis-producing agent (MPA). Aust J Exp Biol Med Sci. 1949;27:123–31.
27. Mylonakis E, Paliou M, Hohmann EL, Calderwood SB, Wing EJ. Listeriosis during pregnancy. A case series and review of 222 cases. Medicine. 2002;81:260–9.
28. Bakardjiev AI, Theriot JA, Portnoy D. *Listeria monocytogenes* traffics from maternal organs to the placenta and back. PLoS Pathogens. 2006;2:e66.
29. Bakardjiev AI, Stacy BA, Portnoy DA. Growth of *Listeria monocytogenes* in the guinea pig placenta and role of cell-to-cell spread in fetal infection. J Infect Dis. 2005;191:1889–97.
30. Ciesielski CA, Hightower AW, Parsons SK, Broome CV. Listeriosis in the United States: 1980–1982. Arch Intern Med. 1988;148:1416–9.
31. Nieman RE, Lorber B. Listeriosis in adults: a changing pattern. Report of eight cases and review of the literature, 1968–1978. Rev Infect Dis. 1980;2:207–27.
32. Schuchat A, Robinson K, Wenger JD, Harrison LH, Farley M, Reingold AL, et al. Bacterial meningitis in the United States in 1995. N Engl J Med. 1997;337:970–6.
33. Safdar A, Armstrong D. Listeriosis in patients at a comprehensive cancer center, 1955–1997. Clin Infect Dis. 2003;37:359–64.
34. Mylonakis E, Hohmann EL, Calderwood SB. Central nervous system infection with *Listeria monocytogenes*. 33 years' experience at a general hospital and review of 776 episodes from the literature. Medicine. 1998;77:313–36.
35. Clauss HE, Lorber B. CNS infection with *Listeria monocytogenes*. Curr Infect Dis Rep. 2008;10:300–6.
36. Brouwer MC, van de Beek D, Heckenberg SG, Spanjaard L, de Gans J. Community-acquired *Listeria monocytogenes* meningitis in adults. Clin Infect Dis. 2006;43:1233–8.
37. Armstrong RW, Fung PC. Brainstem encephalitis (rhombencephalitis) due to *Listeria monocytogenes:* case report and review. Clin Infect Dis. 1993;16:689–702.
38. Alper G, Knepper L, Kanal E. MR findings in listerial rhombencephalitis. AJNR Am J Neuroradiol. 1996;17:593–6.
39. Eckburg PB, Montoya JG, Vosti KL. Brain abscess due to *Listeria monocytogenes*. Five cases and a review of the literature. Medicine. 2001;80:223–35.
40. Cone LA, Leung MM, Byrd RG, Annunziata GM, Lam RY, Herman BK. Multiple cerebral abscesses because of *Listeria monocytogenes*: three case reports and a literature review of supratentorial listerial brain abscess(es). Surg Neurol. 2003;59:320–8.
41. Louria DB, Hensle T, Armstrong D, Collins HS, Blevins A, Krugman D, et al. Listeriosis complicating malignant disease. A new association. Ann Intern Med. 1967;67:261–81.
42. Anaissie E, Kontoyiannis DP, O'Brien S, Kantarjian H, Robertson L, Lerner S, et al. Listeriosis in patients with chronic lymphocytic leukemia who were treated with fludarabine and prednisone. Ann Intern Med. 1992;117:466–9.
43. Rivero GA, Torres HA, Rolston KV, Kontoyiannis DP. *Listeria monocytogenes* infection in patients with cancer. Diagn Microbiol Infect Dis. 2003;47:393–8.
44. Lorber B. Clinical listeriosis-implications for pathogenesis. In: Miller AJ, Smith JL, Somkuti GA, editors. Foodborne listeriosis. New York: Elsevier; 1990. p. 41–9.

45. Dalton CB, Austin CC, Sobel J, Hayes PS, Bibb WF, Graves LM, et al. An outbreak of gastroenteritis and fever due to *Listeria monocytogenes* in milk. N Engl J Med. 1997;336:100–5.
46. Chatzipanagiotou S, Hof H. Sera from patients with high titers of antibody to streptolysin 0 react with listeriolysin. J Clin Microbiol. 1988;26:1066–7.
47. Greisen K, Loeffelholz M, Purohit A, Leong D. PCR primers and probes for the 16S rRNA gene of most species of pathogenic bacteria, including bacteria found in cerebrospinal fluid. J Clin Microbiol. 1994;32:335–51.
48. Kim KS. In vitro and in vivo studies of imipenem – cilastatin alone and in combination with gentamicin against *Listeria monocytogenes*. Antimicrob Agents Chemother. 1986;29:289–93.
49. Stepanović S, Lazarević G, Ješić M, Kos R. Meropenem therapy failure in *Listeria monocytogenes* infection. Eur J Clin Microbiol Infect Dis. 2004;23:484–6.
50. Grumbach NM, Mylonakis E, Wing EJ. Development of listerial meningitis during ciprofloxacin treatment. Clin Infect Dis. 1999;29:1340–1.
51. Viale P, Furlanut M, Cristini F, Cadeo B, Pavan F, Pea F. Major role of levofloxacin in the treatment of a case of *Listeria monocytogenes* meningitis. Diagn Microbiol Infect Dis. 2007;58:137–9.
52. Leiti O, Gross JW, Tuazon CU. Treatment of brain abscess caused by *Listeria monocytogenes* in a patient with allergy to penicillin and trimethoprim-sulfamethoxazole. Clin Infect Dis. 2005;40:907–8.
53. Goulet V. What can we do to prevent listeriosis in 2006? Clin Infect Dis. 2007;44:529–30.
54. Dworkin MS, Williamson J, Jones JL, Kaplan JE. Prophylaxis with trimethoprim-sulfamethoxasole for human immunodeficiency virus-infected patients: impact on risk for infectious diseases. Clin Infect Dis. 2001;33:393–8.
55. Dorman SE, Guide SV, Conville PS, DeCarlo ES, Malech HL, Gallin JI, et al. *Nocardia* infection in chronic granulomatous disease. Clin Infect Dis. 2002;35:390–4.
56. Lerner PI. Nocardiosis. Clin Infect Dis. 1996;22:891–903.
57. Martínez TR, Menéndez VR, Reyes CS, Santos DM, Vallés Tarazona JM, Modesto AM, et al. Pulmonary nocardiosis: risk factors and outcomes. Respirology. 2007;12:394–400.
58. Beaman BL, Beaman L. *Nocardia* species: host-parasite relationships. Clin Microbiol Rev. 1994;7:213–64.
59. Torres HA, Reddy BT, Raad II, Tarrand J, Bodey GP, Hanna HA, et al. Nocardiosis in cancer patients. Medicine. 2002;81:388–97.
60. Chouciño C, Goodman SA, Greer JP, Stein RS, Wolff SN, Dummer JS. Nocardial infections in bone marrow transplant recipients. Clin Infect Dis. 2002;23:1012–9.
61. Van Burik J, Hackman RC, Nadeem SQ, Hiemenz JW, White MH, Flowers ME, et al. Nocardiosis after bone marrow transplantation: a retrospective study. Clin Infect Dis. 1997;24:1154–60.
62. Peleg AY, Husain S, Qureshi ZA, Silveira FP, Sarumi M, Shutt KA, et al. Risk factors, clinical characteristics, and outcome of *Nocardia* infection in organ transplant recipients: a matched case-control study. Clin Infect Dis. 2007;44:1307–14.
63. Byrne E, Brophy BP, Perrett LV. *Nocardia* cerebral abscess: new concepts in diagnosis, management, and prognosis. J Neurol Neurosurg Psychiatry. 1979;42:1038–45.
64. Moylett EH, Pacheco SE, Brown-Elliott BA, Perry TR, Buescher ES, Birhimngham MC, et al. Clinical experience with linezolid for the treatment of Nocardia infection. Clin Infect Dis. 2003;36:313–8.

Chapter 38
Antibacterial Distribution and Drug–Drug Interactions in Cancer Patients

Ursula Theuretzbacher and Markus Zeitlinger

Abstract Cancer as such does not impact distribution of antimicrobials; however, various pathophysiological changes in cancer patients may do so. Neutropenia, cachexia, hypoproteinemia, and effusions are common situations in cancer patients that may change the concentrations of antibiotics in blood and tissues. Such changes should be taken into account and dosage regimens adapted accordingly. As the therapeutic management of cancer patients becomes more complex, drug–drug interactions in oncology are of particular importance. Commonly used antibiotics that are most likely involved in drug–drug interactions are rifampin and its derivates, the macrolides erythromycin and clarithromycin, the fluoroquinolone ciprofloxacin, and trimethoprim/sulfonamide combinations. Knowing the interaction profiles of individual agents and potential outcomes of the interaction allows healthcare providers to minimize the risk.

Keywords Pharmacokinetics • Pharmacodynamics • Distribution • Antibiotics • Interaction • Cancer

Infections are a frequent complication of patients suffering from cancer. Cancer can affect all age groups and may, due to its often progressive character, transform a person with intact organ functions into a critically ill patient. Therefore, the cancer patient requiring antimicrobial therapy might have normal physiology or, in the later stage of the disease, may suffer from severe impairment of body functions including organ dysfunction, sepsis, and shock. In its first part, the present chapter reviews the basic concepts of pharmacokinetics of antibiotics applicable to all patients and then focuses on specific alterations frequently observed in cancer patients.

As patients suffering from cancer often receive a wide range of concomitant medication coincident with their need for antimicrobial therapy, the second part of the chapter will discuss relevant drug–drug interactions in cancer patients requiring antibiotic treatment.

Introduction to Pharmacokinetics

Pharmacokinetics describes the concentration-time profile of a drug within the organism. Its main determinants are dose, absorption, distribution, metabolism, and elimination. Absorption, distribution, metabolism, and elimination (ADME) in turn are influenced by the chemical properties of a drug and by the demographic and physiological characteristics of the organism, resulting in complex organism–drug interactions. Pharmacokinetic profiles can be characterized by a range of pharmacokinetic parameters like bioavailability, plasma protein binding, maximum concentration, area under the concentration-time curve, elimination half life, clearance, and volume of distribution.

- Bioavailability (BA, %): describes the percentage of a drug which becomes systemically available when the drug is not given intravenously.
- Plasma protein binding (PPB, %): is the percentage of a drug which is bound to circulating proteins in plasma. Only the free, unbound fraction (f) of an antibiotic is microbiologically active [1, 2].
- Maximum concentration (C_{max}, g/liter): highest drug concentration achieved during the dosing interval.
- Area under the concentration-time curve (AUC, g·hour/liter): describes the exposure of an organism toward a drug over time.
- Volume of distribution (Vd, liter): represents an approximate value for the distribution of a drug within the organism. As the volume of distribution is calculated only by use of the concentration-time profile in plasma, it is often referred to as "apparent" volume of distribution. This "apparent" volume of distribution can exceed the total volume of the body considerably, indicating accumulation of a drug outside the blood stream. Although volume of distribution can help to describe the penetration

U. Theuretzbacher (✉)
Center for Anti-Infective Agents, Eckpergasse 13, 1180 Vienna, Austria
e-mail: utheuretzbacher@cefaia.com

of a drug from the central compartment (blood) into tissues, the volume of distribution cannot be used to define exact concentrations in individual organs, tissues or tissue compartments.
- Elimination half life ($t_{1/2}$, hour): amount of time during which the concentration in plasma has decreased by 50%.
- Clearance (cl, liter/hour): volume of the body which is totally cleared from drug in a given time. It is an estimation of the potency of the body to eliminate a certain drug from the body. The pharmacological clearance is the sum of renal and extrarenal (mainly hepatic, transdermal and pulmonal) clearance.

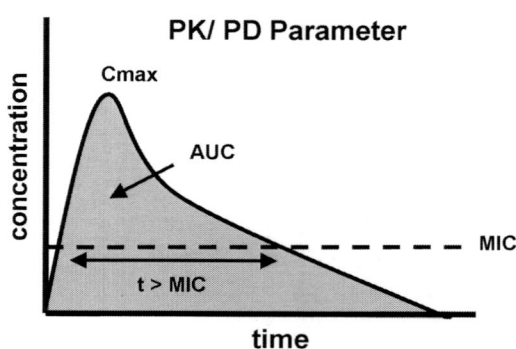

Fig. 38.1 PK/PD Parameters of antimicrobial therapy. Area under the concentration- time curve (AUC) and maximal concentration (C_{max}) divided by the minimal inhibitory concentration (MIC, C_{max}/MIC, AUC/MIC) as well as the time period during which the concentration of the antibiotic exceeds the MIC (t>MIC) of a pathogen are considered the most important PK/PD parameters. The unbound concentration of the drug should be used

Pharmacokinetic/Pharmacokodynamic Indices for Anti-Infective Therapy

Physicians are interested in clinical success or side effects of an antimicrobial agent rather than in its pharmacokinetic profile. In order to predict outcome of an antibacterial treatment by pharmacokinetic parameters they have to be related to pharmacodynamic action by use of pharmacokinetic/pharmacodynamic (PK/PD) indices. The pharmacodynamic action of an antimicrobial is commonly described by the minimal inhibitory concentration (MIC), i.e., the concentration of an antimicrobial drug at which no visible growth of a given bacterial strain can be observed after 24 h of incubation in a growth medium.

fC_{max} and $fAUC_{0-24}$ (free drug AUC over 24 h) to MIC-ratio (fC_{max}/MIC, $fAUC_{0-24}$/MIC) as well as the time (t) the free concentration of the antibiotic exceeds the MIC (ft>MIC) are considered as most important PK/PD indices [3–7]. The relevance of each of these indices for predicting antimicrobial and clinical outcome varies for different antimicrobial classes. For instance, beta-lactam-antibiotics, display a "time-dependent" pattern of activity and ft>MIC is considered most predictive for outcome. For these antibiotics frequent doses, sometimes even continuous infusions lead to best clinical results with lowest side effect rates [8]. In contrast, for antibiotics, such as aminoglycosides, fluoroquinolones, and most other antibiotics, the free drug AUC_{0-24}/MIC-ratio is a good predictive index and determines the antimicrobial efficacy. To achieve fast bacterial eradication, these antibiotics should be given infrequently in high doses as long as this is not precluded by toxicity. However, for aminoglycosides high doses administered once daily not only improves efficacy but also reduces side effects, as aminoglycoside uptake into body cells is saturable and its vestibulotoxicity and nephrotoxicity is higher with a more fractionated dose than with a single bolus [9]. Therefore, PK/PD considerations provide good tools for optimizing the dosage of antibiotics by minimizing toxicity, maximizing activity, and limiting resistance development. Figure 38.1 depicts PK/PD indices for antimicrobial therapy.

Impact of Cancer on Pharmacokinetics of Antimicrobial Agents

Impairment of organs that are responsible for elimination of drugs like kidney or liver impacts the pharmacokinetics of drugs. Although this is also the case for patients suffering from cancer, information on dosing in case of renal or hepatic impairment can be obtained from the approved label of each antibiotic and will not be further discussed here. Nevertheless, it should be noted that, as a general rule, antibiotics with narrow therapeutic index should be used cautiously after cytotoxic chemotherapy has been employed, e.g., aminoglycoside therapy after treatment with cisplatin [10].

Usually, antimicrobial breakpoints are based on pharmacokinetic parameters obtained from blood of healthy subjects during early phases of drug development. However, it is known that disease may alter pharmacokinetics of antibiotics. A wide range of data is available regarding the change of pharmacokinetics of antibiotics in sepsis and septic shock, a disease which alters various functions of the human body [11–13]. Therefore, regulatory authorities like EMA (European Medicines Agency) and FDA (Food and Drug Administration) recommend evaluating pharmacokinetics of antimicrobials in the target population rather than in healthy volunteers [14, 15]. If available, concentrations obtained from the target site of infection should be considered as basis for PK/PD models in order to predict efficacy of antimicrobial therapy in the relevant clinical population [16].

Cancer as such does not impact pharmacokinetics of antimicrobials; however, various pathophysiological changes in cancer patients may do so. For instance, underexposure to an antibiotic might occur because of increased volume of distribution due to oedema, ascites or pleural effusion [17, 18]. In this case ascites or other pathological compartments with high content of water can be considered part of the central compartment when effects of distribution for hydrophilic agents like beta-lactams or aminoglycosides are studied [19, 20]. Another case type is effusions with high protein content. These may bind antibiotics followed by slow back distribution into systemic circulation and prolongation of overall elimination half life [21].

Neutropenia and Neutropenic Fever

Neutropenia is a typical complication of cytostatic chemotherapy. Patients with neutrophil count below 1,000 cells per µl have an increased susceptibility to infection [22]. Antibiotics are frequently prescribed both for treatment of neutropenic fever and prophylactically to reduce the risk of infection.

Beta-lactams show important changes in pharmacokinetics associated with neutropenia [22]. A substantially shorter elimination half life and decreased AUCs of ceftazidime were found in patients with neutropenia compared to healthy elderly patients [23]. Similarly, cefpirome, imipenem, and meropenem showed marked increase in the volume of distribution in patients with neutropenia compared with controls [24, 25]. Due to these pharmacokinetic changes, continuous administration preceded by a loading dose was advocated for beta-lactams in this indication [22].

Various aminoglycoside pharmacokinetic changes have been reported in patients with neutropenia. Amikacin, gentamicin, and tobramycin all showed increased volume of distribution and faster clearance compared to healthy volunteers resulting in reduced average peak concentrations [26–28]. In order to maintain therapeutic drug concentrations, dose adjustment was necessary in some cases [29]. Similar to other indications, once daily administration seems to be comparable or even superior to more frequent dosing of aminoglycosides. An increase of serum creatinine was delayed and less pronounced when amikacin was given once daily compared to once every 8 h [30]. Likewise, higher efficacy and lower toxicity was observed for once vs. thrice daily administration of tobramycin to neutropenic children [31]. Nowadays, the once daily administration of aminoglycoside in neutropenic patients is an accepted dosage regime.

Similar to other antimicrobial classes, increased volume of distribution and clearance was observed for vancomycin and partially also for teicoplanin in neutropenic patients [22, 32, 33]. For vancomycin, substantially reduced elimination half life was reported. Careful monitoring of serum trough concentration is recommended for glycopeptides.

Daptomycin, measured after a standard dose of 6 mg/kg, achieved mean AUC levels in patients with neutropenic fever that where modestly below those observed for healthy volunteers (521 vs. 730 µg×h/mL) [34, 35]. However, high interindividual differences among patients (SD 524 µg×h/mL) seem to be clinically more important. Therefore, in case of a poor clinical response of an individual patient despite in vitro antimicrobial activity of an antibiotic, changed pharmacokinetics should be considered and appropriate modification of the antimicrobial regime initiated.

In contrast, the pharmacokinetics of linezolid in patients with neutropenia did not differ from the overall compassionate use population [36]. We have only insufficient data regarding fluoroquinolones for this indication.

Surgery

Another typical indication for antimicrobial treatment in cancer patients is surgical antimicrobial prophylaxes in elective tumor surgery. Similar to sepsis postsurgical conditions, especially after major interventions, might negatively impact penetration of antibiotics into tissue as demonstrated for piperacillin or levofloxacin [37, 38]. Thus, antibiotics with wide therapeutic index in high doses should be preferred in surgical indications.

Oral bioavailability of ciprofloxacin was reduced in surgery patients on the first days after the intervention. Therefore, intravenous administration of ciprofloxacin in the early period after elective surgery is required [39].

Cachexia

Cachexia may have significant impact on pharmacokinetics of antibiotics [40]. While descriptive pharmacokinetic data are in line with the well documented difficulties for correct dosing of cytostatic chemotherapy in cachectic patients [41, 42], the pathophysiological mechanism is still speculative. Possible changes may include:

- Cachexia and the frequently associated parenteral nutrition may influence the fluid and electrolyte status of the patient [43]. For gentamicin and amikacin, parenteral nutrition resulted in enhanced volume of distribution and reduced peak serum concentration, possibly impacting

effectiveness of these "concentration dependent" antibiotics [26, 43, 44]. Due to the high interindividual differences of aminoglycoside pharmacokinetics, serum concentrations should be frequently measured and the dosing regimen individualized as quickly as possible [26].
- Impact on the absorption process of orally administered drugs: bioavailability of cefuroxime in a cachexia rat model was lower than in animals with normal diet, possibly due to changes in the small intestine [40]. As bioavailability always might be impacted by severe disease, cancer patients with life-threatening infections should get parenteral antibiotics.
- Impaired protein status in malnourished or cachectic patients may lead to higher volume of distribution and modified pharmacodynamic action as unbound drug may more readily diffuse into tissues and interact with targets. In addition, low protein binding might also lead to enhanced renal clearance. As previously discussed, oedema, ascites, and pleural effusion may result in retention of drug in these pathological compartments.
- On the other hand, severely malnourished patients may exhibit decreased oxidative metabolism and reduced glomerular filtration rate leading to higher concentrations in plasma than expected from healthy subjects [42, 45].

These to some extend contradictory mechanisms might explain why cachexia may result both in increase of plasma levels as observed for metronidazole and tetracycline [45, 46] or reduction of AUC as demonstrated for cefuroxime and aminoglycosides [40, 43, 44]. Severity of cachexia, as well as the class of antibiotic influences the pharmacokinetics of the antimicrobial agent.

Hypoproteinemia

Independent of cachexia, changes in protein binding might affect the pharmacokinetics of antibiotics. Numerous conditions such as age (e.g., in neonates), body temperature, plasma pH or a variety of diseases like uremia, hepatitis, hypoalbuminemia, acute viral hepatitis, cirrhosis, nephrotic syndrome, and epilepsy may lead to significant decreases in protein binding [47]. Albumin has the highest binding capacity of all human serum proteins for drugs including antimicrobials [48, 49]. Other proteins which might bind antibiotics include transferrin, lactoferrin, and alpha-1-acid Glycoprotein [50].

Particularly in cases of highly bound antibiotics, pharmacokinetics might be modified by hypoalbuminuriaemia. For ceftriaxone, a cephalosporin that binds strongly to albumin, a significant increase of volume of distribution was detected in steady state conditions. AUC values for free ceftriaxone in these patients were twice as high as for healthy volunteers suggesting favorable antimicrobial activity in these patients.

Table 38.1 Protein binding of selected antimicrobials[a]

Quinolones	Ciprofloxacin: 20–30%
	Levofloxacin: 30–40%
	Moxifloxacin: 40%
Glycopeptides/lipopeptides	Vancomycin: 55%
	Teicoplanin: 90–95%
	Daptomycin: 90%
Aminoglycosides	Gentamicin: <10%
	Amikacin: <10%
	Tobramycin: <10%
Cephalosporins	Cefuroxime: 50%
	Cefotaxime: 25–40%
	Ceftazidime: 10%
	Ceftriaxone: 85–95%
	Cefepime: 19%
Penicillins	Amoxicillin: 17–20%
	Ampicillin: 15%
	Piperacillin: 30%
Carbapenems	Imipenem: 20%
	Meropenem: 2%
	Ertapenem: 92–95%
	Doripenem: 8%
Tetracyclines	Doxycycline: 82%
	Tigecycline: 71–89%
Other	Fosfomycin: 0%
	Linezolid: 31%

[a]Obtained by the respective approved label

On the other hand, for drugs with a narrower therapeutic range but high degree of protein binding (>80%), hypoproteinemia can increase toxicity.

Even in case of antibiotics with low protein binding like amikacin, decreased protein concentration in serum might have a clinical impact. Hypoalbuminemia has been identified as an independent risk factor for aminoglycoside nephrotoxicity [51]. In patients with serum albumin below 3.0 g/dL, amikacin obtained higher peak concentrations and produced significantly more episodes of nephrotoxicity than in patients with albumin level above 3.0 g/dL [51]. However, hypoproteinemia doesn't influence pharmacokinetics or toxicity of all antibiotics as has been shown via experiments in sheep with artificial hypoproteinemia when dosed with minocycline, a tetracycline with moderate protein binding [52]. Table 38.1 provides a list of percentage of protein binding for important parenteral antibiotics.

Tissue Infections

Although the majority of PK/PD models are based on plasma concentrations, many infections do not occur in blood but in tissues. Antimicrobial agents need to reach appropriate target site concentrations to exert their antimicrobial effect. The site of tissue infections, i.e., the location of the bacteria, and thereby the target site of antimicrobial action is represented by the interstitial fluid of tissues and other body fluids such as pleural fluid, bronchial fluid, epithelial lining fluid, middle ear fluid, and cerebrospinal fluid [53]. Homogenized whole tissue samples do not represent the site of infection because bacteria and antibiotics are not distributed evenly in the distinct pharmacological compartments of a tissue. The concentrations of antimicrobials vary in the compartments of complex organs like lung or brain [54, 55] due to the anatomy and the histological structure of the organ and to the physicochemical properties of the drug. For example in case of respiratory tract infections, concentrations may be measured by sampling of sputum, respiratory secretions, pleural fluid, and surgical collection of whole lung tissue and bronchial mucosa, each yielding concentrations for different compartments of the respiratory system and yet none of these may provide adequate information about the site of infection [55, 56]. As for pneumonia, bacteria indeed may be located in the epithelial lining fluid, bronchial mucosa, the interstitial fluid of lung, and in rare cases even within cells. Depending on the pathogen and its location, concentrations of antibiotics should be determined at this infection site and correlated to the pharmacodynamic parameter (usually MIC). In case of pneumonia the site of infection due to extracellular pathogens (pneumococci and most other clinically relevant microorganisms) is the intraalveolar space (epithelial lining fluid) and in later phases, the interstitial fluid of the lung tissue. If intracellular pathogens (Mycobacterium tuberculous, Chlamydia pneumonia) are involved, an additional infection site is represented by alveolar macrophages [55, 57]. The measurement of target site concentrations remains an ongoing challenge, due to methodological obstacles and ethical limitations.

It has been shown that interstitial tissue fluid to plasma equilibration of antimicrobial agents may significantly differ between healthy volunteers and critically ill patients [11, 12, 38]. In addition, high interindividual differences in interstitial tissue fluid penetration should be expected among septic patients, since hemodynamics and treatment strategies substantially vary within this patient group [58, 59]. These high interindividual differences in interstitial tissue fluid penetration might explain the observation that antimicrobial therapy lacks efficiency in some patients, despite documented in vitro susceptibility of the causative pathogen showing that the same pathogen is eradicated in patients with more favorable penetration to the site of infection. Strategies to identify patients with a high risk of not reaching sufficient levels at the site of infection are necessary steps in the successful antimicrobial therapy of critically ill patients [60]. In several in vitro and animal studies, inappropriate target site concentrations have been associated with the development of bacterial resistance [3, 61, 62].

Malignant effusions as a potential factor influencing systemic pharmacokinetics of antimicrobials were discussed above. However, in cancer patients malignant effusions frequently also manifest as a site of potential infections and thus a target site of antimicrobial therapy. Ascites and pleural effusions will be briefly discussed as two important representatives of artificial compartments susceptible to infections.

Pleural effusion usually impacts systemic pharmacokinetics less than ascites due to its smaller amount of fluid. For example, plasma pharmacokinetics of cefoxitin, a cephalosporin used as prophylaxis in surgery, was not impacted by pleural effusion [63]. Although accumulation outside the blood stream is not typical for hydrophilic antimicrobials like cephalosporins, concentrations in pleural fluid for cefuroxime and cefoxitin were comparable or even higher than in systemic circulation [20, 63]. For ascites, maximum concentrations of cefuroxime, a cephalosporin with moderate protein binding, clearly exceeded corresponding concentrations in plasma [20]. In contrast, in pleural effusion fluid concentrations of the highly protein bound ceftriaxone were below than those observed in plasma throughout the dosing interval [21, 64].

Thus, high protein binding seems to prevent sufficient penetration of antibiotics into ascites or pleural fluid. The high amount of protein frequently present in malignant ascites or pleural effusions may additionally reduce the antimicrobial activity at this site. Use of antibiotics with moderate protein binding (below 50%) seems more advisable in this indication.

Drug–Drug Interactions in Cancer Patients

As the therapeutic management of cancer patients becomes more complex, drug interactions in oncology are of particular importance [65]. Unrecognized interactions can lead to overdosing, undertreatment, or potentiation of side effects, each with severe clinical consequences. In addition to cytotoxic chemotherapy, most patients receive supportive care agents such as pain, emesis, depression, seizures, and anti-infective medications. Older oncology patients with multiple comorbidities require medications for comorbid conditions such as cardiovascular, gastrointestinal, and rheumatological diseases and are, thus, at even higher risk of drug–drug interactions [66, 67]. Such medications are most commonly implicated in interactions in cancer patients [68]. According to a study in older oncology outpatients with an average of three comorbid conditions and an average of nine prescription and nonprescription drugs, cardiovascular drugs were the most common medications [69]. Increased availability of over-the-counter (OTC) medication and herbal supplements for self-treatment can all contribute to polypharmacy in this population and is often unknown to the healthcare team [70]. Hanigan et al. reported that 96% of patients took prescription drugs within 3 days prior to chemotherapy, 71% reported taking OTCs, and 69% reported supplement use. On average, patients took 9.6 concomitant medications 3 days prior to chemotherapy. Many of these concomitant medications alter drug metabolism and/or disposition [71]. Additionally, some patients are also exposed to duplicate medications, most often corticosteroids, proton pump inhibitors, or benzodiazepines [68].

Concerning polypharmacy and the chronic use of multiple drugs in patients with cancer and polymorbidities, very limited data exist on their frequency and clinical consequences [72]. To quantify the frequency of potential drug interactions unrelated to chemotherapy in cancer patients and to define risk factors for such interactions, Riechelmann et al. analyzed patient charts [73]. In this study population, 63% of screened patients were at risk for at least one potential drug interaction during their stay and only 25% of these potential interactions were rated as minor. According to this study, the most frequent combinations encountered with potential for interaction were opioids with benzodiazepines, Selective Serotonin Reuptake Inhibitors (SSRI) with opioids, Non-Steroidal Anti-Inflammatory Drugs (NSAID) with low-molecular-weight heparin, dexamethasone with phenytoin, and omeprazole with benzodiazepines. However, not all potential interactions resulted in clinically significant effects [73]. As expected, the potential interactions were found to be more likely to occur in patients with longer hospital stays, those receiving a higher number of medications, and those with risk factors that are more likely to be encountered among older patients with cancer.

For drugs in clinical development, the potential for interactions is usually assessed early on using suitable in vitro probes and careful selection of interacting drugs for early in vivo studies [74]. However, the interaction profile of a drug may not be fully understood until several years after it is introduced onto the market. Given the reality of polypharmacy and the number of clinical problems faced by patients with cancer, a proportion of cancer patients with drug interactions are likely to have serious complications. In addition to case reports, clinical data needs to be generated to raise awareness of this increasingly common problem that may further reduce quality of life of cancer patients.

Management of Potential Drug Interactions

Potential harmful consequences of polypharmacy can only be averted if the mechanism and principles of drug interactions are understood and recognized in advance. As there are rarely well designed clinical studies available, prediction of potential drug interactions must be made based on what is known about the interactive properties of drugs. Being aware of the potential for interactions allows healthcare providers to minimize risk by applying the following principles:

- Avoiding unnecessary polypharmacy including OTC, food additives, and herbs.
- Identifying patients at high risk for developing interactions (i.e., narrow therapeutic range of the medication, decreased hepatic and/or renal function).
- Knowing the interaction profiles of individual agents and potential outcomes of the interaction: Decreased effects may mean a loss of therapeutic effect. Increased effects may mean increased effectiveness, or increased side effects.
- Weighing the risk of the interaction against the benefits of concurrent therapy to the patient.
- Determining if the interaction applies to all drugs within the same class or just a subset.
- Selecting an alternative agent with less interaction potential.
- Actively managing potential interactions by alteration of administration schedules, dosage adjustments, additional patient monitoring.

Usually, antibiotics are used empirically for therapy of acute signs of infections but also used prophylactically for reducing the risk of febrile neutropenia. In general, antibacterial agents – with the exception of rifamycin derivates (rifampin, rifabutin, rifapentine), macrolides (erythromycin and clarithromycin), fluoroquinolones (ciprofloxacin), and trimethoprim/sulfonamide – are rarely implicated in major clinically relevant drug interaction problems. In patients without concurrent tuberculous or other mycobacterial infections, rifamycin derivates and macrolides usually can be avoided. Ciprofloxacin is commonly prescribed for cancer outpatients [75]. The risk of interactions in patients who receive multiple medications needs to be considered including additional monitoring that should be followed if ciprofloxacin can't be avoided. Cotrimoxazole (trimethoprim/sulfamethoxazole) can usually be substituted with other antibiotics for treatment of common bacterial infections.

Principles of Drug Interactions

Drug interactions can be pharmaceutical (in vitro inactivation), pharmacokinetic, or pharmacodynamic. Pharmacodynamic drug interactions may increase or decrease the clinical effects of drugs even without altered drug concentrations. The risk of side effects also may greatly increase.

Drug interactions may have wanted or unwanted effects. The following review will focus on unwanted pharmacokinetic interactions between antibiotics and other drugs that are commonly used in cancer patients. The most important and most common pharmacokinetic drug interactions involving antibiotics are altered drug absorption, inhibition or induction of metabolism, and inhibition of renal excretion. Transporter-based interactions have been increasingly documented such as the inhibition or induction of transport proteins, such as P-glycoprotein (P-gp) by erythromycin [76]. Overlapping substrate specificities with cytochrome P450 enzymes result in complex and sometimes perplexing pharmacokinetic profiles of multidrug regimens [77]. The effects of an interaction may take from several hours to several days to become clinically significant and may last beyond the time period of concurrent administration.

Interactions Affecting Drug Absorption

A number of mechanisms can affect drug absorption including a change in gastric pH, chelation, ion exchange, change in gastric motility, alteration in gut flora, modulation of transport proteins, or inhibition of intestinal enzymes. Indeed bioavailability may be reduced by as much as 90%. Examples in the field of antibiotics include chelation of tetracyclines and quinolones with di-and trivalent cations such as the aluminum or magnesium in antacids, calcium in dairy products, highly buffered drugs, ferrous sulfate in iron replacement agents, and multivitamin preparations with zinc. To prevent chelation of intravenous formulations, quinolones should not be coadministered in the same IV line with a multivalent cation, e.g., magnesium. Even if the impaired absorption and reduced concentration of oral quinolones as a consequence of this absorption interaction is not clinically apparent, it may influence the development of resistance. In a study with over 3,000 patients who received a course of oral levofloxacin, coadministration of divalent, or trivalent cation-containing compounds was significantly associated with subsequent identification of a levofloxacin-resistant isolate [78].

Many absorption interactions can be managed by adjusting the administration schedule to avoid the loss of drug activity. The recommended separation time required between the quinolones and chelating agents varies from two (ciprofloxacin, levofloxacin) to 4 h (moxifloxacin) with antibiotics administered first.

Interactions Based on Drug Metabolism and Transporters

The majority of reported drug interactions are due to drug metabolism inhibition. Cytochrome P450 enzymes are essential for the metabolism of many medications. Although this class has more than 50 enzymes, six of them metabolize 90% of drugs, with the two most significant enzymes being CYP3A4 and CYP2D6 [79]. Individual isoforms are capable of interacting with a wide range of diverse substrates and some CYPs have overlapping substrate specificities. In general, drugs that are metabolized via the cytochrome P450 system should alert clinicians and demand special considerations. Clinicians are encouraged to have a sound knowledge on drugs that behave as substrates, inhibitors, or inducers of CYP3A4, and take proper cautions and close monitoring for potential drug interactions when using such drugs [80, 81].

- P-glycoprotein is a transmembrane protein that controls concentrations of endogenous and exogenous substances across cell membranes by functioning as cellular efflux pumps [82]. Genetic variability in the expression and production of P-gp has a significant effect on the bioavailability and site distribution of many drugs. Both CYP3A4/CYP3A5 and the transporter P-gp are frequently coexpressed in the same cells and share a large number of substrates and modulators. The disposition of such drugs is thus affected by both metabolism and transport.
- A cytochrome P450 inhibitor is any drug that inhibits the metabolism of a cytochrome P450 substrate. Such inhibition may cause reduced metabolism of the substrate and thus increased concentrations with the potential of toxic effects. Clinically, the most important CYP3A4 inhibitors include:
  - HIV protease inhibitors (e.g., ritonavir)
  - Macrolide antibiotics (e.g., erythromycin, clarithromycin)
  - Antidepressants (e.g., fluoxetine and fluvoxamine)
  - Calcium channel blockers (e.g., verapamil, and diltiazem)
  - Antifungals (e.g., ketoconazole, itraconazole)
  - H_2-receptor antagonists (e.g., cimetidine)
  - Steroids and their modulators (e.g., gestodene and mifepristone)
  - Several herbal and dietary components (e.g., grapefruit juice)

- A cytochrome P450 inducer increases the amount of P450 enzyme and may accelerate clearance of a substrate which causes decreased and potentially ineffective concentrations. Typical potent inducers are rifampin, phenytoin, phenobarbital, and ritonavir. St John's Wort induces the expression of P-gp and decreases concentrations of P-gp substrates [83]. The effect of a cytochrome P450 inducer can occur within 24 h up to 1 week after administration [84]. Induction persists for several days.
- A cytochrome P450 substrate is any drug that is metabolized by one or more of the P450 isoenzymes (Table 38.2). A drug that is metabolized by cytochrome P450 isoenzymes becomes vulnerable to interference by other drugs that are either inhibiting or inducing the enzyme system.

Table 38.2 Selected substrates of cytochrome P450 isoenzymes (modified from [76, 77, 79, 80, 84, 107–109])

CYP 3A4 substrates
Antiarrhythmics, benzodiazepines, immune modulators, HIV protease inhibitors, antihistamines, calcium channel blockers, statins, macrolides, itraconazole and ketoconazole

CYP2C9 substrates
NSAIDs, oral hypoglycemic agents, angiotensin II blockers, celecoxib, fluvastatin, naproxen, phenytoin, sulfamethoxazole, tamoxifen, torsemide, warfarin

2B6 substrates
Bupropion, cyclophosphamide, ifosfamide

CYP 2C8 substrates
NSAIDs, oral antidiabetic drugs, warfarin, statins, paclitaxel, digoxin, amiodarone, verapamil, zopiclone, voriconazole

CYP2C19 substrates
Proton pump inhibitors, antiepileptics, amitrptyline, clomipramine, clopidogrel, cyclophosphamide, progesterone, voriconazole

Table 38.3 Influence of antibiotics on Cytochrome P450 isoenzymes and P-gp [76, 105, 108–110]

Drug	Inhibitor	Substrate	Inducer
Rifampin/Rifabutin			3A4, 2C8, 2C9, 2C19, 2B6, P-gp
Erythromycin/Clarithromycin[a]	3A4, P-gp	3A4	
Ciprofloxacin[b]	1A2		
Trimethoprim	2C8		
Sulfamethoxazole	2C9		

[a]Simultaneous reversible and irreversible inhibition effects should be taken into account in a reaction mixture of substrate and multiple inhibitors of CYP3A4 [111]. Azithromycin is not an inhibitor of CYP450 and may be used as substitute if clinically warranted

[b]Levofloxacin and moxifloxacin are weak or no inhibitors of CYP1A2 and may be used as substitute if clinically warranted

Sex differences in cytochrome P450 activity have been reported with increased CYP3A4 activity in women compared with men and CYP1A2 activity being lower in women than in men [85]. Differences in the expression of these enzymes may directly produce interindividual differences in susceptibility to compounds whose toxicity is modulated by these enzymes [86]. Genetic variations can cause a patient to metabolize drugs abnormally fast, abnormally slow, or not at all. Genetic polymorphism is the most common cause of the interindividual differences in metabolism of CYP2D6 substrates. CYP2C9 shows high interethnic and intraethnic variability.

In actual clinical situations with patients taking multiple drugs, clinicians should always consider that metabolic inhibitory effects may be additive and they should be aware that the extent of drug interactions is difficult to predict based on pharmacokinetic studies only examining two drugs [87].

Commonly used antibiotics that are most likely involved in cytochrome P450 mediated drug interactions are: rifampin and its derivates, the macrolides erythromycin and clarithromycin, the fluoroquinolone ciprofloxacin, and trimethoprim/sulfonamide combinations (Table 38.3).

Significant Interactions by Drug Class

Rifamycin Derivates

Rifampin (=Rifampicin) has numerous well documented clinically significant drug interactions associated with its use and new interactions continue to be found. Whenever clinicians prescribe therapy with either rifampin or rifabutin, it is prudent to screen for drug interactions and adjust dosages carefully [87]. Rifampin is indicated as component of a three-drug regimen for treatment of tuberculous and for the treatment of asymptomatic carriers of Neisseria meningitidis and Staphylococcus aureus (not approved in the U.S.). Among the group of antibiotics, rifampin is the most potent inducer of the CYP450 isoenzymes and may cause severe drug interactions if these enzyme induction properties are not considered. The three commercially available rifamycin derivatives – rifampin, rifabutin, and rifapentine – have different CYP3A induction potencies. In vitro data demonstrate that rifampin is the most potent, followed by rifapentine and rifabutin [88]. Although rifabutin interactions are generally less dramatic than rifampin interactions, many are clinically relevant. Rifamycins are essential drugs for the treatment of active tuberculous. In HIV-TB coinfected patients, rifamycins are associated with significant drug interactions with protease inhibitors, Non-Nucleoside Reverse Transcriptase Inhibitors, maraviroc, and raltegravir. Consultation with an HIV expert is recommended [89].

Rifampin induces the isoenzymes CYP3A4, 2C8, 2C9, 2C19, 2B6 and the transporter P-gp [90]. When coadministered with drugs that are substrates of the same enzymes, their metabolism may be accelerated resulting in lower concentrations and less efficacy. The enzyme induction effect is only gradually reduced over a 1–2-week period, and sometimes longer, when rifampin is discontinued. Important CYP 3A4 substrates are listed in Table 38.2. A possible drug interaction between linezolid and rifampin was described by Gephart et al., which resulted in decreased serum linezolid levels, probably caused by increased P-gp expression [91].

Erythromycin/Clarithromycin

Erythromycin and clarithromycin, commonly used macrolides, are known to be substrates and inhibiters of CYP3A4 and P-gp. Complex interactions with potentially serious toxic consequences are known to be caused by this group of antibiotics when combined with CYP 3A4 substrates (Table 38.2). Concurrent administration of clarithromycin and rifabutin has been observed to cause an increased risk of side effects due to elevated rifabutin concentrations [92]. Also, rifampin reduces clarithromycin concentrations. If alternatives are available, erythromycin, and clarithromycin should not be prescribed as part of complex drug regimes.

Ciprofloxacin

The fluoroquinolone ciprofloxacin is an inhibitor of CYP1A2. Coadministration of ciprofloxacin and other drugs primarily metabolized by CYP1A2 (e.g., theophylline, caffeine, tizanidine, clozapine) results in increased plasma concentrations of the coadministered drug (or coffee) and could lead to clinically significant side effects from the coadministered drug [93].

Other quinolones, such as levofloxacin or moxifloxacin, do not show inhibition of CYP1A2 and, thus, don't interfere with theophylline metabolism [94]. Levofloxacin and ciprofloxacin have shown weak inhibition of CYP2C9 in vitro [95], but clinical consequences are not clear.

Ciprofloxacin has been implicated in adverse drug interaction with methotrexate by mechanisms other than CYP450 metabolism [96]. Potential changes of the absorption of ciprofloxacin when extensive mucositis is present have been suspected. Ciprofloxacin also has been shown to interact with phenytoin, sulfonylurea glyburide, cyclosporine, warfarin, and NSAIs [93].

Moxifloxacin and Other Quinolones

Iron and antacids reduce the bioavailability of moxifloxacin (s. above).

Linezolid

Linezolid is a reversible, nonselective inhibitor of monoamine oxidase with interaction potential with adrenergic and serotonergic agents as well as with large amounts of foods or beverages with high tyramine content [97]. It has been well documented in the literature that the combination of linezolid and serotonergic antidepressants such as fluoxetine may cause serotonin syndrome [98, 99].

Aminoglycosides

Due to the ototoxic and/or nephrotoxic potential of aminoglycosides, the concurrent or serial use of other ototoxic or nephrotoxic agents such as vancomycin, amphotericin B, colistin, viomycin, or, cisplatin should be avoided because of the potential for additive effects. They also should not be given concurrently with potent diuretics, such as ethacrynic acid and furosemide as they may enhance aminoglycoside toxicity by altering antibiotic concentrations in serum and tissue.

Vancomycin

Similar to aminoglycosides, the concurrent administration of potentially neurotoxic and/or nephrotoxic drugs should be avoided or carefully monitored. Concomitant administration of vancomycin and anesthetic agents has been associated with erythema and histamine-like flushing and anaphylactoid reactions.

Beta-Lactam Antibiotics

Probenecid inhibits the renal excretion of beta-lactam antibiotics that are mainly eliminated by renal tubular secretion and its use may result in increased and prolonged concentrations.

- Amoxicillin/Clavulanate: The incidence of rashes increases substantially when given with concurrent allopurinol.
- Piperacillin/Tazobactam: The prolongation of the neuromuscular blockade of vecuronium when used concomitantly with piperacillin is not considered clinically important [100]. Case reports suggest that coadministration of methotrexate and piperacillin may reduce the clearance of methotrexate and cause significant increased concentrations of methotrexate [101, 102].
- Carbapenems: Limited data indicates that meropenem may reduce serum levels of valproic acid resulting in impaired seizure control [103]. Concomitant administration of ganciclovir during imipenem therapy should be avoided because of increased risk of seizure.

Metronidazole

Limited or modest interactions with ethanol have been reported for drugs such as metronidazole. Although the possible disulfiram-like reaction (also suggested to be a toxic serotonin syndrome) when metronidazole is combined with alcohol is rare, patients should still be informed about this potential interaction [104].

Trimethoprim-Sulfamethoxazole

Trimethoprim inhibits CYP2C8 and may increase concentrations of CYP2C8 substrates such as NSAIDs, oral antidiabetic drugs, warfarin, statins, paclitaxel, digoxin, amiodarone, verapamil, and zopiclone [105]. Sulfamethoxazole inhibits CYP2C9 and may increase concentrations of CYP2C9 substrates such as warfarin, oral antidiabetic drugs, phenytoin, NSAIDs, angiotensin II receptor blockers [105].

Tigecycline

Tigecycline is not metabolized by the cytochrome P450 system. Nevertheless, concomitant administration with warfarin increases the concentrations of warfarin and monitoring of prothrombin time is advisable [106].

In conclusion, in most cases, significant interactions with antibiotics that are included in complex therapeutic regimes for cancer patients can be avoided by prudent use of antibiotics, substituting rifampin, erythromycin, clarithromycin, ciprofloxacin, and cotrimoxazol by similar antibiotics or by carefully monitoring patients when potential interactions are anticipated.

Acknowledgment We thank all members of the International Society of Anti-Infective Pharmacology (ISAP) and members of the ESCMID PK/PD of Anti-Infectives Study Group (EPASG) who provided valueable advice and discussion during the yearly scientific meetings.

References

1. Kunin CM. Clinical pharmacology of the new penicillins. 1. The importance of serum protein binding in determining antimicrobial activity and concentration in serum. Clin Pharmacol Ther. 1966;7(2):166–79.
2. Beer J, Wagner CC, Zeitlinger M. Protein binding of antimicrobials: methods for quantification and for investigation of its impact on bacterial killing. AAPS J. 2009;11:1–12.
3. Hyatt JM, McKinnon PS, Zimmer GS, Schentag JJ. The importance of pharmacokinetic/pharmacodynamic surrogate markers to outcome. Focus on antibacterial agents. Clin Pharmacokinet. 1995;28(2):143–60.
4. Toutain PL, del Castillo JR, Bousquet-Melou A. The pharmacokinetic-pharmacodynamic approach to a rational dosage regimen for antibiotics. Res Vet Sci. 2002;73(2):105–14.
5. Nicolau DP. Predicting antibacterial response from pharmacodynamic and pharmacokinetic profiles. Infection. 2001;29 Suppl 2:11–5.
6. Frimodt-Moller N. How predictive is PK/PD for antibacterial agents? Int J Antimicrob Agents. 2002;19(4):333–9.
7. Vogelman B, Gudmundsson S, Leggett J, Turnidge J, Ebert S, Craig WA. Correlation of antimicrobial pharmacokinetic parameters with therapeutic efficacy in an animal model. J Infect Dis. 1988;158(4):831–47.
8. Nicolau DP. Pharmacodynamic optimization of beta-lactams in the patient care setting. Crit Care. 2008;12 Suppl 4:S2.
9. Pettorossi VE, Ferraresi A, Errico P, Draicchio F, Dionisotti S. The impact of different dosing regimens of the aminoglycosides netilmicin and amikacin on vestibulotoxicity in the guinea pig. Eur Arch Otorhinolaryngol. 1990;247(5):277–82.
10. Christensen ML, Stewart CF, Crom WR. Evaluation of aminoglycoside disposition in patients previously treated with cisplatin. Ther Drug Monit. 1989;11(6):631–6.
11. Joukhadar C, Klein N, Mayer BX, Kreischitz N, Delle-Karth G, Palkovits P, et al. Plasma and tissue pharmacokinetics of cefpirome in patients with sepsis. Crit Care Med. 2002;30(7):1478–82.
12. Zeitlinger MA, Dehghanyar P, Mayer BX, Schenk BS, Neckel U, Heinz G, et al. Relevance of soft-tissue penetration by levofloxacin for target site bacterial killing in patients with sepsis. Antimicrob Agents Chemother. 2003;47(11):3548–53.
13. Zeitlinger MA, Marsik C, Georgopoulos A, Muller M, Heinz G, Joukhadar C. Target site bacterial killing of cefpirome and fosfomycin in critically ill patients. Int J Antimicrob Agents. 2003;21(6):562–7.
14. FDA. Guidance for Industry. Developing antimicrobial drugs – general considerations for clinical trials. 1998. (wwwfdagov/cder/guidance/2580dftpdf).
15. EMEA. Points to consider on pharmacokinetics and pharmacodynamics in the development of antibacterial medicinal products. 2000. (wwwemeaeuint/pdfs/human/ewp/265599enpdf).
16. Theuretzbacher U. Tissue penetration of antibacterial agents: how should this be incorporated into pharmacodynamic analyses? Curr Opin Pharmacol. 2007;7(5):498–504.
17. Pea F, Viale P, Furlanut M. Antimicrobial therapy in critically ill patients: a review of pathophysiological conditions responsible for altered disposition and pharmacokinetic variability. Clin Pharmacokinet. 2005;44(10):1009–34.
18. Li J, Gwilt P. The effect of malignant effusions on methotrexate disposition. Cancer Chemother Pharmacol. 2002;50(5):373–82.
19. Lanao JM, Dominguez-Gil A, Macias JG, Diez JL, Nieto MJ. The influence of ascites on the pharmacokinetics of amikacin. Int J Clin Pharmacol Ther Toxicol. 1980;18(2):57–61.
20. Lechi A, Arosio E, Xerri L, Mengoli C, Montesi G, Ghidini O. The kinetics of cefuroxime in ascitic and pleural fluid. Int J Clin Pharmacol Ther Toxicol. 1982;20(10):493–6.
21. Benoni G, Arosio E, Cuzzolin L, Vaona B, Raimondi MG, Lechi A. Penetration of ceftriaxone into human pleural fluid. Antimicrob Agents Chemother. 1986;29(5):906–8.
22. Lortholary O, Lefort A, Tod M, Chomat AM, Darras-Joly C, Cordonnier C. Pharmacodynamics and pharmacokinetics of antibacterial drugs in the management of febrile neutropenia. Lancet Infect Dis. 2008;8(10):612–20.
23. Nyhlen A, Ljungberg B, Nilsson-Ehle I. Pharmacokinetics of ceftazidime in febrile neutropenic patients. Scand J Infect Dis. 2001;33(3):222–6.
24. Nyhlen A, Ljungberg B, Nilsson-Ehle I. Pharmacokinetics of meropenem in febrile neutropenic patients. Swedish study group. Eur J Clin Microbiol Infect Dis. 1997;16(11):797–802.
25. Drusano GL, Plaisance KI, Forrest A, Bustamante C, Devlin A, Standiford HC, et al. Steady-state pharmacokinetics of imipenem in febrile neutropenic cancer patients. Antimicrob Agents Chemother. 1987;31(9):1420–2.
26. Davis RL, Lehmann D, Stidley CA, Neidhart J. Amikacin pharmacokinetics in patients receiving high-dose cancer chemotherapy. Antimicrob Agents Chemother. 1991;35(5):944–7.
27. Phillips JK, Spearing RL, Crome DJ, Davies JM. Gentamicin volumes of distribution in patients with hematologic disorders. N Engl J Med. 1988;319(19):1290.
28. Higa GM, Murray WE. Alterations in aminoglycoside pharmacokinetics in patients with cancer. Clin Pharm. 1987;6(12):963–6.
29. Tod M, Padoin C, Petitjean O. Clinical pharmacokinetics and pharmacodynamics of isepamicin. Clin Pharmacokinet. 2000;38(3):205–23.

30. Anon. Efficacy and toxicity of single daily doses of amikacin and ceftriaxone versus multiple daily doses of amikacin and ceftazidime for infection in patients with cancer and granulocytopenia. The International Antimicrobial Therapy Cooperative Group of the European Organization for Research and Treatment of Cancer. Ann Intern Med. 1993;119(7 Pt 1):584–93.
31. Sung L, Dupuis LL, Bliss B, Taddio A, Abdolell M, Allen U, et al. Randomized controlled trial of once- versus thrice-daily tobramycin in febrile neutropenic children undergoing stem cell transplantation. J Natl Cancer Inst. 2003;95(24):1869–77.
32. Fernandez de Gatta MM, Fruns I, Hernandez JM, Caballero D, San Miguel JF, Martinez Lanao J, et al. Vancomycin pharmacokinetics and dosage requirements in hematologic malignancies. Clin Pharm. 1993;12(7):515–20.
33. Le Normand Y, Milpied N, Kergueris MF, Harousseau JL. Pharmacokinetic parameters of vancomycin for therapeutic regimens in neutropenic adult patients. Int J Biomed Comput. 1994;36(1–2):121–5.
34. Bubalo JS, Munar MY, Cherala G, Hayes-Lattin B, Maziarz R. Daptomycin pharmacokinetics in adult oncology patients with neutropenic fever. Antimicrob Agents Chemother. 2009;53(2):428–34.
35. Benvenuto M, Benziger DP, Yankelev S, Vigliani G. Pharmacokinetics and tolerability of daptomycin at doses up to 12 milligrams per kilogram of body weight once daily in healthy volunteers. Antimicrob Agents Chemother. 2006;50(10):3245–9.
36. Smith PF, Birmingham MC, Noskin GA, Meagher AK, Forrest A, Rayner CR, et al. Safety, efficacy and pharmacokinetics of linezolid for treatment of resistant Gram-positive infections in cancer patients with neutropenia. Ann Oncol. 2003;14(5):795–801.
37. Hutschala D, Kinstner C, Skhirtladze K, Mayer-Helm BX, Zeitlinger M, Wisser W, et al. The impact of perioperative atelectasis on antibiotic penetration into lung tissue: an in vivo microdialysis study. Intensive Care Med. 2008;34(10):1827–34.
38. Brunner M, Pernerstorfer T, Mayer BX, Eichler HG, Muller M. Surgery and intensive care procedures affect the target site distribution of piperacillin. Crit Care Med. 2000;28(6):1754–9.
39. Hackam DJ, Christou N, Khaliq Y, Duffy DR, Vaughan D, Marshall JC, et al. Bioavailability of oral ciprofloxacin in early postsurgical patients. Arch Surg. 1998;133(11):1221–5.
40. Gonzalez-Hernandez I, Jung-Cook H, Sotelo A. Effect of malnutrition on the pharmacokinetics of cefuroxime axetil in young rats. J Pharm Pharm Sci. 2008;11(1):9–21.
41. Herrington JD, Tran HT, Riggs MW. Prospective evaluation of carboplatin AUC dosing in patients with a BMI>or=27 or cachexia. Cancer Chemother Pharmacol. 2006;57(2):241–7.
42. Murry DJ, Riva L, Poplack DG. Impact of nutrition on pharmacokinetics of anti-neoplastic agents. Int J Cancer Suppl. 1998;11:48–51.
43. Ronchera-Oms CL, Tormo C, Ordovas JP, Abad J, Jimenez NV. Expanded gentamicin volume of distribution in critically ill adult patients receiving total parenteral nutrition. J Clin Pharm Ther. 1995;20(5):253–8.
44. Tormo C, Abad FJ, Ronchera-Oms CL, Parra V, Jimenez NV. Critically-ill patients receiving total parenteral nutrition show altered amikacin pharmacokinetics. Clin Nutr. 1995;14(4):254–9.
45. Raghuram TC, Krishnaswamy K. Pharmacokinetics of tetracycline in nutritional edema. Chemotherapy. 1982;28(6):428–33.
46. Lares-Asseff I, Cravioto J, Santiago P, Perez-Ortiz B. Pharmacokinetics of metronidazole in severely malnourished and nutritionally rehabilitated children. Clin Pharmacol Ther. 1992;51(1):42–50.
47. Oravcova J, Bohs B, Lindner W. Drug-protein binding sites. New trends in analytical and experimental methodology. J Chromatogr B Biomed Appl. 1996;677(1):1–28.
48. Craig WA, Ebert SC. Protein binding and its significance in antibacterial therapy. Infect Dis Clin North Am. 1989;3(3):407–14.
49. Craig WA, Kunin CM. Significance of serum protein and tissue binding of antimicrobial agents. Annu Rev Med. 1976;27:287–300.
50. Kremer JM, Wilting J, Janssen LH. Drug binding to human alpha-1-acid glycoprotein in health and disease. Pharmacol Rev. 1988;40(1):1–47.
51. Gamba G, Contreras AM, Cortes J, Nares F, Santiago Y, Espinosa A, et al. Hypoalbuminemia as a risk factor for amikacin nephrotoxicity. Rev Invest Clin. 1990;42(3):204–9.
52. Wilson RC, Green NK. Pharmacokinetics of minocycline hydrochloride in clinically normal and hypoproteinemic sheep. Am J Vet Res. 1986;47(3):650–2.
53. Ryan DM. Pharmacokinetics of antibiotics in natural and experimental superficial compartments in animals and humans. J Antimicrob Chemother. 1993;31(Suppl D):1–16.
54. Kearney BP, Aweeka FT. The penetration of anti-infectives into the central nervous system. Neurol Clin. 1999;17(4):883–900.
55. Zeitlinger M, Muller M, Joukhadar C. Lung microdialysis–a powerful tool for the determination of exogenous and endogenous compounds in the lower respiratory tract (mini-review). AAPS J. 2005;7(3):E600–8.
56. Zhanel GG, Dueck M, Hoban DJ, Vercaigne LM, Embil JM, Gin AS, et al. Review of macrolides and ketolides: focus on respiratory tract infections. Drugs. 2001;61(4):443–98.
57. Bergogne-Berezin E. New concepts in the pulmonary disposition of antibiotics. Pulm Pharmacol. 1995;8(2–3):65–81.
58. Joukhadar C, Frossard M, Mayer BX, Brunner M, Klein N, Siostrzonek P, et al. Impaired target site penetration of beta-lactams may account for therapeutic failure in patients with septic shock. Crit Care Med. 2001;29(2):385–91.
59. van Dalen R, Vree TB. Pharmacokinetics of antibiotics in critically ill patients. Intensive Care Med. 1990;16 Suppl 3:S235–8.
60. Zeitlinger BS, Zeitlinger M, Leitner I, Muller M, Joukhadar C. Clinical scoring system for the prediction of target site penetration of antimicrobials in patients with sepsis. Clin Pharmacokinet. 2007;46(1):75–83.
61. Blaser J, Stone BB, Groner MC, Zinner SH. Comparative study with enoxacin and netilmicin in a pharmacodynamic model to determine importance of ratio of antibiotic peak concentration to MIC for bactericidal activity and emergence of resistance. Antimicrob Agents Chemother. 1987;31(7):1054–60.
62. Crokaert F. Pharmacodynamics, a tool for a better use of antibiotics? Intensive Care Med. 2001;27(2):340–3.
63. Otero MJ, Garcia MJ, Barrueco M, Dominguez-Gil A, Gomez F, Portugal Alvarez J. Pharmacokinetics of cefoxitin administered by i.v. infusion to patients with a pleural effusion. Eur J Clin Pharmacol. 1984;26(3):389–92.
64. Goonetilleke AK, Dev D, Aziz I, Hughes C, Smith MJ, Basran GS. A comparative analysis of pharmacokinetics of ceftriaxone in serum and pleural fluid in humans: a study of once daily administration by intramuscular and intravenous routes. J Antimicrob Chemother. 1996;38(6):969–76.
65. Scripture CD, Figg WD. Drug interactions in cancer therapy. Nat Rev Cancer. 2006;6:546–58.
66. Tam-McDevitt J. Polypharmacy, aging, and cancer. Oncology. 2008;22:1052–5. discussion 1055, 1058, 1060.
67. Blower P, de Wit R, Goodin S, Aapro M. Drug-drug interactions in oncology: why are they important and can they be minimized? Crit Rev Oncol Hematol. 2005;55:117–42.
68. Riechelmann RP, Tannock IF, Wang L, Saad ED, Taback NA, Krzyzanowska MK. Potential drug interactions and duplicate prescriptions among cancer patients. J Natl Cancer Inst. 2007;99:592–600.
69. Sokol KC, Knudsen JF, Li MM. Polypharmacy in older oncology patients and the need for an interdisciplinary approach to side-effect management. J Clin Pharm Ther. 2007;32:169–75.
70. Beijnen JH, Schellens JH. Drug interactions in oncology. Lancet Oncol. 2004;5:489–96.
71. Hanigan MH, Dela Cruz BL, Thompson DM, Farmer KC, Medina PJ. Use of prescription and nonprescription medications and

71. supplements by cancer patients during chemotherapy: questionnaire validation. J Oncol Pharm Pract. 2008;14:123–30.
72. Riechelmann RP, Saad ED. A systematic review on drug interactions in oncology. Cancer Invest. 2006;24:704–12.
73. Riechelmann RP, Moreira F, Smaletz O, Saad ED. Potential for drug interactions in hospitalized cancer patients. Cancer Chemother Pharmacol. 2005;56:286–90.
74. Huang SM, Strong JM, Zhang L, Reynolds KS, Nallani S, Temple R, et al. New era in drug interaction evaluation: US Food and Drug Administration update on CYP enzymes, transporters, and the guidance process. J Clin Pharmacol. 2008;48:662–70.
75. Freifeld A, Sankaranarayanan J, Ullrich F, Sun J. Clinical practice patterns of managing low-risk adult febrile neutropenia during cancer chemotherapy in the USA. Support Care Cancer. 2008;16:181–91.
76. Guidance for Industry. Drug Interaction Studies – Study Design, Data Analysis, and Implications for Dosing and Labeling. September 2006. Accessed Feb 2009. http://www.fda.gov/cder/Guidance/6695dft.pdf
77. Pal D, Mitra AK. MDR- and CYP3A4-mediated drug-drug interactions. J Neuroimmune Pharmacol. 2006;1:323–39.
78. Cohen KA, Lautenbach E, Weiner MG, Synnestvedt M, Gasink LB. Coadministration of oral levofloxacin with agents that impair absorption: impact on antibiotic resistance. Infect Control Hosp Epidemiol. 2008;29:975–7.
79. Lynch T, Price A. The effect of cytochrome P450 metabolism on drug response, interactions, and adverse effects. Am Fam Physician. 2007;76:391–6.
80. Zhou SF. Drugs behave as substrates, inhibitors and inducers of human cytochrome P450 3A4. Curr Drug Metab. 2008;9:310–22.
81. Zhou SF. Potential strategies for minimizing mechanism-based inhibition of cytochrome P450 3A4. Curr Pharm Des. 2008;14:990–1000.
82. Brinkmann U, Roots I, Eichelbaum M. Pharmacogenetics of the human drug-transporter gene MDR1: impact of polymorphisms on pharmacotherapy. Drug Discov Today. 2001;6:835–9.
83. Hennessy M, Kelleher D, Spiers JP, Barry M, Kavanagh P, Back D, et al. St Johns wort increases expression of P-glycoprotein: implications for drug interactions. Br J Clin Pharmacol. 2002;53:75–82.
84. Michalets EL. Update: clinically significant cytochrome P-450 drug interactions. Pharmacotherapy. 1998;18:84–112.
85. Brøsen K. Sex differences in pharmacology. Ugeskr Laeger. 2007;169:2408–11.
86. Snawder JE, Lipscomb JC. Interindividual variance of cytochrome P450 forms in human hepatic microsomes: correlation of individual forms with xenobiotic metabolism and implications in risk assessment. Regul Toxicol Pharmacol. 2000;32:200–9.
87. Finch CK, Chrisman CR, Baciewicz AM, Self TH. Rifampin and rifabutin drug interactions. Arch Intern Med. 2002;162:985–92.
88. Weber A, Kaplan M, Chughtai SA, Cohn LA, Smith AL, Unadkat JD. CYP3A inductive potential of the rifamycins, Rifabutin and rifampin, in the rabbit. Biopharm Drug Dispos. 2001;22:157–68.
89. Guidelines for the Use of Antiretroviral Agents in HIV-1-Infected Adults and Adolescents. November 2008. http://aidsinfo.nih.gov/contentfiles/AdultandAdolescentGL.pdf Accessed Feb 2009.
90. Glaeser H, Drescher S, Eichelbaum M, Fromm MF. Influence of rifampicin on the expression and function of human intes-tinal cytochrome P450 enzymes. Br J Clin Pharmacol. 2005;59:199–206.
91. Gebhart BC, Barker BC, Markewitz BA. Decreased serum linezolid levels in a critically ill patient receiving concomitant linezolid and rifampin. Pharmacotherapy. 2007;27:476–9.
92. Hafner R, Bethel J, Power M. Tolerance and pharmacokinetic interactions of rifabutin and clarithromycin in human immunodeficiency virus–infected volunteers. Antimicrob Agents Chemother. 1998;42:631–9.
93. Label information ciprofloxacin (2009) http://www.fda.gov/cder/foi/label/2009/019537s69,19847s43,19857s50,20780s27lbl.pdf. Accessed Feb 2009.
94. Shakeri-Nejad K, Stahlmann R. Drug interactions during therapy with three major groups of antimicrobial agents. Expert Opin Pharmacother. 2006;7:639–51.
95. Zhang L, Wie MJ, Zhao CY, Qi HM. Determination of the inhibitory potential of 6 fluoroquinolones on CYP1A2 and CYP2C9 in human liver microsomes. Acta Pharmacol Sin. 2008;29:1507–14.
96. Dalle JH, Auvrignon A, Vassal G, Leverger G. Interaction between methotrexate and ciprofloxacin. J Pediatr Hematol Oncol. 2002;24:321–2.
97. Label information Linezolid. 2008. http://www.fda.gov/cder/foi/label/2008/021130s016,021131s013,021132s014lbl.pdf. Accessed Feb 2009.
98. Steinberg M, Morin AK. Mild serotonin syndrome associated with concurrent linezolid and fluoxetine. Am J Health Syst Pharm. 2007;64:59–62.
99. Huang V, Gortney JS. Risk of serotonin syndrome with concomitant administration of linezolid and serotonin agonists. Pharmacotherapy. 2006;26:1784–93.
100. Condon RE, Munshi CA, Arfman RC. Interaction of vecuronium with piperacillin or cefoxitin evaluated in a prospective, randomized, double-blind clinical trial. Am Surg. 1995;61:403–6.
101. Zarychanski R, Wlodarczyk K, Ariano R, Bow E. Pharmacokinetic interaction between methotrexate and piperacillin/tazobactam resulting in prolonged toxic concentrations of methotrexate. J Antimicrob Chemother. 2006;58:228–30.
102. de Miguel D, García-Suárez J, Martín Y, Gil-Fernández JJ, Burgaleta C. Severe acute renal failure following high-dose methotrexate therapy in adults with haematological malignancies: a significant number result from unrecognized co-administration of several drugs. Nephrol Dial Transplant. 2008;23:3762–6.
103. Mori H, Takahashi K, Mizutani T. Interaction between valproic acid and carbapenem antibiotics. Drug Metab Rev. 2007;9:647–57.
104. Karamanakos PN, Pappas P, Boumba VA, Thomas C, Malamas M, Vougiouklakis T, et al. Pharmaceutical agents known to produce disulfiram-like reaction: effects on hepatic ethanol metabolism and brain monoamines. Int J Toxicol. 2007;26:423–32.
105. Wen X, Wang JS, Backman JT, Laitila J, Neuvonen PJ. Trimethoprim and sulfamethoxazole are selective inhibitors of CYP2C8 and CYP2C9, respectively. Drug Metab Dispos. 2002;30:631–5.
106. Label information tigecycline (2009) http://www.fda.gov/cder/foi/label/2009/021821s016lbl.pdf. Accessed Feb 2009.
107. Note for guidance on the investigation of drug interactions CPMP/EWP/560/95 1997. http://www.emea.europa.eu/pdfs/human/ewp/056095en.pdf Accessed Feb 2009.
108. Drug Development and Drug Interactions: Table of Substrates, Inhibitors and Inducers. http://www.fda.gov/cder/drug/drugInteractions/tableSubstrates.htm. Accessed Feb 2009.
109. Flockhart DA. Drug Interactions: Cytochrome P450 Drug Interaction Table. Indiana University School of Medicine. 2007. http://medicine.iupui.edu/flockhart/table.htm. Accessed Feb 2009.
110. Granfors MT, Backman JT, Neuvonen M, Neuvonen PJ. Ciprofloxacin greatly increases concentrations and hypotensive effect of tizanidine by inhibiting its cytochrome P450 1A2-mediated presystemic metabolism. Clin Pharmacol Ther. 2004;76:598–606.
111. Zhang X, Jones DR, Hall SD. Prediction of the effect of erythromycin, diltiazem, and their metabolites, alone and in combination, on CYP3A4 inhibition. Drug Metab Dispos. 2009;37:150–60.

Chapter 39
Mycobacterium tuberculous Infection

Michael Glickman

Abstract This chapter will outline various aspects of the diagnosis and treatment of Tuberculous in the cancer patient. We provide a general framework to understand the relationship between immunosuppressive cancer therapy and TB risk. We also review information about the risk of TB with specific malignancies and their treatment. It is our intention that this chapter will provide a cancer-specific supplement the information contained in national guidelines about TB therapy.

Keywords Cancer • Tuberculous • Disseminated disease • Cellular immune defect • Immunotherapy • Chemotherapy • Lymohoma • Solid tumors • Purin analog • Alemtuzumab • Graft versus host disease • T-cell defect

Introduction

In this chapter, we will review Tuberculous in cancer patients. Rather than reviewing basic tenets of Tuberculous diagnosis and therapy, which have been extensively reviewed and codified in national guidelines [1–3], we will focus on aspects of Tuberculous specific to cancer patients. In many cases, specific clinical data about TB in cancer patients is lacking. Therefore, clinical decisions about TB risk, prevention, and therapy in the cancer patient must be made based on extrapolation from data in HIV infected patients, assessment of cancer related immunosuppression, and drug interactions specific to cancer patients. Modern therapy of cancer is in rapid evolution and therapies that suppress immune function are myriad and constantly evolving. We hope to provide a clinical framework to manage Tuberculous in cancer patients that draw on presently available clinical data and can also adapt to the evolution of cancer therapy over time. To understand the epidemiology of TB in cancer patients, it is necessary to examine both the underlying immune response to TB infection and the impact of various cancers and their therapies on the immune system.

Basic Biology of M. tuberculous Infection

Mycobacterium tuberculous is rod shaped bacterium that is acid fast when stained with carbol fuschin and decolorized with acid alcohol. *M. tuberculous* and other slow growing pathogenic mycobacteria have a remarkably slow doubling time in vitro, 18–24 h under optimal conditions. *M. tuberculous* is an obligate human pathogen that passes from person to person by inhalation of aerosolized droplets containing viable bacteria. There is no known environmental reservoir or fomite transmission. Upon deposition in the lung through inhalation, *M. tuberculous* replicates inside host macrophages and can disseminate to almost any organ during early infection. This primary infection is usually asymptomatic in an immunocompetent adult. With the onset of antigen specific immunity and associated granuloma formation, *M. tuberculous* replication is controlled such that bacterial numbers are reduced to uncultivatable levels. The detectable remnants of this primary infection are a delayed type hypersensitivity reaction to *M. tuberculous* antigens, assayed as Tuberculin reactivity or positive Interferon gamma release assay. Some patients will also develop pulmonary scarring and/or lymph node calcification which can be detected on chest radiography but is not specific for TB infection.

The hallmark of *M. tuberculous* infection of humans is latency. Although human immunity is highly effective at controlling *M. tuberculous* during primary infection, in many patients viable bacteria resist complete elimination and persist in a state of clinical and microbiologic dormancy. Latent infection can reactivate to cause active disease, sometimes after decades of latency, but often within the first 5 years after primary infection. In most adult

M. Glickman (✉)
Infectious Diseases Division, Memorial Sloan Kettering Cancer Center, 1275 York Avenue, New York, NY 10065, USA
e-mail: glickmam@mskcc.org

patients, reactivation of latent *M. tuberculous* infection does not occur with a defined defect in immunologic function, although defects in cellular immunity clearly raise the risk of reactivation (discussed further below). Clinical tuberculous in adults is usually the result of reactivation of latent infection and many of our efforts to control Tuberculous in the general population and in cancer patients is based on the detection of latent infection, its elimination by preventative therapy, and surveillance for reactivation in those at risk.

States of Susceptibility to Tuberculous Infection

Control of mycobacterial infection depends on CD4 T cells and cytokines typical of Th1 polarization. This conclusion is based on findings in both humans and mice that establish the critical importance of Interferon gamma, Interleukin 12, and Tumor Necrosis Alpha in defense against mycobacterial infection.

Much of the world receives BCG vaccination at birth. The BCG vaccine is a live, attenuated strain of *Mycobacterium bovis* that is the world's most widely administered vaccine. Although BCG is generally well tolerated, its wide administration has revealed a small subset of the population with inherited susceptibility to mycobacterial infection, manifest by disseminated or progressive localized BCG infection after vaccination. This syndrome, called Mendelian Susceptibility to Mycobacterial disease (MSMD), also confers susceptibility to severe infection with other mycobacteria of low virulence. Characterization of patients with MSMD has defined pathways of antimycobacterial immunity. The mutations that cause MSMD are in either of the two interferon gamma receptors, the signal transduction cascade downstream of the IFN-gamma receptor, the IL-12 cytokine gene, or its receptor [4, 5]. These patients confirm that Th1 immunity is critically important for defense against mycobacterial infection. Experiments using mice deficient in Interferon gamma, TNF, and CD4 T cells confirm these conclusions [6]. Further support for the importance of CD4 T cells and their cytokines on mycobacterial immunity comes from HIV infected patients, who have dramatically elevated rates of reactivation Tuberculous compared to immunocompetent controls [7–9]. Further evidence for the importance of TNF in human antimycobacterial immunity comes from the high rates of Tuberculous in patients receiving therapeutic antibodies that neutralize TNF. In contrast, deficiency of humoral immunity does not seem to predispose patients to Tuberculous.

Cancer and Its Therapy that Produce Deficiencies in Antimycobacterial Immunity

This background provides a framework for understanding the risk of Tuberculous in patients with cancer. Cancer, or cancer therapies, differ widely in the degree and type of immunosuppression that they produce. These differences have significant implications for predicting TB risk. Cancer or its therapy that depletes functional CD4 T cells or impairs their function should confer increased higher risk for TB reactivation than cancers or therapies that deplete only neutrophils or antibodies. For this reason, hematologic malignancies, which impair T cell immunity, should be associated with a higher risk of reactivation Tuberculous than solid tumors that do not specifically impair T cell immunity in the absence of therapy. Similarly, therapeutic interventions that specifically impair T cell function should confer the greatest risk of Tuberculous. Since there is no environmental reservoir of *M. tuberculous*, the chance of either reactivation TB or progressive primary TB after exposure is proportional to the incidence of Tuberculous in the community. In fact, abundant observational data demonstrates that TB rates with cancer or its therapy are proportional to TB prevalence in the surrounding population.

Risk of Tuberculous with Specific Cancers and Cancer Therapies

Several observational studies have examined rates of Tuberculous in cancer patients. The most recent such series examined all cases of Tuberculous at Memorial Sloan Kettering Cancer Center from 1980 to 2004 [10]. The overall rate of microbiologically confirmed Tuberculous was 55/100,000 persons, a rate somewhat higher than the rate recorded in New York City over the same time period. When stratified according to cancer type, hematologic malignancy conferred the highest risk (Hodgkins disease 204/100,000, acute leukemia 120, Non-Hodgkins lymphoma 231) with a lower rate in solid tumors. Among solid tumors, the highest rate of TB was seen in head and neck cancer (135/100,000), a finding that is consistent with earlier studies from MD Anderson and MSKCC [11, 12]. Importantly, when compared to TB rates in the general population, the rate of TB for solid tumor patients born in the US, excluding head and neck cancer, was not higher than rate of the surrounding population. Similar conclusions can be drawn from a review of 30 cancer patients with TB over 10 years from MD Anderson cancer center. Of the 30 TB cases, 19 had hematologic malignancy. Of the 11 solid tumor patients, 4 had head and neck cancer [13].

The impact of birth origin on TB in cancer patients is significant, paralleling the epidemiology of Tuberculous in the United States. Across all tumor types, foreign born cancer patients have TB rates 3–7-fold higher than US born patients[10]. Taken together, these studies indicate that among cancer patients, hematologic malignancy confers the greatest risk of Tuberculous, followed by Head and Neck cancer, and then other solid tumors. It is unclear from this data whether risk of TB is associated with the tumor itself or its treatment.

Bone Marrow Transplantation

Both autologous and allogeneic bone marrow transplantation confer substantial immunosuppression and are often complicated by a wide variety of infections. Allogeneic BMT generally confers a more lasting defect in T-cell function due to measures used to prevent Graft versus host disease (T-cell depletion, pharmacologic immunosuppression) or GVHD itself. Multiple studies have examined rates of Tuberculous following BMT. In a questionnaire based review of mycobacterial infection at European transplant centers, the rate of Tuberculous was 0.09% for autologous and 1.05% for allogeneic transplants [14]. In a series of 8,013 BMTs in Spain, a country with one of the highest rates of Tuberculous in Western Europe (30/100,000), the rate of TB was 101 cases/100,000 patients per year with the rate in allogeneic transplants twice that of autologous transplants. Compared to the rate of the general population, TB was not more common in autologous transplant patients, but occurred in allogeneic patients 3 times as frequently [15]. In both of these European studies, Tuberculous was a late infectious complication, occurring a median of 181 [14] and 324 [15] days after transplant with 8/20 [14] and 4/20 [15] cases presenting with extrapulmonary disease. In a series of 304 allogeneic transplants from India, a high TB incidence country, there were 9 TB cases (2.3%). All of these patients were receiving glucocorticoids for GVHD and five of these cases had disseminated Tuberculous [16]. In a series of 577 allogeneic transplants at Memorial Sloan Kettering Cancer Center, 4 (0.69%) developed Tuberculous, all of whom were foreign born [17]. These studies indicate that Tuberculous is more common in allogeneic transplant patients than autologous patients and that the rate in allogeneic transplants often exceeds the rate in the general population. It is reasonable to conclude that allogeneic BMT patients have an elevated risk of TB, though the risk may vary among regions, and could be considered for screening and prophylaxis (discussed below).

Pharmacologic Cancer Therapy and TB Risk

An increasingly broad array of small molecule and biologic agents are used in the therapy of human malignancy. Many of these agents suppress T cell function or deplete T cell numbers, thereby placing patients at increased risk for infections that require intact T cell function for protection, including Tuberculous. In this section, we will review the risk of Tuberculous that is conferred by these agents.

Alemtuzumab

Alemtuzumab is a humanized monoclonal antibody that binds CD52. Alemtuzumab is FDA approved for salvage therapy of chronic lymphocytic leukemia (CLL), but is also used for therapy of refractory autoimmune disease and to prevent GVHD in allogeneic bone marrow transplantation. CD52 is a surface protein expressed on a wide variety of leukocytes including T cells, B cells, monocytes, and NK cells. As such, Alemtuzumab causes broad immunosuppression that includes T cell depletion that can last 6 months to 1 year after administration. Alemtuzumab has been associated with scattered cases of active Tuberculous when used for bone marrow transplant, hematologic malignancy, and solid organ transplantation. In most reports in the literature, the rates of Tuberculous are low and it is not clear that the incidence is increased by Alemtuzumab compared with alternative therapies or the malignancy itself [18–21]. The highest documented incidence of Tuberculous after Alemtuzumab therapy comes from a series of 27 patients in Hong Kong [22], a high incidence TB area. Seven (26%) developed tuberculous, all but one within 4 months of therapy with Alemtuzumab. In contrast, a British study found only 3/357 cases of TB in Alemtuzumab treated leukemia patients [23], a rate not clearly different from the underlying rate in the hematologic malignancy population. Although these observations are not controlled, they suggest that the risk of TB after Alemtuzumab may depend upon the incidence of latent tuberculous in the treated population and targeted screening and treatment may be reasonable in higher risk patients.

Purine Analogs

Purine nucleoside analogs such as Fludarabine and 2-Chlordeoxyadenosine are commonly used as therapy for CLL, hairy cell leukemia, and in conditioning regimens for allogeneic bone marrow transplantation. The agents produce myelosuppression, including lymphopenia, which can last 1 year from the last administration. In addition to depleting T cell numbers, Fludarabine may also cause functional T cell dysfunction by depleting STAT-1 protein [24], which is required for signal transduction downstream of the Interferon gamma receptor. Thus, purine analogs produce both CD4 T cell depletion and dysfunction. Accordingly, a wide variety of infections have been reported after purine analog therapy including Pneumocystosis, Listeriosis, and reactivation herpesvirus infections, all of which require an intact T cell arm for defense [25]. In a review of 917 patients with hematologic malignancies in Brazil, there were 24 cases of TB. Multivariate analysis of risk factors for development of active Tuberculous included malnutrition, corticosteroids (OR 5.32), and Fludarabine (OR 6.08) [26]. In contrast, in a retrospective review of 18 patients with hairy cell leukemia in Hong Kong, 12 of whom received 2-CDA, there were three cases of Tuberculous. Only one of these cases was in a 2-CDA treated patient [27]. In summary, purine analogs are potent T cell immunosuppressants. The limited clinical data available indicates that they may increase risk for Tuberculous, although the data are not definitive.

Temozolamide

Temozolamide is an oral alkylating agents used in the therapy of glioblastoma and melanoma. This agent produces prolonged and severe CD4 T cell depletion that confers risk of infection. For example, when given to melanoma patients at a dose of 75 mg/m^2, CD4 counts progressively dropped below 200 cells by week 16–20. After two cycles, 64% had CD4<200 [28, 29]. Although such severe CD4 depletion would be predicted to increase rates of TB reactivation, there is only a single case report of TB in a Temozolamide treated patient [30].

TNF Inhibitors

Biologic agents that neutralize Tumor Necrosis Factor confer significant risk of reactivation Tuberculous [31]. Although these agents have not found wide use in cancer therapy, they may find a future role as adjunctive therapy of graft versus host diseases in allogeneic bone marrow transplantation. Early trial of these agents for this purpose have shown some activity [32] and, if they become more widely used, surveillance for reactivation Tuberculous will be warranted as the incidence of active TB after these agents is elevated 4–90-fold depending on comparator group [33, 34].

Diagnosis of Latent Tuberculous in Patients with Cancer

Present strategies for prevention of Tuberculous are based on the identification of people at increased risk, screening for latent TB infection (LTBI) in these populations, and administration of preventative therapy. Having reviewed the risk of TB in different populations of cancer patients, we will now review the use of newer diagnostic tests for LTBI in the cancer population. Recently, assays have become available that use antigen stimulated interferon gamma release (IGRA) from lymphocytes to detect LTBI. These assays use the *M. tuberculous* antigens ESAT-6 and CFP-10 to stimulate peripheral blood lymphocytes to produce Interferon gamma, which is detected by ELISA. Since ESAT-6 and CFP-10 are encoded by genes present in the RD-1 region of the *M. bovis* and *M. tuberculous* chromosomes, which is deleted in BCG, BCG vaccinated patients have negative IGRAs in the absence of true exposure to *M. tuberculous*. As such, these assays are clearly more specific than tuberculin skin testing in BCG vaccinated patients and are potentially useful to determine whether LTBI is present in a PPD positive, BCG vaccinated individual [35]. Their sensitivity for detecting LTBI is likely similar to tuberculin skin testing, although this conclusion is difficult in the absence of a gold standard test to detect LTBI [35]. In contrast to the well validated clinical risk of reactivation conferred by PPD conversion, the risk of active Tuberculous in IGRA positive patients has not been determined. The IGRA marketed under the tradename Quantiferon gold detects soluble Interferon gamma by ELISA. T-spot TB, a similar test that detects IFN-gamma release by ELISPOT, used previously in Europe, was approved for use in the United States in 2008. IGRAs have been recommended by the CDC as a suitable replacement for the PPD in all situations where the PPD is used to diagnose LTBI [36]. As with PPD testing, IGRA positivity is likely to be affected by immune status. Limited clinical data is available about the performance of IGRA in immunosuppressed patients [35, 36]. Additionally, limited clinical data is available about the use of IGRA in cancer patients to diagnose LTBI. The most likely use of these at present would be to screen for LTBI in a cancer patient at high risk for LTBI and reactivation (discussed above) who is PPD positive and BCG vaccinated. A positive IGRA in this circumstance would prove LTBI and make the patient a candidate for preventative therapy. The test is unlikely to be useful in the assessment of a patient with undiagnosed progressive pulmonary infiltrates requiring hospitalization, just as a PPD test is not useful in this setting. A negative IGRA would not be helpful as the sensitivity of these assays in this patient population is unknown [36]. The role of IGRAs in the diagnosis of LTBI is in rapid evolution and more data about their performance in the cancer population will hopefully be forthcoming.

Guidelines for TB Prophylaxis in Cancer Patients

A basic tenet of Tuberculous control is to detect latent infection by tuberculin skin testing in patients at increased risk for reactivation and to administer preventative therapy. This approach is based on large clinical trials demonstrating increased risk of active Tuberculous in patients with positive PPD or radiographic evidence of old TB and reduction of this risk by Isoniazid preventative therapy [37, 38]. As discussed above, many risk factors for reactivation of latent disease have been identified, most prominently HIV infection, gastrectomy, and end-stage renal disease. This paradigm has been extended to apply to certain malignancies that carry an increased risk of Tuberculous. Table 39.1 presents a compilation of relative risk of Tuberculous according to various malignant and nonmalignant risk factors. As presented above, US born solid tumor patients (except head and neck cancer) do not appear to have an increased risk of TB compared to the general population. Patients with hematologic malignancy and head and neck cancer do carry an elevated risk, which is greater in foreign born cancer patients. As a result, the 2000 CDC guidelines for targeted tuberculin testing only identify head and neck cancer and leukemia/lymphoma [2] among cancers as conditions conferring an increased risk of TB. This data supports the CDC recommended screening strategy for LTBI in these populations with a cutoff of 10 mm for Leukemia/Lymphoma/Head and neck cancer [2], although some authors have recommended a cutoff of 5 mm [10]. The PPD positivity cutoff for hematopoietic stem cell transplant patients is 5 mm with prophylactic therapy recommended for HSCT patients either exposed to a source case or with a positive tuberculin skin test [3]. There is also data to suggest that administration of Alemtuzumab, Purine analogs, and Temozolamide would increase a patient's risk of reactivation Tuberculous from known latency. Increased surveillance for reactivation disease and administration of preventative therapy in these patients for PPD positivity is a reasonable strategy.

Table 39.1 Relative risk of TB by clinical condition

Clinical risk factor	Relative risk	PPD cutoff (mm)	Reference
HIV	35–162	5	[2, 7–9]
ESRD	10–25	10	[2]
Gastrectomy	2–5	10	[2]
Hematologic malignancy	8–72	5	[10, 44]
Autologous BMT	1	5	[15]
Allogeneic BMT	3	5	[15]
Head and neck cancer	5–22	10	[10, 44]
Solid tumor US born	Approximately 1	15	[10]

Therapy of Tuberculous in Cancer Patients

The antimicrobial agents used for preventative therapy of latent Tuberculous or treatment of active disease do not differ between cancer and noncancer patients. We will not reiterate these regimens as they are the subject of multiple national guidelines. Several aspects of TB therapy in the cancer patient deserve special emphasis. No controlled clinical trials have been performed specifically in cancer patients with Tuberculous. However, recommendations for HIV patients do differ from immunocompetent TB patients, providing some guidance for management of the immunosuppressed cancer patient. These differences are in the regimens used for the continuation phase of therapy due to concerns about emerging drug resistance and treatment failure. For example, in noncavitary pulmonary disease with a negative sputum smear after the 2 month induction phase, once weekly Isoniazid/Rifapentine can be given to immunocompetent patients to complete 6 months of therapy[1]. This regimen is not recommended in HIV infected patients due to high rates of Rifamycin resistant TB in patients who relapse [39]. Similarly, in HIV patients with CD4 < 100, twice weekly regimens are not recommended due to rifamycin resistance in relapsed patients [40]. Extrapolating this data to the cancer population, it is reasonable to avoid once weekly and twice weekly continuation regimens in cancer patients whose immunosuppression affects CD4 T cells, such those which hematologic malignancies, Allogeneic BMT, or pharmacologic agents that reduce T cell function or number. In these patients, the regimen for the continuation phase should be either 3× per week or daily INH/Rifampin. For Solid tumor patients, standard continuation phase regimens can be used, based on susceptibility testing. For all patients, including cancer patients, the induction regimen does not change and initially includes four drugs (INH, Rifampin, PZA, Ethambutol) until susceptibilities are known.

Important Drug Interactions Relevant to Cancer Patients

Rifampin is a cornerstone of chemotherapy for active tuberculous and therapy of active tuberculous in cancer patient is likely to include this agent. Rifamycins have many significant drug interactions, some of which potentially impact drugs likely to be encountered in the cancer patient. Rifampin induces the metabolism of opiates and therefore lowers the effective levels of opiates. As such, initiation of Rifampin therapy can precipitate painful crises in cancer patients receiving opiates for pain. Careful attention to pain control is necessary when Rifampin is initiated. Rifampin also induces the metabolism of cyclosporin, leading to diminished immunosuppressive effect and elevated risk of GVHD when used in Allogeneic bone marrow transplant. Judgment about the use of Rifampin in the treatment of tuberculous in patients who require one of these medications must be made in conjunction with the patient's oncologist. If dose adjustment in the interacting agent is possible and levels can be monitored (i.e., cyclosporine, Tacrolimus) then Rifampin therapy may be possible. Rifabutin offers a suitable therapeutic alternative to Rifampin [41, 42] and may offer more favorable drug interaction profile for some agents, as has been recommended in therapy of Tuberculous in HIV patients taking protease inhibitors (CDC HIV). If no drug monitoring is available and alternative cancer agents are not available or indicated, a nonrifampin containing TB regimen may be used. This decision has major therapeutic consequences as regimens without rifampin require extension of therapy to 12–18 months, as recommended by national guidelines [43].

Summary

Diagnosis and treatment of TB in the cancer patient is likely to undergo substantial changes in the future. Tuberculous infection remains a significant worldwide health problem with a large reservoir of latent disease. As the array of immunosuppressive cancer therapies expands and are administered to populations with high rates of LTBI, the chance of active Tuberculous in cancer patients is likely to increase. Controlled trials are badly needed to assess the relative risk of TB and its optimal management in the cancer population. As is the case for Tuberculous across all patient groups, new antimicrobials that will allow shortening of TB regimens to less than 6 months are badly needed.

References

1. CDC. Treatment of tuberculosis. MMWR Recomm Rep. 2003;52:1–77.
2. CDC. Targeted tuberculin testing and treatment of latent tuberculosis infection. American Thoracic Society. MMWR Recomm Rep. 2000;49:1–51.
3. CDC. Guidelines for preventing opportunistic infections among hematopoietic stem cell transplant recipients. MMWR Recomm Rep. 2000;49:1–125, CE121–127.
4. Doffinger R, Dupuis S, Picard C, Fieschi C, Feinberg J, et al. Inherited disorders of IL-12- and IFNgamma-mediated immunity: a molecular genetics update. Mol Immunol. 2002;38:903–9.
5. Al-Muhsen S, Casanova JL. The genetic heterogeneity of mendelian susceptibility to mycobacterial diseases. J Allergy Clin Immunol. 2008;122:1043–51.
6. Flynn JL, Chan J. Immunology of tuberculosis. Annu Rev Immunol. 2001;19:93–129.
7. Louie E, Rice LB, Holzman RS. Tuberculosis in non-Haitian patients with acquired immunodeficiency syndrome. Chest. 1986;90:542–5.
8. Vieira J, Frank E, Spira TJ, Landesman SH. Acquired immune deficiency in Haitians: opportunistic infections in previously healthy Haitian immigrants. N Engl J Med. 1983;308:125–9.
9. Selwyn PA, Hartel D, Lewis VA, Schoenbaum EE, Vermund SH, et al. A prospective study of the risk of tuberculosis among intravenous drug users with human immunodeficiency virus infection. N Engl J Med. 1989;320:545–50.
10. Kamboj M, Sepkowitz KA. The risk of tuberculosis in patients with cancer. Clin Infect Dis. 2006;42:1592–5.
11. Feld R, Bodey GP, Groschel D. Mycobacteriosis in patients with malignant disease. Arch Intern Med. 1976;136:67–70.
12. Kaplan MH, Armstrong D, Rosen P. Tuberculosis complicating neoplastic disease. A review of 201 cases. Cancer. 1974;33:850–8.
13. De La Rosa GR, Jacobson KL, Rolston KV, Raad II, Kontoyiannis DP, et al. Mycobacterium tuberculosis at a comprehensive cancer centre: active disease in patients with underlying malignancy during 1990-2000. Clin Microbiol Infect. 2004;10:749–52.
14. Cordonnier C, Martino R, Trabasso P, Held TK, Akan H, et al. Mycobacterial infection: a difficult and late diagnosis in stem cell transplant recipients. Clin Infect Dis. 2004;38:1229–36.
15. de la Camara R, Martino R, Granados E, Rodriguez-Salvanes FJ, Rovira M, et al. Tuberculosis after hematopoietic stem cell transplantation: incidence, clinical characteristics and outcome. Spanish Group on Infectious Complications in Hematopoietic Transplantation. Bone Marrow Transplant. 2000;26:291–8.
16. George B, Mathews V, Srivastava A, Chandy M. Infections among allogeneic bone marrow transplant recipients in India. Bone Marrow Transplant. 2004;33:311–5.
17. Garces Ambrossi G, Jakubowski A, Feinstein MB, Weinstock DM. Active tuberculosis limited to foreign-born patients after allogeneic hematopoietic stem cell transplant. Bone Marrow Transplant. 2005;36:741–3.
18. Abad S, Gyan E, Moachon L, Bouscary D, Sicard D, et al. Tuberculosis due to Mycobacterium bovis after alemtuzumab administration. Clin Infect Dis. 2003;37:e27–8.
19. Baez Y, Giron F, Nino-Murcia A, Rodriguez J, Salcedo S. Experience with Alemtuzumab (Campath-1H) as induction agent in renal transplantation followed by steroid-free immunosuppression. Transplant Proc. 2008;40:697–9.
20. Walsh R, Ortiz J, Foster P, Palma-Vargas J, Rosenblatt S, et al. Fungal and mycobacterial infections after Campath (alemtuzumab) induction for renal transplantation. Transpl Infect Dis. 2008;10:236–9.
21. Peleg AY, Husain S, Kwak EJ, Silveira FP, Ndirangu M, et al. Opportunistic infections in 547 organ transplant recipients receiving alemtuzumab, a humanized monoclonal CD-52 antibody. Clin Infect Dis. 2007;44:204–12.
22. Au WY, Leung AY, Tse EW, Cheung WW, Shek TW, et al. High incidence of tuberculosis after alemtuzumab treatment in Hong Kong Chinese patients. Leuk Res. 2008;32:547–51.
23. Thursky KA, Worth LJ, Seymour JF, Miles Prince H, Slavin MA. Spectrum of infection, risk and recommendations for prophylaxis and screening among patients with lymphoproliferative disorders treated with alemtuzumab*. Br J Haematol. 2006;132:3–12.
24. Frank DA, Mahajan S, Ritz J. Fludarabine-induced immunosuppression is associated with inhibition of STAT1 signaling. Nat Med. 1999;5:444–7.
25. Samonis G, Kontoyiannis DP. Infectious complications of purine analog therapy. Curr Opin Infect Dis. 2001;14:409–13.
26. Silva FA, Matos JO, de Mello QFC, Nucci M. Risk factors for and attributable mortality from tuberculosis in patients with hematologic malignancies. Haematologica. 2005;90:1110–5.
27. Au WY, Kwong YL, Ma SK, Mak YK, Wong KF, et al. Hairy cell leukemia in Hong Kong Chinese: a 12-year retrospective survey. Hematol Oncol. 2000;18:155–9.

28. Rietschel P, Wolchok JD, Krown S, Gerst S, Jungbluth AA, et al. Phase II study of extended-dose temozolomide in patients with melanoma. J Clin Oncol. 2008;26:2299–304.
29. Su YB, Sohn S, Krown SE, Livingston PO, Wolchok JD, et al. Selective CD4+ lymphopenia in melanoma patients treated with temozolomide: a toxicity with therapeutic implications. J Clin Oncol. 2004;22:610–6.
30. de Paiva Jr TF, de Barros ESMJ, Rinck Jr JA, Fanelli MF, Gimenes DL. Tuberculosis in a patient on temozolomide: a case report. J Neurooncol. 2008;92:33–5.
31. Keane J, Gershon S, Wise RP, Mirabile-Levens E, Kasznica J, et al. Tuberculosis associated with infliximab, a tumor necrosis factor alpha-neutralizing agent. N Engl J Med. 2001;345:1098–104.
32. Levine JE, Paczesny S, Mineishi S, Braun T, Choi SW, et al. Etanercept plus methylprednisolone as initial therapy for acute graft-versus-host disease. Blood. 2008;111:2470–5.
33. Seong SS, Choi CB, Woo JH, Bae KW, Joung CL, et al. Incidence of tuberculosis in Korean patients with rheumatoid arthritis (RA): effects of RA itself and of tumor necrosis factor blockers. J Rheumatol. 2007;34:706–11.
34. Gomez-Reino JJ, Carmona L, Valverde VR, Mola EM, Montero MD. Treatment of rheumatoid arthritis with tumor necrosis factor inhibitors may predispose to significant increase in tuberculosis risk: a multicenter active-surveillance report. Arthritis Rheum. 2003;48:2122–7.
35. Pai M, Zwerling A, Menzies D. Systematic review: T-cell-based assays for the diagnosis of latent tuberculosis infection: an update. Ann Intern Med. 2008;149:177–84.
36. Mazurek GH, Jereb J, Lobue P, Iademarco MF, Metchock B, et al. Guidelines for using the QuantiFERON-TB Gold test for detecting Mycobacterium tuberculosis infection, United States. MMWR Recomm Rep. 2005;54:49–55.
37. Ferebee SH. Controlled chemoprophylaxis trials in tuberculosis. A general review. Bibl Tuberc. 1970;26:28–106.
38. WHO. Efficacy of various durations of isoniazid preventive therapy for tuberculosis: five years of follow-up in the IUAT trial. International Union Against Tuberculosis Committee on Prophylaxis. Bull World Health Organ. 1982;60:555–64.
39. Vernon A, Burman W, Benator D, Khan A, Bozeman L. Acquired rifamycin monoresistance in patients with HIV-related tuberculosis treated with once-weekly rifapentine and isoniazid. Tuberculosis Trials Consortium. Lancet. 1999;353:1843–7.
40. CDC. Acquired rifamycin resistance in persons with advanced HIV disease being treated for active tuberculosis with intermittent rifamycin-based regimens. MMWR Morb Mortal Wkly Rep. 2002;51:214–5.
41. Schwander S, Rusch-Gerdes S, Mateega A, Lutalo T, Tugume S, et al. A pilot study of antituberculosis combinations comparing rifabutin with rifampicin in the treatment of HIV-1 associated tuberculosis. A single-blind randomized evaluation in Ugandan patients with HIV-1 infection and pulmonary tuberculosis. Tuber Lung Dis. 1995;76:210–8.
42. Gonzalez-Montaner LJ, Natal S, Yongchaiyud P, Olliaro P. Rifabutin for the treatment of newly-diagnosed pulmonary tuberculosis: a multinational, randomized, comparative study versus Rifampicin. Rifabutin Study Group. Tuber Lung Dis. 1994;75:341–7.
43. American Thoracic Society, CDC, Infectious Diseases Society of America. Treatment of tuberculosis. MMWR Recomm Rep. 2003;52:1–77.
44. Libshitz HI, Pannu HK, Elting LS, Cooksley CD. Tuberculosis in cancer patients: an update. J Thorac Imaging. 1997;12:41–6.

Chapter 40
Nontuberculous Mycobacterial Infections

Amar Safdar

Abstract The spectrum of nontuberculous mycobacterial infections has changed. Improved understanding of the immunopathogenesis of slow growing mycobacerial disease has been accompanied by a higher number of cases in patients with or without cancer. In recent years, difficult-to-treat infections due to rapidly growing mycobacteria are on the rise, this may in part reflect newer molecular identification methods; however, rise in susceptible immunosuppressed patient population and frequently used indwelling prosthetic devices are also important contributors in this trend. Despite resistance to a number of available antimicrobials, newer agents may provide the much-needed treatment options for high-risk cancer patients with nontuberculous mycobacterial infection-disease.

Keywords Rapidly growing mycobacteria • Slow growing mycobacteria • Lady Windermere syndrome • Interferon gamma defect • *Mycobacterium avium* intracellulare

Antimycobacterial Immune Defense

Intact reticuloendothelial system provides the bases of innate immune defense against the invading virulent *Mycobacterium tuberculous* as well as most nonvirulent environmental mycobacterial species other than *M. tuberculous*. However, it is the adaptive cellular immune response that provides effective containment and elimination of intracellular mycobacteria residing within the mononuclear cells [1]. All components of T-lymphocytes including $\gamma\delta$ cells play a role, although CD4 cells are the dominant $\alpha\beta$ lymphocytes that provide the backbone of host's immune response against mycobacterial infections [2, 3]. Interferon gamma (IFN-γ) is the most important proinflammatory cytokine secreted by primed T-helper type-1 (T_H1) lymphocytes, which activates fixed tissue macrophages, recruits peripheral mononuclear cells to the site of infection, and sets in the stage for granuloma formation [4]. The granuloma serves as (a) physical barriers for mycobacterial propagation, (b) promotes unfavorable oxygen and micronutrient deficient environment, and (c) most importantly, creates a milieu in which various components of the immune cells and extracellular cytokines and chemokines interact to enhance effector cell-mediated mycobacterial cell death [5, 6].

The delayed-type hypersensitivity reaction against the invading mycobacterial infection on one hand is critical in effective containment of infection and on the other, via calcification of granulomas, large quantities of caseation necrosis and formation of pulmonary cavities paradoxically enables the intracellular mycobacteria to evade host's immune surveillance [7]. The cytokine that plays important role in antimycobacterial immune defense cascade other than IFN-γ includes interleukin 12, T-cell-derived tumor necrosis factor alpha, and the expending family of TNF-related immunoactive peptides [8–10].

Immunologic Susceptibility to NTM Disease

The host's immune defects in the light of earlier discussion, mostly involve dysregulation of cellular adaptive immune response. A complicated cascade of events is set into effect following exposure to mycobacterial antigens, and organism-specific antigen primed T-cell at the infection site orchestrates events leading to cell death of these intracellular pathogens.

Defects in the protagonist T_H1 cytokine, IFN-γ may either present as deficiency in cytokine production, or dysfunctional cytokine (IFN-γ) specific receptor have been shown to increase difficult-to-treat systemic mycobacteriosis [11–14]. Furthermore, defects in postreceptor cytoplasmic signaling pathways such as signal transducer and activator of transcription 1 (STAT1), signal transducing molecule, nuclear factor (NF)$_\kappa\beta$ essential modulator (NEMO), ancillary cytokines including interleukin-12, interlukine-18, and tumor necrosis factor-α can also lead to enhanced risk of severe disseminated infection due to otherwise nonvirulent mycobacteria [1, 4, 8].

A. Safdar (✉)
Department of Infectious Diseases, Infection Control, and Employee Health, The University of Texas M.D. Anderson Cancer Center, 1515 Holcombe Boulevard, Houston, TX 77030, USA
e-mail: amarsafdar@gmail.com

At present, the consensus to undertake an immunologic work is warranted in only non-HIV-infected patients who present with refractory mycobacterial infections or those with recurring pulmonary nontuberculous mycobacteriosis (NTM) with no known underlying predisposing conditions. The NTM even though is due to organisms with low-disease causing potential, is often in the setting of immunologically intact host, and an extensive immunologic work up at present may not yield clinically relevant information. Although in a select group of patients with unresponsive mycobacterial infection, immunologic investigation may be undertaken in consultation with infectious diseases.

Clinical Characteristics

The scope of mycobacterial infections due to species other than *M. tuberculous* has expanded near-exponentially in the recent past. In part this increase is attributed to the widespread availability of newer molecular identification methods [15]. Most nontuberculous mycobacteria are ubiquitous in nature, and unlike *M. tuberculous* person-to-person spread is not a significant means of transmission of infection. Isolation of these low-virulence mycobacteria is not uncommon and in immunologically intact, nonsusceptible individual they frequently represent either laboratory/environmental contaminant or nondisease-associated colonization of respiratory, orointestinal or genitourinary tracts. In patients with severe adaptive cellular immune defects, these mycobacteria may pose a serious threat.

Another feature that distinguishes these organisms from *M. tuberculous* is that they exhibit variable antimicrobial susceptibility profiles and often not susceptible to the first line antituberculous agents. The NTM is discussed under two broad headings based on the time needed for them to grow in laboratory. Slow-growing mycobacteria (SGM) are somewhat similar to *M. tuberculous* and take between 4 and 8 weeks to grow in enriched culture medium, whereas in case of rapidly growing mycobacteria (RGM) growth becomes evident within 7 days.

Slow-Growing Mycobacteria

Mycobacterium avium-Intracellular

Mycobacterium avium and *Mycobacterium intracellular* were originally differentiated on the bases of virulence to chickens and rabbits, respectively. Human infections were reported in 1943, and during 1980 and 1990s increased appreciation of diseases associated with MAC has been attributed in part due to HIV epidemic, although a higher number of non-HIV-infected patients have also been described as having infectious diseases due to these NTMs.

Pulmonary infections are most common, and isolation of MAC in respiratory tract samples including tracheal aspirate or bronchial samples by itself is not diagnostic of pulmonary MAC infection. Diagnosis requires the presence of a radiographic and clinical disease that is compatible with MAC infection. The radiographic feature suggestive of pulmonary NTM includes small, multicentric nodules, tree-in-bud appearances, and/or small thin-walled cavitary lesions. Cough is the most prominent symptoms, sputum production is relative minimal, except in patients with severe cystic bronchiectasis. Chronic lung disease is a well-recognized predisposing factor in the nonimmunosuppressed patients; these include patients with silicosis, chronic bronchitis, emphysema, and cystic fibrosis. Patients with healed fibrocavitary tuberculous remain at risk for secondary *M. avium-M. intracellular* infection.

Since 1980s, an increasing number of MAC-associated pulmonary NTM cases have been noted in the middle-aged and elderly women with no obvious immune defects. The most common feature of this illness is chronic cough, fatigue, inability to gain weight, depression, and in advance cases multicentric, cystic bronchiectatic pulmonary lesions; fever and night sweats are often not present. The author have described an underlying defect in interferon-gamma production in these patients who were initially mischaracterized as having Lady Windermere syndrome [11, 12]. This defect in the critical cytokine pathway has led the otherwise healthy patients to develop indolent, locally destructive pulmonary lesions due to environmental mycobacteria with low disease-causing potential in otherwise healthy individuals.

MAC infections are difficult to treat due to resistance to several antimicrobial agents; therapeutic regimen comprises of 3–4 drugs to which clinical isolates are susceptible; rifampin, ethambutol, macrolide derivatives such as azithromycin and clarithromycin plus a fluoroquinolone, like ciprofloxacin, moxifloxacin are often used. Clofazimine-based regimens are not suggested due to unacceptable drug toxicity and high mortality seen in HIV seropositive patients with disseminated MAC. The duration of therapy is longer than that for patients with pulmonary tuberculous. Most patients are treated for 18–24 months; in those with extra-pulmonary disease, duration may be extended to 36 months.

Mycobacterium kansasii

Mycobacterium kansasii is antigenically related to *M. tuberculous* and may be associated with false positive PPD due to antigenic cross-reactivity. Most infections in the United States are seen in urban centers situated in the Southeast and Midwestern part of the country. As animal studies suggest, presence of dust by unexplained mechanisms enhances disease-causing potential of *M. kansasii* [16], it is not surprising that patients with pneumoconiosis are more susceptible to *M. kansasii* lung infection compared with general population; infections are fourfold higher in men compared to women. Similarly, infections tend to be common with certain occupations that involve chronic exposure to dust, these include miners, welders, sandblasters, and painters.

Pulmonary infections are slowly progressive although unlike MAC, *M. kansasii* leads to lung involvement difficult to distinguish from tuberculous. Infections frequently involve the upper lung lobes, and thin-wall cavities are seen routinely in patients with *M. kansasii* pulmonary NTM. Treatment is rifampin-based, although rifampin-resistant strains are on the rise, especially in patients with HIV-associated AIDS receiving rifampin prophylaxis [17, 18]. *Mycobacterium kansasii* is intrinsically resistant to pyrazinamide [19], and a large study has shown that isoniazid can be excluded for antimicrobial regimen [20]. Clarithromycin is often added with rifampin plus ethambutol, while awaiting rifampin susceptibility results [21]. Duration of therapy is 12–18 months.

Other Slow-Growing Mycobacteria

Mycobacterium ulcerans, *Mycobacterium marinum*, *Mycobacterium genavense* *Mycobacterium haemophilum*, *Mycobacterium simiae* are occasionally associated with infection in human.

M. haemophilum was almost exclusively seen in patients with severe immune dysfunction either due to HIV-associated AIDS [22] or in recipients of hematopoietic stem cell transplantation [23]. Disseminated infections were common, and predilection for tendon sheaths, bone, and joints was similar to infection seen with RGM.

M. simiae complex includes *M. simiae*, *Mycobacterium lentiflavum*, and *Mycobacterium triplex*; like *M. kansasii* these SGM lead to pulmonary disease that is difficult to distinguish from tuberculous. However, nearly 3/4th of clinical isolates may be associated with no discernable disease [24, 25]. In certain regions of the United States, it has become the second most frequent NTM [25]. Infections tend to be more refractory to antimicrobial therapy, and high-frequency of drug resistance further complicates options for effective drug regimen. Clarithromycin, quinolones, ethambutol, cycloserine, and ethionamide show favorable in vitro activity [26].

Rapidly Growing Mycobacteria

These organisms exhibit prominent growth on solid culture medium within 7 days after incubation. The most recent distribution of pathogenic species includes *Mycobacterium fortuitum* complex, which besides *M. fortuitum*, *Mycobacterium mucogenicum*, and *Mycobacterium septicum*, now also incorporates formerly known species of *Mycobacterium chelonae* complex (*M. chelonae* and *Mycobacterium abscessus*). *Mycobacterium smegmatis* forms the newly described second group, including *M. smegmatis*, *Mycobacterium wolinskyi*, and *Mycobacterium goodii* [27].

Pneumonia. In patients with pulmonary NTM in the United States, RGM are the third common cause of NTM after MAC and *M. kansasii*, respectively. *M. abscessus* is associated with most pulmonary infection in RGM group, whereas infections due to *M. fortuitum*, sub. sp. *fortuitum*, *M. smegmatis* sub. sp. *smegmatis*, and *M. goodii* are less frequent [28]. *M. goodii* has been mostly isolated in patients with aspiration lipoid pneumonia. Similar to SGM, isolation of RGM from respiratory tract samples is not sufficient to make diagnosis of RGM infection; as in most cases, these organisms may represent either colonization or environmental contamination.

To establish RGM's link to pulmonary disease, microbiologic isolation should be accompanied with radiographic and clinically compatible disease [29]. Clinical symptoms of pulmonary NTM, which at best are nonspecific of mycobacterial infection, include chronic, minimally productive cough, low-grade fever, weight loss, and in severe cases hemoptysis may occur [29].

Clinical and microbiological response to antimicrobial therapy for RGM pulmonary mycobacteriosis is less encouraging compared to treatment response in patients with SGM infections [30]. Drug combination including clarithromycin, high-dose cefoxitin plus amikacin has been associated with good clinical response, albeit microbiologically refractory *M. abscessus* infections are not uncommon.

Skin and soft-tissue infection. *M. fortuitum* is the most common RGM that is often associated with skin and soft-tissue infection in immunologically competent patients; most infections occur due to accidental inoculation such as stepping on a nail. Whereas, most infections due to *M. chelonae* are seen in patients with a underlying predisposing condition such as chronic corticosteroid use, rheumatoid arthritis, lupus, and cancer [29, 31].

Health-related infections occur sporadically and have been seen in patients after deep intramuscular injection, sternal wound infection following cardiac surgery, and after a variety of reconstructive and plastic surgical procedures including augmentation mammoplasty, chest wall reconstruction after tumor resection [32].

Catheter-related infections. These infections have become the most common healthcare-related infections due RGM, most infections involve patients with long-term indwelling intravascular catheters, and often catheter-insertion sites are involved. In cancer patients, *M. chelonae* and *M. abscessus* are by far the most common in this setting [33]. Recently identified RGM species are increasingly reported in patients with cancer with catheter-related infection, they include *M. smegmatis* [34], *Mycobacterium neoaurum* [35], *Mycobacterium aurum* [36], *Mycobacterium lacticola* [37], and *Mycobacterium brumae* [38].

It is important to emphasize the fact that the RGM are frequently isolated in hospital and laboratory water supplies, and number pseudo-outbreaks involving contaminated blood culture materials, fiberoptic bronchoscope sterilizing machine contamination have been described [39, 40]. Therefore, strict criteria must be instituted before attributing to these low-virulence ubiquitous nontuberculous mycobacteria as a cause of catheter infection [41]. Treatment includes prompt removal of infected devices, and systemic combination antimicrobial therapy for 6–12 weeks. Selection of antimicrobials depends on RGM species, as a general rule RGM are resistant to most antituberculous agents with the exception of ethambutol. In patients with *M. chelonae-M. abscessus* infections, selection of appropriate drug therapy is even more limited due to high-level of intrinsic drug resistance. Clarithromycin-based regimen is currently recommended, although newer fluoroquinolones, such as gatifloxacin, and moxifloxacin; linezolid in vitro profile also appears promising, albeit further clinical experience is needed before such treatment is recommended. Other agents under investigation include tigecycline, a new glycycline that shows promising activity against most clinical isolates of *M. abscessus* [42].

Summary

The spectrum of nontuberculous mycobacteria is changing rapidly, as immunopathogenesis of SGM continues to improve. In recent years, difficult-to-treat infections due to RGM are on the rise, this may in part reflect newer molecular identification methods; however, rise in susceptible immunosuppressed patient population and frequently used indwelling prosthetic devices are also important contributors in this trend. Despite resistance to a number of available antimicrobials, newer agents may provide the much-needed treatment options for high-risk cancer patients with nontuberculous mycobacterial infection-disease.

References

1. Flynn JL, Chan J. Immunology of tuberculosis. Annu Rev Immunol. 2001;129:93–129.
2. Flynn JL, Goldstein MM, Triebold KJ, Koller B, Bloom BR. Major histocompatibility complex class I-restricted T cells are required for resistance to *Mycobacterium tuberculosis* infection. Proc Natl Acad Sci USA. 1992;89:12013–7.
3. D'Souza CD, Cooper AM, Frank AA, Mazzaccaro RJ, Bloom BR, Orme IM. An anti-inflammatory role for gamma delta T lymphocytes in acquired immunity to *Mycobacterium tuberculosis*. J Immunol. 1997;158:1217–21.
4. Murray HW. Interferon-gamma and host antimicrobial defense: current and future clinical applications. Am J Med. 1994;97:459–67.
5. Algood HMS, Chan J, Flynn JL. Chemokines and tuberculosis. Cytokine Growth Factor Rev. 2003;14:467–77.
6. Patarroyo M. Adhesion molecules mediating recruitment of monocytes to inflamed tissue. Immunobiology. 1994;191:474–7.
7. Kobayashi K, Kaneda K, Kasama T. Immunopathogenesis of delayed-type hypersensitivity. Microsc Res Tech. 2001;53:241–5.
8. Dorman SE, Holland SM. Interferon-γ and interleukin-12 pathway defects and human disease. Cytokine Growth Factor Rev. 2000;11:321–33.
9. Saunders BM, Briscoe H, Britton WJ. T cell-derived tumor necrosis factor is essential, but not sufficient, for protection against *Mycobacterium tuberculosis* infection. Clin Exp Immunol. 2004;137:279–87.
10. Ehlers S, Hölscher C, Scheu S, et al. The lymphotoxin β receptor is critically involved in controlling infections with the intracellular pathogens *Mycobacterium tuberculosis* and *Listeria monocytogenes*. J Immunol. 2003;170:5210–8.
11. Safdar A, White DA, Stover D, Armstrong D, Murray HW. Profound interferon gamma deficiency in patients with chronic pulmonary nontuberculous mycobacteriosis. Am J Med. 2002;113:756–9.
12. Safdar A, Armstrong D, Murray HW. A novel defect in interferon-gamma secretion in patients with refractory nontuberculous pulmonary mycobacteriosis. Ann Intern Med. 2003;138:521.
13. Holland SM, Eisenstin EM, Kuhns DB, et al. Treatment of refractory disseminated nontuberculous mycobacterial infection with interferon gamma. N Engl J Med. 1994;330:1348–55.
14. Dorman SE, Picard C, Lammas D, et al. Clinical features of dominant and recessive interferon gamma receptor 1 deficiencies. Lancet. 2004;364:2113–21.
15. Han XY, Pham AS, Tarrand JJ, Sood PK, Luthra RL. Rapid and accurate identification of mycobacteria by sequencing hypervariable regions of the 16S ribosomal RNA gene. Am J Clin Pathol. 2002;118:796–801.
16. Geruez-Rienx C, Tacquet A, Devulder B. Experimental study of interactions of pneumoconiosis and mycobacterial infections. Ann N Y Acad Sci. 1972;200:106.
17. Klein JL, Brown TJ, French GL. Rifampin resistance in *Mycobacterium kansasii* is associated with rpoB mutations. Antimicrob Agents Chemother. 2001;45:3056–8.
18. Wallace Jr RJ, Dunbar D, Brown BA, et al. Rifampin-resistant *Mycobacterium kansasii*. Clin Infect Dis. 1994;18:736–43.
19. Sun Z, Zhang Y. Reduced pyrazinamidase activity and the natural resistance of *Mycobacterium kansasii* to the antituberculosis drug pyrazinamide. Antimicrob Agents Chemother. 1999;43:537–42.
20. Research Committee, British Thoracic Society. *Mycobacterium kansasii* pulmonary infection: a prospective study of the results of nine months of treatment with rifampin and ethambutol. Thorax. 1994;49:442–5.
21. Yew WW, Piddock LJ, Li MS, Lyon D, Chan CY, Cheng AF. In-vitro activity of quinolones and macrolides against mycobacteria. J Antimicrob Chemother. 1994;34:343–51.
22. Lerner C, Safdar A, Coppel S. *Mycobacterium haemophilum* infection in AIDS. Infect Dis Clin Practice. 1995;4:233–6.
23. White MH, Papadopoulos EB, Small TN, Kiehn TE, Armstrong D. *Mycobacterium haemophilum* infections in bone marrow transplant recipients. Transplantation. 1995;15:957–60.
24. Rynkiewicz DL, Cage GD, Butler WR, Ampel NM. Clinical and microbiological assessment of *Mycobacterium simiae* isolates from a single laboratory in Southern Arizona. Clin Infect Dis. 1998;26:625–30.

25. Valero G, Paters J, Jorgensen JH, Graybill JR. Clinical isolates of *Mycobacterium simiae* in San Antonio, Texas. An 11-yr review. Am J Respir Crit Care Med. 1995;152:1555–7.
26. Valero G, Moreno F, Graybill JR. Activity of clarithromycin, ofloxacin, and clarithromycin plus ethambutol against *Mycobacterium simiae* in murine model of disseminated infection. Antimicrob Agents Chemother. 1994;38:2676–7.
27. Brown BA, Springer B, Steingrube VA, et al. Description of *Mycobacterium wolinskyi* and *Mycobacterium goodii* two new rapidly growing species related to *Mycobacterium smegmatis* and associated with human wound infections: a cooperative study from the International Working Group on Mycobacterial Taxonomy. Int J Syst Bacteriol. 1999;49:1493–511.
28. Griffith DE, Girard WM, Wallace Jr RJ. Clinical features of pulmonary disease caused by rapidly growing mycobacteria: an analysis of 154 patients. Am Rev Respir Dis. 1993;147:1271–8.
29. Jacobson K, Garcia R, Libshitz H, et al. Clinical and radiological features of pulmonary disease caused by rapidly growing mycobacteria in cancer patients. Eur J Clin Microbiol Infect Dis. 1998;17:615–21.
30. Wallace Jr RJ, Cook JL, Glassroth J, et al. Diagnosis and treatment of disease caused by nontuberculous mycobacteria. American Thoracic Society Statement. Am J Respir Crit Care Med. 1997;156 Suppl 1:S1–25.
31. Wallace Jr RJ, Brown BA, Onyi GO. Skin, soft tissue, and bone infections due to *Mycobacterium chelonae chelonae*: importance of prior corticosteroid therapy, frequency of disseminated infections, and resistance to oral antimicrobials other than clarithromycin. J Infect Dis. 1992;166:405–12.
32. Safdar A, Bains M, Polsky B. Clinical microbiological case: refractory chest wall infection following reconstructive surgery in a patient with relapsed lung cancer. Clin Microbiol Infect. 2001;7(563–564):577–9.
33. Engler HD, Hass A, Hodes DS, Bottone EJ. *Mycobacterium chelonei* infection of a Broviac catheter insertion site. Eur J Clin Microbiol Infect Dis. 1989;8:521–3.
34. Skiest DJ, Levi ME. Catheter-related bacteremia due to *Mycobacterium smegmatis*. South Med J. 1998;91:36–7.
35. Woo PC, Tsoi HW, Leung KW, et al. Identification of *Mycobacterium neoaurum* isolated from a neutropenic patient with catheter-related bacteremia by 16S rRNA sequencing. J Clin Microbiol. 2000;38:3515–7.
36. Koranyi KI, Ranalli MA. *Mycobacterium aurum* bacteremia in an immunocompromised child. Pediatr Infect Dis. 2003;22:1108–9.
37. Kiska DL, Turenne CY, Dubansky AS, Domachowske JB. First case report of catheter-related bacteremia due to "*Mycobacterium lacticola*". J Clin Microbiol. 2004;42:2855–7.
38. Lee SA, Raad II, Adachi JA, Han XY. Catheter-related bloodstream infection caused by *Mycobacterium brumae*. J Clin Microbiol. 2004;42:5429–31.
39. Ashford DA, Kellerman S, Yakrus M, et al. Pseudo-outbreak of septicemia due to rapidly growing mycobacteria associated with extrinsic contamination of culture supplement. J Clin Microbiol. 1997;35:2040–2.
40. Fraser VJ, Jones MJ, Murray PR, Medoff G, Zhang Y, Wallace RJ. Contamination of flexible fiberoptic bronchoscopes with *Mycobacterium chelonae* linked to an automated bronchoscope disinfection machine. Am Rev Respir Dis. 1992;145:853–5.
41. Safdar A, Raad II. Management and treatment. In: O'Grady NP, Pittet D, editors. Catheter-related infections in the critically ill. 1st ed. Boston: Kluwer Academic Publishers; 2004. p. 99–112.
42. Wallace RJ, Brown-Elliott BA, Crist CJ, Mann L, Wilson RW. Comparison of the in vitro activity of the glycylcycline tigecycline (formerly GAR-939) with those of tetracycline, minocycline, and doxycycline against isolates of nontuberculous mycobacteria. Antimicrob Agents Chemother. 2002;46:3164–7.

Chapter 41
Parasitic Infections in Cancer Patients: Toxoplasmosis, Strongyloidiasis, and Other Parasites

Brian G. Blackburn and José G. Montoya

Abstract The most important parasitic infections in cancer patients are *Toxoplasma gondii* and *Strongyloides stercoralis*. Both can cause life-threatening disease in immunocompromised patients, where *T. gondii* can present as encephalitis, pneumonia, fever of unknown origin, myocarditis, hepatitis, and chorioretinitis, and *S. stercoralis* as the disseminated hyperinfection syndrome. Effective therapies are available for both, but high case-fatality rates result if these syndromes are not recognized and treated promptly. Excellent preventative measures are available for both parasites, including prophylactic anti-*Toxoplasma* therapy or ivermectin treatment for strongyloidiasis in properly selected patients. Identifying cancer patients at risk for these syndromes is therefore critical, so that these measures can be instituted before life-threatening disease develops.

Keywords Toxoplasmosis • *Strongyloides stercoralis* • *Toxoplasma gondii* • Myocarditis • Hepatitis • Chorioretinitis • Disseminated hyperinfection syndrome

Toxoplasmosis

Introduction

Toxoplasma gondii is a ubiquitous intracellular parasite that infects over one billion people worldwide. In cancer patients, *T. gondii* infection (most commonly reactivation of latent infection) can result in major morbidity and life-threatening syndromes if left untreated. Reactivation of this parasite is usually the result of significantly impaired T-cell mediated immunity. Cancer patients with defects in this arm of the immune system (e.g., lymphoma, acute lymphoblastic leukemia) or who undergo treatments that cause such a defect (e.g., hematopoietic stem cell transplant [HSCT] or alemtuzumab) are at higher risk. Because the organism is so difficult to isolate, laboratory diagnosis is primarily based upon the use of serological, DNA amplification, and immunohistochemical methods. Following early diagnosis, treatment can reverse the initial clinical manifestations of toxoplasmosis, and decrease mortality in immunocompromised patients. Toxoplasmosis in cancer patients should be suspected in patients with fever, pneumonia, hepatitis, myositis, myocarditis or encephalitis, as well as in those with lymphadenopathy, chorioretinitis, and brain abscesses.

Life Cycle and Epidemiology

T. gondii exists in nature primarily in three forms, the tachyzoite, tissue cyst, and oocyst. The *tachyzoite* has a "banana" or "bow" shape, measures 2–3 μm by 5–7 μm, and its presence is pathognomonic for acute or reactivated infection (Fig. 41.1a). Thus, the visualization of tachyzoites in fluids or tissues, using hematoxylin and eosin, Wright-Giemsa, or immunoperoxidase stains, is indicative that a patient's symptoms and signs can be attributed to toxoplasmosis.

Tissue cysts are present in asymptomatic and chronically infected individuals or animals, contain the dormant form called "bradyzoites," and can measure up to 100 μm (Fig. 41.1b). After acute infection, individuals remain infected with *T. gondii* indefinitely, as these tissue cysts persist for life. Tissue cysts in meat are rendered nonviable by γ-irradiation, heating to 67°C (153°F), or freezing for 24 h at ≤−20°C (−4°F). The finding of a tissue cyst in a pathology specimen does not necessarily indicate that a patient's syndrome can be attributed to toxoplasmosis unless a heavy inflammatory reaction and a large number of cysts are also present in the tissue.

Oocysts are present in the gut (and feces) of infected felids (including housecats), contain sporozoites, and measure 10 × 12 μm (Fig. 41.1c). Ten million oocysts per day can be shed by an infected cat, and may remain viable for up to 18 months in moist soil; it takes 1–5 days after excretion into

---
B.G. Blackburn (✉)
Department of Internal Medicine, Division of Infectious Diseases and Geographic Medicine, Stanford University School of Medicine, 300 Pasteur Drive, Room S-101, Stanford, CA 94305, USA
e-mail: blackburn@stanford.edu

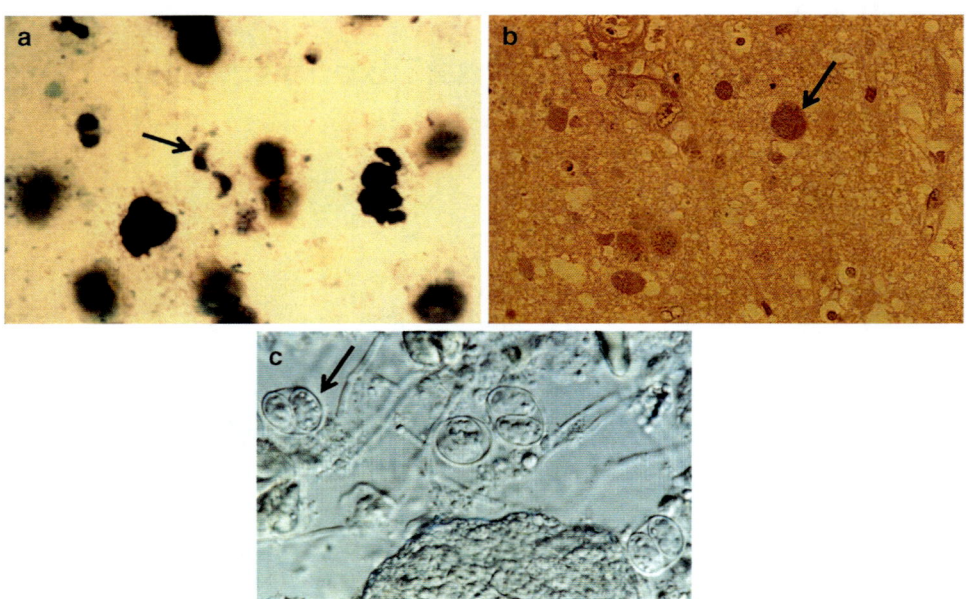

Fig. 41.1 (**a–c**) Main forms of *T. gondii* found in nature (see *arrows*). Tachyzoites (**a**), tissue cysts (**b**) containing bradyzoites, and oocysts (**c**) containing sporozoites

the environment for oocysts to become infective. Felids are the definitive host for *T. gondii*, and it is only in them that the reproductive cycle can be completed and the parasite amplified. Cats shed oocysts for only 1–2 weeks after initial infection with *T. gondii*.

Humans are infected with *T. gondii* primarily via the oral route, either by consuming tissue cysts in meat, or oocysts spread in the environment by cat feces. Although consumption of undercooked or raw infected meat or contact with infected cat feces are the classically recognized sources of infection, more than 50% of recently infected patients do not report either risk factor [1]. Most individuals thus become infected with *T. gondii* in ways less traditionally associated with toxoplasmosis. Therefore, the decision to test patients for *T. gondii* should not be based solely on a history of cat ownership or ingestion of undercooked or raw meat. A recent study performed by the Centers for Disease Control and Prevention (CDC) and the Palo Alto Medical Foundation Toxoplasmosis Serology Laboratory (PAMF-TSL) identified the ingestion of raw oysters, clams, and mussels as a novel risk factor for recent *T. gondii* infection in the United States [2]. Other studies have shown consumption of contaminated water to be an important means of transmission [3–5]. In the U.S., the prevalence of the infection appears to be declining; a recent study demonstrated that the age-adjusted *T. gondii* seroprevalence among persons 6–49 years old was about 11%, significantly decreased from a previous survey [6]. *T. gondii* prevalence increases with age; within the U.S., the seroprevalence also varies widely by geographic locale and by ethnicity; in some cohorts, the prevalence can be as high as 50%. In many countries, persons in lower socioeconomic strata have higher *T. gondii* prevalence rates than their wealthier counterparts [7]. Many countries have much higher *T. gondii* prevalence rates than the U.S., including countries in the developing world and Europe. In certain countries it appears that the prevalence has been sustained for decades or is increasing [7].

The epidemiology, virulence, and clinical manifestations of the parasite may vary by geographical area. It is believed that *T. gondii* has evolved to a few clonal strains (termed types I, II, and III) that are distributed unequally worldwide. The more aggressive type I/III strains appear to be more common in South America, the less virulent type II strain predominates in Europe, and the USA has a mixture of the strains [8].

Clinical Manifestations

Acute *T. gondii* Infection

Most individuals do not experience illness when exposed to *T. gondii* for the first time. When clinical manifestations are present, painless and nonsuppurative lymphadenopathy is the most common presentation in Europe and the U.S. However, recent data indicate that even immunocompetent patients with acute toxoplasmosis in other latitudes (e.g., South America) may present with additional symptoms (e.g., high fever, constitutional symptoms, life-threatening pneumonia) [9]. Thus, cancer patients who travel should be advised regarding prevention and early recognition of toxoplasmosis outside the USA and Europe.

Recent data suggest that chorioretinitis as a result of acute, postnatally acquired *T. gondii* infection occurs more frequently in the USA and Europe than previously thought, particularly in patients older than 50 years of age; older data had suggested that most ocular toxoplasmosis was due to reactivation of congenital infection [5, 10]. Ocular toxoplasmosis causes a retinochoroiditis, and can result in blurred vision, eye pain, decreased visual acuity, floaters, scotoma, photophobia, or epiphora. Other less common but well-documented syndromes have been associated with the acute infection including hepatitis, myositis, and myocarditis.

Toxoplasmosis as a Result of Reactivation of Chronic Infection

Patients who acquire *T. gondii* remain latently infected indefinitely. In patients with cancer, immunosuppressive drugs or stem cell transplants greatly increase the risk of reactivation in latently infected persons. Clinically apparent toxoplasmosis in such patients usually results from reactivation of latent infection rather than from acute infection. In patients with allogeneic stem cell transplants, the presence of graft versus host disease (GVHD) increases the risk for toxoplasmosis, and most of the disease presents between days 31 and 100 (64% of cases) post-transplantation [11].

Several syndromes have been associated with reactivation of the parasite in these patients including encephalitis, chorioretinitis, fever of unknown origin, pneumonia, myocarditis, hepatosplenomegaly, lymphadenopathy, and rash. Brain abscesses can result, causing headache, altered mental status, seizures, coma, and focal neurologic changes (Fig. 41.2). Diffuse encephalitis can also occur, without focal neuroimaging findings, and is associated with a poor prognosis. Meningitis alone is rarely a manifestation of toxoplasmosis. Chorioretinitis can be the sole manifestation of toxoplasmosis in immunocompromised patients and may present with similar symptoms as in acute infections. Other well-documented syndromes occur with toxoplasmosis and are often overlooked. Fever with pneumonia can be the sole manifestation of toxoplasmosis in immunocompromised patients. Toxoplasmic pneumonitis can present with cough, dyspnea, hypoxia, and diffuse bilateral infiltrates. Fever alone has been well described in patients with allogeneic stem cell transplants.

Laboratory Diagnosis

Laboratory diagnosis of *T. gondii* infection and toxoplasmosis can be established by serological methods, polymerase chain reaction (PCR), or immunohistochemistry [12].

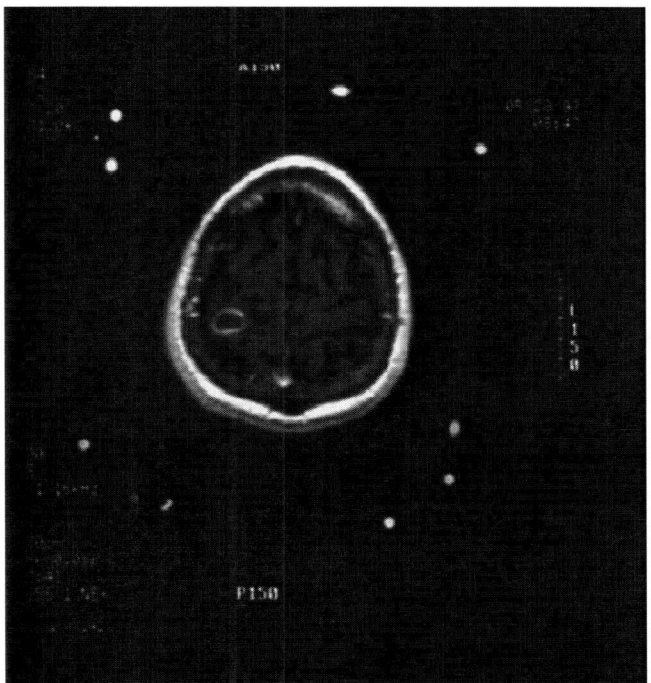

Fig. 41.2 Brain MRI depicting ring-enhancing brain lesion in immunocompromised patient. *T. gondii*-specific immunoperoxidase staining of brain biopsy tissue was diagnostic of toxoplasmic encephalitis

Serological Tests

Initial serological testing for *T. gondii* can be accomplished at nonreference or commercial laboratories, where *Toxoplasma* IgG testing tends to be reliable. IgM results, when negative, are also usually accurate. Positive IgM results, however, should be viewed with caution. Many nonreference laboratories have a high rate of false-positive IgM results when compared against reference *Toxoplasma* laboratories; positive IgM test results should therefore be confirmed at a reference laboratory (see below).

Negative IgG and IgM test results establish that the patient has not been exposed to the parasite (assuming that the patient is capable of producing normal immunoglobulin levels). Positive IgG with negative IgM test results establish that the patient has been infected with the parasite in the past, and is at risk for reactivation. Positive IgM test results (with either positive or negative IgG test results) should raise the suspicion for a recent infection. However, a positive IgM result may indicate not only an acute infection, but also can be observed in the setting of a chronic infection, or may be a false positive result. Positive IgM test results should be confirmed at a reference laboratory (e.g., at PAMF-TSL, http://www.pamf.org/serology/; telephone (650) 853-4828; e-mail, toxolab@pamf.org) [13]. At PAMF-TSL, confirmatory tests include the use of a more specific IgM ELISA (using the "double-sandwich" method invented by Dr. Jack S. Remington), differential agglutination (or AC/HS), IgG avidity testing, IgA ELISA, and IgE ELISA [12].

Because patients chronically infected with *T. gondii* are at risk of reactivating the parasite and toxoplasmosis can be life-threatening, serological testing for toxoplasmosis should be performed in all high risk immunocompromised patients (the more profound the T-cell mediated defect, the higher the risk). The diagnosis of chronic infection is established by a positive IgG test result and a negative IgM test result (additionally, some patients with chronic infection may have a positive IgG and IgM result). Once it has been established that the patient is IgG positive for *Toxoplasma* and that the patient has a chronic infection, there is little or no utility in repeating or performing additional serological testing. Serological testing does not have any role in the diagnosis of toxoplasmosis due to reactivation of a latent infection, and is not useful for following response to therapy. PCR and histological methods are best used in this setting.

Polymerase Chain Reaction

In immunocompromised individuals, PCR of body fluids or tissues is of great value in diagnosing toxoplasmosis. PCR can be performed on almost any body fluid, including cerebrospinal fluid (CSF), bronchoalveolar lavage, vitreous fluid, aqueous humor, and peripheral blood. Positive results usually establish the diagnosis of toxoplasmic encephalitis, pneumonia, chorioretinitis, or disseminated disease, respectively. If feasible and safe, a lumbar puncture should be performed in patients suspected to have toxoplasmic encephalitis. Although the sensitivity of the CSF by PCR has been variable, specificity approaches 100% [14]. Although positive CSF IgM test results have been reported in congenitally infected infants, serological testing of CSF should be discouraged in adults, and PCR testing should be the priority. PCR testing for *T. gondii* is available at PAMF-TSL and other laboratories.

Histological Methods

Tachyzoites and tissue cysts can be demonstrated by the use of Wright-Giemsa staining or immunohistochemistry. Almost any tissue can be examined with the *T. gondii*-specific immunoperoxidase method; this technique has been useful for the diagnosis of toxoplasmic encephalitis. The histological diagnosis of toxoplasmosis requires the demonstration of tachyzoites or multiple tissue cysts near an inflammatory necrotic lesion.

Management

All cancer patients with significant T-cell mediated immunity defects should have *Toxoplasma* serological testing performed and if possible, testing should be done before significant immunosuppressive therapy is begun (e.g., HSCT or immunosuppressive drugs). In patients chronically infected with toxoplasmosis, primary prophylaxis should be considered to prevent reactivation disease, and a low threshold for testing clinically indicated body fluids and tissues for toxoplasmosis (by PCR and immunohistochemistry) should be used when patients fall ill.

Invasive Procedures

Invasive diagnostic procedures should be considered in patients in whom toxoplasmosis is suspected, especially those with fever, pneumonia, myocarditis, brain lesions, encephalitis, chorioretinitis, or rash. Bronchoalveolar lavage or myocardial, brain, vitreous, or skin biopsies should be considered early during the illness and specimens tested by PCR and specialized stains. The empiric use of anti-*Toxoplasma* drugs in patients with multiple brain lesions who are seropositive for *T. gondii* (prior to examining the CSF by PCR or performing a brain biopsy) has not been validated in non-AIDS immunocompromised patients, and if feasible, should be avoided in this patient population. Rather, early consideration should be given to a brain biopsy.

Drugs

Toxoplasmosis should always be treated with combination therapy, and higher doses are indicated for immunocompromised patients (Table 41.1). Pyrimethamine is the most effective agent against *T. gondii* and should be part of the drug regimen if possible. The combination of pyrimethamine/sulfadiazine (with folinic acid to minimize the toxicity of pyrimethamine) is considered the first-line regimen for toxoplasmosis. Limited supply and the lack of an IV formulation have been major barriers for more widespread use. Recent data suggest that trimethoprim/sulfamethoxazole (TMP/SMX) has similar efficacy to pyrimethamine/sulfadiazine in the setting of both toxoplasmic encephalitis and chorioretinitis [15, 16]. TMP/SMX has the additional advantage of being available intravenously. Another effective regimen is pyrimethamine plus clindamycin. Alternatively, pyrimethamine can be used with atovaquone. In extreme cases, when none of the above drugs can be used, clarithromycin, dapsone, or azithromycin can be substituted.

Table 41.1 Recommended drug regimens for immunocompromised patients with toxoplasmosis[a] (primary therapy)

Pyrimethamine (PO)	200 mg loading dose followed by 50 mg (<60 kg) to 75 mg (>60 kg/day)
Folinic acid[b] (PO)	10–20 mg daily (up to 50 mg/day) (during and 1 week after therapy with pyrimethamine)
plus	
Sulfadiazine (PO)	1,000 (<60 kg) to 1,500 mg (>60 kg) every 6 h
or	
Clindamycin (PO or IV)	600 mg every 6 h (up to 1,200 mg every 6 h)
or	
Atovaquone (PO)	1,500 mg orally twice daily
Trimethoprim/sulfamethoxazole (PO or IV)	10 mg/kg/day (trimethoprim component) divided in 2–3 doses (doses as high as 15–20 mg/kg/day have been used)
Pyrimethamine/folinic acid	Same doses as above
plus	
Clarithromycin (PO)	500 mg every 12 h
or	
Dapsone (PO)	100 mg/day
or	
Azithromycin (PO)	900–1,200 mg/day

Preferred combinations: pyrimethamine/sulfadiazine/folinic acid or trimethoprim/sulfamethoxazole
[a]Assistance is available for the diagnosis and management of patients with toxoplasmosis at the Palo Alto Medical Foundation *Toxoplasma* Serology Laboratory, telephone number (650) 853 4828
[b]Folinic acid = leucovorin; folic acid should not be used as a substitute for folinic acid
After the successful use of a combination regimen during the acute/primary therapy phase, same agents at half-does are usually used for maintenance or secondary prophylaxis

Prevention

Seronegative (*Toxoplasma* IgG negative) immunocompromised patients should be advised to avoid exposure to the parasite (http://www.cdc.gov/toxoplasmosis/prevent.html). In addition to the recommendations presented at this website, these patients should also be warned about the possibility of acquiring *T. gondii* by ingesting raw oysters, clams, and mussels.

Seropositive immunocompromised patients should be considered candidates for primary prophylaxis. The most successful agent for this indication has been TMP/SMX (e.g., one double strength [or single strength] tablet daily [assuming normal renal function]). Alternatively, atovaquone can be used (1,500 mg/day) or any of the other drugs listed above, but at half the treatment dose.

Strongyloidiasis

Strongyloidiasis is caused by the intestinal nematode, *Strongyloides stercoralis*. Primarily transmitted in tropical areas, *S. stercoralis* usually causes a chronic gastrointestinal syndrome or can remain asymptomatic for decades [17]. The primary medical importance of this parasite in the developed world lies in its potential to cause the hyperinfection syndrome in immunocompromised patients, wherein larvae may disseminate throughout the body, with mortality rates of up to 70–80% [18–20].

The Organism

The life cycle of *S. stercoralis* is complex, alternating between free-living and parasitic cycles, and includes adult worms, two different larval stages, and eggs. These cycles form the basis for autoinfection and multiplication within the host, features relatively unique among helminths to *Strongyloides* [21, 22].

Soil-living adult worms produce eggs, which give rise to noninfective *rhabditiform larvae*. These either continue the free-living cycle by maturing into adults, or become infective *filariform larvae*. Filariform larvae can penetrate intact human skin, after which they migrate to the lungs. From there, they are expectorated, swallowed, and reach the small intestine; this journey takes about 3–4 weeks. In the intestine, *S. stercoralis* matures into adult worms, which are semi-translucent and about two millimeters long. These produce eggs, which hatch and become rhabditiform larvae. Although most of these larvae exit the gastrointestinal tract via the stool and subsequently develop into adult worms in the soil, a small number directly become infective (filariform) larvae within the gut and penetrate the intestinal mucosa or perianal skin, completing the life cycle without leaving the host. This is termed *autoinfection*, and differentiates *S. stercoralis* from nearly all other helminths in several ways, including indefinite persistence in a host (in the absence of treatment), multiplication in the absence of exogenous re-infection, and potential person-to-person transmission [23].

Epidemiology

Global estimates of strongyloidiasis prevalence vary widely, from 3 to 100 million infected [20, 21, 24]. *S. stercoralis* is less common than other major intestinal nematodes such as *Ascaris*, *Trichuris*, and hookworms [17]. Strongyloidiasis is found throughout the tropics and subtropics and in limited foci of the USA (e.g., Appalachia) and Europe [24]. Because transmission occurs via skin contact with fecally-contaminated soil, transmission is favored where poor hygienic conditions are combined with a warm, moist climate. Primary prevention involves better hygiene and footware use in endemic areas.

Studies based on stool examination in the 1960s and 1970s showed prevalence rates of 0.5–4.0% in differing US cohorts, mostly in the Southeast and Appalachia [21, 24]. Although prevalence has subsequently decreased, infections are still seen in patients from those areas, especially patients who are older than 50 years, institutionalized, of low socioeconomic status, or who have lived in rural areas [24]. In cohorts in developing countries, strongyloidiasis prevalence rates can be striking, for example 25% in Thailand and Nigeria, 28% in Brazil, and 40% in Colombia [21, 24]. Because of the superior sensitivity of serology for diagnosis, seroepidemiology studies generally report higher prevalence rates; in one Peruvian cohort, 9% tested positive by stool examination for *S. stercoralis*, while 72% were seropositive [25]. Prevalence rates in resettled US refugees can be high, with one recent study reporting 46% *S. stercoralis* seroprevalence in a group of resettled Sudanese refugees [26]. Another study found that 39% of asymptomatic refugees in Boston with eosinophilia were *S. stercoralis* seropositive [27]. Given the high prevalence in many tropical and subtropical areas and the lifelong persistence of this parasite in the absence of treatment, physicians should consider strongyloidiasis both in persons with recent exposure to endemic areas, and immigrant or refugee patients in developed countries even if they immigrated decades earlier.

Pathogenesis, Immunity, and the Hyperinfection Syndrome

Strongyloides infection is sustained over time in a given host by a small, stable number of intestinal adult worms. Although these die after a finite lifespan, autoinfection ensures the constant production of new worms, perpetuating the cycle even in the absence of reinfection [28]. In patients with chronic strongyloidiasis, autoinfection is normally well controlled by cell-mediated immunity, and the number of adult worms remains low and stable. With immunosuppression, more autoinfective larvae complete the cycle, and the population of parasitic adult worms increases, causing *hyperinfection* [28]. The large numbers of migrating larvae can disseminate, often associated with polymicrobial sepsis, bronchopneumonia, and meningitis. Untreated, disseminated strongyloidiasis is usually fatal, and even with treatment mortality approaches 25–30% [19, 29].

Both parasite and host factors affect regulation of this cycle. The population size of *S. stercoralis* in a host depends in part on secreted parasite hormones that regulate autoinfection [22, 30]. When the immune response is impaired, larger numbers of autoinfective parasites can develop, as reported in patients with hematologic malignancies, solid organ transplant and HSCT, hypogammaglobulinemia, and severe malnutrition [31–33]. Interestingly, there has been little association between cyclosporine use and hyperinfection syndrome; some evidence suggests cyclosporine may have an antihelminthic effect on *S. stercoralis* [34].

Among HTLV-infected patients, there is a strong association with increased susceptibility to infection with *Strongyloides*, the hyperinfection syndrome, and poor response to treatment. Control of *S. stercoralis* in vivo is most dependent on the Th2 immune response, but the predominant immune response in HTLV-infected patients shifts from Th2 to Th1 [35–37]. There is some suggestion that *S. stercoralis* may hasten the development of leukemia among HTLV co-infected patients [38]. In contrast, there have been surprisingly few reports of hyperinfection among *S. stercoralis*-infected patients with AIDS. Although disseminated strongyloidiasis does occasionally occur in AIDS patients, this disease was removed from the list of AIDS-defining illness by the CDC in 1987 [39, 40].

Corticosteroid use carries a disproportionately high risk for disseminated strongyloidiasis compared to other forms of immunosuppression [41, 42]. Corticosteroids may upregulate growth of *S. stercoralis*, and allow the parasite to develop preferentially into autoinfective filariform larvae, in addition to suppressing immunity [22, 43, 44]. They may also allow nonreproductive adult worms to regain reproductivity [30, 45]. Patients have developed hyperinfection after only a few days of corticosteroid administration [46].

Clinical Findings

Most patients infected with *S. stercoralis* are asymptomatic, or have only mild symptoms. Shortly after infection, some patients develop a localized, erythematous, pruritic rash [29, 47–49]. Pulmonary symptoms and eosinophilia may appear several days later; diarrhea and abdominal pain may follow. Blood is occasionally detected in the stool, but over 50% are asymptomatic. Chronic strongyloidiasis is not generally associated with pulmonary symptoms. Although about 75% of chronically infected patients have eosinophilia, it is usually low-grade (5–15% of the WBC differential) [21, 50]. Migrating larvae may produce *larva currens*, a serpiginous, erythematous, track-like rash. Some chronically infected patients note epigastric pain, nausea, diarrhea, blood loss, and possibly malabsorption. Rarely, heavy infections can cause bowel obstruction. The majority of chronically infected patients are asymptomatic [41]. There has been an association between *S. stercoralis* infection and biliary cancer, but this observation requires confirmation [51].

With hyperinfection, the intestines and lungs harbor many larvae, and diarrhea is common (Fig. 41.3). When dissemination occurs, larvae are found widely, sometimes involving the central nervous system (CNS). Eosinophilia is often absent during hyperinfection. Other gastrointestinal manifestations are common, including abdominal pain, vomiting, and intestinal obstruction. Hemorrhage, peritonitis, or bacteremia can occur. Pneumonitis is common, with cough, respiratory failure, and diffuse interstitial infiltrates or consolidation on radiographs; respiratory secretions often contain the parasite (Fig. 41.4a, b). CNS invasion may cause meningitis and brain abscesses, with larvae in the CSF or tissue. An association with SIADH has been reported [52, 53].

Diagnosis

Uncomplicated strongyloidiasis is diagnosed by finding rhabditiform larvae in microscopic stool examination; it is uncommon to find eggs in the stool. Because few larvae are shed, the sensitivity of a single stool examination is only about 30%; multiple samples should therefore be examined (with concentration techniques). Examination of up to seven stool samples can significantly increase sensitivity [21, 54]. Sampling duodenal fluid or small bowel biopsy can increase sensitivity, but practical issues limit usefulness [55]. Placing stool samples on agar plates to observe tracks left by the motile larvae may be the most sensitive method among the stool examination techniques [56–58].

Because of the difficulty with microscopic diagnosis, serologic tests (which are more sensitive) are often favored, such as the enzyme-linked immunoassay offered by CDC (Atlanta, GA). This is about 95% sensitive in stool-positive patients, although specificity is lower because of cross-reactivity with other helminths [25, 50]. The titer of *Strongyloides* antibodies in infected patients generally begins to decline 6–12 months after cure, as does the peripheral

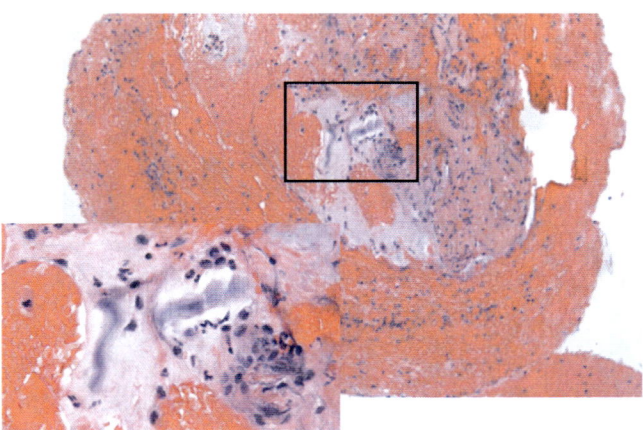

Fig. 41.3 Bronchoscopic biopsy in patient with *Strongyloides* hyperinfection syndrome. Courtesy Chandra Krishnan, MD, Stanford University, Department of Pathology

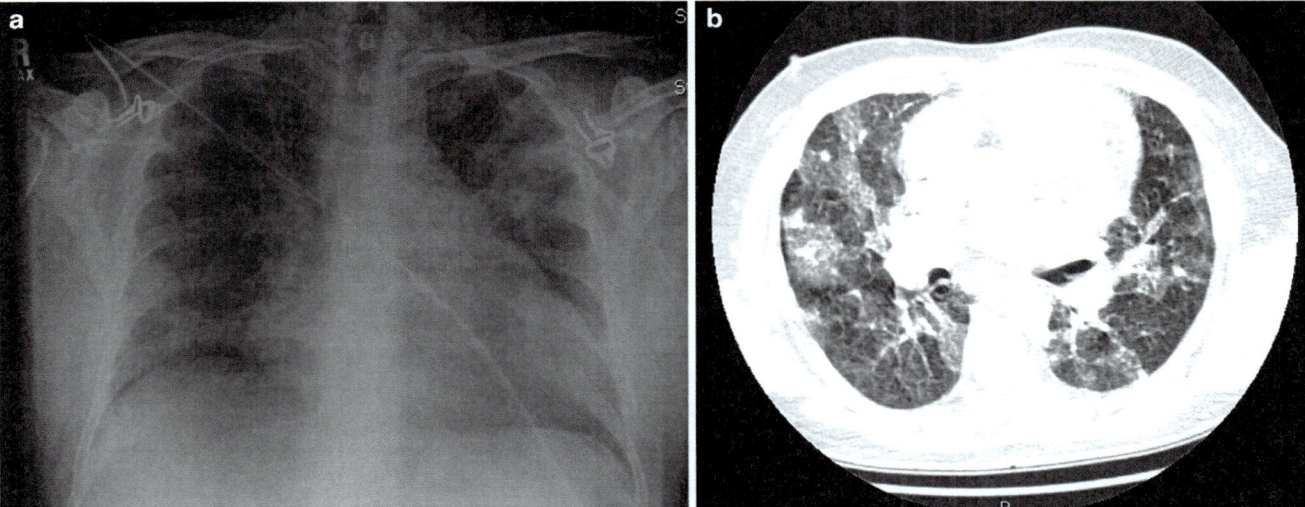

Fig. 41.4 (a) Chest radiograph in patient with *Strongyloides* hyperinfection syndrome. (b) Chest computed tomographic examination in patient with *Strongyloides* hyperinfection syndrome

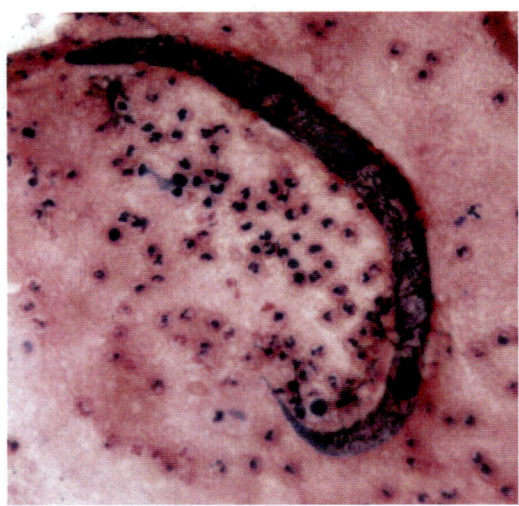

Fig. 41.5 Sputum sample from patient with *Strongyloides* hyperinfection syndrome. Courtesy Stanford University, Microbiology Laboratory

gastrointestinal cancer patients, of whom 24% were infected with *S. stercoralis* [61]. It is also important in nonendemic areas, given the global increase in travel and immigration. One retrospective review at a US cancer center found 2.0 *S. stercoralis* infections per 10,000 leukemia patients, and 0.8 infections per 10,000 cancer patients overall; however, systematic screening was not done, so these are likely underestimates. Among the infected patients, 48% had received systemic corticosteroids, and 36% antineoplastic therapy. Fifty-seven percent had diarrhea, 48% eosinophilia, and 24% developed the hyperinfection syndrome. Both of the patients with hyperinfection syndrome who had received HSCTs died despite appropriate therapy [62].

Although most chemotherapeutic agents have been associated with hyperinfection, the association seems particularly strong for vinca alkaloids [41]. These exert a toxic effect on myenteric neurons, decreasing intestinal motility and increasing larval transit time, perhaps allowing more to become autoinfective filariform larvae.

Treatment

All persons infected with *S. stercoralis* should be treated. The drug of choice for uncomplicated strongyloidiasis is oral ivermectin, 200 µg/kg/day for 2 days, which cures 70–85% of chronically infected patients. One study demonstrated a higher cure rate with two-dose ivermectin regimens compared to previously used single-dose regimens [63, 64]. Alternatives include thiabendazole or albendazole for 3–7 days, although ivermectin appears more effective; thiabendazole is poorly tolerated, and albendazole has the lowest cure rate among these drugs [64–68]. Ivermectin is also preferred for hyperinfection/disseminated strongyloidiasis. It should be administered daily until symptoms have resolved and larvae have not been detected for at least 2 weeks [20, 41]. Several patients with disseminated strongyloidiasis have received veterinary formulations of subcutaneous ivermectin. Although still experimental, this is an alternative for patients poorly tolerant of oral therapy and for those with severe infection [69–72]. Some patients have received a combination of ivermectin and albendazole with success [73]. If possible, immunosuppressive therapy should be stopped (particularly corticosteroids). Some recommend monthly treatment subsequently for patients who require continued immunosuppression [18–20].

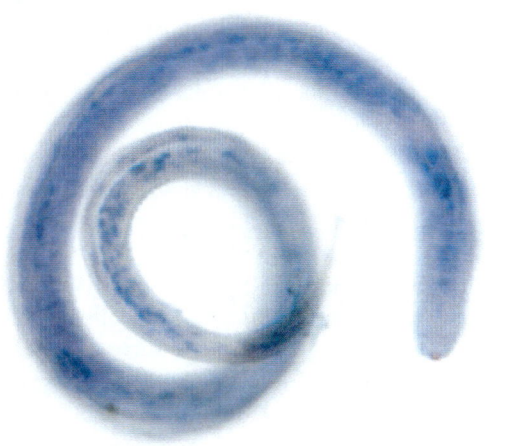

Fig. 41.6 Bronchoalveolar lavage sample showing filariform *S. stercoralis* larvae in patient with hyperinfection syndrome. Courtesy Chandra Krishnan, MD, Stanford University, Department of Pathology

eosinophil count [50, 59, 60]. In contrast to chronic strongyloidiasis, hyperinfection and disseminated strongyloidiasis are easily diagnosed by microscopic stool examination (or other samples, such as sputum), which typically contain many filariform larvae (Figs. 41.5 and 41.6).

Strongyloidiasis in Cancer Patients

Given the risk of hyperinfection syndrome, identifying strongyloidiasis in cancer patients is critical. This is paramount in endemic areas, as evidenced by a Brazilian cohort of

Follow-up stool examinations should be repeated frequently to document cure. For long-term follow-up, serology and eosinophil counts may offer stronger evidence of treatment efficacy. These findings generally begin to normalize 6–12 months after cure [50, 59].

Prevention of Hyperinfection

For all patients who are (or will soon become) immunosuppressed, examination of stool and serologic specimens for *S. stercoralis* should be considered for those who have lived in an endemic area or had other possible exposure to *S. stercoralis* at any time in their life (particularly those infected with HTLV-1 or receiving corticosteroids) [74]. Though most important for persons from highly endemic developing countries, this is also a consideration for residents of the southeastern USA, especially older persons who lived there during childhood. Such screening would be particularly important for those with clinical strongyloidiasis (e.g., eosinophilia, larva currens, abdominal pain). All infected patients should be treated promptly, preferably prior to initiation of immunosuppressive therapy. If a patient's condition requires immunosuppression before *S. stercoralis* diagnostics are available, the risks of empiric antiparasitic therapy for strongyloidiasis must be weighed against the risks of disseminated infection [75].

Other Parasitic Infections of Importance in Cancer Patients

Although *T. gondii* and *S. stercoralis* are the most clinically important parasitic infections in cancer patients, many others also warrant discussion. The clinical relevance of these parasites stems from either (1) increased risk of severe disease in immunocompromised hosts, or (2) association between infection and subsequent malignancy.

Opportunistic Parasites

Trypanosoma cruzi (Chagas' Disease)

Trypanosoma cruzi, a protozoan endemic only to the Americas (mostly limited to the tropics), is transmitted primarily by bloodsucking Triatomine insects [76]. A minority of patients suffer symptoms in the weeks after infection including fever, myocarditis, and meningoencephalitis; although occasionally severe, most patients recover and enter an asymptomatic *indeterminate phase* of infection. *T. cruzi* then persists indefinitely, causing end-organ disease in 20–30%, years-to-decades later [76]. Heart disease is most common (e.g., conduction disease and heart failure) among symptomatic patients, with gastrointestinal disease (megaesophagus or megacolon) also seen; patients with achalasia are at increased risk for esophageal cancer [77]. Diagnosis of chronic infection can be made serologically.

Acute Chagas disease is rarely seen in the USA, but immunocompromised hosts chronically infected with *T. cruzi* are at increased risk for reactivation; this syndrome resembles acute infection, but can be more severe. Atypical manifestations are seen, including *T. cruzi* brain abscesses, skin lesions, and mucosal involvement [78, 79]. Treatment is with either benznidazole or nifurtimox; in the USA, these drugs are available only through CDC. No consensus exists regarding approach to *T. cruzi* infection in oncology patients, but serologic screening should be considered for patients (or HSCT donors) who have lived in endemic areas. Many centers use a presumptive treatment approach in infected, immunocompromised patients, initiating antiparasitic therapy if parasitemia becomes detectable by culture or PCR [80, 81]. Others recommend prophylactic therapy in all infected patients who are currently, or will imminently be, immunosuppressed [82].

Acanthamoeba and *Balamuthia*

Acanthamoeba spp. and *Balamuthia mandrillaris* are free-living, ubiquitous environmental amebae. Although clinically apparent human infection with these organisms is rare, a meningoencephalitis-like syndrome (often with CNS mass lesions) can occur, largely in immunocompromised patients [83]. Disseminated disease can involve the skin, lungs, liver, and bones; typical progression is over weeks to months [84]. Diagnosis typically requires biopsy, although serologic tests exist. Case-fatality rates are high, even with multiple antimicrobials; no consensus treatment regimen exists, but effective antimicrobials include pentamidine, azoles, sulfonamides, macrolides, and flucytosine.

Visceral Leishmaniasis

Leishmania spp. are intracellular protozoans transmitted by sandflies. Most cases of visceral leishmaniasis (VL) are acquired in South Asia, East Africa, or Brazil, although some transmission also occurs in the Mediterranean littoral. A wide clinical spectrum exists for patients, with most infections subclinical. Although immunocompetent patients can progress to symptomatic disease, immunosuppression (such as cancer chemotherapy or HSCT) is an established precipitant of this [85–87]. For patients who become symptomatic, clinical disease can present months or years after initial infection. VL causes protean manifestations, including fever, hepatosplenomegaly, weight loss, skin changes, cytopenias, and hyperglobulinemia. Diagnosis is by biopsy and microscopic examination or culture of involved tissues, although serology can be an adjunct; untreated, progressive VL is usually fatal.

Treatment options include liposomal amphotericin, pentavalent antimony compounds, miltefosine, and paromomycin.

Intestinal Protozoa

Intestinal protozoa such as *Cryptosporidium* spp., *Isospora belli*, and *Cyclospora cayetanensis* can cause severe diarrhea in immunocompromised patients. Recent data suggest *Cryptosporidium* in particular may be a common cause of diarrhea in some oncology cohorts [88, 89]. Diarrhea is generally watery, and diagnosis is by stool studies; all three parasites can be detected through modified acid fast stains, and *Cryptosporidium* can also be detected through sensitive stool immunoassays. Treatment of *Cryptosporidium* is with nitazoxanide, while *Isospora* and *Cyclospora* are treated with trimethoprim-sulfamethoxazole [90].

Microsporida can cause diarrheal disease in immunocompromised patients; they can also disseminate, with involvement of the CNS, lungs, or other organs [91]. Diagnosis is by trichrome staining of the stool, and treatment is with albendazole or fumagillin, depending on the species [90].

Parasites Associated with Carcinogenesis

Liver Flukes

The liver flukes *Clonorchis sinensis* and *Opisthorchis viverrini* are helminths that are acquired by ingestion of undercooked fish. *C. sinensis* is endemic mostly to East Asia and *O. viverrini* to Southeast Asia [92]. These parasites can cause chronic biliary disease, and epidemiologic evidence links infection to the development of cholangiocarcinoma, usually years later. Evidence is best for *O. viverrini*, but is also emerging for *C. sinensis*; a related species, *Opisthorchis felineus*, has been less well studied. Infected persons have a 5–15-fold higher risk of developing cholangiocarcinoma than uninfected persons in endemic areas, depending on the parasite burden and region studied [93, 94]. Diagnosis is generally via stool examination; serologic tests exist, but are not widely available outside endemic areas. Treatment with praziquantel is usually curative, but once cholangiocarcinoma has developed, antiparasitic treatment does not generally affect the course of the malignancy.

Schistosomiasis

Schistosoma spp. are blood flukes acquired through skin contact with infested freshwater. Although several species cause gastrointestinal and hepatic disease, *Schistosoma haematobium* (endemic to Africa and parts of the Middle East), causes primarily genitourinary disease. Chronic infection causes hematuria and urinary obstruction. Infection over many years has been linked epidemiologically with the development of squamous cell bladder carcinoma, an otherwise uncommon malignancy [95]. Diagnosis is classically through stool or urine examinations, but serologic assays are more sensitive. Treatment with praziquantel is usually curative, but does not generally affect the course of the cancer once established.

References

1. Boyer KM, Holfels E, Roizen N, et al. Risk factors for *Toxoplasma gondii* infection in mothers of infants with congenital toxoplasmosis: implications for prenatal management and screening. Am J Obstet Gynecol. 2005;192:564–71.
2. Jones JL, Dargelas V, Roberts J, Press C, Remington JS, Montoya JG. Sources of *Toxoplasma gondii* infection in the United States. In: American Society of Tropical Medicine and Hygiene; 57th annual meeting. New Orleans; 2008.
3. Heukelbach J, Meyer-Cirkel V, Moura RC, et al. Waterborne toxoplasmosis, northeastern Brazil. Emerg Infect Dis. 2007;13:287–9.
4. Aramini JJ, Stephen C, Dubey JP, Engelstoft C, Schwantje H, Ribble CS. Potential contamination of drinking water with *Toxoplasma gondii* oocysts. Epidemiol Infect. 1999;122:305–15.
5. Bowie WR, King AS, Werker DH, et al. Outbreak of toxoplasmosis associated with municipal drinking water. Lancet. 1997;350:173–7.
6. Jones JL, Kruszon-Moran D, Sanders-Lewis K, Wilson M. *Toxoplasma gondii* infection in the United States, 1999 2004, decline from the prior decade. Am J Trop Med Hyg. 2007;77:405–10.
7. Rosso F, Les JT, Agudelo A, et al. Prevalence of infection with *Toxoplasma gondii* among pregnant women in Cali, Colombia, South America. Am J Trop Med Hyg. 2008;78:504–8.
8. Lehmann T, Marcet PL, Graham DH, Dahl ER, Dubey JP. Globalization and the population structure of *Toxoplasma gondii*. Proc Natl Acad Sci U S A. 2006;103:11423–8.
9. Demar M, Ajzenberg D, Maubon D, et al. Fatal outbreak of human toxoplasmosis along the Maroni River: epidemiological, clinical, and parasitological aspects. Clin Infect Dis. 2007;45:e88–95.
10. Stanford MR, Tan HK, Gilbert RE. Toxoplasmic retinochoroiditis presenting in childhood: clinical findings in a UK survey. Br J Ophthalmol. 2006;90:1464–7.
11. Mele A, Paterson PJ, Prentice HG, Leoni P, Kibbler CC. Toxoplasmosis in bone marrow transplantation: a report of two cases and systematic review of the literature. Bone Marrow Transplant. 2002;29:691–8.
12. Montoya JG. Laboratory diagnosis of *Toxoplasma gondii* infection and toxoplasmosis. J Infect Dis. 2002;185 Suppl 1:S73–82.
13. Public Health Service, Department of Health and Human Services (US) and Food and Drug Administration (FDA). FDA public health advisory: limitations of toxoplasma IgM commercial test kits. Rockville: Department of Health and Human Services, Food and Drug Administration; 1997. p. 3.
14. Alfonso Y, Fraga J, Fonseca C, et al. Molecular diagnosis of *Toxoplasma gondii* infection in cerebrospinal fluid from AIDS patients. Cerebrospinal Fluid Res. 2009;6:2.
15. Soheilian M, Sadoughi MM, Ghajarnia M, et al. Prospective randomized trial of trimethoprim/sulfamethoxazole versus pyrimethamine and sulfadiazine in the treatment of ocular toxoplasmosis. Ophthalmology. 2005;112:1876–82.

16. Torre D, Casari S, Speranza F, et al. Randomized trial of trimethoprim-sulfamethoxazole versus pyrimethamine-sulfadiazine for therapy of toxoplasmic encephalitis in patients with AIDS. Antimicrob Agents Chemother. 1998;42:1346.
17. Bethony J, Brooker S, Albonico M, et al. Soil-transmitted helminth infections: ascariasis, trichuriasis, and hookworm. Lancet. 2006;367:1521–32.
18. Lam CS, Tong MK, Chan KM, Siu YP. Disseminated strongyloidiasis: a retrospective study of clinical course and outcome. Eur J Clin Microbiol Infect Dis. 2006;25:14–8.
19. Marcosa LA, Terashimab A, DuPont HL, Gotuzzo E. Strongyloides hyperinfection syndrome: an emerging global infectious disease. Trans Roy Soc Trop Med Hyg. 2008;102:314–8.
20. Maguire JH. Intestinal nematodes (roundworms). In: Mandell GL, Bennett JE, Dolin R, editors. Principles and practices of infectious diseases. 6th ed. Philadelphia: Churchill Livingstone; 2005. p. 3264–6.
21. Siddiqui AA, Berk SL. Diagnosis of Strongyloides stercoralis infection. Clin Infect Dis. 2001;33:1040–7.
22. Siddiqui AA, Genta RM, Berk SL. Strongyloidiasis. In: Guerrant RL, Walker DH, Weller PF, editors. Tropical infectious diseases, 2nd edition – principles, pathogens, & practice. Philadelphia: Churchill Livingstone; 2006. p. 1274–85.
23. Schad GA. Morphology and life history of Strongyloides stercoralis. In: Grove DI, editor. Strongyloidiasis: a major roundworm infection of man. London: Taylor & Francis; 1989. p. 85–104.
24. Genta RM. Global prevalence of strongyloidiasis: critical review with epidemiologic insights into the prevention of disseminated disease. Rev Infect Dis. 1989;11:755–67.
25. Yori PP, Kosek M, Gilman RH, et al. Seroepidemiology of strongyloidiasis in the Peruvian Amazon. Am J Trop Med Hyg. 2006;74:97–102.
26. Posey DL, Blackburn BG, Weinberg M. High prevalence and presumptive treatment of schistosomiasis and strongyloidiasis among African refugees. Clin Infect Dis. 2007;45:1310–5.
27. Seybolt LM, Christiansen D, Barnett ED. Diagnostic evaluation of newly arrived asymptomatic refugees with eosinophilia. Clin Infect Dis. 2006;42:363–7.
28. Neva FA. Biology and immunology of human strongyloidiasis. J Infect Dis. 1986;153:397–406.
29. Grove DI. Human strongyloidiasis. Adv Parasitol. 1996;38:251–309.
30. Genta RM. Dysregulation of strongyloidiasis: a new hypothesis. Clin Microbiol Rev. 1992;5:345–55.
31. Schaeffer MW, Buell JF, Gupta M, Conway GD, Akhter SA, Wagoner LE. Strongyloides hyperinfection syndrome after heart transplantation: case report and review of the literature. J Heart Lung Transplant. 2004;23:905–11.
32. Seet RC, Lau LG, Tambyah PA. Strongyloides hyperinfection and hypogammaglobulinemia. Clin Diagn Lab Immunol. 2005;12:680–2.
33. Morgan JS, Schaffner W, Stone WJ. Opportunistic strongyloidiasis in renal transplant recipients. Transplantation. 1986;42:518–24.
34. Schad GA. Cyclosporine may eliminate the threat of overwhelming strongyloidiasis in immunosuppressed patients. J Infect Dis. 1986;153:178.
35. Carvalho EM, Da Fonseca PA. Epidemiological and clinical interaction between HTLV-1 and Strongyloides stercoralis. Parasite Immunol. 2004;26:487–97.
36. Gotuzzo E, Terashima A, Alvarez H, et al. Strongyloides stercoralis hyperinfection associated with human T cell lymphotropic virus type-1 infection in Peru. Am J Trop Med Hyg. 1999;60:146–9.
37. Hirata T, Uchima N, Kishimoto K, et al. Impairment of host immune response against Strongyloides stercoralis by human T cell lymphotropic virus type 1 infection. Am J Trop Med Hyg. 2006;74:246–9.
38. Plumelle Y, Gonin C, Edouard A, et al. Effect of Strongyloides stercoralis infection and eosinophilia on age at onset and prognosis of adult T-cell leukemia. Am J Clin Pathol. 1997;107:81–7.
39. Viney ME, Brown M, Omoding NE, et al. Why does HIV infection not lead to disseminated strongyloidiasis? J Infect Dis. 2004;190:2175–80.
40. Centers for Disease Control. Revision of the CDC surveillance case definition for acquired immunodeficiency syndrome. MMWR. 1987;36(Suppl):1–15.
41. Keiser PB, Nutman TB. Strongyloides stercoralis in the Immunocompromised population. Clin Microbiol Rev. 2004;17:208–17.
42. Newberry AM, Williams DN, Stauffer WM, Boulware DR, Hendel-Paterson BR, Walker PF. Strongyloides hyperinfection presenting as acute respiratory failure and Gram-negative sepsis. Chest. 2005;128:3681–4.
43. Siddiqui AA, Stanley CS, Skelly PJ, et al. A cDNA encoding a nuclear hormone receptor of the steroid/thyroid hormone-receptor superfamily from the human parasitic nematode Strongyloides stercoralis. Parasitol Res. 2000;86:24–9.
44. Nolan TJ, Megyeri Z, Bhopale VM, et al. Strongyloides stercoralis: the first rodent model for uncomplicated and hyperinfective strongyloidiasis, the Mongolian gerbil (Meriones unguiculatus). J Infect Dis. 1993;168:1479–84.
45. Mansfield LS, Niamatali S, Bhopale V, et al. Strongyloides stercoralis: maintenance of exceedingly chronic infections. Am J Trop Med Hyg. 1996;55:617–24.
46. Fardet L, Généreau T, Poirot JL, Guidet B, Kettaneh A, Cabane J. Severe strongyloidiasis in corticosteroid-treated patients: case series and literature review. J Infect. 2007;54:18–27.
47. Segarra-Newnham M. Manifestations, diagnosis, and treatment of Strongyloides stercoralis infection. Ann Pharmacother. 2007;41:1992–2001.
48. Liu LX, Weller PF. Strongyloidiasis and other intestinal nematode infections. Infect Dis Clin North Am. 1993;7:655–82.
49. Berk SL, Verghese A, Alvarez S, Hall K, Smith B. Clinical and epidemiologic features of strongyloidiasis. A prospective study in rural Tennessee. Arch Intern Med. 1987;147:1257–61.
50. Loutfy MR, Wilson M, Keystone JS, Kain KC. Serology and eosinophil count in the diagnosis and management of strongyloidiasis in a non-endemic area. Am J Trop Med Hyg. 2002;66:749–52.
51. Hirata T, Kishimoto K, Kinjo N, Hokama A, Kinjo F, Fujita J. Association between Strongyloides stercoralis infection and biliary tract cancer. Parasitol Res. 2007;101:1345–8.
52. Reddy TS, Myers JW. Syndrome of inappropriate secretion of antidiuretic hormone and nonpalpable purpura in a woman with Strongyloides stercoralis hyperinfection. Am J Med Sci. 2003;325:288–91.
53. Hayashi E, Ohta N, Yamamoto H. Syndrome of inappropriate secretion of antidiuretic hormone associated with strongyloidiasis. Southeast Asian J Trop Med Public Health. 2007;38:239–46.
54. Nielsen PB, Mojon M. Improved diagnosis of Strongyloides stercoralis by seven consecutive stool specimens. Zentralbl Mikrobiol. 1987;263:616–8.
55. Agrawal V, Agarwal T, Ghoshal UC. Intestinal strongyloidiasis: a diagnosis frequently missed in the tropics. Trans R Soc Trop Med Hyg. 2009;103:242–6.
56. Sato Y, Kobayashi J, Toma H, Shiroma Y. Efficacy of stool examination for detection of Strongyloides infection. Am J Trop Med Hyg. 1995;53:248–50.
57. Hirata T, Nakamura H, Kinjo N, et al. Increased detection rate of Strongyloides stercoralis by repeated stool examinations using the agar plate culture method. Am J Trop Med Hyg. 2007;77:683–4.
58. de Kaminsky RG. Evaluation of three methods for laboratory diagnosis of Strongyloides stercoralis infection. J Parasitol. 1993;79:277–80.

59. Karunajeewa H, Kelly H, Leslie D, Leydon J, Saykao P, Biggs BA. Parasite-specific IgG response and peripheral blood eosinophil count following albendazole treatment for presumed chronic strongyloidiasis. J Travel Med. 2006;13:84–91.
60. Page WA, Dempsey K, McCarthy JS. Utility of serological follow-up of chronic strongyloidiasis after anthelminthic chemotherapy. Trans Royal Soc Trop Med Hyg. 2006;100:1056–62.
61. Machado ER, Teixeira EM, Gonçalves-Pires Mdo R, Loureiro ZM, Araújo RA, Costa-Cruz JM. Parasitological and immunological diagnosis of *Strongyloides stercoralis* in patients with gastrointestinal cancer. Scand J Infect Dis. 2008;40:154–8.
62. Safdar A, Malathum K, Rodriguez SJ, Husni R, Rolston KV. Strongyloidiasis in patients at a comprehensive cancer center in the United States. Cancer. 2004;100:1531–6.
63. Treatment Guidelines from The Medical Letter. Drugs for parasitic infections. Med Lett Drugs Ther. 2007;5(Suppl):e1–15.
64. Igual-Adell R, Oltra-Alcaraz C, Soler-Company E, Sánchez-Sánchez P, Matogo-Oyana J, Rodríguez-Calabuig D. Efficacy and safety of ivermectin and thiabendazole in the treatment of strongyloidiasis. Expert Opin Pharmacother. 2004;5:2615–9.
65. Salazar SA, Berk SH, Howe D, Berk SL. Ivermectin vs thiabendazole in the treatment of strongyloidiasis. Infect Med. 1994;11:50–9.
66. Suputtamongkol Y, Kungpanichkul N, Silpasakorn S, Beeching NJ. Efficacy and safety of a single-dose veterinary preparation of ivermectin versus 7-day high-dose albendazole for chronic strongyloidiasis. Int J Antimicrob Agents. 2008;31:46–9.
67. Datry A, Hilmarsdottir I, Mayorga-Sagastume R, et al. Treatment of *Strongyloides stercoralis* infection with ivermectin compared with albendazole: results of an open study of 60 cases. Trans R Soc Trop Med Hyg. 1994;88:344–5.
68. Marti H, Haji HJ, Savioli L, et al. A comparative trial of a single-dose ivermectin versus three days of albendazole for treatment of *Strongyloides stercoralis* and other soil-transmitted helminth infections in children. Am J Trop Med Hyg. 1996;55:477–81.
69. Pacanowski J, Santos MD, Roux A, et al. Subcutaneous ivermectin as a safe salvage therapy in *Strongyloides stercoralis* hyperinfection syndrome: a case report. Am J Trop Med Hyg. 2005;73:122–4.
70. Chiodini PL, Reid AJ, Wiselka MJ, Firmin R, Foweraker J. Parenteral ivermectin in *Strongyloides* hyperinfection. Lancet. 2000;355:43–4.
71. Turner SA, Maclean JD, Fleckenstein L, Greenaway C. Parenteral administration of ivermectin in a patient with disseminated strongyloidiasis. Am J Trop Med Hyg. 2005;73:911–4.
72. Marty FM, Lowry CM, Rodriguez M, et al. Treatment of human disseminated strongyloidiasis with a parenteral veterinary formulation of ivermectin. Clin Infect Dis. 2005;41:e5–8.
73. Pornsuriyasak P, Niticharoenpong K, Sakapibunnan A. Disseminated strongyloidiasis successfully treated with extended duration ivermectin combined with albendazole: a case report of intractable strongyloidiasis. Southeast Asian J Trop Med Public Health. 2004;35:531–4.
74. Centers for Disease Control and Prevention. Guidelines for preventing opportunistic infections among hematopoietic stem cell transplant recipients. MMWR. 2000;49(RR-10):26–7.
75. Blackburn B. Strongyloidiasis. In: Pickering LK, Baker CJ, Long SS, McMillan JA, editors (American Academy of Pediatrics). Red Book: 2006 report of the committee on infectious diseases. 27th ed. Elk Grove Village: American Academy of Pediatrics; 2006. p. 629–31.
76. Barrett MP, Burchmore RJS, August Stich A, et al. The trypanosomiases. Lancet. 2003;362:1469–80.
77. Brücher BL, Stein HJ, Bartels H, Feussner H, Siewert JR. Achalasia and esophageal cancer: incidence, prevalence, and prognosis. World J Surg. 2001;25:745–9.
78. Fontes Rezende RE, Lescano MA, Zambelli Ramalho LN, et al. Reactivation of Chagas' disease in a patient with non-Hodgkin's lymphoma: gastric, oesophageal and laryngeal involvement. Trans R Soc Trop Med Hyg. 2006;100:74–8.
79. Lury KM, Castillo M. Chagas' disease involving the brain and spinal cord: MRI findings. Am J Roentgenol. 2005;185:550–2.
80. Altclas J, Sinagra A, Dictar M, et al. Chagas disease in bone marrow transplantation: an approach to preemptive therapy. Bone Marrow Transplant. 2005;36:123–9.
81. Dictar M, Sinagra A, Verón MT, et al. Recipients and donors of bone marrow transplants suffering from Chagas' disease: management and preemptive therapy of parasitemia. Bone Marrow Transplant. 1998;21:391–3.
82. Bern C, Montgomery SP, Herwaldt BL, et al. Evaluation and treatment of Chagas disease in the United States: a systematic review. JAMA. 2007;298:2171–81.
83. Visvesvara GS, Moura H, Schuster FL. Pathogenic and opportunistic free-living amoebae: *Acanthamoeba* spp., *Balamuthia mandrillaris*, *Naegleria fowleri*, and *Sappinia diploidea*. FEMS Immunol Med Microbiol. 2007;50:1–26.
84. Kaul DR, Lowe L, Visvesvara GS, Farmen S, Khaled YA, Yanik GA. *Acanthamoeba* infection in a patient with chronic graft-versus-host disease occurring during treatment with voriconazole. Transpl Infect Dis. 2008;10:437–41.
85. Sah SP, Rijal S, Bhadani PP, Rani S, Koirala S. Visceral leishmaniasis in two cases of leukemia. Southeast Asian J Trop Med Public Health. 2002;33:25–7.
86. Fakhar M, Asgari Q, Motazedian MH, Monabati A. Mediterranean visceral leishmaniasis associated with acute lymphoblastic leukemia (ALL). Parasitol Res. 2008;103:473–5.
87. Sirvent-von Bueltzingsloewen A, Marty P, Rosenthal E. Visceral leishmaniasis: a new opportunistic infection in hematopoietic stem-cell transplanted patients. Bone Marrow Transplantation. 2004;33:667–8.
88. Tanyuksel M, Gun H, Doganci L. Prevalence of *Cryptosporidium* sp. in patients with neoplasia and diarrhea. Scand J Infect Dis. 1995;27:69–70.
89. Sulzyc-Bielicka V, Kuźna-Grygiel W, Kołodziejczyk L, et al. Cryptosporidiosis in patients with colorectal cancer. J Parasitol. 2007;93:722–4.
90. Drugs for Parasitic Infections. Treatment Guidelines from The Medical Letter. 2007;5(Suppl):e1–15.
91. Teachey DT, Russo P, Orenstein JM, Didier ES, Bowers C, Bunin N. Pulmonary infection with microsporidia after allogeneic bone marrow transplantation. Bone Marrow Transplant. 2004;33:299–302.
92. Marcos LA, Terashima A, Gotuzzo E. Update on hepatobiliary flukes: fascioliasis, opisthorchiasis and clonorchiasis. Curr Opin Infect Dis. 2008;21:523–30.
93. Lim MK, Ju YH, Franceschi S, et al. *Clonorchis sinensis* infection and increasing risk of cholangiocarcinoma in the republic of Korea. Am J Trop Med Hyg. 2006;75:93–6.
94. Sriamporn S, Pisani P, Pipitgool V, Suwanrungruang K, Kamsa-ard S, Parkin DM. Prevalence of *Opisthorchis viverrini* infection and incidence of cholangiocarcinoma in Khon Kaen, Northeast Thailand. Trop Med Int Health. 2004;9:588–94.
95. Bedwani R, Renganathan E, El Kwhsky F. Schistosomiasis and the risk of bladder cancer in Alexandria. Egypt Br J Cancer. 1998;77:1186–9.

Chapter 42
Zoonoses in Cancer Patients

Donald Armstrong

Abstract Prevention of zoonoses in cancer patients is the theme of this chapter and it is hoped that it will encourage and help doctors caring for such patients to educate them to avoid the infections. Avoidance need not include separation from a pet or occupation or recreation, but the use of caution conditioned by knowledge of the sources of infection and the ways we contact them should lead to effective prevention.

Keywords Zoonoses • Immunocompromised cancer patients • Prevention • Epidemiology • Hygiene • Veterinarians

Zoonoses are defined as infectious diseases, which are transmitted from nonhuman animals to man. According To one study [1] there are 1,415 organisms that infect man and of these 868 (61%) can cause zoonoses. A number of these have a predilection for infecting and for being especially severe in the immunocompromised host [2–4]. Because of this, prevention is extremely important for patients with neoplastic disease and immune defects associated with the neoplasm or its therapy. Immune defects can be categorized as indicated in Table 1.1 [5] and they are discussed extensively in other chapters. This chapter will stress the prevention of zoonoses in patients with neoplastic disease including those who appear to have intact immune responses for that may change with progression of disease or future chemotherapy or irradiation. It must be stressed that pets are extremely important to most humans and often especially to those who are ill. They provide companionship or they can be the objects of biological interest and study. Nonhuman animals provide occupations for large numbers of humans. Contact with various species can result in infections, however, and these can be especially severe in patients with immune defects. There are far too many examples to be included in this chapter, thus the most common will be discussed along with some of the rarer examples, which may be emerging infections and therefore of particular interest. The aim of this chapter is to encourage doctors to educate their patients so that they are aware of these dangers and how best to avoid them.

Unusual contact such as kissing, nuzzling, and even touching [6–8], in an uncontrolled setting, pets and other animals should be discouraged. And, of course, simple hygiene such as hand washing should be stressed. In addition, patient and at times medical doctor contacts with veterinarians is important so that non human animals will receive preventive care as well as care for apparent illnesses.

In addition, in some difficult situations such as a question of whether to initiate rabies vaccine, departments of public health, city or state or the Centers for Disease Control can be very helpful.

Epidemiology

On June 1, 1778, Edward Jenner introduced his paper on vaccination with cowpox to protect against smallpox with the following words [9]. "The deviation of man from the state in which he was placed by nature seems to have proven to him a prolific source of diseases. From the love of splendor, from the indulgences of luxury and from his fondness for amusement, he has familiarized himself with a great number of animals, which may not originally have been intended for his associates. The wolf disarmed of ferocity is now pillowed in the lady's lap. The cat, the little tiger of our island, whose natural home is the forest, is equally domesticated and caressed." I assume Dr. Jenner would be amazed, if not appalled at the number and variety of pets owned by people on his island and world wide – and how pets, wild animals that have contact with pets and people travel, meet and exchange microorganisms. In evaluating the epidemiology of zoonoses there are four major factors to take into account; Geography, the Home, Occupation and together, Habits and Hobbies. Transmission of infections from humans to nonhuman pets has been observed with associated illness. It should be considered especially when either host could be

---

D. Armstrong (✉)
Department of Medicine, Infectious Disease Service, Memorial Sloan-Kettering Cancer Center, 1026 Governor Dempsey Drive, Santa Fe, NM 87501, New York, USA
e-mail: liarm@aol.com

a carrier with reinfection occurring ("ping-pong infections"). Two other methods of exposure, Bioterrorism and xenotransplantation, will not be discussed in this chapter.

Geography

World travel of both people and pets has allowed and continues to present opportunities for spread of zoonoses. Not only people or pets can carry microorganisms but vectors such as mosquitoes can travel by plane and introduce new organisms to a new environment. An example of this is West Nile Virus that came from the Middle East to New York City and then moved across the continent to the west coast of the United States. It has been postulated that the trip across the Atlantic was via mosquitoes on a plane and that the transcontinental trip was by infected crows or humans or other birds. In addition, wild birds migrating over thousands of miles may bring organisms from and to domesticated or wild avian species and thus to humans.

A history of travel of a human should be routinely obtained and should include exposures to pets belonging to the patients and also belonging to friends or neighbors. A pet travel history can be equally important in revealing zoonotic exposures. Vacation plans should be discussed and patients educated about avoiding endemic areas for zoonoses such as the southwestern USA (plague) or babesiosis on islands off the northeastern coast.

Home

Our homes may be shared with mice, rats, and bats among others, each carrying microorganisms that can infect humans and may be lethal particularly in immunocompromised individuals. Some may choose these animals for "pets" including bats by putting out nesting "bat boxes," others may find them as unwelcome "guests." They are difficult to exclude or evict from a home, but it is wise to do so and professional exterminators may be necessary in some instances. Raccoons may make themselves "at home" especially when food may be available in uncovered garbage. Raccoons may bite when they feel cornered or threatened. They may carry rabies. Young raccoons may carry a roundworm parasite, *Baylis ascaris* procyonis that human toddlers may ingest from raccoon feces that can result in brain abscesses.

Occupations

Veterinarians in practice are constantly exposed to pets and farm animals and in some cases to zoo animals. They should be vaccinated against rabies. In the southwestern USA veterinarians have contracted the plague from treating infected cats which are especially prone to be infected or carry fleas from wild rodents. In addition to veterinarians, butchers, abattoir workers, farmers, ranchers, biologists, zoo workers and animal breeders are all liable to be exposed to zoonoses in their daily work. Animal husbandry can expose farmers to three *Brucella* species and Q fever from birth products of cows, goats, and pigs. Microbiologists have been infected with a number of organisms especially *Brucella* spp. and *Mycobacterium tuberculous*.

Habits and Hobbies

Some people are more regularly exposed to the microflora of pets by sleeping with them or kissing them while the pet licks the humans' mouths. Changing cat litter exposes people to toxoplasmosis. In addition sandboxes can be used by neighbors' or feral cats and serve as a source for *Toxoplasma gondii* to infect children. Changing papers from bird cages (as well as handling and kissing birds) may expose owners to ornithosis, salmonellosis, or cryptococcosis, the latter two being well recognized opportunistic pathogens. Hunting and dressing prey can include exposure to tularemia, or brucellosis and even horse back riding can include exposure to mice and rats living with the horses in the stables and shedding their organisms. In addition, *Rhodococcus equi*, is an opportunistic pathogen which has been associated with horse contact

Since dogs, cats, and birds are the most common pets and live closest to their human owners, they will receive the most attention.

Dogs (Table 42.1)

Dog bites frequently result in infections just as human bites do and the mouth flora bacteria causing infection are similar with the exception of *Pasteurella multocida* and *Capnocytophaga canimorsus*, which are more commonly found in dog bites. Both the organisms are sensitive to beta lactams and augmentin. The most important feature of bites, however, is that anaerobes may flourish in the presence of dead tissue so that drainage is all important. Prevention is dependent on education of children and adults about caution with strange dogs and with their own pet dogs, which may bite because of fear often combined with surprise such as stumbling on the pet. Other infections from dogs may be from organisms carried in their gastrointestinal tracts and hygienic measures must be stressed in all potential hosts, but especially those who are immunocompromised. Particular care should be taken with dogs with loose stools. Dog saliva or sputum may carry *Bordetella bronchiseptica*, an opportunistic

Table 42.1 Dogs-associated zoonoses in cancer patients

Organisms	Exposures	Prevention	Diagnosis	Treatment
Bacteria				
Mixed mouth flora including *Streptococcus pyogenes* MSSA or MRSA	Bites	Avoid	Smear and culture	Augmentin, usually empiric, drain when necessary
Pasteurella multocida	Bites	Avoid	Smear and culture	Augmentin, usually empiric, drain when necessary
Capnocytophaga canimorsus	Bites	Avoid	Smear and culture	Augmentin, usually empiric, drain when necessary
Brucella canis	Urine and birth products	Avoid	Smear and blood culture	Tetracycline
Bordetella bronchoseptica[a]	Saliva or sputum	Avoid	Serology, culture and smear	Tetracycline
Salmonella spp. (except *Salmonella typhosa*)[a]	Feces	Avoid	Culture stool and blood	Quinolone, susceptibility prn
Campylobacter spp.[a]	Feces	Avoid	Culture stool and blood	Quinolone or macrolide susceptibility prn
Yersinia pestis[a]	Fleas, sputum	Flea powder	Culture blood and lymph node, sputum	Gentamicin ± quinolone empiric prn
Francisella tularensis	Ticks, skincuts	Carefully remove	Culture blood and skin lesion	Quinolone or aminoglycoside
Leptospira spp.	Urine	Avoid	Serology, PCR	Penicillin, tetracycline
Borrelia burgdorferi	Ticks	Avoid, remove immediately (within 24 h)	Serology	Penicillin
Anaplasma phagocytophilum	Ticks	Avoid, remove immediately	Blood smear, culture PCR	Tetracycline
Ehrlichia spp.	Ticks	Avoid, remove immediately	Blood smear, culture PCR	Tetracycline
Rickettsia rickettsii	Ticks	Avoid, remove immediately	Serology, PCR, skin biopsy	Tetracycline
Fungi				
Blastomyces dermatitidis	Sylvan soil on pets	Keep clean	Smear and culture	Amphotericin B
Microsporon spp.	Hair or lesions	Keep clean and treat	Smear and culture	Topical azole
Trychophyton spp	Hair or lesions	Keep clean and treat	Smear and culture	Topical azole
Parasites				
Giardia lamblia	Feces	Avoid	Stool exam	Metronidazole
Babesia species[a]	Ticks	Remove, tick powder	Blood smear serology	Clindamycin + quinine, atovaquone + azithromycin
Toxocara canis	Feces	Avoid	Smear	Mebendazole or thiabendazole
Dipylidium caninum	Feces, fleas	Avoid feces and fleas	Smear	Niclosamide
Dirofilaria immitis	Mosquitoes	Treat dogs	Serology, lung biopsy	Extirpation
Ecchinococcus granulosus	Feces	Avoid	Smear or biopsy	Albendazole or extirpation
Ancylostoma caninum	Feces	Avoid	Smear or biopsy	Albendazole
Cryptosporidium spp.[a]	Feces	Avoid	Smear	Paramomycin, nitazoxanide, azithromycin
Viruses				
Rabies virus	Bites, saliva	Avoid, vaccine	PM on dog	Presumptive vaccine therapy
LCM virus[a]	Urine	Avoid	Serology, PCR	Supportive
Influenza virus[a]	Respiratory secretions	Avoid, vaccine	Sputum smear serology, PCR	Oseltamivir, zanamavir
Mumps virus	Respiratory secretions	Avoid, vaccine	Saliva	Supportive

[a] Opportunistic pathogen

pathogen, which can produce a whooping cough-like illness in the immunocompromised patient. Dog saliva can also be colonized with *Yersinia pestis*. *Leptospira* spp. can be passed onto humans from dog urine producing leptospirosis. An increase in incidence of this infection has been reported in humans in suburban areas. Dog fleas and ticks should be controlled as indicated in Table 42.1 as part of routine veterinary care and if found should be removed immediately using tweezers or gloves and dropped in alcohol, a toilet or a campfire.

Among the fungi, *Blastomyces dermatiditis* has been associated with dog contact, but it maybe the soil with which both human and dog have contact, which is the vector.

Dermatophytes may cause severe skin infections in patients with T-cell defects and when seen in a dog should be cared for promptly.

Parasites are usually passed from dogs to humans via feces. *Dipylidium caninum*, the dog tapeworm, however, is transmitted by infected fleas, usually ingested by children. *Dirofilaria immitis*, the dog heartworm is transmitted via mosquitoes and can be prevented by prophylaxis of the dog as directed by a veterinarian.

Viruses can be transmitted by various routes, usually respiratory or by saliva. The frequency of spread of influenza viruses to humans is unclear, but should be prevented by immunization of humans. An immunosuppressed patient may not show a normal antibody response, but some protection may result. In the event of a novel influenza virus such as H1N1, when a vaccine is not available, respiratory precautions should be used. Rabies should be considered in any dog bite. If rabies cannot be ruled out in the dog, prophylactic vaccine should be administered to the patient. The regimen should include five inoculations in an immunocompromised host rather than the four now recommended for the normal host [10].

Cats (Table 42.2)

Most infections we get from cats (with the possible exception of bites) are from free roaming cats, which acquire the zoonotic infection from other animals in the wild. Cats carry many of the same organisms as dogs and bites result in the same types of infections. The bites are usually associated with stepping on the cat, startling it in some other fashion or holding it against its will. Cleansing and draining are important just as for dog bites,

Cat scratch disease due to *Bartonella henseleae* has been associated with cat scratches of minimal size as well as larger and sometimes none are apparent at all. Kittens are often the carriers, especially those which roam outside. Feral cats are much more likely to be infected than house cats [11].

Q fever due to *Coxiella burnetii* usually follows exposure to farm animals, but cats – especially farm cats can carry it and pass it to humans through exposure to birth products.

The Plague due to *Y. pestis* can be transmitted to humans by cat fleas or if the cat is sick with pneumonia the organism can be carried in the saliva or sputum. The cats contract the infection or fleas from rodents. The organism is endemic to the USA southwest, but can also be found worldwide. Tularemia due to *Francisella tularensis* can be contracted from direct contact with rabbits or from ticks from cats as well as dogs and is endemic to the southern USA.

The ubiquitous gastrointestinal pathogens *Campylobacter* spp. and *Salmonella* spp. can be transmitted through cat feces.

Among the fungi, *Cryptococcus neoformans* or *Cryptococcus gattii* may be carried by cats especially in nasopharyngeal granulomas. How often they may be passed to humans is uncertain, but nuzzling cats when immunosuppressed should be avoided.

Table 42.2 Cats associated zoonoses in cancer patients

Organisms	Exposures	Prevention	Diagnosis	Treatment
Bacteria				
Mixed mouth flora including *S. pyogenes* and MSSA or MRSA	Bites	Avoid	Smear and culture	Drain prn augmentin
Pasteurella multocida	Bites	Avoid	Smear and culture	Drain prn augmentin
Capnocytophaga spp.	Bites	Avoid	Smear and culture	Drain prn augmentin
Bartonella henselae[a]	Bites scratches	Avoid	Smear and culture serology	Drain prn azithromycin or beta lactam
Coxiella burnetii	Exposure to birth products	Avoid	Blood, lymph node biopsy culture	Tetracycline
Yersinia pestis[a]	Saliva/sputum fleas	Avoid, flea powder	Smear and culture serology	Gentamicin ± quinolone, empiric prn
Francisella tularensis	Ticks, sores, cuts	Remove, tick powder	Smear and culture	Quinolone or aminoglycoside
Campylobacter spp.[a]	Feces	Avoid	Culture feces ± blood	Quinolone or macrolide
Salmonella spp.[a]	Feces	Avoid	Culture feces ± blood	Beta lactam or quinolone
Fungi				
Cryptococcus neoformans[a]	Nasal secretions	See DVM avoid	Smear and culture antigen detection	Amphotericin B + 5FC fluconazole
Dermatophytes	Skin lesions	See DVM avoid	Smear, culture	Topical azoles
Parasites				
Toxoplasma gondii[a]	Feces	Avoid	Serology biopsy	Sulfa pyrimethamine
Ancyclostoma caninum	Feces	Avoid	Stool exam	Albendazole
Echinococcus multilocularis	Feces	Avoid	Stool exam	Albendazole
Viruses				
Rabies virus	Bites, saliva	Avoid, vaccine	Biopsy of contact	Vaccine
Cowpox virus[a]	Skin lesions	Avoid	Smear, culture	Supportive

[a] Opportunistic pathogen

Just as with dogs, cat dermatophytes should be controlled in consultation with a veterinarian.

T. gondii is the most significant opportunistic parasite carried by cats, which takes advantage of T-cell defects. It is widespread in nature, found in mice and other rodents which transmit it to cats, which can then pass it to humans through their feces. In the normal host most infections are asymptomatic or mild, but severe disease including brain abscess may be seen in highly susceptable patients. Since many of the disseminated infections are due to unpredictable reactivation of latent infections it is impractical to use antimicrobial prophylaxis for all patients with antibody indicating previous infection. Very low T cells (<200 cells/µL) should be a consideration for prophylaxis. It is prudent to advise all patients at risk to avoid cat feces and specifically not to empty "kitty litter" boxes. Somebody else in the household should that.

Ancylostma caninum and *Echinococcus multilocularis* can be contracted from cat feces as well as from dogs

Among the viruses, cats can transmit rabies and should be vaccinated and kept up to date just as with dogs.

Cowpox virus can be transmitted to humans from exposure to infected cats [12]. Infections can be severe and persistent in humans and especially in those in the habit of nuzzling the cat's nose where the virus may be carried with or without evident lesions. In humans, the lesions can be destructive locally or in the immunocompromised, disseminate. It is possible that an apparent increase in these infections in Europe is associated with lose of immunity among the general population due to cessation of smallpox vaccinations with vaccinia virus (cowpox) vaccine.

Birds (Table 42.3)

It is not easy to avoid bird feces, especially if the birds are kept as pets. Some one has to clean the cages and it should not be an immunocompromised host. The best known organism is *Chlamydia psittaci*, the cause of parrot fever or psittacosis, which should be called ornithosis because any bird can be a carrier not just psitticine or parrot-like birds. Most birds purchased in pet shops have been quarantined before sale and thus should be cleared of the danger of carrying *C. psittaci*, but regularly birds are sold without this precaution, especially by unauthorized dealers.

Birds may also carry *Campylobacter* and *Salmonella* species.

Very rarely members of the parrot family have carried *M. tuberculous* and infected humans [13]. Such birds are usually symptomatic exhibiting weight loss, ruffled feathers, hoarseness and lymphadenopathy.

Histoplasma capsulatum find the feces of birds a rich source of nourishment and colonize their gastrointestinal tracts as well as the feces. The fungus grows in abundance particularly in the feces of chickens and "blackbirds" including swallows and starlings. Chicken farms and coops, chimneys, blackbird roosts in belfries, or copses should be avoided by the immunocompromised host.

C. neoformans is classically known to flourish in pigeon feces, but also has been isolated from a patient with cryptococcal meningitis and his parakeet with genetically identical fungi [14].

Table 42.3 Birds associated zoonoses in cancer patients

Organisms	Exposures	Prevention	Diagnosis	Treatment
Bacteria				
Chalmydia psittaci	All birds	Avoid feces	Sputum smear, culture	Tetracycline, erythromycin
Salmonella spp.[a]	All birds	Avoid feces	Stool culture	Beta lactam, fluoroquinolone
Campylobacter spp.[a]	All birds	Avoid feces	Stool culture	Azithromycin, fluoroquinolone
Mycobacterium tuberculous[a]	Parrot family	Avoid respiratory secretions	Smear, culture, PCR	Quadruple therapy
Fungi				
Histoplasma capsulatum[a]	Blackbirds, chickens	Avoid feces	Smear, culture, sputum urine antigen	Azoles or amphotericin B
Cryptococcus neoformans[a]	Pigeons, psitticines	Avoid feces	Antigen in CSF or serum smear, culture	Azoles or amphotericin B ± 5FC
Parasites				
Cryptosporidium spp.[a]	Wild or caged birds	Avoid feces	Stool smear	Nitazoxanide
Giardia lamblia[a]	Wild or caged birds	Avoid feces	Stool smear	Metranidazole
Viruses				
Influenza viruses[a]	Ducks, chickens, migrating birds	Vaccine, avoid feces	Sputum smear, culture, PCR	Smear, culture, PCR
Alphaviruses	Migrating birds	Avoid mosquitoes	Culture, serology	Supportive care
Flavoviruses	Migrating birds	Avoid mosquitoes	Culture, serology	Supportive care
West Nile virus[a]	Migrating birds	Avoid mosquitoes	Culture, serology	Supportive care

[a] Opportunistic pathogen

Among the parasites, Cryptosporidia species have been isolated from wild or caged birds and implicated in infecting humans. A rare occurrence has been the finding of *Giardia lamblia* causing diarrheal disease in a patient and his love birds.

Farm birds such as chickens, turkeys, ducks, geese and others, and wild migrating birds of all sorts have proven to be a rich source of viral infection for humans. Many of these infections such as influenza are spread through the feces and others are the result of mosquitoes carrying the virus from birds to humans. These include alphaviruses and flaviviruses causing encephalitis. An excellent example is the West Nile virus, which so readily crossed the North American continent with migrating birds and mosquitoes infecting horses as well as humans.

Less Common Pets or Contacts (Table 42.4)

Mammals

Rodents: The usual pathogens passed from rodents to humans are mouth flora from bites usually including *P. multocida*, and fecal spread of *Campylobacter* spp. and *Salmonella* spp. Mice in the southwestern USA carry Hanta virus, which regularly causes a fatal pneumonia. Mice and hamsters may carry lymphocytic choriomeningitis virus and mice may also harbor mites that carry *Rickettsia akari*, which cause rickettsialpox.

Praire dogs (some people keep as pets) along with other wild rodents may carry plague or tularemia (especially rabbits), and ferrets may carry influenza. Racoons, in addition to rabies, may carry a parasite, *B. ascaris* whose eggs maybe ingested from stools especially by infants playing in dirt, resulting in encephalitis. Pet rats may carry *Streptobacillus moniliformis* [15, 16] resulting in endocarditis in owners.

Bats are the most common carriers of rabies in the USA. They are to be avoided. Fruit bats have been implicated in Australia and Indonesia in transmitting encephalitis viruses that infect horses and humans in the former and pigs and humans in the latter. Bats are also carriers of the SARS corona virus in addition to civet cats and raccoon dogs in Asia.

Beasts of burden: Horses can transmit rabies. They also serve as an intermediate host for encephalitides (Eastern, Western and Venezuelan Equine, and West Nile virus) via mosquitoes to humans. Horse associated *R. equi* can cause severe disease, which manifests by skin and pulmonary lesions in patients with T-cell defects.

Farm animals: Brucellosis can be acquired from cows, pigs, and goats. They are popular in petting zoos and should be handled with special precautions by the zoo keepers and visitors. It is best not to pet them. This includes sheep which may infect humans with orf virus, which cause large pustular skin lesions. Cows may excrete *Escherichia coli* 0157:H4, which can cause lethal disease in humans. Bovine tuberculous due to *Mycobacterium bovis* can cause invasive infection in the immunosuppressed patient. Water buffalo urine can be a rich source of *Leptospira* spp. for human infections.

Nonhuman primates: Even in the immunocompetent, human Herpes simiae infection is close to 100% lethal due to encephalitis. Rhesus, cynomolgus or vervet monkeys should not be kept as pets. They can be asymptomatic carriers of this potentially fatal herpes virus. Animal handlers should be trained to work with monkeys, which should be free from infection before contact. Even so, trained animal handlers have died due to this infection.

The highly lethal Marburg and Ebola viruses can also be transmitted from monkey to man.

Monkey pox virus can cause local lesions in man and even disseminate causing a smallpox like disease. A recent outbreak in the USA was caused by a Gambian rat, which developed monkey pox lesions after arriving in a pet store where the infection was transmitted to American praire dogs, which were sold as pets and resulted in multiple cases in humans. Physicians and public health officials included small pox in the differential diagnosis causing quite a stir in several communities [17].

Chimpanzees have been kept as pets and can infect humans with *M. tuberculous* or carry human malaria. They have become infected with measles, hepatitis A virus, or influenza virus along with *Streptococcus pneumoniae* and *Staphylococcus aureus*. Intestinal pathogens such as giardia and Strongyloides can be excreted by chimpanzees.

Table 42.4 Less common pets or contacts

Mammals
  Rodents: mice, rats, hamsters, gerbils, guinea pigs, rabbits, ferrets, and raccoons
  Beasts of burden: horses, mules, donkeys, oxen, camels, and water buffalo
  Farm animals: cattle, pigs, sheep, goats, and Yaks
  Nonhuman primates: chimps, rhesus, cynomologus macaques, lemurs, and marmosets
  Bats: all species
Birds
  Canaries, finches, parakeets, parrots, and lovebirds
  Chickens, ducks, geese, and turkeys
  Wild birds – at feeders, in shelters, and shot by hunters
Reptiles
  Snakes, lizards, turtles, alligators, and horned toads
Amphibians
  Frogs, toads, salamanders, and newts
Fish
  Aquarium fish, caught, commercial or sport fish, and farmed fish

Note: see text for discussion

Birds

In addition to commonly kept birds, chickens, ducks, turkeys, and geese can carry *C. psittaci* and strains of influenza. The avian flu strain, H3N1 has been isolated from many different birds, but chickens appear to be the primary source of the cases first described. Wild migrating birds often mix with flocks of farmed birds and can carry an organism thousands of miles. Humans who keep bird feeders filled are regularly exposed to bird excreta, which may carry organisms listed in Table 42.3 or in addition to those adenoviruses.

Reptiles

Snakes, lizards, turtles, alligators, or horned toads may all carry enteric pathogens and excrete them into terrarium soil or water sources.

Amphibians

Frogs, Toads, salamanders, or newts may carry the same organisms as reptiles and excrete them into their water or soil.

Fish

Aquarium fish may carry and excrete into their water *Mycobacterium marinum*, which can cause nodular skin lesions or disseminate in immunosuppressed patients. Farmed fish may carry *Vibrio*, vulnificus which causes especially severe gastroenteritis in the presence of immune defects. People handling fish commercially or in home preparation may be exposed to *Streptococcus iniae* or *Erysipelothrix rhusiopathiae*, both of which may cause local skin lesions or disseminate.

Foot Note

For detailed instructions on prevention of infections, which can apply to cancer patients, the CDC has published two compendia [18, 19] on the subject in HIV infected people. These can be applied to children and adults with T-Cell mediated immune defects and these are the patients most likely to develop opportunistic zoonotic infections. These are excellent reference documents.

Summary

Prevention of zoonoses in cancer patients is the theme of this chapter and it is hoped that it will encourage and help doctors caring for such patients in educating them to avoid such infections. Avoidance need not include separation from a pet, or occupation, or recreation, but the use of caution conditioned by knowledge of the sources of infection and the way we may contract them should lead to effective prevention.

References

1. Taylor LH, Latham SM, Woolhouse EJ. Risk factors for human disease emergence. Phil Trans R Soc Lond B. 2001;356:983–9.
2. Murphy FA. Emerging zoonoses. Emerg Infect Dis. 1998;4:429–35.
3. Grant S, Olson CW. Preventing zoonotic diseases in immunocompromised persons: the role of physicians and veterinarians. Emerg Infect Dis. 1999;5:159–63.
4. Zoonotic Diseases Issue. Emerg Infect Dis. 2005;10;2065–2274.
5. Safdar A, Bodey G, Armstrong D. Infections in cancer patients – an overview. In: Safdar A, editor. Principles and practice of cancer infections. New York: Springer; 2010.
6. Armstrong D, Bernard EM. Infections from pets. In: Armstrong D, Cohen J, editors. Infectious diseases. London: Mosby; 1999.
7. Steele JH, Armstrong D. Infections from non domesticated animals. In: Armstrong D, Cohen J, editors. Infectious diseases. London: Mosby; 1999. p. 6.1–6.
8. Centers for Disease Control and Prevention. Compendium of measures to prevent disease associated with animals in public settings National Association of State Public Health Veterinarians, Inc. (NASPHV). MMWM. 2009;58(5):1–21.
9. Jenner E. Vaccination against small pox. Great mind series. Amherst: Prometheus Books; 1996. p. 13.
10. Advisory Committee of on Immunization Practices, CDC. Use of a reduced (4-dose) vaccine schedule for postexposure prophylaxis to prevent human rabies. MMWR. 2010;59(RR-2):1–9.
11. Koehler JE, Glaser CA, Tappero JW. Rochalimaea henselae infection. A new zoonosis with the domestic cat as a reservoir. JAMA. 1994;16(271):531–5.
12. Vorou RM, Papavassiliou VG. Pierroutsakos in cowpox virus infection: an emerging health threat. Curr Opin Infect Dis. 2008;21(2):153–6.
13. Washko RM, Hoefer H, Kiehn TE, Armstrong D, Dorsininville G, Frieden TR. *Mycobacterium tuberculous* infection in a Green-Winged Macaw (Ara chloroptera): report with public health implications. J Clin Microbiol. 1998;36:1101–2.
14. Nosanchuk JD, Shoham S, Fries BC, Shapiro DS, Levitz SM, Casadevall A. Evidence of zoonotic transmission of *Cryptococcus neoformans* from a pet cockatoo to an immunocompromised patient. Ann Intern Med. 2000;132:205–8.
15. Graves MH, Janda JM. Rat bite fever (*Streptobacillus moniliformis*): a potential emerging disease. Int J Infect Dis. 2001;5:151–4.
16. Armstrong D. Zoonoses editorial. Int J Infect Dis. 2001;5:117–8.
17. Centers for Disease Control and Prevention. Multistate outbreak of monkeypox – Illinois, Indiana, Kansas, Ohio, and Wisconsin, 2003. MMWR. 2003;52:561–4.
18. Mofenson LM, Brady MT, Danner SP, Dominguez KL, Hazra R, Handelsman E, et al. Guidelines for the prevention and treatment of opportunistic infections among HIV-exposed and HIV-infected children. MMWR. 2009;58(RR11):1–166.
19. Centers for Disease Control and Prevention. Guidelines for prevention and treatment of opportunistic infections in HIV-infected adults and adolescents. MMWR. 2009;58(RR-4):1–207.

Part IV
Management of Antimicrobial Therapy

Chapter 43
Antimicrobial Stewardship: Considerations for a Cancer Center

Coralia N. Mihu, Alla Paskovaty, and Susan K. Seo

Abstract Since the discovery of penicillin, unbridled enthusiasm for antibiotics has led to their extensive application in medicine, animal care, and agriculture. Injudicious antimicrobial use has also contributed to the emergence and spread of multidrug-resistant bacteria, creating a situation in which there are few or no treatment options for infections due to these organisms. There is increasing awareness that antimicrobial resistance adversely impacts patient safety and public health. In essence, effective antimicrobial stewardship entails the optimal selection, dose, and duration of an antibiotic, resulting in the cure of an infection with minimal toxicity to the patient and minimal impact on selective pressure. A detailed discussion on this important issue is presented in this chapter.

Keywords Multidrug-resistant bacteria • Injudicious antimicrobial use • Optimal antibiotic selection • Duration of antibiotic therapy • Reduced drug toxicity

Introduction

Since the discovery of penicillin, unbridled enthusiasm for antibiotics has led to their extensive application in medicine, animal care, and agriculture [1]. However, representative studies from around the world have shown inappropriate antimicrobial usage in humans between a range of 20 and 50% [2–5]. One unintended outcome has been the selection of pathogenic organisms. An example is *Clostridium difficile*. Although earlier studies showed the value of restricting a specific drug (e.g., clindamycin) to reduce *C. difficile* infection (CDI) and control outbreaks [6–8], the popularity of fluoroquinolones as prescribed agents has been associated with more recent epidemics of CDI [9, 10]. Increased fluoroquinolone resistance among epidemic (i.e., restriction-endonuclease analysis group BI/North American PFGE type I strains) and some nonepidemic strains of *C. difficile* has been described [11].

Injudicious antimicrobial use has also contributed to the emergence and spread of multidrug-resistant bacteria, creating a situation in which there are few or no treatment options for infections due to these organisms. The introduction of newer therapies is not immune to the phenomenon of resistance development, as in the case of tigecycline and *Acinetobacter baumanii* [12] or linezolid and vancomycin-resistant *Enterococcus faecium* (VRE) [13]. Despite a critical need for novel antibacterial agents, there are indications that such drug development programs are declining [14–16]. Emerging resistance is not limited to bacteria since resistant viral, fungal, and parasitic pathogens have also been recognized [17–22].

There is an increasing awareness that antimicrobial resistance adversely impacts patient safety and public health. Resistance can lead to a delay in administering microbiologically effective therapy [23, 24]. In case-control studies, infections due to resistant organisms have been associated with higher rates of mortality, longer hospital stays, and increased medical care costs [24–28]. In 1998, the Institute of Medicine estimated that the annual cost of infections caused by antibiotic-resistant bacteria was $4–5 billion [29]. Finally, drug-associated toxicity is an underappreciated but significant consequence of antimicrobial use. A recent study estimated that >142,000 visits were made annually to United States (US) emergency departments for antibiotic-related adverse events, of which four-fifths were allergic reactions [30]. These findings highlight the tremendous need for judicious use of antimicrobial agents.

In essence, effective antimicrobial stewardship entails the optimal selection, dose, and duration of an antibiotic, resulting in the cure of an infection with minimal toxicity to the patient and minimal impact on selective pressure [31, 32]. While several published surveys demonstrate an increased acceptance on the part of healthcare institutions to establish programs for rational antimicrobial use, it is clear that practices vary considerably and that there is room for improvement

C.N. Mihu (✉)
Department of Infectious Diseases, Infection Control and Employee Health, The University of Texas M.D. Anderson,
1515 Holcombe Blvd. (Unit 1460), Houston, TX 77030, USA
e-mail: CNMihu@mdanderson.org

in both the US and Europe [33–37]. In 2007, the Infectious Diseases Society of America (IDSA) and the Society for Healthcare Epidemiology of America (SHEA) jointly published a statement that outlined the rationale and provided guidelines for development of a formal antimicrobial stewardship program (ASP) by healthcare institutions [38]. How an ASP is implemented will vary from institution to institution, but a comprehensive approach with a full-time dedicated multidisciplinary team appears to be capable of yielding sustained and favorable clinical and economic outcomes [39]. Ideally, each institution should also have an active surveillance system to monitor resistant organisms and an infection control program to minimize secondary transmission of these pathogens [31].

The cancer center represents a distinctive entity, and formation of an ASP should take into account issues that are unique to the cancer center, such as local susceptibility patterns and the complexities of managing infectious complications in patients with varying immunocompromised states. Infection, a common cause of morbidity and mortality in patients with cancer, can result not only from the direct effect of the tumor, but also from the use of foreign devices (e.g., intravascular catheters) to aid in disease management and from cancer treatment (e.g., surgery, chemotherapy, radiation, or combination therapy). Current cancer therapies including tumor necrosis factor antagonists, antimetabolites, and monoclonal antilymphocyte antibodies have become increasingly sophisticated, and their use can add to profound immunosuppression [40–42]. These and other cancer therapies can also influence antimicrobial choice by virtue of their side effect profile (e.g., hepatic or renal toxicity) and potential drug–drug interaction. Another interesting dilemma is the recent influx of new and costly anti-infectives (e.g., mold-active agents like voriconazole and posaconazole, antiviral agents like cidofovir) that may be an incentive to develop an ASP for meaningful cost-containment [39]. The purpose of this chapter is to explore several aspects of coordinating an ASP at a cancer center, including formation of a multidisciplinary team, stewardship strategies, and barriers/challenges.

Table 43.1 Creating a multidisciplinary antimicrobial stewardship program

1. Obtain baseline information
    a. Determine institutional antimicrobial usage and expenditures
    b. Know institutional susceptibilities
    c. Identify problems
2. Select strategies by which to execute antimicrobial stewardship
3. Determine team members and their roles and responsibilities
4. Establish support of hospital administration
5. Build constructive relations with other hospital services and clinicians
6. Devise a fail-safe mechanism for problem-solving
7. Provide feedback to prescribers
8. Conduct audits to monitor effectiveness of program activities

ASP but also for its maintenance [38]. From a practical standpoint, creation of an ASP should involve understanding institutional patterns of antibiotic usage, expenditures, and resistance. Such baseline knowledge is a key to setting goals and quantifying benefits of program activities. Other aims include selecting strategies by which antimicrobial stewardship will be executed in the hospital, determining personnel and means of financial support for the program, and constructing positive relations with the hospital-at-large. The ASP should also provide feedback to prescribers and conduct regular audits to validate the effectiveness of program activities (Table 43.1) [31, 49].

A computer-based infrastructure facilitates stewardship efforts. Utilization of healthcare information technology (IT) in the form of electronic medical records (EMR), computer order entry (COE), and clinical decision-support has the potential to improve prescribing and reduce medication errors as demonstrated by LDS Hospital in Salt Lake City, Utah [50–53]. While the computer surveillance and decision-support system of LDS Hospital is the ideal, conformation of such technology to individual institutions on a broader scale is not yet feasible. Depending on the IT resources available, institutional ASPs can still find ways to efficiently follow local susceptibilities, monitor antimicrobial use, and target antimicrobial interventions [38].

Implementation of ASPs

Effective ASPs can reduce antimicrobial use, improve patient care, and be financially self-supporting in both large academic institutions and small community hospitals [43–47]. Furthermore, the promotion of appropriate antimicrobial use by ASPs is in alignment with a growing emphasis on patient safety and quality assurance [48]. The support of hospital administration, medical staff leadership, and local providers is essential not only for the development of an institutional

The Multidisciplinary Antimicrobial Stewardship Team

The core members of a multidisciplinary ASP are the Infectious Diseases (ID) physician and one or more clinical pharmacists. These members generally have dedicated time precisely for the purpose of antibiotic management and are compensated accordingly. Since antimicrobial stewardship relates to patient safety and is considered to be a medical staff function, the program is usually directed by the ID specialist or codirected by an ID physician and a clinical pharmacist with ID training [38].

Because of the specialized nature of oncologic care, a cancer center is well suited for a multidisciplinary team approach. One of the benefits of collaboration is the ability to develop and disseminate center-wide or malignancy-specific protocols for managing infectious diseases. The ASP team can work with medical and surgical oncologists as well as other allied healthcare specialists (e.g., clinical chemistry and hematology laboratories, microbiology, nursing, pathology, pharmacy, radiation oncology, radiology) as needed to build consensus, educate, monitor implementation, assess compliance and outcomes, and update ID management strategies. Another joint effort would be to work with the hospital pharmacy and therapeutics (P&T) committee to review and modify the formulary, keeping in mind that certain anti-infective classes such as mold-active antifungal agents may be used in high volume for a particular cancer patient population (e.g., patients with acute leukemia) rather than hospital-wide.

Specific to a cancer center, the ID physician with ASP responsibilities should have a broad and deep understanding of the immune defects associated with the underlying malignancy or cancer therapies, the pathogens known to cause infections in the immunocompromised host, and strategies for diagnosis and treatment. Similarly, ASP pharmacists at a cancer center can provide information regarding new or existing chemotherapeutic or antimicrobial agents and their associated pharmacokinetics, dosing schedules, drug–drug interactions, and toxicities. They can also serve as a liaison to hospital pharmacy by providing education to their pharmacy colleagues, monitoring formulary and nonformulary use, and ensuring appropriate antimicrobial selection and dosing.

Although microbiologists and hospital epidemiologists may not be directly involved in the day-to-day activities of the multidisciplinary ASP, they are integral to the functioning of the team. The microbiology laboratory ensures the timely identification of pathogens and the selective reporting of susceptibilities [38, 54]. One trend, however, is the outsourcing of infrequently ordered microbiologic tests to outside reference laboratories as part of cost-containment and quality control efforts [55]. This practice may affect clinical decision-making in high-risk patients, such as those with hematologic malignancies or allogeneic hematopoietic stem cell transplant (HSCT) recipients in whom such tests may be disproportionately ordered. Tracking resistance patterns in the hospital on an annual basis is another important task. Of note, cancer center- or unit-specific antibiograms should be formulated as patterns of antimicrobial use and thus susceptibilities of pathogenic bacteria may differ from the rest of the hospital [56, 57]. If possible, antifungal susceptibilities of *Candida* species should be tabulated, particularly in light of azole prophylaxis in certain cancer patient groups (e.g., allogeneic and autologous HSCT recipients) [58, 59].

Hospital epidemiologists create policies to contain the transmission of resistant pathogens, and they can provide assistance with analyzing the relationship between patterns of antibiotic use and trends in bacterial resistance. Infection control personnel are also well placed to provide continuing education programs to hospital staff [38, 54].

Stewardship Strategies

In general, the ASP team should understand their hospital culture in terms of prescribing practice and choose stewardship strategies that fit within the institutional framework. While there are no randomized, controlled trials in this field, two primary, proactive strategies exist: prior approval (also referred to as preauthorization) and postprescribing review (also called prospective audit with feedback). These are not mutually exclusive, and either approach can be enhanced with supplemental strategies.

The first core strategy links prior approval to a restricted formulary. Most hospitals have a P&T committee that evaluates whether a drug would be suitable for inclusion on the formulary on the basis of therapeutic efficacy, side effect profile, and cost. A well-structured antimicrobial formulary reflects local susceptibilities, minimizes the number of agents available for effective therapy, and avoids duplication [60, 61]. Furthermore, restriction of certain agents with the condition that prescribers call an ID physician or clinical pharmacist for approval has been reported to be effective in reducing inappropriate use and expenditures without detriment to patient care [62–65]. An interesting study performed at the Hospital of the University of Pennsylvania (HUP) in Philadelphia found that recommendations made by the multidisciplinary ASP team were more likely to be in accordance with prescribing guidelines (87 vs. 47%, $p<0.001$) and to result in clinical cure (64 vs. 42%, $p=0.007$) compared with those generated by ID fellows [44]. These findings highlight the need for scheduled time to engage thoughtfully in the approval process as well as staffing by practitioners who are viewed as having expertise in using antibiotics. This system, however, may be viewed as "policing," and clinicians anxious to maintain good relations with their colleagues circumventing it. In addition, prior approval generally only affects initial choice for empiric therapy. This strategy has little influence on duration or modification of therapy once microbiologic and radiographic evidence becomes available.

In postprescribing review, patients already on empiric therapy are identified by computer-generated screening and targeted for evaluation. When an intervention is deemed necessary, the ASP team communicates with the primary service, either verbally or via nonpermanent notes left in the medical record. Examples of interventions include ensuring appropriate dosing, narrowing coverage (also called streamlining or de-escalation), modifying duration, or stopping antibiotics altogether if there is no evidence for infection.

The report by Schentag et al. was one of the earliest to show that clinical pharmacy specialists in conjunction with ID support could effectively handle streamlining and intravenous (IV)-to-oral conversion. By linking the pharmacy and microbiology computer systems, patients could be screened for inappropriate dosing as well as for mismatches between pathogens and drugs. No adverse outcomes were noted in patients whose regimens were modified or stopped, and antibiotic expenditures declined from 31% of the total pharmacy budget to 21.5% in the first year of operation [66]. Improvements in antimicrobial use with associated cost-savings have also been reported by other centers [43, 45]. Moreover, Carling et al. noted concomitant decreased rates of nosocomial infections due to *C. difficile* or resistant Enterobacteriaceae [45]. A significant impact can even be demonstrated at hospitals where daily review is not feasible due to limited resources. At a small community hospital in West Monroe, Louisiana, postprescribing review over a 1-year period by an ID physician and a clinical pharmacist 3 days a week led to a 19% reduction in antimicrobial expenditures [46]. This same report also revealed a potential shortcoming of postprescribing review in that only 69% of 488 suggested interventions were accepted and implemented. By the same token, success or failure of this system rests on the ability and availability of the ASP team members to educate prescribers during the intervention process [67].

Supplemental stewardship strategies include, but are not limited to, education, clinical pathways, streamlining, and IV-to-oral conversion. Depending on the personnel and available institutional resources, an ASP can combine one or more of these with the core stewardship strategy to augment program activities. A full, detailed explanation of these and other supplemental strategies is beyond the scope of this chapter but can be found in other published reviews and guidelines [38, 39, 68].

Briefly, education is the most basic strategy by which to influence clinicians to adopt and maintain good prescribing practices. Initiatives range from one-on-one instruction and formalized educational programs (e.g., lectures, mailings, internet-based learning activities) to utilization review with feedback. Although education is the cornerstone of any ASP, its effectiveness is dependent on the motivation of the clinician to make a behavioral change [69, 70]. Without incorporation of active intervention, education alone is marginally effective and has not demonstrated a sustained impact on prescribing practices [71–73].

Clinical pathways involve the development of peer-reviewed guidelines for commonly encountered infectious diseases. By limiting choice, the process of antibiotic selection for prophylaxis or treatment of an infection is simplified. Examples of national guidelines that would be of relevance to a cancer center include empiric treatment for fever and neutropenia [74], prevention of opportunistic infections in HSCT recipients [75, 76], treatment of aspergillosis [77], treatment of candidiasis [78], and surgical prophylaxis [79, 80]. Standardized antimicrobial order forms, automatic stop orders, and computerized systems can ease the implementation of guidelines [51, 68].

Streamlining is a process that ensures that antimicrobial therapy is matched to culture and susceptibility data within 48–72 h after initiation of treatment. In doing so, prolonged, excessively broad treatment can be avoided. As seen in the management of ventilator-associated pneumonia (VAP), antimicrobial therapy may be shortened [81] or even stopped based on clinical criteria and negative culture results [82, 83]. Singh et al. also found that the rate of subsequent antibiotic-resistant infections was lower in the group receiving short-course treatment for suspected VAP compared to those receiving standard duration (15 vs. 35%, $p=0.017$) [82]. An economic benefit has also been derived from this strategy. In one report, recommendations for streamlining occurred in 54% of antibiotic courses over 7 months, resulting in a projected annual savings of $107,637 [84]. In another report, a pharmacist-based intervention to discontinue unnecessary agents was successful in 134 (98%) of 137 episodes. Potential drug cost-savings and reduction in redundant antibiotic combination days were $10,800 and 584 days, respectively [85].

Finally, a systematic plan for IV-to-oral conversion can decrease hospital length-of-stay (LOS) and healthcare costs. The excellent oral bioavailability of several antimicrobial classes, including the fluoroquinolones, azoles, and oxazolidinones, makes this approach quite feasible. In contrast to oral formulations, IV medications are generally more expensive and can be associated with adverse events like phlebitis and catheter-related infections. Patients also benefit since oral treatment is convenient and easy [86]. This strategy, however, is reserved for those who are hemodynamically stable, have improved clinically within 48 h of prior IV therapy, and have functioning gastrointestinal tracts. Individuals with severe immunodeficiency states or infections like meningitis and endocarditis are not candidates [86, 87]. Representative studies report a positive experience with IV-to-oral conversion in terms of clinical effectiveness and cost savings [88–91].

Barriers and Challenges

A survey of ID physicians conducted by the IDSA Emerging Infections Network (EIN) has identified potential barriers to participation in antimicrobial stewardship [92]. The first barrier is the time and effort needed to develop and maintain an ASP. In 1987, Woodward et al. estimated that more than 100 h per month of combined personnel time were needed to handle telephone requests and antibiotic reviews for just three restricted antibiotic classes at their institution [62]. Nowadays, one can imagine the difficulties in pursing program activities if ASP team members, namely clinical pharmacists, are pulled for assignments elsewhere in the hospital.

Another barrier is recruiting personnel with necessary ID expertise. Hopefully, the growing need for ID-trained pharmacy specialists can be met by encouraging pharmacy schools to support residency training and by training additional preceptors to oversee the instruction of pharmacy residents interested in ID [93]. With respect to the ID physician community, lack of compensation for added work responsibilities and insufficient support by hospital administration are not insignificant issues. In the aforementioned IDSA EIN survey, only 46 (18%) of 250 respondents reported receiving direct remuneration for their participation in antimicrobial stewardship [92]. However, the increasing reluctance of public and private payers to reimburse for healthcare-associated infections (e.g., catheter-related infections) coupled with published data supporting the value of ID specialists in directing institutional antimicrobial stewardship or infection control programs can provide a framework to negotiate appropriate compensation by the hospital [94]. There is also a perception that a particular stewardship strategy, prior approval, may antagonize colleagues in other specialties and potentially lead to lost income due to fewer requests for consultations [92]. This sensitive issue may be of particular concern at nonteaching institutions, but alternative stewardship strategies (e.g., postprescribing review) that do not affect prescribing autonomy can be employed instead [95].

Finally, measuring the full impact of an ASP on clinical outcomes, economics, and resistance is challenging. While a successful ASP can be financially self-supporting, evaluating the true economic benefits can be tough since direct and indirect (i.e., dispensing, administering, monitoring) drug costs represent a fraction of what is affected by optimizing antimicrobial use. One needs to also factor potential cost-savings from avoided adverse drug events, shortened hospital LOS, and decelerated resistance development. While financial savings are typically greatest in the early phases of an ASP, achieving other desirable outcomes such as decreased inappropriate antimicrobial usage and reduced hospital LOS requires continued vigilance [94]. Evaluating the impact of a multidisciplinary ASP on curbing antibiotic resistance is more complicated due to the multifactorial nature of the problem. Theoretically, it is thought that optimizing antibiotic use will minimize selective pressure and maintain or improve bacterial susceptibilities. It is also assumed that this will be accompanied by improvement in survival. Data to support this second notion are sparse, particularly as there are numerous confounders [68, 96]. A more detailed discussion is forthcoming in the next chapter.

Summary

The emergence and spread of multidrug-resistant pathogens coupled with a drying-up antimicrobial pipeline have led to the realization that optimization of currently available agents is an important priority. This has prompted national ID professional societies to advocate for the creation of ASPs by healthcare institutions. Although developing an ASP at a cancer center may seem counterintuitive, cancer patients generally receive multifaceted oncologic care, and a multidisciplinary approach to managing anti-infective therapy is thus complementary. Regardless of the setting, maintenance of an ASP requires processes that are both sustainable and adaptable to the evolving needs of the institution. Frequent assessment of program design is essential to its continued success, and collaboration with other local ASPs is crucial for the benefit of the community-at-large. Joint educational programs are an excellent way to disseminate vital information and promote acceptance of ASP efforts. As more and more hospitals document reductions in unnecessary antimicrobial use, cost-savings, and improvements in patient care, implementation of multidisciplinary ASPs will become more widespread.

References

1. Levy S. The antibiotic paradox: how the misuse of antibiotics destroys their curative powers. 2nd ed. Cambridge: Perseus Publishing; 2002.
2. Yu VL, Stoehr GP, Starling RC, Shogan JE. Empiric antibiotic selection by physicians: evaluation of reasoning strategies. Am J Med Sci. 1991;301:165–72.
3. Gonzales R, Malone DC, Maselli JH, Sande MA. Excessive antibiotic use for acute respiratory infections in the United States. Clin Infect Dis. 2001;33:757–62.
4. Lemmen SW, Becker G, Frank U, Daschner FD. Influence of an infectious disease consulting service on quality and costs of antibiotic prescriptions in a university hospital. Scand J Infect Dis. 2001;33:219–21.
5. Erbay A, Colpan A, Bodur H, Cevik MA, Samore MH, Ergonul O. Evaluation of antibiotic use in a hospital with an antibiotic restriction policy. Int J Antimicrob Agents. 2003;21:308–12.
6. Pear SM, Williamson TH, Bettin KM, Gerding DN, Galgiani JN. Decrease in nosocomial *Clostridium difficile*-associated diarrhea by restricting clindamycin use. Ann Intern Med. 1994;120:272–7.
7. McNulty C, Logan M, Donald IP, et al. Successful control of *Clostridium difficile* infection in an elderly care unit through use of a restrictive antibiotic policy. J Antimicrob Chemother. 1997;40:707–11.
8. Climo MW, Israel DS, Wong ES, Williams D, Coudron P, Markowitz SM. Hospital-wide restriction of clindamycin: effect on the incidence of *Clostridium difficile*-associated diarrhea and cost. Ann Intern Med. 1998;128:989–95.
9. Muto CA, Pokrywka M, Shutt K, et al. A large outbreak of *Clostridium difficile*-associated disease with an unexpected proportion of deaths and colectomies at a teaching hospital following increased fluoroquinolone use. Infect Control Hosp Epidemiol. 2005;26:273–80.

10. Pepin J, Saheb N, Coulombe MA, et al. Emergence of fluoroquinolones as the predominant risk factor for *Clostridium difficile*-associated diarrhea: a cohort study during an epidemic in Quebec. Clin Infect Dis. 2005;41:1254–60.
11. Owens Jr RC, Donskey CJ, Gaynes RP, Loo VG, Muto CA. Antimicrobial-associated risk factors for *Clostridium difficile* infection. Clin Infect Dis. 2008;46 Suppl 1:S19–31.
12. Anthony KB, Fishman NO, Linkin DR, Gasink LB, Edelstein PH, Lautenbach E. Clinical and microbiological outcomes of serious infections with multidrug-resistant gram-negative organisms treated with tigecycline. Clin Infect Dis. 2008;46:567–70.
13. Scheetz MH, Knechtel SA, Malczynski M, Postelnick MJ, Qi C. Increasing incidence of linezolid-intermediate or -resistant, vancomycin-resistant *Enterococcus faecium* strains parallels increasing linezolid consumption. Antimicrob Agents Chemother. 2008;52:2256–9.
14. Payne D, Tomasz A. The challenge of antibiotic resistant bacterial pathogens: the medical need, the market and prospects for new antimicrobial agents. Curr Opin Microbiol. 2004;7:435–8.
15. Spellberg B, Powers JH, Brass EP, Miller LG, Edwards Jr JE. Trends in antimicrobial drug development: implications for the future. Clin Infect Dis. 2004;38:1279–86.
16. Thomson CJ, Power E, Ruebsamen-Waigmann H, Labischinski H. Antibacterial research and development in the 21(st) Century–an industry perspective of the challenges. Curr Opin Microbiol. 2004;7:445–50.
17. Centers for Disease Control and Prevention (CDC). High levels of adamantane resistance among influenza A (H3N2) viruses and interim guidelines for use of antiviral agents – United States, 2005–06 influenza season. MMWR Morb Mortal Wkly Rep. 2006;55:44–6.
18. Morfin F, Thouvenot D. Herpes simplex virus resistance to antiviral drugs. J Clin Virol. 2003;26:29–37.
19. Chou S. Cytomegalovirus UL97 mutations in the era of ganciclovir and maribavir. Rev Med Virol. 2008;18:233–46.
20. Vanden Bossche H, Dromer F, Improvisi I, Lozano-Chiu M, Rex JH, Sanglard D. Antifungal drug resistance in pathogenic fungi. Med Mycol. 1998;36 Suppl 1:119–28.
21. Upcroft P, Upcroft JA. Drug targets and mechanisms of resistance in the anaerobic protozoa. Clin Microbiol Rev. 2001;14:150–64.
22. Plowe CV. The evolution of drug-resistant malaria. Trans R Soc Trop Med Hyg. 2009;103:S11–4.
23. Ibrahim EH, Sherman G, Ward S, Fraser VJ, Kollef MH. The influence of inadequate antimicrobial treatment of bloodstream infections on patient outcomes in the ICU setting. Chest. 2000;118:146–55.
24. Lautenbach E, Patel JB, Bilker WB, Edelstein PH, Fishman NO. Extended-spectrum beta-lactamase-producing Escherichia coli and Klebsiella pneumoniae: risk factors for infection and impact of resistance on outcomes. Clin Infect Dis. 2001;32:1162–71.
25. Bhavnani SM, Drake JA, Forrest A, et al. A nationwide, multicenter, case-control study comparing risk factors, treatment, and outcome for vancomycin-resistant and -susceptible enterococcal bacteremia. Diagn Microbiol Infect Dis. 2000;36:145–58.
26. Carmeli Y, Eliopoulos G, Mozaffari E, Samore M. Health and economic outcomes of vancomycin-resistant enterococci. Arch Intern Med. 2002;162:2223–8.
27. Cosgrove SE, Kaye KS, Eliopoulous GM, Carmeli Y. Health and economic outcomes of the emergence of third-generation cephalosporin resistance in Enterobacter species. Arch Intern Med. 2002;162:185–90.
28. Engemann JJ, Carmeli Y, Cosgrove SE, et al. Adverse clinical and economic outcomes attributable to methicillin resistance among patients with *Staphylococcus aureus* surgical site infection. Clin Infect Dis. 2003;36:592–8.
29. Institute of Medicine. Antimicrobial drug resistance: issues and options. Workshop report. Washington: National Academy Press; 1998.
30. Shehab N, Patel PR, Srinivasan A, Budnitz DS. Emergency department visits for antibiotic-associated adverse events. Clin Infect Dis. 2008;47:735–43.
31. Shlaes DM, Gerding DN, John Jr JF, et al. Society for Healthcare Epidemiology of America and Infectious Diseases Society of America Joint Committee on the Prevention of Antimicrobial Resistance: guidelines for the prevention of antimicrobial resistance in hospitals. Infect Control Hosp Epidemiol. 1997;18:275–91.
32. Polk R. Optimal use of modern antibiotics: emerging trends. Clin Infect Dis. 1999;29:264–74.
33. Klapp DL, Ramphal R. Antibiotic restriction in hospitals associated with medical schools. Am J Hosp Pharm. 1983;40:1957–60.
34. Lesar TS, Briceland LL. Survey of antibiotic control policies in university-affiliated teaching institutions. Ann Pharmacother. 1996;30:31–4.
35. Lawton RM, Fridkin SK, Gaynes RP, McGowan Jr JE. Practices to improve antimicrobial use at 47 US hospitals: the status of the 1997 SHEA/IDSA position paper recommendations. Society for Healthcare Epidemiology of America/Infectious Diseases Society of America. Infect Control Hosp Epidemiol. 2000;21:256–9.
36. Moro ML, Petrosillo N, Gandin C. Antibiotic policies in Italian hospitals: still a lot to achieve. Microb Drug Resist. 2003;9:219–22.
37. Woodford EM, Wilson KA, Marriott JF. Documentation of antibiotic prescribing controls in UK NHS hospitals. J Antimicrob Chemother. 2004;53:650–2.
38. Dellit TH, Owens RC, McGowan Jr JE, et al. Infectious Diseases Society of America and the Society for Healthcare Epidemiology of America guidelines for developing an institutional program to enhance antimicrobial stewardship. Clin Infect Dis. 2007;44:159–77.
39. Paskovaty A, Pflomm JM, Myke N, Seo SK. A multidisciplinary approach to antimicrobial stewardship: evolution into the 21st century. Int J Antimicrob Agents. 2005;25:1–10.
40. Couriel D, Saliba R, Hicks K, et al. Tumor necrosis factor-alpha blockade for the treatment of acute GVHD. Blood. 2004;104:649–54.
41. Virchis A, Koh M, Rankin P, et al. Fludarabine, cytosine arabinoside, granulocyte-colony stimulating factor with or without idarubicin in the treatment of high risk acute leukaemia or myelodysplastic syndromes. Br J Haematol. 2004;124:26–32.
42. Martin SI, Marty FM, Fiumara K, Treon SP, Gribben JG, Baden LR. Infectious complications associated with alemtuzumab use for lymphoproliferative disorders. Clin Infect Dis. 2006;43:16–24.
43. Fraser GL, Stogsdill P, Dickens Jr JD, Wennberg DE, Smith Jr RP, Prato BS. Antibiotic optimization. An evaluation of patient safety and economic outcomes. Arch Intern Med. 1997;157:1689–94.
44. Gross R, Morgan AS, Kinky DE, Weiner M, Gibson GA, Fishman NO. Impact of a hospital-based antimicrobial management program on clinical and economic outcomes. Clin Infect Dis. 2001;33:289–95.
45. Carling P, Fung T, Killion A, Terrin N, Barza M. Favorable impact of a multidisciplinary antibiotic management program conducted during 7 years. Infect Control Hosp Epidemiol. 2003;24:699–706.
46. LaRocco Jr A. Concurrent antibiotic review programs – a role for infectious diseases specialists at small community hospitals. Clin Infect Dis. 2003;37:742–3.
47. Lutters M, Harbarth S, Janssens JP, et al. Effect of a comprehensive, multidisciplinary, educational program on the use of antibiotics in a geriatric university hospital. J Am Geriatr Soc. 2004;52:112–6.
48. Burke JP. Infection control – a problem for patient safety. N Engl J Med. 2003;348:651–6.
49. John Jr JF, Fishman NO. Programmatic role of the infectious diseases physician in controlling antimicrobial costs in the hospital. Clin Infect Dis. 1997;24:471–85.
50. Pestotnik SL, Classen DC, Evans RS, Burke JP. Implementing antibiotic practice guidelines through computer-assisted decision support: clinical and financial outcomes. Ann Intern Med. 1996;124:884–90.

51. Evans RS, Pestotnik SL, Classen DC, et al. A computer-assisted management program for antibiotics and other antiinfective agents. N Engl J Med. 1998;338:232–8.
52. Evans RS, Pestotnik SL, Classen DC, Burke JP. Evaluation of a computer-assisted antibiotic-dose monitor. Ann Pharmacother. 1999;33:1026–31.
53. Mullett CJ, Evans RS, Christenson JC, Dean JM. Development and impact of a computerized pediatric antiinfective decision support program. Pediatrics. 2001;108:E75.
54. Struelens MJ. Multidisciplinary antimicrobial management teams: the way forward to control antimicrobial resistance in hospitals. Curr Opin Infect Dis. 2003;16:305–7.
55. Procop GW, Winn W. Outsourcing microbiology and offsite laboratories. Implications on patient care, cost savings, and graduate medical education. Arch Pathol Lab Med. 2003;127:623–4.
56. Burke JP, Pestotnik SL. Antibiotic use and microbial resistance in intensive care units: impact of computer-assisted decision support. J Chemother. 1999;11:530–5.
57. Binkley S, Fishman NO, LaRosa LA, et al. Comparison of unit-specific and hospital-wide antibiograms: potential implications for selection of empirical antimicrobial therapy. Infect Control Hosp Epidemiol. 2006;27:682–7.
58. Forrest G. Role of antifungal susceptibility testing in patient management. Curr Opin Infect Dis. 2006;19:538–43.
59. Arikan S. Current status of antifungal susceptibility testing methods. Med Mycol. 2007;45:569–87.
60. Marr JJ, Moffet HL, Kunin CM. Guidelines for improving the use of antimicrobial agents in hospitals: a statement by the Infectious Diseases Society of America. J Infect Dis. 1988;157:869–76.
61. Crowe HM, Quintiliani R. Antibiotic formulary selection. Med Clin North Am. 1995;79:463–76.
62. Woodward RS, Medoff G, Smith MD, Gray 3rd JL. Antibiotic cost savings from formulary restrictions and physician monitoring in a medical-school-affiliated hospital. Am J Med. 1987;83:817–23.
63. Coleman RW, Rodondi LC, Kaubisch S, Granzella NB, O'Hanley PD. Cost-effectiveness of prospective and continuous parenteral antibiotic control: experience at the Palo Alto Veterans Affairs Medical Center from 1987 to 1989. Am J Med. 1991;90:439–44.
64. Maswoswe JJ, Okpara AU. Enforcing a policy for restricting antimicrobial drug use. Am J Health Syst Pharm. 1995;52:1433–5.
65. White Jr AC, Atmar RL, Wilson J, Cate TR, Stager CE, Greenberg SB. Effects of requiring prior authorization for selected antimicrobials: expenditures, susceptibilities, and clinical outcomes. Clin Infect Dis. 1997;25:230–9.
66. Schentag JJ, Ballow CH, Fritz AL, et al. Changes in antimicrobial agent usage resulting from interactions among clinical pharmacy, the infectious disease division, and the microbiology laboratory. Diagn Microbiol Infect Dis. 1993;16:255–64.
67. Solomon DH, Van Houten L, Glynn RJ, et al. Academic detailing to improve use of broad-spectrum antibiotics at an academic medical center. Arch Intern Med. 2001;161:1897–902.
68. Bearden DT, Allen GP. Impact of antimicrobial control programs on patient outcomes. Pharmacy perspective. Dis Manage Health Outcomes. 2003;11:723–36.
69. Grimshaw JM, Shirran L, Thomas R, et al. Changing provider behavior: an overview of systematic reviews of interventions. Med Care. 2001;39:II2–45.
70. Gray J. Changing physician prescribing behaviour. Can J Clin Pharmacol. 2006;13:e81–4.
71. Girotti MJ, Fodoruk S, Irvine-Meek J, Rotstein OD. Antibiotic handbook and pre-printed perioperative order forms for surgical antibiotic prophylaxis: do they work? Can J Surg. 1990;33:385–8.
72. Bantar C, Sartori B, Vesco E, et al. A hospitalwide intervention program to optimize the quality of antibiotic use: impact on prescribing practice, antibiotic consumption, cost savings, and bacterial resistance. Clin Infect Dis. 2003;37:180–6.
73. Belongia EA, Knobloch MJ, Kieke BA, Davis JP, Janette C, Besser RE. Impact of statewide program to promote appropriate antimicrobial drug use. Emerg Infect Dis. 2005;11:912–20.
74. Hughes WT, Armstrong D, Bodey GP, et al. 2002 guidelines for the use of antimicrobial agents in neutropenic patients with cancer. Clin Infect Dis. 2002;34:730–51.
75. Guidelines for preventing opportunistic infections among hematopoietic stem cell transplant recipients. MMWR Recomm Rep. 2000;49:1–125; CE1–7.
76. Sullivan KM, Dykewicz CA, Longworth DL, et al. Preventing opportunistic infections after hematopoietic stem cell transplantation: the Centers for Disease Control and Prevention, Infectious Diseases Society of America, and American Society for Blood and Marrow Transplantation Practice Guidelines and beyond. Hematology Am Soc Hematol Educ Program. 2001;1:392–421.
77. Walsh TJ, Anaissie EJ, Denning DW, et al. Treatment of aspergillosis: clinical practice guidelines of the Infectious Diseases Society of America. Clin Infect Dis. 2008;46:327–60.
78. Rex JH, Walsh TJ, Sobel JD, et al. Practice guidelines for the treatment of candidiasis. Infectious Diseases Society of America. Clin Infect Dis. 2000;30:662–78.
79. ASHP Therapeutic Guidelines on Antimicrobial Prophylaxis in Surgery. American society of health-system pharmacists. Am J Health Syst Pharm. 1999;56:1839–88.
80. Bratzler DW, Houck PM. Antimicrobial prophylaxis for surgery: an advisory statement from the National Surgical Infection Prevention Project. Clin Infect Dis. 2004;38:1706–15.
81. Chastre J, Wolff M, Fagon JY, et al. Comparison of 8 vs 15 days of antibiotic therapy for ventilator-associated pneumonia in adults: a randomized trial. JAMA. 2003;290:2588–98.
82. Singh N, Rogers P, Atwood CW, Wagener MM, Yu VL. Short-course empiric antibiotic therapy for patients with pulmonary infiltrates in the intensive care unit. A proposed solution for indiscriminate antibiotic prescription. Am J Respir Crit Care Med. 2000;162:505–11.
83. Kollef MH, Kollef KE. Antibiotic utilization and outcomes for patients with clinically suspected ventilator-associated pneumonia and negative quantitative BAL culture results. Chest. 2005;128:2706–13.
84. Briceland LL, Nightingale CH, Quintiliani R, Cooper BW, Smith KS. Antibiotic streamlining from combination therapy to monotherapy utilizing an interdisciplinary approach. Arch Intern Med. 1988;148:2019–22.
85. Glowacki RC, Schwartz DN, Itokazu GS, Wisniewski MF, Kieszkowski P, Weinstein RA. Antibiotic combinations with redundant antimicrobial spectra: clinical epidemiology and pilot intervention of computer-assisted surveillance. Clin Infect Dis. 2003;37:59–64.
86. Lelekis M, Gould IM. Sequential antibiotic therapy for cost containment in the hospital setting: why not? J Hosp Infect. 2001;48:249–57.
87. Drew RH. Programs promoting timely sequential antimicrobial therapy: an American perspective. J Infect. 1998;37 Suppl 1:3–9.
88. Amodio-Groton M, Madu A, Madu CN, et al. Sequential parenteral and oral ciprofloxacin regimen versus parenteral therapy for bacteremia: a pharmacoeconomic analysis. Ann Pharmacother. 1996;30:596–602.
89. Sevinc F, Prins JM, Koopmans RP, et al. Early switch from intravenous to oral antibiotics: guidelines and implementation in a large teaching hospital. J Antimicrob Chemother. 1999;43:601–6.
90. Ramirez JA, Bordon J. Early switch from intravenous to oral antibiotics in hospitalized patients with bacteremic community-acquired Streptococcus pneumoniae pneumonia. Arch Intern Med. 2001;161:848–50.

91. Wong-Beringer A, Nguyen KH, Razeghi J. Implementing a program for switching from i.v. to oral antimicrobial therapy. Am J Health Syst Pharm. 2001;58:1146–9.
92. Sunenshine RH, Liedtke LA, Jernigan DB, Strausbaugh LJ. Role of infectious diseases consultants in management of antimicrobial use in hospitals. Clin Infect Dis. 2004;38:934–8.
93. Rapp RP. Pharmacy infectious diseases practice. Ann Pharmacother. 2006;40:304–6.
94. McQuillen DP, Petrak RM, Wasserman RB, Nahass RG, Scull JA, Martinelli LP. The value of infectious diseases specialists: non-patient care activities. Clin Infect Dis. 2008;47:1051–63.
95. Rybak MJ. Antimicrobial stewardship. Pharmacotherapy. 2007;27:131S–5S.
96. Phillips I. Prudent use of antibiotics: are our expectations justified? Clin Infect Dis. 2001;33 Suppl 3:S130–2.

Chapter 44
Controversies in Antimicrobial Stewardship

Graeme N. Forrest

Abstract Antimicrobial stewardship programs are recommended by the Infectious Diseases Society of America as a method to control antimicrobial costs and resistance. These programs are usually implemented hospital wide, but there is little evidence on their effects in oncology units. Three controversial areas of antimicrobial stewardship in oncology units include whether these programs decrease antimicrobial resistance when antimicrobial restriction is implemented, the role of antimicrobial cycling on Gram-negative resistance and that these programs rarely control outpatient antimicrobial therapy. This review will discuss these controversial areas with regard to the evidence, strength of trial design, and the generalizability of their outcomes.

Keywords Antimicrobial management • Antimicrobial resistance • Antibiotic cycling • Outpatient antibiotic therapy • VRE • *Clostridium difficile*

Introduction

The preceding chapter discussed the benefits and scope of antimicrobial stewardship in the cancer center. With the costs of prolonged antimicrobial use in patients, especially antifungals and the emergence of multidrug resistant (MDR) bacteria as a threat to patient care, there appears to be a greater urgency to improve antibiotic utilization by controlling their use at an institutional level as a means to control these problems. At present there is very little data on the impact of these programs in cancer centers, with most information based on hospital wide strategies.

As described, establishing an antimicrobial stewardship program is complicated by competing interests all looking for different outcomes. The hospital administration wants to save money through shorter length of stay, decreased pharmacy costs, and lower resistance; infection control is looking for decrease in emergence of resistance in bacteria; pharmacy wants to save money by reducing antimicrobial therapy; microbiology wants to perform less surveillance screening and less susceptibility testing to save money; and lastly infectious disease is expected to develop guidelines, provide staff, and enforcement of the guidelines while getting little in return from the hospital. All these groups have interests in different outcomes, and all these outcomes are usually different from the oncologists who are ultimately responsible for managing the patient and the last thing they want is a patient to die from infection that either was due to ineffective antimicrobial therapy because of either antimicrobial restriction or antimicrobial resistance. It is this conflict of interests that is the basis for the controversies in antimicrobial stewardship.

Fortunately, These conflicts are mitigated in many centers by using a team of specialists to care for oncology patients. This team usually consists of the oncologist, physician assistants or nurse practitioners, infectious disease physician, clinical pharmacists, and the nurses. Subsequently, the group develop guidelines based on evidence when possible and is implemented as a group effort; however there are still areas of controversy that arise even within these guidelines. Several of the controversies to be discussed in this chapter are the impact on antimicrobial resistance by stewardship programs, antimicrobial preauthorization, antibiotic cycling and de-escalation strategies, and outpatient antibiotic management.

Does Antimicrobial Stewardship Impact Antimicrobial Resistance?

From the first combination, antibiotic study in febrile neutropenia [1] followed later by the initiation of empiric antifungal therapy [2] have all contributed to lowering mortality from infection in oncology patients. There are many guidelines for the antimicrobial management of febrile neutropenia in oncology patients in the literature [3–6]. However, antibiotic proliferation within the cancer center has resulted in the emergence of antimicrobial drug resistant organisms, especially vancomycin resistant enterococci (VRE), extended spectrum beta lactamases (ESBL), and of more concern *Klebsiella pneumoniae* carbapenemases (KPC) [7–10]. Therein lies the conundrum; oncology patients need antibiotics often for prolonged periods of time due to their neutropenia [11], but this antibiotic pressure results in the emergence of resistant isolates. If a cancer center does have antimicrobial resistant organisms, this will impact on empiric antimicrobial therapy and result in the selection of either more expensive or more toxic or multiple combinations of antibiotics to ensure adequate coverage [12]. Is there enough evidence that a well-structured antimicrobial program can reduce antimicrobial resistance in a cancer center? This depends on whether the aim of the antimicrobial stewardship program is to arrest an outbreak of a multidrug resistant organism or to have a sustained effect on prevention of resistance [13].

In the oncology setting, the only data supporting antibiotic stewardship programs have been to control outbreaks of multidrug resistant organisms. In particular, the two most common organisms that are targeted are VRE and *Clostridium difficile* [8, 14, 15].

VRE is one of the most common causes of nosocomial blood stream infection in the cancer center, affecting centers worldwide [8, 14, 16–18]. In a cohort study of adult stem cell transplant (ASCT) recipients from the Mayo Clinic, VRE colonization was shown to be associated with increased mortality regardless of other factors at 100 days [19]. Also, Zaas et al. identified vancomycin usage (relative risk [RR] 1.98, Confidence intervals [CI] 1.25–3.14) as a significant risk factor for VRE bloodstream infection in patients with cancer [20]. In recent studies, the risk factors in the cancer center have been identified as aminoglycoside usage within the previous 30 days, while the use of a carbapenem was significantly associated with VR *E. faecium* bacteremia, which had poor outcomes [8]. Prior studies have demonstrated an association with vancomycin either alone or with third generation cephalosporins and sometimes with metronidazole [20–22].

The data supporting the role of vancomycin restriction and reduced acquisition of VRE is unclear. The largest study suggesting that vancomycin was the most significant modifiable risk factor, was performed at 20 hospitals and 50 intensive care units (ICU) where data was adjusted for MRSA colonization. Those ICU's using a directed quality improvement on vancomycin use resulted in a 7.5% reduction in VRE compared to a mean increase of 5.7% ($P<0.001$) in those that did not [23]. As patients with hematologic malignancy due to their illness may be admitted to the ICU, reducing the risk of acquisition in this setting may be very important [24]. Overall, most studies investigating vancomycin usage on VRE colonization and infection have been heterogeneous [25].

All vancomycin intervention studies have been quasi-experimental, pre-post intervention Type A designs at the lowest level of strength of study design as described by Harris et al., and have significant heterogeneity in their study populations [25, 26]. Reflecting their design, many were performed at a single center, lacked a control group, and none removed and reintroduced the interventions [15, 23, 27–35]. Definitions on VRE endemicity versus outbreak are lacking in these studies and most state that VRE have been prevalent for several years [15, 23, 25, 27–35]. Three studies were performed in a cancer center setting [15, 29, 33]. Shaikh et al. interventions were a multifaceted approach at the M.D. Anderson Cancer Center, where they implemented a "vancomycin order form" to decrease empiric vancomycin usage. Simultaneously they implemented infection control policies including hand washing, routine isolation, screening, disposable and dedicated equipment, thorough cleaning of nondisposable equipment, and cohorting [33]. Their interventions over 3 years showed a reduction of total VRE infections from 0.437/1,000 patient days in 1997 to 0.229/1,000 patient days in 1999 ($P=0.008$) and a similar reduction in VRE bloodstream infections and a reduction in vancomycin from 416 g/1,000 patient days to 208 g/1,000 patient days [33]. Montecalvo et al. also performed a multifaceted approach in a cancer center to reduce VRE, reporting a 1-year result, with reduced length of stay and an estimated $189,000 saved with implementing a program [15]. None of the studies looked at mortality reduction, and there has been no long-term follow up to see if these interventions have had long-lasting effects [15, 29, 33].

The rest of the studies on vancomycin use and reduction of VRE were performed in noncancer settings, most commonly ICU's [27, 28, 30–32, 34–36]. All studies demonstrate a reduction in vancomycin usage, either hospital or unit specific. Seven [15, 23, 29–31, 33, 35] of these studies showed statistically significant reductions in VRE infections and colonization ranging from 46 to 83% [25, 29, 33]. The rest [28, 32, 34, 36] were a wash in VRE reduction. The main limitations of these studies is that none controlled for random variables and severity of illness and the main intervention may take time to have an impact on VRE acquisition and similarly the efficacy of the interventions may wane over time [25, 26]. Over the last decade, antibiotics other than vancomycin implicated in causing VRE outbreaks (i.e., ceftazidime, antianaerobic agents) which [27, 30, 37, 38] have changed and reflects that good infection control policies at an institution are important for control of VRE. As good policy though, control of vancomycin usage is as important as good infection control practices in controlling VRE. What are needed are larger multicenter controlled trials to see the true benefit of vancomycin restriction on VRE.

Clostridium difficile associated diarrhea (CDAD) is associated with considerable morbidity in oncology patients [39, 40]. With the emergence of more hypervirulent strains (group B1 toxin) which have a higher mortality, are quinolone resistant, and fail metronidazole therapy more, prevention of this infection has become more imperative [41–43]. The same limitations of the VRE studies inherent in the CDAD data. Although recognized that the importance of antibiotic control, in particular cephalosporins, quinolones, and clindamycin, infection control procedures are just as important, including hand washing, patient isolation, and room disinfection [40, 44–46]. Muto et al. showed how an infection control bundle, which included antibiotic control, especially quinolone use could reduce CDAD with the hypervirulent strain [44, 47]. The greatest importance of preventing this strain is that with the high metronidazole failure, there is increased oral vancomycin usage, which increases costs and may lead to more VRE colonization [42, 48].

The benefit of antimicrobial control appears to be in conjunction with other infection control measures. There appears to be little evidence that either one alone will offer a benefit due to a lack of appropriately controlled studies. Despite this, it just seems prudent that in this era of emerging resistance that all possible measures be implemented to reduce resistant organisms which impact the mortality of cancer patients.

Antibiotic Cycling

There is increasing resistance of Gram-negative (GN) organisms to antibiotics within hospitals, especially within the ICU and cancer center [11, 49–55]. However, there have not been any new classes of antibiotics for the treatment of these MDR GN organisms for many years and there is few if any in the pipeline [56].

Despite the shift towards Gram-postitive organisms causing infections in oncology patients, *Pseudomonas aeruginosa* remains the most common GN infection and is associated with higher mortality [57–59]. The increasing antimicrobial resistance within the GN organisms greatly impacts the selection of empirical antimicrobial therapy in the neutropenic host, which may affect mortality [60–62]. The emergence of carbapenem resistant *P. aeruginosa* and *Acinetobacter* infections means the use of more toxic and less effective antibiotics such as colistin and tigecycline [58, 62, 63].

A method that has developed in the ICU setting is to "cycle" the GN antibiotics, which is the scheduled rotation of antibiotics after an exclusive use for a preset period of 6 or 12 months, as a means to prevent resistance [55]. This was first suggested by Gerding et al., who demonstrated that by rotating gentamicin/tobramycin with amikacin they could increase the susceptibility of GN organisms to all the aminoglycosides, despite the rotation being within the same class of antibiotics [64]. It was this approach that has exciting potential to improve antimicrobial susceptibility and preserve for longer the use of classes of antibiotic agents against GN organisms. However, this approach also is controversial and has not been compared to "antibiotic heterogeneity," which is the use of multiple classes of antibiotics as outlined by the choices in the IDSA febrile neutropenia guidelines [4, 55].

Antibiotic cycling or rotation involves substituting an antibiotic from one class with one or more from different classes, as opposed to replacing with one from the same class [65]. This practice is complicated by the fact that antibiotics that belong to one class may select resistance to one or more unrelated classes as a result of genetic linkages [65]. For example quinolone usage can lead to emergence of imipenem resistant *Pseudomonas* [66, 67].

There have been four studies of antibiotic cycling in a cancer center setting, with three looking at general outcomes and one on VRE [68–71]. A summary of their outcomes is in Table 44.1.

Bradley et al. investigated the impact of cycling antibiotic on hyperendemic VRE in a hematological malignancy unit, which had a baseline prevalence of 50% [71]. They performed a 3 phase study in which phase 1 was a 4 month observational period, phase 2 they substituted ceftazidime for piperacillin/tazobactam (PT), and then phase 3 returned to ceftazidime. In phase 2 they also performed hand-hygiene and infection control actions, which was continued through phase 3. They demonstrated that in phase 1 there was a 57% acquisition of VRE in 6 weeks from admission, compared to 19% in phase 2, and 1% in phase 3, however there was an increase in VRE colonization when ceftazidime was restarted, while vancomycin policy was not changed throughout the study [71]. As described previously, was the effect the cycling or the infection control measures and since there was no randomization, it is difficult to establish causality.

In contrast, Dominguez et al. performed a randomized study of neutropenic patients to one of four regimens cycled over a 2-year period. Of concern from this study, were that only 42% of patients were able to complete their assigned regimen, with 14% having breakthrough bacteremia, and a marked increase in enterococcal infections, but no increase in resistance [70]. A major flaw in this study that is not addressed is that 55% of patients (148/271 evaluable patients) failed their primary regimen and 117 of the 148 (75%) required changing of their antibiotic therapy [70]. The authors importantly do not address what the antibiotic regimens were changed to when deemed a failure, whether there was a crossover of salvage antibiotics into a prior or future regimen or a new antibiotic class altogether, and how long

Table 44.1 Summary of antibiotic cycling studies in oncology centers

Year	H/B	IC	Cycle description	Outcomes
1999 [71]	H	Y	Ceftazadime 4 months – observational Piperacillin/tazobactam 4 months – +IC Ceftazadime 4 months +IC	Reduced VRE Phase 2 > 3 > 1 No change in glycopeptide use No gram-negative resistance data
2000 [70]	H	N	1. Ceftazidime and vancomycin – 6 months 2. Imipenem – 4 months 3. Aztreonam and cefazolin – 5 months 4. ciprofloxacin and clindamycin – 4 months	No difference between groups, however 55% failed regimen and required antibiotic change Increased Enterococci
2007 [68]	B	N	Cefepime – 3 months Piperacillin/tazobactam 3 months For 4 years	No change in gram-negative resistance Increased VRE Comparison group not cycled
2007 [69]	B	N	All received levofloxacin prophylaxis Imipenem – 8 months Cefepime + tobramycin – 8 months Piperacillin/tazobactam + tobramycin – 8 months	Reduced gram-negative bacteremia compared to retrospective cohort Increased VRE

H hematological unit; *B* stem cell transplant unit; *Y* yes; *N* no; *IC* infection control policies implemented; *VRE* vancomycin resistant Enterococci

after starting therapy was the antibiotic change required. With over 50% of patients changing their antibiotic in a cycling study occurring within the cycle, it is most likely we are seeing antibiotic heterogeneity with this study and probably why there was no difference between the groups.

Cadena et al. have the longest time experience of cycling antibiotic therapy in a hematologic unit [68]. They rotated every 3 months PT and cefepime for a 5-year period and compared their profile to a solid organ transplant group. They noted that over this time period there was no increase in GN resistance to either antibiotics and were significant lower than the solid organ transplant group, however VRE increased [68]. Their study is limited as the comparison groups are not similar populations and that the increasing VRE rate again suggests that infection control is just as important issue. Craig et al. also did not see an increase in GN resistance with antibiotic cycling while using levofloxacin prophylaxis, however likewise saw increases in VRE in their unit [69]. Except for Bradley [71], none of the studies implemented infection control practices with the cycling and all studies lack an adequate control group to determine if these outcomes would not have occurred without cycling.

There are many problems that are concerning from these studies. Many patients with hematologic malignancies receive several courses of chemotherapy and require several admissions over their consolidation chemotherapy. No one addresses whether these patients are cycled to different antibiotics from a prior admission, as they could receive the same antibiotic over time and select a resistant organism. The same problem occurs if the patient is transferred to an ICU or to another institution where they may cycle onto a previously seen antibiotic and lastly all these studies demonstrate increases in VRE infections, something that has been shown to increase mortality and costs in the cancer center [8, 19]. At present antibiotic cycling does not appear to worsen GN resistance, but may increase VRE rates and this appears consistent with ICU studies [72]. Importantly, larger better controlled studies are needed to show a true benefit over antibiotic heterogeneity. Unfortunately with the lack of new drug development, strategies are needed to preserve our ability to use antibiotics in oncology patients.

Outpatient Antibiotics: Avoiding the Restriction Process

The previous two sections have focused on controversial inpatient aspects of antimicrobial stewardship programs. Therefore, stewardship programs focus most of their attention on inpatient antibiotic usage as this is where most of them put the time and effort to demonstrate cost-savings, reduced antimicrobial usage, and sometimes resistance. However, since the middle of the 1990s, oncology practices are increasingly using oral antibiotics for febrile neutropenia prevention and infusion centers to give intravenous antibiotics, thereby effectively bypassing antimicrobial stewardship programs [55].

The move to outpatient antibiotic therapy has grown with more guidelines using a risk-based assessment to determine inpatient versus outpatient management [4, 73].

The observation that some patients are at lower risk with febrile neutropenia for serious infection has allowed for more home therapy. This initially was performed using intravenous antibiotics by Talcott et al. and then confirmed in pilot study of 30 patients which showed nine patients required readmission, but unenrolled patients had over 44% higher costs [74, 75]. Due to the cost of either home infusion or even outpatient infusion, the next logical step was to determine if there was a low-risk group of patients that oral antibiotic therapy could be effective in febrile neutropenia. Subsequently, Freifeld et al. performed a randomized, double blind, placebo-controlled study in low-risk patients with fever and neutropenia with duration of less than 10 days [76]. Patients were randomized to either receive oral ciprofloxacin and amoxicillin/clavulinic acid or ceftazidime intravenously and the results demonstrated that the oral regimen was as effective as the intravenous regimen ($P=0.48$) and there were no deaths, but increased intolerance of the oral regimen [76]. There have been many strategies utilized since then, as long as there is careful patient selection and this approach offers decreased hospital costs, risk of acquiring nosocomial infections, and improved patient comfort [73, 77].

With the increased use of outpatient oral antibiotics and intravenous infusions, there is little oversight from antimicrobial stewardship program. While the obvious benefits of home antibiotics for low risk patients have been described, more patients with hematologic malignancies and prolonged neutropenia are being managed as outpatients [77]. The impact on antimicrobial resistance and selection of resistance organisms is unknown, with very little data. Most is extrapolated from inpatient use. Kern et al. showed that a hematology unit at one hospital with high consumption of fluoroquinolones had higher rates of resistant *E. coli* compared to the low user hospital, but there was no difference in activity to *P. aeruginosa* [78].

Fluoroquinolones are the most widely used antibiotic for outpatient febrile neutropenia and for prevention of GN sepsis in leukemia patients. Despite their widespread use in this population, there is little documented resistance and development of carbapenemases [79, 80]. Kern et al. showed over a 6-years period an increase of fluoroquinolone resistant *E. coli* bloodstream isolates to over 50% from patients in their cancer center. They performed a 6-month fluoroquinolone prophylaxis discontinuation trial which showed that the rates of GN bacteremia increased from 8 to 20% in their acute leukemia patients. When they reinitiated the prophylaxis, the rates decreased to 9% again, however *E. coli* resistance returned to 50% again. The benefit appeared to outweigh the risks of resistance, however the inpatient service should be aware of this so that inpatient quinolones are not selected as empiric therapy for sepsis [80]. Fluoroquinolones can select for dual resistance to ciprofloxacin and imipenem in *P. aeruginosa* in vitro via a regulatory gene which can turn on an outer porin [79]. Mueller et al. performed a nested case control study in *P. aeruginosa* isolates with combined imipenem and fluoroquinolone resistance and found that imipenem resistance was strongly associated with imipenem use and not ciprofloxacin use [79]. This is important as carbapenems are frequently used in oncology centers as frontline therapy for sepsis.

The concern of widespread fluoroquinolone usage in the outpatient setting is inadequate empiric antimicrobial therapy especially if the patient presents to an outside hospital where their prior antibiotic therapy may not be known. The emergence of quinolone resistance in *E. coli* and *Klebsiella pneumonia* species is increasing and has been associated with increased mortality [50]. Even in a cohort study by Thom et al., inadequate antimicrobial therapy for these organisms was significantly associated with mortality [81].

The emergence of carbapenem resistant *P. aeruginosa* has not been a major problem from the outpatient setting, however with the presence of ESBL organisms increasing, the use of carbapenems is increasing and this likelihood will increase over time [82, 83]. Although colistin has shown in a single center retrospective review to be effective against MDR *P. aeruginosa*, its long-term toxicity has not been fully addressed in this population [58].

Presently, there is very little information on antimicrobial stewardship with outpatient oncology patients, however despite some reports of increasing GN resistance, the benefits appear to outweigh the risks. Also, most oncology patients receiving outpatient intravenous antibiotics would most likely have been initiated or assessed by an infectious disease specialist who works closely with the oncologists. Awareness of outpatient antimicrobials is important for initiating appropriate antimicrobial therapy when there is a suspicion of sepsis.

Summary

There is very little information on the role of antimicrobial stewardship programs in oncology services, with most data from implementation in general hospital programs. The goals and order of these programs may differ from the aims of the oncology group. Most antibiotic restriction programs in the oncology center are implemented because of an endemic resistance problem or after an outbreak of a resistant organism or *Clostridium difficile*. The supporting data are usually single center quasi-experimental designs without a control group and no ability to determine the washout of their intervention. There is no supporting data that antimicrobial restriction without good infection control practices reduces resistance.

Also, antimicrobial cycling has the same limitations, however has not shown to worsen GN resistance, but has increased VRE in units that have started them.

Lastly, outpatient antibiotic therapy for low-risk patients frequently circumvents antimicrobial programs, but the benefits outweigh the risks, however there is little data on the outcomes of these patients if they present to a treatment center that is not their primary base requiring antimicrobial therapy and whether they receive appropriate therapy.

Despite these controversies and limitations, the hypothetical benefits of monitoring antimicrobial therapy would appear to outweigh the lack of evidence presently available, but larger multicenter trials with a control group would strengthen the data.

References

1. Schimpff S, Satterlee W, Young VM, Serpick A. Empiric therapy with carbenicillin and gentamicin for febrile patients with cancer and granulocytopenia. N Engl J Med. 1971;284:1061–5.
2. Pizzo PA, Robichaud KJ, Gill FA, Witebsky FG. Empiric antibiotic and antifungal therapy for cancer patients with prolonged fever and granulocytopenia. Am J Med. 1982;72:101–11.
3. Akova M, Paesmans M, Calandra T, Viscoli C. A European Organization for Research and Treatment of Cancer-International Antimicrobial Therapy Group Study of secondary infections in febrile, neutropenic patients with cancer. Clin Infect Dis. 2005;40:239–45.
4. Hughes WT, Armstrong D, Bodey GP, Bow EJ, Brown AE, Calandra T, et al. 2002 guidelines for the use of antimicrobial agents in neutropenic patients with cancer. Clin Infect Dis. 2002;34:730–51.
5. Segal BH, Almyroudis NG, Battiwalla M, Herbrecht R, Perfect JR, Walsh TJ, et al. Prevention and early treatment of invasive fungal infection in patients with cancer and neutropenia and in stem cell transplant recipients in the era of newer broad-spectrum antifungal agents and diagnostic adjuncts. Clin Infect Dis. 2007;44:402–9.
6. Cometta A, Viscoli C, Castagnola E, Massimo L, Giacchino R, Gibson B, et al. Empirical treatment of fever in neutropenic children: the role of the carbapenems. International Antimicrobial Therapy Cooperative Group of the European Organisation for Research and Treatment of Cancer and the Gimema Infection Program. Pediatr Infect Dis J. 1996;15:744–8.
7. Deshpande LM, Jones RN, Fritsche TR, Sader HS. Occurrence and characterization of carbapenemase-producing Enterobacteriaceae: report from the SENTRY Antimicrobial Surveillance Program (2000–2004). Microb Drug Resist. 2006;12:223–30.
8. Ghanem G, Hachem R, Jiang Y, Chemaly RF, Raad I. Outcomes for and risk factors associated with vancomycin-resistant Enterococcus faecalis and vancomycin-resistant Enterococcus faecium bacteremia in cancer patients. Infect Control Hosp Epidemiol. 2007;28:1054–9.
9. Mutnick AH, Kirby JT, Jones RN. CANCER resistance surveillance program: initial results from hematology-oncology centers in North America. Chemotherapy Alliance for Neutropenics and the Control of Emerging Resistance. Ann Pharmacother. 2003;37:47–56.
10. Paterson DL, Bonomo RA. Extended-spectrum beta-lactamases: a clinical update. Clin Microbiol Rev. 2005;18:657–86.
11. Pizzo PA, Robichaud KJ, Gill FA, Witebsky FG, Levine AS, Deisseroth AB, et al. Duration of empiric antibiotic therapy in granulocytopenic patients with cancer. Am J Med. 1979;67:194–200.
12. Kollef MH. Providing appropriate antimicrobial therapy in the intensive care unit: surveillance vs. de-escalation. Crit Care Med. 2006;34:903–5.
13. Paterson DL, Rice LB. Empirical antibiotic choice for the seriously ill patient: are minimization of selection of resistant organisms and maximization of individual outcome mutually exclusive? Clin Infect Dis. 2003;36:1006–12.
14. Hachem R, Graviss L, Hanna H, Arbuckle R, Dvorak T, Hackett B, et al. Impact of surveillance for vancomycin-resistant enterococci on controlling a bloodstream outbreak among patients with hematologic malignancy. Infect Control Hosp Epidemiol. 2004;25:391–4.
15. Montecalvo MA, Jarvis WR, Uman J, Shay DK, Petrullo C, Horowitz HW, et al. Costs and savings associated with infection control measures that reduced transmission of vancomycin-resistant enterococci in an endemic setting. Infect Control Hosp Epidemiol. 2001;22:437–42.
16. Junior MS, Correa L, Marra AR, Camargo LF, Pereira CA. Analysis of vancomycin use and associated risk factors in a university teaching hospital: a prospective cohort study. BMC Infect Dis. 2007;7:88.
17. Schmidt-Hieber M, Blau IW, Schwartz S, Uharek L, Weist K, Eckmanns T, et al. Intensified strategies to control vancomycin-resistant enterococci in immunocompromised patients. Int J Hematol. 2007;86:158–62.
18. Worth LJ, Thursky KA, Seymour JF, Slavin MA. Vancomycin-resistant Enterococcus faecium infection in patients with hematologic malignancy: patients with acute myeloid leukemia are at high-risk. Eur J Haematol. 2007;79:226–33.
19. Zirakzadeh A, Gastineau DA, Mandrekar JN, Burke JP, Johnston PB, Patel R. Vancomycin-resistant enterococcal colonization appears associated with increased mortality among allogeneic hematopoietic stem cell transplant recipients. Bone Marrow Transplant. 2008;41:385–92.
20. Zaas AK, Song X, Tucker P, Perl TM. Risk factors for development of vancomycin-resistant enterococcal bloodstream infection in patients with cancer who are colonized with vancomycin-resistant enterococci. Clin Infect Dis. 2002;35:1139–46.
21. Lautenbach E, Bilker WB, Brennan PJ. Enterococcal bacteremia: risk factors for vancomycin resistance and predictors of mortality. Infect Control Hosp Epidemiol. 1999;20:318–23.
22. Lucas GM, Lechtzin N, Puryear DW, Yau LL, Flexner CW, Moore RD. Vancomycin-resistant and vancomycin-susceptible enterococcal bacteremia: comparison of clinical features and outcomes. Clin Infect Dis. 1998;26:1127–33.
23. Fridkin SK, Lawton R, Edwards JR, Tenover FC, McGowan Jr JE, Gaynes RP. Monitoring antimicrobial use and resistance: comparison with a national benchmark on reducing vancomycin use and vancomycin-resistant enterococci. Emerg Infect Dis. 2002;8:702–7.
24. Dubberke ER, Hollands JM, Georgantopoulos P, Augustin K, Dipersio JF, Mundy LM, et al. Vancomycin-resistant enterococcal bloodstream infections on a hematopoietic stem cell transplant unit: are the sick getting sicker? Bone Marrow Transplant. 2006;38:813–9.
25. de Bruin MA, Riley LW. Does vancomycin prescribing intervention affect vancomycin-resistant enterococcus infection and colonization in hospitals? A systematic review. BMC Infect Dis. 2007;7:24.
26. Harris AD, Lautenbach E, Perencevich E. A systematic review of quasi-experimental study designs in the fields of infection control and antibiotic resistance. Clin Infect Dis. 2005;41:77–82.
27. Lautenbach E, LaRosa LA, Marr AM, Nachamkin I, Bilker WB, Fishman NO. Changes in the prevalence of vancomycin-resistant enterococci in response to antimicrobial formulary interventions: impact of progressive restrictions on use of vancomycin and third-generation cephalosporins. Clin Infect Dis. 2003;36:440–6.
28. Morris Jr JG, Shay DK, Hebden JN, McCarter Jr RJ, Perdue BE, Jarvis W, et al. Enterococci resistant to multiple antimicrobial agents, including vancomycin. Establishment of endemicity in a university medical center. Ann Intern Med. 1995;123:250–9.
29. Rubin LG, Tucci V, Cercenado E, Eliopoulos G, Isenberg HD. Vancomycin-resistant Enterococcus faecium in hospitalized children. Infect Control Hosp Epidemiol. 1992;13:700–5.

30. Quale J, Landman D, Saurina G, Atwood E, Ditore V, Patel K. Manipulation of a hospital antimicrobial formulary to control an outbreak of vancomycin-resistant enterococci. Clin Infect Dis. 1996;23:1020–5.
31. Anglim AM, Klym B, Byers KE, Scheld WM, Farr BM. Effect of a vancomycin restriction policy on ordering practices during an outbreak of vancomycin-resistant *Enterococcus faecium*. Arch Intern Med. 1997;157:1132–6.
32. Lai KK. Control of vancomycin-resistant enterococcus. Ann Intern Med. 1997;126:1000–1.
33. Shaikh ZH, Osting CA, Hanna HA, Arbuckle RB, Tarr JJ, Raad II. Effectiveness of a multifaceted infection control policy in reducing vancomycin usage and vancomycin-resistant enterococci at a tertiary care cancer centre. J Hosp Infect. 2002;51:52–8.
34. Patel D, Lawson W, Guglielmo BJ. Antimicrobial stewardship programs: interventions and associated outcomes. Expert Rev Anti Infect Ther. 2008;6:209–22.
35. Guglielmo BJ, Dudas V, Maewal I, Young R, Hilts A, Villmann M, et al. Impact of a series of interventions in vancomycin prescribing on use and prevalence of vancomycin-resistant enterococci. Jt Comm J Qual Patient Saf. 2005;31:469–75.
36. Byers KE, Anglim AM, Anneski CJ, Germanson TP, Gold HS, Durbin LJ, et al. A hospital epidemic of vancomycin-resistant Enterococcus: risk factors and control. Infect Control Hosp Epidemiol. 2001;22:140–7.
37. Noskin GA. Vancomycin-resistant enterococci: clinical, microbiologic, and epidemiologic features. J Lab Clin Med. 1997;130:14–20.
38. Paterson DL, Muto CA, Ndirangu M, Linden PK, Potoski BA, Capitano B, et al. Acquisition of rectal colonization by vancomycin-resistant Enterococcus among intensive care unit patients treated with piperacillin-tazobactam versus those receiving cefepime-containing antibiotic regimens. Antimicrob Agents Chemother. 2008;52:465–9.
39. Palmore TN, Sohn S, Malak SF, Eagan J, Sepkowitz KA. Risk factors for acquisition of *Clostridium difficile*-associated diarrhea among outpatients at a cancer hospital. Infect Control Hosp Epidemiol. 2005;26:680–4.
40. Blot E, Escande MC, Besson D, Barbut F, Granpeix C, Asselain B, et al. Outbreak of *Clostridium difficile*-related diarrhoea in an adult oncology unit: risk factors and microbiological characteristics. J Hosp Infect. 2003;53:187–92.
41. Pepin J, Saheb N, Coulombe MA, Alary ME, Corriveau MP, Authier S, et al. Emergence of fluoroquinolones as the predominant risk factor for *Clostridium difficile*-associated diarrhea: a cohort study during an epidemic in Quebec. Clin Infect Dis. 2005;41:1254–60.
42. Pepin J, Alary ME, Valiquette L, Raiche E, Ruel J, Fulop K, et al. Increasing risk of relapse after treatment of *Clostridium difficile* colitis in Quebec, Canada. Clin Infect Dis. 2005;40:1591–7.
43. Loo VG, Poirier L, Miller MA, Oughton M, Libman MD, Michaud S, et al. A predominantly clonal multi-institutional outbreak of *Clostridium difficile*-associated diarrhea with high morbidity and mortality. N Engl J Med. 2005;353:2442–9.
44. Muto CA, Blank MK, Marsh JW, Vergis EN, O'Leary MM, Shutt KA, et al. Control of an outbreak of infection with the hypervirulent *Clostridium difficile* BI strain in a university hospital using a comprehensive "bundle" approach. Clin Infect Dis. 2007;45:1266–73.
45. Khan R, Cheesbrough J. Impact of changes in antibiotic policy on *Clostridium difficile*-associated diarrhoea (CDAD) over a five-year period in a district general hospital. J Hosp Infect. 2003;54:104–8.
46. McNulty C, Logan M, Donald IP, Ennis D, Taylor D, Baldwin RN, et al. Successful control of *Clostridium difficile* infection in an elderly care unit through use of a restrictive antibiotic policy. J Antimicrob Chemother. 1997;40:707–11.
47. Muto CA, Pokrywka M, Shutt K, Mendelsohn AB, Nouri K, Posey K, et al. A large outbreak of *Clostridium difficile*-associated disease with an unexpected proportion of deaths and colectomies at a teaching hospital following increased fluoroquinolone use. Infect Control Hosp Epidemiol. 2005;26:273–80.
48. Pepin J. Vancomycin for the treatment of *Clostridium difficile* Infection: for whom is this expensive bullet really magic? Clin Infect Dis. 2008;46:1493–8.
49. Brahmi N, Blel Y, Kouraichi N, Lahdhiri S, Thabet H, Hedhili A, et al. Impact of ceftazidime restriction on gram-negative bacterial resistance in an intensive care unit. J Infect Chemother. 2006;12:190–4.
50. Lautenbach E, Metlay JP, Bilker WB, Edelstein PH, Fishman NO. Association between fluoroquinolone resistance and mortality in *Escherichia coli* and *Klebsiella pneumoniae* infections: the role of inadequate empirical antimicrobial therapy. Clin Infect Dis. 2005;41:923–9.
51. Lautenbach E, Weiner MG, Nachamkin I, Bilker WB, Sheridan A, Fishman NO. Imipenem resistance among *Pseudomonas aeruginosa* isolates: risk factors for infection and impact of resistance on clinical and economic outcomes. Infect Control Hosp Epidemiol. 2006;27:893–900.
52. Patterson JE. Multidrug-resistant gram-negative pathogens: multiple approaches and measures for prevention. Infect Control Hosp Epidemiol. 2006;27:889–92.
53. Pitout JD, Le P, Church DL, Gregson DB, Laupland KB. Antimicrobial susceptibility of well-characterised multiresistant CTX-M-producing *Escherichia coli*: failure of automated systems to detect resistance to piperacillin/tazobactam. Int J Antimicrob Agents. 2008;32:333–8.
54. Poirel L, Pitout JD, Nordmann P. Carbapenemases: molecular diversity and clinical consequences. Future Microbiol. 2007;2:501–12.
55. Rolston KV. Challenges in the treatment of infections caused by gram-positive and gram-negative bacteria in patients with cancer and neutropenia. Clin Infect Dis. 2005;40 Suppl 4:S246–52.
56. Boucher HW, Talbot GH, Bradley JS, Edwards JE, Gilbert D, Rice LB, et al. Bad bugs, no drugs: no ESKAPE! An update from the Infectious Diseases Society of America. Clin Infect Dis. 2009;48:1–12.
57. Zinner SH. Changing epidemiology of infections in patients with neutropenia and cancer: emphasis on gram-positive and resistant bacteria. Clin Infect Dis. 1999;29:490–4.
58. Hachem RY, Chemaly RF, Ahmar CA, Jiang Y, Boktour MR, Rjaili GA, et al. Colistin is effective in treatment of infections caused by multidrug-resistant *Pseudomonas aeruginosa* in cancer patients. Antimicrob Agents Chemother. 2007;51:1905–11.
59. Wisplinghoff H, Bischoff T, Tallent SM, Seifert H, Wenzel RP, Edmond MB. Nosocomial bloodstream infections in US hospitals: analysis of 24,179 cases from a prospective nationwide surveillance study. Clin Infect Dis. 2004;39:309–17.
60. Glasmacher A, von Lilienfeld-Toal M, Schulte S, Hahn C, Schmidt-Wolf IG, Prentice A. An evidence-based evaluation of important aspects of empirical antibiotic therapy in febrile neutropenic patients. Clin Microbiol Infect. 2005;11 Suppl 5:17–23.
61. Safdar A, Rodriguez GH, Balakrishnan M, Tarrand JJ, Rolston KV. Changing trends in etiology of bacteremia in patients with cancer. Eur J Clin Microbiol Infect Dis. 2006;25:522–6.
62. Anthony KB, Fishman NO, Linkin DR, Gasink LB, Edelstein PH, Lautenbach E. Clinical and microbiological outcomes of serious infections with multidrug-resistant gram-negative organisms treated with tigecycline. Clin Infect Dis. 2008;46:567–70.
63. Paterson DL, Doi Y. A step closer to extreme drug resistance (XDR) in gram-negative bacilli. Clin Infect Dis. 2007;45:1179–81.
64. Gerding DN, Larson TA. Aminoglycoside resistance in gram-negative bacilli during increased amikacin use. Comparison of experience in 14 United States hospitals with experience in the Minneapolis Veterans Administration Medical Center. Am J Med. 1985;79:1–7.
65. Brown EM, Nathwani D. Antibiotic cycling or rotation: a systematic review of the evidence of efficacy. J Antimicrob Chemother. 2005;55:6–9.

66. Gasink LB, Fishman NO, Weiner MG, Nachamkin I, Bilker WB, Lautenbach E. Fluoroquinolone-resistant *Pseudomonas aeruginosa*: assessment of risk factors and clinical impact. Am J Med. 2006;119(526):e19–25.
67. Paterson DL. The epidemiological profile of infections with multidrug-resistant *Pseudomonas aeruginosa* and *Acinetobacter* species. Clin Infect Dis. 2006;43 Suppl 2:S43–8.
68. Cadena J, Taboada CA, Burgess DS, Ma JZ, Lewis JS, Freytes CO, et al. Antibiotic cycling to decrease bacterial antibiotic resistance: a 5-year experience on a bone marrow transplant unit. Bone Marrow Transplant. 2007;40:151–5.
69. Craig M, Cumpston AD, Hobbs GR, Devetten MP, Sarwari AR, Ericson SG. The clinical impact of antibacterial prophylaxis and cycling antibiotics for febrile neutropenia in a hematological malignancy and transplantation unit. Bone Marrow Transplant. 2007;39:477–82.
70. Dominguez EA, Smith TL, Reed E, Sanders CC, Sanders Jr WE. A pilot study of antibiotic cycling in a hematology-oncology unit. Infect Control Hosp Epidemiol. 2000;21:S4–8.
71. Bradley SJ, Wilson AL, Allen MC, Sher HA, Goldstone AH, Scott GM. The control of hyperendemic glycopeptide-resistant Enterococcus spp. on a haematology unit by changing antibiotic usage. J Antimicrob Chemother. 1999;43:261–6.
72. Masterton RG. Antibiotic cycling: more than it might seem? J Antimicrob Chemother. 2005;55:1–5.
73. Rolston KV. New trends in patient management: risk-based therapy for febrile patients with neutropenia. Clin Infect Dis. 1999;29:515–21.
74. Talcott JA, Whalen A, Clark J, Rieker PP, Finberg R. Home antibiotic therapy for low-risk cancer patients with fever and neutropenia: a pilot study of 30 patients based on a validated prediction rule. J Clin Oncol. 1994;12:107–14.
75. Talcott JA, Finberg R, Mayer RJ, Goldman L. The medical course of cancer patients with fever and neutropenia. Clinical identification of a low-risk subgroup at presentation. Arch Intern Med. 1988;148:2561–8.
76. Freifeld A, Marchigiani D, Walsh T, Chanock S, Lewis L, Hiemenz J, et al. A double-blind comparison of empirical oral and intravenous antibiotic therapy for low-risk febrile patients with neutropenia during cancer chemotherapy. N Engl J Med. 1999;341:305–11.
77. Kern WV. Outpatient management in patients with neutropenia after intensive chemotherapy – is it safe? Ann Oncol. 2005;16:179–80.
78. Kern WV, Steib-Bauert M, de With K, Reuter S, Bertz H, Frank U, et al. Fluoroquinolone consumption and resistance in haematology-oncology patients: ecological analysis in two university hospitals 1999–2002. J Antimicrob Chemother. 2005;55:57–60.
79. Mueller MR, Hayden MK, Fridkin SK, Warren DK, Phillips L, Lolans K, et al. Nosocomial acquisition of *Pseudomonas aeruginosa* resistant to both ciprofloxacin and imipenem: a risk factor and laboratory analysis. Eur J Clin Microbiol Infect Dis. 2008;27:565–70.
80. Kern WV, Klose K, Jellen-Ritter AS, Oethinger M, Bohnert J, Kern P, et al. Fluoroquinolone resistance of *Escherichia coli* at a cancer center: epidemiologic evolution and effects of discontinuing prophylactic fluoroquinolone use in neutropenic patients with leukemia. Eur J Clin Microbiol Infect Dis. 2005;24:111–18.
81. Thom KA, Schweizer ML, Osih RB, McGregor JC, Furuno JP, Perencevich EN, et al. Impact of empiric antimicrobial therapy on outcomes in patients with *Escherichia coli* and *Klebsiella pneumoniae* bacteremia: a cohort study. BMC Infect Dis. 2008;8:116.
82. Tacconelli E, Tumbarello M, Bertagnolio S, Citton R, Spanu T, Fadda G, et al. Multidrug-resistant *Pseudomonas aeruginosa* bloodstream infections: analysis of trends in prevalence and epidemiology. Emerg Infect Dis. 2002;8:220–1.
83. Nicasio AM, Kuti JL, Nicolau DP. The current state of multidrug-resistant gram-negative bacilli in North America. Pharmacotherapy. 2008;28:235–49.

Chapter 45
Prevention of Antimicrobial Resistance: Current and Future Strategies

Cesar A. Arias and Adolf W. Karchmer

Abstract Antibiotic-resistant organisms are now commonly found in centers dedicated to the care of cancer patients, but most worrisome, have been increasingly reported as a cause of serious infections in community settings, even in healthy individuals with no apparent contacts with the health system. The discovery and development of antimicrobial agents is one of the most significant advances in the history of clinical medicine. The delivery of aggressive invasive and immunosuppressive medical care, as occurs with cutting edge therapies today, will not be possible in the absence of effective antimicrobial agents. This concept is particularly crucial in the care of cancer patients who receive complex chemotherapeutic regimens that damage their immune system. The emergence of increasingly multidrug resistance bacteria is a limiting challenge to successful cancer therapy and is accentuated by the absent development of new antimicrobials that are active against the most recalcitrant bacterial species. A concerted and integrated effort among clinicians, hospital epidemiologists, academic medical centers, pharmaceutical companies and government agencies is essential if the "tide" of antimicrobial resistant microorganisms that threaten the future of modern medical care is to be arrested.

Keywords Antibiotic resistance • Multidrug resistant gram negative bacteria • Carbapenemases • *E. faecium* • MRSA • *Enterobacteriaceae* • Mathematical models • Prevention of antibiotic resistance

The Emerging Threat of Antimicrobial Resistance

It is certainly difficult to imagine the care of a cancer patient in the absence of antimicrobial compounds since the therapies directed to destroy and eradicate cancer cells often have important effects in the immune system predisposing these patients to acquire a variety of infections. The success achieved in cancer chemotherapy relies in part on the capability to prevent and treat infectious complications during the course of therapy, an ability that has now been seriously threatened by the emergence of antibiotic resistance in both Gram-positive and Gram-negative bacteria. Antibiotic-resistant organisms are now commonly found in centers dedicated to the care of cancer patients, but most worrisome, have been increasingly reported as a cause of serious infections in community settings, even in healthy individuals with no apparent contacts with the health system [1].

Among the Gram-positive bacteria, infections produced by methicillin-resistant *Staphylococcus aureus* (MRSA) and vancomycin-resistant *Enterococcus faecium* (VRE) are by far the most critical clinical challenges in hospitalized patients (Table 45.1). Recent data from the National Health Care Safety Network from the Centers of Diseases Control and Prevention (CDC) indicate that *S. aureus* is the second most common nosocomial pathogen isolated in the USA (after coagulase-negative *Staphylococcus* spp.) and the number one cause of ventilator-associated pneumonias and skin and soft tissue infection in US hospitals (2006–2007) [2]. In the same study, 56.2% of *S. aureus* nosocomial isolates were resistant to oxacillin (e.g., MRSA), indicating that the frequency of MRSA isolation in the USA continues to be very high. Also, MRSA organisms are now increasingly being reported as the cause of severe infections in patients with no contact with healthcare institutions (community-associated [CA] MRSA). A single clone of CA-MRSA (designated USA300) is responsible for the vast majority of skin and soft-tissue infections seen in US emergency rooms [3] and now appears to be replacing hospital-associated clones in hospitals all over the world [1, 3–8].

E. faecium is another example of the evolution of a nosocomial pathogen; considered initially as an organism of low virulence and the cause of sporadic infections, *E. faecium* has been able to evolve and become a major clinical problem (Table 45.1). These organisms are now one of the most

---

C.A. Arias (✉)
Department of Internal Medicine, Division of Infectious Diseases
University of Texas Medical School at Houston,
6431 Fannin St, MSB 2.112 Houston, TX 77030, USA
e-mail: cesar.arias@uth.tmc.edu

Table 45.1 Selected multiresistant bacterial organisms causing major clinical problems and prevalence

Organism	Antibiotic resistance	Common mechanism of resistance	Antimicrobial resistance percentages in US hospitals[a]
S. aureus	Oxacillin (MRSA)	Acquisition of the *mecA* gene encoding penicillin binding protein (PBP)	56.2
	Vancomycin		–
	VISA	Thickening of the cell wall (not fully elucidated)	
	VRSA	Change in the last amino acid of peptidoglycan precursors	
	Daptomycin	Associated with changes in cell wall and cell membrane (not fully elucidated)	–
	Linezolid	Mutations in the 23S rRNA genes	–
		Acquisition of a methyl transferase gene (*cfr*)	–
Enterococcus faecium	Vancomycin	Change in the last amino acid of peptidoglycan precursors	80
	Ampicillin (common)	Mutation and over-expression of *pbp5*	90.4
	HLR to aminoglycosides	Acquisition of aminoglycoside modifying enzymes	–
	Linezolid	Mutations in the 23S rRNA genes	–
	Daptomycin	Unknown	–
	Q/D	Enzymes that inactivate Q/D, target modification	
Klebsiella pneumoniae/	Oxyimino cephalosporins	Extended-spectrum β-lactamase	27.1/8.1[b]
Escherichia coli	Carbapenems	Carbapenemases, decreased permeability	10.8/0.9[b]
Acinetobacter spp.	Carbapenems	Decreased permeability, efflux, and carbapenemases	29.2[b]
Pseudomonas aeruginosa	Carbapenems	Decreased permeability, efflux, and carbapenemases	23[b]

VISA S. aureus with intermediate susceptibility to vancomycin; *VRSA* vancomycin-resistant *S. aureus*; *HLR* high-level resistance; *VR* vancomycin-resistant; *Q/D* quinupristin/dalfopristin; *HD* high-dose
[a] Data from Hidron et al., 2008 [2]
[b] Percentages relate to central-line-associated bloodstream infections as reported by Hidron et al. [2]
Modified from Arias CA & Murray BE [1]

common bacterial species isolated from nosocomial infections in 2006–2007 and, more worrisome, greater than 80% of *E. faecium* in the US hospitals are resistant to vancomycin and ampicillin, two of the most important antienterococcal antibiotics. This phenomenon has been attributed to the ability of a genetic lineage of *E. faecium* (often designated clonal cluster 17) to acquire virulence, colonization, and antibiotic resistance determinants that increase their ability to cause disease in the hospital setting [9, 10].

The situation with Gram-negative organisms is even more dire since therapeutic options for these bacteria are more limited and new compounds appear to be far in the horizon of clinical development. Members of the *Enterobacteriaceae* family are the most common Gram-negative pathogens in humans, but *Pseudomonas aeruginosa* and *Acinetobacter* have a prominent role as infectious agents in cancer patients [11] (Table 45.1). Until recently, clinically important multi-drug resistance in Gram-negative organisms was mainly mediated by the presence of acquired genes encoding extended-spectrum β-lactamase enzymes (ESBLs) and β-lactamases mediated by chromosomal genes. These β-lactamases precluded the use of penicillin derivatives and potent cephalosporins, and substantially limited the therapeutic options for treatment of infections caused by the resistance Gram-negative organisms. The ESBL-producing enterobacteria have been increasingly reported in hospitals (e.g., 27% of *Klebsiella pneumoniae* associated with central-line bloodstream infections in the US are likely to harbor ESBLs [2]) and are now present in community settings [12]. However, most concerning, is the emergence and dissemination of carbapenemases in members of the *Enterobacteriaceae* family, *Pseudomonas aeruginosa* and *Acinetobacter* spp [12]. The genes coding for the carbapenemase enzymes (which effectively hydrolyze all the available carbapenems) are usually carried on transferable plasmids that often harbor other resistance factors as well. As a result, no reliable treatment is currently available for many of these organisms. Since members of the *Enterobacteriaceae* family are part of the normal human intestinal flora, the potential of spread of these enzymes by the fecal-oral route is enormous; moreover, bacteria carrying carbapenamases can persist for years. These genes could also spread to the healthy population in the community following the pattern we are currently seeing with the ESBLs [12, 13].

Clinicians taking care of cancer patients are now facing this gloomy picture and are challenged with "nonstandardized" decisions, particularly in treating certain infections caused by multidrug-resistance *E. faecium*, *Pseudomonas aeruginosa*, and *Acinetobacter* spp. The problem is exacerbated by the absence from pharmaceutical pipeline of new antimicrobials with reliable bactericidal activity against the latter microorganims. Also, the costs of treating infections caused by antibiotic resistant bacteria place additional stresses on the health-care system. A recent estimate indicated that an important number of invasive infections were caused by MRSA in 2005, and that their treatment cost billions of dollars [14]; similarly, in 1998, an estimated 4.5 billion dollars were spent in treating nosocomial infections [15, 16]. In this dire scenario, prevention and control of the spread of antibiotic resistant bacteria in clinical settings, particularly those dealing with highly complex and vulnerable cancer patients, becomes of paramount importance. We will discuss some theoretical and practical strategies to counteract the emergence of antibiotic-resistant organisms in hospital settings. We will not include any comment on strategies directed to control the use of antibiotics in hospitals such as antibiotic restriction and stewardship programs since these topics will be discussed extensively in other chapters of this book.

Strategies to Prevent Antibiotic Resistance

Mathematical Models and Prevention of Antibiotic Resistance

Modeling of infectious diseases has become an important tool of public-health decision making including HIV/AIDS, pandemic influenza and, more recently, antibiotic resistance [17, 18]. These mathematical models have been constructed to attempt the identification of critical factors responsible for the increasing trends of antimicrobial resistance in nosocomial pathogens. The rationale for the use of these models is that they can potentially predict the factors that contribute to the emergence and dissemination of drug resistance and may help in designing and implementing strategies to control these factors [16, 19]. More than 60 modeling articles have been published on bacterial resistance to antibiotics since 2003 [20] and a detailed description of these models is beyond the scope of this chapter, although a few examples are worth mentioning. In 2000, a mathematical model was designed to evaluate the transmission dynamics of any one of several species of antibiotic-resistant bacteria which are usually commensals of the gastro-intestinal or respiratory tracts or the skin of humans [19]. This model assumes that bacteria are transmitted in hospitals via direct contact between patients, through contamination of the hospital environment or via human "vectors" (mostly health-care workers) [19]. Based on numerical assumptions related to the dynamics of transmission and the effect of the use of antimicrobials, several conclusions were drawn: (1) inferences related to individual risk factors for the development of resistance to one particular antibiotic may be completely different for a different antibiotic; (2) nonspecific interventions that reduce transmission of all bacteria in the hospital would also reduce the prevalence of colonization by resistant bacteria, and (3) changes in the epidemiology of resistant bacteria in a given hospital after a successful intervention may occur over weeks to months but would be faster than in the community [19]. This model emphasizes that the introduction of antibiotic resistant bacteria into the community will potentially cause an influx of these bacterial species into the hospital until an "equilibrium" is reached with the net final result being the replacement of the hospital flora by CA antibiotic-resistant bacteria. A mathematical model using MRSA as an example has predicted that the CA-MRSA USA300 strain will replace hospital-associated clones and that this highly virulent organism will become the predominant clone in hospitals across the USA [21]; in fact, some studies suggest this process is occurring [4–8].

More recently, another model was designed to study the epidemiology of antibiotic-resistant bacteria in hospitals. The key elements in hospital-acquired infections caused by resistant bacteria were quantified and presented in a two-level analysis [22]. The model offered an ecological view of the evolution of antibiotic resistance by correlating the interaction of these two levels of bacterial populations [22]. This mathematical approach shows that the endemicity of antibiotic-resistant bacteria depends on the balance of bacterial populations with and without the corresponding resistance trait and that the rates of infection with multidrug resistant bacteria are proportional to the total bacterial load of each resistant strain [22]. Thus, controlling the number of infected patients and bacterial loads in the hospital setting appear to be the best strategies to curtail transmission.

Subsequently, and based on the above conclusions, the same group developed a different model designed to assess the effectiveness of interventions to control the emergence and spread of bacterial resistance in the hospital and included several key additional factors contributing to resistance, including the effects of the immune system, acquisition of resistance genes, and antimicrobial exposure [16]. The findings suggested the following: (1) shorter lengths of antibiotic therapy and early interruption appear to provide an advantage for the resistant strains, (2) early initiation of antibiotics is the most important strategy that prevents the emergence of resistant strains and (3) combination therapy with two antibiotics prevents the emergence of resistance strains in contrast to adding sequentially new antimicrobials.

The use of combination therapy to prevent the emergence of bacterial resistance has also been supported by a different model, which numerically evaluated different treatment protocols [23] and similarly concluded that when more than one antibiotic is used, sequential use of different antibiotics in the population is always inferior to treatments where equal fractions of the population receive different antimicrobials simultaneously [23].

Although approaches defined by modeling have gained acceptance in recent years, they have elicited heavy criticism due to the fact that sometimes the calculations are based on simplistic assumptions whereas the dynamics of actual events are more complex [17, 24, 25]. Nonetheless, mathematical modeling is a useful resource with which to examine a public health problem whose inherent variability is difficult to standardize for clinical studies and the conclusions generated by models may suggest hypotheses that can be tested in well-designed clinical trials.

Infection Control Strategies

The "Search and Destroy" Approach

In the Netherlands and Scandinavian countries, a strategy designated "search and destroy" has been used successfully to control the spread of MRSA. This approach involves actively screening patients and health-care workers for MRSA and is complemented by strict isolation policies of known and suspected carriers and treatment of infection in high-risk patients with antimicrobials effective against MRSA until cultures results are available [26]. This program was established in 1980 and has managed to maintain the prevalence of MRSA in hospitals at very low levels compared to other parts of the world, including neighboring countries in Europe [27]. To control the spread of MRSA with the "search and destroy" strategy, the hospital population is divided in four groups: (1) the higher risk group include known carriers of MRSA (patients and health-care workers) or those who have a positive culture after screening; (2) patients who have been transferred to a Dutch or Scandinavian hospital from other countries, patients who shared a room with known carriers or were hospitalized in wards known to have a higher transmission of MRSA (including nursing homes and long-term care facilities, among others); (3) health-care workers involved in the management of known MRSA carriers, hospital staff who have worked in hospitals abroad, and dialysis patients who received treatment abroad, and (4) individuals who have no known risk factors [27]. Individuals in group (1) are always isolated with strict contact precautions and health-care workers are excluded from patient contact until their cultures are negative. Groups (2) and (3) are isolated until their MRSA status is confirmed and individuals in group (4) are cultured but not isolated preemptively [27]. The effectiveness of the "search and destroy" strategy has been validated in epidemiological studies [27] and mathematical models [28] support this kind of intervention. However, this approach has been questioned due to the costs associated with the implementation of this policy [29]; for example, in a 700 bed hospital in the Netherlands, the yearly cost of the "search and destroy" policy between 1999 and 2001 was € 280,000 [30]. By 2004, a Dutch hospital reported spending € 1,383,200 to search for MRSA (search component) and € 2,736,762 for isolation and eradication (destroy component) [27]. Additionally, quality of patient care may be reduced [31] by the strict limitations and regulations applied to hospital staff and also the availability of hospital beds could be limited by the isolation of patients in single rooms and the need to close wards temporarily [28]. Moreover, this policy assumes the availability and use of rapid diagnostic tests to detect the resistant microorganisms to avoid unnecessary isolation. Although rapid diagnostic tests are available for MRSA, their use is also limited by costs. Interestingly, in a screening study using routine microbiological tests to detect MRSA in the Netherlands, 95% of patients were unnecessarily isolated for an average of 5 days [32].

The Centers for Disease Control and Prevention (CDC) Campaign to Prevent Antimicrobial Resistance

In 2002, the CDC developed an integrated campaign using evidence – based guidelines with the aim of preventing the emergence of antimicrobial resistance in nosocomial settings [33, 34]. The strategy included a 12-step approach (Table 45.2)

Table 45.2 Twelve steps to prevent antimicrobial resistance among hospitalized patients

Prevent infection
1. Vaccinate
2. Get the catheters out

Diagnose and treat infection effectively
3. Target the pathogen
4. Access the experts

Use antimicrobials wisely
5. Practice antimicrobial control
6. Use local data
7. Treat infection, NOT contamination
8. Treat infection NOT colonization
9. Know when to say "no" to vancomycin
10. Stop treatment when infection is cured or unlikely

Prevent transmission
11. Isolate the pathogen
12. Break the chain of control

Adapted from Centers for Disease Control and Prevention, campaign to prevent antimicrobial resistance [34]

which encompasses four main objectives: (1) prevent infections, (2) optimize the diagnostic tools and treat infections effectively, (3) use the appropriate antibiotics, and (4) prevent transmission of antibiotic-resistant organisms. This strategy has been evaluated and shown to be successful [35, 36] since the key elements can be easily tailored to fit the needs of any institution, regardless of size, affiliation or specialty. Additionally, the approach is flexible and can be implemented as a single step, as a broad strategy with multiple steps or as a "package" with the introduction of all 12 steps [35].

The CDC also released guidelines for the prevention of intravascular catheter-related infections and hand hygiene [37, 38]. The prevention of catheter related infection guidelines emphasize training in the proper insertion and maintenance of catheters using full barrier methods, preference for chlorhexidine skin preparation and selection of patients for the insertion of central venous lines [37]. Antiseptic or antibiotic impregnated central venous catheters were recommended if rates of catheter-related infections were high in an institution [37]. The catheter management is an important part of the 12-step campaign encouraging physicians to remove catheters as soon as they are not needed, avoid culturing catheter tips, and treat catheter-related bacteremia and not colonization [34]. In this regard, a collaborative cohort study performed in intensive care units assessed the effectiveness of implementing evidence-based interventions to decrease the rates of catheter-associated bloodstream infections [39]. The study showed that the implementation of such interventions (e.g., sustained education to health-care personnel, availability of a central-line cart, use of a checklist and feedback sessions on quality of practice, among others) resulted in a large and sustained reduction in rates of catheter-associated bacteremia during the study period (18 months) [39].

Another important component is hand hygiene procedures which encompass a core element of the CDC campaign and, in general, of efforts to prevent nosocomial infections and the dissemination of antibiotic-resistant organisms. Nonetheless, many health-care workers are noncompliant with optimal hand hygiene and it is performed in less than 50% of patient encounters [40–42]. Reasons for this behavior have been thoroughly investigated and include forgetfulness, fear of skin damage, time limitations due to other priorities in patient care, and lack of adequate access to hand-rub sanitizers or sinks [42–44]. To address this problem, the World Health Organization (WHO Global Safety Challenge "Clean Care is Safer") and the University of Geneva Hospitals developed a user-centered approach, which incorporates strategies of cognitive behavior, social marketing and human factors engineering, followed by an iterative prototype test phase within a target population [42]. This program, designated "my five moments for hand hygiene," systematically engages the moments of contact between health-care workers and patients and evokes ownership and commitment to the hand hygiene process through a complete understanding of the dynamics of transmission [42, 45]. The model defines two specific areas, (1) a patient's zone, defined as the patient's intact skin and the immediate surroundings colonized by the patient's own flora, and (2) the health-care's zone, which contains all other surfaces [42]. Each moment is defined according to the interaction of the health-care worker and a zone: the *first* moment occurs between the last hand-to-surface contact with an object belonging to the health-care zone and the first within the patient zone; in other words, the moment crossing the virtual line between the two zones. Hand hygiene at this point will prevent cross-colonization of the patient and sometimes, exogenous infection [42]. The *second* moment occurs before an aseptic task develops within the patient zone and includes hand exposure to patient's clothes, skin, or any object, usually with the health-care worker engaging in an aseptic task such as giving an injection, performing wound care or handling a venous access. Hand hygiene at this point aims to prevent colonization and a subsequent health-care associated infection [42]. The *third* moment happens after body fluid exposure risk; this moment is associated with the risk of exposing hands to a fluid contaminated site, occurs within the patient's zone and requires immediate hand hygiene before any hand-to-surface exposure within the patient zone. These measures aim to reduce the risk of colonization or infection of a health-care worker with highly infectious organisms and decrease the transmission of bacteria from an infected or colonized body site to a potentially clean site on the same patient [42]. Immediate action is required at this moment since hands are not sufficiently protected by gloves and additional hand hygiene is required after glove removal [46]. The *fourth* moment occurs after patient contact; this moment happens when leaving the patient zone and before touching an object in the health-care zone. Hand hygiene at this point substantially reduces contamination of health-care worker's hands with the patient's flora and intends to prevent the risk of dissemination to the health-care environment (mostly in the health-care worker zone) [42]. Finally, the *fifth* moment occurs after contact with patient surroundings and is a variant of moment *four*, occurring after hand exposure to any surface in the patient zone but without touching the patient. The moment involves objects contaminated by the patient's flora which are removed from the patient's zone and are taken to the health-care zone in order to be decontaminated or discarded. Due to hand exposure to these objects, hand hygiene is absolutely required at this time.

This strategy and multistep approach to hand hygiene behavior had been noted to be the most efficient technique to increase patient safety and decrease the risk of nosocomial infections [40, 46–49]. Thus, the understanding of the critical moments of hand hygiene helps in designing infection control programs by reducing the dissemination of multidrug resistant microorganisms in the hospital environment with the objective of preventing nosocomial infections. A comprehensive approach for this "five moments" includes the training of health-care personnel, the designing of medical units, and a thorough performance assessment.

Treatment Based Strategies

Antibiotic Cycling

This strategy is based on the rationale that withdrawing a class of antibiotics or a specific compound for a defined period and reintroducing it at a later time can prevent the emergence of resistant bacteria to the particular antimicrobial class or agent [50]. The theoretical advantage of this approach is that it may increase the number of antibiotics active against multidrug resistant bacteria and maintain antibiotic "heterogeneity," a practice whereby multiple antibiotic classes are used in a clinical setting (i.e., intensive care or cancer unit) with the aim of reducing the emergence of resistant bacteria that otherwise might occur as a result of using a single or limited number of antibiotic classes [50]. A biological justification for the using of antibiotic cycling rests on the assumption that cyclic exposure to a homogeneous antimicrobial class or compound creates an environment of reduced antibiotic resistance because resistant strains may have a growth disadvantage when selective pressure is withdrawn and because exposure to a new class of antibiotics (assuming no cross-resistance) is presumed to eliminate the resistant organisms selected during the previous cycle [51]. Three methods have been advocated to achieve this goal: (1) mixing of antibiotic classes, (2) scheduled changes of antibiotic classes and (3) rotation of antibiotics [50].

The first clinical evaluation of this strategy was performed by Gerding et al. [52], who cycled aminoglycosides over a 10-year period in a Minneapolis Veterans Affairs hospital. Using cycles of 12–51 months, the investigators found significantly reduced resistance to gentamicin when amikacin was used, but a return of resistance with the rapid reintroduction of gentamicin. Thus, the researchers decided to reintroduce gentamicin more gradually and were able to prevent the emergence of gentamicin resistant strains [52]. Kollef et al. [53] evaluated the influence of scheduled antibiotic changes on the incidence of nosocomial infections among patients undergoing cardiac surgery. The investigators cycled third generation cephalosporins with fluoroquinolones for a period of 6 months each. The overall incidence of ventilator-associated pneumonia was significantly reduced in the second 6-month period, compared with that in the first 6-month period. This effect was mainly due to a significant reduction in the incidence of ventilator-associated pneumonia attributed to antibiotic-resistant Gram-negative bacteria [53]. In a similar investigation, different classes of antibiotics were cycled for the treatment of suspected or documented Gram-negative infections during three consecutive 6 months periods in intensive-care units and involving more than 3,600 patients [54]. The researchers found that the hospital mortality rate significantly decreased during the third antibiotic cycle for the most critically ill patients [54] supporting some benefit of cycling. Raymond et al., published the results of a 2-year study analyzing the effect of specific antibiotic rotation schedules for the treatment of pneumonia and intra-abdominal infections [55]. Outcome analysis revealed significant reductions in the incidence of infection due to resistant Gram-positive and Gram-negative bacteria and mortality in the study population [50, 55]. Another more recent study cycled linezolid and vancomycin every 3 months for a period of 2 years in a surgical intensive-care unit [56]. During 4 years prior to cycling, 543 infections with Gram-positive organisms were documented, including 105 by MRSA (8.8./1,000 patient days) and 21 by VRE (1.8/1,000 patient-days). In the 2 years after implementation of cycling, the rate of MRSA infections dropped to 1.8/1,000 patient days ($p<0.00001$) whereas VRE infections remained the same, suggesting that quarterly cycling of linezolid and vancomycin may help reduce the rates of MRSA infection in particular units. The cycling strategy has also been evaluated in a bone marrow transplant unit. Cadena et al. studied the effect of cycling in a hematology-oncology unit over a period of 5 years from January 1999 to June 2004, alternating piperacillin-tazobactam and cefepime in 3 months periods [57]. During this study, the rates of susceptibility among Gram-negatives to cefepime and piperacillin-tazobactam remained stable, but the rates of isolation of vancomycin and ampicillin-resistant *Enterococcus* spp. increased.

Several caveats should be noted when interpreting these studies since important methodological limitations are present in the majority of them: (1) due to the complexity of the issue, the real effect of a single intervention can only be determined when all variables (including infection control practices) are controlled or accounted for in complex statistical analysis (which has not been always the case and it is difficult to ascertain in the studies), (2) the dynamics of antibiotic-resistance in critical care units depend on different factors including the natural fluctuations of colonized patients [58, 59]; the often rapid turnover of ICU patients could influence enormously the rates of colonization and subsequent infection, (3) several of these studies have used only historical controls. Another important issue to consider is the biology of antibiotic resistance; a susceptible bacterial species can become resistant either by undergoing mutational changes or by horizontal acquisition of resistance genes. Some of the genetic units carrying resistance genes also harbor genes that make the bacteria more "fit" to colonize human tissues and produce disease and these genes are not necessarily selected by antibiotics. For example, *Enterococcus faecium* from clonal cluster 17 appear to recruit in the same plasmid determinants that enhance their ability to colonize the gastro-intestinal tract, produce disease, and become resistant to antibiotics. Releasing the antimicrobial pressure or changing it will do little to prevent the dissemination of these plasmids in the hospital environment since other factors are at play in the survival of the organism. Finally, mathematical models have repeatedly predicted that antibiotic cycling might paradoxically create the opposite effect: create more resistance [21, 60], a fact that has been supported by some clinical studies [61, 62]. Thus, it seems unlikely that cycling will ever prevent the resistance problems in nosocomial settings.

Shorter Antibiotic Courses, Narrow Spectrum and Combination Therapies

Although large prospective-randomized studies assessing the optimal duration of antimicrobials in clinical practice are still lacking in many infections, the sustained and prolonged use of antimicrobials beyond the recommended duration is a common practice among physicians, particularly those caring for critically ill patients. The unnecessary use of antimicrobials has been shown to be a major risk factor for the development of multidrug resistant bacteria [63, 64]. Shorter courses of antimicrobial therapy have been shown to prevent the emergence of resistance and thus have been advocated as a strategy to ameliorate antibiotic resistance. For example, a prospective randomized double-blinded clinical trial was conducted in 151 intensive care units in France to determine whether 8 days of antimicrobial therapy was as effective as 15 days for the treatment of ventilator-associated pneumonia (1999–2002). The overall conclusion was that in nonbacteremic patients receiving initial appropriate empirical therapy, the 8-day regimen was clinically comparable to the 15-day regimen with the possible exception of nonfermenting Gram-negative organisms [65]. Furthermore, among those who developed recurrent pulmonary infection, multidrug resistant pathogens emerged less frequently in those receiving 8 days of antibiotic therapy compared to patients receiving the longer course of antibiotic therapy. Similar studies have been performed in other diseases such as urinary tract infections, pyelonephritis [66] and community acquired pneumonia [67], but more studies are required to reach consensus.

An alternative strategy is to use narrow-spectrum antibiotics and several well-conducted studies suggest that certain infections such as nonlife threatening community-acquired pneumonia can be successfully treated with narrow-spectrum antibiotics such as doxycycline [68]. In a randomized prospective trial, the efficacy of intravenous doxycycline with other routinely used antibiotic regimens was assessed in 87 patients admitted with the diagnosis of community-acquired pneumonia. The mean interval between starting an antibiotic and the clinical response and the mean length of hospitalization were significantly decreased in the doxycycline group compared with the other group. Thus, it was concluded that doxycycline was an effective and inexpensive therapy for the empirical treatment of hospitalized patients with mild to moderately severe community-acquired pneumonia. Similarly, the use of narrow-spectrum agents such as penicillin, trimethoprim, and gentamicin (instead of cephalosporins) plus infection control measures have been shown to decrease the occurrence of *Clostridium difficile* infections [69]. Thus, the use of narrow-spectrum compounds for specific infections should be further explored in future studies and appropriate clinical settings.

Finally, the use of combination therapies is yet another approach that may be useful in the prevention of the emergence of antimicrobial resistance. The clinical efficacy of combination antimicrobial therapies for the treatment of severe bacterial infections has been a matter of debate. The rationale for the use of combination antibiotic therapies is that this approach may offer increased synergistic activity to the treatment strategy and thus, may prevent the emergence of antibiotic resistance; a hypothesis that has been supported by mathematical modeling studies (see above) [16]. The majority of studies have included the combination of a β-lactam and an aminoglycoside antibiotic; a recent Cochrane collaboration review performed to assess the efficacy of β-lactam monotherapy vs. β-lactam plus aminoglycoside combination therapy in sepsis (64 trials, randomizing 7,568 patients) concluded that the addition of the aminoglycoside did not offer any additional benefit and the all-cause fatality was unchanged; moreover, aminoglycoside use increased the risk of nephrotoxicity [70]. Similarly, several clinical studies in bacteremia also found no significant reduction in mortality when using the combination (β-lactam plus aminoglycoside) vs. monotherapy (β-lactam only) [71–73]. Nonetheless, reduced mortality has been documented using the aminoglycoside-/β-lactam combination for treatment of patients with bloodstream infections caused by *Pseudomonas aeruginosa* [73–75], *Klebsiella* species [76], and in the setting of bacteremia cause by Gram-negative bacilli in neutropenic patients [72, 77]. A meta-analysis showed similar mortality, more favorable clinical outcomes and less nephrotoxicity using the combination of ciprofloxacin plus β-lactams compared to β-lactams plus aminoglycosides to treat patients with febrile neutropenia [78]. The use of the combination of the β-lactam/fluoroquinolones is supported by in vitro and in vivo studies that confirm the synergistic effect of the combination [79, 80]. A recent retrospective cohort analysis that included 398 and 304 unique patients with bacteremia caused by Gram-negative bacillus who received single and combination antibiotic therapy, respectively, found that combination therapy with β-lactams and fluoroquinolones was associated with a reduction in 28-day all-cause mortality among less severely ill patients, but there was no difference in critically ill patients [81]. Overall, combination therapy is most likely of clinical benefit when treating bacteremia caused by *P. aeruginosa*, Gram-negative bacilli bacteremia in neutropenic patients and when used to assure treatment with at least one agent that is active against the organism in vitro (provide adequate therapy). Importantly, *P. aeruginosa* bacteremia among patients on admission to the hospital is significantly more likely among immunocompromised patients with central venous catheters (the cancer patient receiving chemotherapy) than immunocompetent persons [82]. Of note, the above studies have evaluated clinical efficacy and not prevention of resistance, thus, it is not clear that combination therapy will be an effective strategy to prevent the emergence of antimicrobial resistant bacteria.

Future Perspectives

Containing the spread of antibiotic resistance organisms is a major public health priority, since advances in clinical medicine can only be achieved if we maintain an upper hand against these bacteria. The dearth of antibacterial compounds in development for the treatment of emerging resistant pathogens calls for new strategies to combat this problem. The "ideal" scenario would be to have a vaccine available (including active and passive immunization strategies) for each "superbug," a prospect that is not realistic at the present time. An interesting and potentially suitable approach is the use of bacteriophages (or their products) to eradicate colonizing and infecting multidrug resistant bacteria [83]. Phages are the most abundant biological entities on earth and most significantly, they destroy half of the world's bacterial population every 48 h [84]. Phages are very specific for their host, kill bacteria efficiently, and have been used in the clinic for decades [85]. Moreover, the Food and Drug Administration approved in 2006, a "cocktail" of six individual purified phages as treatment for *Listeria monocytogenes* contamination of ready-to-eat meat and poultry products [83].

Several approaches for the phage-based therapy have been evaluated including the use of lysis-deficient phages [86], which can kill bacterial cells without lysis thus avoiding release of endotoxin and precipitating shock [86], and the use of whole phages as transport vehicles for delivery of lethal genes [87] or chemically linked antibiotics for specific bacterial species [88]. However, important drawbacks to the use of phages for therapy include the rapid development of resistance to phage attachment, the release of bacterial cell wall products that can trigger a systemic inflammatory response in humans leading to shock [86] and the production of neutralizing antibodies upon extended or repeated treatment of the same individual [89]. A variation of the phage-based therapy is the utilization of phage products (instead of the whole phage) to kill bacteria. Fischetti et al., have successfully used phage enzymes as therapeutic tools against some bacteria including *Streptococcus pyogenes* [90, 91], pneumococci [91], and *Bacillus anthracis* [92]. These peptidoglycan degrading enzymes (designated lysins) are highly evolved molecules that quickly destroy the bacterial cell wall. Nanograms quantities can kill up to 10^7 bacteria in a matter of seconds [93]. Animal models have corroborated the potential of these enzymes as agents to eradicate colonization. For example, animals were rapidly (48 hrs) cleared of the colonizing strains of streptococci or pneumococci after the administration of small amounts of lysins; however, the lysins were not able to eradicate infecting intracellular bacteria [90, 91]. Such a strategy could be useful in the eradication from patients of colonizing antibiotic-resistant bacteria and thus decrease the risk of developing a subsequent infection.

Summary

The discovery and development of antimicrobial agents is one of the most significant advances in the history of clinical medicine. The delivery of aggressive invasive and immunosuppressive medical care, as occurs with cutting edge therapies today, will not be possible in the absence of effective antimicrobial agents. This concept is particularly crucial in the care of cancer patients who receive complex chemotherapeutic regimens that damage their immune system. The emergence of increasingly multidrug resistance bacteria is a limiting challenge to successful cancer therapy and is accentuated by the absent development of new antimicrobials that are active against the most recalcitrant bacterial species. A concerted and integrated effort among clinicians, hospital epidemiologists, academic medical centers, pharmaceutical companies and government agencies is essential if the "tide" of antimicrobial resistant microorganisms that threaten the future of modern medical care is to be arrested.

References

1. Arias CA, Murray BE. Antibiotic-resistant bugs in the 21st century – a clinical super-challenge. N Engl J Med. 2009;360:439–43.
2. Hidron AI, Edwards JR, Patel J, et al. NHSN annual update: antimicrobial-resistant pathogens associated with healthcare-associated infections: annual summary of data reported to the National Healthcare Safety Network at the Centers for Disease Control and Prevention, 2006-2007. Infect Control Hosp Epidemiol. 2008;29:996–1011.
3. Moran GJ, Krishnadasan A, Gorwitz RJ, et al. Methicillin-resistant *S. aureus* infections among patients in the emergency department. N Engl J Med. 2006;355:666–74.

4. Reyes J, Rincon S, Diaz L, et al. Dissemination of methicillin-resistant *Staphylococcus aureus* USA300 sequence type 8 lineage in Latin America. Clin Infect Dis. 2009;49:1861–7.
5. Popovich KJ, Weinstein RA, Hota B. Are community-associated methicillin-resistant *Staphylococcus aureus* (MRSA) strains replacing traditional nosocomial MRSA strains? Clin Infect Dis. 2008;46:787–94.
6. Seybold U, Kourbatova EV, Johnson JG, et al. Emergence of community-associated methicillin-resistant *Staphylococcus aureus* USA300 genotype as a major cause of health care-associated blood stream infections. Clin Infect Dis. 2006;42:647–56.
7. Patel M, Waites KB, Hoesley CJ, Stamm AM, Canupp KC, Moser SA. Emergence of USA300 MRSA in a tertiary medical centre: implications for epidemiological studies. J Hosp Infect. 2008;68:208–13.
8. Carleton HA, Diep BA, Charlebois ED, Sensabaugh GF, Perdreau-Remington F. Community-adapted methicillin-resistant *Staphylococcus aureus* (MRSA): population dynamics of an expanding community reservoir of MRSA. J Infect Dis. 2004;190:1730–8.
9. Arias CA, Panesso D, Singh KV, Rice LB, Murray BE. Cotransfer of antibiotic resistance genes and a hylEfm-containing virulence plasmid in *Enterococcus faecium*. Antimicrob Agents Chemother. 2009;53:4240–6.
10. Willems RJ, Homan W, Top J, et al. Variant *esp* gene as a marker of a distinct genetic lineage of vancomycin-resistant Enterococcus faecium spreading in hospitals. Lancet. 2001;357:853–5.
11. Walsh TJ. Advances and challenges in infectious diseases supportive care of patients with hematologic malignancies, hematopoietic stem cell transplantation, and severe aplastic anemia. Semin Hematol. 2009;46:191–7.
12. Schwaber MJ, Carmeli Y. Carbapenem-resistant *Enterobacteriaceae*: a potential threat. JAMA. 2008;300:2911–3.
13. Rodriguez-Bano J, Alcala JC, Cisneros JM, et al. Community infections caused by extended-spectrum beta-lactamase-producing *Escherichia coli*. Arch Intern Med. 2008;168:1897–902.
14. Klevens RM, Morrison MA, Nadle J, et al. Invasive methicillin-resistant *Staphylococcus aureus* infections in the United States. JAMA. 2007;298:1763–71.
15. Cassell GH, Mekalanos J. Development of antimicrobial agents in the era of new and reemerging infectious diseases and increasing antibiotic resistance. JAMA. 2001;285:601–5.
16. D'Agata EM, Dupont-Rouzeyrol M, Magal P, Olivier D, Ruan S. The impact of different antibiotic regimens on the emergence of antimicrobial-resistant bacteria. PLoS One. 2008;3:e4036.
17. Kermack WO, McKendrick AG. A contribution of to the mathematical theory of epidemics. Proc R Soc London. 1927;115:700–21.
18. Anderson RM. The pandemic of antibiotic resistance. Nat Med. 1999;5:147–9.
19. Lipsitch M, Bergstrom CT, Levin BR. The epidemiology of antibiotic resistance in hospitals: paradoxes and prescriptions. Proc Natl Acad Sci U S A. 2000;97:1938–43.
20. Temime L, Hejblum G, Setbon M, Valleron AJ. The rising impact of mathematical modelling in epidemiology: antibiotic resistance research as a case study. Epidemiol Infect. 2008;136:289–98.
21. D'Agata EM, Webb GF, Horn MA, Moellering Jr RC, Ruan S. Modeling the invasion of community-acquired methicillin-resistant *Staphylococcus aureus* into hospitals. Clin Infect Dis. 2009;48:274–84.
22. Webb GF, D'Agata EM, Magal P, Ruan S. A model of antibiotic-resistant bacterial epidemics in hospitals. Proc Natl Acad Sci USA. 2005;102:13343–8.
23. Bonhoeffer S, Lipsitch M, Levin BR. Evaluating treatment protocols to prevent antibiotic resistance. Proc Natl Acad Sci USA. 1997;94:12106–11.
24. Kitching RP, Thrusfield MV, Taylor NM. Use and abuse of mathematical models: an illustration from the 2001 foot and mouth disease epidemic in the United Kingdom. Rev Sci Tech. 2006;25:293–311.
25. May RM. Uses and abuses of mathematics in biology. Science. 2004;303:790–3.
26. Nulens E, Broex E, Ament A, et al. Cost of the methicillin-resistant *Staphylococcus aureus* search and destroy policy in a Dutch university hospital. J Hosp Infect. 2008;68:301–7.
27. Wertheim HF, Vos MC, Boelens HA, et al. Low prevalence of methicillin-resistant *Staphylococcus aureus* (MRSA) at hospital admission in the Netherlands: the value of search and destroy and restrictive antibiotic use. J Hosp Infect. 2004;56:321–5.
28. Bootsma MC, Diekmann O, Bonten MJ. Controlling methicillin-resistant *Staphylococcus aureus*: quantifying the effects of interventions and rapid diagnostic testing. Proc Natl Acad Sci U S A. 2006;103:5620–5.
29. Vriens M, Blok H, Fluit A, Troelstra A, Van Der Werken C, Verhoef J. Costs associated with a strict policy to eradicate methicillin-resistant *Staphylococcus aureus* in a Dutch University Medical Center: a 10-year survey. Eur J Clin Microbiol Infect Dis. 2002;21:782–6.
30. Kunori T, Cookson B, Roberts JA, Stone S, Kibbler C. Cost-effectiveness of different MRSA screening methods. J Hosp Infect. 2002;51:189–200.
31. Stelfox HT, Bates DW, Redelmeier DA. Safety of patients isolated for infection control. JAMA. 2003;290:1899–905.
32. Kaiser AM, Schultsz C, Kruithof GJ, Debets-Ossenkopp Y, Vandenbroucke-Grauls C. Carriage of resistant microorganisms in repatriates from foreign hospitals to The Netherlands. Clin Microbiol Infect. 2004;10:972–9.
33. Stephenson J. CDC campaign targets antimicrobial resistance in hospitals. JAMA. 2002;287:2351–2.
34. Centers for Disease Control and Prevention. 12 steps to prevent antimicrobial resistance among hospitalized patients: campaign to prevent antimicrobial resistance. 2010. http://www.cdc.gov/drugresistance/healthcare/ha/12steps_HA.htm. Accessed 19 June 2010.
35. Brinsley K, Srinivasan A, Sinkowitz-Cochran R, et al. Implementation of the campaign to prevent antimicrobial resistance in healthcare settings: 12 steps to prevent antimicrobial resistance among hospitalized adults – experiences from 3 institutions. Am J Infect Control. 2005;33:53–4.
36. Cosgrove SE, Patel A, Song X, et al. Impact of different methods of feedback to clinicians after postprescription antimicrobial review based on the centers for disease control and prevention's 12 steps to prevent antimicrobial resistance among hospitalized adults. Infect Control Hosp Epidemiol. 2007;28:641–6.
37. Boyce JM, Pittet D. Guideline for hand hygiene in health-care settings: recommendations of the Healthcare Infection Control Practices Advisory Committee and the HICPAC/SHEA/APIC/IDSA Hand Hygiene Task Force. Infect Control Hosp Epidemiol. 2002;23:S3–40.
38. O'Grady NP, Alexander M, Dellinger EP, et al. Guidelines for the prevention of intravascular catheter-related infections. Infect Control Hosp Epidemiol. 2002;23:759–69.
39. Pronovost P, Needham D, Berenholtz S, et al. An intervention to decrease catheter-related bloodstream infections in the ICU. N Engl J Med. 2006;355:2725–32.
40. Pittet D, Hugonnet S, Harbarth S, et al. Effectiveness of a hospital-wide programme to improve compliance with hand hygiene. Infection Control Programme. Lancet. 2000;356:1307–12.
41. Larson EL, Cimiotti J, Haas J, et al. Effect of antiseptic handwashing vs alcohol sanitizer on health care-associated infections in neonatal intensive care units. Arch Pediatr Adolesc Med. 2005;159:377–83.
42. Sax H, Allegranzi B, Uckay I, Larson E, Boyce J, Pittet D. 'My five moments for hand hygiene': a user-centred design approach to understand, train, monitor and report hand hygiene. J Hosp Infect. 2007;67:9–21.
43. Pittet D, Mourouga P, Perneger TV. Compliance with handwashing in a teaching hospital. Infection Control Program. Ann Intern Med. 1999;130:126–30.
44. Larson E, Killien M. Factors influencing handwashing behavior of patient care personnel. Am J Infect Control. 1982;10:93–9.

45. Evans HL, Sawyer RG. Preventing bacterial resistance in surgical patients. Surg Clin North Am. 2009;89:501–19.
46. World Health Organization. WHO guidelines on hand hygiene in health care. Geneva: World Health Organization; 2009.
47. Pessoa-Silva CL, Hugonnet S, Pfister R, et al. Reduction of health care associated infection risk in neonates by successful hand hygiene promotion. Pediatrics. 2007;120:e382–90.
48. Aboelela SW, Stone PW, Larson EL. Effectiveness of bundled behavioural interventions to control healthcare-associated infections: a systematic review of the literature. J Hosp Infect. 2007;66:101–8.
49. Trick WE, Vernon MO, Welbel SF, Demarais P, Hayden MK, Weinstein RA. Multicenter intervention program to increase adherence to hand hygiene recommendations and glove use and to reduce the incidence of antimicrobial resistance. Infect Control Hosp Epidemiol. 2007;28:42–9.
50. Kollef MH. Is antibiotic cycling the answer to preventing the emergence of bacterial resistance in the intensive care unit? Clin Infect Dis. 2006;43 Suppl 2:S82–8.
51. Bonten MJ, Weinstein RA. Antibiotic cycling in intensive care units: the value of organized chaos? Crit Care Med. 2006;34:549–51.
52. Gerding DN, Larson TA, Hughes RA, Weiler M, Shanholtzer C, Peterson LR. Aminoglycoside resistance and aminoglycoside usage: ten years of experience in one hospital. Antimicrob Agents Chemother. 1991;35:1284–90.
53. Kollef MH, Vlasnik J, Sharpless L, Pasque C, Murphy D, Fraser V. Scheduled change of antibiotic classes: a strategy to decrease the incidence of ventilator-associated pneumonia. Am J Respir Crit Care Med. 1997;156:1040–8.
54. Kollef MH, Ward S, Sherman G, et al. Inadequate treatment of nosocomial infections is associated with certain empiric antibiotic choices. Crit Care Med. 2000;28:3456–64.
55. Raymond DP, Pelletier SJ, Crabtree TD, Evans HL, Pruett TL, Sawyer RG. Impact of antibiotic-resistant Gram-negative bacilli infections on outcome in hospitalized patients. Crit Care Med. 2003;31:1035–41.
56. Smith RL, Evans HL, Chong TW, et al. Reduction in rates of methicillin-resistant Staphylococcus aureus infection after introduction of quarterly linezolid-vancomycin cycling in a surgical intensive care unit. Surg Infect (Larchmt). 2008;9:423–31.
57. Cadena J, Taboada CA, Burgess DS, et al. Antibiotic cycling to decrease bacterial antibiotic resistance: a 5-year experience on a bone marrow transplant unit. Bone Marrow Transplant. 2007;40:151–5.
58. Austin DJ, Bonten MJ, Weinstein RA, Slaughter S, Anderson RM. Vancomycin-resistant enterococci in intensive-care hospital settings: transmission dynamics, persistence, and the impact of infection control programs. Proc Natl Acad Sci USA. 1999;96:6908–13.
59. Bonten MJ, Bergmans DC, Speijer H, Stobberingh EE. Characteristics of polyclonal endemicity of Pseudomonas aeruginosa colonization in intensive care units. Implications for infection control. Am J Respir Crit Care Med. 1999;160:1212–9.
60. Bergstrom CT, Lo M, Lipsitch M. Ecological theory suggests that antimicrobial cycling will not reduce antimicrobial resistance in hospitals. Proc Natl Acad Sci U S A. 2004;101:13285–90.
61. van Loon HJ, Vriens MR, Fluit AC, et al. Antibiotic rotation and development of gram-negative antibiotic resistance. Am J Respir Crit Care Med. 2005;171:480–7.
62. Warren DK, Hill HA, Merz LR, et al. Cycling empirical antimicrobial agents to prevent emergence of antimicrobial-resistant Gram-negative bacteria among intensive care unit patients. Crit Care Med. 2004;32:2450–6.
63. Dennesen PJ, van der Ven AJ, Kessels AG, Ramsay G, Bonten MJ. Resolution of infectious parameters after antimicrobial therapy in patients with ventilator-associated pneumonia. Am J Respir Crit Care Med. 2001;163:1371–5.
64. Ibrahim EH, Ward S, Sherman G, Schaiff R, Fraser VJ, Kollef MH. Experience with a clinical guideline for the treatment of ventilator-associated pneumonia. Crit Care Med. 2001;29:1109–15.
65. Chastre J, Wolff M, Fagon JY, et al. Comparison of 8 vs 15 days of antibiotic therapy for ventilator-associated pneumonia in adults: a randomized trial. JAMA. 2003;290:2588–98.
66. Talan DA, Stamm WE, Hooton TM, et al. Comparison of ciprofloxacin (7 days) and trimethoprim-sulfamethoxazole (14 days) for acute uncomplicated pyelonephritis pyelonephritis in women: a randomized trial. JAMA. 2000;283:1583–90.
67. Dunbar LM, Wunderink RG, Habib MP, et al. High-dose, short-course levofloxacin for community-acquired pneumonia: a new treatment paradigm. Clin Infect Dis. 2003;37:752–60.
68. Ailani RK, Agastya G, Ailani RK, Mukunda BN, Shekar R. Doxycycline is a cost-effective therapy for hospitalized patients with community-acquired pneumonia. Arch Intern Med. 1999;159:266–70.
69. McNulty C, Logan M, Donald IP, et al. Successful control of Clostridium difficile infection in an elderly care unit through use of a restrictive antibiotic policy. J Antimicrob Chemother. 1997;40:707–11.
70. Paul M, Grozinsky S, Soares-Weiser K, Leibovici L. Beta-lactam antibiotic monotherapy versus beta lactam aminoglycoside antibiotic combination therapy for sepsis. Cochrane Database Syst Rev. 2006;1:CD003344.
71. Klibanov OM, Raasch RH, Rublein JC. Single versus combined antibiotic therapy for gram-negative infections. Ann Pharmacother. 2004;38:332–7.
72. Leibovici L, Paul M, Poznanski O, et al. Monotherapy versus beta-lactam-aminoglycoside combination treatment for gram-negative bacteremia: a prospective, observational study. Antimicrob Agents Chemother. 1997;41:1127–33.
73. Safdar N, Handelsman J, Maki DG. Does combination antimicrobial therapy reduce mortality in Gram-negative bacteraemia? A meta-analysis. Lancet Infect Dis. 2004;4:519–27.
74. Chamot E, Boffi El Amari E, Rohner P, Van Delden C. Effectiveness of combination antimicrobial therapy for Pseudomonas aeruginosa bacteremia. Antimicrob Agents Chemother. 2003;47:2756–64.
75. Hilf M, Yu VL, Sharp J, Zuravleff JJ, Korvick JA, Muder RR. Antibiotic therapy for Pseudomonas aeruginosa bacteremia: outcome correlations in a prospective study of 200 patients. Am J Med. 1989;87:540–6.
76. Korvick JA, Bryan CS, Farber B, et al. Prospective observational study of Klebsiella bacteremia in 230 patients: outcome for antibiotic combinations versus monotherapy. Antimicrob Agents Chemother. 1992;36:2639–44.
77. EORTOC. Ceftazidime combined with a short or long course of amikacin for empirical therapy of gram-negative bacteremia in cancer patients with granulocytopenia. The EORTC International Antimicrobial Therapy Cooperative Group. N Engl J Med. 1987;317:1692–8.
78. Bliziotis IA, Michalopoulos A, Kasiakou SK, et al. Ciprofloxacin vs an aminoglycoside in combination with a beta-lactam for the treatment of febrile neutropenia: a meta-analysis of randomized controlled trials. Mayo Clin Proc. 2005;80:1146–56.
79. Drago L, De Vecchi E, Nicola L, Legnani D, Lombardi A, Gismondo MR. In vitro synergy and selection of resistance by fluoroquinolones plus amikacin or beta-lactams against extended-spectrum beta-lactamase-producing Escherichia coli. J Chemother. 2005;17:46–53.
80. Piccoli L, Guerrini M, Felici A, Marchetti F. In vitro and in vivo synergy of levofloxacin or amikacin both in combination with ceftazidime against clinical isolates of Pseudomonas aeruginosa. J Chemother. 2005;17:355–60.
81. Al-Hasan MN, Wilson JW, Lahr BD, et al. Beta-lactam and fluoroquinolone combination antibiotic therapy for bacteremia caused by gram-negative bacilli. Antimicrob Agents Chemother. 2009;53:1386–94.

82. Schechner V, Nobre V, Kaye KS, et al. Gram-negative bacteremia upon hospital admission: when should *Pseudomonas aeruginosa* be suspected? Clin Infect Dis. 2009;48:580–6.
83. Fischetti VA, Nelson D, Schuch R. Reinventing phage therapy: are the parts greater than the sum? Nat Biotechnol. 2006;24:1508–11.
84. Hendrix RW. Bacteriophages: evolution of the majority. Theor Popul Biol. 2002;61:471–80.
85. Sulakvelidze A, Alavidze Z, Morris Jr JG. Bacteriophage therapy. Antimicrob Agents Chemother. 2001;45:649–59.
86. Matsuda T, Freeman TA, Hilbert DW, et al. Lysis-deficient bacteriophage therapy decreases endotoxin and inflammatory mediator release and improves survival in a murine peritonitis model. Surgery. 2005;137:639–46.
87. Westwater C, Kasman LM, Schofield DA, et al. Use of genetically engineered phage to deliver antimicrobial agents to bacteria: an alternative therapy for treatment of bacterial infections. Antimicrob Agents Chemother. 2003;47:1301–7.
88. Yacoby I, Shamis M, Bar H, Shabat D, Benhar I. Targeting antibacterial agents by using drug-carrying filamentous bacteriophages. Antimicrob Agents Chemother. 2006;50:2087–97.
89. Dabrowska K, Switala-Jelen K, Opolski A, Weber-Dabrowska B, Gorski A. Bacteriophage penetration in vertebrates. J Appl Microbiol. 2005;98:7–13.
90. Nelson D, Loomis L, Fischetti VA. Prevention and elimination of upper respiratory colonization of mice by group A streptococci by using a bacteriophage lytic enzyme. Proc Natl Acad Sci USA. 2001;98:4107–12.
91. Loeffler JM, Nelson D, Fischetti VA. Rapid killing of *Streptococcus pneumoniae* with a bacteriophage cell wall hydrolase. Science. 2001;294:2170–2.
92. Schuch R, Nelson D, Fischetti VA. A bacteriolytic agent that detects and kills *Bacillus anthracis*. Nature. 2002;418:884–9.
93. Fischetti VA. Using phage lytic enzymes to control pathogenic bacteria. BMC Oral Health. 2006;6 Suppl 1:S16.

Part V
Infection Prevention: Antimicorbial Prophylaxis and Immunization

Chapter 46
Antibacterial, Antifungal, and Antiviral Prophylaxis in High-Risk Cancer and Stem Cell Transplant Population

Marcio Nucci and John R. Wingard

Abstract Infection represents a major cause of morbidity and mortality in hematopoietic stem cell transplant (HSCT) recipients and cancer patients. Antimicrobial prophylaxis is justifiable in these immunosuppressed patients, but its benefits may be offset by potential problems such as the selection for resistant organisms, an increase in toxicity and cost. Therefore, any attempt to administer an antimicrobial agent should be accompanied by a reflection of the potential benefits and risks of prophylaxis. This chapter reviews the rationale and current recommendations for antimicrobial prophylaxis of infections in HSCT recipients and in high-risk cancer patients, the latter group represented mostly by patients with hematologic malignancies, including those with acute leukemia, multiple myeloma, and lymphoma.

Keywords Prophylaxis • Antibacterial • Antifungal • Antiviral • Resistance • Prevention

Introduction

Infection represents a major cause of morbidity and mortality in hematopoietic stem cell transplant (HSCT) recipients and cancer patients. This chapter will focus on antimicrobial prophylaxis of infections in HSCT recipients and in high-risk cancer patients. The latter group is represented mostly by patients with hematologic malignancies, including those with acute leukemia, multiple myeloma, and lymphoma. These patients are usually severely immunosuppressed by the underlying disease and its treatment, and strategies to prevent the occurrence of infection include the use of antimicrobial agents.

M. Nucci (✉)
Department of Internal Medicine, Hematology Unit Head, Mycology Laboratory, Hospital Universitário Clementino Fraga Filho – Federal University of Rio de Janeiro, Rua Professor Rodolpho Paulo Rocco 255 Sala 4A 12, 21941-913 Rio de Janeiro, Brazil
e-mail: mnucci@hucff.ufrj.br

Antimicrobial prophylaxis is justifiable in these immunosuppressed hosts due to various reasons. First, infections are frequent; second, clinical signs of infection are subtle, making their early diagnosis (critical for the success of therapy) a great challenge; third, response to treatment is usually suboptimal mostly because recovery of host defenses is a key factor for resolution of infection. On the other hand, the use of antimicrobial agents for prophylaxis of infection is not devoid of problems. Its wide use may increase the possibility of the development of resistance; it may select for resistant organisms; it may increase toxicity and may increase the cost. Therefore, any attempt to administer an antimicrobial agent should be accompanied by a reflection of the potential benefits and risks of prophylaxis. In general, the higher is the incidence of infection the more beneficial is likely to be antimicrobial prophylaxis. However, the prediction of an incidence of infection is not simple, and requires an analysis of various factors including patient's prior exposure to pathogens, underlying disease, previous and current treatment, geographic area, and others.

Antimicrobial prophylaxis may be primary, when prevention targets an individual who has not been infected in the past, and secondary, when prevention is used to avoid recurrence of infection in an individual who has been previously infected.

Antibacterial Prophylaxis

Prophylaxis in Neutropenic Patients

Infection is a common complication of myelosuppression caused by antineoplastic chemotherapy. Neutropenic fever requires antibiotics and frequently costly hospitalization and may result in impairment in quality of life, toxicity, life-threatening complications, or death. Even when well controlled, infection may necessitate interruptions in the antineoplastic treatment regimen. Bacteria are by far the most common infectious pathogens during neutropenia.

Fever is often the only manifestation of bacterial infection during neutropenia, and thus considerable efforts have been directed toward management of neutropenic fever. Likewise, there has been considerable study of ways to prevent infection to reduce its complications.

Who Is at Risk?

Key to a prophylactic strategy is the identification of those patients at high risk for infection. The duration and depth of neutropenia are the most prominent risk factors both for any bacterial infection but also serious bacterial infection. In addition, the disease, treatment regimen, and host characteristics also influence the risk for neutropenic bacterial infection. Acute leukemia is associated with substantially higher risk for bacterial infection than solid tumors. Even for solid tumors, many chemotherapy regimens are associated with a very low (<10%) risk for neutropenic infection. Examples of chemotherapy regimens with low risks for neutropenic infection are listed in several reviews [1, 2]. Indeed, it is estimated that only 10–15% of patients treated for solid tumors have sufficient risk for infection to warrant consideration for prophylaxis [3]. There is considerable heterogeneity in the risk for infection within groups of patients with similar risk factors. Increasingly, it is recognized that polymorphisms in immune responses account for at least some of this heterogeneity.

Prevention Strategies

Two strategies to prevent infection during neutropenia have been evaluated: antibiotics and myeloid growth factors. The intent of the two strategies differs: antibiotics are intended to reduce tissue invasion and bloodstream dissemination of pathogens colonizing mucosal and integumentary surfaces while myeloid growth factors are intended to reduce the risk for infection by shortening the at-risk interval. Antibiotics have been mostly evaluated as prophylaxis in the patients at greatest risk: patients with hematologic malignancies with prolonged neutropenia. Myeloid growth factors have been best evaluated in patients with solid tumors, a group at lower risk for serious infections.

Antibiotic Prophylaxis

Numerous trials have evaluated antibiotic prophylaxis with a variety of antibiotics, but most studies have used a fluoroquinolone. A variety of benefits have been noted in single trials, and these benefits have been assessed in meta-analyses [4–8]. Benefits documented include a reduction in febrile episodes,

Table 46.1 Parameters affected by antibiotic prophylaxis

Parameter	Odds ratio	95% Confidence interval
Febrile episodes	0.67	0.56–0.81
Clinically documented infections	0.53	0.36–0.80
Microbiologically documented Infections	0.50	0.35–0.70
Infections due to gram negative organisms	0.26	0.20–0.35
Infections due to gram positive organisms	0.29	0.22–0.38
Bacteremia	0.64	0.52–0.77
Infection-related deaths	0.58	0.55–0.81
Mortality	0.67	0.55–0.81

From [6]

fewer clinically and microbiologically documented infections by both Gram-positive and Gram-negative organisms, lower likelihood of bacteremia, and fewer infection-related deaths (Table 46.1). A survival benefit has also been noted [6]. Two trials in patients receiving cyclic chemotherapy for solid tumors and lymphoma demonstrated reduced infections and infectious complications [9, 10], but the magnitude of benefit in these patients was less than in patients with hematologic malignancy. For example, the number of patients needed to treat to prevent one febrile episode was 5 for patients with hematologic malignancies, but 23 for solid tumor/lymphoma patients. Some trials also showed a reduction in the need for empiric antibiotics [11] and a shorter treatment course of empiric antibiotics [12, 13]. The fluoroquinolones have been associated with less toxicity than trimethoprim-sulfamethoxazole (TMP-SMX) [6] and have activity against *Pseudomonas aeruginosa* in contrast to the TMP-SMX and thus have become preferred agents for prophylaxis. Some studies indicate a benefit for combinations of antibiotics over single agent therapy as prophylaxis, but the benefits have not been consistent and no survival benefit has been shown.

One of the concerns with antibiotic prophylaxis is the potential for antibiotic resistance, which may compromise patient safety and thwart the effectiveness of the prophylactic regimen but also compromise the effectiveness of other antibiotic regimens not only for the individual patient but also the entire population of patients. Fluoroquinolone resistance has been increasing [14]. A nonsignificant increase in resistant colonizing Gram-negative organisms has been noted in patients given fluoroquinolone prophylaxis [6], although no increase in resistant infecting organisms has been noted as yet. One meta-analysis did not show any trends to increases in resistant organisms [7]. Another concern is the risk for an increase in *Clostridium difficile* infections. Again, this has not been seen to date [4]. Yet another concern is a higher rate of Gram-positive infections, but this too has not been a consistent finding [4]. Important to note is that although these concerns have not been realized at present, ongoing surveillance is necessary.

Myeloid Growth Factors

Infection results in accelerated destruction of neutrophils and the release of proinflammatory cytokines, which may slow neutrophil production and temporarily counter the endogenous stimulatory signals to increase neutrophils. Thus, the net effect of infection is typically prolongation of neutropenia longer than otherwise expected. Exogenously administered myeloid growth factors are uniquely suited to speed neutrophil recovery. Given prophylactically, multiple trials demonstrate convincingly that granulocyte colony-stimulating factor (G-CSF) and granulocyte-macrophage colony-stimulating factor (GM-CSF) can substantially shorten neutropenia resulting from multiple solid tumor chemotherapy regimens. As a consequence, there are fewer febrile episodes, fewer infection-related deaths, and improved overall survival benefits [15] (Table 46.2).

In solid tumor therapy, most regimens are given in timed cycles, and adherence to the scheduled treatment regimen without treatment delays or reduction in chemotherapy doses has been found to be associated with antineoplastic effectiveness. A number of studies have examined the ability of myeloid growth factors to maintain chemotherapy dose intensity and have found G-CSF to permit better maintenance (95 vs. 87%, $p < 0.001$) [15].

As noted earlier, there is considerable heterogeneity in the risk for neutropenic fever or infection according to the chemotherapy regimen. Most studies of myeloid growth factors have been conducted in solid tumor patient populations receiving chemotherapy regimens associated with a high risk of neutropenic fever (risk of 40% or higher). In recent years, examination of their use in regimens associated with lower risks of infection (20–40%) [16, 17] has documented similar benefits of myeloid growth factors. It is important to note that most patients (>80%) with solid tumors receive chemotherapy regimens associated with neutropenic infection risks substantially less than 20% [3]. Consensus panels recommend that in low-risk patients (risk less than 10%) myeloid growth factors are not justified since they are associated with high costs, toxicity, and some inconvenience of administration [1, 2, 18, 19]. For patients receiving chemotherapy regimens associated with a risk of neutropenic fever between 10 and 20%, the presence of comorbidities that increase risk provides justification of the use of myeloid growth factors.

For leukemia therapy, myeloid growth factors have some benefits during induction therapy, but there are no effects on remission and survival and thus their usefulness is marginal. However, their use has been associated with reduced febrile episodes and hospitalizations for infection during postremission consolidation therapy.

Combinations of Myeloid Growth Factors and Antibiotics

Several studies have noted that the combination of growth factors and antibiotics is more effective than either alone with reductions in neutropenic febrile episodes [15, 20, 21].

Which Is Appropriate for Individual Patients?

When the decision is made that the patient's treatment is associated with sufficient risk to warrant consideration for infection prophylaxis, one should weigh what the goal is. If the most important consideration is chemotherapy dose intensity, then G-CSF is preferable. This would be applicable when the therapeutic intent is curative. If the goal is primarily to protect the patient from neutropenic infection, antibiotics are a suitable alternative, or alternatively, a reduction in the chemotherapy doses. In a setting in which there is a high rate of fluoroquinolone resistance, antibiotic prophylaxis would be much less desirable.

Prophylaxis for Nonneutropenic Patients

Patients with Impaired Humoral Immunity

Hypogammaglobulinemia is a frequent accompaniment of chronic lymphocytic leukemia and multiple myeloma as well as other hematologic malignancies and contributes to the susceptibility for infection, particularly by encapsulated bacteria, and life-threatening infectious complications. Multiple studies have shown that the administration of intravenous immunoglobulin (IVIG) can be beneficial in reducing the risk of clinically and microbiologically documented infection rates, and meta-analyses have confirmed these single studies [22]. IVIG has been given at 2–4-week intervals in various studies, and the optimal dose schedule has not been adequately established. The role for IVIG prophylaxis in patients with lymphoproliferative disorders seems most suitable for those with recurrent infections associated with hypogammaglobulinemia. An alternative strategy would be antibiotic prophylaxis by agents active against the encapsulated organisms, but no comparative trials have been performed.

Table 46.2 Parameters affected by myeloid growth factors

Parameter	Risk reduction	95% Confidence interval
Febrile episodes	0.54	0.43–0.67 (11)
Documented infections	0.51	0.36–0.73 (10)
Infection-related deaths	0.55	0.33–0.90 (11)
Early mortality	0.60	0.43–0.83 (11)

From [15, 84]

Splenectomy

Patients who have undergone splenectomy or who have conditions that result in hyposplenism are susceptible for serious infections by polysaccharide encapsulated bacteria, especially *Streptococcus pneumoniae*. Immunization with vaccines for *S. pneumoniae, H. influenzae*, and *N. meningitidis* prior to elective splenectomy is advisable when possible since immune responses after splenectomy are impaired. Nevertheless, immunization after splenectomy should be performed although one should recognize that protection may not be complete. Antibiotic prophylaxis with antibiotics active against the encapsulated bacteria should be given, with choice determined by local susceptibility patterns. The optimal drug, duration, and dose schedule have not been established. Young age and the early period after splenectomy appear to be associated with greater risks for infection [23].

Chronic Graft Versus Host Disease (GVHD)

Patients with chronic GVHD are susceptible for serious pneumococcal disease. Pneumococcal vaccination should be given to all HSCT patients, but since responses often are impaired, antibiotic prophylaxis is also recommended during active therapy for chronic GVHD [24].

Antifungal Prophylaxis

Prophylaxis in Neutropenic Patients

Risk Assessment

Neutropenia is a risk factor for invasive fungal infections (IFI). In patients not receiving antifungal prophylaxis, invasive candidiasis (yeast) and aspergillosis (mold) account for more than 80% of IFI in neutropenic patients [25]. Other pathogens include yeast of the genus *Trichosporon* [26] and the molds *Fusarium* species [27, 28] and Zygomycetes [29]. While candidiasis may occur early in the course of neutropenia, invasive aspergillosis (IA) and other mold infections occur almost exclusively in patients with prolonged (>2 weeks) and profound (<100/mm^3) neutropenia [28]. This distinction is very important because most chemotherapy regimens are not associated with prolonged and profound neutropenia and do not require antimold prophylaxis. Table 46.3 lists the most frequent situations associated with prolonged and profound neutropenia. Other important risk factors for candidiasis are gastrointestinal mucositis and the presence of a central venous catheter. By contrast, neutropenic patients at high risk to develop mucosal candidiasis are those with severe oral and gastrointestinal mucositis.

Primary Prophylaxis, *Candida*

Prophylaxis against invasive candidiasis is not indicated in all neutropenic patients. In allogeneic HSCT recipients, two randomized clinical trials (RCTs) showed that fluconazole reduced the frequency of superficial and systemic candidiasis, as well as infection-related mortality [30, 31]. In both trials, fluconazole was given at a dose of 400 mg/day. Considering these two trials and the drug profile (good compliance, few side effects), fluconazole is considered the drug of choice for the prophylaxis of invasive candidiasis before engraftment in allogeneic HSCT recipients, and may be started from the beginning or just after the end of the conditioning regimen. A lower dose of fluconazole (200 mg/day) was also effective in preventing superficial and systemic candidiasis in one RCT [32].

Fluconazole is not effective in preventing infection caused by all *Candida* species. *Candida krusei* is intrinsically resistant

Table 46.3 Duration of neutropenia according to different chemotherapy regimens for high-risk cancer patients and hematopoietic stem cell transplantation

Disease/type of HSCT	Treatment/stem cell source	Duration of neutropenia (days)	Additional risk factors for IFI
AML	Induction "7+3" or HDARAC	20–30	Mucositis, catheter
AML	Postremission consolidation with HDARAC	10–15	Mucositis, catheter
ALL	Induction	15–30	Corticosteroids
Large cell NHL[a]	Salvage treatment regimens	7–15	Corticosteroids, mucositis
Pediatric lymphoma	Various regimens	7–10	Corticosteroids, mucositis, catheter
Allogeneic HSCT	Peripheral blood	10–15	Corticosteroids, cyclosporine, mucositis, catheter, acute GVHD
Allogeneic HSCT	Cord blood	20–60	Corticosteroids, cyclosporine, mucositis, catheter, acute GVHD
Autologous HSCT	Peripheral blood	7–10	Corticosteroids, mucositis

HSCT hematopoietic stem cell transplantation; *IFI* invasive fungal infection; *AML* acute myeloid leukemia; *HDARAC* high-dose cytarabine; *ALL* acute lymphoid leukemia; *NHL* non-Hodgkin's lymphoma; *GVHD* graft versus host disease
[a]Primary treatment for large cell NHL is usually associated with neutropenia of short duration (<7 days)

to fluconazole, and *Candida glabrata* exhibits minimal inhibitory concentrations (MIC) higher than other species. As a consequence, fluconazole has shown to select for these less-susceptible *Candida* species [33, 34], and is not recommended for the prevention of infection due to these two species.

In addition to preventing invasive candidiasis, fluconazole administered concurrently with cyclophosphamide may be associated with less hepatic and renal toxicities because of a possible protective effect of fluconazole in the hepatic metabolism of cyclophosphamide, caused by its inhibition of cytochrome P450 2C9 [35].

Other than fluconazole, itraconazole oral solution (but not capsules) [36–38], voriconazole [39], and micafungin [40] effectively prevent the occurrence of invasive candidiasis in HSCT recipients during the preengraftment period. Itraconazole is less well tolerated than the other azoles [36, 38].

The incidence of invasive candidiasis is not homogeneous across all types of allogeneic HSCT. Transplants with myeloablative conditioning regimens are associated with severe neutropenia and mucositis, and are likely to benefit from anti-*Candida* prophylaxis during neutropenia. By contrast, some conditioning regimens of nonmyeloablative HSCT do not induce mucositis and are associated with neutropenia lasting <7 days. Although usually prescribed, anti-*Candida* prophylaxis may not be necessary in these instances. The same is true for most autologous HSCT recipients in which routine anti-*Candida* prophylaxis may be not indicated. However, even without strong evidence from RCTs, most experts recommend anti-*Candida* prophylaxis for autologous HSCT recipients who have underlying hematologic malignancies who will receive intense conditioning regimens associated with severe mucositis, or with an expected prolonged neutropenia due to graft manipulation.

The evidences for prophylaxis for invasive candidiasis during neutropenia in other settings are not as solid as in allogeneic HSCT. One meta-analysis examined 16 trials including more than 3,700 patients receiving fluconazole or placebo, no treatment or oral polyenes as prophylaxis during neutropenia, and found that outside the setting of HSCT, fluconazole was effective in preventing superficial fungal infections but not systemic fungal infections or fungal-related death. However, in studies with >15% incidence of IFI, fluconazole was effective [41]. Therefore, the ineffectiveness of fluconazole in non-HSCT neutropenic patients is probably related to the heterogeneity of the populations of neutropenic patients studied (with different incidences of invasive candidiasis) rather than an absence of efficacy. In general, the higher is the risk for the patient to develop severe mucositis during neutropenia, the higher is the risk for invasive candidiasis.

Primary Prophylaxis, *Aspergillus*

Prophylaxis for IA is indicated for patients with expected duration of neutropenia >14 days. This typically occurs in induction remission of acute myeloid leukemia (AML) and in allogeneic HSCT transplants with bone marrow or cord blood as the source of stem cells. By contrast, recipients of autologous transplantation and allogeneic HSCT with non-myeloablative conditioning are expected to have neutropenia of shorter duration and are at very low risk to develop IA. An intermediate group of risk is represented by allogeneic HSCT recipients receiving peripheral blood stem cells, patients with acute lymphoid leukemia (ALL) in induction remission and AML patients receiving consolidation treatment. These patients may develop prolonged neutropenia but in the majority of instances neutropenia last <14 days. However, severe T-cell-mediated immunodeficiency may be present and add as an important risk factor for IA in such patients.

In allogeneic HSCT, micafungin given from conditioning until engraftment was associated with a trend suggesting ability to prevent aspergillosis. In this trial, the incidence of IA was 0.2% among 425 patients receiving micafungin and 1.5% among 457 patients receiving fluconazole ($p=0.07$) [40].

The use of itraconazole oral solution in HSCT recipients resulted in a reduction in the frequency of IPA in two RCTs, but about 25% of patients discontinued itraconazole because of gastrointestinal side effects [36, 38]. In patients with AML, a reduction in the incidence of IA was not observed in trials comparing itraconazole with fluconazole, and itraconazole was associated with more adverse events [42, 43]. A recent meta-analysis of itraconazole trials suggest that there is a reduction in *Aspergillus* infections, but only if a certain threshold of bioavailable dosing is used [44]. Its ability to prevent IFI has been associated with trough itraconazole concentrations >500 ng/mL, best achieved with the IV formulation (followed by the oral solution if the gastrointestinal function is intact). The oral capsule formulation suffers from erratic bioavailability and is best avoided.

Posaconazole was tested in patients with AML or myelodysplasia receiving induction therapy, and shown to be as effective as fluconazole, with good tolerability [45]. This study also showed that posaconazole was effective in preventing aspergillosis, with a reduction in fungal-related mortality. A limitation of this study is the fact that in the majority of cases of IA in the fluconazole arm, the diagnosis was based on the results of serum galactomannan. The lower number of cases of IA in the posaconazole arm could be due to the fact that serum galactomannan has a low performance in patients receiving mold-active azoles.

Taken together, the results of these studies using mold-active azoles and their impact in reducing the incidence of IPA are appealing [46]. These findings, however, should be balanced against our significantly improved ability for the early detection of fungal infections and the potential undesirable consequences including toxicities, drug–drug interactions, costs, and emergence of resistance [47]. Finally, it is important to keep in mind the limitations of global prophylaxis defined as prophylaxis to all patients with a certain diagnosis (e.g., all patients undergoing therapy for acute leukemia). Indeed, the risk among these patients is variable. It is highest among patients with relapsed/refractory disease who should probably receive primary yeast and mold prophylaxis; the risk is somewhat lower among patients undergoing remission induction chemotherapy and in whom yeast prophylaxis and a surveillance guided diagnostic-based preemptive strategy is best. The lowest risk for IFI is during consolidation therapy. These patients may not even require systemic prophylaxis.

A randomized trial in patients with prolonged neutropenia showed no benefit for nebulized amphotericin B [48]. More recently, in a double-blind placebo-controlled trial, the frequency of IPA was lower in patients receiving nebulized liposomal amphotericin B (4 vs. 14%, $p=0.005$). However, discontinuation of prophylaxis due to poor compliance was frequent [49].

Secondary Prophylaxis

Because the risk of reactivation of IMIs is high following resumption of immunosuppression, secondary prophylaxis is indicated in such patients [50]. A recent review of secondary antifungal prophylaxis included 197 patients with previous proven or possible IA who received additional cytotoxic chemotherapy or HSCT while receiving secondary prophylaxis with amphotericin B, itraconazole, or flucytosine or combinations of these agents. Documented relapse of IA was only 16% (31 of 197) who received prophylaxis compared to 62% (26 of 42) who did not ($p<0.0001$) [51]. In allogeneic HSCT patients with history of aspergillosis, the risk of reactivation is lower if treatment was given for >30 days and radiographic abnormalities resolved [52]. In another series of HSCT recipients, among 129 patients with prior history of IA, reactivation of infection was more likely to occur in patients with longer duration of neutropenia before transplant, advanced status of the underlying disease, and short period (<6 weeks) between IA and HSCT. The risk of IA early after HSCT (within 30 days) was higher in transplants with myeloablative conditioning regimens, while Cytomegalovirus (CMV) disease, bone marrow or cord blood transplant, and grades II–IV acute GVHD increased the risk of IA occurring 30 days posttransplant [53]. Options for secondary prophylaxis include amphotericin B and its lipid formulations, caspofungin, itraconazole, voriconazole, and lipid amphotericin B followed by voriconazole [51, 54–56]. In addition to secondary chemoprophylaxis, strategies to abbreviate the duration of neutropenia, such as the use of reduced-intensity conditioning regimens and peripheral blood stem cells, and the use of granulocyte transfusions may be employed [57, 58].

Prophylaxis in Nonneutropenic Patients

IFI occur in allogeneic HSCT recipients who develop severe GVHD. Although the number of neutrophils is normal in these patients, there is a paucity of inflammatory cells in lung tissues, indicating that these patients are functionally neutropenic [59].

Whereas invasive candidiasis may occur in this period, HSCT recipients with severe GVHD are at very high risk for invasive mold infections (aspergillosis, fusariosis, zygomycosis, and others). Similar to the early posttransplant period (during neutropenia), fluconazole is the drug of choice for the prevention of invasive candidiasis. In one RCT, fluconazole was given from conditioning until day +75 posttransplant [31]. A post-hoc analysis of this trial has shown that fluconazole was associated with prolonged protection against invasive candidiasis, even beyond the period of prophylaxis [60]. Options form anti-*Candida* prophylaxis in the postengraftment period include itraconazole oral solution (with the limitations of poor gastrointestinal tolerance) [36, 38], posaconazole [61], and voriconazole [39].

For antimold prophylaxis, the two RCT of itraconazole oral solution showed a benefit in reducing the incidence of IA, but again, the ~25% discontinuation for gastrointestinal side effects offsets its benefit [36, 38]. In one RCT, posaconazole was compared with fluconazole in patients with GVHD. There was a trend toward a lower incidence of IFI in patients receiving posaconazole, and a significant reduction in the incidence of IA (2% in patients receiving posaconazole vs. 7% in fluconazole recipients, $p=0.006$) [61]. In another study, voriconazole was compared to fluconazole in a double-blind RCT. Patients received prophylaxis from conditioning until day +100 (or +180 if patients developed GVHD). In addition, serum galactomannan monitoring was performed twice a week in the first 60 days, and once a week thereafter (unless patients developed GVHD). There were no differences in the incidence of IFI, but there was a trend for a lower incidence of IA (5.4% in the voriconazole arm and 7% in the fluconazole arm, $p=0.05$) [39].

As mentioned before, the results of these studies using mold-active azoles indicate that they indeed reduce the incidence of IA. However, the trial comparing fluconazole and voriconazole suggests that active monitoring with biweekly serum galactomannan and chest CT scan is an alternative to the use of a mold-active azole. Therefore, several factors should be taken into consideration in determining if prophylaxis is appropriate at a specific treatment center, for a given patient or patient population to target a specific infection, or if prophylaxis should be withheld and a diagnostic-based preemptive strategy used instead.

Antiviral Prophylaxis

Prophylaxis in Neutropenic Patients

Herpes Simplex Virus (HSV)

Active infection by HSV is common in patients with cancer undergoing antineoplastic therapy [62]. Most HSV infections are due to reactivation of latent virus from an infection much earlier in life; namely, seropositive patients are those chiefly at risk. Thus, HSV serology offers a good way to determine if the patient is at risk. The likelihood of reactivation is influenced by the intensity of cytotoxic treatment. Reactivation occurs in approximately 70% of patients undergoing induction chemotherapy for AML or those receiving intensive conditioning regimens for HSCT. Randomized trials have demonstrated the effectiveness of acyclovir to prevent recurrent infection in AML and HSCT patients [62]. Prophylaxis is generally given until neutrophil recovery. It is important to note that acyclovir does not totally prevent reactivation, but rather delays its occurrence during antiviral administration. Generally, reactivation after neutrophil recovery occurs but its occurrence once host defenses are more robust results in milder disease or is subclinical.

Prophylaxis in Other Settings

Cytomegalovirus (CMV) After HSCT

CMV seropositive patients undergoing allogeneic HSCT are at risk for reactivation, and serious disease typically occurs after engraftment during the second or third month after HSCT. Asymptomatic viremia generally occurs 1–2 weeks before onset of clinical disease, which is most commonly in the form of interstitial pneumonia, or less frequently, enterocolitis. Ganciclovir, acyclovir, and valacyclovir have been shown to be associated with a reduction in the risk for CMV disease in seropositive patients [63–65]. Because of its myelosuppressive effects, ganciclovir is generally begun at time of engraftment in patients at risk. The course of prophylaxis is given during the chief risk period, until day 100–120. An alternative strategy is monitoring patients by testing blood samples weekly with the pp65 antigen assay or CMV quantitative PCR to detect virus activation, and then once viremia is detected, antiviral therapy is initiated with ganciclovir (or foscarnet) "preemptively," to prevent subsequent development of clinical disease.

Seropositive patients undergoing autologous HSCT can also experience reactivation of CMV but CMV disease is infrequent in contrast to allogeneic HSCT; thus, similar prophylaxis and preemptive strategies are not necessary. However, in patients who have T-cell depletion of the stem cell graft, or who have received immunosuppressive therapies such as purine analogs, alemtuzumab, rituximab, or chronic corticosteroids, CMV disease can occur and routine CMV monitoring and preemptive therapy if reactivation is detected are advisable [66, 67].

CMV seronegative patients are also at risk for CMV infection from virus transmitted from the donor stem cell graft or blood products from CMV seropositive donors. A stem cell graft from a seronegative donor (when feasible) and blood products from CMV seronegative donors should be given to negate the risk of CMV transmission.

Varicella-Zoster Virus (VZV)

VZV reactivation in seropositive patients is common after both autologous and allogeneic HSCT [62]. Onset of disease occurs several months after HSCT (median onset 5 months). Acyclovir prophylaxis is effective in prevention of reactivation and should be given for 1 year since shorter duration (6 months) has been associated with rebound overt zoster after discontinuation [68–70]. Valacyclovir can be substituted for acyclovir. Patients with chronic GVHD should continue acyclovir beyond 1 year for at least the duration of active immunosuppressive therapy but perhaps longer until lymphocyte recovery. Bortezomib given for therapy of multiple myeloma has also been associated with reactivation of VZV in approximately 13% of patients [71]. The reason for this is not known, but is perhaps related to its inhibition of production of NFκB, which is necessary for T-cell activation.

Epstein–Barr Virus (EBV)

EBV activation can occur after allogeneic HCT, and patients with profound T-cell immunodeficiency are especially vulnerable to EBV disease, which typically occurs during the first 9 months after HCT. The most common and serious manifestation of EBV is lymphoproliferative disease. The risk is mostly in patients with profound T-cell deficiency, such as seen after T-cell depletion of the stem cell graft, use of anti-T-cell antibodies, cord blood as stem cell source, and after mismatched or haploidentical transplantation. Monitoring EBV load by assaying blood samples for EBV DNA by quantitative PCR can identify patients at greatest risk for lymphoproliferative disease. In patients with high titres of EBV, a reduction of immunosuppression (if possible) can be useful or rituximab can be given preemptively [72].

Other Pathogens

Antipneumocystis

Risk groups in which prophylaxis should be considered against *Pneumocystis jirovecii* include lymphoreticular cancers and myeloablative therapy with HSCT in which treatment regimens result in suppression of T-lymphocyte immunity (e.g., corticosteroids, purine analogs, monoclonal antibodies directed against T cells, and others) [73]. Infection can be prevented by TMP-SMX, which can be given as one double strength tablet (160 mg TMP plus 800 mg SMX) once or twice daily, but 2 or 3 times weekly also is effective [74]. Aerosolized pentamidine given once monthly at a 300-mg dose or dapsone (100 mg/day orally) are alternatives, but they are less effective. A retrospective study in 327 HSCT recipients, failure of prophylaxis was observed in 4 of 44 patients receiving pentamidine, 1 of 31 receiving dapsone, and in none of 105 patients receiving TMP-SMX [75]. In HSCT recipients, prophylaxis is usually started just after engraftment, and continued for 6 months posttransplant, or until discontinuation of immunosuppressive therapy.

Antiparasitic

Toxoplasmosis

Toxoplasmosis in cancer patients occurs as reactivation of primary infection, in the context of severe depression of T-cell-mediated immunity (GVHD, chronic use of corticosteroids, use of purine analogs, alemtuzumab, and others) [76, 77]. In allogeneic HSCT recipients who were seropositive for toxoplasmosis, PCR screening in the serum showed positive tests in 16% of patients [78]. PCR screening has been recommended in recipients of cord blood graft who develop GVHD and are not receiving TMP-SMX. Indeed, although reactivation has been rarely reported in patients receiving TMP-SMX, this is the drug of choice for prophylaxis against toxoplasmosis.

Strongyloidiasis

Strongyloides stercoralis is endemic in a large area in the globe (in general moist temperature areas such as the tropics, sub-tropics, and southeast of Europe and the USA). The great concern about strongyloidiasis is the possibility for the occurrence of hyperinfection and the frequently fatal disseminated syndrome. The later occurs in patients with T-cell immunodeficiency, but it is difficult to select a group of immunosuppressed patients at higher risk since there are reports of its occurrence in patients receiving topical corticosteroids [79]. In addition, considering the high incidence of strongyloidiasis in endemic areas, the disseminated syndrome seems to be quite rare. A retrospective study in 253 patients with hematologic malignancies from a single center in Brazil reported an incidence of 21% of strongyloidiasis, but only one case of disseminated syndrome [80]. In a prospective study from the same institution, 13% of 164 hematologic patients who were screened with three stool examinations had at least one positive exam. No patient developed the disseminated syndrome [81]. Taking these data into consideration, it is difficult to make formal recommendations regarding prophylaxis, especially in endemic areas. In nonendemic areas, it has been suggested that patients with unexplained eosinophilia or who have resided in or traveled to an endemic area should be screened for strongyloidiasis with an enzyme-linked immunosorbent assay (ELISA). In immunocompromised patients living in an endemic region, the ELISA test showed sensitivity, specificity, positive, and negative predictive values of 68, 89, 48, and 95%, respectively [81]. The use of an antiparasitic drug for patients with positive screening test is tempting, but there is no support in the literature. In a randomized study in Brazil, 103 patients with hematologic malignancies and negative stool examinations received thiabendazole (50 mg/kg/day for 2 days) or placebo every month. Five patients had strongyloidiasis, four in the placebo and one in the thiabendazole arm ($p > 0.05$) [82]. The use of ivermectin (200 µg/kg/day for 2 days; repeated after 2 weeks) has been suggested in patients from nonendemic areas and positive screening tests [83].

References

1. Aapro MS, Cameron DA, Pettengell R, Bohlius J, Crawford J, Ellis M, et al. EORTC guidelines for the use of granulocyte-colony stimulating factor to reduce the incidence of chemotherapy-induced febrile neutropenia in adult patients with lymphomas and solid tumours. Eur J Cancer. 2006;42:2433–53.
2. Smith TJ, Khatcheressian J, Lyman GH, Ozer H, Armitage JO, Balducci L, et al. 2006 update of recommendations for the use of white blood cell growth factors: an evidence-based clinical practice guideline. J Clin Oncol. 2006;24:3187–205.
3. Crawford J, Dale DC, Kuderer NM, Culakova E, Poniewierski MS, Wolff D, et al. Risk and timing of neutropenic events in adult cancer patients receiving chemotherapy: the results of a prospective nationwide study of oncology practice. J Natl Compr Canc Netw. 2008;6:109–18.
4. Leibovici L, Paul M, Cullen M, Bucaneve G, Gafter-Gvili A, Fraser A, et al. Antibiotic prophylaxis in neutropenic patients: new evidence, practical decisions. Cancer. 2006;107:1743–51.

5. Imran H, Tleyjeh IM, Arndt CA, Baddour LM, Erwin PJ, Tsigrelis C, et al. Fluoroquinolone prophylaxis in patients with neutropenia: a meta-analysis of randomized placebo-controlled trials. Eur J Clin Microbiol Infect Dis. 2008;27:53–63.
6. Gafter-Gvili A, Fraser A, Paul M, Leibovici L. Meta-analysis: antibiotic prophylaxis reduces mortality in neutropenic patients. Ann Intern Med. 2005;142:979–95.
7. Gafter-Gvili A, Paul M, Fraser A, Leibovici L. Effect of quinolone prophylaxis in afebrile neutropenic patients on microbial resistance: systematic review and meta-analysis. J Antimicrob Chemother. 2007;59:5–22.
8. Engels EA, Lau J, Barza M. Efficacy of quinolone prophylaxis in neutropenic cancer patients: a meta-analysis. J Clin Oncol. 1998;16:1179–87.
9. Bucaneve G, Micozzi A, Menichetti F, Martino P, Dionisi MS, Martinelli G, et al. Levofloxacin to prevent bacterial infection in patients with cancer and neutropenia. N Engl J Med. 2005;353:977–87.
10. Cullen M, Steven N, Billingham L, Gaunt C, Hastings M, Simmonds P, et al. Antibacterial prophylaxis after chemotherapy for solid tumors and lymphomas. N Engl J Med. 2005;353:988–98.
11. Gilbert C, Meisenberg B, Vredenburgh J, Ross M, Hussein A, Perfect J, et al. Sequential prophylactic oral and empiric once-daily parenteral antibiotics for neutropenia and fever after high-dose chemotherapy and autologous bone marrow support. J Clin Oncol. 1994;12:1005–11.
12. Bow EJ, Loewen R, Vaughan D. Reduced requirement for antibiotic therapy targeting gram-negative organisms in febrile, neutropenic patients with cancer who are receiving antibacterial chemoprophylaxis with oral quinolones. Clin Infect Dis. 1995;20:907–12.
13. de MS, van den Broek PJ, Willemze R, van FR. Strategy for antibiotic therapy in febrile neutropenic patients on selective antibiotic decontamination. Eur J Clin Microbiol Infect Dis. 1993;12:897–906.
14. Cometta A, Calandra T, Bille J, Glauser MP. Escherichia coli resistant to fluoroquinolones in patients with cancer and neutropenia. N Engl J Med. 1994;330:1240–1.
15. Kuderer NM, Dale DC, Crawford J, Lyman GH. Impact of primary prophylaxis with granulocyte colony-stimulating factor on febrile neutropenia and mortality in adult cancer patients receiving chemotherapy: a systematic review. J Clin Oncol. 2007;25:3158–67.
16. Timmer-Bonte JN, Adang EM, Smit HJ, Biesma B, Wilschut FA, Bootsma GP, et al. Cost-effectiveness of adding granulocyte colony-stimulating factor to primary prophylaxis with antibiotics in small-cell lung cancer. J Clin Oncol. 2006;24:2991–7.
17. Vogel CL, Wojtukiewicz MZ, Carroll RR, Tjulandin SA, Barajas-fueroa LJ, Wiens BL, et al. First and subsequent cycle use of pegfilgrastim prevents febrile neutropenia in patients with breast cancer: a multicenter, double-blind, placebo-controlled phase III study. J Clin Oncol. 2005;23:1178–84.
18. Crawford J, Althaus B, Armitage J, Balducci L, Bennett C, Blayney DW, et al. Myeloid growth factors. Clinical practice guidelines in oncology. J Natl Compr Canc Netw. 2007;5:188–202.
19. Pagliuca A, Carrington PA, Pettengell R, Tule S, Keidan J. Guidelines on the use of colony-stimulating factors in haematological malignancies. Br J Haematol. 2003;123:22–33.
20. Timmer-Bonte JN, de Boo TM, Smit HJ, Biesma B, Wilschut FA, Cheragwandi SA, et al. Prevention of chemotherapy-induced febrile neutropenia by prophylactic antibiotics plus or minus granulocyte colony-stimulating factor in small-cell lung cancer: a Dutch Randomized Phase III. Study J Clin Oncol. 2005;23:7974–84.
21. von MG, Kummel S, du BA, Eiermann W, Eidtmann H, Gerber B, Hilfrich J, Huober J, Costa SD, Jackisch C, Grasshoff ST, Vescia S, Skacel T, Loibl S, Mehta KM, Kaufmann M. Pegfilgrastim +/- ciprofloxacin for primary prophylaxis with TAC (docetaxel/doxorubicin/cyclophosphamide) chemotherapy for breast cancer. Results from the GEPARTRIO study. Ann Oncol. 2008;19:292–8.
22. Raanani P, Gafter-Gvili A, Paul M, Ben-Bassat I, Leibovici L, Shpilberg O. Immunoglobulin prophylaxis in hematological malignancies and hematopoietic stem cell transplantation. Cochrane Database Syst Rev. 2008;CD006501.
23. Price VE, Blanchette VS, Ford-Jones EL. The prevention and management of infections in children with asplenia or hyposplenia. Infect Dis Clin North Am. 2007;21:697–ix.
24. Engelhard D, Cordonnier C, Shaw PJ, Parkalli T, Guenther C, Martino R, et al. Early and late invasive pneumococcal infection following stem cell transplantation: a European Bone Marrow Transplantation survey. Br J Haematol. 2002;117:444–50.
25. Saral R. Candida and Aspergillus infections in immunocompromised patients: an overview. Rev Infect Dis. 1991;13:487–92.
26. Kontoyiannis DP, Torres HA, Chagua M, Hachem R, Tarrand JJ, Bodey GP, et al. Trichosporonosis in a tertiary care cancer center: risk factors, changing spectrum and determinants of outcome. Scand J Infect Dis. 2004;36:564–9.
27. Nucci M, Marr KA, Queiroz-Telles F, Martins CA, Trabasso P, Costa S, et al. Fusarium infection in hematopoietic stem cell transplant recipients. Clin Infect Dis. 2004;38:1237–42.
28. Gerson SL, Talbot GH, Hurwitz S, Strom BL, Lusk EJ, Cassileth PA. Prolonged granulocytopenia: the major risk factor for invasive pulmonary aspergillosis in patients with acute leukemia. Ann Intern Med. 1984;100:345–51.
29. Chayakulkeeree M, Ghannoum MA, Perfect JR. Zygomycosis: the re-emerging fungal infection. Eur J Clin Microbiol Infect Dis. 2006;25:215–9.
30. Goodman JL, Winston DJ, Greenfield RA, Chandrasekar PH, Fox B, Kaizer H, et al. A controlled trial of fluconazole to prevent fungal infections in patients undergoing bone marrow transplantation. N Engl J Med. 1992;326:845–51.
31. Slavin MA, Osborne B, Adams R, Levenstein MJ, Schoch HG, Feldman AR, et al. Efficacy and safety of fluconazole prophylaxis for fungal infections after marrow transplantation – a prospective, randomized, double-blind study. J Infect Dis. 1995;171:1545–52.
32. MacMillan ML, Goodman JL, DeFor TE, Weisdorf DJ. Fluconazole to prevent yeast infections in bone marrow transplantation patients: a randomized trial of high versus reduced dose, and determination of the value of maintenance therapy. Am J Med. 2002;112:369–79.
33. Marr KA, Seidel K, White TC, Bowden RA. Candidemia in allogeneic blood and marrow transplant recipients: evolution of risk factors after the adoption of prophylactic fluconazole. J Infect Dis. 2000;181:309–16.
34. Wingard JR, Merz WG, Rinaldi MG, Johnson TR, Karp JE, Saral R. Increase in Candida krusei infection among patients with bone marrow transplantation and neutropenia treated prophylactically with fluconazole. N Engl J Med. 1991;325:1274–7.
35. Upton A, McCune JS, Kirby KA, Leisenring W, McDonald G, Batchelder A, et al. Fluconazole coadministration concurrent with cyclophosphamide conditioning may reduce regimen-related toxicity postmyeloablative hematopoietic cell transplantation. Biol Blood Marrow Transplant. 2007;13:760–4.
36. Marr KA, Crippa F, Leisenring W, Hoyle M, Boeckh M, Balajee SA, et al. Itraconazole versus fluconazole for prevention of fungal infections in patients receiving allogeneic stem cell transplants. Blood. 2004;103:1527–33.
37. Oren I, Rowe JM, Sprecher H, Tamir A, Benyamini N, Akria L, et al. A prospective randomized trial of itraconazole vs fluconazole for the prevention of fungal infections in patients with acute leukemia and hematopoietic stem cell transplant recipients. Bone Marrow Transplant. 2006;38:127–34.
38. Winston DJ, Maziarz RT, Chandrasekar PH, Lazarus HM, Goldman M, Blumer JL, et al. Intravenous and oral itraconazole versus intravenous and oral fluconazole for long-term antifungal prophylaxis in allogeneic hematopoietic stem-cell transplant recipients. A multicenter, randomized trial. Ann Intern Med. 2003;138:705–13.

39. Wingard JR, Carter SL, Walsh TJ, Kurtzberg J, Small TN, Gersten ID, et al. Results of a randomized, double-blind trial of fluconazole (FLU) vs. voriconazole (VORI) for the prevention of invasive fungal infections (IFI) in 600 allogeneic blood and marrow transplant (BMT) patients. Blood. 2007;110:163.
40. van Burik JA, Ratanatharathorn V, Stepan DE, Miller CB, Lipton JH, Vesole DH, et al. Micafungin versus fluconazole for prophylaxis against invasive fungal infections during neutropenia in patients undergoing hematopoietic stem cell transplantation. Clin Infect Dis. 2004;39:1407–16.
41. Kanda Y, Yamamoto R, Chizuka A, Hamaki T, Suguro M, Arai C, et al. Prophylactic action of oral fluconazole against fungal infection in neutropenic patients. A meta-analysis of 16 randomized, controlled trials. Cancer. 2000;89:1611–25.
42. Glasmacher A, Cornely O, Ullmann AJ, Wedding U, Bodenstein H, Wandt H, et al. An open-label randomized trial comparing itraconazole oral solution with fluconazole oral solution for primary prophylaxis of fungal infections in patients with haematological malignancy and profound neutropenia. J Antimicrob Chemother. 2006;57:317–25.
43. Vardakas KZ, Michalopoulos A, Falagas ME. Fluconazole versus itraconazole for antifungal prophylaxis in neutropenic patients with haematological malignancies: a meta-analysis of randomised-controlled trials. Br J Haematol. 2005;131:22–8.
44. Glasmacher A, Prentice A, Gorschluter M, Engelhart S, Hahn C, Djulbegovic B, et al. Itraconazole prevents invasive fungal infections in neutropenic patients treated for hematologic malignancies: evidence from a meta-analysis of 3,597 patients. J Clin Oncol. 2003;21:4615–26.
45. Cornely OA, Maertens J, Winston DJ, Perfect J, Ullmann AJ, Walsh TJ, et al. Posaconazole vs. fluconazole or itraconazole prophylaxis in patients with neutropenia. N Engl J Med. 2007;356:348–59.
46. Segal BH, Almyroudis NG, Battiwalla M, Herbrecht R, Perfect JR, Walsh TJ, et al. Prevention and early treatment of invasive fungal infection in patients with cancer and neutropenia and in stem cell transplant recipients in the era of newer broad-spectrum antifungal agents and diagnostic adjuncts. Clin Infect Dis. 2007;44:402–9.
47. Lewis RE, Prince RA, Chi J, Kontoyiannis DP. Itraconazole preexposure attenuates the efficacy of subsequent amphotericin B therapy in a murine model of acute invasive pulmonary aspergillosis. Antimicrob Agents Chemother. 2002;46:3208–14.
48. Schwartz S, Behre G, Heinemann V, Wandt H, Schilling E, Arning M, et al. Aerosolized amphotericin B inhalations as prophylaxis of invasive aspergillus infections during prolonged neutropenia: results of a prospective randomized multicenter trial. Blood. 1999;93:3654–61.
49. Rijnders BJ, Cornelissen JJ, Slobbe L, Becker MJ, Doorduijn JK, Hop WC, Ruijgrok EJ, Lowenberg B, Vulto A, Lugtenburg PJ, de MS. Aerosolized liposomal amphotericin B for the prevention of invasive pulmonary aspergillosis during prolonged neutropenia: a randomized, placebo-controlled trial. Clin Infect Dis. 2008;46:1401–18.
50. Offner F, Cordonnier C, Ljungman P, Prentice HG, Engelhard D, De BD, Meunier F, de PB. Impact of previous aspergillosis on the outcome of bone marrow transplantation. Clin Infect Dis. 1998;26:1098–03.
51. Sipsas NV, Kontoyiannis DP. Clinical issues regarding relapsing aspergillosis and the efficacy of secondary antifungal prophylaxis in patients with hematological malignancies. Clin Infect Dis. 2006;42:1584–91.
52. Fukuda T, Boeckh M, Guthrie KA, Mattson DK, Owens S, Wald A, et al. Invasive aspergillosis before allogeneic hematopoietic stem cell transplantation: 10-year experience at a single transplant center. Biol Blood Marrow Transplant. 2004;10:494–503.
53. Martino R, Parody R, Fukuda T, Maertens J, Theunissen K, Ho A, et al. Impact of the intensity of the pretransplantation conditioning regimen in patients with prior invasive aspergillosis undergoing allogeneic hematopoietic stem cell transplantation: a retrospective survey of the Infectious Diseases Working Party of the European Group for Blood and Marrow Transplantation. Blood. 2006;108:2928–36.
54. Allinson K, Kolve H, Gumbinger HG, Vormoor HJ, Ehlert K, Groll AH. Secondary antifungal prophylaxis in paediatric allogeneic haematopoietic stem cell recipients. J Antimicrob Chemother. 2008;61:734–42.
55. Cordonnier C, Maury S, Pautas C, Bastie JN, Chehata S, Castaigne S, et al. Secondary antifungal prophylaxis with voriconazole to adhere to scheduled treatment in leukemic patients and stem cell transplant recipients. Bone Marrow Transplant. 2004;33:943–8.
56. de FP, Spagnoli A, Di BP, Locasciulli A, Cudillo L, Milone G, Busca A, Picardi A, Scime R, Bonini A, Cupelli L, Chiusolo P, Olivieri A, Santarone S, Poidomani M, Fallani S, Novelli A, Majolino I. Efficacy of caspofungin as secondary prophylaxis in patients undergoing allogeneic stem cell transplantation with prior pulmonary and/or systemic fungal infection. Bone Marrow Transplant. 2007;40:245–9.
57. Grigull L, Schrauder A, Schmitt-Thomssen A, Sykora K, Welte K. Efficacy and safety of G-CSF mobilized granulocyte transfusions in four neutropenic children with sepsis and invasive fungal infection. Infection. 2002;30:267–71.
58. Dignani MC, Anaissie EJ, Hester JP, O'brien S, Vartivarian SE, Rex JH, et al. Treatment of neutropenia-related fungal infections with granulocyte colony-stimulating factor-elicited white blood cell transfusions: a pilot study. Leukemia. 1997;11:1621–30.
59. Stergiopoulou T, Meletiadis J, Roilides E, Kleiner DE, Schaufele R, Roden M, et al. Host-dependent patterns of tissue injury in invasive pulmonary aspergillosis. Am J Clin Pathol. 2007;127:349–55.
60. Marr KA, Seidel K, Slavin MA, Bowden RA, Schoch HG, Flowers ME, et al. Prolonged fluconazole prophylaxis is associated with persistent protection against candidiasis-related death in allogeneic marrow transplant recipients: long-term follow-up of a randomized, placebo-controlled trial. Blood. 2000;96:2055–61.
61. Ullmann AJ, Lipton JH, Vesole DH, Chandrasekar P, Langston A, Tarantolo SR, et al. Posaconazole or fluconazole for prophylaxis in severe graft-versus-host disease. N Engl J Med. 2007;356:335–47.
62. Wingard JR, Leather HL. Viral infections among patients with hematological malignancies. In: Wiernik PH, Goldman JM, Dutcher JP, et al., editors. Neoplastic diseases of the blood. 4th ed. Cambridge: Cambridge University Press; 2003. p. 968–1005.
63. Goodrich JM, Bowden RA, Fisher L, Keller C, Schoch G, Meyers JD. Ganciclovir prophylaxis to prevent cytomegalovirus disease after allogeneic marrow transplant. Ann Intern Med. 1993;118:173–8.
64. Ljungman P, de La CR, Milpied N, Volin L, Russell CA, Crisp A, et al. Randomized study of valacyclovir as prophylaxis against cytomegalovirus reactivation in recipients of allogeneic bone marrow transplants. Blood. 2002;99:3050–6.
65. Prentice HG, Gluckman E, Powles RL, Ljungman P, Milpied N, Fernandez Ranada JM, et al. Impact of long-term acyclovir on cytomegalovirus infection and survival after allogeneic bone marrow transplantation. European Acyclovir for CMV Prophylaxis Study Group. Lancet. 1994;343:749–53.
66. Lee MY, Chiou TJ, Hsiao LT, Yang MH, Lin PC, Poh SB, et al. Rituximab therapy increased post-transplant cytomegalovirus complications in Non-Hodgkin's lymphoma patients receiving autologous hematopoietic stem cell transplantation. Ann Hematol. 2008;87:285–9.
67. Lin PC, Lee MY, Lin JT, Hsiao LT, Chen PM, Chiou TJ. Virus reactivation in high-risk non-Hodgkin's lymphoma patients after autologous CD34+ -selected peripheral blood progenitor cell transplantation. Int J Hematol. 2008;87:434–9.
68. Thomson KJ, Hart DP, Banerjee L, Ward KN, Peggs KS, Mackinnon S. The effect of low-dose aciclovir on reactivation of varicella zoster

virus after allogeneic haemopoietic stem cell transplantation. Bone Marrow Transplant. 2005;35:1065–9.
69. Boeckh M, Kim HW, Flowers ME, Meyers JD, Bowden RA. Long-term acyclovir for prevention of varicella zoster virus disease after allogeneic hematopoietic cell transplantation – a randomized double-blind placebo-controlled study. Blood. 2006;107:1800–5.
70. Erard V, Guthrie KA, Varley C, Heugel J, Wald A, Flowers ME, et al. One-year acyclovir prophylaxis for preventing varicella-zoster virus disease after hematopoietic cell transplantation: no evidence of rebound varicella-zoster virus disease after drug discontinuation. Blood. 2007;110:3071–7.
71. Chanan-Khan A, Sonneveld P, Schuster MW, Stadtmauer EA, Facon T, Harousseau JL, et al. Analysis of herpes zoster events among bortezomib-treated patients in the phase III APEX study. J Clin Oncol. 2008;26:4784–90.
72. Meerbach A, Wutzler P, Hafer R, Zintl F, Gruhn B. Monitoring of Epstein–Barr virus load after hematopoietic stem cell transplantation for early intervention in post-transplant lymphoproliferative disease. J Med Virol. 2008;80:441–54.
73. Green H, Paul M, Vidal L, Leibovici L. Prophylaxis of Pneumocystis pneumonia in immunocompromised non-HIV-infected patients: systematic review and meta-analysis of randomized controlled trials. Mayo Clin Proc. 2007;82:1052–9.
74. Ohata Y, Ohta H, Hashii Y, Tokimasa S, Ozono K, Hara J. Intermittent oral trimethoprim/sulfamethoxazole on two non-consecutive days per week is effective as Pneumocystis jiroveci pneumonia prophylaxis in pediatric patients receiving chemotherapy or hematopoietic stem cell transplantation. Pediatr Blood Cancer. 2009;52:142–4.
75. Vasconcelles MJ, Bernardo MV, King C, Weller EA, Antin JH. Aerosolized pentamidine as pneumocystis prophylaxis after bone marrow transplantation is inferior to other regimens and is associated with decreased survival and an increased risk of other infections. Biol Blood Marrow Transplant. 2000;6:35–43.
76. Martin SI, Marty FM, Fiumara K, Treon SP, Gribben JG, Baden LR. Infectious complications associated with alemtuzumab use for lymphoproliferative disorders. Clin Infect Dis. 2006;43:16–24.
77. Pagano L, Trape G, Putzulu R, Caramatti C, Picardi M, Nosari A, et al. Toxoplasma gondii infection in patients with hematological malignancies. Ann Hematol. 2004;83:592–5.
78. Martino R, Bretagne S, Einsele H, Maertens J, Ullmann AJ, Parody R, et al. Early detection of Toxoplasma infection by molecular monitoring of Toxoplasma gondii in peripheral blood samples after allogeneic stem cell transplantation. Clin Infect Dis. 2005;40:67–78.
79. Genta RM. Dysregulation of strongyloidiasis: a new hypothesis. Clin Microbiol Rev. 1992;5:345–55.
80. Nucci M, Portugal R, Pulcheri W, Spector N, Ferreira SB, de Castro MB, et al. Strongyloidiasis in patients with hematologic malignancies. Clin Infect Dis. 1995;21:675–7.
81. Schaffel R, Nucci M, Carvalho E, Braga M, Almeida L, Portugal R, et al. The value of an immunoenzymatic test (enzyme-linked immunosorbent assay) for the diagnosis of strongyloidiasis in patients immunosuppressed by hematologic malignancies. Am J Trop Med Hyg. 2001;65:346–50.
82. Portugal R, Schaffel R, Almeida L, Spector N, Nucci M. Thiabendazole for the prophylaxis of strongyloidiasis in immunosuppressed patients with hematological diseases: a randomized double-blind placebo-controlled study. Haematologica. 2002;87:663–4.
83. Keiser PB, Nutman TB. Strongyloides stercoralis in the immunocompromised population. Clin Microbiol Rev. 2004;17:208–17.
84. Lyman GH, Kuderer NM, Djulbegovic B. Prophylactic granulocyte colony-stimulating factor in patients receiving dose-intensive cancer chemotherapy: a meta-analysis. Am J Med. 2002;112:406–11.

Chapter 47
Controversies in Antimicrobial Prophylaxis

Ben de Pauw and Marta Stanzani

Abstract The risk of life-threatening infection in association with chemotherapy-induced neutropenia coincided miraculously with the development of a second generation of antimicrobial agents. Even after having randomized more than 10,000 patients in clinical trials on prophylaxis during neutropenia, there is still no convincing scientific evidence to support the apparently attractive strategy. Even trials that at first glance appear to provide a positive answer do not survive a meticulous dissection. Two major factors are accountable for this unfortunate situation: a lack of trials with an adequate number of patients and a shortage of reliable diagnostic tools to establish infections in neutropenic patients. Meta-analysis has become a fashionable approach to meet the problem of low numbers to a certain extent, but the outcome has to be interpreted with caution. Trials that do not include statistically significant findings tend to be rejected by peer-reviewed journals, which may lead to an overestimation of the prophylactic effect. A comprehensive discussion of controversies related to antimicrobial prophylaxis is provided in this chapter.

Keywords Prophylaxis • Neutropenia • Fungal infection • Antifungals

Introduction

Gerald Bodey's description of the risk of life-threatening infection in association with chemotherapy-induced neutropenia coincided miraculously with the development of a second generation of antimicrobial agents [1]. The oldtimers, sulphonamides, penicillin, and gentamicin were replaced by more potent and less toxic compounds that, with due restrictions, even could be administered orally. Without delay, these new antibiotics were introduced into the standard management of patients treated for malignant disease who had acquired an infection. Unfortunately, the overall impact of the new drugs was rather disappointing because, before therapy was started, infections were often already in a stage beyond cure. Late recognition of serious infections was related to the absence of typical signs and symptoms of infection in neutropenic patients in conjunction with a lack of sensitive diagnostic tools. A typical standard diagnostic program consisted of chest X-ray and culturing of blood and material from any clinically suspicious lesion. Against this background, earlier initiation of antibiotic therapy seemed an attractive option to prevent rapidly fatal infections. When it became clear that approximately 80% of the bacterial pathogens responsible for infection during neutropenia originated from patients' own endogenous flora, half of them acquired during hospitalization, the idea of prophylaxis, i.e., warding off an overwhelming event, was born and numerous prophylactic regimens of increasing complexity were designed [2]. The ultimate schemes included a protected environment program with high-efficiency particulate air (HEPA) filtration, strict patient isolation, special water-purification systems, special handling of patients washes, and food restrictions to prevent acquisition of exogenous organisms in combination with so-called "intestinal decontamination." This strategy implied administration of nonadsorbable antibiotics aiming at complete suppression of the endogenous intestinal bacterial flora and at prevention of acquiring exogenous organisms. The most common antibiotics for that purpose were gentamicin, vancomycin, framycetin, colistin, neomycin/polymyxin. A limited patient's compliance was the major obstacle to success of such programs. Moreover, the protective effect remained at least questionable. Elimination of the complete microbial flora of the digestive system obviously created space for colonization of the gut by aggressive micro-organisms during the hospitalization, whenever the carefully constructed protective barrier was broken. As a result, the majority of infections that occurred in chemotherapy-induced neutropenic patients were caused by these difficult-to-treat nosocomial pathogens. Subsequently, "selective decontamination," eradication of Gram-negative aerobic organisms

M. Stanzani (✉)
Institute of Haematology and Clinical Oncology "Lorenzo e Ariosto Seràgnoli", Sant'Orsola-Malpighi Hospital, University of Bologna, Via Massarenti, 9, 40138 Bologna, Italy
e-mail: marta.stanzani2@unibo.it

from the digestive tract while leaving the commensal nonpathogenic anaerobic flora untouched, became popular. This concept, based on several studies in immunocompromised mice, offered promise in a few small randomized trials in patients who were treated for cancer, but a statistically convincing trial was never conducted [3]. Shortly after its introduction in clinical practice, clinicians started to use trimethoprim/sulfamethoxazole, usually given together with oral polymyxin and nystatin or amphotericin B, for prophylactic purposes. In fact this approach combined selective decontamination of the gut with systemic antibiotic cover, since trimethoprim/sulfamethoxazole is well absorbed and does achieve therapeutic blood levels. In many centers trimethoprim/sulfamethoxazole containing regimens, which also protected the patients against pneumocystosis, became the regimens of choice until the arrival of the fluoroquinolones. The spectrum of activity of these antibiotics that were well tolerated generated a myriad of industry-sponsored large clinical trials on their use in a prophylactic setting. When the dust of these trials settled, fluoroquinolone-based schedules appeared as the new standard for antibacterial prophylaxis. Antifungal prophylaxis evolved more or less along the same route. Mouth rinsing with and/or swallowing of either amphotericin B or nystatin were poorly tolerated by patients who experienced a remarkable similarity between these drugs and sticky sand. The first azoles, miconazole and ketoconazole, were hardly better appreciated and their use was often accompanied by allergic reactions. The availability of fluconazole and itraconazole seemed to change the scene but, alike the situation with fluoroquinolones for antibacterial prophylaxis, the cumulative data from all clinical trials were not sufficiently convincing to gain antimicrobial prophylaxis an unequivocal positive recommendation in the current guidelines from the Infectious Diseases Society of America [4]. To see what went wrong in the assessment of the feasibility of antimicrobial prophylaxis that remains intuitively attractive to a large majority of clinicians we need to scrutinize the pivotal data.

Clinical Trials on Antibacterial Prophylaxis

Soon after their introduction in the 1980s, the fluoroquinolones became the most fashionable antibiotics in the prophylaxis of bacterial infections in neutropenic patients. There were many reasons for this popularity. Fluoroquinolones show clinical activity against most Gram-negative and many Gram-positive micro-organisms, as well as against atypical mycobacteria. After oral administration of the fluoroquinolones, high levels are achieved in the gastrointestinal tract, which results in an almost complete suppression of the Gram-negative enterobacteria without interfering with the endogenous anaerobic flora. This class of drugs has an excellent bioavailability, an excellent tolerance, a limited number of side effects and interactions, and does not cause myelosuppression. In 8 out of 9 placebo-controlled clinical trials that were conducted between 1983 and 1993 and included almost 1,000 patients, ciprofloxacin and norfloxacin were found safer and appeared to be more effective in reducing the incidence of Gram-negative bacteremia than their comparators, principally trimethoprim/sulfamethoxazole. Conversely, no differences in overall mortality and episodes of fever were found. Streptococci became the most frequently isolated pathogens, and extensive use of the quinolones did raise the concern of the development of resistances against enterobacteriaceae, especially *Escherichia coli*. The introduction of levofloxacin, a fluoroquinolone with improved Gram-positive coverage, fostered two new large clinical studies in more than 2,300 patients who were treated for a hematological malignancy. The results of these two large, multi-center, randomized, double-blind, placebo-controlled trials were published in prominent medical journals [5, 6]. Cullen et al. addressed the potential of orally administered levofloxacin, given once daily at a dose of 500 mg for 7 days, to cover low-risk patients against infection during neutropenia ($<0.5 \times 10^9$/L) induced by standard chemotherapy for solid tumors or malignant lymphoma. In this placebo-controlled study, which included 1,565 patients, levofloxacin reduced the incidence of clinically documented infections during the first cycle of chemotherapy from 8 to 3.5% ($p<0.001$), while, considering the whole course of chemotherapy, the rate of febrile episodes was reduced from 15 to 11% ($p=0.01$). No difference was found with regard to infection-related mortality and overall mortality or in the development of antibacterial resistance [5]. The second trial by Bucaneve and his group comprised 760 patients with hematological malignancies who underwent aggressive antineoplastic therapy with an anticipated profound and protracted neutropenia ($<1.0 \times 10^9$/L for more than 7 days). The occurrence of fever was 85% in the placebo group to 65% in the levofloxacin group ($p=0.001$). In fact, the data generated by this trial was quite similar to those from previous trials on quinolone prophylaxis with a statistically significant decrease in the rate of microbiologically documented infections from 39 to 22% with a reduction in the number of bacteremias sustained by Gram-negative bacteria ($p<0.001$). However, once more, no difference was observed in infection-related mortality and overall mortality [6]. In the same year, Gafter-Gvili et al. performed a meta-analysis on 14 randomized, controlled trials of antibiotic prophylaxis that included more than 1,200 neutropenic patients and that compared quinolones to either a placebo or no treatment. The study populations consisted mainly of patients who were treated for an acute leukemia or who received an autologous bone marrow transplantation. It was concluded that prophylactic administration of a quinolone would result in a reduction of the rate of febrile neutropenia and documented bacterial infections, and lower mortality. Moreover, there seemed to be no increase in the number of fluoroquinolone-resistant bacteria. Unfortunately, the quality of some of the trials that were included in this analysis was not sufficient to allow a firm conclusion [7]. The biggest and most recent meta-analysis on 101 clinical trials, which comprised around 12,600 neutropenic patients, the majority suffering from hematological malignancies, performed by the same group demonstrated that prophylaxis significantly reduces the overall mortality when compared to placebo or no intervention [8].

Clinical Trials on Antifungal Prophylaxis

More than 25 years ago, the rationale for chemoprophylaxis of fungal infections appeared already persuasive enough to initiate clinical trials on this subject. The poor tolerance and limited efficacy of orally administered polyenes have abandoned this approach. The trend-setting paper by Goodman et al. on fluconazole given as prophylaxis in bone marrow transplant recipients showed a reduced rate of proven invasive candidal infections [9]. In a reaction to this publication fluconazole was widely introduced as a safe drug for prophylactical purposes, and the choice for this strategy appeared to be endorsed by the improved overall survival registered in a similar trial conducted by the Seattle bone marrow transplant team [10]. Van Burik et al. reviewed 355 autopsies performed in Seattle between 1990 and 1994. Among transplanted individuals who had been protected by fluconazole prophylaxis, Candida infections amounted to 8% as compared with 27% in those without [11]. However, a follow-up of the Slavin study learned that the superior survival registered in the fluconazole arm was maintained, but this advantage could not be attributed to a decreased fungal infection-related death rate only [12]. Disappointingly, even 38 comparative trials were not enough to establish a positive impact of fluconazole on candidiasis-related mortality in patient populations other than bone marrow transplant recipients unequivocally. The way out of this labyrinth of statistically underpowered trials was meta-analysis; it showed a convincing beneficial effect of prophylactic fluconazole among certain subgroups such as patients who are colonized by Candida species and received highly dosed remission-induction therapy for acute myelogenous leukemia [13, 14]. This observation makes sense as disseminated candidiasis is supposed to be preceded by colonization of the gastrointestinal tract in combination with immunosuppression and damage of the mucosal lining by cytotoxic therapy [15]. Orally administered fluconazole both reduces the Candida burden in the gut and eliminates the organisms if they gain access to the bloodstream. This explanation helped to grant the label of evidence-based medicine to what already had become common practice.

In the endeavor to prevent infections by Aspergillus species and other molds, the focus was directed at itraconazole as soon as it became available for clinical use. For many reasons, the results were not as good as was hoped for. First of all, the drug was poorly tolerated and had an erratic bioavailability, although this was improved by the introduction of an oral suspension. After a few negative clinical trials, a British and American group of investigators found itraconazole to protect neutropenic patients better against invasive aspergillosis than did fluconazole in the comparative arms [16–19]. Unfortunately, the difference in infections due to Aspergillus species in British trial was related to an outbreak at one institution. The population of the American study consisted of allogeneic bone marrow transplant recipients. Three of 71 patients given itraconazole (4%) and 8 of 67 patients given fluconazole (12%) acquired aspergillosis; this difference was not statistically significant, and prophylaxis with itraconazole did not result in an improved survival. A similar trial by the Seattle corroborated these findings and indicated that itraconazole might interfere with the metabolism of cytostatic drugs like cyclophosphamide [20]. Posaconazole has in vitro activity against a wide range of molds including Aspergillus species and it also appeared well tolerated and safe. This new azole featured as the main comparator in two randomized prophylactic trials. In the first study among patients undergoing chemotherapy for hematological malignancies, the incidence of invasive aspergillosis was 1% after posaconazole compared with 7% after alternative prophylaxis without there being a difference in survival. The second study was done among stem cell transplant recipients on immunosuppressive therapy for graft-versus-host disease. In the posaconazole arm, 2% of cases showed evidence of proven or probable invasive aspergillosis as compared to 7% in the fluconazole arm. In addition, there were fewer deaths among those receiving posaconazole that was well tolerated. It needs to emphasize that most of the probable aspergillosis cases were based on a positive galactomannan antigen test, whereas it is a fact that mold-active antifungal drugs lower concentrations of this antigen. Remarkably, these studies were performed without posaconazole having first won its spurs as primary therapy of invasive aspergillosis. A prophylactic trial in bone marrow transplant recipients that compared voriconazole with fluconazole learned that invasive aspergillosis occurred in 5% of the fluconazole-treated patients and in 2% of the voriconazole group, a result similar to that obtained with posaconazole in a different setting [21].

As the airways serve as main portal of entry for Aspergillus spores, there was a rationale to explore the role of inhalation of antifungals. Aerosolized particles of Amphotericin B of a size to similar Aspergillus conidia are supposed to travel the same route, which was supposed to prevent colonization of the airways by molds. The hypothesis is appealing, but the results obtained in the only prospective randomized study were disappointing; the aerosol of amphotericin B offered no advantage with respect to the number of documented infections or overall survival. Moreover, intolerance forced about one third of patients to discontinue inhalations prematurely. Tolerance appeared better with aerosolized liposomal amphotericin B, which resulted in a lower rate of proven aspergillosis without a survival benefit in comparison with a placebo [22].

The use of intravenous amphotericin B for prophylactic purposes has been limited, presumably due to its inherent toxicity. This scene changed with the introduction of the lipid preparations, but so far none of these drugs have been evaluated in landmark trials on antifungal prophylaxis. As a rule, the trials were small and none the amphotericin B formulations did produce results, such as a reduction in the number of cases with invasive aspergillosis or a lower mortality rate that would urge a modification of standard treatment schedules. The use of low doses of polyenes may be a major reason for the disappointing outcome. Enthusiasm for this strategy was generated by the observation that low-dose amphotericin B prophylaxis, alone or in combination with nasal amphotericin B, seemed to decrease the incidence of aspergillosis in bone marrow transplant recipients as compared with historical controls. However, none of the prospective, randomized trials could confirm these hope giving findings [23, 24]. The interest in low doses of intravenous amphotericin B, such as 0.10 mg/kg daily or 0.5 mg/kg three times a week, or liposomal amphotericin B, 3 mg/kg 3 days a week, is astonishing. Where the lack of success of itraconazole is commonly attributed to poor tolerance and difficulty in achieving satisfactory serum and tissue levels, found investigators motivation to test a homoiopathic dose of amphotericin B. If lower toxicity constitutes a valuable argument to use a suboptimal dose of amphotericin B, completely refraining from this type of prophylaxis to avoid all toxicity would be the next logical step.

Caspofungin and micafungin, the latest arrivals to the antifungal armamentarium, were shown to be as effective as their azole comparators, itraconazole and fluconazole, respectively [25, 26]. The studies showed indeed that candins are effective in this setting, but the need for these compounds for prophylactic purposes is rather limited given the availability of equally efficacious, cheaper oral antifungal drugs. Moreover, the large micafungin study in bone transplant recipients did not cover the fungal-prone episode of graft-versus-host disease, which precludes a genuine assessment.

Considerations

Even after having randomized more than 10,000 patients in clinical trials on prophylaxis during neutropenia, there is still no convincing scientific evidence to support the apparently attractive strategy [27]. The discussion sections of the papers written on these trials accentuate the investigators' disappointment by way of detailed explanations for the failure to show a benefit of the intervention. Even trials that at first glance appear to provide a positive answer do not survive a meticulous dissection. One single study showing that a particular regimen was superior to another would end the controversy on the value of prophylaxis. As this is not the case, the question raises whether all regimens are equally good or equally bad. Two major factors are accountable for this unfortunate situation: a lack of trials with an adequate number of patients and a shortage of reliable diagnostic tools to establish infections in neutropenic patients. A small sample size, typically around a 100 patients per arm where more than 1,000 are required, will result in an insignificant finding due to a type II error. Besides, recruiting large numbers of unselected patients will hardly improve the situation, because it implies inclusion of many low-risk cases, which only will make the analysis more difficult. Meta-analysis has become a fashionable approach to meet the problem of low numbers to a certain extent, but the outcome has to be interpreted with caution. Trials that do not include statistically significant findings tend to be rejected by peer-reviewed journals, which may lead to an overestimation of the prophylactic effect. Moreover, meta-analysis do not account for flaws in the original trial designs, such as cover of the wrong risk episode and selective exclusion of a category of patients. Lack of reliable diagnostic tools is responsible for the fact that there is no generally accepted endpoint for clinical studies on prophylaxis. Success is usually defined as a survival of the neutropenic episode without infections that require broad-spectrum antimicrobial therapy and no need for interruption of the prophylactic drugs. Hence, parameters of outcome like fever, culture results, antigen levels, CT abnormalities, overall survival, infection-related death, infection, administration of broad-spectrum antimicrobials or antifungal agents, and side effects feature prominently in reports on clinical trials. However, each of these parameters has serious shortcomings. At first glance, overall mortality may appear a sensitive, unbiased measure of the effect of prophylaxis, but other independent factors such as the type of cytotoxic therapy, patient age, or status of the underlying disease do have their impact on the risk of death. Infection-related death is difficult to establish, particularly when no autopsies are performed. Indeed, in spite of systematic diagnostic workup with cultures, antigen testing and CT scans, more than half of the fatal invasive aspergillosis and candidiasis cases remain undetected [28]. Finally, broad-spectrum antibiotics and antifungals are usually instituted on suspicion of infection, a subjective parameter but cherished by clinicians who are minimally interested in colonization rates.

Drawing up the sheet on antimicrobial prophylaxis must include an assessment of the likely negative effects, i.e., toleration, toxicity, costs, and development of resistance to the involved antimicrobial drugs. Antibiotics appear to be more safe than antifungal drugs, which are, depending on the class, nephrotoxic or hepatotoxic and display numerous interactions with possible comedication due to their P-450-dependent metabolism in the liver. Development of resistance is an issue with the extensive use of fluoroquinolones and other bacterials but less so with antifungals. Widespread introduction of fluconazole as anti-*Candida* prophylaxis in neutropenic patients was associated with the appearance of *Candida* species other than *Candida albicans* and an increased *Aspergillus*-related mortality from 18 to 29% in the autopsy study by Van Burik et al. These changes are rather due to selection as a result of elimination of susceptible strains and, presumably, a prolonged survival that may dispose toward acquisition of other fungal infections [11, 29]. The same mechanism may play a role in the emergence of Zygomycetes during or after the use of voriconazole. Likewise, even a huge meta-analysis on the effect of quinolone prophylaxis does not allow definite conclusions on the rate of occurrence of bacterial resistance in neutropenic patients [30]. Several observational studies examined the impact of suspending the use of antibacterial prophylaxis when a high incidence of resistance to fluoroquinolones was documented, but the results of this strategy were not consistent and, therefore, the validity of this approach remains questionable [31–34].

It is clear that prophylaxis does not make the clinician's life easier because the strategy is not foolproof and has some serious pitfalls. On the other hand, using our knowledge of the pathophysiology of infections in neutropenic patients, supported by the results of subgroup analysis, it has become clear that it is possible to protect patients at high risk against rapidly fatal infections by bacterial and fungal pathogens (see Table 47.1).

Table 47.1 Situations to consider the use of prophylaxis

Prevention of bacterial infections
- Prolonged chemotherapy-induced neutropenia
- (Functional) asplenia

Prevention of fungal infections
- *Candida* species
  - Colonization gastrointestinal tract and/or skin
  - Radio/chemotherapy-related mucosal damage
  - Central venous line
  - Prolonged use of antibacterial agents
- *Aspergillus* species
  - Depressed cellular immunity, as in graft-versus-host disease
  - Prolonged chemotherapy-induced neutropenia
  - Prolonged use of corticosteroids or other immunosuppressive agents
  - Cytomegalovirus infection in a transplant recipient

Guidelines for Clinical Practice in Neutropenic Patients

McQuay and Moore proposed four questions that need to be considered before a reasonable decision on the use of prophylaxis can be made [35]. First, would the event we are trying to prevent, i.e. overwhelming infection, be difficult to treat if it occurred? Second, is an overwhelming infection a serious event in a neutropenic cancer patient? Third, is prophylaxis safe and well tolerated? Fourth, is the prophylaxis effective, i.e., is the number needed to treat to save one patient relatively low such as <20, i.e., is the incidence of the infectious complication high? A firm "yes" would be the answer to first three questions, albeit that the adverse events associated with the use of antifungals are not neglectable but without appropriate therapy the mortality would exceed 90%. On the other hand, given the availability of the modern powerful antibiotics and antifungal compounds, the answer to the first question depends on local diagnostic facilities since early detection would allow a timely treatment of a disseminated infection. The answer would be different for centers vigilantly pursuing a preemptive approach with structured diagnostic surveillance and for centers that do not have the facilities or the means to do so [36]. Answering the fourth question is extremely complicated and probably responsible for most of the controversies that surround the employment of antimicrobial prophylaxis in neutropenic patients.

An ideal prophylactic antimicrobial agent should be safe to be administered over long periods of time, effective against those pathogens that cause life-threatening infections, available in both oral and intravenous formulations, inexpensive, and associated with a very low propensity to emergence of resistance. As there are no drugs that meet all these criteria, individual clinicians have to make up the balance between advantages and disadvantages of prophylaxis.

Taking Gram-negative sepsis for a target, the number-of-needed-to-treat patients to prevent the event may be as low as 2. This looks impressive but in general it does not translate into an improved survival since nowadays all clinicians adhere to prompt empirical cover by very efficacious broad-spectrum antibiotics at the onset of fever. However, if the focus is directed at the use of antibacterial prophylaxis in high-risk patients, the situation is quite different. A recent meta-analysis of studies that included only patients who received high-dose chemotherapy for acute leukemia or stem cell transplantation indicated a reduced death rate among individuals on prophylaxis with fluoroquinolones [37]. So, high-risk patients should be considered as candidates for antibacterial prophylaxis with quinolones. Prophylaxis should commence at the start of chemotherapy and stop at the resolution of the neutropenia or when fever occurs. Similarly, there is a reasonable consensus on the value of fluconazole prophylaxis in patients at high risk for invasive *Candida* infection. This high-risk population also consists of patients with expected protracted and profound neutropenia and severe mucositis. Indwelling central venous access devices pose an additional risk factor. Based on previous findings, it appears that body surveillance cultures may help to determine the subset of patients who are most likely to develop hematogenous candidiasis. Antibacterial and anticandidal prophylaxis should be terminated after recovery from neutropenia.

The prevention of infections by *Aspergillus* species and other molds is a more complicated issue. Neutropenia is not the leading risk factor. A depressed cellular immunity is more important and this implies the time that the risk period stretches from the start of bone marrow suppression until the tapering of immunosuppressive drugs at the resolution of graft-versus-host disease. Keeping this in mind, it is perplexing that anti-*Aspergillus* prophylaxis under these extremely risky circumstances does not ensure a survival benefit among bone marrow transplant recipients treated for graft-versus-host disease [38]. Secondly, aspergillosis is an airborne disease. Since spores of *Aspergillus* are ubiquitous in nature, the patient may acquire infection both during his hospital stay and while at home. This explains why the protective influence of HEPA filtration is rather unsatisfactory. Furthermore, the incidence of invasive aspergillosis varies highly between centers and ranges from 0% to as high as 25% or more, which makes a universally applicable guideline on the use of prophylaxis difficult. When prophylaxis is deemed necessary, the flexibility afforded by the parenteral and oral formulations of anti-*Aspergillus* azoles is a most attractive feature, since it allows patients to leave the hospital while continuing therapy.

In summary, the decision in favor of prophylaxis hinges around incidence and risk factors. If we accept this conclusion, we have left the field of prophylaxis *strictu sensu*, i.e., giving an antibacterial or antifungal drug to an unselected cohort of patients with a defined underlying disease who undergo a specified cytoreductive therapy. Concentration on specific risk groups means that we have turned to targeted prophylaxis, in between a prophylactic and a preemptive strategy. A preemptive approach is a treatment of early, subclinical disease when therapy would be maximally effective [39]. The major advantage of this strategy is that patients who do not need therapy are not exposed to potentially toxic drugs. The cornerstones of its success are careful clinical and laboratory examination of the patient in conjunction with understanding of the temporal sequence of microbial events after transplantation or intensive chemotherapy. Applications of the new diagnostic tools that have a rapid turn-around time are vital to the feasibility of this strategy. If antigen testing, PCR techniques, high-resolution CT-scanning, and extensive clinical experience are not available, one should rather rely on prophylaxis and empirical therapy to avoid confrontation with an infection in a stage beyond cure. So, the choice of the most appropriate strategy does not only depend on the prevalence of a given infection but also on the local circumstances. It might be expected that improvement of disease markers will further decrease the need for prophylaxis [40, 41]. Toll-like receptors are essential components of the immune response to fungal pathogens. Seropositivity for cytomegalovirus in donors or recipients or in both, as compared with negative results, was associated with an increase in the 3-year probability of invasive aspergillosis (12 vs. 1%). Development of immunogenic vaccine would change the scene completely, but the prospects of having a safe and effective vaccine are not bright [42].

The role of antimicrobial drugs clarified leaves the question of dosing. The official registration of fluconazole refers to 400 mg daily, the dosage used in the hope to cover *Aspergillus* species during the initial trials, while subsequent studies suggested that lower doses suffice for *Candida* species [43]. Anyhow, a therapeutic dose of the prophylactic compound is mandatory since it is not likely that respective pathogens are more sensitive to the antimicrobial agents when they are about to enter the body.

Secondary prophylaxis is a completely different issue. Patients with a proven or probable invasive fungal infection run a high risk when they must undergo further cycles of chemotherapy or a bone marrow transplant. Without additional precautions, reactivation rates as high as 50% have been reported. Hence, this group of patients should receive a therapeutic dose of a systemically active antifungal when the next course of chemotherapy is started. This, in fact, preemptive strategy proved effective in the prevention of recrudescence in the majority of patients. An oral azole might be considered for bridging the period between two consecutive neutropenic episodes.

To conclude, Benjamin Franklin is supposed to have said that "an ounce of prevention is worth a pound of cure." It is not known in which context this brilliant man made his statement, but it is hardly imaginable that he was referring to the prophylactic use of antimicrobial agents in immunocompromised patients.

References

1. Bodey GP, Buckley M, Sathe YS, Freireich EJ. Quantitative relationships between circulating leukocytes and infection in patients with acute leukemia. Ann Intern Med. 1966;64(2):328–40.
2. Schimpff SC, Young VM, Greene WH, Vermeulen GD, Moody MR, Wiernik PH. Origin of infection in acute nonlymphocytic leukemia. Significance of hospital acquisition of potential pathogens. Ann Intern Med. 1972;77(5):707–14.
3. Guiot HF, van den Broek PJ, van der Meer JW, van Furth R. Selective antimicrobial modulation of the intestinal flora of patients with acute nonlymphocytic leukemia: a double-blind, placebo-controlled study. J Infect Dis. 1983;147(4):615–23.

4. Hughes WT, Armstrong D, Bodey GP, Bow EJ, Brown AE, Calandra T, et al. Guidelines for the use of antimicrobial agents in neutropenic patients with cancer. Clin Infect Dis. 2002;34(6):730–51.
5. Cullen M, Steven N, Billingham L, Gaunt C, Hastings M, Simmonds P, et al. Antibacterial prophylaxis after chemotherapy for solid tumors and lymphomas. N Engl J Med. 2005;353(10):988–98.
6. Bucaneve G, Micozzi A, Menichetti F, Martino P, Dionisi MS, Martinelli G, et al. Gruppo Italiano Malattie Ematologiche dell'Adulto (GIMEMA) Infection Program. Levofloxacin to prevent bacterial infection in patients with cancer and neutropenia. N Engl J Med. 2005;353(10):977–87.
7. Gafter-Gvili A, Fraser A, Paul M, Leibovici L. Meta-analysis: antibiotic prophylaxis reduces mortality in neutropenic patients. Ann Intern Med. 2005;142:979–95.
8. Gafter-Gvili A, Fraser A, Paul M, van de Wetering M, Kremer L, Leibovici L. Antibiotic prophylaxis for bacterial infections in afebrile neutropenic patients following chemotherapy. Cochrane Database Syst Rev. 2005;4:CD004386.
9. Goodman JL, Winston DJ, Greenfield RA, Chandrasekar PH, Fox B, Kaizer H, et al. A controlled trial of fluconazole to prevent fungal infections in patients undergoing bone marrow transplantation. N Engl J Med. 1992;326:845–51.
10. Slavin MA, Osborne B, Adams R, Levenstein MJ, Schoch HG, Feldman AR, et al. Efficacy and safety of fluconazole prophylaxis for fungal infections after marrow transplantation – a prospective, randomized double blind study. J Infect Dis. 1995;171:1545–52.
11. Van Burik J-AH, Leisenring W, Myerson D, Hackman RC, Shulman HM, Sale GE, et al. The effect of prophylactic fluconazole on the clinical spectrum of fungal diseases in bone marrow transplant recipients with special attention to hepatic candidiasis. An autopsy study of 355 patients. Medicine. 1998;77:246–54.
12. Marr KA, Seidel K, Slavin M, Bowden R, Schoch HG, Flowers MED, et al. Prolonged fluconazole prophylaxis is associated with persistent protection against candidiasis-related death in allogeneic marrow transplant recipients: long-term follow-up of a randomized, placebo-controlled trial. Blood. 2000;96:2055–61.
13. Kanda Y, Yamamoto R, Chizuka A, Hamaki T, Suguro M, Arai C, et al. Prophylactic action of oral fluconazole against fungal infection in neutropenic patients. A meta-analysis of 16 randomized, controlled trials. Cancer. 2000;89:1611–25.
14. Bow EJ, Laverdiere M, Lussier N, Rotstein C, Cheang MS, Ioannou S. Antifungal prophylaxis for severely neutropenic chemotherapy patients. A meta-analysis of randomized-controlled clinical trials. Cancer. 2002;94:3230–46.
15. Uzun O, Anaissie EJ. Antifungal prophylaxis in patients with hematological malignancies: a reappraisal. Blood. 1995;86:2055–61.
16. Vreugdenhil G, Van Dijke BJ, Donnelly JP, Novakova IRO, Raemaekers JMM, Hoogkamp-Korstanje MAA, et al. Efficacy of itraconazole in the prevention of fungal infections among neutropenic patients with hematological malignancies and intensive chemotherapy. A double blind, placebo controlled study. Leuk Lymphoma. 1993;11:353–8.
17. Menichetti F, Del Favero A, Martino P, Bucaneve G, Micozzi A, Girmenia C, et al. GIMEMA Infection Program. Itraconazole oral solution as prophylaxis for fungal infections in neutropenic patients with hematologic malignancies: a randomized, placebo-controlled, double-blind, multicenter trial. Clin Infect Dis. 1999;28:250–5.
18. Morgenstern GR, Prentice AG, Prentice HG, Ropner JE, Schey SA, Warnock DW. A randomized controlled trial of itraconazole versus fluconazole for the prevention of fungal infections in patients with haematological malignancies. Brit J Haematol. 1999;105:901–11.
19. Winston DJ, Maziarz RT, Chandrasekar PH, Lazarus HM, Goldman M, Blumer JL, et al. Intravenous and oral itraconazole versus intravenous and oral fluconazole for long-term antifungal prophylaxis in allogeneic hematopoietic stem-cell transplant recipients. A multicenter, randomised trial. Ann Intern Med. 2003;138:705–13.
20. Marr KA, Crippa F, Leisenring W, Hoyle M, Boeckh M, Blajee SA, et al. Itraconazole versus fluconazole for the prevention of fungal infections in patients receiving allogeneic stem cell transplants. Blood. 2004;103:1527–33.
21. Wingard JR, Carter SL, Walsh TJ, Kurtzberg J, Small TN, Gersten ID, et al. Results of a randomized, double-blind trial of fluconazole (FLU) vs. voriconazole (VORI) for the prevention of invasive fungal infections (IFI) in 600 allogeneic blood and marrow transplant (BMT) patients. Blood 2008;110(11):55–6a, Abstract #163.
22. Rijnders BJ, Cornelissen JJ, Slobbe L, Becker MJ, Doorduijn JK, Hop WCJ, et al. Aerosolized liposomal amphotericin B for the prevention of invasive pulmonary aspergillosis during prolonged neutropenia: a randomized, placebo-controlled trial. Clin Infect Dis. 2008;46:1401–8.
23. Mattiuzzi GN, Estey E, Raad I, Giles F, Cortes J, Shen Y, et al. Liposomal amphotericin B versus the combination of fluconazole and itraconazole as prophylaxis for invasive fungal infections during induction chemotherapy for patients with acute myelogenous leukaemia and myelodysplastic syndrome. Cancer. 2003;97:450–6.
24. Kelsey SM, Goldman JM, McCann S, Newland AC, Scarffe JH, Oppenheim BA, et al. Liposomal amphotericin B (AmBisome) in the prophylaxis of fungal infections in neutropenic patients: a randomised, double-blind placebo-controlled study. Bone Marrow Transpl. 1999;23:163–8.
25. Mattiuzzi GN, Alvarado G, Giles FJ, Ostrosky-Zeichner L, Cortes J, O'Brien S, et al. Open-label, randomised comparison of itraconazole versus caspofungin for prophylaxis in patients with hematological malignancies. Antimicrob Agents Chemother. 2006;50:143–7.
26. Van Burik J-A, Ratanatharathorn V, Stepan DE, Miller CB, Lipton JH, Vesole DH, et al. National Institute of Allergy and Infectious Diseases Mycoses Study Group. Micafungin versus fluconazole for prophylaxis against invasive fungal infections during neutropenia in patients undergoing hematopoietic stem cell transplantation. Clin Infect Dis. 2004;39:1407–16.
27. Bow EJ. Considerations in the approach to invasive fungal infection in patients with haematological malignancies. Brit J Haematol. 2008;140:133–52.
28. Sinko J, Csomor J, Nikolova R, Lueff S, Krivan G, Remenyi P, et al. Invasive fungal disease in allogeneic hematopoietic stem cell transplant recipients: an autopsy-driven survey. Transpl Infect Dis. 2008;10:106–9.
29. Trick WE, Fridkin SK, Edwards JR, Hajjeh RA, Gaynes RP, National Nosocomial Infections Surveillance System Hospitals. Secular trend of hospital-acquired candidemia among intensive care unit patients in the United States during 1989–1999. Clin Infect Dis. 2002;35:627–30.
30. Gafter-Gvili A, Paul M, Fraser A, Leibovici L. Effect of quinolone prophylaxis in afebrile neutropenic patients on microbial resistance: systematic review and meta-analysis. J Antimicrob Chemother. 2007;59:5–22.
31. Kern WV, Klose K, Jellen-Rittre AS, Octhnger M, Bohnert J, Kern P, et al. Fluoroquinolone resistance of Escherichia coli at cancer center: epidemiologic evolution and effects of discontinuating prophylactic fluroquinolone use in neutropenic patients with leukemia. Eur J Clin Microbiol Infect Dis. 2005;24:111–8.
32. Reuter S, Kern WV, Sigge A, Döhner H, Marre R, Kern P, et al. Impact of fluoroquinolone prophylaxis on reduced infection-related mortality among patients with neutropenia and hematologic malignancies. Clin Infect Dis. 2005;40(8):1087–93.
33. Martino R, Subira M, Altés A, López R, Sureda A, Domingo-Albós A, et al. Effect of discontinuing prophylaxis with norfloxacin in patients with hematologic malignancies and severe neutropenia. A matched case-control study of the effect on infectious morbidity. Acta Haematol. 1998;99(4):206–11.

34. Gomez L, Garau J, Estrada C, Marquez M, Dalmau D, Xercavins M, et al. Ciprofloxacin prophylaxis in patients with acute leukemia and granulocytopenia in an area with a high prevalence of ciprofloxacin-resistant *Escherichia coli*. Cancer. 2003;97(2):419–24.
35. McQuay HJ, Moore RA. Using numerical results from systematic reviews in clinical practice. An Intern Med. 1997;126:712–20.
36. De Pauw BE, Donnelly JP. Prophylaxis and aspergillosis – has the principle been proven? N Engl J Med. 2007;356:409–11.
37. Leibovici L, Paul M, Cullen M, Bucaneve G, Gafter-Gvili A, Fraser A, et al. Antibiotic prophylaxis in neutropenic patients. New evidence, practical decisions. Cancer. 2006;107:1743–51.
38. Ullmann AJ, Lipton JH, Vesole DH, Chandrasekar P, Langston A, Tarantolo SR, et al. Posaconazole or fluconazole for prophylaxis in severe graft-versus-host disease. N Engl J Med. 2007;356:335–47.
39. Rubin RH. Preemptive therapy in immunocompromised hosts. N Engl J Med. 1991;324:1057–8.
40. Ostrosky-Zeichner L. Biomarkers for diagnosis and disease monitoring. J Inv Fungal Dis. 2008;2:42–5.
41. Bochud PY, Chien JW, Marr KA, Leisenring WM, Upton A, Janer M, et al. Toll-like receptor 4 polymorphisms and aspergillosis in stem-cell transplantation. N Engl J Med. 2008;359:1766–77.
42. Spellberg B. Vaccine prospects for invasive fungal disease. J Inv Fungal Dis. 2008;2:18–24.
43. MacMillan ML, Goodman JL, DeFor TE, Weisdorf DJ. Fluconazole to prevent yeast infections in bone marrow transplantation patients: a randomized trial of high versus reduced dose, and determination of the value of maintenance therapy. Am J Med. 2002;112:369–79.

Chapter 48
Infection Prevention – Protected Environment and Infection Control

J. Peter Donnelly

Abstract In our daily life, we all encounter a range of microorganisms by breathing, eating and drinking and by direct contact with each other and the objects around us. This routine occasionally leads to infection. By contrast, patients who are given chemotherapy to treat cancer can succumb dramatically when confronted with these commonplace infections. Moreover when death ensued it was all the more tragic since in many cases it might have been avoided altogether had effective treatment been instituted early enough or, better still, if the infection had been prevented in the first place. In this chapter, an overview of infection control measures including protected environment for severely immunocompromised cancer patients is presented.

Keywords Infection control • Hand hygiene • Universal protection • Airborne protection • Prophylactic topical oral non-absorbable antimicrobials • Protected environment

In our daily life, we all encounter a range of microorganisms by breathing, eating and drinking and by direct contact with each other and the objects around us. This routine occasionally leads to infection. We acquire viral infections by inhalation and ingestion, bacterial infections through cuts and abrasions and occasionally through contaminated food and drink. Any infection that ensues is usually short-lived, often self-limiting and if medical care is needed it is usually straightforward and simple. By contrast, patients who are given chemotherapy to treat cancer can succumb dramatically when confronted with these commonplace infections. Moreover when death ensued it was all the more tragic since in many cases it might have been avoided altogether had effective treatment been instituted early enough or, better still, if the infection had been prevented in the first place.

J.P. Donnelly (✉)
Department of Haematology and Nijmegen Institute for Infection, Inflammation and Immunity, Radboud University Nijmegen Medical Centre, Geert Grooteplein Zuid 8, 6525 GA Nijmegen, The Netherlands
e-mail: p.donnelly@usa.net

Infections Risks

Fifty years ago it was already apparent that patients with leukaemia were exquisitely vulnerable to infectious complications arising from a state of compromised immunity induced by their underlying disease and, more crucially, the therapy employed to treat them. Fever was the signal but could only be explained in about half of cases by microbiologically defined infections and clinically defined infections [1]. The causes of infection identified were found to be common or garden bacteria such as *Escherichia coli*, *Klebsiella pneumoniae* and *Staphylococcus aureus* and an unusually high proportion were due to *Pseudomonas aeruginosa*, a known resident of the hospital environment (Fig. 48.1). It was clear to the early pioneers that the source of these opportunistic pathogens was either the patient (endogenous origin) or his or her immediate environment (exogenous origin). *Candida* and *Aspergillus* (respectively endogenous and exogenous opportunistic pathogens) were also known even then to pose a threat [2]. What was termed "fever of undetermined origin" was thought likely to be related to tissue injury. This together with the absence of neutrophils rendered some, though not all patients, particularly susceptible to some of his or her own normal commensal flora as well as to some of the interlopers that had taken up residence on the skin and mucosal surfaces primarily of the oral cavity and gastrointestinal tract. This hypothesis lead naturally to a two-pronged approach namely, decontamination of the body surfaces and protection from the environment. Within a decade, the "Life Island" was born and experiments with antibiotics to sterilise the gastrointestinal tract had lead to the choice of a cocktail of antibiotics know as GVN (gentamicin, vancomycin and nystatin) to suppress Gram-negative bacilli, Gram-positive bacteria and yeasts [3, 4]. With uncanny prescience, it was also appreciated that the use of antibiotics was likely to be attended by a shift of infecting agents to those that were more resistant and of "low-order pathogenicity" and that the approach may suffer from diminishing returns [2]. This was because the normal commensal flora loses its ecological balance under the selective pressure of antibiotics allowing free

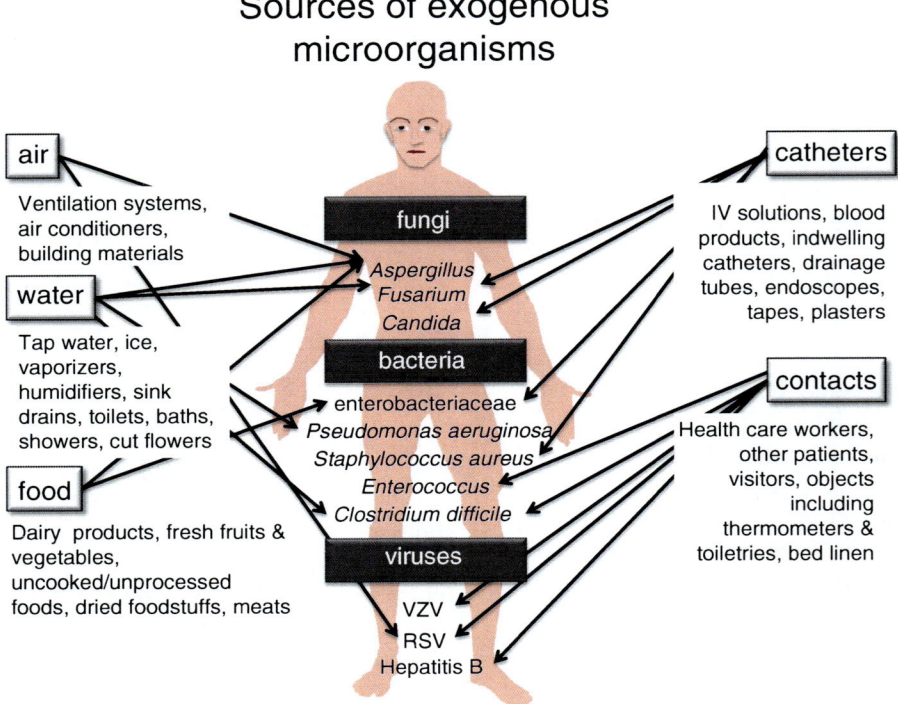

Fig. 48.1 Sources of exogenous microorganisms that can be cause infection

access to exogenous organisms that readily take up residence on the mucosa. The partnership was established between antimicrobial prophylaxis and the physical means of protecting patients from acquiring microorganism from the environment. Indeed, they became, and still are, inextricably bound up with each other to this day.

Basic Principles of Infection Control

Before considering measures that pertain to the patient with cancer it is useful to consider the basic principles of infection control (Table 48.1). Many of these are plain common sense such as good hygiene. Others such as limiting contact with potentially pathogenic microorganisms are considered essential. Others such as a double door entry to the ward to restrict traffic and help exclude outside air are considered desirable if not always possible. However, there are surprisingly few studies that have examined every aspect of physical infection prevention listed in the table and none that have investigated the relative importance of each one in a multifactorial way. The knowledge that exists was due to the energy and insight of a few pioneers who were driven by the desire to show deaths due to infection was avoidable and that prevention was indeed better than cure.

The Protected Environment

The early pioneers of cytostatic chemotherapy knew how devastating infection could be and took the intuitive step of instituting preventative measures drawn up to reduce exogenously acquired infections and minimise the endogenous variety. The notion of the protective environment combined with prophylactic antibiotics (PEPA) was born [3, 5–8]. This required building units in which physical contact was minimised, food was sterilised, the air was filtered and the patients oral cavity and gastrointestinal tract was coated with an antibiotic cocktails to suppress potential pathogens. Small early studies supported the efficacy of the measures insofar as they reduced at least bacteraemia though they failed to improve overall remission rates [9]. Other problems were tackled as and when they arose. Water needed to be filtered to remove harmful bacteria particularly *P. aeruginosa*, the then undisputed queen of the hospital pathogens. Moreover, keeping sinks free of this bacterium also required unusual measures such as heating the drain. Floors had to be sealed and patients were either housed in laminar flow rooms or sealed tents such as the "Life Island." All objects entering the tent were sterilised or disinfected and were passed through a lock system. There were dividends, but also costs among which were psychological feelings of being isolated. Moreover Life Islands were very expensive to purchase and maintain. Opinions were also divided about their true utility

Table 48.1 Prevention and control of infections

Accommodation	Single occupancy wherever possible
Ventilation	Adequate number of air exchanges
	No air from outside
	HEPA filtration
	Directed airflow
	Positive air pressure from room to corridor
	Continuous monitoring of pressure
	Anteroom
	Self closing doors
	Double door entry at the main entrance to the ward
Furnishing	No carpets
	Smooth, nonporous surfaces that are easily cleaned
Water supply	Fungal free, *Pseudomonas* free
Sanitation	Separate sinks in room and anteroom
	On-suite toilet and shower
	Separate toiletries and toothbrush
Equipment	Keep clean and dust-free
Cleaning	Remove dust safely
	Highest level of cleaning
	Disinfection of surface as necessary
Decorations	No fresh cut flowers
	No potted plants
Laundry	Fresh laundered clothing and bedding
Hygiene	Hand-washing
	Protective clothing if necessary
Food & drink	Low-microbial content e.g. cooked foods, pasteurised dairy products, no lettuce or other raw vegetables, only fruit and vegetables that can be washed and disinfected before being peeled, bottled water for drinking and rinsing of the mouth
	Ice cubes from filtered water

and the studies designed to show their efficacy often lacked power due to small numbers [10]. This is not a rebuke by any means since few centres had such facilities and studies of sufficient power as would be demanded nowadays proved impossible to mount and complete. More importantly the advances in antibiotic development were more effective and treatment and drugs for effective prophylaxis were beginning to appear (see previous chapter) offering an effective alternative.

However, isolation did not disappear entirely. The idea of cohorting patients in to separate wards was ingrained and enshrined in the discipline. Moreover dedicated nursing staff was a *sine qua non*. It was also considered plain common sense to nurse neutropenic patients in well ventilated rooms with a supply of filtered air to remove bacteria and fungi. Also using dedicated equipment as far as possible was already becoming a standard of care and minimising contact between patients was considered a necessary precaution. Patients at high risk of infection were essentially confined to their protected space until the risk diminished, which could be several weeks.

Hence although many studies of antimicrobial prophylaxis have been done, most take some degree of protective isolation so much for granted that they do not think it worth mentioning in the reports.

Protected Environment and Prophylactic Antibiotic Programmes

Protected environment (PE) and prophylactic antibiotic programmes (PEPA) were developed to reduce the incidence of infections due to exogenous and endogenous opportunistic pathogens during periods of high risk and incorporated a raft of measures. These included HEPA filter air supply, strict patient isolation, water purification, special handling of waste matter including that produced by the patient and food restrictions [11]. As early as 1971, a 5-year analysis of protective isolation showed that exogenous organisms could be virtually eliminated as a source of risk, thus increasing the chances of recovery or remission from disease [12]. However, it was also clear that endogenous pathogens presented the greatest risk [13]. This observation was confirmed by others as some aetiological agents of infection such as *P. aeruginosa* could be identified in surveillance samples before the onset of infection [14–16]. In some cases, the opportunistic pathogen was acquired from the environment and it colonised the patients before causing infection [17]. None the less, interest in preventing bacterial infections by relying partly on protective isolation waned especially once the clear effectiveness of empirical broad spectrum antibacterial therapy became widely accepted [18–24]. However, it was appreciated that HEPA filtered air could still reduce exposure to unwelcome mould spores and, given the meagre choices of drugs available for prophylaxis and therapy it was considered prudent, if not essential, to maintain a PE for this purpose.

The availability of patient PEs in the form of isolation units plus the development of prophylactic topical and oral non-absorbable antimicrobial regimens (PA) led to studies of the efficacy of such PEPA programmes. These programmes were generally designed to make the patient and his environment as free of micro-organisms as possible.

The first PE was essentially a bed surrounded by a plastic canopy with gauntlets attached to the canopy to access the patient [8]. All items entering the unit were sterilised, food was prepared aseptically and the air was HEPA filtered. Subsequently, permanently installed and semi-portable laminar air flow (LAF) units were utilised [25]. These were rooms with one entire wall consisting of HEPA filters, providing high rates of minimally turbulent air exchange. Special water and toilet facilities were provided. Personnel dressed in sterile attire when they entered the units and all items placed in the rooms were sterilised.

Institutions utilising LAF units developed individualised programmes for microbiological monitoring of patients and their environment. Usually, environmental monitoring included air sampling, floor and surface sampling and settling plates. In a study comparing results obtained from LAF rooms with those from regular hospital rooms, none of the air samples from hospital rooms were sterile whereas 53% of samples from LAF rooms were sterile. Only 1% of air samples from LAF rooms contained potential pathogens compared to 59% from regular hospital rooms [26].

Patient culture specimens were collected 1–2 times weekly from ears, nose, throat, stool, urine and skin (and other body sites at some institutions). Special techniques were developed to obtain semi-quantitative throat and total body skin culture specimens. Some of these procedures were time-consuming and eventually had to be discontinued. A study of the effects of the oral antimicrobial regimen in 91 patients demonstrated that a majority of aerobic bacteria were no longer cultured during prophylaxis [27]. A substantial number of persistent organisms were non-pathogenic. Despite the administration of large doses of antifungal agents, most isolates of *Candida* spp. persisted or increased in concentration during prophylaxis and a substantial number of new isolates were cultured. Weekly cultures of stool specimens demonstrated that although some bacteria could not be isolated during antibiotic prophylaxis, they rapidly reappeared when prophylaxis was discontinued, indicating that they had only been suppressed. Only a few of these persistent organisms had developed resistance to the PA regimen. In a study conducted by Klastersky et al. of PEPA vs. PA only, they concluded that isolation did not reduce the frequency of persistent bacteria from patient cultures which suggested that these persistent bacteria originated from the faecal flora rather than the environment [28]. Unlike the previous study they found that persistent bacteria were more resistant to PA.

Persistent organisms were likely to be the cause of the infections occurring in patients on the PEPA program [29]. In a study of 102 patients there were 68 single organism bacterial infections. Fifty were caused by organisms cultured before entry on the program, including 13 of 18 *Pseudomonas* infections. Klastersky et al. noted that Gram-negative bacilli that were cultured repeatedly from patients on PA were often responsible for subsequent infections [28]. Schimpff et al. reported that patients receiving PA who discontinued the regimen while still on ant leukaemic therapy were at substantial risk of morbidity and mortality from infection [30].

The first study comparing outcomes of patients receiving antileukaemic chemotherapy on the PEPA program with controls was a case-controlled, but not randomised study [9]. The complete remission rate was not significantly higher (61 vs. 48%) for the PEPA group, but the duration of remission and survival were significantly longer in the PEPA group, which was most likely because the PEPA patients received more intensive chemotherapy. Three prospective randomised comparative studies of PEPA programmes were conducted in patients with acute leukaemia in the USA. All of the studies included a third group who received only PA [30–32]. The remission rates between PEPA and control patients were not statistically significant in two of the studies. However, in the study of Schimpff et al. the complete remission rates were significantly higher in the PEPA and PA alone groups than in the controls (54, 63 and 24%, $p < 0.05$). The median survival was also nearly twice as long in the PEPA and PA groups.

All of the studies demonstrated some beneficial effect from the PEPA program on infection. Bodey et al. [9] found that the proportion of days on study with severe infection was higher among the controls and the difference was statistically significant for those infections when the number of neutrophils was $<1 \times 10^9/L$ ($<1,000/mm^3$), but not when it was $<0.1 \times 10^9/L$ ($<100/mm^3$). Levine [32] found that the numbers of episodes of severe infection per 100 days on study were 0.67 for PEPA patients, 1.73 for PA patients, and 1.88 for controls, differences that were statistically significant ($p < 0.025$). Deaths due to infection occurred in 0, 24 and 25% respectively ($p < 0.05$). In the study of Schimpff et al. [30], PEPA, PA only and control patient groups spent equivalent times with severe neutropenia. The patients assigned to PEPA and PA contracted half as many severe infections as control patients. Only 17% of PEPA patients died of infection compared to 32% of PA and 52% of controls ($p < 0.05$). The complete remission rates were 54, 63 and

24% ($p<0.05$). The median duration of survival was half as long for control patients than the other two groups.

During the early 1970s, seven European hospitals conducted a prospective randomised trial of PEPA in 137 evaluable patients undergoing anti-leukaemic chemotherapy [68]. There was a great diversity in age, chemotherapy regimens, number of prior regimens, isolation units and prophylactic antimicrobial regimens. Groups A consisted of 42 patients assigned to PEPA, Group B consisted of 44 patients assigned to PE only and the 51 patients in Group C received routine hospital care. Patients in Groups B and C received oral amphotericin B or nystatin, but no antibacterial agents. The proportion of days spent with <100 PMN/mm^3 were 25, 29 and 19%, respectively.

The number of episodes of severe infection and frequency of fever were essentially the same in the three groups. Only 14% of patients in Group A were free of potential pathogens in their gastrointestinal flora during the entire induction period and none in the other two groups. Patients in Group A had a greater proportion of infections caused by Gram-positive cocci which responded better to therapy. Lower respiratory tract infections were significantly more frequent in Group C (6, 7, and 24%, respectively) suggesting some benefit from isolation. The complete remission rates of 69, 61 and 49% were not significantly different and the differences were more likely due to the chemotherapy than the prophylactic measures. Survival at 30 days after end of therapy was 79, 79 and 75%. The authors concluded that the program was not effective in preventing infection.

Subsequently, studies were initiated in other malignancies, such as small cell carcinoma of the lung and breast carcinoma. Randomised trials were designed for patients with lymphoma and soft tissue sarcoma (tumours which were susceptible to chemotherapy regimens) to determine if the reduction in risk of infections during periods of neutropenia accomplished by the PEPA program would permit dosage escalation of chemotherapeutic agents [33, 34]. Also, did dosage escalation improve remission rates and duration of remission and survival? Unfortunately, the results were not sufficiently encouraging to justify continuing such investigations. For example, in the lymphoma study, patients on the PEPA program had more prolonged severe neutropenia (255 vs. 147 days) and a lower proportion of days with major infection (2 vs. 10%) [33].

Full dosage escalation was achieved in 96% of PEPA patients compared to 77% of controls ($p<0.09$). Unfortunately, despite these benefits, the complete remission rate among patients who received full dosage escalation was only modestly higher than for those with no dosage escalation.

The PEPA program was very labour intensive and expensive, hence, programmes at most institutions were discontinued or extensively modified. LAF rooms were replaced by HEPA filtered units, and cooked food for sterile food. Trimethoprim-sulphamethoxazole and, later, fluoroquinolones were used for anti-bacterial prophylaxis with and without patient isolation [35]. Unfortunately, the benefits of such prophylaxis have been offset by emergence of resistant organisms at some institutions.

Letters and articles began to appear questioning whether it was all necessary especially after the almost universal acceptance of the principle of promptly starting therapy with broad spectrum antibiotics as soon as a patient became febrile [18, 19]. Proponents of PEPA also divided into different camps with the Europeans, in particular the Netherlands, advancing the cause of selective gut decontamination as being the most effective measure for reducing infection. The introduction of cotrimoxazole and later the broad-spectrum quinolones such as ciprofloxacin seemed to spell the demise of PEPA. However, as stated above, even the most comprehensive study of antimicrobial prophylaxis is predicated on their being an advanced degree of protective isolation – single rooms, HEPA filtered air, good ventilation, contact restrictions, low microbial content food and drink, etc.

HEPA filtration relies on the use of fibres arranged at random that remove at least 99.97% of airborne particles of bigger than 0.3 μm diameter (Aspergillus spores are 2.5–3.5 μm in diameter). Strictly speaking particles are not filtered, but rather are trapped by sticking to the fibres. The air flow is set to achieve at least 12 exchanges of air every hour. Originally developed for the Manhattan project to prevent dissemination of radioactive particles they have found uses across industry from aerospace to the pharmaceutical industry, computer manufacturing to nuclear power plants as well as in health care and even the humble vacuum cleaner. The main purpose now of HEPA filtration is to rescue the number of extraneous mould spore in the patient's immediate environment. That the system works in principle was shown many years ago. Indeed it has been shown that spores can be reduced dramatically such that the acquisition by the patient is minimal.

A recent systematic review of the value of HEPA in preventing fungal infection concluded that "The placement in protected areas of patients with haematological malignancies with severe neutropenia or patients with bone marrow transplants appears to be beneficial, but no definitive conclusion could be drawn from the data available" [36]. In a rebuttal, Bodey pointed out that *Aspergillus* was airborne and a reasonable endpoint to consider whereas *Candida* is transmitted by contact and was, in fact, more predominant than the mould. Hence, PEPA would be expected to have an impact on the incidence of aspergillosis, but not candidiasis. The flaw in the meta-analysis was the result of lumping two different disease entities into the same category simply because the microorganisms in question belong to the fungal domain [11]. Intriguingly, Eckmanns et al. complained that none of the studies on HEPA filtration they analysed had been blinded. Quite how this idealised state could be achieved was not mentioned, but it suffices to say that the logistics of such a study alone would defeat even the avid adherent of the approach. The meta-analysis was not all bad as it did suggest that HEPA filtration was beneficial in preventing fungi despite the lack of definitive evidence, the paucity of studies, the discordant end-points and other deficiencies [36]. A recent meta-analysis identified 20 studies that reported randomised or nonrandomised controlled studies of protective isolation and showed that PEPA led to reduced clinically and microbiologically defined infections and also to a lower mortality [37]. However, the authors emphasised that prophylactic antibiotics within a PE provided the greatest effect. This essentially confirms that PEPA works when coupled with prophylactic antibiotic therapy. The authors also concluded that these measures had little effect on mould infections. This supports the results of an earlier systematic review of the influence of HEPA filtration on the mortality and fungal infections [36]. The review failed to discover any significant advantages of HEPA filtration in reducing mortality among patients with haematological malignancies with severe neutropenia. However, the study was not with its critics [11]. The studies reviewed by Eckmanns et al. used data of studies designed to examine the whole PEPA programmes and not just those focussed on air control. They also made the conceptual error of including *Candida* infections among the fungal infections when HEPA is not expected to have any impact whatsoever on yeast infections that are not transmitted through air. Indeed single centre studies have reported an impressive reduction in the incidence of invasive aspergillosis after patients were relocated from LAF rooms to a facility that implemented positive pressure isolation [38]. Clearly the subject remains as contentious as ever as there is no study involving multiple centres of sufficient size and power to prove the case conclusively. None the less it does not seem unreasonable to mange high risk patients in an environment of clean air devoid of as many spores as possible.

Whether or not HEPA filtration impacts on the incidence of invasive aspergillosis under normal circumstances, it has been shown effective in reducing the incidence of invasive aspergillosis in the setting of an outbreak [39]. HEPA filtration has also be shown to reduce spore counts arising from building activities and other measures such as enhanced cleaning, sealing of windows and antifungal prophylaxis also have a role [40, 41] especially when building works are going on, a common fact of life. One way to ensure a relatively safe environment is to conduct air sampling to establish that the ventilation system is working, but not to use it to predict infection [41, 42]. Others have also shown that HEPA filtration alone is insufficient to prevent invasive aspergillosis during building renovation, which requires other measures such as sealing off the building site, wetting the rubble and work area, and limiting traffic in wards housing patients are also necessary [43]. Hence, on balance, it seems reasonable to recommend maintaining PEs for those at high risk of developing invasive mould diseases. Who is at high risk will depend upon the mix of patients and the treatment they receive, but recipients of an allogeneic HSCT following myeloablative therapy certainly fall into this category for as long as they remain neutropenic. Other high-risk patients may include those receiving intensive remission induction therapy for acute myeloid leukaemia or myelodysplastic syndrome in those centres that use PEs.

Water and Moulds

Air is not the only potential source of moulds as *Aspergillus* has been found in hospital water in centres in the USA as well as in Europe [44–46]. Other moulds such as *Fusarium* have been identified in water in certain centres [47]. This emphasises the fact that even though water from the community supply meets standards for potable water it may not meet the requirements of the patient at high risk of developing mould infections. However, given that the problem may be a local concern, it can be identified by examining the water from taps and showers and dealing with it using appropriate measures as and when needed rather than adopting a blanket measures. Moreover DNA may be more likely found in kitchen sinks in the community than in hospital water supplies [48].

There is also evidence that patients may be entering the hospital already colonised with *Aspergillus* conidia. which can be distinguished from those found in the air in and around the hospital [49]. Also, finding *Aspergillus* conidia in the air of transplant units may be completely unrelated to infection [50]. Indeed the latter authors abandoned microbiological surveillance opting for the emphasis to be placed on maintaining the ventilation system, ensuring the integrity of the unit and good environmental cleanliness.

Ideally what is needed is a large randomised controlled trial of protected isolation alone vs. prophylactic antimicrobial agents vs. both vs. neither. However, such a trial is unlikely to take place practically as much as any other reasons.

Infection Control

Control of infection should be achieved by adhering to the guidelines propagated by the CDC, SHEA and WIP that apply to any hospital supplemented by any measures.

Hand Hygiene

In these days of unabated hospital acquired infections, this simple measure cannot be emphasised enough. From Pontius Pilate to Lady Macbeth, hand washing has been seen as a rite of purification. It took an almost obsessive pursuit by Ignatius

Semmelweis to discover the reason behind this. In his hospital in Vienna, in the 1840s, maternal deaths due to puerperal infections were 2–4 fold higher in one of the maternity clinics, where he worked, than in the other. He eliminated meticulously all other conceivable explanations for this difference and concluded sombrely that he and his colleagues as well as medical students were unwittingly carrying the contagion from autopsies back to their patients. Serendipity also played her role insofar as his friend died after being accidentally stabbed by a scalpel while performing a post-mortem. The pathological findings were enough to convince Semmelweis of the connection between the cause of his friend's demise and that of many of the women in labour. Hands were the obvious culprit so he introduced hand washing in bleach, which lead to a dramatic fall in the death rate to almost zero in a matter of months. Evidence enough one would think that hand disinfection could reduce infectious mortality dramatically. However, the medical world remained sceptical as the conventional wisdom favoured the notion that diseases spread in the form of miasmas or rather pollution of the air and water. Vested interests could simply not countenance the idea that germs that had not yet been proven to exist could possibly be necessary and sufficient to explain sepsis, contagions and major outbreaks of diseases like cholera. In Glasgow, a fellow surgeon, Joseph Lister, introduced an alternative method disinfection using carbolic acid and achieved similar impressive results even with compound fractures and other injuries. Unlike Semmelweis, Lister had the advantage that time was at his side as the Germ Theory was beginning to win converts. Still it took the efforts of Florence Nightingale to effect the radical change necessary for hygiene to become a mainstream. During the Crimean war, she arrived at the British barracks in Scutari to find wounded soldiers being badly cared for by overworked medical staff trying to cope with insurmountable problems in the face of official indifference. Medicines were in short supply, hygiene virtually absent and 10 times more soldiers were dying of disease than from battle wounds. Cleaning the sewers and improving ventilation brought down death rates sharply. She insisted on adequate lighting, a proper diet and, importantly, on cleanliness, now known as hygiene, as it alone was a major barrier to infection. Her activities and mobilisation of the establishment proved a tipping point leading ultimately to the clean and sterile techniques of modern medicine. She was also instrumental in helping Linda Richards to become the first professionally trained American nurse who established nursing training programmes in the USA as well as in Japan. She is also credited with creating the first system of keeping individual medical records for patients in hospitals.

Curiously, despite being fully aware of the fact that microorganisms are the cause of such diseases we seem no better now at washing our hands than our forbears were. Why should this be so is beyond the scope of this chapter, but it is worth reflecting on the fact that we subject ill patients to complex and expensive therapies and yet still risk the entire enterprise by failing to wash our hands enough thereby allowing infection to loom.

Food and Drink

It was recognised early that food and drink could allow patients to become colonised with potential pathogens [51, 52]. Indeed the risk of uncooked foods such as salads was already known [53]. Attempts at serving sterile foods were made, but these were not exactly appetising and gave way to the notion of serving foods with low-microbial content. These were essentially freshly cooked meals served while hot, fresh fruits whose skins were disinfected before peeling and serving only pasteurised dairy products. A survey of transplant centres conducted in 1999 showed that the majority served sterile foods, although 1 in 5 used a microwave to disinfect foods and half restricted normal foods [54]. This sort of diet has been dubbed the "Neutropenic diet." A survey done among 156 institutions belonging to the Association of Community Cancer Centres showed 120 (78%) placed patients with neutropenia on restricted diets with 9 in 10 starting once neutropenia had occurred, while only 9% of institutions restricted diets when cancer treatment was initiated [55]. The most commonly restricted foods were fresh fruits and juices, fresh vegetables, and raw eggs although few restricted tap water. A more recent study of given remission induction therapy for AML or high-risk MDS explored the issue in a trial of cooked diet vs. one that allowed fresh fruit and vegetables washed in tap water and found no difference in the incidence of major infections involving bacteraemia and pneumonia [56]. All patients were nursed in a protected environment, received prophylaxis with levofloxacin and an antifungal agent with activity against moulds, and were given empiric therapy at the onset of fever. Hence it seems fair to conclude that any impact on the potential infection through consuming the raw foods was likely to minimal given the activity of levofloxacin against the sort of enteric gram-negative bacilli known to contaminate fruit vegetables.

Similarly the availability of the microwave oven makes it possible to serve hot, wholesome meals that are palatable as well as safe. The quality and abundance of bottled water also makes obviates the need for relying on the sometimes variable quality of water, which may be potable under normal circumstances but unsuitable for patients who are severely immunocompromised and may also be suffering from oral mucositis. Restrictions on the consumption of uncooked vegetables is a necessary precaution given that these can be imported from all over the world including from countries that allow raw sewage sludge to be used as fertiliser. Indeed the complexities of the modern food supply chain and the recurrent outbreaks associated with salad vegetables make it impossible to be sure of product safety [57–60]. Hence complete avoidance of lettuces and ready made fresh salads is prudent given the concern that plants might be more important as a carrier for human enteric pathogens like *E. coli* O157:H7 and *Salmonella enterica* serovars [61]. The same *E. coli* has also been implicated in several outbreaks traced back to the ground beef used for commercial hamburgers [62–65]. Other foodstuffs are a potential source of fungal contamination including dried pepper, tea and the like.

Future Perspectives

The treatment of cancers has never been better with new therapies that are more specific and therefore less likely to lead to collateral damage to the immune defences [66]. Modalities to prepare for haematopoietic stem cell transplants are also less myeloablative so should lead to less injury to the bone marrow and mucosal barrier. There are many national and international guidelines for the prevention of infection e.g. the National Comprehensive Cancer Network *Prevention and Treatment of Cancer-related Infections* (http://www.nccn.org/professionals/physician_gls/PDF/infections.pdf), and international collaborations such as the European Conference on Infection in Leukaemia organised under the auspices of the Infectious Diseases Group of the European Organisation for Research and Treatment of Cancer (EORTC), the Infectious Diseases Working Party of the European Group for Blood and Bone Marrow Transplantation (EBMT), the Supportive Care Group of the European LeukaemiaNet (ELN) and the International Immunocompromised Host Society (ICHS) [67] are also widely available and are moving towards presenting a common approach. However offering comprehensive guidelines in a weighty document is one thing. Spreading the message to all health care workers is another. The basis of infection prevention can perhaps be summarised as shown in Fig. 48.2 – finger tips – minimise contact, know the patient, remain alert, clean the hands and maintain the highest standards of care. Each of these is the tip of the iceberg and presuppose a knowledge base, adequate resources, trained personnel, regular evaluation, and continuous education. Risks for infection and perhaps the causes of infection may change with the disease and its treatment. But the basic principles remain the same.

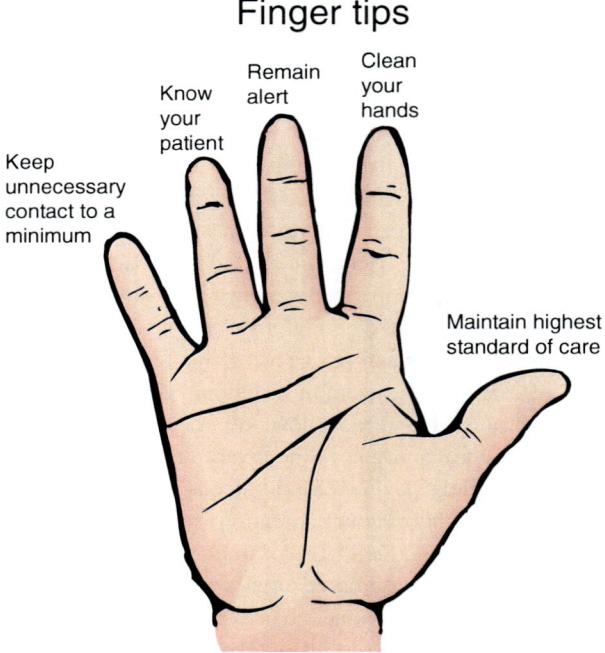

Fig. 48.2 Finger tips as an aid to reducing infections

References

1. Silver RT, Utz JP, Frei III E, Mc CN. Fever, infection and host resistance in acute leukemia. Am J Med. 1958;24(1):25–39.
2. Frei III E, Levin RH, Bodey GP, Morse EE, Freireich EJ. The nature and control of infections in patients with acute leukemia. Cancer Res. 1965;25(9 Pt 1):1511–5.
3. Levitan AA, Perry S. The use of an isolator system in cancer chemotherapy. Am J Med. 1968;44(2):234–42.
4. Preisler HD, Goldstein IM, Henderson ES. Gastrointestinal "sterilization" in the treatment of patients with acute leukemia. Cancer. 1970;26(5):1076–81.
5. Levitan AA, Perry S. Infectious complications of chemotherapy in a protected environment. N Engl J Med. 1967;276(16):881–6.
6. Bodey GP, Hart J, Freireich EJ. Prolonged survival of a leukemic patient in a protected environment. Am J Med Sci. 1968;256(2):112–21.
7. Bodey GP, Loftis J, Bowen E. Protected environment for cancer patients. Effect of a prophylactic antibiotic regimen on the microbial flora of patients undergoing cancer chemotherapy. Arch Intern Med. 1968;122(1):23–30.
8. Hazen JG, Levitan AA, Bourgeois LD. Patient isolator systems in cancer chemotherapy. The use of high-dose "nonabsorable" antibiotics in the reduction of bowel flora. Am J Gastroenterol. 1968;50(3):195–201.
9. Bodey GP, Gehan EA, Freireich EJ, Frei III E. Protected environment-prophylactic antibiotic program in the chemotherapy of acute leukemia. Am J Med Sci. 1971;262(3):138–51.
10. Nauseef WM, Maki DG. A study of the value of simple protective isolation in patients with granulocytopenia. N Engl J Med. 1981;304(8):448–53.
11. Bodey GP, Freireich EJ. Influence of high-efficiency particulate air filtration on mortality and fungal infection: a rebuttal. J Infect Dis. 2006;194(11):1621–2; author reply 2–3.

12. Lynch J, Jameson B, Gamble DR, Kay HE. Five-year analysis of protective isolation. Lancet. 1971;1(7708):1034–40.
13. Schneider M, Schwarzenberg L, Amiel JL, Cattan A, Schlumberger JR, Hayat M, et al. Pathogen-free isolation unit – three years' experience. Br Med J. 1969;1(5647):836–9.
14. Schimpff SC, Moody M, Young VM. Relationship of colonization with *Pseudomonas aeruginosa* to development of *Pseudomonas bacteremia* in cancer patients. Antimicrob Agents Chemother (Bethesda). 1970;10:240–4.
15. Schimpff SC. Surveillance cultures. J Infect Dis. 1981;144(1):81–4.
16. Newman KA, Schimpff SC, Young VM, Wiernik PH. Lessons learned from surveillance cultures in patients with acute nonlymphocytic leukemia. Usefulness for epidemiologic, preventive and therapeutic research. Am J Med. 1981;70(2):423–31.
17. Schimpff SC, Young VM, Greene WH, Vermeulen GD, Moody MR, Wiernik PH. Origin of infection in acute nonlymphocytic leukemia. Significance of hospital acquisition of potential pathogens. Ann Intern Med. 1972;77(5):707–14.
18. Schimpff S, Satterlee W, Young VM, Serpick A. Empiric therapy with carbenicillin and gentamicin for febrile patients with cancer and granulocytopenia. N Engl J Med. 1971;284(19):1061–5.
19. Klastersky J, Henri A, Hensgens C, Daneau D. Gram-negative infections in cancer. Study of empiric therapy comparing carbenicillin-cephalothin with and without gentamicin. JAMA. 1974;227(1):45–8.
20. Gaya H, Klastersky J, Schimpff SC, Fiere D, Widmaier S, Nagel G. Prospective randomly controlled trial of three antibiotic combinations for empirical therapy of suspected sepsis in neutropenic cancer patients. Eur J Cancer. 1975;11(Suppl):5–8.
21. Klastersky J, Hensgens C, Debusscher L. Empiric therapy for cancer patients: comparative study of ticarcillin-tobramycin, ticarcillin-cephalothin, and cephalothin-tobramycin. Antimicrob Agents Chemother. 1975;7(5):640–5.
22. Schimpff SC, Landesman S, Hahn DM, Standiford HC, Fortner CL, Young VM, et al. Ticarcillin in combination with cephalothin or gentamicin as empiric antibiotic therapy in granulocytopenic cancer patients. Antimicrob Agents Chemother. 1976;10(5):837–44.
23. Klastersky J, Debusscher L, Weerts-Ruhl D, Prevost JM. Carbenicillin, cefazolin, and amikacin as an empiric therapy for febrile granulocytopenic cancer patients. Cancer Treat Rep. 1977;61(8):1433–9.
24. Schimpff SC, Aisner J. Empiric antibiotic therapy. Cancer Treat Rep. 1978;62(5):673–80.
25. Bodey GP, Freireich EJ, Frei III E. Studies of patients in a laminar air flow unit. Cancer. 1969;24(5):972–80.
26. Bodey GP, Johnston D. Microbiological evaluation of protected environments during patient occupancy. Appl Microbiol. 1971;22(5):828–36.
27. Bodey GP, Rosenbaum B. Effect of prophylactic measures on the microbial flora of patients in protected environment units. Medicine (Baltimore). 1974;53(3):209–28.
28. Klastersky J, Debusscher L, Weerts D, Daneau D. Use of oral antibiotics in protected units environment: clinical effectiveness and role in the emergence of antibiotic-resistant strains. Pathol Biol (Paris). 1974;22(1):5–12.
29. Bodey GP, Rodriguez V. Infections in cancer patients on a protected environment-prophylactic antibiotic program. Am J Med. 1975;59(4):497–504.
30. Schimpff SC, Greene WH, Young VM, Fortner CL, Cusack N, Block JB, et al. Infection prevention in acute nonlymphocytic leukemia. Laminar air flow room reverse isolation with oral, nonabsorbable antibiotic prophylaxis. Ann Intern Med. 1975;82(3):351–8.
31. Yates JW, Holland JF. A controlled study of isolation and endogenous microbial suppression in acute myelocytic leukemia patients. Cancer. 1973;32(6):1490–8.
32. Levine AS. Protected environment – prophylactic antibiotic programmes; clinical studies. Clin Haematol. 1976;5(2):409–24.
33. Bodey GP, Rodriguez V, Cabanillas F, Freireich EJ. Protected environment-prophylactic antibiotic program for malignant lymphoma. Randomized trial during chemotherapy to induce remission. Am J Med. 1979;66(1):74–81.
34. Bodey GP, Rodriguez V, Murphy WK, Burgess A, Benjamin RS. Protected environment – prophylactic antibiotic program for malignant sarcomas: randomized trial during remission induction chemotherapy. Cancer. 1981;47(10):2422–9.
35. Gurwith MJ, Brunton JL, Lank BA, Harding GK, Ronald AR. A prospective controlled investigation of prophylactic trimethoprim/sulfamethoxazole in hospitalized granulocytopenic patients. Am J Med. 1979;66(2):248–56.
36. Eckmanns T, Ruden H, Gastmeier P. The influence of high-efficiency particulate air filtration on mortality and fungal infection among highly immunosuppressed patients: a systematic review. J Infect Dis. 2006;193(10):1408–18.
37. Schlesinger A, Paul M, Gafter-Gvili A, Rubinovitch B, Leibovici L. Infection-control interventions for cancer patients after chemotherapy: a systematic review and meta-analysis. Lancet Infect Dis. 2009;9(2):97–107.
38. Benet T, Nicolle MC, Thiebaut A, Piens MA, Nicolini FE, Thomas X, et al. Reduction of invasive aspergillosis incidence among immunocompromised patients after control of environmental exposure. Clin Infect Dis. 2007;45(6):682–6.
39. Hahn T, Cummings KM, Michalek AM, Lipman BJ, Segal BH, McCarthy Jr PL. Efficacy of high-efficiency particulate air filtration in preventing aspergillosis in immunocompromised patients with hematologic malignancies. Infect Control Hosp Epidemiol. 2002;23(9):525–31.
40. Humphreys H. Positive-pressure isolation and the prevention of invasive aspergillosis. What is the evidence? J Hosp Infect. 2004;56(2):93–100; quiz 63.
41. Falvey DG, Streifel AJ. Ten-year air sample analysis of Aspergillus prevalence in a university hospital. J Hosp Infect. 2007;67(1):35–41.
42. Anttila VJ, Nihtinen A, Kuutamo T, Richardson M. Air quality monitoring of HEPA-filtered hospital rooms by particulate counting. J Hosp Infect. 2009;71(4):387–8.
43. Cornet M, Levy V, Fleury L, Lortholary J, Barquins S, Coureul MH, et al. Efficacy of prevention by high-efficiency particulate air filtration or laminar airflow against Aspergillus airborne contamination during hospital renovation. Infect Control Hosp Epidemiol. 1999;20(7):508–13.
44. Warris A, Klaassen CH, Meis JF, De Ruiter MT, De Valk HA, Abrahamsen TG, et al. Molecular epidemiology of Aspergillus fumigatus isolates recovered from water, air, and patients shows two clusters of genetically distinct strains. J Clin Microbiol. 2003;41(9):4101–6.
45. Warris A, Voss A, Abrahamsen TG, Verweij PE. Contamination of hospital water with *Aspergillus fumigatus* and other molds. Clin Infect Dis. 2002;34(8):1159–60.
46. Anaissie EJ, Stratton SL, Dignani MC, Summerbell RC, Rex JH, Monson TP, et al. Pathogenic Aspergillus species recovered from a hospital water system: a 3-year prospective study. Clin Infect Dis. 2002;34(6):780–9.
47. Anaissie EJ, Kuchar RT, Rex JH, Francesconi A, Kasai M, Muller FM, et al. Fusariosis associated with pathogenic fusarium species colonization of a hospital water system: a new paradigm for the epidemiology of opportunistic mold infections. Clin Infect Dis. 2001;33(11):1871–8.
48. Vesper SJ, Haugland RA, Rogers ME, Neely AN. Opportunistic Aspergillus pathogens measured in home and hospital tap water by quantitative PCR (QPCR). J Water Health. 2007;5(3):427–31.
49. Leenders AC, van Belkum A, Behrendt M, Luijendijk A, Verbrugh HA. Density and molecular epidemiology of Aspergillus in air and relationship to outbreaks of Aspergillus infection. J Clin Microbiol. 1999;37(6):1752–7.

50. Rupp ME, Iwen PC, Tyner LK, Marion N, Reed E, Anderson JR. Routine sampling of air for fungi does not predict risk of invasive aspergillosis in immunocompromised patients. J Hosp Infect. 2008;68(3):270–1.
51. Watson P, Bodey GP. Sterile food service for patients in protected environments. J Am Diet Assoc. 1970;56(6):515–20.
52. Newman KA, Schimpff SC. Hospital hotel services as risk factors for infection among immunocompromised patients. Rev Infect Dis. 1987;9(1):206–13.
53. Remington JS, Schimpff SC. Occasional notes. Please don't eat the salads. N Engl J Med. 1981;304(7):433–5.
54. Kruger WH, Hornung RJ, Hertenstein B, Kern WV, Kroger N, Ljungman P, et al. Practices of infectious disease prevention and management during hematopoietic stem cell transplantation: a survey from the European group for blood and marrow transplantation. J Hematother Stem Cell Res. 2001;10(6):895–903.
55. Smith LH, Besser SG. Dietary restrictions for patients with neutropenia: a survey of institutional practices. Oncol Nurs Forum. 2000;27(3):515–20.
56. Gardner A, Mattiuzzi G, Faderl S, Borthakur G, Garcia-Manero G, Pierce S, et al. Randomized comparison of cooked and noncooked diets in patients undergoing remission induction therapy for acute myeloid leukemia. J Clin Oncol. 2008;26(35):5684–8.
57. Nygard K, Lassen J, Vold L, Andersson Y, Fisher I, Lofdahl S, et al. Outbreak of Salmonella Thompson infections linked to imported rucola lettuce. Foodborne Pathog Dis. 2008;5(2):165–73.
58. Gupta SK, Nalluswami K, Snider C, Perch M, Balasegaram M, Burmeister D, et al. Outbreak of Salmonella braenderup infections associated with Roma tomatoes, northeastern United States, 2004: a useful method for subtyping exposures in field investigations. Epidemiol Infect. 2007;135(7):1165–73.
59. Takkinen J, Nakari UM, Johansson T, Niskanen T, Siitonen A, Kuusi M. A nationwide outbreak of multiresistant *Salmonella typhimurium* in Finland due to contaminated lettuce from Spain, May 2005. Euro Surveill. 2005;10(6):E050630.1.
60. Horby PW, O'Brien SJ, Adak GK, Graham C, Hawker JI, Hunter P, et al. A national outbreak of multi-resistant *Salmonella enterica* serovar Typhimurium definitive phage type (DT) 104 associated with consumption of lettuce. Epidemiol Infect. 2003;130(2):169–78.
61. Franz E, van Bruggen AH. Ecology of *E. coli* O157:H7 and *Salmonella enterica* in the primary vegetable production chain. Crit Rev Microbiol. 2008;34(3–4):143–61.
62. King LA, Mailles A, Mariani-Kurkdjian P, Vernozy-Rozand C, Montet MP, Grimont F, et al. Community-wide outbreak of *Escherichia coli* O157:H7 associated with consumption of frozen beef burgers. Epidemiol Infect. 2009;137(6):889–96.
63. Strachan NJ, Dunn GM, Locking ME, Reid TM, Ogden ID. *Escherichia coli* O157: burger bug or environmental pathogen? Int J Food Microbiol. 2006;112(2):129–37.
64. Chapman PA, Siddons CA, Cerdan Malo AT, Harkin MA. A one year study of *Escherichia coli* O157 in raw beef and lamb products. Epidemiol Infect. 2000;124(2):207–13.
65. Centers for Disease control and prevention. Escherichia coli O157:H7 infections associated with eating a nationally distributed commercial brand of frozen ground beef patties and burgers – Colorado, 1997. MMWR Morb Mortal Wkly Rep. 1997;46(33):777–8.
66. Winer E, Gralow J, Diller L, Karlan B, Loehrer P, Pierce L, et al. Clinical cancer advances 2008: major research advances in cancer treatment, prevention, and screening – a report from the American Society of Clinical Oncology. J Clin Oncol. 2009;27(5):812–26.
67. Meunier F, Lukan C. The first European conference on infections in leukaemia – ECIL1: a current perspective. Eur J Cancer. 2008;44(15):2112–7.
68. Dietrich M, Gaus W, Vossen J, van der Waaij D, Wendt F. Protective isolation and antimicrobial decontamination in patients with high susceptibility to infection. A prospective cooperative study of gnotobiotic care in acute leukemia patients. I: clinical results. Infect. 1977;5(2):107–14.

Chapter 49
Prevention of Tropical and Parasitic Infections: The Immunocompromised Traveler

Francesca F. Norman and Rogelio López-Vélez

Abstract The number of immunocompromised travelers is increasing and persons with significant preexisting medical conditions may be exposed to infectious diseases at their destination of choice. The risks of developing severe disease are increased and advising these complex patients may be challenging for health care professionals. Recommendations for prevention of specific travel-related infections and vaccination in immunocompromised patients as well as general advice for the cancer patient wishing to travel are outlined.

Keywords Travel medicine • Immunocompromise • Cancer • Transplant • Vaccination

Introduction

The dramatic increase in international travel which has occurred over the last few decades with the massive increase in tourism and international migration has also had an impact on the quality of travel, as more people visit remote and exotic destinations and activities become more adventurous [1]. As limits to travel disappear and new therapeutic approaches for many illnesses develop, persons with significant preexisting medical conditions are now more able to travel and may be exposed to a variety of infections at their destination [2–5]. The risk of developing certain geographically restricted infectious diseases tends to diminish after abandoning endemic areas, but some infections may persist for decades and reactivation of dormant infection may occur particularly in the immunocompromised [1].

Immunocompromised patients who wish to travel constitute a special risk group who often do not seek or do not receive adequate travel advice [6]. These travelers are therefore a particular challenge for health care professionals advising on the varied aspects of travel medicine as "safe" travel becomes a priority [7]. Health promotion and education are essential and advice for this group of travelers should be tailored according to individual needs and should be planned well in advance, preferably at least 2 months prior to departure and at specialized clinics.

Immunosuppressed individuals have a potentially increased susceptibility for many infections and for each patient the benefits of possible interventions, such as vaccination or prophylaxis for specific infections, should be balanced against the risks involved.

Special Considerations for Immunocompromised Travelers

For practical purposes, immunocompromised travelers may be divided into categories according to the degree or cause of the immune suppression [8]. This chapter deals with severely immunocompromised patients (non-HIV) and more specifically with oncological patients including those with associated conditions resulting from the disease or its treatment. Patients with active leukemia or lymphoma, generalized malignancy, aplastic anemia, persons who have received recent radiotherapy or chemotherapy, solid organ transplant (particularly in the first post-transplant year) or bone marrow transplant (especially first 2 years post-transplantation or longer but with graft versus host disease) are all considered to have severe immunocompromise. Solid organ transplantation may be a therapeutic option in the management of certain solid tumors such as hepatocellular carcinoma and transplant patients have also been shown to have an increased risk for developing malignant tumors secondary to the immune suppression; so recommendations for transplant patients will also be reviewed [9, 10]. For solid organ recipients the degree of immune suppression may vary depending

R. López-Vélez (✉)
Tropical Medicine and Clinical Parasitology Unit,
Department of Infectious Diseases, Ramón y Cajal Hospital,
Instituto Ramón y Cajal de Investigación Sanitaria (IRYCIS),
Madrid 28034, Spain
e-mail: rlopezvelez.hrc@salud.madrid.org

on the organ involved (less severe immune suppression for renal than for cardiac or liver transplants, with pulmonary and small intestine transplants requiring the most profound suppression). Immunosuppression is maximal during the first 3–6 months after transplantation and usually diminishes after 1 year, but a degree of suppression persists long-term and this should be taken into account when considering recommendations in this subset of patients.

Medication which may cause significant immunosuppression includes high dose of corticosteroids (dose of ≥2 mg/kg or 20 mg/day of prednisone or equivalent when administered for ≥2 weeks, so that live vaccines should be administered at least 1 month after discontinuing this therapy) and most chemotherapy agents: alkylating agents (e.g., cyclophosphamide, cisplatin, carboplatin), antimetabolites (e.g., azathioprine, mercaptopurine), plant alkaloids and terpenoids (e.g., vinblastine, paclitaxel), anthracyclines (e.g., doxorubicin, daunorubicin), topoisomerase inhibitors (e.g., irinotecan, etoposide), transplant-related immunosuppressive drugs (e.g., cyclosporine, tacrolimus, sirolimus, mycophenolate mofetil), monoclonal antibodies (e.g., rituximab) and methotrexate [8, 11–13].

Situations not associated with significant immunologic compromise include the use of low dose, topical or inhaled steroid treatment or local steroid injections, patients in remission after leukemia, lymphoma or cancer and at least 3 months after last chemotherapy treatment, patients who are longer than 2 years post-bone marrow transplant, without graft versus host disease and who are not on immunosuppressor drugs, and patients on chronic hormonal therapies (e.g., tamoxifen, gonadotrophin release inhibitors) [8].

Certain conditions which may arise during the management of cancer patients may be associated with only limited immune deficits, but may predispose to specific complications of infections acquired during travel. Asplenia increases the risk of meningococcal disease, *Streptococcus pneumoniae* and *Hemophilus influenza B* infection, severe malaria or babesiosis [14, 15]. Patients with underlying thrombocytopenia may be at increased risk of hemorrhagic complications due to dengue infection [16]. Patients with chronic liver disease would be at increased risk of severe disease and complications if travel-related hepatitis A infection is contracted [17].

For most cancer patients the main period of immunocompromise is during or immediately after therapy (chemotherapy or radiation) and most are unlikely to travel at this time [18]. However, patients should be advised against traveling immediately post chemotherapy or radiotherapy, at least until treatment is complete, blood counts have stabilized and the patient is not requiring transfusions. In the case of solid organ transplant or bone marrow transplant recipients, travel should be postponed if possible beyond 6–12 months especially if proposed travel is to developing areas of the world [19].

General Recommendations for Immunocompromised Travelers

For travelers with preexisting medical conditions, gathering additional information regarding travel health insurance, insurance for repatriation if significant illness while abroad and the addresses of health clinics at the destination of choice would be useful prior to departure. Sufficient medication should be carried to last the entire duration of the trip, and if possible, this should be distributed between hand and checked luggage. Patients should be advised not to purchase medication while abroad, especially in developing countries, due to the possibility of unknowingly acquiring counterfeit drugs. In specific cases, a physician's letter, translated if applicable, specifying the patient's medical history and treatment, should be given to the patient. High risk patients may wish to carry a supply of antibiotics for standby self-treatment in circumstances such as prolonged traveler's diarrhea or respiratory infections with specific instructions on appropriate use.

Recommendations for Prevention of Specific Infections

The risk of acquisition of certain infections varies depending on the geographical area visited. Knowledge of world distribution of infectious diseases and agents facilitates risk assessment. Relevant infectious risks for travelers according to world area are shown in Map 49.1 and Table 49.1.

Enteric pathogens: Immunocompromised individuals are at increased risk for food and waterborne infections and advice should be given regarding the necessary precautions to minimize this risk. Raw or undercooked food (including fruit, vegetables, dairy products, seafood and meat) should not be consumed. Special emphasis should be made on the importance of consuming safe water (generally bottled), avoiding drinks prepared with tap water, and avoiding the consumption of ice (made with tap water). During specific activities, such as teeth brushing or swimming, water should not be swallowed. Hands should be washed often and especially after any contact with animals. Children may be particularly at risk if they have been playing with dirt or sand. Infections caused by *Salmonella* spp., *Campylobacter* spp., *Listeria* spp., *Vibrio* spp., *Cryptosporidium* spp., *Yersinia enterocolitica*, and *Toxoplasma* spp. may be transmitted in this way and may cause severe, acute, and in some cases, chronic infections in these patients.

Diarrhea is the most common illness in travelers and constitutes an important health problem affecting up to 40% of individuals traveling from low-risk countries to high-risk developing areas. High-risk regions of the world for acquiring

49 Prevention of Tropical and Parasitic Infections: The Immunocompromised Traveler

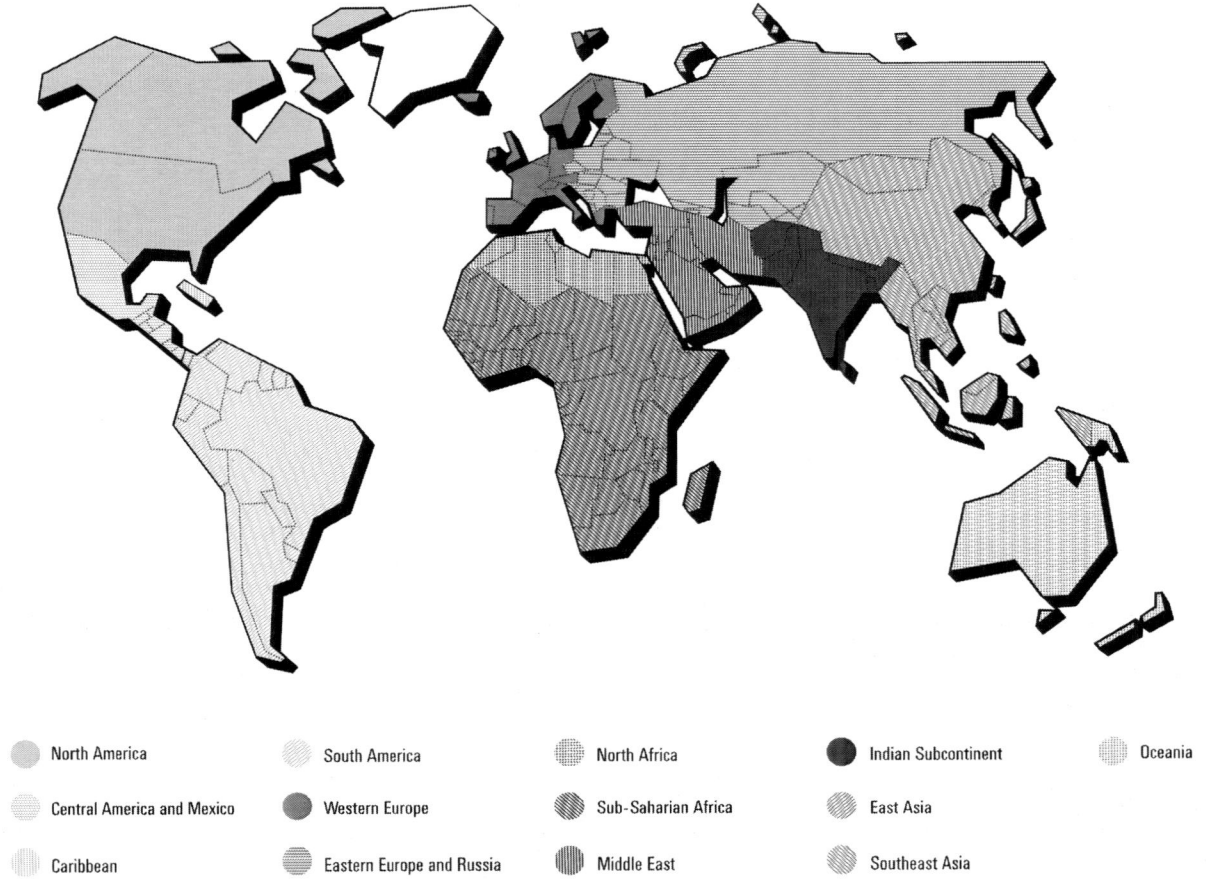

Map 49.1

Table 49.1 Geographical distribution of infectious diseases and agents

Geographical area	Countries	Infectious disease
North Africa	Algeria, Egypt, Libya, Morocco, and Tunisia	Dengue, West Nile virus, rabies, hepatitis A/E, tuberculous (TB), leptospirosis, typhoid fever, malaria (very low risk), leishmaniasis, schistosomiasis (Nile delta), and lymphatic filariasis (Nile delta)
Sub-Saharan Africa	Angola, Benin, Botswana, Burkina Faso, Burundi, Cameroon, Cape Verde Islands, Central African Republic, Chad, Congo, Democratic Republic of Congo (Zaire), Djibouti, Equatorial Guinea, Eritrea, Ethiopia, Gabon, Gambia, Ghana, Guinea, Guinea-Bissau, Ivory Coast, Kenya, Lesotho, Liberia, Madagascar, Malawi, Mali, Mauritania, Mozambique, Namibia, Niger, Nigeria, Reunion Islands (France), Rwanda, Senegal, Seychelles, Sierra Leone, Somalia, South Africa, Sudan, Swaziland, Togo, Sao Tome and Principe, Tanzania, Uganda, Western Sahara, Zambia, and Zimbabwe	Dengue, HTLV-I (in certain countries), West Nile virus, rabies, yellow fever, polio (outbreaks in certain countries), hepatitis A/B/E, typhoid fever, rickettsiosis, cholera (outbreaks in some countries), TB, meningococcal meningitis (African meningitis belt), histoplasmosis, malaria, human African trypanosomiasis, filariasis, leishmaniasis, schistosomiasis, and strongyloidiasis
North America	Canada, and USA (including Hawaii)	West Nile virus, rabies, rickettsiosis, Lyme disease, TB (sporadic cases), leptospirosis (Hawaii), coccidioidomycosis, histoplasmosis, blastomycosis, strongyloidiasis, and babesiosis
Central America and Mexico	Belize, Costa Rica, El Salvador, Guatemala, Honduras, Mexico, Nicaragua, and Panamá	Dengue, West Nile virus, rabies, hepatitis A/B/E, leptospirosis, TB, coccidioidomycosis, histoplasmosis, paracoccidioidomycosis, malaria (mainly *Plasmodium vivax*, risk of *Plasmodium falciparum* in Panama), leishmaniasis, Chagas disease, and strongyloidiasis

(continued)

Table 49.1 (continued)

Geographical area	Countries	Infectious disease
Caribbean	Antigua and Barbuda, Aruba, Bahamas, Barbados, Bermuda (UK), Cayman Islands (UK), Cuba, Dominica, Dominican Republic, Grenada, Guadeloupe (including St. Barthelemy and St. Martin), Haiti, Jamaica, Martinique (France), Montserrat (UK), Netherlands Antilles (Bonaire, Curaçao, Saba, St. Eustatius, St. Maarten), Puerto Rico (US), St. Vincent and the Grenadines, St. Kitts and Nevis, St. Lucia, Trinidad and Tobago, Virgin Islands (British), and Virgin Islands (USA)	Dengue, HTLV-I, hepatitis A/B/E, leptospirosis, TB, histoplasmosis, malaria (*P. falciparum* in Haiti, isolated cases in Dominican Republic, Jamaica and Bahamas/Great Exuma), lymphatic filariasis (Haiti and Dominican Republic), leishmaniasis, and schistosomiasis
South America	Argentina, Bolivia, Brazil, Chile, Colombia, Ecuador, French Guiana, Guyana, Paraguay, Peru, Suriname, Uruguay, and Venezuela	Dengue, HTLV-I, rabies, yellow fever (specific areas), hepatitis A/B, typhoid fever, TB, cholera, histoplasmosis, coccidioidomycosis, paracoccidioidomycosis, malaria (except Chile and Paraguay), leishmaniasis, Chagas disease, lymphatic filariasis (in certain countries), strongyloidiasis, and schistosomiasis
Western Europe	Andorra, Austria, Belgium, Denmark, Finland, France, Germany, Greece, Iceland, Ireland, Italy, Liechtenstein, Luxembourg, Malta, Monaco, Netherlands, Norway, Portugal, San Marino, Spain, Sweden, Switzerland, and United Kingdom	Rabies, tick-borne encephalitis, TB, brucellosis, leishmaniasis (Mediterranean basin), and babesiosis
Eastern Europe and Russia	Albania, Armenia, Azerbaijan, Belarus, Bosnia-Herzegovina, Bulgaria, Croatia, Czech Republic, Estonia, Georgia, Hungary, Kazakhstan, Kyrgyzstan, Latvia, Lithuania, Moldova, Montenegro, Poland, Slovakia, Slovenia, Romania, Russia, Serbia, Tajikistan, Turkmenistan, Ukraine, and Uzbekistan	West Nile virus, rabies, hepatitis A/B, tick-borne encephalitis, diphtheria (outbreaks in some countries of the former Soviet Union), typhoid fever, TB, malaria (in certain countries), and leishmaniasis
Middle East	Bahrain, Cyprus, Iraq, Iran, Israel, Jordan, Kuwait, Lebanon, Oman, Qatar, Saudi Arabia, Syria, Turkey, United Arab Emirates, and Yemen	Dengue, HTLV (in certain areas of Iran), West Nile virus, rabies, hepatitis A/B/E, cholera, typhoid fever, meningococcal meningitis (pilgrims to Mecca), brucellosis, TB, malaria (in certain countries), leishmaniasis, filariasis (Yemen), and schistosomiasis (in certain countries)
East Asia	China (including Hong Kong and Macau), Japan, Mongolia, North Korea, South Korea, and Taiwan	Dengue, Japanese encephalitis, HTLV-I, West Nile virus, rabies, hepatitis A/B/E, TB, leptospirosis, rickettsiosis, typhoid fever, penicilliosis, malaria (in certain countries), leishmaniasis, schistosomiasis, strongyloidiasis, filariasis, and food borne trematodiasis
Indian Subcontinent	Afghanistan, Bangladesh, Bhutan, India, Maldives, Nepal, Pakistan, and Sri Lanka	Dengue, rabies, Japanese encephalitis, hepatitis A/B/E, typhoid fever, TB, leptospirosis, meningococcal meningitis (Afghanistan and Nepal), malaria (except Maldives), leishmaniasis, lymphatic filariasis, and schistosomiasis
Southeast Asia	Brunei, Burma (Myanmar), Cambodia, East Timor, Indonesia, Laos, Malaysia, Philippines, Singapore, Thailand, and Vietnam	Dengue, rabies, Japanese encephalitis, hepatitis A/B/E, typhoid fever, TB, penicilliosis, malaria, lymphatic filariasis, schistosomiasis, strongyloidiasis, and food borne trematodiasis
Oceania (Pacific area)	Australia, Fiji, French Polynesia, Kiribati, Marshall Islands, Micronesia, Nauru, Niue (NZ), New Caledonia (France), New Zealand, Palau, Papua New Guinea, Samoa, Solomon Islands, Tokelau (NZ), Tonga, Tuvalu, Vanuatu, Wallis and Futuna	Dengue, Japanese encephalitis, HTLV-1, hepatitis A, TB, leptospirosis, malaria (in certain countries), lymphatic filariasis, and strongyloidiasis

traveler's diarrhea include developing countries of Africa, Asia, Latin America, and parts of the Middle East [20]. Bacterial pathogens are the most important etiologic agents of traveler's diarrhea, with enterotoxigenic *Escherichia coli*, *Campylobacter* spp., *Salmonella* spp., *Shigella* spp., *Aeromonas* spp., *Plesiomonas shigelloides*, and noncholera vibrios accounting for the majority of infections. Viruses (mainly norovirus, rotavirus, and enteric adenoviruses) have also been isolated in cases of traveler's diarrhea. Diarrhea caused by parasites (*Giardia intestinalis*, *Entamoeba histolytica*, *Cryptosporidium parvum*, and *Cyclospora cayetanensis*) is less frequent in travelers and tends to be chronic, affecting long-term travelers visiting developing countries [21].

Traveler's diarrhea usually resolves without treatment within a few days, but in a proportion of cases the infection causes significant morbidity, immunocompromised individuals being at specific risk. The use of appropriate antimicrobials for self-treatment in the event of diarrhea lasting more than 1–2 days especially if there is associated vomiting, fever and/or bloody stools would be recommended in these patients [19]. Suitable agents would be fluoroquinolones (e.g., ciprofloxacin 500 mg orally every 12 h for 3–5 days) or short courses of azithromycin mg (500 mg) every 24 h for 1–3 days. The nonabsorbable drug rifaximin may also be an option, although the role of this drug in the management of traveler's diarrhea is still being reviewed. In specific cases, short-term prophylaxis for traveler's diarrhea may also be considered, usually with one of the fluoroquinolones, although side effects such as the development of *Clostridium difficile*-associated diarrhea preclude long-term or widespread use in all immunocompromised travelers [22, 23].

Respiratory pathogens: Respiratory infections are the second most common infections which may affect travelers [24]. Seasonal influenza is currently the second most frequent vaccine-preventable infection in travelers [25]. In tropical and subtropical countries, the risk of influenza is year-round whereas in the Southern hemisphere the risk peaks from May to October, opposite to that of the Northern hemisphere. Yearly influenza immunization should be considered for all adults in at risk groups, including persons who have immunosuppression or chronic pulmonary, cardiovascular, renal, hepatic or hematologic disorders, especially if traveling to at risk areas [26]. Outbreaks of influenza with high transmission have also been documented in cruise ships [25]. Endemic mycoses (histoplasmosis, penicilliosis, and coccidioidomycosis) may also be acquired by this route and immunocompromised patients are at particular risk of severe disseminated disease. Certain activities, such as visiting caves, having contact with bats or birds and excavating, have been associated with a higher risk of transmission and these should be avoided, especially as protective gear has been demonstrated to have only a limited effect [27]. Due to the risk of tuberculous, including multi-drug resistant and extremely drug resistant tuberculous particularly in developing countries [28], documenting a baseline tuberculin test should be considered in these patients prior to travel, especially in the case of long-stay travelers and if certain risk activities are planned. Repeating the test 4–6 weeks post-travel would enable early detection of conversion so that any necessary therapeutic measures may be established.

Infections transmitted by arthropod bites: Mosquitoes, ticks and flies are the main vectors for transmission of tropical or geographically-restricted infections such as malaria, leishmaniasis, yellow fever, dengue, trypanosomiasis, filariasis, specific rickettsial diseases, borreliosis, and viral encephalitis. Effective vaccinations exist for some of these infections and specific prophylaxis may be used to minimize the risk of malaria, but for the majority no specific prevention measures exist, or these, such as the yellow fever vaccine cannot be used in immunocompromised patients. Some vaccines may offer limited protection in the immunocompromised as demonstrated by a study, which found decreased seroconversion rates in heart transplant patients compared with healthy subjects following tick-borne encephalitis virus vaccine [29]. All travelers to risk areas should be advised to avoid bites through the use of insect repellents, protective clothing (impregnated with insecticide if possible) and insecticide-treated bed nets.

Malaria and dengue are the most frequent infections transmitted by arthropods in travelers. In the healthy host, most clinical cases of dengue are self-limiting and there is currently insufficient data regarding complications in immunosuppressed individuals. Malaria is a significant risk for all types of travelers. There are no specific data regarding increased malaria risk in immunocompromised hosts [19, 30]. However, splenectomized patients do have an increased risk of severe malaria [14, 15]. Choice of malaria prophylaxis will depend, amongst other factors, on destination and specific itinerary. Chloroquine would be the first choice in areas of the world with chloroquine-sensitive malaria (mainly in Central America and Caribbean). Chloroquine may increase cyclosporine levels in transplant patients and drug levels should be carefully monitored. For areas with chloroquine-resistant malaria the options are atovaquone-proguanil, mefloquine and doxycycline. The latter two drugs may also interact with some of the common immunosuppressant drugs and drug levels should be monitored accordingly. Co-medication commonly used by travelers such as antidiarrheals, cardiovascular drugs, and analgesics do not appear to have a significant clinical impact on safety and effectiveness of mefloquine and chloroquine prophylaxis [31]. Caution is advised in diabetic travelers using mefloquine due to the possibility of hypoglycemia in certain situations [32]. Folic acid supplements should be given to patients taking proguanil who are on other antifolate medication such as trimethoprim-sulphamethoxazole. Before initiating malaria prophylaxis, important side effects such as the possibility of cardiac toxicity associated with chloroquine and mefloquine use in patients with chronic cardiac disease should also be considered, bearing in mind that these may be particularly harmful in patients with underlying disease. Indications, recommendations, and side effects of the main drugs used for malaria prophylaxis are shown in Table 49.2.

Infections transmitted through skin and mucous membranes: Patients should avoid swimming in fresh water and walking barefoot due to the risk of infections like schistosomiasis, leptospirosis, and geohelminthiasis (ancylostomiasis and strongyloidiasis). Schistosomiasis is endemic in Sub-Saharan

Table 49.2 Main drugs used for malaria prophylaxis

Drug	Dose	Indication	Side effects	Precautions
Chloroquine Tablets with 150 mg base (250 mg salt)	Adult patient 40–80 kg: 2 tablets (300 mg base), orally, once a week Children: 5 mg/kg base, orally, once a week, up to max. adult dose of 300 mg base Start 1 week prior to travel and continue for 1 month after return	Areas with chloroquine sensitive *Plasmodium* May be used in children and during pregnancy	Mild reactions (5–10%): abdominal pain, nausea, vomiting, diarrhea May worsen symptoms of psoriasis Agranulocytosis, neutropenia, thrombocytopenia, aplastic anemia Rare: psychosis, convulsions, retinopathy when used at prophylactic doses	Contraindicated if chloroquine hypersensitivity or retinopathy Use with caution if: G6PD deficiency CNS disease Myasthenia gravis Epilepsy Psychosis Impaired hearing Hematologic disease Liver disease
Atovaquone+Proguanil (Malarone®) Adult tablets: 250 mg atovaquone+100 mg proguanil Pediatric tablets: 62.5 mg atovaquone+25 mg proguanil	1 adult tablet every day if >40 kg Children 5–10 kg: ½ pediatric tablet every day; 11–20 kg: 1 pediatric tablet a day; 21–30 kg: 2 pediatric tablets a day; 31–40 kg: 3 pediatric tablets a day Start 1–2 days before departure, take daily and continue for 1 week after return	Areas with chloroquine-resistant *Plasmodium* and areas with multi-drug resistant *P. falciparum*	Abdominal pain, vomiting Headache, occasionally difficulty in sleeping Fever Rash	Contraindicated in children <5 kg, should not be used in pregnancy (insufficient data), and if severe renal failure (creatinine clearance<30 mL/min)
Mefloquine 250 mg (salt) tablets	5 mg/kg salt in children >5 kg and older than 3 months (once a week) In adults: 1 tablet per week Start 1 week prior to departure and continue for 1 month after return	Areas with chloroquine resistance (areas in Southeast Asia with reported mefloquine-resistant *P. falciparum*) Recommended in children 3 months or older and >5 kg, appears to be safe in pregnancy	Neurologic: may affect the central and peripheral nervous system (headache, dizziness, vertigo, and convulsions) Psychiatric: changes in sleep patterns, anxiety, mood changes Severe neuropsychiatric symptoms are rare Gastrointestinal symptoms	Contraindicated in psychiatric patients, epilepsy, and ventricular arrhythmias Caution if used with other potentially cardiotoxic drugs Caution when used by professionals who require great dexterity (e.g., pilots)
Doxycycline 100 mg tablets	100 mg daily Start 1 day before entering at-risk area and continue for 1 month on return	Areas with chloroquine resistance and with multi-drug resistant *P. falciparum* (no reported resistance to doxycycline)	Photosensitivity (4–16%) Gastrointestinal symptoms: nausea, abdominal pain and esophagitis Vaginal candidiasis	Contraindicated in children <8 years and in pregnancy Caution if liver failure

Africa, in Asia, and in restricted areas of America. Areas associated with greatest risk for tourists/short-term travelers are the Dogon country in Mali and Lake Malawi. *Strongyloides stercoralis*, which may cause severe complications such as the hyperinfestation syndrome in immunocompromised hosts, may also be transmitted by direct contact with bare skin.

Infections transmitted by animal bites: Depending on the type of travel and the activities undertaken whilst traveling, patients may have greater exposure and contact with animals than in their home environment. Immunocompromised hosts are at risk for severe life-threatening infection with *Capnocytophaga canimorsus* (DF2 bacillus) following a dog bite. *Bartonella henselae*, *Pasteurella multocida* and *Mycobacterium marinum* may also be transmitted through animal contact [28]. Canine rabies is prevalent among stray dogs in India, several countries of Southeast Asia and Latin America. Indications for rabies vaccine are outlined below. Patients should take pertinent precautions and avoid contact with animals if necessary while traveling abroad.

Sexually and parenterally transmitted infections: Sexual activity may increase during travel [8] and so the possibility of sexually transmitted infections also increases if adequate protective measures are not used. Infections which may be transmitted through sexual contact include HIV, hepatitis B and C, *Neisseria gonorrhoeae*, *Chlamydia trachomatis*, *Treponema pallidum* (syphilis), *Haemophilus ducreyi*, *Calymmatobacterium* (*Klebsiella*) *granulomatis*, *Herpes simplex* type II, human papillomavirus, and *Trichomonas vaginalis*, and these all constitute a risk for immunocompromised patients. Hepatitis B or C, HIV, and other sexually transmitted infections have a high prevalence in developing countries. As well as advising on the practice of safe sex, travelers should also be aware of the risks of particular infections (mainly HIV, hepatitis B and C) associated with other practices such as piercing, tattooing, acupuncture, or dental procedures and these should be avoided while abroad. The importance for cancer patients of traveling only once blood counts are stable and transfusions are not required should be stressed. The safety of blood transfusions whilst abroad, particularly in developing counties, may not be guaranteed (higher prevalence of some transmissible agents such as HIV in the general population and substandard screening of the blood supply), exposing these patients to an increased risk of blood-borne infectious agents [33–35].

Vaccination in the Immunocompromised Traveler

Immunocompromised individuals may benefit from pretravel vaccination for certain conditions. Infections normally prevented by vaccination may be life-threatening in the immunocompromised host and may even contribute to graft rejection in transplant patients [19, 36]. Although there have been reports of graft rejection temporally associated with vaccination, data from other studies do not support this association [37–39]. With respect to healthy travelers, vaccine responses may be suboptimal and immune responses may wane more rapidly in the immunocompromised, so that protection may be decreased and additional vaccine doses may be necessary [8, 18, 19]. Travelers with severe immunocompromise cannot be given live virus or bacterial vaccines [8, 36, 40, 41]. The majority of vaccines with killed and attenuated microorganisms may be safely used in immunocompromised individuals with minimal reported side effects. Vaccine response appears to be best if given prior to immune suppression with chemotherapy, radiotherapy, or high dose corticosteroids (administer preferably more than 2 weeks before these therapies) or at least 3 months after completion of chemotherapy and/or radiotherapy. Live vaccines should be avoided within 3 months of last chemotherapy and should only be used if in remission or no significant immunocompromise [18, 42, 43]. Patients with hypogammaglobulinemia and certain hematologic malignancies such as chronic lymphatic leukemia may respond particularly poorly to vaccines, but response has been shown to improve for certain vaccines if administered at an early stage of the disease [44]. In the case of solid organ transplant recipients, where immunosuppressive medication is maintained long-term, vaccination should be undertaken when immunosuppression is at baseline levels, but live vaccines should not be used. Patients with post-transplant hypogammaglobulinemia have an increased frequency of recurrent infections and may have a poor response to vaccination [45–47]. Although there are no specific guidelines on when to restart immunizations in transplant patients, a minimum period of 6–12 months post-transplant would seem reasonable [48].

For immunocompromised patients who wish to travel before these specified time periods, concerns may be raised about vaccine coverage and passive immunization for certain infections by utilizing specific immunoglobulins may be a possibility. The administration of immunoglobulins in patients with IgA deficiency would be contraindicated due to the possible risk of anaphylaxis [49].

Specific Recommendations for Vaccination in Immunocompromised Travelers

Before undertaking any vaccination in immunocompromised patients the recommendations outlined above should be taken into account.

Routine vaccines: During the pretravel consultation enquiries can be made regarding immunization status of routine vaccines, schedules may be completed and any necessary booster doses may be administered. Specifically, the risk of exposure to vaccine-preventable infections such as diphtheria and polio may be increased for travelers to certain geographical areas due to recent outbreaks in some countries. Measles is prevalent in many areas of the developing world: as live vaccines are contraindicated in immunocompromised patients, the administration of specific measles immunoglobulin should be considered in susceptible travelers. Vaccines for special risk groups such as the influenza and pneumococcal vaccine should also be recommended as per official guidelines [18, 26, 50].

Specific vaccines for travelers: For immunocompromised travelers the use of hepatitis A, hepatitis B, meningococcal, rabies, tick-borne encephalitis, and parenteral typhoid fever vaccine should be evaluated according to specific travel destination, itinerary, planned activities, and other risk factors. Recommended vaccines for travelers and indications for use are outlined in Table 49.3 [19, 51, 52].

Table 49.3 Vaccination recommendations in immunocompromised travelers

Vaccine	Indication	Recommendation[a]
Routine killed (inactivated) vaccines		
Tetanus-diphtheria-pertussis (Td or Tdap)	Non immune traveler. Diphtheria may be a specific risk in areas with epidemic outbreaks (areas of eastern Europe and countries of the former Soviet Union)	Booster indicated every 10 years. Same schedule may be used in immunocompetent and immunocompromised children
Inactivated poliovirus (parenteral IPV)	Non immune traveler. Consider booster dose in high risk travelers	Use recommended schedule based on age and time before departure. Oral polio vaccine (OPV) is *contraindicated* in immunocompromised hosts and in household contacts of these patients
Killed (inactivated) vaccines with special indications		
Pneumococcal (23-v polysaccharide or 7-v conjugate vaccines)	In high risk groups	May be given and is recommended in immunocompromised patients and in other patients with specific chronic medical conditions also associated with an increased risk of pneumococcal disease (e.g., chronic pulmonary, hepatic, renal or cardiovascular disease, diabetes mellitus, functional or anatomic asplenia: if elective splenectomy vaccinate ≥2 weeks before surgery). Pneumococcal conjugate vaccine recommended for children <5 years, consider use of polysaccharide vaccine in children >2 years with certain medical conditions[a]
Influenza (inactivated)	In high risk groups	Indicated yearly in immunocompromised patients >6 months of age. Live intranasal influenza vaccine is *contraindicated* in immunosuppressed patients
Inactivated vaccines for travelers		
Hepatitis A	Non immune traveler, especially if long-term travel in high-risk endemic areas	A single dose offers protection 1 month after vaccination and at least during 6 months, a second dose at 6–12 months may offer protection of longer duration. In immunocompromised patients the same schedule may be used as for healthy hosts but additional booster doses may be necessary, due to decreased response. If no time for vaccination prior to departure or poor response to vaccination immunoglobulin may be administered (protects for 3–6 months)
Hepatitis B (viral recombinant particles)	Long-stay travelers, health professionals/cooperation work, travelers with behavioral indications (sexually active not in a monogamous relationship, intravenous drug users, etc.)	May be administered to immunosuppressed patients. Test for anti-HB-Abs response after vaccination and revaccinate accordingly. High dose hepatitis B vaccination may increase seroconversion rates in patients with higher rates of vaccine failure such as certain immunocompromised hosts (CCDR)
Meningococcal (polysaccharide or conjugate)	Travelers to Mecca during the annual Hajj and to areas within the "meningitis belt" in Sub-Saharan Africa, especially from December to June	Either one of the vaccines may be used (Quadrivalent ACYW135 conjugate vaccine preferably). Proof of vaccination required by the government in Saudi Arabia for travelers to Mecca during the Hajj
Rabies	Pre-exposure immunization in long-term travelers and those with risk of occupational exposure	May be used in immunocompromised patients although response may be diminished in certain patients (e.g., patients with lymphoma) (Hay et al. [51]). Vaccine may be administered intradermally although a better response is achieved in immunosuppressed patients if the im route is used. When used as postexposure prophylaxis concomitant use of immunosuppressant medication should be avoided
Japanese encephalitis	Travelers to certain rural areas of Asia, especially if staying >1 month during the Monsoon season	May be administered to immunocompromised patients. New inactivated vaccine currently licensed
Tick-borne encephalitis	Travelers to central and eastern Europe, especially during the Summer months and in forest areas	May be administered to immunocompromised patients but response may be decreased
Typhoid (Vi)	At risk travelers especially if long-term or areas with potential outbreaks	May be used in immunocompromised patients. The oral live vaccine (Ty21a) is *contraindicated* in immunocompromised patients

(continued)

Table 49.3 (continued)

Vaccine	Indication	Recommendation[a]
Cholera (inactivated bacteria + recombinant B subunit)	Not routinely indicated in travelers. May be indicated if traveling to area with major ongoing outbreak, but only confers brief/incomplete immunity	May be used in immunocompromised hosts
Live vaccines CONTRAINDICATED in immunocompromised host		
BCG	Not routinely indicated in travelers	Contraindicated in immunocompromised patients
MMR (Measles Mumps Rubella)	Nonimmune travelers	Consider MMR vaccine prior to immunosuppression if favorable immunologic situation. May use specific Ig (measles) in susceptible immunocompromised travelers traveling to endemic countries
Varicella	High-risk nonimmune travelers	Consider vaccination prior to immunosuppression if favorable immunologic situation
Yellow fever	Traveler to endemic areas. Subject to international legislation	Very few studies evaluating risk of yellow fever vaccination among severely immunocompromised but vaccine contraindicated in these patients. Some governments allow entry with an official vaccination waiver letter but other countries will not accept entry without vaccination. Official sites for the proposed country of destination should be consulted prior to departure

[a] See official Advisory Committee on Immunization Practices (ACIP) recommendations for specific doses and timing [26, 50]

Summary

- Pretravel advice for special risk groups such as immunocompromised travelers should be individually tailored and should be planned in advance (at least 2 months prior to departure).
- During the immediate post radiotherapy or chemotherapy period, travel to developing countries should be avoided if possible.
- Patients given any pretravel vaccine doses ≥2 weeks before start of immune suppression need not be revaccinated, unless additional doses are required as per schedule.
- Live vaccines are contraindicated in patients considered to have severe immunosuppression.
- For cancer patients with persistent immunologic compromise such as in the case of disseminated malignancy, active hematologic malignancy, or if undergoing active treatment, killed vaccines may be used, but response may be suboptimal and additional booster doses may be necessary.
- For cancer patients in remission, administration of vaccines (both live and killed) should be deferred for at least 3 months after completion of chemotherapy or radiotherapy to ensure safe administration (in the case of live vaccines) and to optimize response.
- For solid organ transplant patients live vaccines should not be used and appropriate killed vaccines should be deferred until at least 6 months post-transplantation or when immunosuppression has been reduced.
- Stem cell transplant recipients, longer than 2 years post-transplant, not on immunosuppression regimes and without graft versus host disease are considered to have no significant immunologic compromise, so both live and killed vaccines may be used as indicated in normal host.
- Monitoring antibody levels to determine if adequate protective levels have been achieved following vaccination may be useful in specific circumstances.
- The use of nonpharmacological protective measures to avoid infections while traveling abroad should be emphasized: immunocompromised patients may be less than adequately protected by vaccinations and the risk of potential drug interactions may be minimized.
- If a patient becomes ill, even years after returning, the possibility of infections acquired during travel should be considered, bearing in mind that infections may run an atypical course with severe complications in immunocompromised individuals.

References

1. Martín-Dávila P, Fortún J, Lopez-Velez R, Norman F, Montes de Oca M, Zamarron P, et al. Transmission of tropical and geographically restricted infections during solid-organ transplantation. Clin Microbiol Rev. 2008;21:60–96.
2. Kotton CN. Zoonoses in solid-organ and hematopoietic stem cell transplant recipients. Clin Infect Dis. 2007;44:857–66.
3. Boggild AK, Sano M, Humar A, Salit I, Gilman M, Kain KC. Travel patterns and risk behavior in solid organ transplant recipients. J Travel Med. 2004;11:37–43.
4. Kofidis T, Pethig K, Ruther G, Simon AR, Strueber M, Leyh R, et al. Traveling after heart transplantation. Clin Transplant. 2002;16:280–4.
5. Mileno MD, Bia FJ. The compromised traveler. Infect Dis Clin North Am. 1998;12:369–412.
6. Uslan DZ, Patel R, Virk A. International travel and exposure risks in solid-organ transplant recipients. Transplantation. 2008;86:407–12.

7. Perdue C, Noble S. Foreign travel for advanced cancer patients: a guide for healthcare professionals. Postgrad Med J. 2007;83:437–44.
8. Centers for Disease Control and Prevention. Health information for international travel 2008. Atlanta: US Department of Health and Human Services, Public Health Service; 2007.
9. Neuberger J. Liver-cell cancer and transplantation. Lancet Oncol. 2009;10:5–7.
10. Zafar SY, Howell DN, Gockerman JP. Malignancy after solid organ transplantation: an overview. Oncologist. 2008;13:769–78.
11. Lu TY, Jonsdottir T, van Hollenhoven RF, Isenberg A. Prolonged B-cell depletion following rituximab therapy in systemic lupus erythematosus: a report of two cases. Ann Rheum Dis. 2008;67:1493–4.
12. Hudson E, Westmoreland D, Gorman C, Poynton CH, Lester JF, Maughan TS. Severe prolonged immunosuppression following fludarabine and rituximab combination therapy. Chemotherapy. 2008;54:242–4.
13. Liossis SN, Sfikakis PP. Rituximab-induced B cell depletion in autoimmune diseases: potential effects on T-cells. Clin Immunol. 2008;127:280–5.
14. Davidson RN, Wall RA. Prevention and management of infections in patients without a spleen. Clin Microbiol Infect. 2001;7:657–60.
15. Lipman HM. Preventing severe infection after splenectomy: risk of malaria and meningitis increases with asplenia. BMJ. 2005;331:576.
16. Strobel M, Muller P, Lamaury I, Rouet F. Dengue fever: a harmful disease in patients with thrombocytopenia? Clin Infect Dis. 2001;33:580–1.
17. Lefilliatre P, Villeneuve JP. Fulminant hepatitis A in patients with chronic liver disease. Can J Public Health. 2000;91:168–70.
18. An Advisory Committee Statement (ACS). The immunocompromised traveller. Can Commun Dis Rep. 2007;33:1–24.
19. Kotton CN, Ryan ET, Fishman JA. Prevention of infection in adult travelers after solid organ transplantation. Am J Transplant. 2005;5:8–14.
20. Diemert DJ. Prevention and self-treatment of traveler's diarrhea. Clin Microbiol Rev. 2006;19:583–94.
21. Reinthaler FF, Feierl G, Stunzner D, Marth E. Diarrhea in returning Austrian tourists: epidemiology, etiology and cost-analyses. J Travel Med. 1998;5:65–72.
22. Norman FF, Perez-Molina JA, de Perez A, Jimenez BC, Navarro M, Lopez-Velez R. *Clostridium difficile*-associated diarrhea after antibiotic treatment for traveler's diarrhea. Clin Infect Dis. 2008;46:1060–3.
23. Dupont HL, Haake R, Taylor DN, Ericsson CD, Jiang ZD, Okhuysen PC, et al. Rifaximin treatment of pathogen-negative travelers' diarrhea. J Travel Med. 2007;14:16–9.
24. Ryan ET, Kain KC. Health advice and immunizations for travelers. N Engl J Med. 2000;342:1716–25.
25. Marti F, Steffen R, Mutsch M. Influenza vaccine: a travelers' vaccine? Expert Rev Vaccines. 2008;7:679–87.
26. Centers for Disease Control and Prevention. Recommended adult immunization schedule – United States, 2009. MMWR. 2009;57(53):Q1–4.
27. Lyon GM, Bravo AV, Espino A, Lindsley MD, Gutierrez RE, Rodriguez I, et al. Histoplasmosis associated with exploring a bat-inhabited cave in Costa Rica, 1998–1999. Am J Trop Med Hyg. 2004;70:438–42.
28. Trevejo RT, Barr MC, Robinson RA. Important emerging bacterial zoonotic infections affecting the immunocompromised. Vet Res. 2005;36:493–506.
29. Dengler TJ, Zimmermann R, Meyer J, Sack FU, Girgsdies O, Kubler WE. Vaccination against tick-borne encephalitis under therapeutic immunosuppression. Reduced efficacy in heart transplant recipients. Vaccine. 1999;17:867–74.
30. Conlon CP. The immunocompromised traveler. In: Steffen R, editor. Textbook of travel medicine and health. Hamilton: B.C. Decker; 2001. p. 464–9.
31. Handschin JC, Wall M, Steffen R, Stürchler D. Tolerability and Effectiveness of malaria chemoprophylaxis with mefloquine or chloroquine with or without co-medication. J Travel Med. 1997;4:121–7.
32. Assan R, Perronne C, Chotard L, Larger E, Vilde JL. Mefloquine-associated hypoglycaemia in a cachectic AIDS patient. Diabetes Metab. 1995;21:54–7.
33. Yee TT, Lee CA. Transfusion-transmitted infection in hemophilia in developing countries. Semin Thromb Hemost. 2005;31:527–37.
34. Dhingra N, Hafner V. Safety of blood transfusion at the international level: the role of WHO. Transfus Clin Biol. 2006;13:200–2.
35. Luban NL. Transfusion safety: where are we today? Ann N Y Acad Sci. 2005;1054:325–41.
36. Duchini A, Goss JA, Karpen S, Pockros PJ. Vaccinations for adult solid-organ transplant recipients: current recommendations and protocols. Clin Microbiol Rev. 2003;16:357–64.
37. Ballout A, Goffin E, Yombi JC, Vandercam B. Vaccinations for adult solid organ transplant recipient: current recommendations. Transplant Proc. 2005;37:2826–7.
38. Blumberg EA, Fitzpatrick J, Stutman PC, Hayden FG, Brozena SC. Safety of influenza vaccine in heart transplant recipients. J Heart Lung Transplant. 1998;17:1075–80.
39. Kobashigawa JA, Warner-Stevenson L, Johnson BL, Moriguchi JD, Kawata N, Drinkwater DC, et al. Influenza vaccine does not cause rejection after cardiac transplantation. Transplant Proc. 1993;25:2738–9.
40. Avery RK, Ljungman P. Prophylactic measures in the solid-organ recipient before transplantation. Clin Infect Dis. 2001;33 Suppl 1:S15–21.
41. Molrine DC, Hibberd PL. Vaccines for transplant recipients. Infect Dis Clin North Am. 2001;15:273–305.
42. McCarthy AE, Mileno MD. Prevention and treatment of travel-related infections in compromised hosts. Curr Opin Infect Dis. 2006;19:450–5.
43. Suh KN, Mileno MD. Challenging scenarios in a travel clinic: advising the complex traveler. Infect Dis Clin North Am. 2005;19:15–47.
44. Sinisalo M, Vilpo J, Itälä M, Väkeväinen M, Taurio J, Aittoniemi J. Antibody response to 7-valent conjugated pneumococcal vaccine in patients with chronic lymphocytic leukaemia. Vaccine. 2007;26:82–7.
45. Goldfarb NS, Avery RK, Goormastic M, Mehta AC, Schilz R, Smedira N, et al. Hypogammaglobulinemia in lung transplant recipients. Transplantation. 2001;71:242–6.
46. Mawhorter S, Yamani MH. Hypogammaglobulinemia and infection risk in solid organ transplant recipients. Curr Opin Organ Transplant. 2008;13:581–5.
47. Yamani MH, Avery RK, Mawhorter SD, Young JB, Ratliff NB, Hobbs RE, et al. Hypogammaglobulinemia following cardiac transplantation: a link between rejection and infection. J Heart Lung Transplant. 2001;20:425–30.
48. National Advisory Committee on Immunization. Canadian immunization guide. Ontario: Public Health Agency of Canada, Infectious Disease and Emergency Preparedness Branch; 2006.
49. Ericsson CD. Travellers with pre-existing medical conditions. Int J Antimicrob Agents. 2003;21:181–8.
50. Centers for Disease Control and Prevention. Recommended immunization schedules for persons aged 0 through 18 years – United States, 2010. MMWR. 2010;57(51&52)1–4.
51. Hay E, Derazon H, Bukish N, Scharf S, Rishpon S. Post-exposure rabies prophylaxis in a patient with lymphoma. JAMA. 2001;285:166–7.
52. Wyplosz B, Van der Vliet D, Consigny PH, Calmus Y, Mamzer-Bruneel MF, Guillemain R, et al. Vaccinations for the traveling adult solid organ transplant recipient (excluding hematopoietic stem cell transplant recipients). Med Mal Infect. 2008. doi:10.1016/j.medmal.2008.11.006

Chapter 50
Prophylactic Vaccination of Cancer Patients and Hematopoietic Stem Cell Transplant Recipients

William Decker and Amar Safdar

Abstract Prophylactic immunization in cancer patients is safe and cost-effective in reducing the disease burden and complications arising from vaccine preventable infections. For maximal effectiveness, patients should be vaccinated with inactivated vaccines at least 2 weeks prior or 3 months subsequent to myeloablative chemotherapy. Hematopoietic stem cell transplant recipients should similarly be vaccinated 6–12 months posttransplant, immune reconstitution permitting. Vaccination of patients with B-cell malignancies is more problematic, but difficulties can be somewhat ameliorated by applying higher doses of vaccine in greater frequencies than would be typical for immunocompetent individuals. Live vaccines are typically considered to be unsafe for oncology patients, but may be safely administered to HSCT recipients who are >2 years posttransplant. While many common infections can be managed through a strategy of conscientious vaccination, there are many other serious infections that specifically afflict immunocompromised patient populations and for which effective vaccines do not yet exist. While vaccines that will address some of these infectious conditions are currently in development, it is unlikely that all important oncological infections will ultimately be addressed by a vaccine approach as market-based development strategies are unlikely to target infections with a negligible impact upon immunocompetent populations. In this chapter, we present a comprehensive review of vaccination in oncology patients.

Keywords Vaccines • Cancer • Transplant • Influenza • Pneumococcus • Varicella • Bioimmune adjuvant • Immune suppression • Chemotherapy • Graft versus host disease • Stem cell transplantation

Cancer patients and recipients of hematopoietic stem cell transplant (HSCT) are unusually susceptible to infectious disease due to the potent one-two punch of immunosuppressive disease and immunoablative treatment regimens. Given this increased susceptibility, patient morbidity and mortality can be favorably impacted by prophylactic vaccination against a myriad of infectious diseases, even diseases for which most individuals possess preexisting immunity from childhood vaccination. Clinical experience with a variety of vaccines including influenza, pneumococcal, meningococcal, HiB, hepatitis B, herpes zoster, and polio has indicated that prophylactic vaccination of cancer patients should be a routine part of standard of care treatment [1–3]. It is further suggested that HSCT patients be revaccinated with MMR and DPT childhood vaccines at 12 months posttransplant, immune reconstitution permitting [4]. Results from existing cancer patient vaccination programs suggest that morbidity and mortality will continue to be impacted favorably as new vaccination strategies are developed for pathogens that are particularly detrimental to immunocompromised patient populations and for which vaccines do not currently exist. This list of pathogens could include CMV, EBV, community-acquired respiratory viruses (RSV, parainfluenza virus, rhinovirus), adenovirus, and polyomavirus as well as a variety of eukaryotic molds, yeasts, and fungi that do not typically infect immunocompetent individuals [5].

Effects of Neoplastic Disease upon Immunity

Many different tumor types are known to actively subvert immune surveillance via an extremely broad and diverse array of mechanisms (Table 50.1). While some such mechanisms subvert immune detection in an antigen-specific fashion via the generation of tumor-specific regulatory T-cells or myeloid-derived suppressor cells [6–11], others more broadly and nonspecifically suppress global immunity by inducing dendritic cell dysfunction or by a general skewing of adaptive immunity away from Th-1, thereby dampening the cell-mediated responses that typically govern tumor immunity. Tumors may acquire the ability to secrete a wide variety of pleiotropic

W. Decker (✉)
Department of Blood and Marrow Transplantation, The University of Texas M.D. Anderson Cancer Center, 1515 Holcombe Boulevard (Unit 0065), Houston, TX 77030, USA
e-mail: wkdecker@mdanderson.org

Table 50.1 Tumor-derived factors implicated in functional modulation of dendritic cells

Factor	Effect on DC
Cytokines	
IL-10	Impairment of differentiation, maturation, and function in vitro and in vivo
	Increased apoptosis in vitro
IL-6	Impairment of differentiation and maturation in vitro and in vivo
M-CSF	Inhibition of differentiation from CD34+ progenitors in vitro
GM-CSF	Generation of immature APC with inhibitory role in vitro and in vivo
VEGF	Alteration of differentiation of multiple lineages including DC in vitro and in vivo
	Accumulation of immature cells with inhibitory function in vitro and in vivo
Other mediators	
Gangliosides	Impairment of phenotypic and functional differentiation in vitro
	Phenotypic alteration and apoptosis in vitro
Prostanoids	Impairment of maturation and activity in vitro
NO	Induction of apoptosis in vitro
Hyaluronan	Induction of apoptosis through induction of NO in vitro
Polyamines	Induction of altered maturation in vitro
Tumor antigens	
MUC1	Impairment of maturation and function in vitro
PSA	Alteration of differentiation and maturation in vitro
HER-2/neu	Alteration of antigen processing function in vitro

Table derived from Pinzon-Charry et al. [19]
HER-2/neu HER-2/neu oncogene product; *MUC1* tumor-derived mucin; *NO* nitric oxide; *PSA* prostate-specific antigen; *VEGF* vascular endothelial growth factor

factors that impact dendritic cell differentiation, maturation, function, and longevity. Cytokines such as IL-10, IL-6, IL-4, or TGF-β inhibit the generation of Th-1 responses by skewing T-cell responses toward a Th-2 or toward a regulatory phenotype [6, 8, 9, 12–21]. Other cytokines such as M-CSF, GM-CSF, or VEGF prevent development and differentiation of dendritic cells or produce DC with impaired functional capacities [17, 19, 22–30]. Other tumor-derived molecules such as gangliosides, prostanoids, nitric oxide, hyaluronan, and polyamines can inhibit function or accelerate the induction of programmed cell death [19, 31–38]. Even certain tumor-specific antigens such as PSA, MUC-1, and HER-2/neu are known to inhibit DC function by a variety of mechanisms [19, 39–41]. Indoleamine 2,3-dioxygenase (IDO), the expression of which is frequently elevated in cancers, is also known to play an important and potent role in immune suppression [42, 43]. Tumors may even avoid immune detection in the absence of T-cell suppressive factors via the downregulation of MHC class I (i.e., HLA-A, B, and C) on the cell surface with the concomitant upregulation of NK cell suppressive factor HLA-G [44, 45]. Tumor-related B-cell immunodeficiencies exist as well, chiefly evidenced by the hypogammaglobulinemia observed among many patients afflicted with chronic lymphocytic leukemia (CLL). Th-1 responses are also negatively impacted in CLL patients [46].

The net results of altered DC differentiation, maturation, function, and longevity become manifest, not only by the failure of the immune system to recognize and eradicate tumors but also through the inability of memory T-cells to respond to recall antigens [26]. This inability to respond to recall antigens can be further exacerbated by myeloablative chemotherapy, which may result in apoptosis of dividing lymphocyte subsets and suppression of de novo hematopoiesis by marrow stem cell populations. The degree of myelosuppression between different chemotherapeutic agents is not uniform, varying significantly by class and mechanism of action; however, acute myelosuppression, neutropenia, and/or pancytopenia typically reach nadirs 7–14 days post therapy with significant recoveries observed 3–4 weeks post therapy. Accordingly, nearly all vaccination protocols stipulate administration of the vaccine no later than 2 weeks prior to initiation of myeloablative chemotherapy and no sooner than 3 months after cessation [1].

Clinical Experience with Vaccination in Oncology Populations

There are a variety of important reasons to vaccinate oncology patients against community-acquired infectious diseases or to revaccinate them against common childhood diseases. The incidence of disease among cancer patients is not necessarily higher than that of the general population for all infections; however, once a cancer patient develops clinically relevant disease, incidence of morbidity and mortality are almost always more severe than in the population at large. Additionally, long-term survivors of HSCT will find themselves in need of revaccination against the common childhood diseases as their emerging, naïve immune systems become fully reconstituted. Clinical experience with the vaccination of oncology patients has indicated that, though these patients tend to respond is a less robust fashion than healthy controls, significant clinical benefit may frequently be achieved.

Influenza

There is an exceptional amount of clinical experience with influenza vaccination in patients with solid malignancies, those undergoing myeloablative chemotherapy, and those who have received HSCT for hematologic malignancy. Clinical studies have demonstrated that case fatality rates among these high-risk patient groups can be quite high, exceeding 30% in one study [3, 47–57]. Table 50.2 outlines ten clinical studies that report significantly elevated mortality rates among various different oncology populations. Given the high case fatality rate, influenza vaccination of cancer patients should be considered standard of care treatment, and a number of studies have demonstrated that cancer patients, when vaccinated appropriately, can achieve rates of seroconversion nearly as high as those of healthy controls [1, 58–62] (i.e., selected studies in Table 50.3). In general, seroconversion is poor when vaccination occurs less than 2 weeks prior to myeloablative chemotherapy or less than 3 months after myeloablative chemotherapy [1, 63–66], when vaccination of HSCT patients is attempted sooner than 6 months posttransplant [1, 67, 68], or when patients are suffering from malignancies like CLL or multiple myeloma that severely impact B-cell function [1, 69–71]. Recent work by Safdar et al. indicated that rates of enhanced seroconversion among non-Hodgkin's lymphoma patients given a ninefold higher dose of a subunit vaccine could be up to 50% higher than patients receiving standard dose levels (135 vs. 15 μg); nevertheless, seroconversion was still relatively poor, indicating that prophylactic approaches other than traditional vaccination will likely be needed in order to adequately protect this patient population [72].

Herpes Zoster

Transplant recipients or those with hematologic malignancies exhibit reactivation rates of herpes zoster that are several times higher than the population at large, and persons with certain types of leukemia exhibit reactivation rates up to 100 times higher than those of the general population. While the live varicella vaccine is contraindicated in stem cell transplant or leukemic patients, it is the presence of varicella-specific antibody titers that most directly correlates with reactivation, hence the heat-inactivated varicella vaccine may be administered in the oncology setting [2, 4, 73–75]. A number of studies have demonstrated that the timing of vaccine administration is crucial to its success. Two studies in which HSCT patients received vaccine within 6 months of transplant demonstrated no differences in the incidence of herpes zoster reactivation than among control subjects [2, 76];

Table 50.2 Influenza frequency and case fatality in HSCT and cancer patients

	Population and setting	Influenza years	Number of patients under observation	Frequency of influenza[a]	Case fatality
Couch	HSCT, hospitalized, single center	1992–1995	[b]	[b]	5/20 (25%)
	Leukemia, hospitalized, single center	1992–1995	[b]	[b]	9/27 (33%)
Ljungman	HSCT, single center[c]	1989–1996	545	15 (2.8%)	2/15 (13%)
	Allogeneic HSCT, 37 European centers[c]	1997–1998	819	14 (1.7%)	4/14 (29%);
	Autologous HSCT, 37 European centers[c]		1154	2 (0.2%)	0/2 (0%);
	Allogeneic HSCT, 37 European centers[c]	1997–2000	More than 819	[a]	7/30 (23%);
	Autologous HSCT, 37 European centers[c]		More than 1,154	[a]	2/9 (22%)
Hassan	Allogeneic HSCT, single center[c]	1996–2001	230	5 (2.2%)	1/5 (20%)
	Autologous HSCT, single center[c]		396	0 (0%)	
Nichols	HSCT, 120 days within transplantation date only, single center	1989–2002	4,797	62 (1.3%)	6/62 (10%)
Machado	HSCT, respiratory symptoms present, single center[c]	2001–2002	179	41/179 (23%)	0/41 (0%)[d]
Whimbey	HSCT, hospitalized, local influenza epidemic present, respiratory symptoms present, single center	1991–1992	28	8/28 (29%)	1/8 (13%)
Yousuf	Leukemia, hospitalized, local influenza epidemic present, respiratory symptoms present, single center	1993–1994	45	15/45 (33%)	4/15 (27%)
Schepetiuk	Nosocomial outbreak in oncology ward, single center	1997	19		2/19 (11%)
Elting	Leukemia, local influenza epidemic present, respiratory symptoms present, single center	1991–1992	37	4/37 (11%)	1/4 (25%)

Table derived from Kunisaki and Janoff [3]
[a]Frequencies are those reported during the total observation period (influenza years)
[b]Not reported
[c]Outpatient or inpatient status not specified
[d]Only reported mortality from pneumonia, not all-cause mortality

Table 50.3 Overview of clinical studies evaluating influenza vaccine in oncology patients

References	Population	No.	Seroconversion
Ortbals et al. [62]	Malignant diseases	42 cancer; 96 controls	Fourfold increase in antibody titer 71% cancer patients; 94% controls
Ganz et al. [60]	Various cancers	17 cancer patients; 15 controls	No significant difference in antibody response
Gross et al. [65]	Children with various malignancies	120 cancer	HI antibody titer >40; 30% on chemotherapy within 1 month; 89% off chemotherapy by 1 month
Hodges et al. [69]	Hematology patients	31 cancer; 41 controls	Fourfold increase in titer to H1N1 16/31 (52%); (78% in healthy volunteers)
Lange et al. [66]	Children with ALL	22 on chemotherapy; 16 no chemotherapy	Children off chemotherapy had three times the antibody titers after first vaccine administration compared to those on chemotherapy
Schafer et al. [71]	Hematologic malignancies	52 cancer; 28 control	Fourfold increase in antibody titer 26/52 (50%) cancer patients; 23/28 (82%) controls
Anderson et al. [58]	Lung cancer patients	59 cancer; 0 controls	Fourfold increase in antibody titer 49/59 (83%) cancer patients
Robertson et al. [70]	Multiple myeloma	48 cancer	HI antibody titer >40; 9 (19%) cancer
Brydak et al. [59]	Women with breast cancer	9 cancer; 19 controls	HI antibody titer >40; 88.8% cancer; 100% controls
Chisholm et al. [64]	Children with various malignancies	42 cancer patients	
Nordoy et al. [61]	Various cancers	35 cancer; 38 controls	Antibody titer >40; 72% cancer; 87% controls

Table derived from Sommer et al. [1]

Table 50.4 Overview of clinical studies evaluating pneumovax-23 in oncology patients

References	Population	No.	Valent	Seroconversion
Levine et al. [79]	Hodgkin disease	24 cancer; 24 controls	14	12% response rate after prior chemotherapy 14% response rate after prior radiation treatment 9% response rate after both chemotherapy and radiation
Siber et al. [81]	Hodgkin disease	53 cancer; 10 controls	11	49% 6-month response rate
Siber et al. [82]	Hodgkin disease	51 cancer; 4 controls	14	25% response rate
Molrine et al. [78]	Hodgkin disease	70 cancer; 20 controls	23	75% of control response rate 95% of control response rate
Robertson et al. [70]	Multiple myeloma	43 cancer	23	24/43 (56%) response rate
Hartkamp et al. [80]	Chronic lymphocytic leukemia	24 cancer	23	5 (22%) patients responded to vaccine
Nordoy et al. [61]	Various malignancies	35 cancer; 38 controls	23	73.7% response rate

Table derived from Sommer et al. [1]

however, a subsequent study demonstrated that vaccine given 30 days prior to transplant was extremely effective in preventing viral reactivation. In this study, the incidence of reactivation among vaccinated transplant recipients was 13% whereas the incidence among subjects receiving a placebo vaccine was 33% [2, 77].

Pneumococcal Pneumonia

The pneumococcal vaccine is a multivalent conjugate vaccine that protects recipients against infection from the most clinically relevant strains of *Streptococcus pneumoniae*, a common source of infection and sepsis in oncology populations. In two studies, administration of the vaccine to cancer patients resulted in antibody titers that were nearly comparable to those of healthy adults [1, 61, 78]; however, vaccination during radiation therapy and myeloablative chemotherapeutic treatment regimens [1, 79] or vaccination of patients with B-cell malignancies [1, 70, 80–82] tended to result in suboptimal response rates in a majority of patients (Table 50.4). As with other vaccination strategies, it appears to be important that patients are vaccinated more than 2 weeks prior to the start of myeloablative chemotherapy or more than 3 months after cessation. In the transplant setting, where incidence of pneumococcal infection has been estimated to be as high as 36%, it is recommended that patients receive the vaccine between 6 and 12 months post transplant [4, 83–85].

Haemophilus influenzae B

Haemophilus influenzae type B (HiB) is another opportunistic pathogen that commonly afflicts oncology populations, and broad-based themes and vaccination strategies for HiB infection follow the same general guidelines as preceding infections. Vaccination for HiB should occur more than 2 weeks prior to or more than 3 months subsequent to myeloablative chemotherapy and/or radiation therapy. When these guidelines are followed, cancer patients have been shown to achieve protective antibody titers at levels similar to those of healthy adults [1, 70, 86]. The US transplant guidelines stipulate the administration of the HiB vaccine at 12 months post transplant [4]. Further, repeated or booster doses of vaccine have been shown to significantly increase the percentage of post-transplant individuals who are able to achieve protective antibody titers, generally considered to be 1 μg/mL [4, 87, 88].

Hepatitis B Virus

A large number of studies have demonstrated that responses to the hepatitis B virus (HBV) vaccine are very poor, on the order of only 20%, when the vaccine is administered concomitantly with myeloablative chemotherapy (Table 50.5) [1, 89–95]; however, Hovi et al. [1, 96] demonstrated that, similar to other vaccines, seroconversion to the HBV vaccine among cancer patients can occur with equal frequency as healthy controls when the vaccine is not administered during an active chemotherapeutic regimen. Subsequently, Zignol et al. [1, 97] demonstrated that a booster dose given 1 year following myeloablative chemotherapy was successful in recovering protective HBV titers in 91% of individuals whose titers diminished during active chemotherapy. For patients who must be vaccinated during myeloablative chemotherapy, a high-dose formulation exists, and booster doses should be given until antibody titers reach the protective threshold of 10 mIU/mL [1]. In transplant populations, Jaffe et al. evaluated immunity to the standard three dose HBV vaccine regimen among patients who met minimum eligibility requirements including a CD4$^+$ T-cell count of >200 cells/μL, a circulating IgG concentration of >5 mg/mL, and who were no longer taking immunosuppressive medications. In this study, mean time to vaccination was 23.4 months, and seroconversion occurred among 64% (187/292) of participants [4, 98].

Poliovirus

While the risk of contracting polio infection is low in the US and Western Europe, revaccination is still recommended for transplant and other oncology populations, especially those individuals who might be at elevated risk for exposure. There are few studies demonstrating the efficacy of inactivated poliovirus vaccine among oncology populations; however, in a long-term follow-up study, Ljungman et al. determined that the probability of transplant patients retaining immunity to poliovirus at 10 years post vaccination was 94%, provided that the vaccine had been administered at the conclusion of active treatment [1, 99]. Predictably, Bosu et al. also determined that vaccination of ALL patients with inactivated poliovirus vaccine during myeloablative chemotherapy typically produced antibody titers that were suboptimal and inadequate to mediate immunity [1, 100].

In addition to standard inactivated vaccines that may be administered to oncology populations, there is also a need to rebuild immunity to childhood diseases among transplant recipients who have acquired new immune systems. Two vaccines that may be considered in the transplant setting are the diphtheria-pertussis-tetanus (DPT) vaccine and the measles-mumps-rubella (MMR) vaccine, given the severity of pertussis and measles infections among adult populations. There is very little information regarding the incidence or severity of pertussis among transplant recipients, with information in the literature limited to anecdotal case reports [4, 101–103]. Nevertheless, given the safety profile of the vaccine, there appears to be little argument for withholding the DPT vaccine from transplant recipients, at least until such time that contraindicating data might arise. The MMR vaccine is a live, heavily attenuated virus vaccine, and as such is not appropriate for administration within 2 years of transplant unless a specific outbreak has developed. In the absence of an outbreak, the vaccine has been used successfully and safely >2 years posttransplant, and administration at this time point has become the standard recommendation [4, 104–106].

Table 50.5 Overview of clinical studies evaluating HBV vaccine in oncology patients

References	Population	No.	Seroconversion
Locasciulli et al. [90]	Children with leukemia	38 ALL; 11 ANLL	12.2% (6/49) response rate
Weitberg et al. [94]	Various malignancies	26 cancer	42% (5/11) responded to vaccine
Rosen et al. [91]	Breast cancer	32 cancer; 7 controls	6/32 (19%) cancer; 6/7 (86%) controls
Hovi et al. [96]	Children with various malignancies	51 on chemotherapy; 114 no chemotherapy	67% on chemotherapy; 97% off chemotherapy
Goyal et al. [89]	ALL	152 cancer	16/152 (10.5%) cancer
Somjee et al. [92]	ALL	111 cancer	21/111 (19%)
Yetgin et al. [95]	ALL	94 cancer	33/94 (35%) response rate
Somjee et al. [93]	ALL	29 cancer	5/29 (21%) response rate
Zignol et al. [97]	Children with various malignancies	67 cancer	35/67 (52%) lost protective antibody titers after chemotherapy; 29/32 (91%) recovered protective antibody titers after booster dose >1 year after chemotherapy

Table derived from Sommer et al. [1]

Unmet Needs: Oncology-Associated Infections for Which Vaccines Do Not Exist

While vaccination of oncology patients can ameliorate morbidity and mortality of diseases that are common among all patient populations, there are a number of serious infections that are observed almost exclusively among immunocompromised individuals. Accordingly, vaccines that might offer protection from these uncommon infections do not currently exist, yet their ultimate production, in some form or fashion, might be able to greatly alleviate a significant amount of morbidity among oncology populations. The kinds of infectious agents that can be deadly to cancer patients but relatively harmless to the general population tend to be either viral or eukaryotic (i.e., yeasts, molds, fungi) in nature.

Viral Infections

Cytomegalovirus (CMV) reactivation is thought to occur in 80% of seropositive patients following HSCT, though a wide variety of prophylactic treatments including acyclovir, valacyclovir, ganciclovir, and foscarnet can be used to prevent the onset and/or ameliorate symptoms [5]. Some investigators have suggested that universal CMV vaccination would be a cost-effective prophylactic enterprise for society as a whole by virtue of the cost savings that would be accrued from the treatment of symptomatic infants and, later in life, from adult HSCT recipients [107]. Accordingly, a significant amount of effort and resources have been placed upon vaccine development, and it is anticipated that CMV vaccination could be relatively commonplace in the future [108, 109]. In 2009, Pass et al. reported that administration of an adjuvanted recombinant CMV envelope glycoprotein B vaccine achieved about 50% efficacy in seronegative adults and also seemed to have some efficacy in preventing viral transmission from seropositive mothers to newborn infants [110].

Epstein–Barr virus (EBV), the causative agent of mononucleosis, is acquired by over 90% of individuals in industrialized Western nations by the age of 40. Like CMV, it is never wholly cleared by the immune system and can be reactivated following HSCT or myeloablative chemotherapy, resulting in a spectrum of uncontrolled lymphoproliferative diseases. Though the condition is known as posttransplant lymphoproliferative disease (PTLD) in the transplant setting, it can occur under any circumstance in which immune suppression exists. Treatment of EBV-associated PTLD consists primarily of reducing immunosuppressive treatment regimens; there are however, a number of other active therapies including adoptive immunotherapy, chemoprophylaxis (i.e., with acyclovir or ganciclovir), α-interferon, anti-B-cell antibodies, and anti-IL-6 antibodies [5]. The presence of EBV-associated disease among healthy individuals (i.e., mononucleosis) and the association of EBV infection with a variety of malignancies suggest that the population at large could benefit from an efficacious vaccine, and efforts at vaccine development are apparent in the literature [111–113].

Community acquired respiratory viruses such as respiratory syncytial virus (RSV), influenza, parainfluenza, and rhinovirus play a very significant role in morbidity and mortality of the immunocompromised host. Clinical experience at the Fred Hutchinson Cancer Research Center, the University of Texas MD Anderson Cancer Center, and The European Group for Blood and Marrow Transplantation indicates that mortality can approach 63% following RSV infection, 43% following influenza infection, 16% following parainfluenza infection, and 31% following rhinovirus infection among oncology populations [5, 50, 114–121]. While the development of vaccination strategies for large subgroups of multivalent vectors is an inherently challenging proposition, some progress is being made toward the development and implementation of universal RSV vaccination [122] and parainfluenza virus vaccination [123] among pediatric populations. Even if such efforts are slow to result in a vaccine that might be appropriate for immunocompromised oncology populations, enhancements to herd immunity should dramatically reduce the incidence of infection among all populations. Nonetheless, given the ubiquity and infectiousness of these broad groups of viruses, infection control strategies will necessarily play a crucial role in the prevention of acquisition and transmission for the foreseeable future.

Other important viruses that may affect immunocompromised oncology populations include adenovirus and polyomavirus. Adenovirus infection has been reported in up to 21% of HSCT recipients and is a major contributor to mortality in about 10% of these patients. Common serotypes isolated from oncology patients include 1, 2, and 5; however, the existence of nearly 50 clinically relevant serotypes confounds reasonable efforts at vaccine production [5, 124–129]; moreover, adenoviral infections are of limited pathological relevance in immunocompetent populations. The two clinically relevant polyomaviruses, JC virus and BK virus, ubiquitously infect most individuals by adolescence, establishing latent infections in kidney, blood, and brain. Polyomavirus reactivation following HSCT most commonly presents as progressive multifocal leukoencephalopathy (PML), interstitial nephritis, or hemorrhagic cystitis (HC) [5]. As with adenovirus, there do not appear to be any serious candidate polyomavirus vaccines currently in the clinical development pipeline.

Eukaryotic Infections

The profound neutropenia and mucosal toxicity induced by myeloablative chemotherapy and/or cytotoxic conditioning regimens allow a number of yeasts to establish opportunistic infections in oncology patients. *Candida, Trichosporon*, and *Malassezia* species may be observed among individuals with immune suppression. Individuals with prolonged immune suppression including recipients of HSCT and chronic corticosteroid use are also susceptible to infection by *Cryptococcus neoformans* and endemic dimorphic fungi like *Histoplasma, Blastomyces,* and *Coccidioides* species. Systemic disseminated candidiasis may have an associated mortality as high as 60%, despite aggressive intervention and chemoprophylaxis with a variety of antifungal drugs [5, 130–133]. Closely related to yeast species, molds are another eukaryotic pathogen that are very important in the oncology setting. Most invasive mold infections are caused by *Aspergillus*, particularly *A. fumigatus*, but *Scedosporium, Fusarium,* and zygomycotic fungi of the *Rhizopus, Mucor,* and *Rhizomucor* genera are also important clinical pathogens. As with yeast species, chemoprophylaxis is the mainstay of prevention and treatment in immunosuppressed patient populations. Aspergillosis is a common complication following HSCT with mortality exceeding 80% in leukemic patients with refractory cancer and prolonged neutropenia [5, 134]. Mortality following infection with *Scedosporium* and *Fusarium* species is also exceedingly high with few, if any, neutropenic or myelosuppressed patients recovering in the absence of immune reconstitution and recovery of immune function [5, 135–138]. Yet in spite of the clear need for alternative treatment regimens to eukaryotic pathogens, eukaryotic vaccine development appears limited primarily to preclinical efforts [139].

Summary

Prophylactic vaccination of oncology patients is a safe an extremely cost-effective way to manage common infections that play a significant role in morbidity and mortality. For maximal effectiveness, patients should be vaccinated with inactivated vaccines at least 2 weeks prior or 3 months subsequent to myeloablative chemotherapy. Hematopoietic stem cell transplant recipients should similarly be vaccinated at least 2 weeks prior to transplant or 6–12 months posttransplant, immune reconstitution permitting. When these guidelines are followed, seroconversion among oncology patients rivals that of healthy controls, and immunity to disease can be fairly robust. Vaccination of patients with B-cell malignancies is more problematic, but difficulties can be somewhat ameliorated by applying higher doses of vaccine in greater frequencies than would be typical for immunocompetent individuals. Live vaccines are typically considered to be inappropriate for oncology patients, but may be safely administered to HSCT recipients who are >2 years posttransplant. While many common infections can be managed through a strategy of conscientious vaccination, there are many other serious infections that specifically afflict immunocompromised patient populations and for which effective vaccines do not yet exist. While vaccines that will address some of these infectious conditions are currently in development, it is unlikely that all important oncological infections will ultimately be addressed by a vaccine approach as market-based development strategies are unlikely to target infections with a negligible impact upon immunocompetent populations. For these niche infections, it will be a continuing challenge for physicians and scientists to apply innovative and cost-effective approaches to disease management.

References

1. Sommer AL, Wachel BK, Smith JA. Evaluation of vaccine dosing in patients with solid tumors receiving myelosuppressive chemotherapy. J Oncol Pharm Pract. 2006;12:143–54.
2. Cohen JI. Strategies for herpes zoster vaccination of immunocompromised patients. J Infect Dis. 2008;197 Suppl 2:S237–41.
3. Kunisaki KM, Janoff EN. Influenza in immunosuppressed populations: a review of infection frequency, morbidity, mortality, and vaccine responses. Lancet Infect Dis. 2009;9:493–504.
4. Wilck MB, Baden LR. Vaccination after stem cell transplant: a review of recent developments and implications for current practice. Curr Opin Infect Dis. 2008;21:399–408.
5. Transplant Infections, 3rd edition, Bowden RA, Ljungman P, and Snydman DR, eds. Lippincott, Williams, and Wilkins, Philadelphia; 2010.
6. Chen W, Wahl SM. TGF-beta: the missing link in CD4+CD25+ regulatory T cell-mediated immunosuppression. Cytokine Growth Factor Rev. 2003;14:85–9.
7. Humphries W, Wei J, Sampson JH, Heimberger AB. The role of tregs in glioma-mediated immunosuppression: potential target for intervention. Neurosurg Clin N Am. 2010;21:125–37.
8. Kirkbride KC, Blobe GC. Inhibiting the TGF-beta signalling pathway as a means of cancer immunotherapy. Expert Opin Biol Ther. 2003;3:251–61.
9. Li MO, Flavell RA. TGF-beta: a master of all T cell trades. Cell. 2008;134:392–404.
10. Nagaraj S, Gabrilovich DI. Tumor escape mechanism governed by myeloid-derived suppressor cells. Cancer Res. 2008;68:2561–3.
11. Pan PY, Ma G, Weber KJ, et al. Immune stimulatory receptor CD40 is required for T-cell suppression and t regulatory cell activation mediated by myeloid-derived suppressor cells in cancer. Cancer Res. 2009;70(1):99–108.
12. Allavena P, Piemonti L, Longoni D, et al. IL-10 prevents the differentiation of monocytes to dendritic cells but promotes their maturation to macrophages. Eur J Immunol. 1998;28:359–69.
13. Beckebaum S, Zhang X, Chen X, et al. Increased levels of interleukin-10 in serum from patients with hepatocellular carcinoma correlate with profound numerical deficiencies and immature phenotype of circulating dendritic cell subsets. Clin Cancer Res. 2004;10:7260–9.
14. Buelens C, Verhasselt V, De GD, et al. Interleukin-10 prevents the generation of dendritic cells from human peripheral blood mononuclear cells cultured with interleukin-4 and granulocyte/macrophage-colony-stimulating factor. Eur J Immunol. 1997;27:756–62.
15. Enk AH, Angeloni VL, Udey MC, Katz SI. Inhibition of Langerhans cell antigen-presenting function by IL-10. A role for IL-10 in induction of tolerance. J Immunol. 1993;151:2390–8.

16. Ludewig B, Graf D, Gelderblom HR, et al. Spontaneous apoptosis of dendritic cells is efficiently inhibited by TRAP (CD40-ligand) and TNF-alpha, but strongly enhanced by interleukin-10. Eur J Immunol. 1995;25:1943–50.
17. Menetrier-Caux C, Montmain G, Dieu MC, et al. Inhibition of the differentiation of dendritic cells from CD34(+) progenitors by tumor cells: role of interleukin-6 and macrophage colony-stimulating factor. Blood. 1998;92:4778–91.
18. Park SJ, Nakagawa T, Kitamura H, et al. IL-6 regulates in vivo dendritic cell differentiation through STAT3 activation. J Immunol. 2004;173:3844–54.
19. Pinzon-Charry A, Maxwell T, Lopez JA. Dendritic cell dysfunction in cancer: a mechanism for immunosuppression. Immunol Cell Biol. 2005;83:451–61.
20. Ratta M, Fagnoni F, Curti A, et al. Dendritic cells are functionally defective in multiple myeloma: the role of interleukin-6. Blood. 2002;100:230–7.
21. Cohen N, Mouly E, Hamdi H, et al. GILZ expression in human dendritic cells redirects their maturation and prevents antigen-specific T lymphocyte response. Blood. 2006;107:2037–44.
22. Gabrilovich D, Ishida T, Oyama T, et al. Vascular endothelial growth factor inhibits the development of dendritic cells and dramatically affects the differentiation of multiple hematopoietic lineages in vivo. Blood. 1998;92:4150–66.
23. Gottfried E, Kreutz M, Mackensen A. Tumor-induced modulation of dendritic cell function. Cytokine Growth Factor Rev. 2008;19:65–77.
24. Kusmartsev S, Nefedova Y, Yoder D, Gabrilovich DI. Antigen-specific inhibition of CD8+ T cell response by immature myeloid cells in cancer is mediated by reactive oxygen species. J Immunol. 2004;172:989–99.
25. Lissoni P, Malugani F, Bonfanti A, et al. Abnormally enhanced blood concentrations of vascular endothelial growth factor (VEGF) in metastatic cancer patients and their relation to circulating dendritic cells, IL-12 and endothelin-1. J Biol Regul Homeost Agents. 2001;15:140–4.
26. Pak AS, Wright MA, Matthews JP, et al. Mechanisms of immune suppression in patients with head and neck cancer: presence of CD34(+) cells which suppress immune functions within cancers that secrete granulocyte-macrophage colony-stimulating factor. Clin Cancer Res. 1995;1:95–103.
27. Saito H, Tsujitani S, Ikeguchi M, Maeta M, Kaibara N. Relationship between the expression of vascular endothelial growth factor and the density of dendritic cells in gastric adenocarcinoma tissue. Br J Cancer. 1998;78:1573–7.
28. Serafini P, Carbley R, Noonan KA, et al. High-dose granulocyte-macrophage colony-stimulating factor-producing vaccines impair the immune response through the recruitment of myeloid suppressor cells. Cancer Res. 2004;64:6337–43.
29. Takahashi A, Kono K, Ichihara F, et al. Vascular endothelial growth factor inhibits maturation of dendritic cells induced by lipopolysaccharide, but not by proinflammatory cytokines. Cancer Immunol Immunother. 2004;53:543–50.
30. Young MR, Wright MA, Lozano Y, et al. Increased recurrence and metastasis in patients whose primary head and neck squamous cell carcinomas secreted granulocyte-macrophage colony-stimulating factor and contained CD34+ natural suppressor cells. Int J Cancer. 1997;74:69–74.
31. Bonham CA, Lu L, Li Y, et al. Nitric oxide production by mouse bone marrow-derived dendritic cells: implications for the regulation of allogeneic T cell responses. Transplantation. 1996;62:1871–7.
32. Della BS, Gennaro M, Vaccari M, et al. Altered maturation of peripheral blood dendritic cells in patients with breast cancer. Br J Cancer. 2003;89:1463–72.
33. Kanto T, Kalinski P, Hunter OC, Lotze MT, Amoscato AA. Ceramide mediates tumor-induced dendritic cell apoptosis. J Immunol. 2001;167:3773–84.
34. Peguet-Navarro J, Sportouch M, Popa I, et al. Gangliosides from human melanoma tumors impair dendritic cell differentiation from monocytes and induce their apoptosis. J Immunol. 2003;170:3488–94.
35. Shurin GV, Shurin MR, Bykovskaia S, et al. Neuroblastoma-derived gangliosides inhibit dendritic cell generation and function. Cancer Res. 2001;61:363–9.
36. Sombroek CC, Stam AG, Masterson AJ, et al. Prostanoids play a major role in the primary tumor-induced inhibition of dendritic cell differentiation. J Immunol. 2002;168:4333–43.
37. Yang L, Yamagata N, Yadav R, et al. Cancer-associated immunodeficiency and dendritic cell abnormalities mediated by the prostaglandin EP2 receptor. J Clin Invest. 2003;111:727–35.
38. Yang T, Witham TF, Villa L, et al. Glioma-associated hyaluronan induces apoptosis in dendritic cells via inducible nitric oxide synthase: implications for the use of dendritic cells for therapy of gliomas. Cancer Res. 2002;62:2583–91.
39. Aalamian M, Tourkova IL, Chatta GS, et al. Inhibition of dendropoiesis by tumor derived and purified prostate specific antigen. J Urol. 2003;170:2026–30.
40. Hiltbold EM, Vlad AM, Ciborowski P, Watkins SC, Finn OJ. The mechanism of unresponsiveness to circulating tumor antigen MUC1 is a block in intracellular sorting and processing by dendritic cells. J Immunol. 2000;165:3730–41.
41. Monti P, Leone BE, Zerbi A, et al. Tumor-derived MUC1 mucins interact with differentiating monocytes and induce IL-10highIL-12low regulatory dendritic cell. J Immunol. 2004;172:7341–9.
42. Muller AJ, Prendergast GC. Indoleamine 2, 3-dioxygenase in immune suppression and cancer. Curr Cancer Drug Targets. 2007;7:31–40.
43. Munn DH, Mellor AL. Indoleamine 2, 3-dioxygenase and tumor-induced tolerance. J Clin Invest. 2007;117:1147–54.
44. Bukur J, Seliger B. The role of HLA-G for protection of human renal cell-carcinoma cells from immune-mediated lysis: implications for immunotherapies. Semin Cancer Biol. 2003;13:353–9.
45. Pistoia V, Morandi F, Wang X, Ferrone S. Soluble HLA-G: are they clinically relevant? Semin Cancer Biol. 2007;17:469–79.
46. Hamblin AD, Hamblin TJ. The immunodeficiency of chronic lymphocytic leukaemia. Br Med Bull. 2008;87:49–62.
47. Couch RB, Englund JA, Whimbey E. Respiratory viral infections in immunocompetent and immunocompromised persons. Am J Med. 1997;102:2–9.
48. Elting LS, Whimbey E, Lo W, et al. Epidemiology of influenza A virus infection in patients with acute or chronic leukemia. Support Care Cancer. 1995;3:198–202.
49. Hassan IA, Chopra R, Swindell R, Mutton KJ. Respiratory viral infections after bone marrow/peripheral stem-cell transplantation: the Christie hospital experience. Bone Marrow Transplant. 2003;32:73–7.
50. Ljungman P. Respiratory virus infections in bone marrow transplant recipients: the European perspective. Am J Med. 1997;102:44–7.
51. Ljungman P. Respiratory virus infections in stem cell transplant patients: the European experience. Biol Blood Marrow Transplant. 2001;7(Suppl):5S–7.
52. Machado CM, Boas LS, Mendes AV, et al. Low mortality rates related to respiratory virus infections after bone marrow transplantation. Bone Marrow Transplant. 2003;31:695–700.
53. Nichols WG, Guthrie KA, Corey L, Boeckh M. Influenza infections after hematopoietic stem cell transplantation: risk factors, mortality, and the effect of antiviral therapy. Clin Infect Dis. 2004;39:1300–6.

54. Schepetiuk S, Papanaoum K, Qiao M. Spread of influenza A virus infection in hospitalised patients with cancer. Aust NZ J Med. 1998;28:475–6.
55. Whimbey E, Elting LS, Couch RB, et al. Influenza A virus infections among hospitalized adult bone marrow transplant recipients. Bone Marrow Transplant. 1994;13:437–40.
56. Yousuf HM, Englund J, Couch R, et al. Influenza among hospitalized adults with leukemia. Clin Infect Dis. 1997;24:1095–9.
57. Chemaly RF, Ghosh S, Bodey GP, et al. Respiratory viral infections in adults with hematologic malignancies and human stem cell transplantation recipients: a retrospective study at a major cancer center. Medicine (Baltimore). 2006;85:278–87.
58. Anderson H, Petrie K, Berrisford C, et al. Seroconversion after influenza vaccination in patients with lung cancer. Br J Cancer. 1999;80:219–20.
59. Brydak LB, Guzy J, Starzyk J, Machala M, Gozdz SS. Humoral immune response after vaccination against influenza in patients with breast cancer. Support Care Cancer. 2001;9:65–8.
60. Ganz PA, Shanley JD, Cherry JD. Responses of patients with neoplastic diseases to influenza virus vaccine. Cancer. 1978;42:2244–7.
61. Nordoy T, Aaberge IS, Husebekk A, et al. Cancer patients undergoing chemotherapy show adequate serological response to vaccinations against influenza virus and *Streptococcus pneumoniae*. Med Oncol. 2002;19:71–8.
62. Ortbals DW, Liebhaber H, Presant CA, Van III AA, Lee JY. Influenza immunization of adult patients with malignant diseases. Ann Intern Med. 1977;87:552–7.
63. Chisholm J, Howe K, Taj M, Zambon M. Influenza immunisation in children with solid tumours. Eur J Cancer. 2005;41:2280–7.
64. Chisholm JC, Devine T, Charlett A, Pinkerton CR, Zambon M. Response to influenza immunisation during treatment for cancer. Arch Dis Child. 2001;84:496–500.
65. Gross PA, Lee H, Wolff JA, et al. Influenza immunization in immunosuppressed children. J Pediatr. 1978;92:30–5.
66. Lange B, Shapiro SA, Waldman MT, Proctor E, Arbeter A. Antibody responses to influenza immunization of children with acute lymphoblastic leukemia. J Infect Dis. 1979;140:402–6.
67. Engelhard D, Nagler A, Hardan I, et al. Antibody response to a two-dose regimen of influenza vaccine in allogeneic T cell-depleted and autologous BMT recipients. Bone Marrow Transplant. 1993;11:1–5.
68. Gandhi MK, Egner W, Sizer L, et al. Antibody responses to vaccinations given within the first two years after transplant are similar between autologous peripheral blood stem cell and bone marrow transplant recipients. Bone Marrow Transplant. 2001;28:775–81.
69. Hodges GR, Davis JW, Lewis Jr HD, et al. Response to influenza A vaccine among high-risk patients. South Med J. 1979;72:29–32.
70. Robertson JD, Nagesh K, Jowitt SN, et al. Immunogenicity of vaccination against influenza, *Streptococcus pneumoniae* and *Haemophilus influenzae* type B in patients with multiple myeloma. Br J Cancer. 2000;82:1261–5.
71. Schafer AI, Churchill WH, Ames P, Weinstein L. The influence of chemotherapy on response of patients with hematologic malignancies to influenza vaccine. Cancer. 1979;43:25–30.
72. Safdar A, Rodriguez MA, Fayad LE, et al. Dose-related safety and immunogenicity of baculovirus-expressed trivalent influenza vaccine: a double-blind, controlled trial in adult patients with non-Hodgkin B cell lymphoma. J Infect Dis. 2006;194:1394–7.
73. Grant RM, Weitzman SS, Sherman CG, et al. Fulminant disseminated Varicella Zoster virus infection without skin involvement. J Clin Virol. 2002;24:7–12.
74. Stratman E. Visceral zoster as the presenting feature of disseminated herpes zoster. J Am Acad Dermatol. 2002;46:771–4.
75. Tauro S, Toh V, Osman H, Mahendra P. Varicella zoster meningoencephalitis following treatment for dermatomal zoster in an alloBMT patient. Bone Marrow Transplant. 2000;26:795–6.
76. Redman RL, Nader S, Zerboni L, et al. Early reconstitution of immunity and decreased severity of herpes zoster in bone marrow transplant recipients immunized with inactivated varicella vaccine. J Infect Dis. 1997;176:578–85.
77. Hata A, Asanuma H, Rinki M, et al. Use of an inactivated varicella vaccine in recipients of hematopoietic-cell transplants. N Engl J Med. 2002;347:26–34.
78. Molrine DC, George S, Tarbell N, et al. Antibody responses to polysaccharide and polysaccharide-conjugate vaccines after treatment of Hodgkin disease. Ann Intern Med. 1995;123:828–34.
79. Levine AM, Overturf GD, Field RF, et al. Use and efficacy of pneumococcal vaccine in patients with Hodgkin disease. Blood. 1979;54:1171–5.
80. Hartkamp A, Mulder AH, Rijkers GT, van Velzen-Blad H, Biesma DH. Antibody responses to pneumococcal and haemophilus vaccinations in patients with B-cell chronic lymphocytic leukaemia. Vaccine. 2001;19:1671–7.
81. Siber GR, Weitzman SA, Aisenberg AC. Antibody response of patients with Hodgkin's disease to protein and polysaccharide antigens. Rev Infect Dis. 1981;3(Suppl):S144–59.
82. Siber GR, Gorham C, Martin P, Corkery JC, Schiffman G. Antibody response to pretreatment immunization and post-treatment boosting with bacterial polysaccharide vaccines in patients with Hodgkin's disease. Ann Intern Med. 1986;104:467–75.
83. Engelhard D, Cordonnier C, Shaw PJ, et al. Early and late invasive pneumococcal infection following stem cell transplantation: a European Bone Marrow Transplantation survey. Br J Haematol. 2002;117:444–50.
84. Kulkarni S, Powles R, Treleaven J, et al. Chronic graft versus host disease is associated with long-term risk for pneumococcal infections in recipients of bone marrow transplants. Blood. 2000;95:3683–6.
85. Sheridan JF, Tutschka PJ, Sedmak DD, Copelan EA. Immunoglobulin G subclass deficiency and pneumococcal infection after allogeneic bone marrow transplantation. Blood. 1990;75:1583–6.
86. Ek T, Mellander L, Hahn-Zoric M, Abrahamsson J. Intensive treatment for childhood acute lymphoblastic leukemia reduces immune responses to diphtheria, tetanus, and Haemophilus influenzae type b. J Pediatr Hematol Oncol. 2004;26:727–34.
87. Barra A, Cordonnier C, Preziosi MP, et al. Immunogenicity of Haemophilus influenzae type b conjugate vaccine in allogeneic bone marrow recipients. J Infect Dis. 1992;166:1021–8.
88. Guinan EC, Molrine DC, Antin JH, et al. Polysaccharide conjugate vaccine responses in bone marrow transplant patients. Transplantation. 1994;57:677–84.
89. Goyal S, Pai SK, Kelkar R, Advani SH. Hepatitis B vaccination in acute lymphoblastic leukemia. Leuk Res. 1998;22:193–5.
90. Locasciulli A, Santamaria M, Masera G, et al. Hepatitis B virus markers in children with acute leukemia: the effect of chemotherapy. J Med Virol. 1985;15:29–33.
91. Rosen HR, Stierer M, Wolf HM, Eibl MM. Impaired primary antibody responses after vaccination against hepatitis B in patients with breast cancer. Breast Cancer Res Treat. 1992;23:233–40.
92. Somjee S, Pai S, Kelkar R, Advani S. Hepatitis B vaccination in children with acute lymphoblastic leukemia: results of an intensified immunization schedule. Leuk Res. 1999;23:365–7.
93. Somjee S, Pai S, Parikh P, et al. Passive active prophylaxis against Hepatitis B in children with acute lymphoblastic leukemia. Leuk Res. 2002;26:989–92.
94. Weitberg AB, Weitzman SA, Watkins E, et al. Immunogenicity of hepatitis B vaccine in oncology patients receiving chemotherapy. J Clin Oncol. 1985;3:718–22.

95. Yetgin S, Tunc B, Koc A, et al. Two booster dose hepatitis B virus vaccination in patients with leukemia. Leuk Res. 2001;25:647–9.
96. Hovi L, Valle M, Siimes MA, Jalanko H, Saarinen UM. Impaired response to hepatitis B vaccine in children receiving anticancer chemotherapy. Pediatr Infect Dis J. 1995;14:931–5.
97. Zignol M, Peracchi M, Tridello G, et al. Assessment of humoral immunity to poliomyelitis, tetanus, hepatitis B, measles, rubella, and mumps in children after chemotherapy. Cancer. 2004;101:635–41.
98. Jaffe D, Papadopoulos EB, Young JW, et al. Immunogenicity of recombinant hepatitis B vaccine (rHBV) in recipients of unrelated or related allogeneic hematopoietic cell (HC) transplants. Blood. 2006;108:2470–5.
99. Ljungman P, Aschan J, Gustafsson B, et al. Long-term immunity to poliovirus after vaccination of allogeneic stem cell transplant recipients. Bone Marrow Transplant. 2004;34:1067–9.
100. Bosu SK, Ciudad H, Sinks LF, Ogra PI. Antibody response to poliovirus immunization in childhood leukemia. Med Pediatr Oncol. 1975;1:217–25.
101. Florax A, Ehlert K, Becker K, Vormoor J, Groll AH. Bordetella pertussis respiratory infection following hematopoietic stem cell transplantation: time for universal vaccination? Bone Marrow Transplant. 2006;38:639–40.
102. Kochethu G, Clark FJ, Craddock CF. Pertussis: should we vaccinate post transplant? Bone Marrow Transplant. 2006;37:793–4.
103. Suzuki N, Mizue N, Hori T, et al. Pertussis in adolescence after unrelated cord blood transplantation. Bone Marrow Transplant. 2003;32:967.
104. Ljungman P, Fridell E, Lonnqvist B, et al. Efficacy and safety of vaccination of marrow transplant recipients with a live attenuated measles, mumps, and rubella vaccine. J Infect Dis. 1989;159:610–5.
105. Ljungman P, Engelhard D, de la Cámara R, et al. Vaccination of stem cell transplant recipients: recommendations of the Infectious Diseases Working Party of the EBMT. Bone Marrow Transplant. 2005;35:737–46.
106. Machado CM, de Souza VA, Sumita LM, et al. Early measles vaccination in bone marrow transplant recipients. Bone Marrow Transplant. 2005;35:787–91.
107. Griffiths PD. CMV vaccine trial endpoints. J Clin Virol. 2009;46 Suppl 4:S64–7.
108. Schleiss MR. Cytomegalovirus vaccines: at last, a major step forward. Herpes. 2009;15:44–5.
109. Dekker CL, Arvin AM. One step closer to a CMV vaccine. N Engl J Med. 2009;360:1250–2.
110. Pass RF, Zhang C, Evans A, et al. Vaccine prevention of maternal cytomegalovirus infection. N Engl J Med. 2009;360:1191–9.
111. Lockey TD, Zhan X, Surman S, Sample CE, Hurwitz JL. Epstein–Barr virus vaccine development: a lytic and latent protein cocktail. Front Biosci. 2008;13:5916–27.
112. Moutschen M, Leonard P, Sokal EM, et al. Phase I/II studies to evaluate safety and immunogenicity of a recombinant gp350 Epstein–Barr virus vaccine in healthy adults. Vaccine. 2007;25:4697–705.
113. Sokal EM, Hoppenbrouwers K, Vandermeulen C, et al. Recombinant gp350 vaccine for infectious mononucleosis: a phase 2, randomized, double-blind, placebo-controlled trial to evaluate the safety, immunogenicity, and efficacy of an Epstein–Barr virus vaccine in healthy young adults. J Infect Dis. 2007;196:1749–53.
114. Bowden RA. Respiratory virus infections after marrow transplant: the Fred Hutchinson Cancer Research Center experience. Am J Med. 1997;102:27–30.
115. Champlin RE, Whimbey E. Community respiratory virus infections in bone marrow transplant recipients: the M.D. Anderson Cancer Center experience. Biol Blood Marrow Transplant. 2001;7(Suppl):8S–10.
116. Ghosh S, Champlin RE, Englund J, et al. Respiratory syncytial virus upper respiratory tract illnesses in adult blood and marrow transplant recipients: combination therapy with aerosolized ribavirin and intravenous immunoglobulin. Bone Marrow Transplant. 2000;25:751–5.
117. Ljungman P, Ward KN, Crooks BN, et al. Respiratory virus infections after stem cell transplantation: a prospective study from the Infectious Diseases Working Party of the European Group for Blood and Marrow Transplantation. Bone Marrow Transplant. 2001;28:479–84.
118. Nichols WG, Gooley T, Boeckh M. Community-acquired respiratory syncytial virus and parainfluenza virus infections after hematopoietic stem cell transplantation: the Fred Hutchinson Cancer Research Center experience. Biol Blood Marrow Transplant. 2001;7(Suppl):11S–5.
119. Nichols WG, Corey L, Gooley T, Davis C, Boeckh M. Parainfluenza virus infections after hematopoietic stem cell transplantation: risk factors, response to antiviral therapy, and effect on transplant outcome. Blood. 2001;98:573–8.
120. Whimbey E, Champlin RE, Couch RB, et al. Community respiratory virus infections among hospitalized adult bone marrow transplant recipients. Clin Infect Dis. 1996;22:778–82.
121. Whimbey E, Englund JA, Couch RB. Community respiratory virus infections in immunocompromised patients with cancer. Am J Med. 1997;102:10–8.
122. Schickli JH, Dubovsky F, Tang RS. Challenges in developing a pediatric RSV vaccine. Hum Vaccin. 2009;5:582–91.
123. Sato M, Wright PF. Current status of vaccines for parainfluenza virus infections. Pediatr Infect Dis J. 2008;27:S123–5.
124. Flomenberg P, Babbitt J, Drobyski WR, et al. Increasing incidence of adenovirus disease in bone marrow transplant recipients. J Infect Dis. 1994;169:775–81.
125. Howard DS, Phillips II GL, Reece DE, et al. Adenovirus infections in hematopoietic stem cell transplant recipients. Clin Infect Dis. 1999;29:1494–501.
126. La Rosa AM, Champlin RE, Mirza N, et al. Adenovirus infections in adult recipients of blood and marrow transplants. Clin Infect Dis. 2001;32:871–6.
127. Shields AF, Hackman RC, Fife KH, Corey L, Meyers JD. Adenovirus infections in patients undergoing bone-marrow transplantation. N Engl J Med. 1985;312:529–33.
128. Wasserman R, August CS, Plotkin SA. Viral infections in pediatric bone marrow transplant patients. Pediatr Infect Dis J. 1988;7:109–15.
129. Yolken RH, Bishop CA, Townsend TR, et al. Infectious gastroenteritis in bone-marrow-transplant recipients. N Engl J Med. 1982;306:1010–2.
130. Anaissie EJ, Kontoyiannis DP, O'Brien S, et al. Infections in patients with chronic lymphocytic leukemia treated with fludarabine. Ann Intern Med. 1998;129:559–66.
131. Bodey GP, Mardani M, Hanna HA, et al. The epidemiology of *Candida glabrata* and *Candida albicans* fungemia in immunocompromised patients with cancer. Am J Med. 2002;112:380–5.
132. Edwards Jr JE, Bodey GP, Bowden RA, et al. International conference for the development of a consensus on the management and prevention of severe Candidal infections. Clin Infect Dis. 1997;25:43–59.
133. Viscoli C, Girmenia C, Marinus A, et al. Candidemia in cancer patients: a prospective, multicenter surveillance study by the Invasive Fungal Infection Group (IFIG) of the European Organization for Research and Treatment of Cancer (EORTC). Clin Infect Dis. 1999;28:1071–9.
134. Baddley JW, Stroud TP, Salzman D, Pappas PG. Invasive mold infections in allogeneic bone marrow transplant recipients. Clin Infect Dis. 2001;32:1319–24.
135. Berenguer J, Rodriguez-Tudela JL, Richard C, et al. Deep infections caused by *Scedosporium prolificans*. A report on 16 cases in

Spain and a review of the literature. Scedosporium Prolificans Spanish Study Group. Medicine (Baltimore). 1997;76:256–65.
136. Boutati EI, Anaissie EJ. Fusarium, a significant emerging pathogen in patients with hematologic malignancy: ten years' experience at a cancer center and implications for management. Blood. 1997;90:999–1008.
137. Maertens J, Lagrou K, Deweerdt H, et al. Disseminated infection by *Scedosporium prolificans*: an emerging fatality among haematology patients. Case report and review. Ann Hematol. 2000;79:340–4.
138. Musa MO, Al EA, Halim M, et al. The spectrum of Fusarium infection in immunocompromised patients with haematological malignancies and in non-immunocompromised patients: a single institution experience over 10 years. Br J Haematol. 2000;108:544–8.
139. Ito JI, Lyons JM, az-Arevalo D, Hong TB, Kalkum M. Vaccine progress. Med Mycol. 2009;47 Suppl 1:S394–400.

Index

A

Abdominal infections, 12
Acanthamoeba spp., 477
Acinetobacter baumannii, 427–428, 491
Acneiform eruptions, 240
Acne keloidalis, 251
Acute generalized exanthematous pustulosis (AGEP), 238
Acute myeloid leukemia (AML), 525
    gemtuzumab ozogamicin, 57
    invasive mold infections, 264–265
Acyclovir
    antiviral resistance, HSV, 398
    varicella-zoster virus, 399–400
    VZV, 362–364
Adaptive immunity, CMV, 341–342
Adenovirus
    clinical presentation, 377
    diagnosis, 378
    HSCT recipients, 377–378
    immunocompromised patients, 377–378
    leukemia patients, 377–378
    prevention/vaccination, 378
    solid organ transplant patients, 378
    treatment, 378
Adoptive immunotherapy, CMV, 350–351
Aerobic gram-negative bacilli
    definition, 423–424
    enterobacteriaceae
        Escherichia coli, 424–426
        Klebsiella pneumoniae, 426
        Klebsiella species, 425
        magnetic resonance imaging, 425
        Serratia marcescens, 425
        spectrum of infections, 425
    nonfermentative
        Acinetobacter baumannii, 427–428
        antimicrobial stewardship, 429–430
        Chryseobacterium species, 428
        documented infections therapy, 429
        empiric therapy, 429
        frequency of infections, 426
        moderate-to-high-grade bacteremia frequency, 427
        Pseudomonas aeruginosa, 426–427
        Pseudomonas fluorescens, 428
        Stenotrophomonas maltophilia, 427
        treatment, 428
        trimethoprim/sulfamethoxazole (TMP/SMX), 427
    proportions, 424
Airway mucus impaction, 162–163
Alanine aminotransferase (ALT), HBV and HCV reactivation, 190, 191

Alemtuzumab, 457
    CLL, phase III clinical trials in, 55, 56
    CMV reactivation, 55–56
    prophylaxis, 56
    viral infections, 56
Allogeneic hematopoietic stem cell transplant (aHSCT)
    early posttransplant period
        antimicrobial therapy in, 19–20
        diagnostic procedures, 18–19
        fungal infections, 20
        neutropenia, epidemiology of infections, 17–18
        pulmonary infections and noninfectious complications, 19
    fever and infection, 17, 18
    intermediate posttransplant period
        bacterial and fungal infections, 21
        epidemiology of infections, 21
    late posttransplant period, epidemiology of infections, 22
    viral infections
        early, 20–21
        late, 22
Aminoglycosides, drug class, 451
Amphotericin B (AMB), 285
    antimicrobial prophylaxis, 536
    deoxycholate (dAMB), 307
    lipid complex (ABLC), 307, 308
Anaerobic gram-negative bacilli, 430
Angiogenin 4, 177
Anidulafungin, 323, 324
Antibacterial distribution
    antimicrobial agents, impact of cancer
        beta-lactams, 445
        breakpoints, 444–445
        cachexia, 445–446
        hypoproteinemia, 446
        impairment of organs, 444
        neutropenia and neutropenic fever, 445
        protein binding, 446
        surgery, 445
    drug–drug interactions
        drug absorption affection, 449
        drug class, 450–452
        drug metabolism and transporters, 449–450
        polypharmacy, 448
        potential drug interaction management, 448
        principles, 448–449
        therapeutic management, 447–448
    malignant effusions, 447
    pharmacokinetic/pharmacodynamic (PK/PD) indices, 444
    pharmacokinetics, 443–444
    tissue infections, 446–447

Antibacterial prophylaxis, 534–535
  neutropenic patients
    antibiotic prophylaxis, 522–523
    high risks patients, 522
    infection, 521–522
    myeloid growth factors, 523
    parameters affected, 522
    prevention strategies, 522, 523
    treatment, 523
  nonneutropenic patients
    chronic graft versus host disease (GVHD), 524
    impaired humoral immunity, 523
    splenectomy, 524
Antibiotic-coated catheter, 117–118
Antibiotics
  cycling
    antimicrobial resistance, 512–513
    ASP, 501–502
  neutropenic patient
    prophylaxis, antibacterial, 522–523
    therapy, 7–8
Anti-CD2 antibodies, 58
Anti-CD3 antibodies, 58
Anti-CD4 antibodies, 57–58
Anti-CD20 antibodies
  radioimmunoconjugates, 54
  rituximab, 48–54
  second-generation, 54, 55
Anti-CD22 antibodies, 57
Anti-CD23 antibodies, 57
Anti-CD33 antibodies, 57
Anti-CD52 antibodies, 54–56
Antifungal drug resistance
  anidulafungin, 323, 324
  breakthrough infections, 324
  caspofungin, 323–325
  echinocandin
    drugs, 323
    resistance, 324
  elevated MICs, 325
  Erg11, 318
  Fks
    mediated resistance, 325
    mutations, 324
    non-Fks mechanisms, 325
  fungal susceptibility, 318–320, 323
  glucan synthase, 323–325
  invasive fungal infections, 317
  itraconazole, 322
  mechanisms, 318, 320
  micafungin, 323, 324
  minimal inhibitory concentration (MIC), 324
  newer triazole antifungals
    CYP51p, 318, 320
    systemic, 318, 319
  pharmacokinetic variability
    posaconazole, 322–323
    voriconazole, 320–322
  in vitro susceptibilities, 324
Antifungal prophylaxis, 535–536
  antimold prophylaxis, 527
  Candida krusei, 524–525
  neutropenic patients
    acute myeloid leukemia (AML), 525
    Aspergillus, primary, 525–526
    candidiasis, primary, 524–525
    chemotherapy regimens, duration of, 524
    fluconazole, 524–525
    invasive fungal infections (IFI), 524
    posaconazole, 525
    risk assessment, 524
    secondary prophylaxis, 526
  nonneutropenic patients, 526–527
Antifungal susceptibility testing, in vitro
  Aspergillus species
    Aspergillus fumigatus, 305–306
    Aspergillus terreus, 306
    echinocandins, 306
    MIC distributions, 305, 306
    resistance mechanisms, 306
  Candida species
    amphotericin B (AMB), 305
    Candida krusei, 304
    CLSI standardized method, 305
    drugs, 305
    fluconazole treatment, 304
    MIC interpretative criteria, 304
  moulds, 305
  non-Aspergillus moulds, 307
Antifungal therapies. See also Antifungal drug resistance
  cryptococcal disease, 294–295
  histoplasmosis, 298
  invasive aspergillosis (IA)
    clinical data, 311–312
    clinical trials, 309, 310
    preclinical data, 309, 311
Antiinfective-impregnated catheters, catheter salvage, 129
Antiinfective lock solutions, catheter salvage, 129–130
Antiinfective lock therapy (ALT), catheter salvage
  adjunctive treatment, studies of, 133
  concentrations of, 134
Antiinfective luer-activated devices, catheter salvage, 130
Anti-interleukin-2 receptor antibodies, hematologic malignancies
  basiliximab, 59
  daclizumab, 58–59
  denileukin diftitox, 58
Anti-interleukin-6-receptor antibodies, hematologic malignancies, 59
Antimicrobial prophylaxis
  amphotericin B, 536
  Aspergillus species, 535, 538
  Candida infections, 535, 538
  caspofungin, 536
  clinical trials
    antibacterial prophylaxis, 534–535
    antifungal prophylaxis, 535–536
    guidelines, neutropenic patients, 537–538
  considerations, 536–537
  drugs role, 538
  fatal infections, 537
  fungal infections, 535, 537
  gram-negative sepsis, 537
  life-threatening infection, 533
  micafungin, 536
  neutropenia, 538
Antimicrobial resistance
  ASP
    Clostridium difficile associated diarrhea (CDAD), 501
    febrile neutropenia, 499–500
    Klebsiella pneumoniae carbapenemases (KPC), 500
    vancomycin resistant enterococci, 500
  prevention
    antibiotic cycling, 512–513

carbapenemases, 508
CDC, 510–512
Enterobacteriaceae, 508
Enterococcus faecium, 507–508
gram-negative organisms, 508
gram-positive bacteria infections, 507
hospitalized patients, 510, 511
infection control strategies, 510–512
Listeria monocytogenes, 514
mathematical models, antibiotic resistance, 509–510
methicillin-resistant *Staphylococcus aureus* (MRSA), 507
multiresistant bacterial organisms, 507, 508
nanograms, 514
narrow spectrum, 513–514
organisms, 507
phage-based therapy, 514
search and destroy approach, 510
shorter antibiotic courses, 513–514
strategies, 509–510
treatment, 512–514
Antimicrobials
agents, impact of cancer
beta-lactams, 445
breakpoints, 444–445
cachexia, 445–446
hypoproteinemia, 446
impairment of organs, 444
neutropenia and neutropenic fever, 445
protein binding, 446
surgery, 445
coating, of catheters, 116
peptides, 177–178
therapy, aHSCT
duration of, 20
neutropenic fever, 19–20
Antimicrobial stewardship
neutropenia, 101, 102
NFGNB, 429–430
Antimicrobial stewardship program (ASP)
Acinetobacter baumannii, 491
antibiotic cycling, 501–502
antimicrobial resistance
Clostridium difficile associated diarrhea (CDAD), 501
febrile neutropenia, 499–500
Klebsiella pneumoniae carbapenemases (KPC), 500
vancomycin resistant enterococci, 500
barriers and challenges, 494–495
Clostridium difficile infection (CDI), 491
computer-based infrastructure, 492
emerging infections network (EIN), 494–495
fluoroquinolones, 503
gram-negative (GN) organisms, 501
implementation of, 492
infectious diseases (ID), 492
injudicious antimicrobial use, 491
multidisciplinary team, 492–493
outpatient antibiotic therapy, 502–504
postprescribing review, 493–494
Pseudomonas aeruginosa, 501
strategies of, 493–494
streamlining, 494
Antimold prophylaxis, 527
Antimycobacterial immunity, *Mycobacterium tuberculosis* infection
alemtuzumab, 457
biology of, 455–456
bone marrow transplantation, 457

cancer therapies, 456–457
pharmacologic cancer therapy, 457
purine analogs, 457–458
risk factors, 456–457
states of susceptibility, 456
temozolamide, 458
TNF inhibitors, 458
Antiparasitic prophylaxis, 528
Antipneumocystis, 528
Antiseptic catheters, 117
Anti-TNFa monoclonal antibodies, hematologic malignancies, 59–60
Antiviral prophylaxis
CMV, 346–347
cytomegalovirus (CMV), 527
Epstein-Barr virus (EBV), 527–528
herpes simplex virus (HSV), 527
neutropenic patients, 527
varicella-zoster virus (VZV), 527
VZV, 364–365
Antiviral resistance
cytomegalovirus
ganciclovir, 400–401
hematopoietic stem cell transplantation, 400
prevention, 401
rheumatoid arthritis, 401
valganciclovir, 400
genotypic resistance, 397, 398
hepatitis B virus
lamivudine-resistant mutants, 403
prophylactic and therapeutic strategies, 402
vaccination, 403
herpes simplex virus
acyclovir, 398
cidofovir, 399
definition, 397–398
diagnosis, 399
leflunomide, 399
rheumatoid arthritis, 399
risk factors, 398–399
therapy, 399
toxicity, 399
influenza viruses
antiviral therapy, 401–402
diagnosis, 402
oseltamivir, 402
zanamivir, 402
varicella-zoster virus, 399–400
Apolizumab (Hu1D10), 60
Arthropod bites, immunocompromised traveler, 555, 556
Aseptic meningitis, 211–212
ASP. See Antimicrobial stewardship program (ASP)
Aspergillosis, 9, 257, 258, 287–288. See also Invasive aspergillosis (IA)
invasive fungal diseases, 331, 332
Aspergillus, antifungal prophylaxis, 525–526
Aspergillus fumigatus, 150, 283, 305–306
Aspergillus spp.
antifungal prophylaxis, 535
Aspergillus fumigatus, 305–306
Aspergillus terreus, 306
echinocandins, 306
infective endocarditis, 228
MIC distributions, 305, 306
neutropenic patients, 538
resistance mechanisms, 306
Autoimmune bullous dermatoses, 236–237

B

Bacillus Calmette-Guerin (BCG), 43
Bacteremia, 198
Bacterial colonization and host immunity
    gastrointestinal mucosa and intestinal immune responses
        adaptive immunity, 178
        antimicrobial peptides, 177–178
        dendritic cells (DCs), 177
        effector compartment, 178
        epithelial cells, types of, 176
        IgA and cytokines, 178–179
        initiation compartment, 178
    microbiota, 175–176
Bacterial infections, 7
    aHSCT, 21
Bacterial meningitis, acute, 211
Balamuthia mandrillaris, 477
Bartonella henseleae, 484
Basiliximab, 59
Behçet disease (BD), 239, 240
Beta-D-glucan assay, 284
    candidiasis, 263
    invasive candidiasis, 275
    invasive mold infections, 267
Beta-lactam antibiotics, 451
Bevacizumab, colon cancer, 42
BK virus (BKV)
    definition, 387
    hemorrhagic cystitis (HC)
        associated disease, 388–389
        cidofovir, 390
        clinical results, 390, 392
        definition, 388
        diagnosis, 389
        HCT recipients, 390
        intravenous immunoglobulin (IVIg), 390
        leflunomide, 390
        nephritis, 392
        organ manifestations, 392
        treatment, 389–391
    transmission and pathogenesis, 388
    viremia, 388
    virologic aspects, 387–388
Blastomyces dermatitidis, 294, 483
Blastomycosis
    Blastomyces dermatitidis, 296
    clinical symptoms, 296, 297
    diagnosis, 296
    immunosuppression, 296
Blood cultures, invasive candidiasis, 275
Bone marrow transplantation, 457
Bowel-associated dermatosis-arthritis syndrome, 239
Brain abscess
    clinical presentation, 213
    diagnosis and management of, 213
    etiology and risk factors, 212–213
    listeriosis, 438
Brain cancer, postoperative infections
    diagnosis of, 68
    etiology of, 68
    incidence of, 67–68
    prevention, 68
    risk factors, 68
    treatment of, 68
Brain stem encephalitis, 437–438

Breast cancer, 41–42
    breast cellulitis, 42
    interventions, surgical site infections
        diagnosis of, 71
        etiology of, 71
        incidence of, 70
        prevention, 71
        risk factors, 70–71
        treatment of, 71
Bronchial obstruction, pneumonia, 147–148
Bronchiolitis obliterans organizing pneumonia (BOOP), 158, 159
Bronchopleural fistula (BPF), 72
Bullous drug eruptions, 235–236
Bullous graft-*versus*-host-disease (GVHD), 235
Bullous insect bite reaction, 235
Bullous pemphigoid, 237

C

Cachexia, antimicrobial agents, 445–446
Calciphylaxis, 244
Candida infections
    antifungal prophylaxis, 535
    neutropenic patients, 535
Candida krusei, 304, 524–525
Candida spp., 9
    amphotericin B (AMB), 305
    Candida krusei, 304, 524–525
    catheter salvage, 135
    CLSI standardized method, 305
    CRBSI, 119
    drugs, 305
    echinocandin drugs, 323
    Fks-mediated resistance, 325
    fluconazole treatment, 304
    infective endocarditis, 227–228
    MIC interpretative criteria, 304
Candidemia
    and acute disseminated candidiasis, 278–279
    clinical presentation, 276
Candidiasis, 257
    antifungal prophylaxis, 524–525
    candidemia, diagnosis of
        beta-D-glucan assay, 263
        microbiology and culture, 262–263
        PCR, 263–264
    clinical syndromes, 262
    disseminated maculopapular skin rash, 262
    hepatosplenic, diagnosis of, 264
Capnocytophaga canimorsus, 482
Carbapenemases, antimicrobial resistance, 508
Cardiogenic (hydrostatic) pulmonary edema, 153–154
Caspofungin
    antifungal drug resistance, 323–325
    antimicrobial prophylaxis, 536
Catheter-related blood stream infection (CRBSI)
    CVCs, 113
    diagnosis of, 114
    genitourinary tract infections, 199
    management of
        Candida species, 119
        CoNS, 118
        gram negative bacilli, 119

Index

guide wire, exchange, 119–120
Micrococcus species, 119
Staphylococcus aureus, 119
maximal sterile barrier
antibiotic-coated catheter, 117–118
antimicrobial coating of, 116
antimicrobial lock solutions, 118
antiseptic catheters, 117
elements, 116
tunneling, 116
pathogenesis, 113
systemic catheter infections, 114
Catheter-related infections, 12–13, 465–466. *See also* Catheter-related blood stream infection (CRBSI)
biofilm, 118
with catheter removal, diagnostic tests
comparison of, 115
quantitative segment culture, 116
semiquantitative roll-plate culture, 115
clinical manifestations and definitions, 114
prevention of, 116, 117
without catheter removal, diagnostic tests
comparative quantitative blood culture, 114
differential time to positivity, 115
Catheter salvage, IVDR BSI
in prevention
antiinfective-impregnated catheters, 129
antiinfective lock solutions, 129–130
antiinfective luer-activated devices, 130
catheter securement, 130
chlorhexidine bathing, 129
chlorhexidine-impregnated insertion site dressings, 129
cutaneous antisepsis, 126
HICPAC guidelines, 125, 126
insertion site, 128
institutional systems, 131–132
intensive insulin therapy, 130–131
maximal barrier precautions, 128
simulation-based training, 128
strategies for, 127
topical antimicrobials, 126–128
treatment
antiinfective lock therapy, 133–134
Candida spp., 135
CoNS, 136
gram-negative bacilli, 136
guidewire exchange, 134
long-term cuffed and tunneled central venous catheter, 132
pathogen-specific recommendations, 134–135
Staphylococcus aureus, 135–136
urokinase, 134
Cat scratch disease, 484
Cell-mediated immunity, nocardiosis, 439–440
Cellular immune dysfunction, hematologic malignancies, 33, 34
Cellulitis, 201–202
Centers for Disease Control and Prevention (CDC), antimicrobial resistance, 510–512
Central nervous system (CNS)
cancer, 43–44
cryptococcal disease, 294
diagnosis, methodical approach, 207–208
histoplasmosis, 298
infectious syndromes and management
brain abscess, 212–213
encephalitis, 208–210

meningitis, 210–212
postoperative infections, 214
listeriosis, infection, 437
noninfectious problems
GVHD, 215
neoplastic meningitis, 214–215
PNS, 215
RPLS, 215
stem cell transplantation (SCT), 207
zygomycete infection, 308
Central venous catheters (CVCs), 79, 113
Chagas' disease, 477
Chemotherapy
Mycobacterium tuberculosis infection, 459–460
and radiation-related genitourinary tract infections
bacteremia, 198
catheter-related bloodstream infection, 199
febrile neutropenia, 198–199
Chemotherapy-induced acral blisters and erythema, 248
Chemotherapy-induced lung injury (CILI)
diagnosis, 154
drug toxicity, chronic manifestations of, 154
histopathologic changes in, 155
radiographic changes in, 155
steroid therapy, 156
Chest
computed tomographic hyperinfection syndrome, 475
computed tomography, 344
radiography, 344
Staphylococcus aureus, CT, 411
Children, postoperative infections
age, 78
blood transfusion, 79
CVCs, 79
minimally invasive surgery (MIS), 79
neutropenia, 79
nutrition, 79
type of tumor, 78–79
Chlamydia psittaci, 487
Chlorhexidine, catheter salvage, 129
Chronic lymphocytic leukemia (CLL), 35
Cidofovir
antiviral resistance, HSV, 399
BKV, 390
CMV, 348, 350
Ciprofloxacin, 451
Clarithromycin, 451
Clostridial bacteremia, 198
Clostridial myonecrosis, 203
Clostridium difficile associated diarrhea (CDAD), 501
Clostridium difficile infection (CDI), 491
diagnosis, 185
epidemiology and risk factors, 184–185
management, 186
pathogenesis, 185
prevention and control, 186
transplantation, 185
CNS. *See* Central nervous system (CNS)
Coagulase-negative staphylococci (CoNS), 412
catheter salvage, 136
CRBSI, 118
infective endocarditis, 226
Coccidiodes immitis, 295

Coccidioidomycosis
    azole antifungals, 296
    Coccidiodes immitis, 295
    diagnosis, 296
    T-cell immunity, 295
    unifocal/multifocal pulmonary disease, 295
Colon cancer, 42, 43
Colony stimulating factors (CSF), 333–334
Coma bullae, 234
Community-acquired pneumonia (CAP), 146
Computed tomography (CT) scan
    invasive mold infections, 264–265
    neutropenic enterocolitis, 183
Congestive heart failure, 153–154
Coronavirus
    clinical presentation, 380
    diagnosis, 381
    immunocompromised patients, 380
    prevention, 381
    treatment, 381
Cowpox virus, 485
Coxiella burnetii, 484
CRBSI. *See* Catheter-related blood stream infection (CRBSI)
C reactive protein (CRP), 107
Critically ill cancer patients
    critical care utilization
        diagnostic approach, 88–89
        life-threatening complications, 88
        scoring systems, 88
        therapy, 89
    ICU
        oncologists and infectious disease specialists, 87–88
        patient's goals, 88
    infectious complications, prevention of, 90
Cryptococcal disease
    AIDS epidemic, 293
    antifungal therapy, 294–295
    cancer patients, 295
    central nervous system, 294
    clinical findings, 293–295
    Cryptococcus neoformans, 293
    Cryptococcus species, 294
    infections, 293
    respiratory mycosis, 294
Cryptococcosis, 9
Cryptococcus neoformans, 293, 485
Cryptococcus species, 294
Cryptogenic organizing pneumonitis (COP), 160–161
Cryptosporidium spp., 478
Cutaneous antisepsis, catheter salvage, 126
Cutaneous T-cell lymphoma, 243
Cytochrome P450 isoenzymes, 449, 450
Cytokines, immunotherapy, 335, 336
Cytomegalovirus (CMV)
    adoptive immunotherapy, 350–351
    antiviral prophylaxis, 527
    antiviral resistance, 349–350
        ganciclovir, 400–401
        hematopoietic stem cell transplantation, 400
        prevention, 401
        rheumatoid arthritis, 401
        valganciclovir, 400
    chest computed tomography, 344
    chest radiography, 344
    cidofovir, 348, 350
    clinical manifestations, 344–345
    diagnosis
        anti-CMV immunostaining, 343
        hematoxylin and eosin (H&E) stain, 343
        methods, 342
        mRNA detection, 344
        quantitative polymerase chain reaction (qPCR), 343
        shell vial technique, 343
    foscarnet, 348
    ganciclovir-resistant, 349–350
    host immunity
        adaptive immunity, 341–342
        immune evasion, 342
        innate immunity, 342
    HSCT, 21
    less, 342
    management of, 350
    natural killer (NK) cells, 342
    non-HCT setting, 351
    pneumonia, 151, 344
    prevention
        antiviral agents, 347–348
        antiviral prophylaxis and pre-emptive therapy, 346–347
        immunoprophylaxis, 346
        monitoring and pre-emptive therapy, 348
        posttransplant risk reduction, 346–347
        pretransplant risk reduction, 346
        special populations, 348
    retinitis, 344–345
    risk factors
        after allogeneic HCT, 345
        allogeneic HCT recipients, 345
        autologous HCT, 346
        nonmyeloablative HCT, 345
        umbilical cord blood transplantation, 346
    rituximab, 52–53
    stem cell transplantation, 346
    structure and replication, 341
    vaccination, 350
    valganciclovir-resistant, 348, 349

D

Daclizumab, 58–59
Defensins, 177
Delayed pulmonary toxicity syndrome, 162
Dendritic cells (DCs), 177
Denileukin diftitox, 58
Dermatitis
    acute, 233
    irritant dermatitis, 241, 242
    radiation dermatitis, with erythema, 242
Diabetic blisters, 235
Diffuse alveolar damage (DAD), 157
Diffuse alveolar hemorrhage (DAH), 160
Dimorphic fungi, 331, 332
Dipylidium caninum, 484
Dirofilaria immiti, 484
Disseminated candidiasis
    acute, 278–279
    chronic, 279
    skin lesions in, 276
Disseminated intravascular coagulation (DIC), 244
Documented infections therapy, 429
Drug–drug interactions
    cytochrome P450 inhibitor, 449

cytochrome P450 isoenzymes, 449, 450
drug absorption affection, 449
drug class
  aminoglycosides, 451
  beta-lactam antibiotics, 451
  ciprofloxacin, 451
  erythromycin/clarithromycin, 451
  linezolid, 451
  metronidazole, 451
  moxifloxacin, 451
  rifamycin derivates, 450
  tigecycline, 452
  trimethoprim-sulfamethoxazole, 452
  vancomycin, 451
drug metabolism and transporters, 449–450
P-glycoprotein, 449
polypharmacy, 448
potential drug interaction management, 448
principles, 448–449
therapeutic management, 447–448

E

EBV. *See* Epstein-Barr virus (EBV)
Echinocandins, 278, 279, 285–286
  Aspergillus species, 306
  drugs, 323
  resistance, 324
  zygomycosis, 308
Edema and lymphedema bullae, 235
EGFR-induced acneiform pustulosis, 240
Emerging infections network (EIN), 494–495
Empiric therapy
  antibiotic, 98–100
  antifungal, 108–109, 287
  antimicrobial, 417
  febrile neutropenia, controversies in, 105–109
  NFGNB, 429
Encephalitis
  clinical manifestations of, 208
  diagnosis, 209
  immunocompetent host, 208, 210
  immunosuppressed host, 208–210
  parainfectious encephalitides, 208
  post-infectious/post-immunization, 209
  septic encephalopathy, 209
  treatment recommendations, 209–210
Endemic mycosis
  blastomycosis
    Blastomyces dermatitidis, 296
    clinical symptoms, 296, 297
    diagnosis, 296
  coccidioidomycosis
    azole antifungals, 296
    Coccidiodes immitis, 295
    diagnosis, 296
    T-cell immunity, 295
    unifocal/multifocal pulmonary disease, 295
  histoplasmosis
    antifungal therapy, 298
    central nervous system, 298
    clinical findings, 297
    culture of, 297
    Histoplasma antigen, 297
    Histoplasma capsulatum, 297
Endocarditis, 277. *See also* Infective endocarditis (IE)

Endophthalmitis, 276
End-organ infection, 12
Engraftment syndrome (ES), 159
Enteric pathogens, 552, 554–555
Enterobacteriaceae, 508
  Escherichia coli, 424–426
  Klebsiella pneumoniae, 426
  Klebsiella species, 425
  magnetic resonance imaging, 425
  Serratia marcescens, 425
  spectrum of infections, 425
Enterococcus
  clinical presentation/diagnosis, 416
  epidemiology, 416
  infective endocarditis, 227
  treatment, 416–417
Enterococcus faecium, 507–508
Enterovirus
  clinical presentation, 381
  diagnosis, 381
  immunocompromised patients, 381
  prevention, 381
  treatment, 381
Eosinophilic dermatoses, 249
Eosinophilic folliculitis, 240
Epithelial innate immunity, 168–169
Epstein-Barr virus (EBV)
  antiviral prophylaxis, 527–528
  B cell, 365
  immunocompromised hosts, 365–366
  transmission, 365
  treatment, 366
Erythema
  annulare centrifugum, 247–248
  and chemotherapy-induced acral blisters, 248
  gyratum repens, 247–248
  multiforme (EM), 246–247
  nodosum (EN), 245–246
Erythematous lesions
  chemotherapy-induced acral blisters and erythema, 248
  EM/SJS and TEN, 246–247
  eosinophilic dermatoses, 249
  erythema annulare centrifugum, 247, 248
  erythema gyratum repens, 247–248
  granuloma annulare, 248–249
  necrolytic migratory erythema, 248
  urticaria and angioedema, 246
Erythromycin, 451
Escherichia coli, 424–426
Esophageal cancer, postoperative infections
  diagnosis of, 73
  incidence of, 72
  prevention, 72
  risk factors, 72–73
  treatment of, 73
Esophagitis, invasive candidiasis, 276
Eukaryotic infections, 566–567

F

Febrile neutropenia
  algorithm for, 101
  ASP, 499–500
  empiric therapy, controversies in, 105
    acute phase protein responses, 107
    antibiotic regimen, 106

Febrile neutropenia (*cont.*)
    antifungal therapy, 107–109
    cause of, negative blood cultures, 106–107
    high risk for, 109
    genitourinary tract infections, 198–199
    low-risk
        antibiotic regimens in, 98
        outpatient management of, 99
        treatment options for, 98
Fks
  mediated resistance, 325
  mutations, 324
  non-Fks mechanisms, 325
Fluconazole, antifungal prophylaxis, 524–525
Fluoroquinolones, ASP, 503
Food and drink, infection prevention, 547–548
Foscarnet, CMV, 348
Friction blister, 234
Fungal infections, 8–10, 258. *See also* Invasive mold infections (IMIs)
  aHSCT, 20
  antifungal susceptibility testing, in vitro
    Aspergillus species, 305–307
    Candida species, 304–305
    moulds, 305
    non-*Aspergillus* moulds, 307
  antimicrobial prophylaxis, 535, 537
  combination antifungal therapy, 309–312
  invasive, 317
    preemptive therapy, 287
    risk factors, 284
  invasive aspergillosis (IA)
    clinical data, 311–312
    clinical trials, 309, 310
    micafungin (MICA), 311
    preclinical data, 309, 311
  therapeutic drug monitoring (TDM)
    parameters, 301, 302
    posaconazole, 303–304
    voriconazole, 301–303
  zygomycosis treatment
    adjunctive therapy, 309
    AMB deoxycholate (dAMB), 307
    animal data, 308
    antifungal agents, 307
    clinical data, 308–309
    in vitro data, 308
Fungal susceptibility, antifungal drug resistance, 318–320, 323
Fungi, infective endocarditis
  Aspergillus species, 227
  Candida species, 227–228
Fusariosis, 288
Fusarium spp., 9

G

Galactomannan
  EIA antigen, invasive mold infections, 266–267
  test, 284
Ganciclovir
  antiviral resistance, CMV, 400–401
  CMV, 349–350
Gastrointestinal mucosa and intestinal immune responses, bacterial colonization
  adaptive immunity, 178
  antimicrobial peptides, 177–178
  dendritic cells (DCs), 177
  effector compartment, 178
  epithelial cells, types of, 176
  IgA and cytokines, 178–179
  initiation compartment, 178
Gastrointestinal (GI) tract interventions, postoperative infections
  diagnosis of, 74
  etiology of, 74
  incidence of, 73
  microorganisms, 74
  prevention, 74–75
  risk factors, 73–74
  treatment of, 74
Gemtuzumab ozogamicin, 57
Genital and urinary tract neoplasms, postoperative infections
  diagnosis of, 76
  etiology of, 76
  gynecologic procedures, 75
  incidence of, 75
  prevention, 76–77
  risk factors, 75–76
  treatment of, 76
  vaginal cuff infection, 75
Genitourinary tract infections
  bowel preparation, 200
  chemotherapy and radiation-related
    bacteremia, 198
    catheter-related bloodstream infection, 199
    febrile neutropenia, 198–199
  factors, 195
  fever, noninfectious causes of, 204
  implantable device infections, 199
  microflora, 195
  peritonitis and intraabdominal abscess, 200–201
  predisposing risk factors and infections in, 196
  septic pelvic thrombophlebitis, 203–204
  surgery-related
    intraabdominal and pelvic abscess, 197–198
    wound infection, 197
  surgical infection, prevention of, 200
  tumor-related, 196
  wound infections
    cellulitis, 201–202
    clostridial myonecrosis, 203
    necrotizing fasciitis, 202–203
Glucan synthase, 323–325
Graft-*versus*-host-disease (GVHD)
  basiliximab, 59
  chronic, 524
  daclizumab, 58–59
  HSCT, 22
  Nikolsky sign and epidermal detachment, 235
Gram-negative bacilli
  aerobic
    definition, 423–424
    enterobacteriaceae, 424–426
    nonfermentative, 426–430
    proportions, 424
  anaerobic, 430
  catheter salvage, 136
  CRBSI, 119
  multi-drug-resistant (MDR), 423
Gram-negative (GN) organisms
  antimicrobial resistance, 508
  ASP, 501
Gram-positive bacteria infections, antimicrobial resistance, 507

Index

Gram-positive bacterial disease management
　invasive bacterial disease, 409, 410
　pathogens, 409, 410
　staphylococci
　　coagulase negative staphylococci, 412
　　Staphylococcus aureus, 409–412
　streptococci
　　definition, 412–413
　　empiric antimicrobial therapy, 417
　　enterococcus, 416–417
　　b-hemolytic streptococci, 414–415
　　Streptococcus pneumoniae, 415–416
　　viridans group streptococci, 413
Granulocyte transfusions, 334–335
Granuloma annulare, 248–249
Grover disease, 241
GU cancers, 43

H

Haemophilus influenzae type B (HiB), 564–565
Hair and scalp lesions, 250
Hand hygiene, 546–547
Head and neck cancer interventions, postoperative infections
　diagnosis of, 69
　etiology of, 69
　incidence of, 69
　prevention, 70
　risk factors, 69
　treatment of, 69–70
Healthcare Infection Control Practices Advisory Committee (HICPAC) guidelines, 125, 126
Hematologic malignancies
　acute leukemia, 34–35
　cellular immune dysfunction, 33, 34
　chronic lymphocytic leukemia, 35
　humoral immune dysfunction, 33–34
　immune defects in, 34, 35
　immune host-defects in
　　host defenses role, patient response, 28
　　infections control, 28
　　predominant pathogen association with, 29
　lymphoma, 36
　monoclonal antineoplastic therapy (*see* Monoclonal antineoplastic therapy, hematologic malignancies)
　mucosal impairment, 34
　myeloma, 35–36
　neutropenia
　　antifungal prophylaxis, 31
　　bacterial infections, epidemiology of, 30
　　candidemia, incidence of, 31
　　disseminated aspergillosis, 32
　　fungal infections, incidence of, 28, 30
　　hepatosplenic candidiasis, 29, 31
　　influenza and mucor pneumonia, 32
　　MRI of, 30
　　severe infection episodes, circulating neutrophils, 30
　qualitative phagocyte defects, 30–31
　splenic dysfunction, 34
Hematopoietic stem cell transplantation (HSCT). *See also* Allogeneic hematopoietic stem cell transplant (aHSCT)
　antiviral resistance, CMV, 400
　BKV, 387
　lung infiltrates, noninfectious complications of
　　early-onset, 159–160
　　late-onset, 160–162
　vaccination (*see* Prophylactic vaccination, HSCT)
　VZV, 360–362
Hematoxylin and eosin (H&E) stain, 343
b-Hemolytic streptococci
　clinical manifestations/diagnosis, 414
　definition, 414
　epidemiology, 414
　treatment, 414–415
Hemorrhagic cystitis (HC), BKV
　associated disease, 388–389
　cidofovir, 390
　clinical results, 390, 392
　definition, 388
　diagnosis, 389
　HCT recipients, 390
　intravenous immunoglobulin (IVIg), 390
　leflunomide, 390
　nephritis, 392
　organ manifestations, 392
　treatment, 389–391
Hepatitis B virus (HBV)
　antiviral resistance
　　lamivudine-resistant mutants, 403
　　prophylactic and therapeutic strategies, 402
　　vaccination, 403
　reactivation, antineoplastic therapy
　　definition, 189
　　frequency of, 189
　　management of, 190
　　pathogenesis and clinical manifestations, 189–190
　　risk factors, 190
　rituximab, 52
　vaccine, 565
Hepatitis C virus (HCV)
　reactivation, antineoplastic therapy
　　management of, 192
　　pathogenesis and clinical manifestations, 191–192
　　risk factors, 192
　rituximab, 52
Hepatosplenic candidiasis, 31, 264, 276
Herpes simplex virus (HSV)
　antiviral prophylaxis, 527
　antiviral resistance
　　acyclovir, 398
　　cidofovir, 399
　　definition, 397–398
　　diagnosis, 399
　　leflunomide, 399
　　rheumatoid arthritis, 399
　　risk factors, 398–399
　　therapy, 399
　　toxicity, 399
Herpes viruses
　Epstein-Barr virus (EBV)
　　B cell, 365
　　immunocompromised hosts, 365–366
　　transmission, 365
　　treatment, 366
　HHV-6, 365
　HHV-8, 366–367
　infection phases, 359
Herpes zoster vaccine, 563–564
Histoplasma antigen, 297
Histoplasma capsulatum, 297, 485

Histoplasmosis
  antifungal therapy, 298
  central nervous system, 298
  clinical findings, 297
  culture of, 297
  Histoplasma antigen, 297
  Histoplasma capsulatum, 297
  immunosuppression, 297
  in *Nocardia* pneumonia, 148–149
HLA-DR antibody, hematologic malignancies, 60
Hospital-acquired pneumonia (HAP), 146–147
Human herpes virus–6 (HHV–6), 365
Human herpes virus–8 (HHV–8), 366–367
Human metapneumovirus (hMPV)
  clinical presentation, 380
  diagnosis, 380
  immunocompromised patients, 380
  Paramyxoviridae family, 379
  prevention, 380
  treatment, 380
Humoral immune dysfunction, hematologic malignancies, 33–34
Hydrostatic pulmonary edema, 153–154
Hypereosinophilic syndrome, 249
Hypoproteinemia, antimicrobial agents, 446

I
Ibritumomab tiuxetan, 54
Idiopathic pneumonia syndrome (IPS), 159–160
IMIs. *See* Invasive mold infections (IMIs)
Immune evasion, CMV, 342
Immune system, monoclonal antibodies interaction, 47–48
Immunocompromised traveler
  considerations for, 551–552
  prevention, recommendations for
    animal bites, 556
    arthropod bites, 555, 556
    enteric pathogens, 552, 554–555
    geographical distribution of, 553–554
    respiratory pathogens, 555
    sexually and parenterally transmitted infections, 556–557
    skin and mucous membranes, 555–556
  recommendations for, 552
  vaccination in, 557
    recommendations, 557–559
Immunological factors, 4–6
Immunotherapy
  antifungal agents, 335–336
  chronic granulomatous disease (CGD), 332
  cytokines, 335, 336
  graft-*versus*-host disease (GVHD), 331, 332
  host defense deficits, 331, 332
  immune augmentation strategies, 333
  immunologic effect, antifungals, 336
  immunomodulators, 335–336
  invasive fungal diseases
    aspergillosis and moulds, 331, 332
    yeasts and dimorphic fungi, 331, 332
  neutrophil number augmentation
    colony stimulating factors (CSF), 333–334
    granulocyte transfusions, 334–335
  principles and challenges, 332–333
  recombinant interferon-g, 335
  toll-like receptors (TLR), 335–336
Impaired humoral immunity, 523
Implantable device infections, 199

Infection prevention, 548
  and contol, principles of, 542, 543
  food and drink, 547–548
  hand hygiene, 546–547
  protected environment, 542–543
    and PEPA, 543–546
  risks, 541–542
  water and moulds, 546
Infective endocarditis (IE)
  clinical presentation, 220–221
  CoNS, 226
  diagnosis and investigation
    antibiotics, 221
    blood cultures, 221
    echocardiography, 221
    modified Duke criteria, 221, 222
  enterococci, 227
  epidemiology
    incidence of, 219
    studies of, 219, 220
  etiologic agents, 224
  fungi, 227–228
  management
    surgery, 224
    treatment regimens, 222, 224
  NBTE, 228–229
  risk factors for, 220
  Staphylococcus aureus, 224–226
  streptococci, 226–227
Infliximab, 59–60
Influenza viruses
  antiviral resistance
    antiviral therapy, 401–402
    diagnosis, 402
    oseltamivir, 402
    zanamivir, 402
  antiviral resistance pattern, 375
  clinical presentation, 374
  diagnosis, 375
  hemagglutinins (HA), 374
  HSCT recipients, 374
  immunocompromised patients, 374–375
  leukemia patients, 374
  neuraminidase (NA), 374
  prevention/vaccination, 375–376
  solid organ transplant patients, 375
  treatment, 375
  vaccination
    clinical studies, 564
    frequency and case fatality in, 563
Innate immunity, CMV, 342
Inotuzumab ozogamicin, 57
Intensive care unit (ICU). *See also* Critically ill cancer patients
  oncologists and infectious disease specialists, 87–88
  patient's goals, 88
Intensive insulin therapy, catheter salvage, 130–131
Interferon gamma (IFN-g), 335
  NTM, 463
Intestinal protozoa, 478
Intraabdominal and pelvic abscess, 197–198
Intravascular catheter-related blood stream infections (IVDR BSI)
  catheter salvage (*see* Catheter salvage, IVDR BSI)
  microbiology, 125
  pathogenesis of
    mortality of, 124
    percutaneous IVD, sources of infection, 124
    pulsed-field gel electrophoresis, 125

Intravenous immunoglobulin (IVIg)
    BKV, 390
    parvovirus B19, 392
Invasive aspergillosis (IA), 264–266
    clinical data, 311–312
    clinical trials, 309, 310
    micafungin (MICA), 311
    preclinical data, 309, 311
Invasive candidiasis, 257
    Candida species in, 273
    candidemia and acute disseminated candidiasis, 278–279
    chronic disseminated candidiasis, 279
    clinical presentation
        candidemia, 276
        disseminated, skin lesions in, 276
        endocarditis, 277
        esophagitis, 276
        hepatosplenic, 276
        intra-abdominal infections, 277
        ocular infection, 276–277
        trombophlebitis, 277
        urinary tract, 277
    diagnosis
        blood cultures, 275
        definitions, 275
        nonculture-based methods, 275
        radiological signs, 275–276
    epidemiology, 273–274
    mucocutaneous, 278
    pathogenesis, 274
    prophylaxis, 277
    resistance patterns, 274
    risk factors, 274–275
    systemic agents, 278
    treatment, 277–278
Invasive fungal disease
    aspergillosis and moulds, 331, 332
    drugs, 257
    immunopathogenesis of, 257–258
    immunotherapy for, 258
    sinus disease, 267–268
    yeasts and dimorphic fungi, 331, 332
Invasive fungal infections (IFIs)
    antifungal prophylaxis, 524
    diagnosis of, 261
        candidiasis, 262–264
        mold infections, 264–268
    preemptive therapy, 287
    risk factors, 284
Invasive mold infections (IMIs)
    amphotericin B (AMB), 285
    Aspergillus fumigatus, 283
    1,3-beta-D-glucan test, 284
    clinical syndromes, 264
    conventional diagnostic methods, 284
    diagnosis of
        beta-D-glucan assay, 267
        galactomannan antigen, 266–267
        histopathology and microbiology, 265–266
        imaging, 264–265
        invasive fungal sinus disease, 267–268
        PCR, 267
    diagnostics, 283–284
    echinocandins, 285–286
    empiric antifungal treatment, 287
    epidemiology of, 283, 284
    galactomannan test, 284
    lipid formulations, 285, 286
    polymerase chain reaction (PCR), 284
    posaconazole, 285
    preemptive therapy, 287
    prevention and prophylaxis, 286–287
    radiologic methods, 284
    salvage antifungal therapy, 288
    second-generation triazoles, 285
    therapies
        aspergillosis, 287–288
        fusariosis, 288
        phaehyphomycosis, 288
        scedosporiosis, 288
        zygomycosis, 288
    voriconazole, 285
Invasive pulmonary mycosis. *See* Pulmonary mycosis
Itraconazole, antifungal drug resistance, 322

J
JC virus, 392, 393

K
Klebsiella pneumoniae, 426
Klebsiella pneumoniae carbapenemases (KPC), 500

L
Lady Windermere syndrome, 464
Lamivudine, 190
Late-onset neutropenia (LON), rituximab, 53
Leflunomide
    antiviral resistance, HSV, 399
    BKV, 390
Leukemia
    acute, 34–35
    neutropenic enterocolitis, 181, 182
Leukocytoclastic vasculitis, 243–244
Limb interventions, postoperative infections, 77
Linezolid, 451
Lipid formulations, 285, 286
Lipodermatosclerosis, 246
Liposomal amphotericin B (LAMB), 307, 308
Listeria monocytogenes, 435, 436, 438, 514
Listeriosis
    in cancer patients, 438
    clinical settings, 438
    clinical syndromes
        bacteremia, 437
        brain abscess, 438
        brain stem encephalitis, 437–438
        CNS infection, 437
        infection, in pregnancy, 436–437
        meningitis, 437
        neonatal period, 436–437
    CNS, 436
    diagnosis, 438–439
    epidemiology, 436
    listeriae, 436
    listerial meningitis, 437
    Listeria monocytogenes, 435, 436, 438
    pathogenesis, 435–436
    prevention, 439
    rhombencephalitis, 437–438
    treatment, 439
Liver flukes, 478

Lumiliximab, 57
Lung cancer, 40–41
  interventions, postoperative infections
    diagnosis of, 72
    etiology of, 72
    incidence of, 72
    prevention, 72
    risk factors, 72
    treatment of, 72
  pneumonia, 41
Lung infiltrates, cancer patient
  CILI, 154–158
  HSCT, noninfectious complications of
    early-onset, 159–160
    late-onset, 160–162
  hydrostatic pulmonary edema, 153–154
  nonhydrostatic pulmonary edema, 154
  radiation-induced lung injury, 158–159
  small airway mucus impaction, 162–163
  TRALI, 162
Lymphoma, 36

M

Magnetic resonance imaging (MRI), hematologic malignancies, 30
Malaria prophylaxis, 555, 556
Mannose binding lectin (MBL), 109
Marantic endocarditis. *See* Nonbacterial thrombotic endocarditis (NBTE)
Mechanical blisters, 234–235
Meningitis
  acute bacterial meningitis, 211
  Candida, 212
  chronic, 212
  listeriosis, 437
  non-infectious causes of, 212
  viral (aseptic) meningitis, 211–212
Methicillin-resistant *Staphylococcus aureus* (MRSA), 70, 147, 507
Metronidazole, 451
Micafungin (MICA)
  antifungal drug resistance, 323, 324
  antimicrobial prophylaxis, 536
  invasive aspergillosis, 311
Microbiota, bacterial colonization and host immunity, 175–176
Micrococcus species, CRBSI, 119
Miliaria crystallina, 238
Miliaria rubra, 241
Mold infections. *See* Invasive mold infections (IMIs)
Monkey pox virus, 486
Monoclonal antibodies, colon cancer, 42, 43
Monoclonal antineoplastic therapy, hematologic malignancies
  anti-CD2 antibodies, 58
  anti-CD3 antibodies, 58
  anti-CD4 antibodies, 57–58
  anti-CD20 antibodies
    radioimmunoconjugates, 54
    rituximab, 48–54
    second-generation, 54, 55
  anti-CD22 antibodies, 57
  anti-CD23 antibodies, 57
  anti-CD33 antibodies, 57
  anti-CD52 antibodies, 54–56
  anti-interleukin–2 receptor antibodies
    basiliximab, 59
    daclizumab, 58–59
    denileukin diftitox, 58
  anti-interleukin–6-receptor antibodies, 59
  anti-TNFa monoclonal antibodies, 59–60
  HLA-DR antibody, 60
  infections and complications, 49
  interaction of, 47–48
Moulds, infection prevention, 546
Moxifloxacin, 451
mRNA detection, 344
Mucocutaneous candidiasis, 278
Mucosal barrier injury (MBI) and infections
  cytotoxic therapy-induced mucositis, 169
  epithelial innate immunity, 168–169
  inflammatory response, 170
  neutropenia, 167–168
  neutropenic enterocolitis (NE), 170, 171
  primary host defence, disintegration of, 167
Mucosal impairment, hematologic malignancies, 34
Multi-drug-resistant (MDR), 423
Multinational Association for Supportive Care in Cancer (MASCC) risk-index for neutropenic patients, 98
Multiple myeloma, 35
Mupirocin prophylaxis, 127–128
Muromonab, 58
Mycobacterial infections, 8
Mycobacterium avium, 464
Mycobacterium haemophilum, 465
Mycobacterium intracellular, 464
Mycobacterium kansasii, 464–465
Mycobacterium marinum, 487
Mycobacterium simiae, 465
Mycobacterium tuberculosis, 486
  biology of, 455–456
  deficiencies in antimycobacterial immunity
    alemtuzumab, 457
    bone marrow transplantation, 457
    cancer therapies, 456–457
    pharmacologic cancer therapy, 457
    purine analogs, 457–458
    risk factors, 456–457
    solid tumors, 456, 457
    states of susceptibility, 456
    temozolamide, 458
    TNF inhibitors, 458
  diagnosis, 458
  graft *versus* host diseases, 456, 458
  guidelines, TB prophylaxis
    chemotherapy, 459–460
    clinical condition risk, 459
    drug interactions, 459–460
    therapy, 459
  T-cell defect, 457
Mycosis fungoides and cutaneous T-cell lymphoma, 243
Myeloid growth factors, 523
Myeloma, 35–36

N

Neck cancer interventions, postoperative infections, 69–70
Necrolytic migratory erythema, 248
Necrotizing fasciitis, 202–203
Neoplastic disease, patient infections
  abdominal infections, 12
  antibiotic therapy, in neutropenic patient, 7–8
  bacterial infections, 7
  catheter-related infections, 12–13
  diagnostic evaluation of, 6–7

Index

end-organ infection, 12
epidemiological factors, 4
factors in, 3
fungal infections, 8–10
history of, 3
hosts' susceptibility, 4
immunological factors, 4–6
mycobacterial infections, 8
parasitic infections, 10–12
pathogens of, 7
pneumonia, 12
viral infections, 10, 11
Nephritis, BKV, 392
Neutropenia
  aHSCT
    epidemiology of infections, 17–18
    fever, antimicrobial therapy, 19–20
  antibacterial prophylaxis
    antibiotic prophylaxis, 522–523
    high risks patients, 522
    infection, 521–522
    myeloid growth factors, 523
    parameters affected, 522
    prevention strategies, 522, 523
    treatment, 523
  antibiotic therapy, 7–8
  antifungal prophylaxis
    acute myeloid leukemia (AML), 525
    Aspergillus, primary, 525–526
    candidiasis, primary, 524–525
    chemotherapy regimens, duration of, 524
    fluconazole, 524–525
    invasive fungal infections (IFI), 524
    posaconazole, 525
    risk assessment, 524
    secondary prophylaxis, 526
  antimicrobial prophylaxis, 537–538
  antiviral prophylaxis, 527
  bacterial infections, distribution of, 96
  in children, 79
  epidemiology of infections
    bacterial pathogens in, 96, 97
    Candida spp., 97
  febrile episodes, nature of, 95, 96
  fever, management of
    antibiotic regimens, 101, 102
    empiric antibiotic therapy, 98–100
    evaluation of response and duration of therapy, 100–101
    febrile episode, ambulatory management of, 99, 100
    risk assessment and risk-based therapy, 97–98
  hematologic malignancies
    antifungal prophylaxis, 31
    bacterial infections, epidemiology of, 30
    candidemia, incidence of, 31
    disseminated aspergillosis, 32
    fungal infections, incidence of, 28, 30
    hepatosplenic candidiasis, 29, 31
    influenza and mucor pneumonia, 32
    MRI of, 30
    severe infection episodes, circulating neutrophils, 30
  immune defects, 5–6
  initial assessment of, 97
  invasive candidiasis, 278
  meningitis, 211
  mucosal barrier injury and infections, 167–168
  protected environment for, 5

risk of infection, 4
  white blood cell (WBC) transfusions, 4–5
Neutropenic enterocolitis (NEC), 170, 171
  CT scan findings, 183
  diagnosis
    diarrhea, 182, 183
    fever, 182, 183
  epidemiology, 181–182
  management, 183–184
  pathogenesis of, 182
Neutrophilic eccrine hidradenitis, 241
Neutrophil number augmentation
  colony stimulating factors, 333–334
  granulocyte transfusions, 334–335
NFGNB. See Nonfermentative gram-negative bacilli (NFGNB)
Nocardia abscessus, 148
Nocardia pneumonia, 148–149
Nocardiosis
  in cancer patients, 440
  cell-mediated immunity, 439–440
  clinical syndromes, 440
  diagnosis, 440
  nocardia species, 439
  treatment, 440
Nodular vasculitis, 245, 246
Nonbacterial thrombotic endocarditis (NBTE)
  incidence of, 228
  vs. infective endocarditis, 229
  treatment of, 229
Nonfermentative gram-negative bacilli (NFGNB)
  Acinetobacter baumannii, 427–428
  antimicrobial stewardship, 429–430
  Chryseobacterium species, 428
  documented infections therapy, 429
  empiric therapy, 429
  frequency of infections, 426
  moderate-to-high-grade bacteremia frequency, 427
  Pseudomonas aeruginosa, 426–427
  Pseudomonas fluorescens, 428
  Stenotrophomonas maltophilia, 427
  treatment, 428
  trimethoprim/sulfamethoxazole (TMP/SMX), 427
Noninfectious lung infiltrates. See Lung infiltrates, cancer patient
Non-neutropenic patients
  antibacterial prophylaxis
    chronic graft *versus* host disease (GVHD), 524
    impaired humoral immunity, 523
    splenectomy, 524
  antifungal prophylaxis, 526–527
Nontuberculous mycobacteriosis (NTM), 149
  antimycobacterial immune defense, 463
  clinical characteristics, 464
  immunologic susceptibility, 463–464
  interferon gamma (IFN-g), 463
  Lady Windermere syndrome, 464
  Mycobacterium avium, 464
  Mycobacterium intracellular, 464
  rapidly growing mycobacteria
    catheter-related infections, 465–466
    pneumonia, 465
    skin and soft-tissue infection, 465
  slow-growing mycobacteria
    mycobacterium avium-intracellular, 464
    Mycobacterium haemophilum, 465
    Mycobacterium kansasii, 464–465
    Mycobacterium simiae, 465

Nosocomial meningitis, 211
NTM. *See* Nontuberculous mycobacteriosis (NTM)

O

Ocular infection, invasive candidiasis, 276–277
Oseltamivir antiviral resistance, influenza viruses, 402
Outpatient antibiotic therapy, 502–504

P

Pancreatic panniculitis, 245
Paneth cells, 177, 178
Panniculitis
  cold, 245
  differential diagnosis, 245
  nodular vasculitis, 245, 246
  pancreatic, 245
  sclerosing, 246
Papulosquamous lesions
  dermatitis, 241–242
  mycosis fungoides and cutaneous T-cell lymphoma, 243
  pityriasis rosea, 243
  pityriasis rubra pilaris, 243
  psoriasis, 242, 243
Parainfluenza viruses (PIV)
  clinical presentation, 376
  diagnosis, 376–377
  HSCT recipients, 376
  immunocompromised patients, 376
  leukemia patients, 376
  prevention/vaccination, 377
  solid organ transplant patients, 376
  treatment, 377
Paraneoplastic autoimmune multiorgan syndrome, 236
Paraneoplastic neurological syndromes (PNS), 215
Paraneoplastic pemphigus, 236, 237
Parasitic infections, 10–12
  Acanthamoeba spp., 477
  Balamuthia mandrillaris, 477
  Chagas' disease, 477
  Cryptosporidium spp., 478
  intestinal protozoa, 478
  liver flukes, 478
  Schistosoma spp., 478
  schistosomiasis, 478
  strongyloidiasis
    in cancer patients, 476
    clinical findings, 474–475
    diagnosis, 475–476
    epidemiology, 474
    hyperinfection prevention, 477
    hyperinfection syndrome, 474
    organism, 473
    pathogenesis and immunity, 474
    treatment, 476
  toxoplasmosis
    clinical manifestations, 470–471
    diagnosis, 471–472
    life cycle and epidemiology, 469–470
    management, 472, 473
    prevention, 473
  Trypanosoma cruzi, 477
  visceral leishmaniasis (VL), 477–478
Parvovirus B19, 392, 393
Pasteurella multocida, 482

Pattern recognition receptors (PRRs), 168
Pelvic abscess, 197–198
Pemphigus, 236, 237
Peptide nucleic acid fluorescent in situ hybridization (PNA-FISH) test, 263
Peritonitis and intraabdominal abscess, genitourinary tract infections, 200–201
Petechiae, 245
Phaehyphomycosis, invasive mold infections, 288
Phagocyte defects, hematologic malignancies, 30–31
Pharmacokinetics
  antibacterial distribution, 443–444
  parameters, 443–444
Pharmacokodynamic (PD) indices, for anti-infective therapy, 444
Pharmacologic cancer therapy, 457
Pityriasis rosea, 243
Pityriasis rubra pilaris, 243
PIV. *See* Parainfluenza viruses
Plague, 484
Pneumococcal vaccine, 564
Pneumocystis jerovici pneumonia (PCP), 43, 44
Pneumocystis pneumonia, 149
Pneumonia, 11, 12
  immune defects, 143
    aspiration and bronchial obstruction, 147–148
    community-acquired pneumonia, 146
    hospital-acquired pneumonia, 146–147
    infections in, 144
    neutropenia, 145
    neutrophils, 145
    Pseudomonas lung abscess, 145
    septic emboli, 148
  pathogens
    histoplasmosis in, 148
    invasive pulmonary mycosis, 150–151
    nocardiosis, 148–149
    nontuberculous mycobacteriosis, 149
    Pneumocystis, 149
    tuberculosis, 149
    viruses, 151
Poliovirus, 565
Polymerase chain reaction (PCR), 284
  candidiasis, 263–264
  empiric antifungal therapy, 108–109
  invasive mold infections, 267
  parvovirus B19, 392
Polyomavirus
  BK virus
    definition, 387
    hemorrhagic cystitis, 388–392
    transmission and pathogenesis, 388
    virologic aspects, 387–388
  JC virus, 392, 393
  parvovirus B19, 392, 393
Porphyria cutanea tarda (PCT), 237
Posaconazole
  antifungal prophylaxis, 525
  clinical trials, 303
  drug interactions, 302, 303
  hepatic dysfunction, 303
  invasive mold infections (IMIs), 285
  pharmacokinetic variability, 322–323
  toxicity, 303–304
Postoperative infections
  brain cancer, 67–68
  breast cancer interventions, surgical site infections, 70–71

central nervous system
  external ventricular drains (EVDs), 214
  postcraniotomy infections, 214
  shunt infections, 214
 in children, 77–80
 esophageal cancer, 72–73
 genital and urinary tract neoplasms, 75–77
 GI tract interventions, 73–75
 head and neck cancer interventions, 69–70
 limb interventions, 77
 lung cancer interventions, 71–72
 surgery infections, prevention and management for, 77
Posttransplantation constrictive bronchiolitis (PTCB), 161–162
Posttransplantation lymphoproliferative disorder (PTLD), 162
Pre-emptive therapy, CMV, 346–347
Procalcitonin (PCT), 107
Progressive multifocal leukoencephalopathy (PML), 10, 209, 392
 rituximab, 53
Prophylactic antibiotic programmes (PEPA) and PE
 airborne protection, 545
 exogenous and endogenous opportunistic pathogens, 543
 HEPA filtration, 545–546
 patient culture specimens, 544
 prophylactic topical and oral non-absorbable antimicrobials, 544
 randomised trial of, 545
 remission rates, 544
 universal protection, 545
Prophylactic vaccination, HSCT
 chemotherapy, 562
 eukaryotic infections, 566–567
 Haemophilus influenzae type B, 564–565
 hepatitis B virus, 565
 herpes zoster, 563–564
 immune suppression, 562
 influenza, 563, 564
 pneumococcal pneumonia, 564
 poliovirus, 565
 tumor-derived factors, dendritic cells, 561, 562
 viral infections
  adenovirus and polyomavirus, 566
  CMV and EBV, 566
  respiratory viruses, 566
Protected environment (PE), 542–543. *See also* Prophylactic antibiotic programmes (PEPA) and PE
Pseudomonas aeruginosa, 426–427, 501
Pseudomonas fluorescens, 428
Pseudomonas lung abscess, 145
Pseudoporphyria cutanea tarda, 237, 238
Psoriasis, 242, 243
Pulmonary alveolar proteinosis (PAP), 160, 161
Pulmonary edema
 HSCT, early-onset noninfectious complications of, 159
 hydrostatic, 153–154
 nonhydrostatic, 154
Pulmonary mycosis
 fungal infections diagnosis, 150
 incidence of, 150
 treatment of, 151
Pulmonary nocardiosis, lymphoma, 33
Pulmonary veno-occlusive disease (PVOD), 160
Pulsed-field gel electrophoresis, IVDR BSI, 125
Purine analogs, 457–458
Purpuric and petechial lesions
 calciphylaxis, 244
 DIC, 244
 leukocytoclastic vasculitis, 243–244
 petechiae, 245
 superficial thrombophlebitis, 244
Pustular lesions
 acneiform eruptions, 240
 AGEP, 238
 eosinophilic folliculitis, 240
 Grover disease, 241
 miliaria rubra, 241
 neutrophilic eccrine hidradenitis, 241
 reactive neutrophilic dermatoses, 239–240
Pyoderma gangrenosum, 239, 240

Q

Q fever, 484
Quantitative polymerase chain reaction (qPCR), 343

R

Radiation-induced lung injury, lung infiltrates, 158–159
Radiation pneumonitis, 158
Radioimmunoconjugates, anti-CD20, 54
Rapidly growing mycobacteria (RGM)
 catheter-related infections, 465–466
 lung disease, 8
 pneumonia, 465
 skin and soft-tissue infection, 465
Reactive neutrophilic dermatoses, 239–240
Recombinant interferon-g, 335
Respiratory mycosis, cryptococcal disease, 294
Respiratory pathogens, immunocompromised traveler, 555
Respiratory syncytial virus (RSV)
 clinical presentations, 372
 diagnosis, 373
 HSCT recipients, 372–373
 immunocompromised patients, 372–373
 leukemia patients, 372–373
 prevention/vaccination, 374
 solid organ transplant recipients, 373
 treatment, 373
Respiratory viruses
 acute infectious illness, 381–382
 adenovirus
  clinical presentation, 377
  diagnosis, 378
  HSCT recipients, 377–378
  immunocompromised patients, 377–378
  leukemia patients, 377–378
  prevention/vaccination, 378
  solid organ transplant patients, 378
  treatment, 378
 coronavirus
  clinical presentation, 380
  diagnosis, 381
  immunocompromised patients, 380
  prevention, 381
  treatment, 381
 enterovirus
  clinical presentation, 381
  diagnosis, 381
  immunocompromised patients, 381
  prevention, 381
  treatment, 381
 human metapneumovirus (hMPV)
  clinical presentation, 380
  diagnosis, 380

Respiratory viruses (cont.)
    immunocompromised patients, 380
    Paramyxoviridae family, 379
    prevention, 380
    treatment, 380
  infections, 371, 372
  influenza viruses
    antiviral resistance pattern, 375
    clinical presentation, 374
    diagnosis, 375
    hemagglutinins (HA), 374
    HSCT recipients, 374
    immunocompromised patients, 374–375
    leukemia patients, 374
    neuraminidase (NA), 374
    prevention/vaccination, 375–376
    solid organ transplant patients, 375
    treatment, 375
  parainfluenza viruses (PIV)
    clinical presentation, 376
    diagnosis, 376–377
    HSCT recipients, 376
    immunocompromised patients, 376
    leukemia patients, 376
    prevention/vaccination, 377
    solid organ transplant patients, 376
    treatment, 377
  respiratory syncytial virus (RSV)
    clinical presentations, 372
    diagnosis, 373
    HSCT recipients, 372–373
    immunocompromised patients, 372–373
    leukemia patients, 372–373
    prevention/vaccination, 374
    solid organ transplant recipients, 373
    treatment, 373
  rhinovirus
    clinical presentation, 379
    diagnosis, 379
    immunocompromised patients, 379
    Picornaviridae family, 378–379
    prevention, 379
    treatment, 379
  syndromes, 371, 372
Retinitis, CMV, 344–345
Reversible posterior leukoencephalopathy syndrome (RPLS), 215
Rheumatoid arthritis, antiviral resistance
  CMV, 401
  HSV, 399
Rhinovirus
  clinical presentation, 379
  diagnosis, 379
  immunocompromised patients, 379
  Picornaviridae family, 378–379
  prevention, 379
  treatment, 379
Rhizopus multicentric cavitary pneumonia, 150
Rhombencephalitis, 437–438
Ribavirin, 192
Rifamycin derivates, 450
Rituximab
  associated infection
    cytomegalovirus, 52–53
    hepatitis B and C, 52
    HIV1-associated conditions, 51
    indications, 53–54
    late-onset neutropenia (LON), 53
    phase III randomized controlled trials, 50, 51
  B-cell depletion, 49
  maintenance therapy, 50
  side effects of, 50
RSV. *See* Respiratory syncytial virus (RSV)

S

Salvage antifungal therapy, 288
Scalp lesions, 250
Scedosporiosis, 288
Schistosoma haematobium, 478
Schistosoma spp., 478
Schistosomiasis, 478
Septal panniculitis, 245–246
Septic encephalopathy, 209
Septic pelvic thrombophlebitis, 203–204
Serratia marcescens, 425
Sexually and parenterally transmitted infections, 556–557
Single nucleotide polymorphisms (SNPs), 168–169
Siplizumab, 58
Skin
  lesions, disseminated candidiasis, 276
  and soft-tissue infection, 465
Skin disorders
  erythematous lesions
    chemotherapy-induced acral blisters and erythema, 248
    EM/SJS and TEN, 246–247
    eosinophilic dermatoses, 249
    erythema annulare centrifugum, 247, 248
    erythema gyratum repens, 247–248
    granuloma annulare, 248–249
    necrolytic migratory erythema, 248
    urticaria and angioedema, 246
  hair and scalp lesions, 250
  panniculitis
    cold, 245
    differential diagnosis, 245
    nodular vasculitis, 245, 246
    pancreatic, 245
    sclerosing, 246
  papulosquamous lesions
    dermatitis, 241–242
    mycosis fungoides and cutaneous T-cell lymphoma, 243
    pityriasis rosea, 243
    pityriasis rubra pilaris, 243
    psoriasis, 242, 243
  purpuric and petechial lesions
    calciphylaxis, 244
    DIC, 244
    leukocytoclastic vasculitis, 243–244
    petechiae, 245
    superficial thrombophlebitis, 244
  pustular lesions
    acneiform eruptions, 240
    AGEP, 238
    eosinophilic folliculitis, 240
    Grover disease, 241
    miliaria rubra, 241
    neutrophilic eccrine hidradenitis, 241
    reactive neutrophilic dermatoses, 239–240
  ulcerative lesions and skin tumors, 249–250
  vesiculobullous lesions
    acute dermatitis, 233
    autoimmune bullous dermatoses, 236–237

bullous drug eruptions, 235–236
bullous GVHD, 235
bullous insect bite reaction, 235
diabetic blisters, 235
edema and lymphedema bullae, 235
mechanical blisters, 232
miliaria crystallina, 238
porphyria cutanea tarda (PCT), 237
pseudoporphyria cutanea tarda, 237, 238

Slow-growing mycobacteria (SGM)
   mycobacterium avium-intracellular, 464
   Mycobacterium haemophilum, 465
   Mycobacterium kansasii, 464–465
   Mycobacterium simiae, 465

Solid tumor patients
   breast cancer, 41–42
   CNS cancer, 43–44
   colon cancer, 42, 43
   GU cancers, 43
   vs. hematologic malignancy, 39, 40
   infection risks and pathogens, 39–40
   lung cancer, 40–41
   Mycobacterium tuberculosis infection, 456, 457
   neutropenia, 39
   treatment regimens, 41

Splenectomy, 524
Splenic dysfunction, hematologic malignancies, 34
Staphylococci
   coagulase negative staphylococci, 412
   Staphylococcus aureus
      chest computerized tomography, 411
      clinical manifestations, 410–411
      diagnosis, 410–411
      epidemiology, 409–411
      treatment, 411–412

Staphylococcus aureus
   antibiotic treatment, 411
   catheter salvage, 135–136
   chest computerized tomography, 411
   clinical manifestations, 410–411
   CRBSI, 119
   diagnosis, 410–411
   epidemiology, 409–411
   infective endocarditis
      daptomycin, 225–226
      neutropenia, 225
      TEE, 225
      vancomycin, 225, 226
   treatment, 411–412

Stem cell transplantation (SCT), HBV and HCV reactivation, 189–192
Stenotrophomonas maltophilia, 427
Stevens–Johnson syndrome (SJS), 246–247
Streamlining, ASP, 494
Streptococci
   definition, 412–413
   empiric antimicrobial therapy, 417
   enterococcus
      clinical presentation/diagnosis, 416
      epidemiology, 416
      treatment, 416–417
   b-hemolytic streptococci
      clinical manifestations/diagnosis, 414
      definition, 414
      epidemiology, 414
      treatment, 414–415
   infective endocarditis
      penicillin, minimal inhibitory concentration, 226–227
      Streptococcus bovis, 227
      Streptococcus pneumoniae
         clinical presentations/diagnosis, 415
         epidemiology, 415
         treatment, 415–416
      viridans group streptococci, 413

Streptococcus aureus, mupirocin prophylaxis, 127–128
Streptococcus pneumoniae
   clinical presentations/diagnosis, 415
   epidemiology, 415
   treatment, 415–416

Strongyloides stercoralis. *See* Strongyloidiasis
Strongyloidiasis, 528
   bronchoalveolar lavage, 476
   bronchoscopic biopsy, 475
   in cancer patients, 476
   clinical findings, 474–475
   diagnosis, 475–476
   epidemiology, 474
   hyperinfection prevention, 477
   hyperinfection syndrome, 474
   organism, 473
   pathogenesis and immunity, 474
   sputum, 476
   treatment, 476

Sulfamethoxazole (SMX), 427
Suppurative pelvic thrombophlebitis, 203–204
Surgical infection, genitourinary tract, 200
Surgical site infections (SSIs). *See* Postoperative infections
Sweet syndrome, acute febrile neutrophilic dermatosis, 239
Systemic catheter infections, CRBSI, 114

T

TDM. *See* Therapeutic drug monitoring (TDM)
Temozolomide, 44, 458
Therapeutic drug monitoring (TDM)
   parameters, 301, 302
   posaconazole
      clinical trials, 303
      drug interactions, 302, 303
      hepatic dysfunction, 303
      toxicity, 303–304
   voriconazole
      blood levels, tests for, 302–303
      clinical trials, 301–302
      criterias, 303
      drug interactions, 301, 302
      hepatic metabolism, 301
      toxicity, 302
   voriconazole, pharmacokinetic variability, 322

Thrombophlebitis, 244
Tigecycline, 452
Tissue infections, 446–447
Tocilizumab, 59
Toll-like receptors (TLR), 335–336
Topical antimicrobials, catheter salvage, 126–128
Toxic epidermal necrolysis (TEN), 246–247
Toxoplasma encephalitis, 209
Toxoplasma gondii
   acute infection, 470–471
   forms of, 470
   zoonoses, 485

Toxoplasmosis, 528
  clinical manifestations
    acute infection, 470–471
    chronic infection, 471
  diagnosis
    histological methods, 472
    polymerase chain reaction, 472
    serological tests, 471–472
  drugs, 472, 473
  invasive procedures, 472
  life cycle and epidemiology
    oocysts, 469–470
    tissue cysts, 469, 470
  management, 472, 473
  prevention, 473
Transfusion-related acute lung injury (TRALI), 162
Transthoracic echocardiography (TTE), 221
Travel medicine, 551
Triazoles, 318–320
Trimethoprim (TMP), 427
Trimethoprim-sulfamethoxazole, 452
Trombophlebitis, invasive candidiasis, 277
Trypanosoma cruzi, 477
Tuberculosis, 149
  deficiencies in antimycobacterial immunity
    alemtuzumab, 457
    bone marrow transplantation, 457
    cancer therapies, 456–457
    pharmacologic cancer therapy, 457
    purine analogs, 457–458
    risk factors, 456–457
    states of susceptibility, 456
    temozolamide, 458
    TNF inhibitors, 458
  diagnosis, 458
  guidelines, TB prophylaxis
    clinical condition risk, 459
    drug interactions, 459–460
    therapy, 459
  Mycobacterium tuberculosis, 455–456
  T-cell defect, 457
Tumor necrosis factor (TNF) inhibitors, 458
Typhlitis. *See* Neutropenic enterocolitis (NEC)

U

Ulcerative lesions and skin tumors
  chronic leg ulcers, 250
  leukemia cutis, 251
  metastatic breast carcinoma, 250
Umbilical cord blood transplantation, 346
Urinary tract
  candidiasis, 277
  infection, 199
  neoplasms, postoperative infections, 75–77
Urokinase, catheter salvage, 134
Urticaria and angioedema, 246

V

Vaccination
  HSCT (*see* Prophylactic vaccination, HSCT)
  immunocompromised traveler, 557
    recommendations, 557–559

Valacyclovir, VZV, 363
Valganciclovir
  antiviral resistance, CMV, 400
  CMV, 348, 349
Vancomycin, 451
Vancomycin resistant enterococci (VRE), 500
Varicella vaccine, 364, 563
Varicella zoster virus (VZV)
  acyclovir, 362–364
  antiviral prophylaxis, 364–365, 527
  antiviral resistance, 399–400
  antivirals, 364
  atypical generalized zoster, 362
  cell-mediated, 360
  clinical manifestations, 362
  epidemiology, 360
  hematopoietic stem cell transplant (HSCT) recipients, 360–362
  HSCT, 22
  humoral immunity, 363
  immunodeficiency, 360
  laboratory diagnosis, 362
  prevention and infection control, 363–364
  risk factors, 360
  treatment, 362–363
  vaccination, 364
  valacyclovir, 363
  varicella vaccine, 364
  zoster vaccine, 364
Vesiculobullous lesions
  acute dermatitis, 233
  autoimmune bullous dermatoses, 236–237
  bullous drug eruptions, 235–236
  bullous GVHD, 235
  bullous insect bite reaction, 235
  diabetic blisters, 235
  edema and lymphedema bullae, 235
  mechanical blisters, 232
  miliaria crystallina, 238
  porphyria cutanea tarda (PCT), 237
  pseudoporphyria cutanea tarda, 237, 238
Viremia, BKV, 388
Viridans group streptococci (VGS), 413
Viruses
  aseptic meningitis, 211–212
  infections, 10, 11, 566
    aHSCT, 20–22
  pneumonia, 151
Visceral leishmaniasis (VL), 477–478
Voriconazole
  blood levels, tests for, 302–303
  clinical trials, 301–302
  criterias, 303
  drug interactions, 301, 302
  hepatic metabolism, 301
  invasive mold infections (IMIs), 285
  pharmacokinetic variability
    CYP2C19, 320–321
    intra-and interpatient, 321
    logistic regression analysis, 321
    plasma drug exposures, 321
    polymorphisms, 320–321
    therapeutic drug monitoring, 322
  toxicity, 302
VZV. *See* Varicella zoster virus (VZV)

W

Wells syndrome, 249
Wound infection, genitourinary tract infections
- cellulitis, 201–202
- clostridial myonecrosis, 203
- necrotizing fasciitis, 202–203
- surgery-related, 197

Y

Yeasts, 331, 332
Yersinia pestis, 483

Z

Zanamivir antiviral resistance, influenza viruses, 402
Zanolimumab, 57–58
Zoonoses
- *Bartonella henseleae*, 484
- bats, 486
- beasts of burden, 486
- *Blastomyces dermatiditis*, 483
- *Capnocytophaga canimorsus*, 482
- chimpanzees, 486
- *Chlamydia psittaci*, 487
- cowpox virus, 485
- *Coxiella burnetii*, 484
- *Cryptococcus neoformans*, 485
- definition, 481
- *Dipylidium caninum*, 484
- *Dirofilaria immiti*, 484
- epidemiology, 481–482
- farm animals, 486
- geography, 482
- habits and hobbies
  - amphibians, 487
  - birds, 485–487
  - cats, 484–485
  - dog bites, 482–484
  - fish, 487
  - mammals, 486
  - reptiles, 487
- *Histoplasma capsulatum*, 485
- home, 482
- monkey pox virus, 486
- *Mycobacterium marinum*, 487
- *Mycobacterium tuberculosis*, 486
- nonhuman primates, 486
- occupations, 482
- *Pasteurella multocida*, 482
- rodents, 486
- *Toxoplasma gondii*, 485
- veterinarians, 482
- *Yersinia pestis*, 483

Zoster vaccine, 364
Zygomycosis, 265
- invasive mold infections (IMIs), 288
- treatment
  - adjunctive therapy, 309
  - AMB deoxycholate (dAMB), 307
  - animal data, 308
  - antifungal agents, 307
  - clinical data, 308–309
  - echinocandins, 308
  - in vitro data, 308